D1283800

THE SURGERY
OF INFANCY
AND CHILDHOOD

Its Principles and Techniques

By ROBERT E. GROSS, M.D., D.Sc.

William E. Ladd Professor of Children's Surgery

The Harvard Medical School

Chief of Surgical Service

The Children's Hospital, Boston

With 1488 Illustrations on 567 Figures
Drawings by Etta Piotti

W. B. SAUNDERS COMPANY

PHILADELPHIA & LONDON

Preface

The writing of this book concerning general surgery of infancy and childhood could not have been accomplished in its present form without certain advantages and assets which by good fortune have come to me during the last two decades. These have been in the form of academic and hospital positions and privileges which have permitted the study of a large number of patients in a special field of surgery, providing a body of material which is unique. It is a pleasure to express to the Harvard Medical School and to the Children's Hospital of Boston my deep appreciation for the extraordinary opportunities which they have afforded me to work in this field. This volume constitutes, in part, a report of stewardship and a summary of progress which has been attained.

It was largely due to the vision and pioneering efforts of Dr. William E. Ladd that the surgical service of the Boston Children's Hospital was set up and firmly established as a separate unit. Coming from this service, the substance of this book represents a practical experience in pediatric surgery, summarizing observations and results of operations on thousands of babies and children. The handling of this case load would not have been possible without the untiring efforts of a most superb staff of house officers, nurses, anesthetists, and medical confreres, all of whom have carried a huge portion of the burden in caring for these patients. We are most appreciative of all their help through the years: the report which appears in this volume is largely a record of their magnificent work.

The subject matter presented herewith could not have been gathered without the generous efforts of my colleagues who, without the slightest restraint, have cheerfully and graciously allowed me to include illustrations which bear on our surgical cases. Dr. Edward B. D. Neuhauser has long been an authoritative and most helpful roentgenologist, upon whom we have leaned heavily in the study and care of patients; he has provided the films which are used so extensively in the various chapters. Dr. Sidney Farber has always been our mainstay in the field of pathology; we have used his guidance constantly and we have drawn heavily on his vast store of excellent records to provide the various photographs of specimens which are used unstintingly. To them both go my deepest thanks.

In the study of so large a body of clinical matter, great reliance has been placed upon the investigations and analyses by a score of members of our house and visiting staffs, all of whom have helped me enormously. Dr. Robert M. Smith has contributed the chapter on anesthesia and Dr. Donald W. MacCollum has included his treatment for hypospadias and wringer-arm injuries. The studies and the manuscript could not have been completed without the secretarial assistance of Mrs. Virginia Dunn, Mrs. Hollis Wiseman, Miss Marie Dresser, and Miss Edith Pierson. Mr. Ferdinand R.

Harding and Mr. Russell B. Harding have photographed the patients, the pathologic specimens, and the roentgenograms. To each and all of these co-workers I would like to express my deep appreciation and indebtedness.

Finally, it is a pleasure to thank the W. B. Saunders Company for warm cooperation in this joint effort and for its contribution in bringing forth a volume which is in keeping with the highest standards of the publisher's art.

ROBERT E. GROSS, M.D.

Boston, Massachusetts

CHAPTER 17

Duplications of the Alimentary Tract 221

CHAPTER 18

Foreign Bodies in the Alimentary Tract 246

CHAPTER 19

Appendicitis. 253

CHAPTER 24

Malformations of the Anus and Rectum 348

CHAPTER 25

Rectal Bleeding in Infants and Children 369

CHAPTER 26

Omental Cysts and Mesenteric Cysts 377

CHAPTER 27

Primary Peritonitis 384

CHAPTER 42

Miscellaneous Conditions of the Liver and Biliary Passages . 524

CHAPTER 43

Diseases of the Spleen 542

CHAPTER 44

Hypoglycemia 574

CHAPTER 58

Cysts and Primary Tumors of the Thorax 762

CHAPTER 59

Bronchiectasis 785

CHAPTER 60

The Patent Ductus Arteriosus 806

CHAPTER 61

Coarctation of the Aorta 828

CHAPTER 1

The Field of Children's Surgery

In writing a textbook on children's surgery, there immediately comes to mind the question, "What is children's surgery?" It is a field which is impossible to define exactly; it is easier to tell what it is not. Children's surgery is not limited to an anatomical area of the body, such as the thorax or the abdomen. It is not the encompassment of diseases of a single system, such as urologic surgery. It has no standing as a circumscribed and well defined field recognized by all physicians. It has no regularized programs of training, widely available in teaching centers throughout the country. There are no special boards which can certify those men who would like to practice this type of surgery. The field of pediatric surgery has little of the éclat which surrounds the well developed fields of special surgery which have sprung up in the last half century.

In the American system of medical education and practice, there is little if any need of adding further encumbrance by the addition of another specialty; already we have departmentalized and isolated too many areas of our teaching and routine care of human illnesses. I am firmly convinced that no effort should be made, either now or in the future, to set aside or split off the surgery of childhood as a specialty; yet the fact remains that in many communities it is frequently true that a baby or young child with a surgical ailment receives woefully inadequate care. He often falls somewhere between the general surgeon and a surgical specialist, neither one of whom regards the situation as being entirely within his sphere of work. Those who daily operate upon adults, even with the greatest of skill, are sometimes appalled—or certainly are not at their best—when called upon to operate upon and care for a tiny patient. Something more than diminutive instruments or scaled-down operative manipulations are necessary to do the job in a suitable manner. Vitally necessary is a special knowledge of the pathology which will be encountered and a familiarity with the best methods of correcting the condition which is found. Once at the operating table, there is no opportunity to read or consult about the problem at hand, and not infrequently procedures are carried out which are far from optimum in giving a child the best chance of survival. It is a common attitude to feel that poor results or excessive mortality rates are always a concomitant of surgical undertakings in the young.

A study of the literature, and the gathering of many personal communications from physicians in different parts of the country, regarding failures and deaths which do not get recorded in medical writings, leave little doubt that much can yet be accomplished in the betterment of surgical treatment for the young patient. To gain desirable improvements it is not necessary to create a new surgical specialty, but it is quite evident that our larger communities and many of our academic centers can support a man, or a small group of men, who are particularly interested in these problems and the devising of ways for treating them.

There is little use in trying to snatch from the jaws of death a baby who—with a multitude of anomalies—will be hopelessly deformed or retarded in spite of the fact

Table 1

Summary of General Surgical Operations
Procedures in 1950, Boston Children's Hospital

Abdominal Procedures

Appendectomy	197
Pyloromyotomy	84
Gastrostomy	23
Suture, gastric perforation	3
Suture, duodenal perforation	1
Lysis of adhesions	14
Gastrojejunostomy	4
Esophagogastrostomy	1
Duodenojejunostomy	6
Jejunojejunostomy	1
Ileo-ileostomy	4
Ileostomy	16
Closure of ileostomy	13
Meckel's diverticulectomy	3
Closure, perforation of bowel	2
Excision, duplication of bowel	4
Reduction, intussusception	41
Reduction, volvulus	2
Ladd's procedure	5
Removal of foreign body	5
Colectomy	1
Colostomy	15
Closure of colostomy	16
Abdominoperineal resection	39
Removal, intestinal polyp	2
Removal, rectal or colonic polyp	11
Proctoscopy	25
Anoplasty	11
Excision of anal fistula	5
Dilatation of anal stenosis	4
Resection of sigmoid	1
Biliary exploration	20
Splenectomy	21
Pancreatectomy	2
Removal, abdominal neoplasm	13
Exploratory laparotomy	23
Splenorenal anastomosis	1
Inguinal herniorrhaphy	504
Excision, hydrocele	73
Femoral herniorrhaphy	1
Epigastric herniorrhaphy	2
Umbilical herniorrhaphy	54
Diaphragmatic herniorrhaphy	8
Repair of omphalocele	5
Excision of umbilical cyst	4
Closure of evisceration	3
Exploration wound	1
Drainage, subdiaphragmatic abscess	3

Thoracic Operations

Excision, cystic hygroma	2
Esophagoscopy	1
Dilatation of esophagus	53

Anastomosis for esophageal atresia	22
Closure, tracheo-esophageal fistula	4
Excision, esophageal duplication	1
Thoracotomy	8
Thymectomy	2
Removal, lung cyst	1
Excision of tumor	4
Repair, perforation of lung	1
Lobectomy	10
Pneumonectomy	1
Angiocardiography	4
Division, patent ductus arteriosus	67
Potts procedure for tetralogy	40
Blalock procedure for tetralogy	8
Division of vascular rings	8
Excision of coarctation	46
Thoracolumbar sympathectomy	2

Neck and Face Operations

Repair of hare lip	71
Repair cleft palate	128
Rhinoplasty	3
Plastic procedure to mouth	5
Plastic to ears	20
Removal, stone Stenson's duct	1
Excision, cystic hygroma of neck	13
Removal, submaxillary cyst	2
Plastic to neck	1
Tonsillectomy and adenoidectomy	1
Excision, cervical lymph nodes	10
Excision, cervical cyst or sinus	31
Radical neck dissection	3
Excision of frontal sinus	1

Genito-Urinary Procedure

Nephrectomy	17
Nephrostomy	3
Plastic, ureteropelvic stricture	3
Ureteropyelostomy	1
Ureterosigmoidostomy	7
Incision of ureterocele	8
Cystectomy	2
Biopsy, bladder tumor	1
Repair, rectovesical fistula	2
Repair, recto-urethral fistula	2
Suprapubic cystostomy	27
Urethral dilatation	12
Excision, urethral fistula	2
Urethroplasty	17
Orchiectomy	1
Excision, testicualr tumor	1
Excision, scrotal tumor	1
Orchidopexy	42

Table 1 (*Continued*)

Circumcision	16	Suture of lacerations	29
Cystoscopy	79	Removal, superficial foreign body	5
		Z plastic procedure	7
Gynecological Procedures		Excision of scars	7
		Burn dressing	38
Oophorectomy	4	Skin graft	41
Closure, rectovaginal fistula	4	Incision and drainage, abscess	16
Colpohysterectomy for tumor	1	Biopsy	25
Hymenotomy	3	Plastic to web fingers	15
Biopsy, gonads	4	Removal of extra digits	14
Plastic to double vagina	1	Tenoplasty	4
		Repair of trigger thumb	2
Skeletal and Muscular Procedures		Marrow biopsy	5
		Removal, sacrococcygeal tumor	3
Fusion of knee	1	Excision of varicosities	1
Sequestrectomy	2	Removal of toe nails	2
Application of hip spica	6	Total	2735*
Open reduction, mandibular fracture	1		
Removal of ganglion	7		
Myotomy for torticollis	1		
Closed reduction of fracture	4		
Amputation	2		

Miscellaneous Procedure

Excision, superficial tumor or cyst......... 166
    Simple cysts............ 66
    Angiomas............. 39
    Nevi................. 35
    Baker's cyst........... 9
    Sinus tracts............ 17

that some single malformation in the urinary tract, the intestinal system, or the cardio-vascular apparatus has been nicely repaired. Fortunately, the vast majority of babies or children who have come under our care have had some single abnormality, the correction of which results in an individual who can be a useful and happy citizen. There are few satisfactions that are greater than the operative correction of an anomaly which restores a child to perfect health—a feat which can be accomplished in a surprisingly high percentage of cases.

At the Children's Hospital of Boston there has grown up through the years a division of responsibility for surgical cases which is unique and indeed peculiar, but which has been quite effective as far as patient-care is concerned. There are four main surgical divisions: neurosurgical, orthopedic, otolaryngological, and general surgical. The scopes of work for the first three are obvious enough and they follow generally accepted specialty lines; the general surgical service takes whatever is left. But this tail of the animal is by no means its smallest part. To give an idea of the relative size of these various fields, the Hospital figures for in-patient operations are summarized for the year 1950 as follows:

Neurosurgical	407
Orthopedic	494
Otolaryngological	1873
Dental	111
Eye	64
General surgical	2447
Total	5396

* There were 2735 procedures in 2447 operations, some patients having more than 1 procedure during an operation.

4

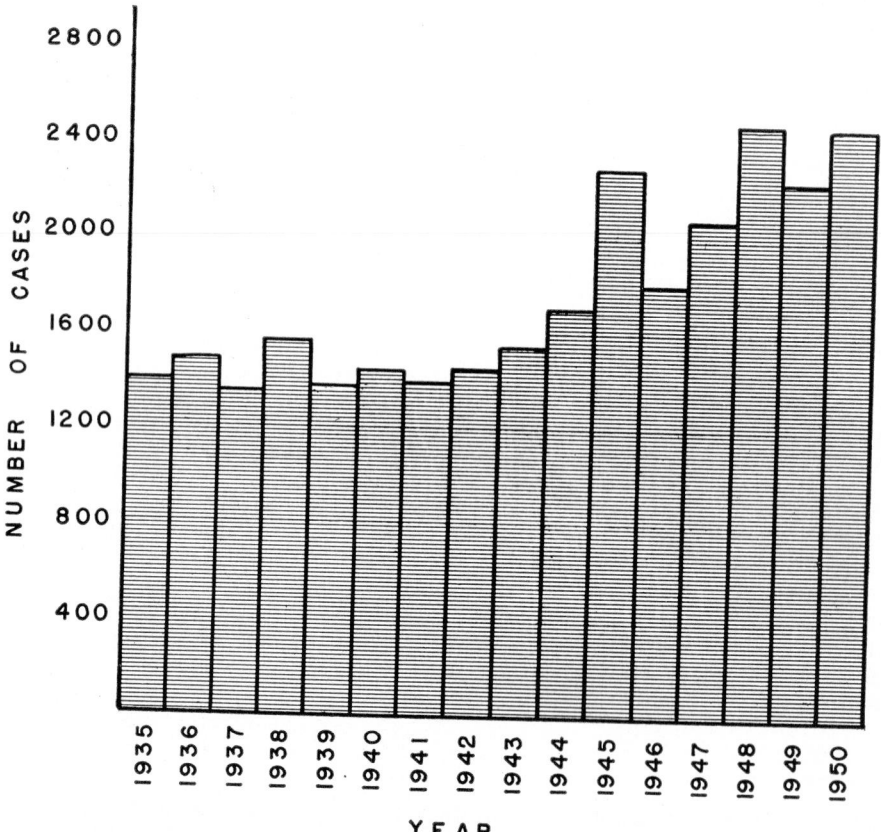

Fig. 1. Number of patients operated upon each year on the General Surgical Service of the Boston Children's Hospital. (This does not include operations of a neurosurgical, orthopedic, otolaryngological, dental, or ophthalmologic nature—all of which are handled on other services.)

The 2447 operations performed by the Surgical Service are itemized in Table 1. During this year, the anesthesia department had to provide, in addition to the above, for out-patient minor operations in various departments, certain x-ray treatments under general anesthesia, reduction of fractures in the out-patient department, encephalograms, et cetera, making a total of 5741 general anesthesias.

It is apparent that the field of children's surgery has rather indefinite borders which shift according to: (1) The material which is available in any particular community. (2) The activities of a staff in developing certain segments of the work. (3) The facilities which are available in the hospital, and other factors. Therefore, the list shown in Table 1 is no indication of what we think the field should encompass; it is merely a record of the material which it has been our good fortune to handle; any predominance of particular subjects reflects the inclinations and interests of our doctors. Without doubt, lists from other institutions would show quite dissimilar groups of cases and fields of emphasis.

The purposes of this book are twofold: First, to sum up the material that we in the Surgical Service have been called upon to treat. By making an objective appraisal of results, we gain an accurate knowledge concerning the methods of surgical procedures which have been good and those which have been poor. Only by such a critical analysis can we hope to improve the results on the Service in the future. Second, to make available to the medical profession whatever we have learned about various surgical conditions in infancy and childhood. No effort has been made to include and discuss all controversial views which are represented in the literature. In writing this volume, we do not wish to minimize the importance of the writings of others who have contributed to the field; our desire is merely to describe the forms of therapy and management which we have come to feel are the ones most suitable for handling the various diseases and abnormalities.

From the outset, it is obvious that this book is incomplete; it lacks discussion of many subjects which are a part of our daily surgical practice. Yet the line of practicality has to be drawn somewhere; we have included only those chapters which might be of widest interest and greatest help to other students and physicians.

CHAPTER 2

Preoperative and Postoperative Care

Advances which have been made in the preoperative and postoperative care of infants and children have contributed greatly to the increasing success of pediatric surgery. This newer knowledge has also made it possible to perform with creditable results certain operative procedures which in the past were thought to be impractical or even impossible. Some of the special considerations related to various diseases are discussed in the following chapters. In this section it is our intention to outline general but practical guides to therapy, which must be modified to meet specific conditions which are encountered.

The Art of Surgery

In a book on pediatric surgery, the most difficult chapter to write is that concerning preoperative and postoperative care. It is possible to put in writing certain policies and well defined techniques which might be helpful to readers, and knowledge of which will allow adequate handling of the routine problems which are encountered. However, the care of children requires in addition a certain indefinable something which is well-nigh impossible to describe and transmit to others by spoken or written word. This factor might well be called the "art" of pediatric surgery; it cannot be measured, quantitated, or characterized any more than one can describe adequately the tints of Titian, the bold strokes of Michelangelo or the chiaroscuro of Sargent.

To those of us who have the responsibility of directing an active surgical service, this "extra something" is a priceless attribute which is most sought for in members of the visiting and house staffs. Its value was impressed upon me thoroughly during the war years, when it became our lot to have a chief resident whose training was seemingly inadequate for this post but who was available because an active duodenal ulcer kept him from military duty. He possessed a real fondness and affection for children; he was indefatigable in his efforts to make them comfortable and happy; he was almost constantly at the bedside of those who were desperately ill so that the drainage tubes, the infusions, or the medications could be supervised or altered to best advantage; after most other personnel had gone to bed he arose and made rounds again to make sure that things were in order and that nothing went amiss in those quiet and sometimes tragic hours which can come between midnight and dawn. Such interest and selfless attention to the job paid handsome dividends. Children who were old enough to appreciate the situation left the service without fear; they had developed a real devotion to the man. More important still, a larger number of children and babies than ever before left the service alive. In spite of the fact that our staff coverage was but a fraction of what it had been before the war, and the case load had risen greatly, the mortality rates in several types of surgical conditions were actually reduced. It is impossible to praise too highly these qualities in a physician which are so hard to define and yet are so important in the care of patients. Fortunate is the staff which is able to attract individuals of such character, understanding, and industry; we are fully conscious of our debt to them.

In the present chapter we can set forth only some of the routines, practices, and opinions which have been found to be of value in the surgical care of young subjects; in between the lines should be added the many personal attentions and supervisions which cannot be put in writing, but which are so vitally important.

RESPONSIBILITY FOR THE SURGICAL CASE

It is our opinion that the best results in pediatric surgery are obtained when a surgical service functions as an independent unit, and when patients with surgical conditions are the responsibility of such a staff during their preoperative and postoperative course. This plan, effected at the Boston Children's Hospital by Dr. William E. Ladd, has functioned with clear advantage since 1927, and is based on certain principles: (1) There should be no possible doubt regarding who is in charge of the case. (2) The first-hand information which the surgeon and his operating team possess about the surgical pathology or the surgical procedure which has been performed is usually of great importance in proper handling of the patient. (3) The acquisition of knowledge (required for good preoperative and postoperative care of patients) should interest surgeons operating upon children just as much as it does those who operate upon adults.

The policy which we believe to be best in the management of infants and children who require surgery does not deny the very considerable assistance which other services or physicians can bring when unusual problems arise. We feel, however, that such help should be obtained on a consultation basis, keeping management of the case in the hands of the surgeon or the surgical service. Needless to say, to make this system work effectively, the surgeon and his team must take cognizance of the problems which are encountered, and must have the time and facilities to analyze and direct the solution of them. The results of such an organization should be assayed frequently by the presentation of representative cases before the entire hospital staff in open and frank discussion. In this way, knowledge originating from many sources becomes available and can be applied with clear understanding when the surgical conditions must be treated subsequently in other patients.

It is fully realized that in some communities pediatric surgical conditions are encountered only infrequently and that the surgeon is desirous of undertaking only the technical parts of an operation, preferring to leave the management of a baby or growing child to the general practitioner or pediatrician who has much greater familiarity with the various problems of young subjects. Under these circumstances, combined authority is the most practical way of caring for the child and his illness. Nevertheless, it is our belief that as surgical material accumulates in increasing quantity, there comes a time when pediatric surgery receives its greatest impetus by placing a youngster under the supervision of one individual or one service. The constant goal should be to seek lower fatality rates and to attain quicker and more satisfactory results for those who survive surgical procedures. These ends will be approached more closely by those surgeons who devote their major energies to the field and who are willing to assume supervision before and after the technical exercise. Furthermore, when the volume of material becomes great, the pediatrician and practitioner generally prefer to be relieved of the handling of postoperative details. Within the last two decades, nearly 100,000 patients have been operated upon in the Boston Children's Hospital by the orthopedic, neurosurgical, otolaryngological, and general surgical services. The medical men have not desired to be swamped by the mass of treatments and the supervisory burden of caring for such a large number of patients after surgery. The pediatricians have had plenty to do in the study of these cases before operation and in their care after hospital discharge!

PREOPERATIVE CARE

Psychic Preparation

It is an all-too-common practice for parents to tell a child nothing of what is to be done (or to deliver him to the hospital on some pretext) and then abandon him in an atmosphere which is foreign, exciting, and mysterious. This can seriously undermine the faith of a child in his mother and father; he is very apt to develop a feeling of not knowing when or where he will be left subsequently by his family. The child faces a great unknown; cooperation from him may become impossible. The worries and nightmares which often follow such a profound and terrifying experience can produce lasting mental distortions.

Infants and very small children cannot be prepared mentally for hospitalization and surgery, but with older children the parents can help tremendously in allaying fears and in preventing psychic disturbances which might arise after hospitalization has passed. In the majority of instances, surgery is elective and there is time for stories or games of "hospital," "nurse," or "doctor" which can be told or played at home. The child becomes a bit familiar with hospital ways or routine, and when finally taken to such a place can be admitted unafraid and cooperative. Even in acute illness or injury, a word of explanation by parents does much to gain the child's confidence and eliminate anxiety. In all cases, a simple explanation of what is to come should be made, and should precede that of the surgeon, so that the child continues his feeling of trust and of closeness to his mother and father.

To gain rapport, the surgeon should always talk with a child and explain that it is necessary to "fix up" or "make well" the condition which exists. Certain words connote terrible things, and therefore should never be used. Even though nitrous oxide induction or anesthesia is contemplated, it should never be stated that the child is going to "have gas." To a child "gas" means just one thing—that horrible smelly stuff that comes out of a kitchen stove and which can kill people! It is better to explain that he is going to breathe a little something, is going to have a good sleep, and will *wake up in about an hour*. Likewise, the word "operation" is apt to suggest a great cut, a lot of blood, or a procedure which is fatal. It is better to omit the word, explaining in a few simple terms that the stomach ache has to be fixed, that the lump has to be made better, or that the break has to be mended. It is very convincing to a child to point to a girl in the next bed and say that she has had the same trouble and is now getting well, or that the boys across the ward were just as sick but will now be waiting to see him when he wakes up. Better than any word or explanation, glances at these other children rapidly assure a newcomer that it is possible to live through his difficulties. It is important to give a fair statement of how long it will be before leaving the hospital; the youngster then tends to minimize the operative undertaking and to focus upon the happy day when he will be going home.

Preoperative Feeding

An *infant* is usually fed every four hours; the rate of metabolism is so rapid that withholding of feedings not only makes a baby hungry and restless, but also depletes his store of glycogen. Therefore, an infant's feedings should not be omitted any longer than necessary before operation. The last bottle, which is given approximately four hours before operation, consists of sweetened water or orange juice. The stomach of an infant (when there is no obstruction) is so active that within two hours it is completely empty; therefore, the possibilities of vomiting and aspiration during anesthesia are very slight. *Older children*, accustomed to passing through the night without food, do not usually require nourishment after the evening meal. It is permissible to allow them to drink any "clear" fluid (water, orange juice, ginger ale) which is desired up to 2 A.M. If a lengthy or difficult surgical procedure is contemplated, it will be tolerated better if 10 per cent glucose in water is administered intravenously before or during the first part of the operation.

Vitamin Therapy

Vitamin K (for example, Hykinone 2.5 to 5.0 mg. daily) should be administered preoperatively to all newborn infants since they commonly have a mild bleeding tendency as a result of transient hypoprothrombinemia. Vitamin C (25 to 100 mg. by mouth or by subcutaneous injection daily) should be given to depleted patients to promote good wound healing.

Antibiotic Therapy

Because of the high incidence of pulmonary complications in newborn infants and also in some older children undergoing thoracic surgery, we generally give all of these patients prophylactic penicillin therapy. Probably much of this is unnecessary, but without doubt it sometimes helps to kill off bacteria lurking in the respiratory tract which could give rise to serious infection following general anesthesia or during the immobilization which accompanies a major surgical undertaking.

For operation on the urinary tract, when there has been pyuria, much can be gained by the use of appropriate antibiotics which have a wide spectrum of activity, such as aureomycin or terramycin. While such drugs can suppress bacterial infection and tend to minimize a postoperative spread, they can hardly be expected to clear the urine completely, since this is generally impossible until one corrects surgically the underlying abnormality, obstruction, or defect.

When children have lesions of the alimentary tract requiring elective surgery, such as removal of a megacolon or closure of a colostomy, we rely mostly upon cleansing irrigations to prepare the bowel. Many surgeons use Sulfathalidine, streptomycin, or neomycin before all elective surgery on the colon or ileum; these preparations may be helpful and they do no harm, provided that vitamin K is simultaneously administered. We place little emphasis or reliance upon these drugs for reducing the bacterial flora of the intestinal contents.

Antibiotic and Chemotherapeutic 24-Hour Dosage

	Orally	Parenterally
Gantrisin	60 mg. per lb.	
Sodium Gantrisin		60 mg. per lb.
Sulfadiazine	60 mg. per lb.	30 mg. per lb.
Sulfathalidine (or Sulfasuxidine)	100 mg. per lb.	
Penicillin		5000–10000 units per lb.
Streptomycin	20 mg. per lb.	10–20 mg. per lb.
Aureomycin	10 mg. per lb.	3 mg. per lb.
Terramycin	20 mg. per lb.	3–6 mg. per lb.

Repletion for Seriously Ill Patients

Infants and children who have been seriously ill are frequently dehydrated or mal-nourished; balance should be restored as well as possible in the time available before surgery. Dehydration due to fever, poor intake, or vomiting must be corrected, at least partially, by the administration of parenteral fluids. By intravenous injection of glucose, ketosis should always be completely overcome (the urine being made free of ketone substances) before anesthesia is started. Minor degrees of electrolyte imbalance are common in sick children, but it is not necessary to remedy them before surgery. However, in seriously ill children, some attempt must be made to shift the imbalances pre-operatively, fully realizing that total correction is impractical at this time. The over-coming of dehydration and the surgical correction of the underlying pathology are more effective in restoring blood chemistries to normal than are attempts at complicated preoperative intravenous electrolyte replacement. Any hemoglobin levels below 10 to 12 gm. per 100 cc. should be treated preoperatively by transfusion of whole blood or packed red cells.

Reduction of Fever

Children with high fevers withstand anesthesia and surgery poorly; operation upon a child with marked pyrexia is apt to be accompanied by exceedingly high pulse rate, collapse, or convulsions. We make it a rule that surgery (as for appendectomy, treat-ment of peritonitis, or the like) will not be performed until the temperature is brought below 102° per rectum. If a feverish child is sedated, is given aspirin by rectum (or sodium salicylate 0.5 to 1 gm. intravenously), sponged with alcohol or tepid water, fanned, re-hydrated with intravenous fluids, and given antibiotics, fever is lowered rapidly (Fig. 144). This regimen may require several hours, but the time spent is extremely effective in reducing the hazards of anesthesia and operation.

Aspirin Dosage

0– 2 yrs.	50–100 mg.
0– 5 yrs.	100–300 mg.
5–12 yrs.	300–600 mg.

(Given orally or per rectum, and may be repeated in two to four hours for several doses, as needed.)

Enema

There seems to be some sort of archaic belief that all patients who undergo anes-thesia and elective surgery should have an enema the evening before; this is mostly non-sense. Used as a routine, it accomplishes little. It certainly upsets the child and it greatly increases the work of the nursing staff. Without doubt, it is desirable to deflate the bowel if fecal masses can be felt in the sigmoid, but for the vast majority of children an enema is completely unnecessary. If there is any question about the sluggishness of the bowel, it is far better before operation (for herniorrhaphy or the like) to give a tablespoon of mineral oil or milk of magnesia the evening before operation. This will begin to work its way through the intestinal tract and insure that movements a day or two after surgery will not be difficult to pass.

When planning some intra-abdominal procedure which is near the colon and which requires maximum exposure, much can be accomplished by washing the bowel with a soapsuds enema prior to surgery and by the placement of a rectal tube during operation, so that the colon is deflated properly.

When some operation is to be performed within the lumen of the rectum or colon (such as removal of a polyp), it is of utmost importance to clean the bowel thoroughly beforehand by irrigations, the last one of which should be given about two hours before operation. Whenever a resection is to be performed (such as for Hirschsprung's disease), cleansing and removal of fecal concretions may require literally days of washings; this step is such an important part of the management that surgery must be deferred until the bowel is thoroughly cleared.

Matching of Blood

Whenever a long or extensive operation is to be performed, it is always advisable to type the child's blood and have blood matched before the procedure is started. This eases the burden on blood bank personnel, and it avoids confusion in the operating room which is apt to arise if typing and cross-matching are left until the patient is on the table and is in trouble.

Sedation

Children vary tremendously in their reactions and in their excitability. Some show little concern when coming into a hospital; others are very apprehensive. Some have serious illnesses which understandably make them fussy, irritable, or even uncontrollable. One of the greatest acts of kindness the doctor can perform is the prompt and adequate use of sedatives. For the quieting of a "nervous" or tense child, one of the barbiturates, given by mouth in suitable doses every six to eight hours is very helpful. When a child has pain, or must be subjected to disturbing procedures or manipulations before operation, it is better to use morphine by subcutaneous injection each three or four hours. Average doses are shown in the following list; these are only guides and may have to be varied somewhat according to the circumstances in any given case.

Sedatives for Infants and Children

Age	Average Weight lb.	Phenobarbital or Nembutal mg.	Morphine mg.	Demerol mg.
Newborn	7			
6 mos.	16	30		
1 yr.	21	50	1.0	10
2 yrs.	27	60	1.4	20
4 yrs.	35	90	2.4	25
6 yrs.	45	100	4.0	40
8 yrs.	55	120	5.4	45
10 yrs.	65	150	6.0	50
12 yrs.	80	200	8.0	50

Orders for any preanesthetic sedative must be given with consideration for other drugs which have been administered in the hours immediately preceding it. When a patient is taken to an operating room, his preoperative sedation should be sufficient to cause him to be asleep, or at least be drowsy and unafraid.

OPERATIVE CARE

Prevention of Heat Loss

During transportation to the operating suite chilling should be avoided, a point of special importance when dealing with babies. Our operating rooms are maintained at temperatures of 68–70° F.; to conserve an infant's body heat, the legs and arms are swathed in cotton sheet-wadding. Occasionally, a well wrapped hot water bottle is laid under the infant. Warmed blankets are used routinely both before and after surgery.

Aspiration of Stomach

Any child undergoing abdominal surgery should have a Levin tube passed and the stomach evacuated prior to the induction of anesthesia.

Placement of Intravenous Needle

Sick children for whom major procedures are planned require supportive intravenous fluids and blood during operation. These can be given satisfactorily in most older subjects (who have large and readily accessible veins) through a percutaneous intravenous needle. In all babies and in most of the smaller children, it is far better to "cut down" on a vein (Fig. 9) and tie into place a cannula or a polyethylene plastic tube (No. 19 for babies, No. 14 for large children). This allows fluid or blood to be injected very rapidly, if required. Furthermore, it gives great assurance that the system will work satisfactorily if called upon in an emergency. It requires ten to fifteen minutes to insert a "cut-down" into an arm, or preferably an ankle vein, but this is time well spent. In seriously ill patients, this can be done under local procaine infiltration, prior to the induction of general anesthesia, in this way reducing the length of the anesthesia time. In general, we perform a "cut-down" just after a patient has gone to sleep; during the period that a vein cannula is being inserted, the anesthetist has opportunity to deepen the plane of anesthesia gradually, so that in ten or fifteen minutes the child is completely relaxed and is ready for starting the operation.

After insertion of a cannula or plastic catheter into a vein, it has attached to it a "set" consisting of a graduated burette (open at the top) and tubing in the path of which are provided a drip chamber and below this a three-way stopcock with an open side arm (Fig. 4). This system has many important features: (1) At any time, blood or any kind of fluid can be poured into the open reservoir. (2) At a glance, markings (down to 5 cc.) on a slender burette clearly show how much fluid has gone into the patient, a point of tremendous importance in babies and small children where a flood must be avoided. (3) With the glass drip chamber, fluid can be allowed to run by gravity and the rate of flow can be seen in the drip glass (the rate can be adjusted by a Hoffman clamp placed upon, and partially compressing, the rubber tube above the drip chamber). (4) The three-way stopcock is generally left in a position so that fluid (or blood) flows through it (using the gravity method). However, in an emergency, a 10 or 20 cc. Luer-Lok syringe can be attached to the open side arm of the valve, and with appropriate turnings of the valve and pumping of the syringe, fluid (or blood) can be drawn from the reservoir and then pumped rapidly into the vein. This system has the theoretical disadvantage of being open at the top and thereby possibly inviting contamination. However, we have had no known infection during the thousands of cases in which it has been employed in the last twenty-five years; its advantages are so outstanding that we have no desire to change it in any way.

(A cannula or plastic tube should seldom be left more than thirty-six to forty-eight hours in one vein; longer lodgement is too apt to be followed by disturbing phlebitis or thrombosis. If the child's condition is still so critical that a vein cannula is desired for a greater period, it should be shifted to another vessel.)

Measurement of Blood Loss

During extensive procedures, especially cardiovascular surgery, it is sometimes difficult for the surgeon to estimate the blood loss with any degree of correctness; he is therefore in a poor position to determine the amount needed for replacement. We have found it very helpful to measure blood which is withdrawn from the field through the suction apparatus (by viewing the amount which appears in the graduated collecting bottle on the floor) and by weighing all blood-soaked sponges which are discarded. For this latter purpose, sponges of a uniform dry weight are employed (so that they do not have to be individually weighed beforehand) and a scale is used (Fig. 486) which rapidly indicates how much blood is in the soiled sponges. The amount of blood which has been lost is almost always much more than the surgeon would have estimated! After measuring the loss, the circulating nurse or anesthetist can guide and prescribe the amount of blood which should be given intravenously; in this way, a patient can be kept on a stable plane, even though the operation is long and the blood loss is great.

GENERAL POSTOPERATIVE CARE

Dressings

Bandages and dressings must be well secured, else the child will remove or disturb them. For most surgical wounds, wide strips of adhesive tape which cover the dressing completely will suffice. For abdominal wounds, binders are seldom necessary. Wounds of the neck must be protected from spilled feedings and vomitus; those of the lower abdomen, back, or thigh must be protected from urine and feces. Pliofilm, or rubber dam, serves as satisfactory waterproof covering for dressings in any of these locations. This impervious cover should not be tacked down around its entire periphery because the underlying skin will sweat and the wound become macerated; it is best to cover the gauze dressing only with a flap or bib. Wounds upon fingers and hands must usually be splinted, or else encased in some sort of a dressing which immobilizes them; also they must be well protected from soiling. We cover all such bandages with tight-fitting stockinette which not only effectively protects, but can easily be changed without disturbing the underlying bandage if external soiling should occur. Great care must be taken in the anchorage of gastrostomy, chest, or bladder catheters, since even the smallest of infants have demonstrated considerable skill in the removal of these essential tubes.

Sedation

Directions for adequate sedation should always be included in the postoperative orders. Small doses of phenobarbital are given as needed to most infants, while for older children morphine in appropriate amounts is generally preferable. For patients who are not very ill, such orders can be written for every three or four hours "as needed." For seriously ill or excited children, sedation should be given "by the clock," calculating the dose rather carefully so that the child will be kept at a subdued level and will have the quiet and rest which are so beneficial.

Restraints

While restraints are to be avoided whenever possible, in certain circumstances they are essential. For example, following harelip repairs, infants are placed in special jackets, the sleeves of which are securely pinned to the diaper; thus the infant cannot scratch or otherwise interfere with the lip repair. The arms of postoperative cleft-palate patients are maintained in extension (at the elbow) by means of *Welcome sleeves*. With these in place, the child cannot suck his thumb nor can he place hard, undesirable objects in his mouth, yet he can comfortably move about in bed and can walk.

When infants are to have sutures removed, or are to be given parenteral fluid therapy, they are restrained either by "bundling" (Fig. 5) or by tying down their arms and legs. Older children require restraints less frequently, but during intravenous therapy we always splint the arm or leg, and fasten it to the bed (Fig. 7).

Nursing Care

Following anesthesia, all children are kept under close watch until full consciousness has returned. This, of course, is no different from care given to adults, but the frequency of pulmonary aspiration in children is such that extra precautions must be taken. Complications in infants and children can occur so rapidly that all seriously ill patients should receive constant nursing care. Because the complications are predominantly respiratory in nature, it is well to have suction apparatus immediately available at all times. An infant's laryngoscope and intratracheal tubes of suitable size are also kept close at hand for use in the event of an emergency.

Temperatures of all infants and children are routinely taken by rectum, except following anal or perianal operations, when axillary readings are employed. High temperatures can occur, particularly following bladder and kidney procedures or in the presence of peritonitis; in these patients temperature readings are taken frequently.

Following the majority of procedures, patients are encouraged to move around in bed as much as possible. Small and sick infants tend to lie flat on their backs. In this position, pulmonary drainage is poor and a dependent type of pneumonia frequently appears; an infant should be turned every few hours. Following some operative procedures, it is necessary that a patient be maintained in one certain position if proper wound healing is to occur. For example, following excision of a sacrococcygeal teratoma, the infant should be kept face down, with the buttocks uppermost and exposed to the air. In this situation, the nursing care of the baby is greatly facilitated by placing the child on a small Bradford frame (this frame holds the child 10 to 12 inches above the mattress. A hole in the central part of the canvas which covers the frame allows urine and feces to drop through into a bed pan which is placed directly under this area).

A severely burned patient, immobilized in copious dressings, poses a difficult problem in nursing care. Such a child is placed on a Stryker frame, which allows turning every few hours, so that he alternately lies in face-up and face-down positions.

To avoid pressure sores, the delicate cutaneous tissues of infants must be continually protected from irritation and pressure. All arm boards or splints must be thickly padded.

Following anoplasty, or establishment of an ileostomy, excoriation of the surrounding skin may be severe. It is much easier to avoid this than to treat it after it has developed. Frequent cleansing and application of a soothing ointment (compounded of castor oil, zinc oxide, and Aristol) are of much value.

Convulsions

Convulsions in infants and children on general surgical wards are most commonly caused by high fevers; other etiologic factors are cerebral damage due to anoxia, thrombosis, or intracranial hemorrhage. When convulsions do occur, every effort must be made to reduce any fever, and the child should be kept heavily sedated with phenobarbital. Sometimes twitchings, or even convulsions, are due to cerebral edema from overhydration and are signs of impending disaster. If such seems to be the case, any administration of parenteral fluids must be stopped immediately; in some situations, attempts at dehydration by intravenous injection of 50 per cent glucose are indicated.

Antibiotic and Chemotherapy

Prophylactic Therapy. There is little to recommend the routine use of antibiotics following clean surgery. It is not only painful and expensive, but may be harmful in that sensitization occurs, or else resistant bacterial strains become dominant. There are, however, certain rather clear indications for prophylactic therapy in pediatric surgery: (1) Because of the high incidence of pulmonary infection, drugs should be given prophylactically to newborn infants who have undergone surgery, and to all patients who have had intrathoracic procedures. (2) Following plastic surgery, where the cosmetic result might be compromised by infection, antibiotics should be used liberally. (3) In cases in which it is possible that there has been peritoneal contamination, antibiotics should be intensively employed. (4) Following operations upon the urinary tract, particularly when indwelling catheters or struts have been left in place, prophylactic therapy is desirable. The most commonly employed agent is penicillin, and it is usually administered postoperatively for a period of five to seven days. When mixed types of infections might be anticipated, other drugs such as Gantrisin, aureomycin, or terramycin can be used advantageously to give a broader spectrum of protection against gram-positive and gram-negative organisms.

Treatment of Infections. Penicillin is the most widely used agent in the treatment of surgical infections, but when certain organisms are present, other drugs are much more efficacious. *Streptomycin* is usually potent against gram-negative bacteria. *Aureomycin* and *terramycin* are of great use, especially when the patient can take these substances by mouth; when injected intravenously, their use is often complicated by thrombosis. When they are given by mouth for any length of time, vitamin K should be administered concurrently since their inhibitory effect upon intestinal flora is known to cause hypoprothrombinemia.

One complication of oral antibiotic therapy, frequently encountered in infants, is the development of thrush. Most antibiotics enhance the growth of monilia, and when thrush appears, their administration must be stopped. In such instances, and if infection is still to be combated, sulfonamides are particularly valuable.

Sulfadiazine is a most useful drug in pediatric surgery. Its low cost, its ease of administration, its effectiveness against a wide range of bacteria, and its relatively low toxicity make it an exceedingly desirable agent. It can be given orally or the sodium salt can be injected parenterally. When used intravenously or subcutaneously, the concentration should not be above 5 per cent. For optimum results, a blood sulfadiazine level of approximately 10 mg. per 100 cc. should be maintained. When patients are receiving sulfadiazine, care must be taken to insure an adequate fluid intake, and preferably the urine should be kept basic. Urine specimens should be examined frequently for blood and sulfadiazine crystals. Possessing the same superiority as sulfadiazine, but having the added advantage of greater solubility in the urine, Gantrisin is coming into great favor and we find that we are using it with increasing frequency. The sodium salt is also available when parenteral administration is necessary.

Certain combinations of drugs have synergistic actions of greater effectiveness than when the drugs are given singly. Penicillin with sulfadiazine or with streptomycin has been very satisfactory in the treatment of peritonitis. Para-aminosalicylic acid (90 mg.

per pound of body weight per 24 hours, orally, divided into 4 doses) has been found of particular value in aiding the treatment of tuberculous infections by streptomycin.

Other newer antibiotics such as bacitracin, polymyxin, and neomycin are not without serious nephrotoxic and neurotoxic effects when administered parenterally. Topically, their use appears to be safe, and when indicated, they are of considerable value. Bacitracin is particularly helpful in treatment of penicillin-resistant staphylococcus infections, and of necrotizing bacterial gangrene. Polymyxin B sulfate is especially effective against pseudomonas and other gram-negative organisms, so that it may help in the treatment of contaminated wounds and burns. Neomycin has a broad spectrum of activity. It is absorbed only slightly when taken orally, and has been shown to be extremely potent for bowel "sterilization."

Postoperative Intestinal Distention

In infants and children, the dangers of tracheal aspiration during vomiting are extremely high. Particularly when a youngster is in a debilitated state and when there has been an intra-abdominal operation, can aspiration produce an immediate fatality or a very serious pulmonary complication. Therefore, vomiting should always be kept at a minimum; it is best prevented by keeping the stomach deflated with a gastric suction tube. For babies, a No. 10 or 12 urethral catheter (with several holes cut in that part which rests in the stomach) is satisfactory; for larger children, a Levin tube must be employed. Suction from a Bell apparatus is practical and is easy to manage. When greater suction is required (in older children), it is our custom to employ the hospital (piped) suction system, but to introduce between this and the patient's aspiration bottle a reducing valve, by means of which the negative pressure can be constantly and automatically regulated. Whenever a child has gastric suction, a daily record must be kept of the amount of fluid aspirated and the character of the material withdrawn (brown, dark green, light green, colorless). The color of the gastric juice will give an indication when the tube can be removed safely.

The use of a Miller-Abbott tube (or Cantor tube) is seldom practical for children under two years of age. Even for some patients in the range from two to four years, it can be exceedingly difficult to get a tube started down properly; continuing efforts to make the tube enter the duodenum may do more harm than good. Beyond three to four years of age, a small Cantor tube (size 12) can generally be inserted and made to progress satisfactorily. All gastric or intestinal tubes should be irrigated every two hours with small amounts of normal saline to keep them open and functioning properly.

Intestinal tubes should be left in place until abdominal distention abates, until auscultation reveals that peristaltic activity is returning, and until flatus is passed per rectum. *Gastric* tubes should be left in place as long as there is any green material coming up the tube (indicating that reverse peristalsis is still present in the small intestine).

In the handling of inlying gastric tubes, there is a widespread practice of not allowing patients to drink water, for fear of washing excessive amounts of chloride out of the stomach; to us this seems almost brutal. With a tube in place, a patient's nose, mouth, pharynx, and esophagus become dry and irritated. If the child is conscious (and hence has little danger of aspiration), it is far better to allow drinking of water so the mouth and pharynx can be kept moist, letting this fluid which reaches the stomach suck back immediately through the tube. The patient is much more comfortable this way; to compensate for the increased chloride losses, additional amounts of saline can be added to the parenteral fluid which he is receiving. Without doubt, if water is allowed to remain for long in a stomach, osmotic activity permits escape of great quantities of gastric electrolytes into it. However, if swallowed water sucks back quickly through a tube, electrolyte loss is negligible.

Drugs such as Pitressin or neostigmine should never be used when there is any suspicion of an existing peritonitis or when there has been any suture line in the intestine or colon. These drugs are of occasional value for mild ileus following retroperitoneal procedures, or when abdominal operations have been undertaken but the bowel has not been opened.

The intermittent insertion of a rectal tube for relief of gaseous distention of the large bowel often does much to bring comfort to a patient.

In combating abdominal distention, a considerable portion of the material in the intestinal lumen is inert nitrogen, which has come from the room air which has been swallowed. It is possible to remove some of this nitrogen by placing the individual in a tent containing an atmosphere which is very low in nitrogen and very high in oxygen. Such a therapeutic adjunct is not very satisfactory for adults, but seems to be of considerable help in babies and small children; it is of particular assistance in these age groups in which it is difficult or impossible to pass an intestinal suction tube to decompress the lower alimentary tract. To have any real effectiveness, the tent must be closed tightly so the concentration of oxygen can be maintained at 90 to 95 per cent. Besides any beneficial effects which it might have on the intestine, the high concentration oxygen is helpful in other ways, particularly in facilitating a greater oxygen uptake by lungs which are embarrassed in any manner. In no case have we seen harmful effects of high concentration oxygen, even when continued for many days.

Postoperative Feeding

Except after major intra-abdominal procedures, oral feeding can usually be resumed six to eight hours following surgery. *Children* are first given clear fluids to drink, then are rapidly advanced to normal diets; generally, they are taking full nourishment by the following day. *Infants* are started off on water, then sweetened orange juice, following which they resume their preoperative feeding schedule, generally within twelve hours.

For most infants, up to four or five months of age, who do not have special feeding problems, we use one of the following formulas. While a wide variety of other formulas are quite suitable, we have generally found that one of these is satisfactory for routine cases. By largely limiting ourselves to the use of these two, it is possible to cut down greatly the burden on the diet kitchen which prepares the infant feedings.

1. Evaporated milk . . . . 6 oz.
   Water . . . . 8 oz.
   50% Karo (red label) . . . . 1 oz.
   (= approximately 20 cal. per oz.)

2. Whole milk . . . . 16 oz.
   Water . . . . 2½ oz.
   50% Karo (red label) . . . . 1½ oz.
   (= approximately 20 cal. per oz.)

Feedings are usually given on a four-hour schedule in amounts to supply 2½ to 3 oz. (50 to 60 calories) per pound of body weight per twenty-four hours. Infants older than two months do not usually have a feeding at 2 A.M., but if the infant is hungry, for a few nights following surgery it is advisable to give this bottle to insure adequate fluid and caloric intake.

Variations in formula are required in special circumstances. A few infants tolerate fat poorly, in which case low-fat or fat-free formulas are helpful. (Whole milk has 4 per cent fat. Two per cent milk is made of one-half fat-free milk and one-half whole milk.)

3. 2% milk.. 18 oz.
   50% Karo (red label)................................. 2 oz.
   (= approximately 19 cal. per oz.)

4. Fat-free milk... 18 oz.
   50% Karo (red label)................................. 4 oz.
   (= approximately 19 cal. per oz.)

Infants suffering from pancreatic fibrosis absorb fats and proteins poorly. Often they do quite well on a protein hydrolysate formula:

5. Nutramigen .... 10 tbsp.
   Water... $16\frac{1}{2}$ oz.
   (= approximately 19 cal. per oz.)

If Nutramigen mixture is irritating to the intestinal tract and produces diarrhea (as is so often the case), it is better to give the child a standard formula (such as No. 1 above) and add about $\frac{1}{8}$ teaspoonful of Viokase* (a pancreatic extract) to each bottle just before the feeding (the pancreatic extract cannot be added during preparation of the formula because it is destroyed by heat).

A formula of Nutramigen, because of its low residue, is frequently of value for a few days for infants following intestinal anastomosis and anoplasty.

Thickened feedings are occasionally of some use in cases of pyloric stenosis or of chalasia of the esophagus; rice pablum is employed for thickening. One part of it is added to 15 or 20 parts of formula. This mixture is not too thick to pass through an average nipple.

Gavage or Tube Feeding

All premature babies, and indeed some full-term infants, are too weak to suck properly and they should be fed by gavage. A small tube is inserted down the mouth or nostril into the stomach, all air is aspirated, the formula is allowed to run in slowly, the tube is withdrawn, and the baby is allowed to drop off to sleep.

Tube feeding is employed for the alimentation of certain older children with poor appetites (e.g., burned patients) or with surgical conditions in which oral feedings are contraindicated (e.g., electrical burns of the mouth). In these, a small-sized polyethylene tube† is passed through the nose into the stomach, and a slow drip of high-protein, high-caloric feeding is given. Large quantities may be administered by this method, but care must be taken to prevent overdistention of the stomach and the attendant risk of vomiting and pulmonary aspiration.

---

* Viobin Corporation, Monticello, Illinois.

† Polyethylene Medical Tubing PE 190. Inner diameter 0.047 inch; outer diameter 0.067 inch. This will fit over a No. 18 needle.

Vitamins

All children should receive daily, supplemental, vitamin therapy. The best preparation to use is a water-miscible one. It is available as prepared by several companies. Each 0.6 cc. (0.3 to 0.6 cc. is the standard daily dose for infants) contains not less than

Vitamin A	5000 units
Vitamin D	1000 units
Thiamine chloride	1.0 mg.
Riboflavin	0.4 "
Ascorbic acid	50.0 "
Nicotinamide	2.0 "

For babies it may be added to the formula after sterilization; for older children it can be given directly by spoon or in any fluid which the child likes.

FLUID THERAPY

The Necessity for Fluid

Water is the largest single component of the body and in spite of its inert quality is one of the most important constituents. It is necessary for maintaining many normal functions of the living organism, among which the following are the most prominent: acting as a medium for the digestive processes of the alimentary tract, adding to the blood volume to give proper hemodynamics for the circulation, transportation of nutritious substances and vital elements in the blood stream and through the body structures, maintenance of the excretory mechanism of the kidneys, moistening of the various mucous membranes, and cooling of the body surfaces.

In health, fluid requirements of the body are met and held in a nice balance by the free ingestion of food and water and by the elimination of excesses through the urinary system. In surgical diseases, the balances are disturbed by reduction of oral intake, by excessive losses (vomiting, enterostomy, diarrhea, and so on), by increased demands (fever, exudates), and possibly by distortions of renal function. If these various aberrations are mild and are temporary, the reserves of the body can be adjusted in a compensatory manner. If the dislocations are great, it is impossible for adequate shifts to take place; those body functions which depend on water begin to lag, and more severe illness or even death can supervene unless fluids are given by some appropriate means, which generally implies that water must be supplied through parenteral routes.

The Problem of Fluid Therapy

Three general statements are in order regarding the handling of fluid therapy for surgical patients in childhood and infancy. *First*, a considerable proportion of surgical patients do not need any supplemental administration of water intravenously, hypodermically, or by rectal taps. Many operations, such as inguinal herniorrhaphy, excision of branchiogenic or thyroglossal sinuses, removal of cutaneous lesions, and a host of other procedures are in no way accompanied by disturbances of the intestinal tract before the surgery or after the nausea of anesthesia has passed. Mild shifts and water deficits will be tolerated and compensated for rapidly and safely as soon as the child begins to drink in a few hours after operation.

Second, severe water deficiencies in seriously ill children demand prompt, adequate, and sustained replacements by parenteral routes, regardless of whether the excessive loss occurred *previously* (starvation, vomiting, diarrhea), is taking place *currently* (vomiting, gastric suction, enterostomy), or is expected in the *immediate future* (intestinal siphonage which shows little promise of diminishing, uncontrollable efflux from an enterostomy, continuing pyrexia, polyuria of renal failure, or the like). A child can be kept in better condition if fluid balances are *corrected* as early as possible and are kept in a reasonable state throughout the illness than if great deficits are permitted to occur and then heroic efforts made to correct them.

Third, in children and particularly in babies with surgical conditions, it is just as important to recognize the dangers of water retention as those of fluid deficit. Kidneys of young subjects have a very limited capacity for excreting excess fluid, particularly when this is accompanied by unnecessary amounts of salt which have been injected into the body. These limitations of the kidney become all the more apparent during a major illness or following an anesthesia; temporary depressions of renal function can permit water to dam up in the body and not only can produce annoying disturbances of peripheral edema and retardation of wound healing but can also bring fatality from alveolar filling of the lung, edema of the cardiac musculature, or waterlogging of the brain. The inability of the kidneys of children and babies to excrete large amounts of unwanted and dangerous water becomes very apparent when the circulation has been flooded inadvertently by solutions which have been injected by parenteral routes. It is so easy to give water through needles into the subcutaneous tissues and especially into veins, that an unwary doctor can easily give too much. While tremendous advances have been made in surgery during the last few decades by providing adequate fluid therapy, it must be realized that the intravenous needle can also be one of our most dangerous tools if used indiscriminately. More children and babies have died of overhydration than have died of dehydration! It is essential to realize that fluid therapy is important in saving life, but if overdone can rapidly produce a fatality.

Amounts of Fluid Required

While the amounts of fluid required daily by adults have been widely appreciated, the amounts to be used for children and especially babies are often poorly understood. In general, there is a tendency to give too much when dealing with very small subjects. If excess amounts are injected, troublesome or even fatal complications can appear. Conversely, if amounts slightly below optimum figures are given, one can still supply a little more fluid at a subsequent time, the situation thereby being handled in a perfectly safe manner. It is much better to err on the side of not giving enough fluid than to infuse too much.

The chart shown in Figure 2 provides a rough guide for the amount of fluid required (by parenteral routes) by normal subjects of various weights. For surgical patients, these must be increased to cover any abnormal losses which are occurring from excessive sweating, vomiting, alimentary suction, enterostomy leakage, et cetera. After calculating the amount of fluid which is to be used in a twenty-four hour period, care must be taken that this is not all given at once; it must be divided and given at intervals of each twelve or preferably each eight hours. To overload the circulation at any one time may be fatal; to distribute the incoming fluid around the hours of the day and night gives only a minimal load which the weakened circulation can stand.

After one determines the total amount of fluid which is to be given in a given day, the figure may have to be altered subsequently by those highly important observations which one makes on the patient's condition. Peripheral edema, rapidly increasing weight (by daily weighing), moisture in the lungs, cerebral edema (twitching) are all fiindngs

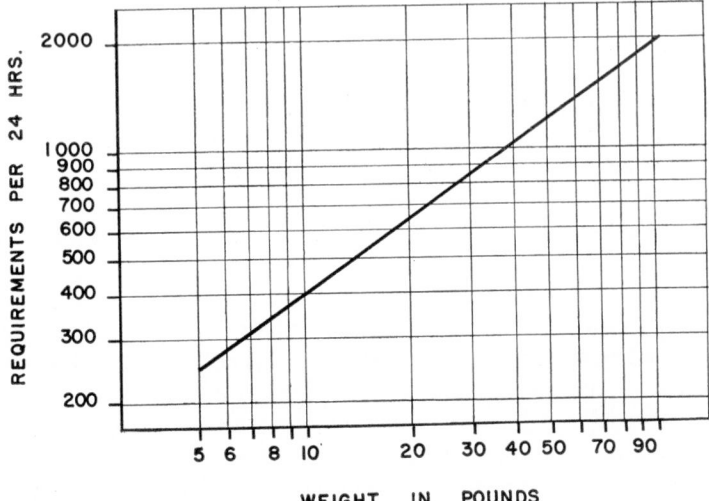

Fig. 2. Graph showing parenteral fluid requirements for maintenance of young subjects, in whom there are no preexisting deficits or current abnormal losses.

which indicate that the supply of fluid should be reduced promptly; if the various factors are marked, disaster is averted by withdrawing fluid from the body by stimulating the kidneys with 50 per cent glucose intravenously. Conversely, decreased elasticity of the skin, dryness of the oral membranes, sunken appearance of the eyes, lethargy, oliguria, or high concentration of urine are indications for increasing the amounts of fluid which will be employed. For the severely ill child, nothing can supplant proper bedside supervision each six or eight hours, at each of which visits the physician in charge sums up all the observations available and then clearly gives the orders which are to be carried out during the subsequent interval.

Methods of Fluid Administration

There is no perfect substitute for the oral intake of water and other nutritious fluids. Generally, natural appetite and thirst are the best measures of the body demands. Unfortunately, the severely ill surgical patient generally has derangements of the gastro-

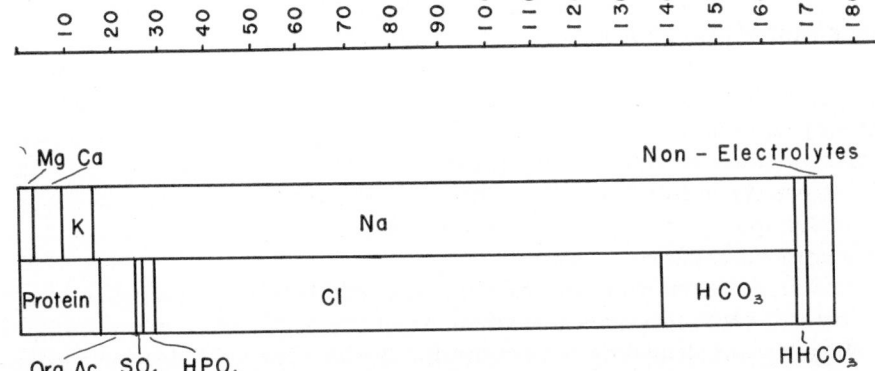

Fig. 3. Electrolyte composition of human plasma. (From Gamble: Chemical Anatomy, Physiology, and Pathology of Extracellular Fluid).

intestinal tract which prohibit taking food and fluid by mouth, at least for a critical period. It becomes necessary to supply these by other routes.

Rectal Taps. Fluid can be taken into the body when given by instillation of small amounts of water into the rectum every two or three hours, or by inserting into the rectum a small catheter through which water is allowed to drip slowly and constantly. These methods were widely used in the past, but now are almost entirely supplanted by hypodermoclysis or venoclysis which allows greater amounts to be given and also has the particular advantage of permitting one to be quite sure of how much the patient actually receives.

Hypodermoclysis is a fairly safe way of introducing fluids but has limitations which greatly reduce its usefulness. It produces discomfort, which, however, is not serious if the material is not injected too quickly or in too large amounts. The rate of uptake is slow, but can be augmented by addition of hyaluronidase to the solution. Solutions which are too weak or are too strong are dangerous; the concentration must be kept within a rather narrow range for the fluid to be absorbed and to avoid regional tissue damage. Sites available for injection are limited to the back and the thighs. The former is impractical after operation when the child will be lying on its back or has a large dressing or binder around an abdominal wound. Not infrequently, the thighs are being used for multiple injections of antibiotics and it is disturbing to also use them for infusion of fluids. Furthermore, hypodermoclysis almost always requires the services of a nurse or attendant during the period that fluid is being run in—coverage which is sometimes difficult to obtain. We find that we are using hypodermoclysis with greatly diminishing frequency, preferring to infuse most fluids by vein. However, under some circumstances hypodermoclysis is still a most valuable method. The substances which can be injected thus are physiologic saline or a mixture of one part physiologic saline and one part 5 per cent glucose in water; stronger or more hypotonic solutions should never be given. Fifteen cubic centimeters per pound are about all that should be given at one time.

Venoclysis. For older children, whose veins are prominent and accessible, the problems of introducing intravenous fluids are no different from those of adults. However, for small children, and particularly babies, considerable skill is required to introduce a needle properly into the tiny and fragile veins, to keep it there while fluid is running in, and at the same time prevent leakage of the solution out into surrounding tissues where it might do harm. We have been most fortunate in having house staffs who enjoy the challenge of intravenous therapy, and have developed an amazing knack for performing these tasks. Their willingness and their ability to do this job have been responsible more than any other single factor in pulling a large number of critically ill patients through desperate postoperative struggles.

In infants, veins of the scalp are most commonly used for intravenous therapy. In malnourished infants, other vessels such as those on the back of the hand are prominent and may be utilized. We have a firm rule that fluids should never be injected into the superior longitudinal sinus or into a femoral vein; in either place the risk of damage to nearby structures is enormous. For older children, veins on the back of the hand, in the antecubital space, or on the anteromedial aspect of the ankle are the ones most readily accessible and easiest to use.

To facilitate intravenous infusions, it is extremely helpful to the patient, the nurse, and the doctor if some provision is made to quiet the child before and during the procedure. Wiggling and struggling can disrupt the whole affair, dislodge the needle, make it necessary to start over again, and thoroughly test the patience of all concerned. Conversely, if the patient is sedated adequately, the infusion goes quickly, effectively, and with a minimum of effort.

For a *single* intravenous infusion, some limit must be placed upon the amount of fluid which can be given, the rate of injection, and the frequency with which the treatment can be repeated. Ordinarily, the amount should not exceed 10 cc. per pound of body weight and for small babies should take at least fifteen to twenty minutes to run in; when dealing with children beyond a year or two of age, the infusion should be given slowly over the course of an hour or two. Infusions should seldom be given more than twice, or certainly not more than three times per twenty-four hours.

For *continuous* intravenous work, in which fluid is allowed to go in slowly over a long period, the apparatus should have in its tubing a glass drip chamber so that the rate of infusion can be carefully adjusted (by compression of the tube with a Hoffman clamp) to the number of drops per minute which are desired. Ordinarily, it is not practical to keep a flow going at a rate less than 8 drops (0.5 cc.) per minute. With this set-up there is little if any danger of producing an undesirable surge of fluid into the circulation, but there is some risk of running in too great a total over a period of time. Therefore, when continuous intravenous drips are being used in babies and small children, close supervision is necessary and clear orders must be given about the total, which the nurse or attendant must not exceed in any six or eight-hour stretch.

Materials Available for Fluid Therapy

A considerable variety of fluids can be used for getting water, electrolytes, and nourishment into the body. Which one is used depends upon the current needs of the patient and the route which is available through which fluids can be given.

For *oral* ingestion, one's hands are often tied because the patient has some disturbance which throws the alimentary tract out of function temporarily. However, there comes a time when some material can be taken in this way, even though it fills only a part of the needs. While other substances might not yet be tolerated, water in small amounts can possibly be taken and retained. If this can be kept down, mixtures of saline and glucose (half physiologic saline, half 10 per cent glucose) supply some salt and a few calories. As things improve, Nutramigen mixtures are helpful since they are easy to digest, have a very fine curd and low residue; they supply amino acids and some protein. Orange, grapefruit, and tomato juices are high in potassium content; they are palatable and helpful liquids whenever potassium deficiency lurks in the background. While the totals taken by mouth might be small, they are important in getting the gastro-intestinal tract to function again, and they reduce the amounts which have to be supplied by intravenous or subcutaneous routes.

For *subcutaneous* injection, physiologic saline is the fluid most commonly used. When the need for salt is less and the demand for calories is greater, a mixture (equal parts of physiologic saline and of 5 per cent glucose in water) can be given. Solutions of lower osmotic tension should not be employed; they may actually draw electrolytes into the area (from the circulation) and therefore have damaging systemic effects. Likewise, solutions of higher osmotic tension are dangerous since they give regional necrosis and may draw into the area water from the circulation.

For *intravenous* injection, the most commonly used solutions are physiologic saline or glucose (5 or 10 per cent) in water. While it is known that 10 per cent glucose is followed by some spillage of sugar in the urine, and indeed this concentration might have a slightly dehydrating effect, it is felt that the material, if not injected too rapidly, probably gives a higher caloric uptake than 5 per cent glucose in water and is therefore preferred. These substances (the saline or the glucose solution) can be stored in 500 or 1000 cc. flasks; they are our mainstay in fluid therapy, *and the vast majority of cases can be handled with these solutions alone.* For those unusual situations when a more concentrated sodium chloride solution is necessary (which is very rare) or when potassium is required, these can be added in the open burette as desired.

Blood is widely used for those situations when the red blood count or the hemoglobin level is depressed to any appreciable extent. Unless there is concurrent hemorrhage, blood is not administered to infants and small children in amounts exceeding

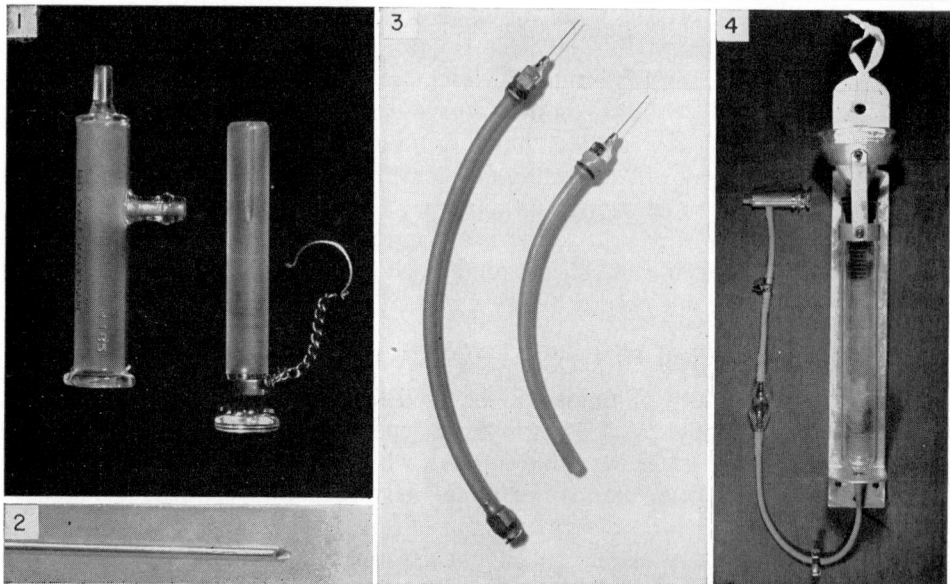

Fig. 4. Pieces of apparatus which are very useful for intravenous infusions of fluid or blood to children and babies. 1. Chamberlain modification of a Kaufman Syringe. The plunger contains a groove which, when turned toward the side-arm, allows fluid to enter the barrel. Therefore, it is not necessary to withdraw a barrel-full of blood through the needle when withdrawing the plunger to admit the injection fluid to enter from the side-arm of the syringe. 2. Intravenous needle with a very short bevel. This minimizes the protrusion of the needle through the back wall of a vein. 3. Needles fitted directly on to sections of rubber, particularly useful for placement into tiny scalp veins of babies when the infusion is to be continued for a long period of time. The needle can be strapped with adhesive tape to the scalp; the soft rubber segment absorbs any movements and therefore minimizes chances of dislodgment of the needle. 4. Burette for intravenous infusion. In the tube beyond the burette is a glass bulb with a central drip core, so the rate of infusion can be seen. Beyond this is a three-way stopcock to the side of which a Luer-Lok syringe can be attached if fluid has to be pumped under pressure. At the end of the tube is a Kaufman syringe (Chamberlain modification).

10 cc. per pound of body weight at any one time. Plasma is used generously if there is any important depression of the serum-protein level, the hemoglobin value being satisfactory.

Apparatus

For use in babies and in small children, those types of infusion apparatus which are so commonly employed for adults are completely unsatisfactory. In most of these one cannot tell whether the fluid is running except by noticing a fall in the fluid level of the flask or by seeing from time to time bubbles of air passing from a side-arm up through the fluid. These are sufficient in adults when large quantities of fluid are being infused, but in tiny subjects when the amounts injected are quite small, such observations are misleading; all too often it is impossible to tell whether any fluid is running into the patient at any one particular moment.

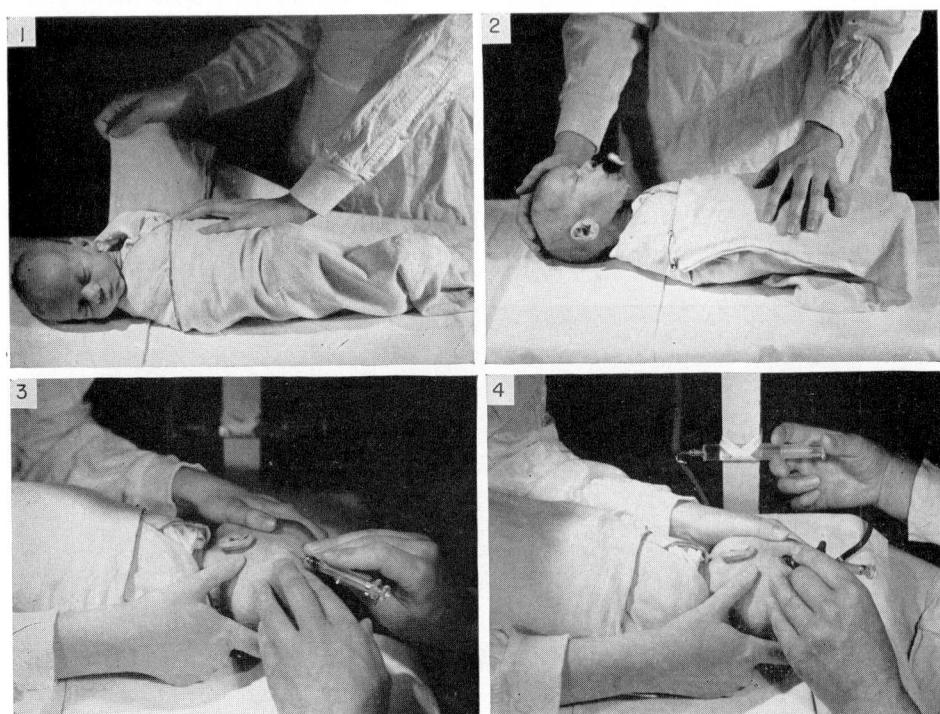

Fig. 5. Intravenous injection of fluids into a baby, employing a scalp vein. 1. Bundling the baby with a sheet or blanket to immobilize the legs and arms. 2. Bundling is completed. The baby is quieted with a sugar-nipple. 3. Scalp shaved. Position of the nurse (at left) as she immobilizes the child's head. Physician (at right) directing the needle, mounted on a Kaufman syringe, into a vein. 4. Needle in vein. Barrel of Kaufman plunger withdrawn. With his right hand, the doctor can pump the Luer-Lok syringe and thus inject the fluid under pressure. (Above the field is hung a burette, as shown in Figure 4.) The infusion can be completed in 15 to 20 minutes.

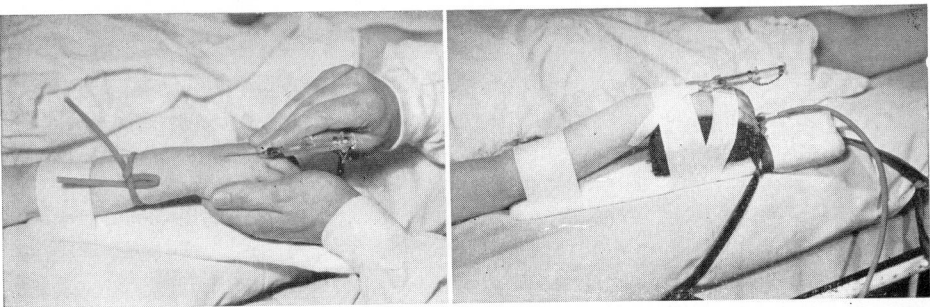

Fig. 6. Intravenous infusion in hand of a child. *Left*, Arm-board ready. Tourniquet on forearm. Needle, mounted on a Kaufman syringe, being inserted. *Right*, Infusion running. Hand immobilized over pad or sponge rubber to arm-board. Needle strapped into place. Arm-board tied to side of bed.

Types of apparatus for parenteral fluid therapy which we have found to be practical are illustrated in Figure 4. We routinely use a 250 cc. (or 100 cc.) burette of heat-resistant glass, open at the top, which can receive a one-hole stopper carrying a three-inch heat-resistant glass funnel. The burette is graduated in 5 cc. markings. The lower end of the burette is fitted with rubber tubing, in the course of which are successively, a screw (Hoffman) clamp, a glass Murphy drip bulb, a three-way stopcock, and finally a Chamberlain type Kaufman side-arm syringe, to which a fine needle can be fitted. Theoretically, such an apparatus has the objection of having an open top which might allow contamination, but with scrupulous technique we have never had this occur. The open-top burette has the enormous advantage of permitting addition of fluids from time to time if more are needed, and also permits making mixtures at the bedside by adding small amounts of concentrated stock solutions (potassium chloride, sodium chloride, et cetera). We have used this arrangement for more than twenty-five years at the Children's Hospital; it has been so satisfactory that we have no desire to change it in any way.

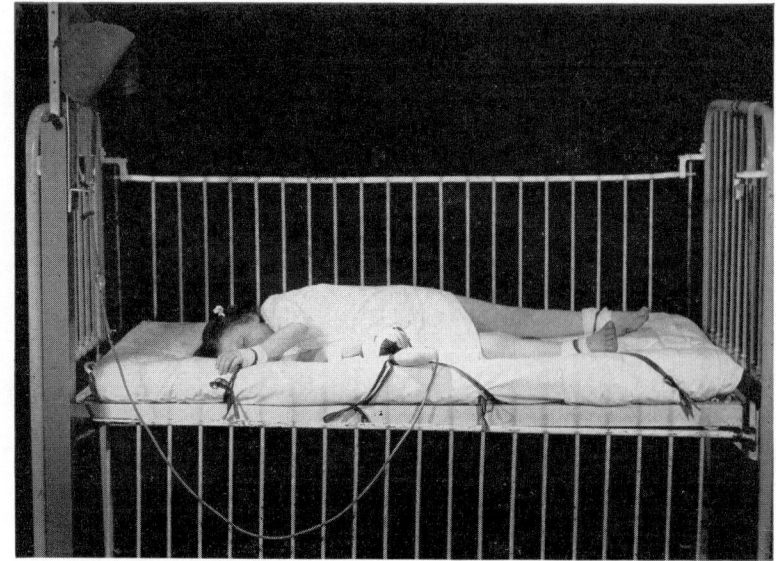

Fig. 7. Child in bed, receiving intravenous infusion. She is turned on her side. Wrist, ankles, and armboard are restrained. Sedation is essential.

In performing a venipuncture on a small child or baby, it is completely unsatisfactory to have a needle mounted on a straight glass connector at the end of rubber tubing, as is so commonly used for adults. With such an arrangement, it is difficult or impossible to know just when the needle has entered the vein; furthermore, fluid is very apt to escape into the perivascular tissues before the vein is punctured and the tiny vessel is then lost to view. For injecting fluids into veins of a small child or baby, it is essential to have a Kaufman side-arm syringe, onto which the fine needle is mounted. With this equipment, the needle can be deliberately maneuvered and inserted into the tiniest of veins; a test can then be made by withdrawing the plunger a millimeter or so to see if blood comes back into the barrel. When this has been attained, the plunger is fully withdrawn and fluid flows from the side-arm in through the infusing needle. An excellent modification of the Kaufman syringe is the Chamberlain adaptation, which provides a single longitudinal groove on the surface of the plunger. This groove is kept turned away from the side-arm while the needle is being directed into a vein, which position is proved by gently withdrawing the plunger a millimeter or two to see if blood comes back into the barrel. Now holding the needle steadily in place, the plunger is rotated on its long axis so the longitudinal groove on the plunger comes over against the side-arm, permitting fluid to fill the barrel of the syringe as the plunger is slowly withdrawn. It is thus possible to start the infusion without aspirating as much blood as is required when using a standard Kaufman syringe, a point of great significance when dealing with babies, from whom it is difficult to withdraw much blood.

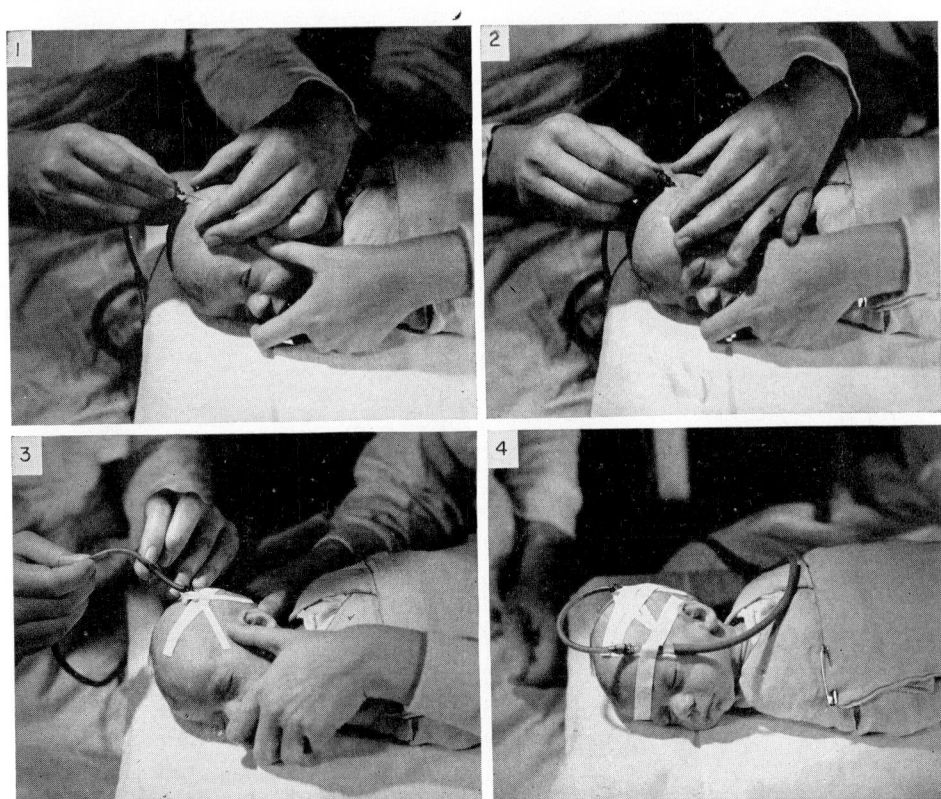

Fig. 8. Arrangement for long-continued drip of intravenous fluids to a baby. 1. The child is bundled. Small needle, carrying a soft rubber connector, being inserted into vein. 2. Needle in vein. 3. Needle strapped into place with adhesive tape. 4. The rubber connector attached to the infusion apparatus (the burette of which hangs on a nearby pole). With an arrangement of this sort, infusion can be continued for many hours. With luck, the needle will stay in place for 12 to 18 hours. When the child is placed back in its crib, sand-bags can be placed in front of the forehead and behind the occiput to limit movements of the head. With this sort of continuous infusion in the scalp, the baby should not be fed by mouth; there is too much danger of vomiting and aspiration, since the child cannot move its head adequately to clear the throat.

It is extremely helpful to have a Murphy drip glass mounted in the tubing. As fluid drops from the mechanism in the center of this chamber, one can see at a glance whether fluid is running properly, can easily estimate the rate of flow, and if necessary can adjust the rate of flow by partially compressing the rubber tube above with a Hoffman clamp.

The three-way stopcock in the rubber tubing is extremely useful when there is a call to inject fluids rapidly in emergency situations or when very small intravenous needles are being used and gravity is insufficient to give a satisfactory flow. A 10 or 20 cc. Luer-Lok syringe can be attached to the open arm of this three-way stopcock. By turning the valve into an appropriate position, fluid can be drawn down from the burette into the syringe; the valve is then turned in a direction which allows dejection of fluid from the syringe into the infusion apparatus. It is a very simple matter to manipulate alternately the stopcock and syringe to give a pumping action so that fluids can be injected with great speed or under high pressure when these features are desired.

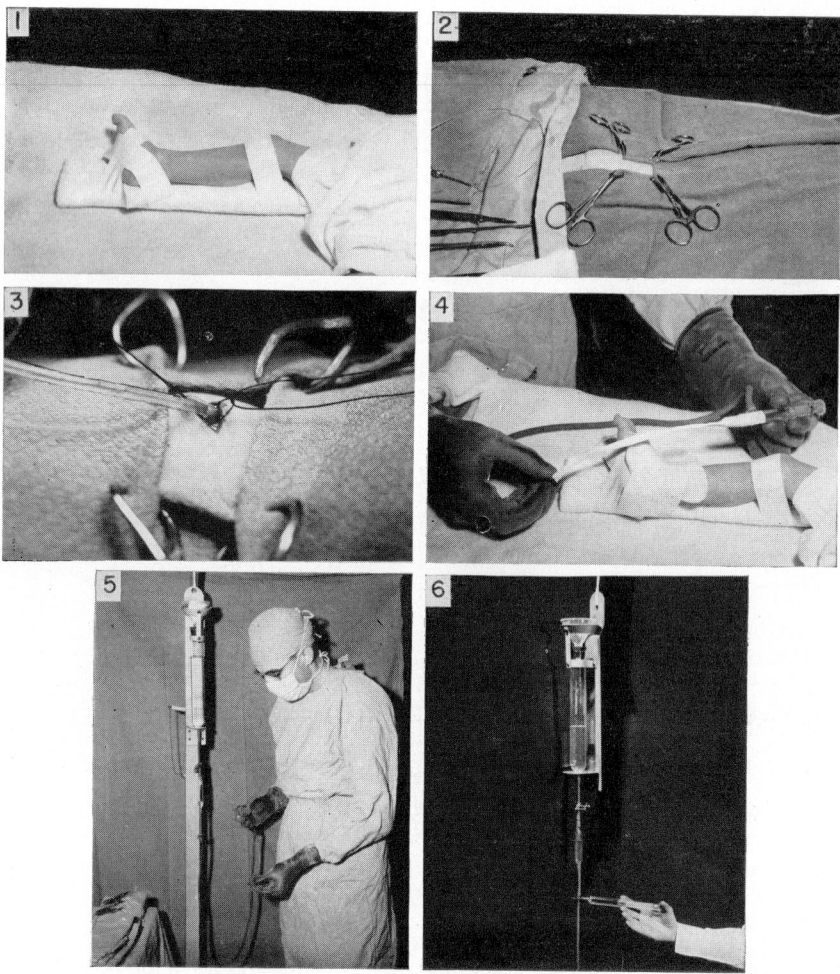

Fig. 9. Method for placing a "cut-down" for intravenous infusions or transfusions during operation, or to critically ill children. 1. Lower leg and foot strapped to a padded board; a piece of sponge rubber under the ankle to prevent pressure sores. 2. Skin prepared with antiseptic, and drapes placed around the field. 3. Skin opened, vein exposed. Polyethylene tube run into vein. It will be tied in the vein with a silk thread. 4. Dressing applied. The polyethylene tube has been fitted to a needle on the Kaufman syringe. Adhesive tape is run along the syringe, needle, and plastic tube to hold them together. 5. The reservoir and infusion apparatus. Hanging on the pole is a burette (with a funnel at its top). The long tubing runs to the Kaufman syringe which the doctor is holding. 6. Close-up view of the burette and its attachments. Below the burette is a dripper-glass, which allows visualization of the rate at which fluid is passing. Below is a three-way stop cock, carrying a Luer-Lok syringe which can be used to inject fluid or blood rapidly if an emergency arises.

Because the veins of a small child or an infant are delicately thin and because babies are prone to squirm, it is exceedingly difficult to keep an ordinary needle in place for a very long time without its sharp point piercing the vein wall or becoming dislodged. To minimize these accidents, the points of needles should be ground to have short bevels; the short-bevel point is sharp enough to penetrate the overlying skin and the vein wall, but is much less likely to pierce the opposite vein wall once it is in place. For babies, a No. 24 needle is used.

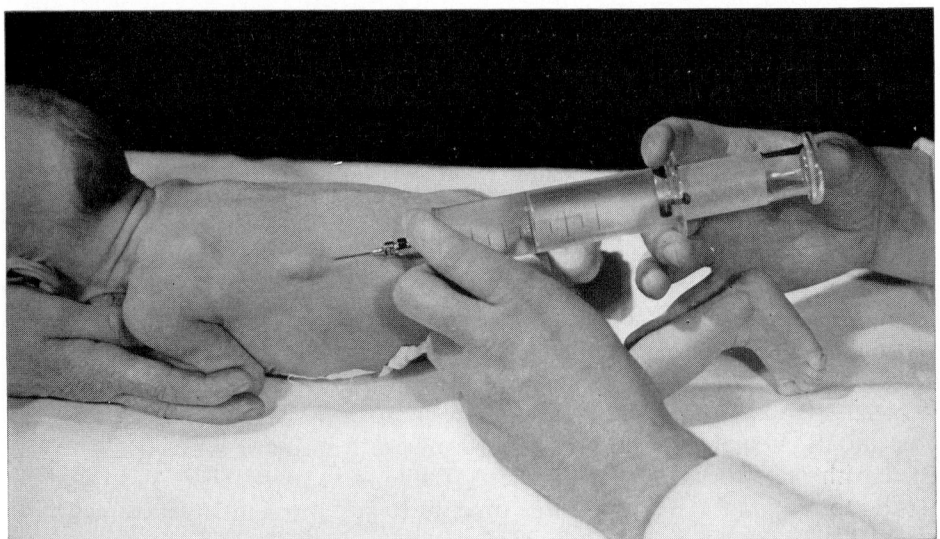

Fig. 10. Hypodermoclysis into tissues of back of a small baby, employing a needle and syringe

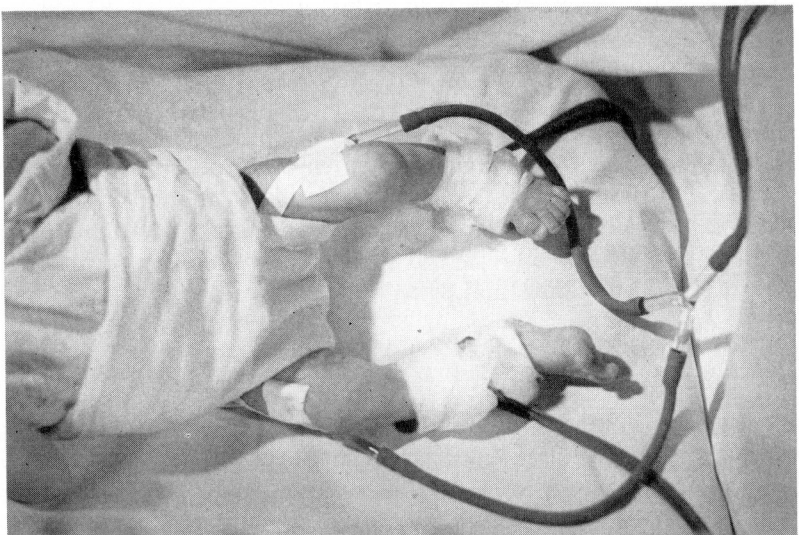

Fig. 11. Common method of giving hypodermoclysis in thighs of babies. The ankles are restrained. Needles inserted and strapped to each thigh.

Aims of Fluid Therapy

It is the main goal of parenteral fluid therapy to tide the child over a crisis until fluids can be ingested and retained through the normal processes of alimentation. For basic needs, sufficient fluid must be given to maintain the vital excretory functions of the kidney, to supply that which is used for the insensible pulmonary and cutaneous evaporations, and to keep the tissues of the body in a reasonable state of hydration. In addition, if depletions have *already* occurred, these must be corrected to bring the fluid status back to something approaching normalcy. If losses are *currently taking place* or are *expected to continue*, sufficient fluid must be given to provide for these and thereby prevent further robbing of the body tissues. From the clinical course of the patient and his disease process, it is generally possible to predict from day to day what the fluid needs will be, which is a summation of those normally used by a patient of the given weight and those which are necessary to cover the abnormal losses. Rather than let a patient slip into a state of marked dehydration and then attempt to retrieve him, it is far better to supply adequate fluids from day to day, and thereby keep the subject in a fairly stable water balance.

If there is any question about the amount of fluid which should be administered, it is preferable to err on the side of underhydration rather than overhydration. If too much fluid is administered, pulmonary moisture, cardiac failure, or cerebral edema can lead rapidly to overwhelming disaster. Conversely, if it is found that a child is a little on the "dry" side, this does no great harm and can be corrected easily by supplying a little more fluid in some form. In a small child or a baby, the dangers of overhydration are exceedingly great; many fatalities have occurred because of overenthusiasm in ordering parenteral fluids. There are few things more devastating to a baby than a flood of water into its circulation. It is essential to realize that there are limits which cannot be exceeded with safety. Once an intravenous needle is in place, there is a tremendous temptation to run in all the fluids at one time, or to add just a little extra fluid for good measure. This is very apt to be a lethal act.

For seriously ill children, it is quite necessary to make a daily list or chart which gives a running summary of the various fluid losses and the various fluid administrations. This balance sheet, combined with clinical observations of the child's status of hydration, is the best guide for outlining or altering fluid therapy.

While parenteral fluid therapy is often a lifesaving measure, every effort should be made to terminate it as quickly as possible, tapering this off as soon as the alimentary tract is able to take over its vital functions. Parenteral injections are extraordinarily expensive in the use of physician, nurse, and attendant's time, and furthermore they are not without some risk. No laboratory test or clinical acumen can handle the delicate matter of fluid balance by artificial injection as well as can a child who has a clear mind, an open gullet, a functioning intestinal tract, and free access to water and food.

PROVISION FOR CALORIC NEEDS

Caloric Requirements

Operations which bring about mild and short-term disturbances of the alimentary tract (such as herniorrhaphy, treatment of congenital abnormalities of the neck, removal of certain cutaneous lesions, and many others) need cause no concern about a temporary loss of intake. The period of starvation is only for a day or a fraction thereof, which deficiency is insignificant and can be readily cared for by drawing upon the abundant stores of the body.

Those illnesses (such as peritonitis, intestinal obstruction, conditions requiring intestinal resection, et cetera) which bring serious disruption of the intestinal functions imply that starvation will be an important factor; strong efforts should be made by appropriate measures to meet the caloric needs of the body as far as possible. In all instances, it is possible to keep the metabolic fires burning brightly by abolishing (or preventing) ketosis. Theoretically, it would be desirable to supply all of the calories which the patient needs for production of heat and energy; from a practical standpoint this cannot be done fully with the various substances which are available today. Therefore, the best that can be offered is to make the supply as generous as possible, fully realizing that this will leave a deficit which must be covered by breakdown of protein and fat depots of the body. We attempt to minimize this wasting and thereby reduce the job of rebuilding these stores in the subsequent period of rehabilitation and convalescence.

Materials Available for Parenteral Use

While very weak *glucose solutions* can be injected subcutaneously, most of the fluids that have any important nutrient value must be given intravenously. Foremost on this list is 5 per cent glucose in distilled water, or preferably *10 per cent glucose in water*. The latter is our principal material and it is used unstintingly, the only limit to the total amount injected being that figure beyond which the volume of fluid should not go. *Plasma* has an important place in those situations in which there is starvation for more than three or four days and in which the plasma protein level is beginning to fall or is expected to fall. Plasma should not be injected in amounts greater than 10 cc. per pound in any single twenty-four hour period. Because of the higher risks of transmitting the virus of hepatitis, *pooled* plasma should never be used. *Human albumin* (salt-poor) is an exceedingly valuable addition to our armamentarium for providing protein. It is available in 20 per cent suspension (about three times normal plasma concentration). If diluted in distilled water to the concentration of plasma albumin, it has little advantage over plasma infusion in most circumstances. When it is injected as a concentrated solution (up to three times normal), it has a dehydrating effect and also provides a large amount of protein without augmenting greatly the fluid intake. When given to babies in the concentrated form (20 per cent suspension) amounts of 1 to 2 cc. per pound of body weight are well tolerated. We use this material extensively in newborn babies who are critically ill or who have undergone some major procedure, such as repair of esophageal atresia. *Amino acid* preparations have been studied by numerous investigators in the hopes of providing building blocks from which the body can synthesize proteins; without doubt some of this material is utilized. On occasion we have used these substances intravenously but have not been very favorably impressed by the results; we now give these mixtures but rarely. *Emulsified fats* are receiving considerable study and should have the feature of supplying a much higher caloric intake, compared gram for gram to protein and carbohydrate. Apparently the fat can be burned by the body. The problems of preparing and storing the materials have not yet been simplified to the point where they are available for general use; our experience with them has been limited. It is hoped that in the future emulsified fats can be prepared in ways which will make them practical for routine intravenous administration.

While there are some who have strongly advocated the use of amino acid solutions or emulsified fats for intravenous therapy, we have not used these to any extent. It has been our practice to get in as much glucose as possible, and also each day give some blood, some plasma, or some human albumin to piece together a therapeutic program which—while it has obvious deficiencies—does permit one to drag desperately ill children through very dark valleys and eventually get them on the road to recovery.

ELECTROLYTE THERAPY

General Considerations

There are many mild shifts in electrolyte pattern which do not require active measures directed toward replacement of the losses. Short periods of starvation which are incurred after a large number of operations (such as herniorrhaphy, plastic operations, removal of congenital anomalies of the neck, treatment of cutaneous lesions) can almost always be disregarded as far as electrolyte disturbances are concerned; these will be eliminated rapidly as soon as the patient again takes food.

There are other conditions in which there has been actual *loss* of electrolytes from the body (for example, with vomiting in typical cases of unruptured appendicitis) but in which the loss is small and has taken place within a day or two. Under these circumstances it is seldom necessary to give replacement therapy; the imbalances will correct themselves within a few days after the offending lesion has been treated and the patient begins to take food and fluid by mouth.

In *contrast* are those situations (peritonitis, intestinal obstruction, and so on) in which there has been starvation for some days, and already a considerable loss of gastric and intestinal juices, superimposed upon which a major operation will be performed. In addition there will be a period of many days during which electrolyte losses will continue and may be enormous (in sweat, in urine, and in gastric and intestinal siphonage); in all of these cases the electrolyte shifts assume great prominence and may greatly tax or even exceed the capacity of the body in making adjustments. Improvement of the patient (and even his survival) demands active measures for correction of electrolyte deviations. If great deficits are allowed to mount up, it may be utterly impossible to correct them; conversely, if an adequate running supply is provided, the patient's life will probably be spared.

Units of Measurement

"Milliequivalents per liter" has become the standard unit of measure for the various chemical components of the body fluids. This value is obtained by dividing milligrams per liter by atomic weight and multiplying by valency. The CO_2 content of blood can be changed from volumes per cent to milliequivalents by dividing by 2.2. While it has been common practice in the past to measure the various elements in terms of "milligrams per cent" or "volumes per cent," it is far better to change all of these to "milliequivalents per liter," since this gives better comprehension of the electrolyte pattern and facilitates calculation of the therapy.

Normal values for blood constituents or components are as follows:

Component	Normal Values	
Sodium	138–144	mEq/L
Chloride	100–106	mEq/L
Potassium	4–7	mEq/L
CO_2	22–28	mEq/L
pH	7.35–7.45	

In the electrolyte pattern of human plasma (Fig. 3) the sum of the cations is equal to the sum of the anions; this provides electrical equality. The normal proportion of carbonic acid (H_2CO_3) to bicarbonate (HCO_3) is 1:20. The ratio of these two substances is the fundamental determinant of pH of the blood. In derangements of acid-base balance, values for either H_2CO_3 or HCO_3 may be normal, increased, or decreased. A change in blood pH toward the acid side may be produced by either an increase in H_2CO_3 or a decrease in the HCO_3 fraction. A change in blood pH toward the alkaline side may be produced by either a decrease in the H_2CO_3 or an increase in the amount of HCO_3 in the blood. Either alkalosis or acidosis can be "compensated," in which instance blood CO_2 levels are abnormal, but the pH is not.

Abnormal States

While there are a wide variety of combinations representing abnormal states, there are certain ones of particular importance because of the frequency with which they are found and because of the profound disturbances which they can bring about.

Alkalosis is the most common shift of total electrolyte pattern which is encountered in surgical patients. It is most commonly brought about by long-continued vomiting or by removal of gastric or intestinal juices (pyloric obstruction, intestinal obstruction, peritonitis, enterostomy). The more rapid loss of chloride ions than of sodium ions in vomitus gives a relative depression of the chloride anion in the plasma electrolyte pattern; compensation is accomplished by a rise in the bicarbonate fraction, thereby producing a shift of pH to the alkaline side of 7.4.

Aciaosis. In the surgical diseases of children, acidosis is much less common than alkalosis. It is most frequently encountered when there are interferences with the regulatory mechanism of the kidney or of the respiratory apparatus. Renal damage can disrupt the selective processes of elimination by the kidney. An example of this is seen in the hyperchloremic acidosis which can occur after transplantation of ureters into the sigmoid and when, in addition, there is damage to the kidneys. Continuing reabsorption of urinary products from the bowel increases the total amount of electrolytes which the kidneys must excrete. Being unable to remove selectively proper amounts of chloride, this builds up in the blood, is followed by a compensatory fall in the plasma bicarbonate and a marked reduction in the carbonic acid; there is onset of acidosis. Prolonged anesthesia, particularly with closed systems, may be accompanied by poor absorption of carbon dioxide by the apparatus, allowing this substance to build up to high levels in the alveoli and producing high carbonic acid levels in the blood; the blood pH can shift to 7.2 or even as far as 7.0. Such temporary and extreme acidosis almost certainly accounts for many of the cardiac irregularities or even arrests which have occurred under anesthesia.

Sodium Deficiency. Sodium is a major component of the body fluids; heavy losses of stomach or intestinal juices may cause rapid sodium depletion. Replacement of this loss by using only glucose and water results in a further washing out of sodium and a reduction of concentration of this ion in the plasma and various body fluids. Mild lowering of the plasma sodium concentration, possibly to 130 to 135 milliequivalents, may be inconsequential. Depressions 10 to 15 milliequivalents below normal should bring considerable concern and also attempts at correction; but if there is edema (and the fluid compartment of the body is thereby increased), the total body sodium may not be depressed as far as the plasma value would seem to indicate. Depressions below concentration of 120 milliequivalents per liter are extremely serious, produce marked lethargy and weakness, and certainly call for speedy and intensive replacements. In such situations, one is usually dealing with complicated problems, all facets of which must be taken into account when planning the therapy.

Potassium Deficiency. Potassium deficiencies occur very commonly in surgical patients, but generally they can be completely ignored because the shifts are minimal; most subjects have adequate stores of potassium (which can shift from cells out into the fluid compartment) and it is seldom necessary to supply potassium parenterally, the patient making up the deficit in an adequate way as soon as food can be taken by mouth. However, when losses of gastric juice, succus entericus, or urine are prolonged over a period of many days, and potassium is not supplied by parenteral routes, *hypokalemia* occurs; the patient shows marked lassitude, weakness of the extremities, tachycardia, a depression of the plasma potassium level, and possibly electrocardiographic deviations, indicated by a lowering and prolongation of the T-waves, and possibly inversion of T-waves. Because other conditions can produce similar electrocardiographic changes, relevant clinical data are of great importance in interpreting electrocardiographic abnormalities.

The most important clinical signs of potassium deficit from a diagnostic standpoint are: (1) The therapeutic refractoriness of metabolic alkalosis and acidosis to specific corrective measures. (2) Silent ileus. (3) The failure to achieve an appreciable gain in strength by administering sodium salt solutions of appropriate tonicity.

Replacement of potassium by injection, based merely on a low plasma figure, might seriously overload the patient and bring about disastrous results. Parenteral replacement of potassium must always be made with caution.

Hyperkalemia. Rises of potassium above normal in the plasma and body tissue can occur during renal failure and retention, during excessive tissue breakdowns (burns or trauma, when accompanied by oliguria), from hemolytic crises, from transfusion reactions, or from too rapid injection of potassium during some therapeutic program. Above the normal levels, potassium virtually becomes a poison and may rapidly produce irritability, cardiac irregularity, and death.

Properly read and controlled electrocardiograms are considered by many to be more accurate measures of potassium poisoning than are plasma levels, since the changes in the electrical potential of the myocardium are believed to reflect both intracellular and extracellular concentrations. If a base-line tracing is available for comparison, electrocardiograms can indicate potassium intoxication (in possibly 80 per cent of cases) fairly well when plasma levels are above 6.5 and reliably so when the levels are above 7 mEq/L. The T-waves are high and the S-T segments depressed; more advanced signs are disappearance of T-waves and onset of heart block.

Salt Retention. Under some circumstances, retention of salt by the body is a normal process, most commonly seen in the first twenty-four or forty-eight hours after operation when the pituitary-adrenal cortical response acts to conserve body fluids; there is a diminution in excretion of sodium, chloride, and water by the kidneys. Cognizance should be taken of this factor and injection of salt solutions should not be made in amounts which overload the kidneys. This does not mean that the supply of water and salt should always be kept low during the first day or two after surgery. If, during this time, there are high losses of an extrarenal sort (as from marked gastric suction or from enterostomy leakage) the need for parenteral fluid and electrolyte therapy may be great.

Aside from the normal hormonal reaction occurring within the first few days after surgery, the kidneys of children, and especially babies, simply do not have the capacity to eliminate excessive amounts of salt if this has been injected in an indiscriminate way; salt can be retained in the tissues and edema will develop. While this is not particularly harmful in extremities or in other subcutaneous areas, it can greatly interfere with the healing of a wound or an intestinal anastomosis and can rapidly lead to breakdown of suture lines. Edema fluid is particularly dangerous when it accumulates in the alveolar spaces, in the myocardium, or in the brain, with the possibility of producing death rapidly by anoxemia, cardiac insufficiency, or respiratory failure respectively.

Materials Available for Replacement Therapy

During the past few decades the important findings of many investigators have focused attention on the particular distortions of electrolyte pattern which can occur in various combinations of defects. To treat these particular situations, electrolyte solutions of appropriate composition have been devised for parenteral therapy, including Hartmann's, Darrow's, Ringer's, and Butler's formulas. More recently, polyionic solutions are being prepared by commercial houses for clinical use. Without doubt there is merit in these various mixtures for treatment of particular sets of imbalances, but we are much inclined to believe that their use can sometimes also be harmful in that unneeded elements (e.g., potassium) can be given in excess. We have completely given up using these complex electrolyte solutions, feeling that it is more practical and economical to use as the main body of fluid for the infusion a physiologic saline or else 10 per cent glucose in distilled water; to these, small amounts of various additional electrolytes can be added at the bedside as desired. For such purpose, it is our practice to have stored and on hand small 75 cc. flasks* containing concentrated electrolyte solutions. The first is a 1 M KCl solution (1 cc. of which furnishes 1 milliequivalent of potassium as potassium chloride). The solution is dyed blue so that when added to intravenous solutions the attendant personnel can tell at a glance that potassium is being administered. The second (but rarely used) is a 4.6 M NaCl solution (1 cc. of which provides 4.6 milliequivalents of sodium; 3.3 cc. of the solution diluted up to 100 cc. gives a "physiologic" saline; 10 cc. diluted up to 100 cc. gives a 3 per cent solution of sodium chloride). Either of these substances (or both) can be added to the burette of physiologic solution (or glucose solution) which is the main body of the material being injected intravenously.

Aims of Electrolyte Therapy

There is little point in attempting to correct minor deviations in electrolyte patterns which undoubtedly occur in many mild illnesses. However, when electrolyte distortion becomes marked, corrective measures should always be instituted to compensate for them before crises arise. Furthermore, it is important to anticipate losses which are known to be occurring and which probably will continue unabated for some days. For example, if intestinal siphonage, or leakage from an enterostomy, is proceeding at a rate which shows little evidence of letdown, it is much better to keep supplying salt solution and prevent depletion than it is to allow serious shifts to occur and then invoke last-minute heroic measures to try to correct them.

There are few aberrations in electrolyte shifts which cannot be overcome by parenteral injection of physiologic saline. When one is presented with laboratory evidence of marked depletion of sodium chloride, there is a common tendency to want to use hypertonic solution to correct this promptly. In general, we have found that most of the marked dislocations can be handled adequately by physiologic saline alone. Rather than proceed too quickly, it usually seems better and probably safer to make the adjustments more slowly, even though it might require several days to reach the desired goal. However, on rare occasions when confronted with hyponatremia and impending circulatory collapse with renal shutdown, we have used hypertonic salt solution with good effect. (After having gotten into such situations, reflection and a review of therapy of the previous days often made us feel that the crisis had been iatrogenic; not enough electrolyte had been supplied during times when losses had been great.)

It is not necessary to take specific steps aimed directly at correcting an abnormal pH of the plasma (in the presence of normally functioning kidneys). We use the laboratory evidence of altered blood carbon dioxide or pH as a mere indicator of the severity of any dislocations in the direction of acidosis or alkalosis; marked shifts imply that intensive and continued supervision must be given to the electrolyte therapy, which is simply a

---

* Manufactured by Macalaster Bicknell Co., 243 Broadway, Cambridge, Mass.

replacement of cation and anion deficits. It is almost always found that focus on measures to correct any low levels of sodium and chloride will eventually and satisfactorily bring correction of the acidosis or alkalosis.

In general, for those patients who have to be supported for many days on parenteral therapy, the basic requirements are given empirically (after estimating the total fluid needed) with one-third as physiologic saline and two-thirds as 10 per cent glucose in water through the twenty-four hours. If electrolyte depletions are great, more salt can be added while the dextrose solution is being run in.

From a practical point of view, in dealing with those subjects who will require parenteral therapy for only two or possibly three days, there is little need of incurring the expense and trouble of performing blood chemical studies; the minor variations which almost certainly exist will correct themselves quickly as the patient begins to eat. Conversely, when dealing with complicated cases, and certainly in all those in which parenteral therapy is being given beyond three days, it is essential to have blood chemical studies at appropriate intervals to give an index of the patient's condition and to guide the replacement program. Even so, complete reliance must never be made on figures from a laboratory. To sum up the whole picture, it is also very important to take into account clinical observations on the patient and the course of his disease.

The above statements and generalities concerning electrolyte and fluid therapy apply only if a patient's renal function is normal. In the presence of anuria (or marked oliguria) from lower nephron degeneration, therapy must be radically different and closely supervised. The patient cannot excrete electrolytes or waste products of metabolism; the only fluid exchanged is the "insensible loss" which occurs from the lungs and skin. Therefore, only very small amounts of fluid are required; no electrolytes should be given and every effort should be made to reduce tissue breakdown which releases nitrogenous products and the dangerous potassium. To achieve this tissue-protein sparing effect, limited amounts of 10 per cent dextrose in water are given, making certain that the amount of fluid given is low enough to prevent formation of edema. The patient is tided along in this precarious manner in the hope that kidney function will return, which it does in a considerable proportion of cases.

In recent years, various studies of potassium metabolism have made many clinicians potassium-conscious and have led to therapeutic efforts in correction of minor deviations, which, for the most part, are completely unnecessary. For the vast majority, a small potassium deficit can be ignored because this will be corrected spontaneously in a satisfactory way as soon as the child begins to drink and eat. However, when extraordinary losses are occurring beyond a three- or four-day period, it is important to take cognizance of any potassium deficiency which can contribute greatly to the picture of exhaustion; appropriate steps must be taken to supply this element. Because of the risk of potassium poisoning, certain limits must be imposed upon the concentration of solutions which are used and on the rate with which potassium is supplied to the body. Concentrations greater than 3 or 4 mEq per 100 cc. of fluid should seldom be given, even when body depletions are great. Replacement should never be too rapid, and in no instance (except in very unusual cases) should the material be supplied in excess of 2 mEq per pound of body weight per twenty-four hours.

As one views the whole problem of supplying sick patients with calories, vitamins, water, and electrolytes, it becomes evident that it is almost impossible to supply by parenteral means all of the calories which are needed, but that it is completely possible for the physician to supply all of the vitamins, water, and electrolytes. So easy is it to inject the latter two substances, that one must constantly guard against the danger of giving too much water or salt, or both. These considerations are particularly pertinent when dealing with frail, postoperative patients in the first year or two of life.

No problem encountered in the care of infants and children can be more perplexing at times than the determination of electrolyte requirements and the management of these in ways that are safe. Unusually complicated cases tax the ingenuity of the surgeon and his medical consultants; therapy can become extremely intricate and must be individualized to fit the needs of the case. While it is obvious that no general statements can possibly apply in all situations, our experience over a number of years with a very large series of surgical cases has demonstrated that the vast majority of patients can be handled by adherence to fairly simple regimens. Through the long hours of tribulation, it becomes very clear that even the sickest of patients can be pulled through if appropriate laboratory tests are done and frequent clinical observations are made for guiding the therapy along those treacherous paths which eventually lead upward toward the high-road of recovery.

CHAPTER 3

Anesthesia for Pediatric Surgery

General Considerations

There are certain characteristics of the response of children to anesthesia and surgery which differ from those of adults and which must be borne in mind by both surgeon and anesthetist. An intelligent approach to the choice and management of anesthesia can be made only if one knows of the special hazards involved and the complications which are most frequently encountered.

Small Size. The most obvious feature of the pediatric patient, of course, is his small size. It might be assumed erroneously that small patients are weak, and that a higher operative and anesthetic mortality is to be encountered for this reason, but it has been our experience that any child who comes to operation in good condition may be expected to withstand anesthesia and surgery of considerable magnitude, provided that care is taken to observe the basic principles of oxygenation and maintenance of fluid balance. Excepting possibly very tiny premature infants, no mortality that occurs in pediatric surgery should be excused merely on the basis of small size or young age of a patient.

Anatomically, there are disproportions and weaknesses of structure that are of some disadvantage to the young child, especially in respect to respiratory activity. The neck and chest have poor musculature, and the bony structure of the thorax is elastic and unstable. The abdomen can be large and bulky, and can impede the motions of the diaphragm. For these various reasons, the respiratory exchange is easily depressed. The heavy head, large tongue, narrow airway, short neck, and actively secreting mucus glands increase the tendency toward respiratory obstruction. The architecture of the infant lung provides a relatively small alveolar surface and a large dead space, making for decreased efficiency of ventilation.

Physiologically, the typical reactions of the young child are rapid, variable, and extreme. This is due to a high metabolic activity and to an incomplete development. Lack of mature control of body systems gives exaggerated responses to stimuli. Changes in depth of anesthesia are abrupt and they come without warning. The rate of respiration may accelerate to 100, and as quickly slow to 20, with bizarre gasping rhythms occurring at any time. Heavy metabolic demands of the body call for a large oxygen supply, consequently any anoxia is poorly tolerated. Heart action tends to be regular, but varies widely in rate. In infants under ether anesthesia, the average rate may run normally as high as 180, while that of older children can be from 140 to 160. Fluid exchange is also rapid; dehydration or blood loss leads to development of shock with considerable speed. Heat regulation is poor; the body temperature of a small infant can readily fall to 92° in a cool operating room, or rise to 105° in an overheated one.

The high metabolic activity of children is shown in the response of their nervous system. Emotionally, they are unstable and often uncontrollable. If a child is improperly prepared, fear gives way to excitement, screaming, or frenzied struggling—all of which makes a hazardous introduction to anesthesia and surgery. There is frequently a tendency toward convulsions, which is heightened in the presence of fever or acidosis. Excessive epinephrine secretion in infants is in large degree responsible for the excessive heart rate, and the pronounced reflex irritability. It has been found that infants under anesthesia are particularly prone to develop acidosis; this can be traced to overactivity of the sympathetic nervous system and to excessive formation of lactic acid. All these factors are characteristic of children; the younger the patient, the more they are exaggerated.

Handicaps Can Be Overcome. In spite of the above-mentioned differences between a child and an adult, general anesthesia can be given safely to any youngster. Once properly medicated, a child beyond two years of age is a good subject for anesthesia. Though variable and tricky in his reactions, his heart has considerable strength, and there is a reasonable margin of safety. A wide variety of anesthetic agents and methods can be used; there are few problems that arise that cannot be readily handled. With small infants,

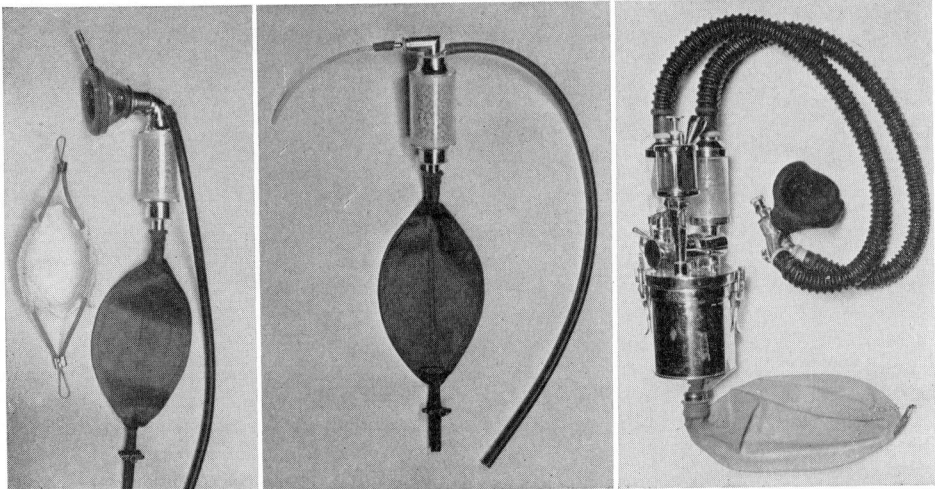

Fig. 12. *Left,* Small to and fro apparatus suitable for a baby, equipped with face mask. *Miadle,* Same apparatus fitted to intratracheal tube. The close coupling is important for reducing the dead air space to a minimum. *Right,* For comparison, an adult-sized circle apparatus.

however, the situation is quite different. Though they are strong if handled deftly, there is little margin of reserve; once upset, the infant may get into serious danger immediately. Choice of anesthetic agents and techniques is limited; the methods and the apparatus must be suited to the special requirements of each small patient.

ANESTHETIC EQUIPMENT

No anesthesia should be started unless the anesthetist has immediately at hand oxygen, suction, oral airway, laryngoscope, and endotracheal tubes of appropriate size. Since the patients treated on a pediatric surgical service may vary in size from a three-pound premature infant to an oversized adolescent of two hundred pounds, a wide variety of airways, laryngoscopes, and endotracheal tubes must be available. For open drop ether it is sufficient to have two sizes of masks, an infant and the standard Yankauer mask. These are covered with four and eight layers of gauze respectively. The Richardson bottle is an excellent device for vaporizing ether which is to be insufflated or blown to the patient through a mouth hook or an endotracheal tube. For endotracheal anesthesia for surgery not involving an open chest, insufflation anesthesia via a simple metal Y tube (Fig. 15) and the Stephen-Slater non-rebreathing valve are both accepted methods of great value.

Closed-system anesthesia may be administered by using any of the standard anesthesia machines; equipment for both "to and fro" and "circle" absorption should be on hand, as each arrangement has a field of usefulness. The same masks are used in both systems.

For to and fro absorption technique, small soda-lime canisters are necessary; these may be obtained in 100 and 300 cc. sizes. Two-liter rebreathing bags are used for infants. Fittings and tubings should be chosen to reduce the dead space to a minimum, as carbon dioxide accumulation is a major hazard; these are considerations of prime importance when dealing with small children and especially babies.

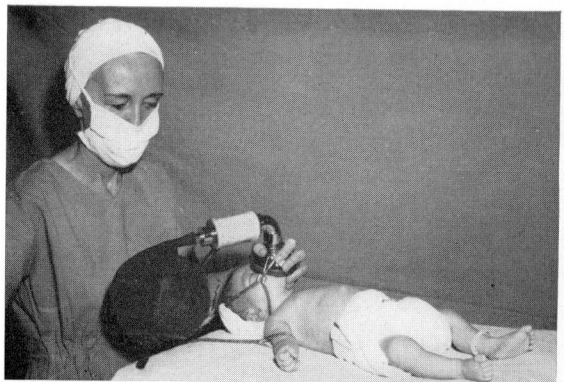 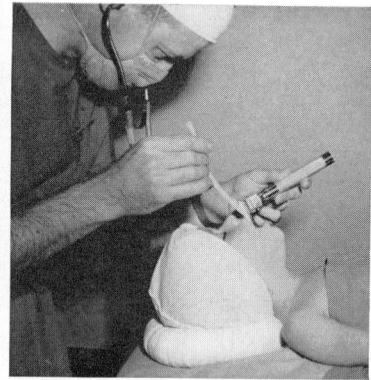

Fig. 13. *Left*, Closed system for administration of cyclopropane to babies. This arrangement, with a tightly fitting face mask, is the one we generally prefer, but in some intrathoracic procedures the face mask can be discarded and the system connected directly to an intratracheal tube. *Right*, Laryngeal intubation. Optimum position and alignment of head for laryngoscopy and insertion of the tube.

For circle absorption technique, special small-sized canisters and tubes have been utilized, but experience has convinced us that the size of the canister is not extremely important. Our practice has been to use an adult-sized canister, shorten the length of the conduit tubes, and reduce the size of the yoke adapter to a minimum. The greatest hazard of the circle system lies in resistance of the valves. Much care should be used to keep valves clean and thus prevent sluggish action.

Although closed-system anesthesia involves great danger of building up resistance or increasing the accumulation of carbon dioxide, it may be indicated for the purpose of greater oxygenation, administration of cyclopropane or nitrous oxide, or for giving positive pressure anesthesia. We find the to and fro system preferable in small infants because it eliminates the resistance of the valves. The circle system has become more successful in older children, because of better elimination of carbon dioxide. Respiration is assisted in all patients throughout closed-system anesthesia by intermittently compressing the rebreathing bag.

PREOPERATIVE PREPARATION

Children who come to operation excited and poorly prepared may not only suffer real emotional complications, but carry a definitely higher rate of morbidity and mor-

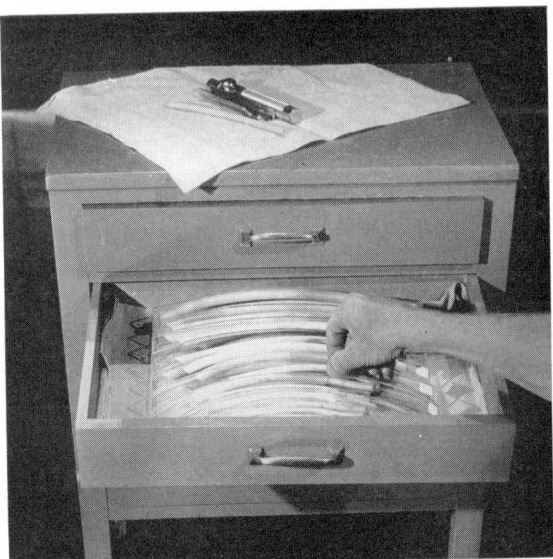

Fig. 14. Cabinet (mounted on wheels) which is very handy for storage and quick accessibility of endotracheal tubes and equipment. By use of precautions in cleansing, handling, and storing of equipment, tracheitis from contamination can be prevented.

tality. Respiratory irregularities, aspiration of vomitus, convulsions, and cardiac arrest all occur more frequently in patients who have had inadequate preparation and a stormy induction.

Emotional State

The emotional preparation of children who are old enough to understand can be initiated at home. Parents should reassure the child about what he will see, and about the treatment he is to get. It is important to bring the patient to the hospital in adequate time for a preoperative work-up. Excepting emergencies, he should not be rushed to a

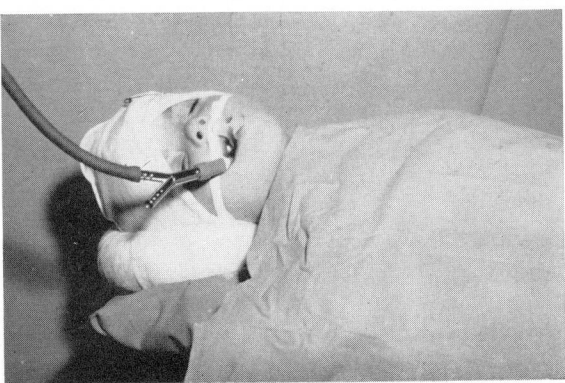

Fig. 15. A useful way of administering anesthetic gas mixture to a small patient. To the tracheal tube is connected a Y tube, one arm of which receives the gas which is gently flowing through the rubber tube, the other arm being left open to the room air. The arrangement is simple and yet very effective. If the child is in a precarious state, any period of apnea can be managed by intermittent placement of a finger tip over the open arm; this gives very gentle, intermittent inflation of the lungs. This arrangement is also useful for administering oxygen to some patients after operation, and before they are extubated.

hospital just before operation, nor should he be subjected to a barrage of examinations on the eve of a major surgical procedure.

Correction of Deficiencies

It is of course essential that the child be in the best possible physical condition for operation. It is the responsibility of both the surgeon and the anesthetist to make sure that correctable defects are tended to before operation. Children on whom surgery is contemplated not infrequently have upper respiratory infections, diarrhea or intestinal upsets, persistent fever, or anemia. If possible, these should be controlled before accepting the subject for anesthesia. The red blood count should be 4 million or more, the hemoglobin above 10 grams per cent, and the urine free of ketone bodies. In acutely ill patients, high fever, dehydration, electrolyte imbalance, or even shock may be encountered; while these cannot be alleviated completely before surgery which is urgently required, it has been shown that anesthetic and surgical mortality rates are reduced markedly if there is a delay until antibiotics, hydration, and electrolyte therapy have gained some control over these situations.

Feeding

If the intestinal tract is functioning normally, routine preoperative care should provide feeding until four hours before operation. As much as possible, one should avoid upsetting feeding schedules of infants. Patients who are to be operated upon late in the morning may be given sweetened orange juice at breakfast time; those to be operated upon in the afternoon should have a full breakfast. When long and exhausting operative procedures are contemplated, these will be tolerated better if the patient is given 10 per cent glucose intravenously just before operation or during the first part of the procedure.

Anesthetist's Evaluation

For all elective procedures, it is important on the day before operation to have an anesthetist visit the child to check his general physical condition and to size up his emotional state. Much can be done at this time in preparation for the trip to the operating room; a few minutes spent in getting acquainted with the youngster, and in gaining his confidence, will be well repaid. Details of the coming procedure need not be offered unless questions are asked; if queries are made, honest, reassuring information should be given. If the child is unusually apprehensive, appropriate sedative should be ordered to insure a full night's sleep before the surgery.

Preoperative Medication

Some writers state that children do not need preoperative sedation and that it is preferable to reason with them and thus gain their cooperation. Although a few can be kept quiet by this method, most children above two or three years of age will not yield to an approach of simple reasoning, and they will merely become more excited and uncontrollable when faced with the foreign and sinister atmosphere of the operating room. Older children who may appear to cooperate, do so only by extreme self-control in the presence of repressed fear which is released as soon as the anesthesia begins. It is our firm belief that it is safer and less trying for all concerned to give sedation which dispels the anxiety of children and renders them drowsy and relaxed before leaving their rooms. When properly prepared, they should have no remembrance of their trip to the operating room.

In addition to quieting a patient, medication lowers metabolic activity and provides mild analgesia, so that less anesthesia will be required. A belladonna derivative is always used to depress salivation and to block excessive vagal activity.

Scopolamine is used commonly because it is superior as a drying agent and in addition is slightly depressant; for small infants, atropine is preferable because it does not depress respirations. For all thoracic surgery, atropine is chosen because of its better vagolytic action.

The accompanying table represents medication schedules we currently use for average children in good condition; reductions must be made for patients who are debilitated:

Preoperative Medication for Infants and Children

Age	Average Weight lbs.	Nembutal or Phenobarbital mg.	Morphine mg.	Demerol mg.	Scopolamine mg.	Atropine mg.
Newborn	7	—	—	—	—	0.1
6 mos.	16	30	—	—	—	0.2
1 yr.	21	50	1.0	10	0.1	0.3
2 yrs.	27	60	1.4	20	0.2	0.3
4 yrs.	35	90	2.3	25	0.2	0.4
6 yrs.	45	100	4.0	40	0.2	0.4
8 yrs.	55	120	5.4	45	0.3	0.4
10 yrs.	64	150	6.0	50	0.3	0.4
12 yrs.	80	200	8.0	50	0.4	0.6

For infants under nine or ten months of age, sedatives are too apt to produce marked respiratory depression or apnea during anesthesia, and hence should always be omitted. Beyond such ages, anesthesia will always be more satisfactory if preoperative sedation is given. For this purpose, morphine by hypodermic injection is the drug of choice; to attain reasonable effect, it should be given an hour before operation. For a child who is unduly apprehensive or active, it is very helpful to give Nembutal or phenobarbital two or three hours before the morphia. Barbiturates can be given by mouth in corn syrup, with a few swallows of water to get them down.

Children who are going to be operated upon late in the morning should not be permitted to go through the waiting hours hungry, crying, and excited. It is best to give them orally at 6:00 A.M. a barbiturate, possibly with sweetened orange juice, which will make them drowsy or sleepy until the time for surgery; atropine and morphine are then given hypodermically an hour before operation.

CHOICE OF ANESTHETIC AGENTS AND TECHNIQUES

The type of anesthesia is determined by the age of the patient, his preoperative condition, and the kind of operation to be performed. Although most of the agents employed for adult anesthesia find some use in pediatric work, a general anesthetic is indicated for the great majority of cases. The variability of infants and children in their response to narcotics makes it safer to give controllable and easily eliminated inhalation agents in preference to single-dose, longer-acting drugs given by injection. An appreciable number of operations can be performed under rectal or intravenous administration of drugs when special circumstances demand it. If local, block, or spinal techniques are employed for young patients, they will usually be so restless and apprehensive that they require sedation which borders on general anesthesia itself; it is safer and more efficient to give a general anesthetic in the first place.

Ether of Prime Importance

The position of ether as the most reliable all-round anesthetic for pediatric anesthesia has never been seriously questioned. The ordeal of induction may be avoided or minimized by use of less irritating agents. Once ether anesthesia is established, it affords ample relaxation for the surgeon, and a wide margin of safety for the patient. Since it acts as a respiratory and cardiovascular stimulant in the usual plane of anesthesia, it has definite advantage over most other anesthetics, especially in young patients whose respiratory effort is easily embarrassed. Children tolerate ether very well, and they eliminate it rapidly with less postoperative nausea than adults. In the hands of the average anesthetist, who deals only occasionally with infants undergoing major surgery, ether should be the common anesthetic which is employed. Other drugs should be reserved for unusual clinical conditions. The preference for ether still allows for many variations in type of induction and in the techniques of administration, with or without other agents.

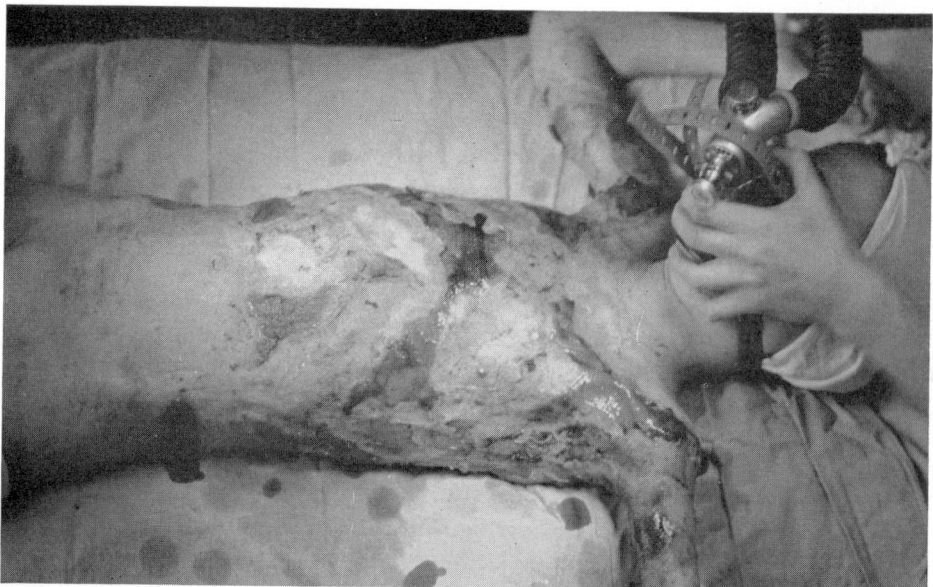

Fig. 16. Anesthesia for changing of dressings of a severely burned child. With removal of the bandages, the subject is placed on a sterile sheet, after which cleansing or skin grafting and application of fresh dressings are done. For these procedures we prefer cyclopropane anesthesia. Generally, fluids are being currently administered through an intravenous needle in an unburned extremity; into this system intravenous Pentothal can also be added if desired.

Cyclopropane

Cyclopropane has proven to be very useful for some major surgical procedures in newborn babies, such as correction of esophageal atresia, repair of diaphragmatic hernia, or relief of intestinal obstruction. It is also extremely valuable, and probably less toxic than ether, when treating very ill, older subjects for such conditions as intussusception, appendicitis with peritonitis, or severe burns. Cyclopropane is less irritating than ether, but more potent than nitrous oxide; it affords adequate relaxation for most pediatric surgery. Evidence of cardiac irritability under cyclopropane is seldom seen in children. Its administration requires greater skill on the part of the anesthesiologist than does ether or some of the other more commonly used agents. It might qualify as an ideal anesthetic agent for children were it not for its explosive hazard and also its broncho-constrictive action, which at times can lead to severe respiratory obstruction in small patients.

Vinyl Ether

Vinethene (divinyl ether) is especially useful as an induction agent for young children. It is rapid in action, less offensive than ether, and is quickly eliminated. It is good for short minor procedures and for various examinations which have to be done under anesthesia. It has proved to be toxic when used throughout long major procedures, and hence should be limited to those which are not over ten to fifteen minutes in length. Care should be taken to administer it more slowly than ether, as it is taken up more readily. It should always be given on an open mask and always with ample air, the mask not being fitted closely on the face. If patients build up a high concentration rapidly, characteristic rolling of the eyes and generalized stiffening will be followed by convulsive motions until the mask is removed and air or oxygen is given. Such a manifestation is due to high concentration of Vinethene, and not to an underlying state of acidosis or fever, as with ether convulsions. If the anesthetist recognizes the early signs of hyperventilation and fixed, staring eyes, he can quickly give more air and thereby avoid tremors.

Avertin

In selected cases Avertin (tribromoethanol) may be given rectally to induce deep sedation or "basal anesthesia." This may be indicated in patients who are extremely hard to manage, or in cases in which it is especially necessary to prevent excitement, as in neurosurgical patients with elevated intracranial pressure. In our hands Avertin has proved to be preferable to the barbiturates for this purpose, because of its greater predictability and its bronchodilating effect. Avertin is used in dosage of 80 to 100 mg. per kilogram of body weight. When it is used, morphine and Nembutal are always omitted. Avertin has been used extensively at this hospital and has not resulted in toxicity or other untoward complications. It is not used in patients under a month of age, or in extremely ill children. We have found it to be a safe, reliable, and very desirable basal anesthetic. It can be administered by rectal tube to a child while in his own bed, so that he is completely asleep while being transported to the operating suite. Its one big disadvantage is that it requires the services of an anesthetist for a protracted period during the induction, and before operation is actually begun. This is an important consideration when trying to run a busy and complicated operating room schedule. Because of this excessive drain on the anesthesiology staff, we have now limited the use of Avertin to a relatively small group of patients, in whom basal anesthesia is highly desirable (as in operations about the palate, jaws, et cetera).

Local Anesthesia

It is almost never satisfactory to employ local anesthesia for surgery in childhood (except possibly for removal of small cutaneous lesions), and only on rare occasions is it necessary for surgery in infancy. There are, however, some procedures in debilitated babies, and particularly prematures, in which abdominal procedures can well be carried out under infiltration of the abdominal wall with 1 or 2 per cent procaine. For babies, mild sedation may be given in the form of one to three mixture of brandy in 10 per cent glucose solution, administered 15 minutes before operation. Two to 3 cc. of the mixture per pound usually makes the infant quiet and relaxed. During abdominal operations, closure of the peritoneum may require brief administration of cyclopropane for additional relaxation. While we formerly used local anesthesia rather frequently in small or premature babies undergoing abdominal operations, we have now largely turned away from it in favor of cyclopropane.

Intravenous Anesthesia

Rapid-acting barbiturates have definite application in pediatric anesthesia. Induction is facilitated if an intravenous needle is already in place. In combination with nitrous oxide, Pentothal sodium offers excellent anesthesia for operations which require little relaxation. Reduction of fractures, cystoscopic work, and prolonged orthopedic and plastic procedures (away from the mouth) may be performed under this combination. The patient has a rapid and pleasant recovery, and is more willing to return if further surgery is needed later. When x-ray apparatus or the cautery must be employed, Pentothal-nitrous oxide anesthesia is safe from the point of view of preventing explosions.

Muscle Relaxants

Curare and related agents have been used successfully in several clinics doing pediatric anesthesia, but in general there has been hesitancy in using them for infants. Curare does not have wide application in pediatric work since relaxation is usually adequate under inhalation agents. Difficulties associated with use of curare agents in infants and children make them exceedingly dangerous, and we therefore believe that they should never be used under any circumstances. Their use should be thoroughly condemned.

Tracheal Intubation

An inlying tracheal tube plays an important part in pediatric anesthesia. It maintains a free airway, allows suction removal of any bronchial secretions, and facilitates control of respiration by the anesthetist. Definite indications for its use are:

1. Neurosurgery, in which the patient's face and airway will be inaccessible to the anesthetist.

2. Surgery requiring the prone position, with resultant depressed respiration and inaccessible airway.

3. Surgery involving opening of the chest and temporary collapse of a lung.

4. Any operation upon patients who might vomit undigested food and aspirate it during anesthesia.

Some anesthetists employ endotracheal anesthesia for nearly all types of surgery. Since reports have appeared listing tracheitis, edema, and even death due to intubation, we feel that it should not be used without real justification. In our practice, these complications have been largely eliminated by keeping endotracheal apparatus scrupulously clean and by use of gentle atraumatic technique in introducing the tube.

When operations do not involve opening the chest, endotracheal anesthesia can be administered by way of a metal Y tube (Fig. 15), the patient inhaling the anesthetic through one arm of the Y, and exhaling through the other. No valves are involved; the system is simple and practically foolproof. Even small infants tolerate this method for hours without respiratory disturbance.

INDUCTION

Most infants cry and resist induction momentarily, but apparently with little more emotional disturbance than the crying occasioned by hunger. With older children who come to the operating room quiet, cooperative, or dozing, induction should not involve arousing them and then forcing them back to sleep with rough, frightening maneuvers. By simply blowing over the face of a child an 80:20 mixture of nitrous oxide and oxygen at 20 liters per minute, even a fully alert child will become drowsy, then unconscious, without alarm or struggle. A mask may then be used for further induction with Vinethene or ether by open or closed system.

Nitrous oxide induction with ether sequence may be carried out as with adults, if children are first reassured about the anesthesia machine and the mask. After such explanation, children may agree to hold the mask themselves, pretending they are talking into a telephone. Induction with cyclopropane has the advantage of being pleasant and more rapid than with nitrous oxide, but if children are resistant, sudden motions entail some danger of static electricity and explosion.

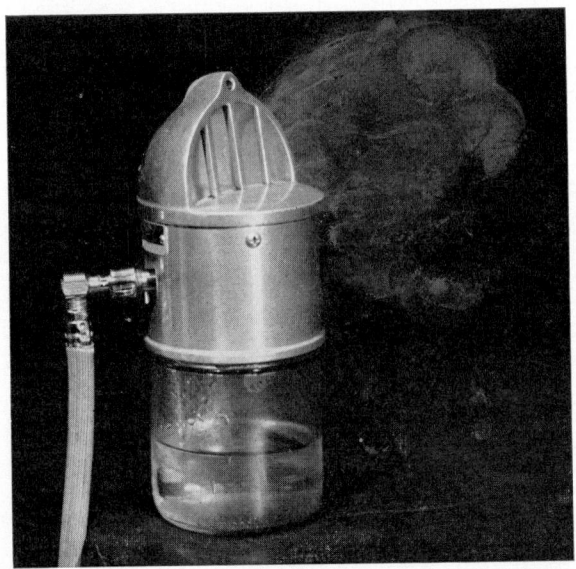

Fig. 17. A Mistogen apparatus for supplying nebulized water into a closed space, such as an oxygen tent or an incubator. The rubber tube brings compressed air or oxygen, which activates the nebulizer, producing a fine moist mist. The apparatus requires very little care for maintenance. It is extremely useful for postoperative patients in whom there has been irritation of the air passages by bronchoscopy, by tracheal intubation, or by operative procedure on or adjacent to the trachea (such as for esophageal surgery).

Intravenous Pentothal affords fast, easy induction once the venipuncture has been performed. However, most children are quite upset by needles and prefer a mask; the difficulties involved by puncturing a small vein in a squirming patient make intravenous induction of questionable advantage. If a patient happens to have an intravenous infusion already running, as may be the case in sick children who have been receiving preoperative hydration therapy, Pentothal induction is excellent. It is very simple and pleasant to induce the anesthesia with Pentothal, given via the infusion.

Small infants who are ill or toxic, but are still quite active, require general anesthesia which will afford gentle, rapid induction, will not disturb them physiologically, and will not be followed by prolonged depression. They are especially difficult to induce with the volatile agents such as Vinethene or ether, because they have extremely active laryngeal reflexes. Irritant vapors provoke severe breath-holding, laryngeal spasm, and induction which is prolonged and harmful. Cyclopropane induction is to be preferred.

When infants come to surgery in good contition and are strong and active, as those entering for herniorrhaphy, pyloromyotomy, or harelip repair, it is felt that Vinethene induction followed by open ether is best. Although volatile anesthetics are irritating and induction more disturbing, these patients tolerate the procedure well, and are not subjected to the greater explosive danger associated with cyclopropane. Usually nitrous oxide is blown over the faces of children before Vinethene is begun, and they are made so drowsy that they make little resistance to the addition of Vinethene.

MAINTENANCE

The maintenance of anesthesia can be accomplished by open drop, insufflation, semi-closed, or closed inhalation methods, by intravenous and other techniques. The open drop method has the advantage of simplicity; it eliminates valves, resistance, and mechanical detects which are inherent in all machines. Carbon dioxide accumulation may still occur, especially in heavily covered masks which are allowed to become wet. Oxygen should be introduced under masks of infants and weak children.

Open-drop ether anesthesia is satisfactory for most general surgery. For operations about the head, face, and neck, however, the anesthetist must use other methods, for a

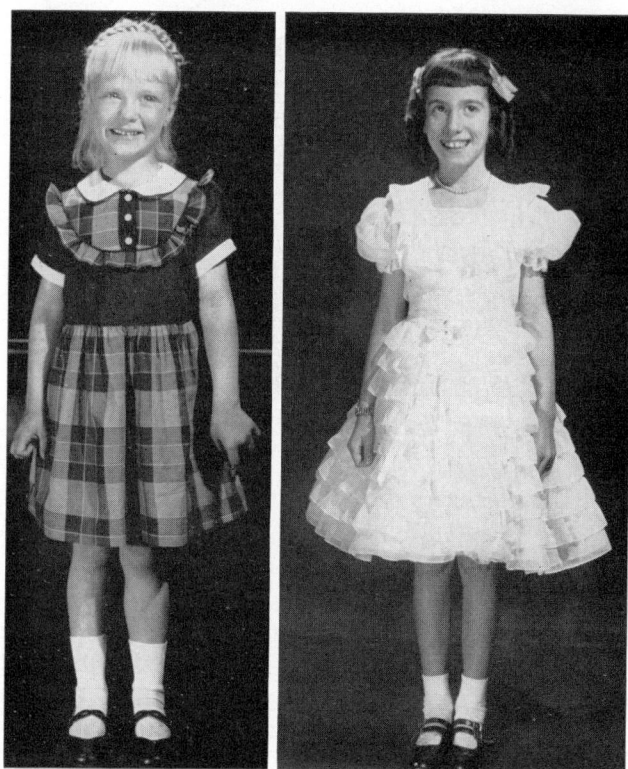

Fig. 18. Typical patients, to demonstrate that anesthesias can be used repeatedly without harmful or toxic effects on the liver and other organs. Furthermore, if patients are adequately prepared and the anesthetic is properly administered, there need be no fear, psychic trauma, or damage to the personality. *Left,* This child had had severe burns of 40 per cent of the body, requiring grafting. She has had ten general anesthesias. Now, following her rehabilitation, she is a happy, cheerful, and effervescent youngster. *Right,* A child who sustained a lye stricture of the entire esophagus at two years. During a period of seven years she has had 59 general anesthesias for esophageal dilation. She is a happy, cheerful, and cooperative girl.

mask is in the operator's way. For tonsillectomy, harelip, cleft palate, dental and ocular surgery, ether may be vaporized at a distance from the patient in a Richardson bottle or standard anesthesia machine insufflated into the pharynx by oral hook or airway, or carried into the lungs by an endotracheal tube. Our practice has been to use pharyngeal insufflation for tonsil, harelip, and palate surgery, and endotracheal insufflation for dental and ocular surgery.

The stages of anesthesia in children are more difficult to differentiate than in adults. Infants betray light plane of anesthesia by first flexing elbows, then clenching their fists. Eye signs are unreliable. Respiration, though often rapid and irregular, is the most valuable guide to follow. An even, rhythmic exchange is the best sign of a well administered anesthetic. The use of a stethoscope strapped to the patient's chest enables the anesthetist to follow heart and respiration accurately throughout the operation, a point of particular interest in a baby or small child who will be extensively covered by surgical drapes.

CHAPTER 4

Disruption of Abdominal Wounds

Personal communications from many surgeons indicate that improper healing of abdominal-wall wounds in children and especially in babies constitutes a problem of considerable magnitude and frequency of occurrence. It is a great disappointment to perform successfully some intra-abdominal procedure, only to have the child or baby succumb from evisceration. Fortunately, the incidence of disruption can now be reduced to a negligible figure, and fatalities from this cause can almost be abolished.

Our observations and policies regarding closure and treatment of abdominal-wall wounds have been made over a period of twenty years, from 1931 through 1950, during which time focus on the care of the abdominal wound has paid tremendous dividends in improved healing and in a continually decreasing incidence of dehiscence.

FACTORS CONTRIBUTING TO GOOD WOUND HEALING

There are a number of items, each of which is of some importance in producing or handling a wound which will heal with nicety and strength. No one of these factors should be emphasized to the exclusion of others; all have some place in the proper management of abdominal-wall wounds. If due regard is taken of all of them, the operator can be assured with great certainty that the closure of the abdominal wall will be followed by rapid and complete healing. Fortunately, all of the factors can be controlled in most cases by the surgeon if he is meticulous in his treatment at the operating table and is careful in his supervision of the case during the first week thereafter.

The Choice of an Incision

In general, the shorter an incision, the less are the chances of disruption following its closure, but this in no way alters the fact that incisions of great length will unite well if properly repaired. Certainly, a wound should not be made unnecessarily short in the hope of avoiding difficulties after its closure; a very short wound limits the exposure too much, does not give the optimum conditions for proper performance of the intra-abdominal manipulations, and indeed by repeated and forceful retraction of the wound edges produces such damage that healing of it might be impaired. It is far better to have an opening which is properly placed with relation to the intra-abdominal lesion, and of sufficient length that the operation can be carried out without hauling and pulling on the wound margins.

Transverse Abdominal Wounds have been particularly useful for exposures in the subhepatic fossa when exploring the extrahepatic biliary tree or for transabdominal approach to the renal fossa for removal of large embryomas of the kidney or neuroblastomas of the retroperitoneal structures. Transverse wounds have an advantage in that they can be extended for long distances if the need arises for more liberal exposure. They heal with great strength and we have seldom encountered important complications from them.

Gridiron Incisions have the disadvantage of providing a limited exposure, but have the enormous superiority of healing with maximum strength when the overlapping meshworks of muscles and fascial layers fall back into place when retractors are removed and the wound is closed. The various fascial and muscle bundles make a latticework which becomes even more tight as the abdominal wall contracts after recovery from anesthesia. Gridiron wounds do not allow easy enlargement of an abdominal wall opening, hence they should be avoided when exploratory laparotomy is contemplated or whenever there is doubt concerning the type of lesion which is going to be encountered. This type of wound is particularly useful when the nature of the lesion is known with great certainty before operation, and when only a small opening is required over a well localized process. The best examples of such situations are the use of a McBurney incision for removal of an appendix and the similar Robertson incision in the right upper quadrant for treatment of hypertrophic pyloric stenosis. During the last fifteen years, during which we have used the McBurney incision almost routinely for acute appendicitis (with or without rupture), there have been virtually no important wound problems. During the last ten years, during which the Robertson incision has been used for almost all of the pyloric stenosis cases, there has not been a single instance of dehiscence in this type of wound.

Rectus Incision, with Medial Retraction. In some localities it is common practice in removing an appendix to retract the rectus muscle belly medially (Battle incision), giving an opening which is nicely located over the organ. In children and infants this approach should never be used; there are such short gaps between the nerves supplying the rectus muscle that damage to these is very apt to lead to subsequent wound weakness or herniation.

Rectus-Splitting Incision. This incision is very easy to make and can be rapidly extended if necessary, but it gives a repaired wound which is weaker than all others in the abdominal wall. It has been widely used, and is, I believe, responsible for much of the grief which has come from wound disruptions. While it gives quick and extensive exposure, its repair implies that all of the lines of closure (peritoneum, muscle, fascia, etc.) lie in a single plane, so that any peritoneal disruption allows a wedge of intestine to be aimed outward directly at the weakest zone of each layer of the abdominal wall. The number of catastrophes which we have had in the past make us feel emphatically that a rectus-splitting incision should *never* be used on a baby or a small child whenever extensive abdominal exploration is to be carried out. We have completely abandoned it except for very short incisions for quite simple procedures such as establishment of a gastrostomy or a transverse colostomy.

Rectus Incision with Lateral Retraction. While requiring a little more time to open the wound, and necessitating a somewhat longer incision to obtain a given exposure, a rectus incision with lateral retraction of the muscle belly has outstanding superiority because the wound provided by its closure has far greater strength than one in which the rectus muscle has been split. When a muscle belly (which had been retracted laterally) is allowed to drop back into alignment, it interposes a broad structure between the suture lines of the peritoneum and of the anterior rectus fascia. This provides a barrier to any loop of intestine which might possibly break through the peritoneum. Furthermore, the interposed muscle gives extensive surfaces which can seal posteriorly and anteriorly, the adherence of which rapidly give strength to the wound. The lateral-retracting rectus incision is the one we have come to use most commonly for extensive intraabdominal procedures such as exploration, intestinal resection, reduction of malrotation, colectomy, removal of renal tumors, abdomino-perineal pull-through of the rectosigmoid for

Hirschsprung's disease or imperforate anus with a high rectal pouch. We believe it is the abandonment of muscle-splitting incisions and the more liberal use of lateral-retracting rectus incisions which have been largely responsible for the great fall in our number of wound disruptions in the last ten years.

Closure of Abdominal Wounds

For the closure of abdominal wounds in children and babies, stay sutures through all layers of the abdominal wall should not be employed. They are brutal, unnecessary, and certainly do not give the best healing. It is far better to make an accurate and careful closure, layer by layer. For the peritoneum of children 000 chromic catgut, in a continuous suture, is quite satisfactory. The remaining layers are best repaired with 0000 Deknatel silk. For babies, the peritoneal suture can be made with 0000 chromic catgut and for the remaining layers 00000 silk employed. It is highly important to avoid tissue damage arising from unnecessary clamping of structures, brutal handling of tissues with forceps, and tying of sutures too tightly.

The only indication we accept for use of stay sutures is for secondary closure of wounds (which have been intentionally reopened, or which have disrupted) wherein the anatomical structures are obscured, edematous, hemorrhagic, and friable. Under these circumstances, mass sutures obviously give the best chance of producing a solid abdominal wall.

Whenever intestine or colon is exteriorized, it is extremely important to close the peritoneum (with interrupted silk sutures) around the entire periphery of the loop which is brought out through the abdominal wall. Children and babies are apt to strain, cry, or wiggle during the postoperative period and there is a very considerable chance of pushing a loop of small intestine out alongside of the ileostomy (or colostomy) unless this possibility has been prevented by complete and proper closure of the peritoneal layer.

Treatment, or Avoidance, of Abdominal Distention

Abdominal distention is a constant threat to the healing of a wound in the parietes; if allowed to persist, it can end in disaster by disrupting the wound, forcing intestines out into the subcutaneous tissues or into the dressing. When already present, important degrees of distention must be treated by gastric suction or by intestinal intubation. If the distention is largely gaseous, much benefit can be attained by placing the patient in an atmosphere of very high oxygen concentration[1] (90% or more), employing for this a tent which is tightly closed.

It is of great importance to *avoid* distention in procedures which are apt to be followed by large accumulations of gas or fluid in the intestinal tract. Patients who have had extensive abdominal exploration, or who are known to have peritonitis, should be placed on constant gastric suction for some days to *prevent* dangerous collections in the alimentary tract. Nowhere in surgery can it be more rightfully said that an ounce of prevention is worth a pound of cure!

Nutritional Status

To insure proper wound healing, certain abnormal body states must not be allowed to occur postoperatively or, if present, must be corrected as quickly as possible. *Anemia* must be rectified or prevented by blood transfusions. *Hypoproteinemia* discourages healing and it is essential that such a state be alleviated by intravenous infusions of plasma, albumin, or blood. *Chemical imbalance* frequently results in edematous and boggy tissues, and wound healing is deterred. Intravenous fluids administered judiciously will help correct imbalance, but fluids must not be given in amounts sufficient to produce or increase edema, the presence of which contributes so greatly to faulty union of tissues. Saline solutions should never be given promiscuously; they should be injected only when there is sodium or chloride depletion, as in cases with diarrhea, persistent vomiting, or malfunctioning ileostomy. Such statements are particularly pertinent for the small child or baby, whose kidneys are generally unable to excrete excess amounts of chlorides. *Supplemental vitamin C* administration is particularly useful in cases in which there is malnourishment. This antiscorbutic factor is essential in the formation of intercellular substances which give strength to a healing wound.

TREATMENT OF DEHISCENCE OR EVISCERATION

Wound dehiscence (separation) and evisceration (protrusion of abdominal viscera) fortunately occur but rarely. Such complications are emergencies which require immediate operative replacement of the viscera and reclosure of the abdominal opening. When dehiscence is incomplete and involves only one or two layers of the wall, the wound may be treated expectantly but with the warning in mind that evisceration may occur at any moment. Should such a wound heal, an incisional hernia will frequently follow which will require correction at a later date. The sudden appearance of serous fluid on an abdominal wound dressing must always be immediately investigated for the possibility of evisceration.

Treatment of Evisceration

When evisceration has occurred, exposed loops of bowel should be covered with sterile warm saline-soaked gauze pads, and a sterile binder applied over these. Atropine and morphine are given in suitable dosage for preoperative medication and the child immediately taken to the operating room. The choice of anesthetic agent depends upon the patient's condition. Ether is probably the safest in most cases, and gives good abdominal relaxation. In the very sick, the use of cyclopropane may be of advantage. With sterile technique, the dressing is carefully removed, the viscera held out of the way, and the skin of the abdominal wall prepared with a mild antiseptic solution, such as aqueous Zephiran chloride (1:1000) solution. Drapes are suitably arranged. The exposed viscera are cleaned with warm saline and are returned to the abdominal cavity. Old suture material should be removed and the wound edges freshened. Because the abdominal wall layers are frequently frayed and torn, it is generally impossible to close the wound in layers with any degree of satisfaction. However, when possible, structures should be brought together by interrupted silk sutures. Wound closure is now undertaken, generally by means of through-and-through sutures of heavy silk, silkworm gut, or steel wire. These sutures go through all layers, including peritoneum, and are later tied over short segments of rubber tubing to prevent undue cutting of the skin. For the reapproximation of the skin edges, interrupted silk sutures are placed between the through-and-through sutures. Skin sutures may be removed on the seventh or eighth postoperative day, but the stay sutures should be left untouched until the twelfth or fourteenth day. To combat peritonitis, active measures should be used as required, including intestinal suction-decompression, oxygen tent, intensive chemotherapy, parenteral alimentation, and so on.

STATISTICS

During the twenty years from 1931 onward, 8319 major abdominal operations have been performed at the Boston Children's Hospital. This figure is exclusive of all herniorrhaphies and cystotomies, but does include all intra-abdominal procedures and kidney surgery. By years, and by five-year periods, the numbers of cases were as follows:

```
1931................................................... 294 ⎫
1932................................................... 299 ⎪
1933................................................... 277 ⎬ 1528
1934................................................... 313 ⎪
1935................................................... 345 ⎭
1936................................................... 314 ⎫
1937................................................... 316 ⎪
1938................................................... 415 ⎬ 1877
1939................................................... 434 ⎪
1940................................................... 398 ⎭
1941................................................... 425 ⎫
1942................................................... 483 ⎪
1943................................................... 397 ⎬ 2131
1944................................................... 401 ⎪
1945................................................... 425 ⎭
1946................................................... 460 ⎫
1947................................................... 502 ⎪
1948................................................... 594 ⎬ 2783
1949................................................... 599 ⎪
1950................................................... 628 ⎭
```

During the twenty-year period from 1931 onward there have been 75 eviscerations: data concerning these are listed in Table 2:

Table 2

Evisceration Data by Five-Year Periods

Five-Year Periods	Number of Intra-abdominal Operations	Number of Eviscerations	Incidence of Evisceration %	Deaths in Evisceration Cases	Mortality in Evisceration Cases %
1931–1935	1528	20	1.31	11	55
1936–1940	1877	31	1.76	14	45
1941–1945	2131	13	0.61	6	46
1946–1950	2783	11	0.39	3	27

A study of Table 2 clearly shows that, despite an increasing number of intra-abdominal procedures, eviscerations have been diminishing. Furthermore, in those patients with evisceration, the mortality rate has fallen to about half of its former figure, a fact which is attributed to more careful supervision of the patient who has sustained this complication and to the recent availability of various antibiotics.

The problem of evisceration is largely one of infancy. Of the 75 cases we have encountered, 64 of the subjects were less than two years of age while the remaining 11 were beyond this age group. These facts emphasize that the principles of wound care above described are of particular importance when the surgeon is treating patients in the first year or two of life.

REFERENCES

1. Fine, J., Banks, B. M., Sears, J. B. and Hermanson, L.: The Treatment of Gaseous Distention of the Intestine by the Inhalation of Ninety Five Percent Oxygen. Ann. Surg., *103*:375, 1936.
2. Gross, R. E.: A New Method for Surgical Treatment of Large Omphaloceles. Surgery, *24*:277, 1948.
3. Gurd, F. B.: Transverse Incision of the Abdomen—the Laparotomy Wound of Choice. Canad. M.A.J., *42*:10, 1940.
4. Gurd, F. B.: Anatomical Principles Involved in Abdominal Incisions. S. Clin. North America, *25*:271, 1945.
5. Gurd, F. B.: Fundamentals of Technique in the Transverse Abdominal Incision. Surgery, *20*:217, 1946.
6. Gurd, F. B.: Abdominal Incisions. In Bancroft, F. W. and Wade, P. A.: Surgical Treatment of the Abdomen, p. 389. J. B. Lippincott Company, Philadelphia, 1947.
7. Hiatt, R. B.: Surgical Treatment of Congenital Megacolon. Ann. Surg., *133*:321, 1951.
8. Lanman, T. H. and Ingalls, T. H.: Vitamin C Deficiency and Wound Healing. An Experimental and Clinical Study. Ann. Surg., *105*:616, 1937.
9. McBurney, C.: The Incision Made in the Abdominal Wall in Cases of Appendicitis, with a Description of a New Method of Operating. Ann. Surg., *20*:38, 1894.
10. Ravdin, I. S.: Hypoproteinemia and Its Relation to Surgical Problems. Ann. Surg., *112*:576, 1940.
11. Robertson, D. E.: Congenital Pyloric Stenosis. Ann. Surg., *112*:687, 1940.

CHAPTER 5

Surgery in Premature Infants

While the surgery of an infant or small child requires certain considerations which differ from those of surgery in adults, it is obvious that surgery in a *premature* baby calls for *especial handling and delicacy* because of the smallness and fragility of the tiny subject and also because of physiologic variations which are known to exist. It is important to recognize these physiologic immaturities, and to compensate for them appropriately when handling these diminutive patients. As is generally recognized by physicians, a premature baby who has no congenital abnormality requires ideal hospital facilities to have any reasonable chance of survival. The problems of care demand even greater attention and special consideration when a premature baby possesses some congenital malformation which requires surgical correction.

While the combination of prematurity and a serious anatomical defect might seem to be overwhelming and even incompatible with survival, it is becoming increasingly clear that in a reasonably high percentage of cases such a deformed baby can be operated upon, the anomaly corrected, and the child can come through the ordeal sound in mind and body. Our observations on surgery of premature infants are gathered from operations upon 159 premature babies between January 1, 1936, and December 31, 1951. Not all of these were actually premature in the sense that their period of gestation was shortened, nor did all of them necessarily weigh less than 5 pounds at birth. However, all in the series weighed 5 pounds or less at the time of operation, and hence for the purposes of this study were classified as being "premature." These 159 premature infants are dealt with in the various chapters (and statistics thereof) concerning esophageal atresia, intestinal atresia, malrotation, and so on, elsewhere in this book. Therefore, the cases listed here are *not* in addition to those listed in other chapters.

To describe surgery in premature babies, three general aspects of the problem will be presented: (1) Physiologic aberrations in the premature child (who has no anatomical defect). (2) Principles in the surgical care of premature babies who must be operated upon for correction of congenital malformations. (3) Statistical summary of results of surgery in premature infants.

ALTERED PHYSIOLOGY OF THE PREMATURE BABY

In the premature infant there are several systems which function in ways which are quite dissimilar to those of full-term and larger babies. While this physiology can be regarded as normal for the premature infant, the variations must be enumerated and emphasized to guide us in the intelligent post-delivery care of a premature baby, especially one who also has a congenital abnormality. Some of the more important and obvious alterations in the various systems can be pointed out as follows. For a complete review of the subject, the reader is referred to the excellent monograph "The Physiology of the Newborn Infant" by Smith,[3] from which much of this material is gathered.

Regulation of Body Temperature

While the body weight of a *normal full-term infant* is about 5 per cent of that of the average adult, the body surface area is approximately 15 per cent. In the *premature infant*, the body surface area is proportionately even greater, and hence there is much more apt to be serious heat loss. Furthermore, there is a paucity of insulating subcutaneous fat, a lack of vasomotor vascular control, and an inadequacy of the sweating and shivering reactions. The production of body heat is at a low level. These various factors combine to make the temperature of the premature infant quite unstable; it varies widely from very low to high ranges, depending upon the environment to which the individual is subjected.

Respiratory System

When the respiratory minute-volume exchange is related to body surface area, the figures obtained for premature and full-term infants approximate those obtained for adults. However, this equality is accomplished by the premature infant at the expense of a vastly greater respiratory exertion, this effort reaching such a point that only slight respiratory reserve remains. The respiratory movements of the newborn are almost entirely diaphragmatic; if respirations are hampered by abdominal distention, diaphragmatic hernia, atelectasis, or pneumonia, the premature infant has little or no respiratory reserve to fall back upon. The breathing of a premature infant is frequently jerky or of the Cheyne-Stokes type in character. In some this is thought to be due to mild anoxia and will frequently disappear when additional oxygen, above the concentration of room air, is administered.

It has long been known that the brain of a full-term baby will survive more severe episodes of anoxia than will the central nervous system of an adult; furthermore, it is generally believed that the brain of a premature baby can withstand more severe and longer episodes of anoxia than will the brain of a full-term infant. Nevertheless, every effort should be made to abolish anoxia, or reduce it to a minimum, so that brain damage in the premature infant can be avoided.

Cardiovascular System

The blood volume of a full-term baby is proportionately similar to that of an adult, amounting to about 8 per cent of the body weight, but it can vary within wide ranges, amounting to as much as one-fourth or one-third of its total amount, depending upon the time when the umbilical cord is clamped (before or after cessation of pulsations within it).

When compared to a full-term baby, the premature infant tends to have a slightly higher pulse rate, a lower blood pressure, a lower erythrocyte count, a lower hemoglobin level, and yet has to meet the demands of a relatively larger body surface area; this demand is met by a greater cardiac output, a compensation which is accomplished by reducing the cardiac reserve. A depleted cardiovascular reserve, combined with a poor vasomotor peripheral control, makes the premature infant particularly vulnerable to changes in blood volume, such as those occurring in shock or overhydration.

The plasma protein levels of premature infants are universally low. This deficiency is more evident in the globulin than in the albumin fraction. The resulting diminution of plasma protein osmotic pressure, when combined with the increased capillary permeability which is such an outstanding feature of prematurity, facilitates formation of edema.

Low globulin levels, coupled with low leukocyte counts, contribute to high susceptibility to infection.

Blood coagulation is usually normal or slightly prolonged at birth, but transient hypoprothrombinemia within the subsequent few days commonly leads to the development of hemorrhages in various organs of the body.

Alimentary System

Because of the incomplete development of supporting musculature, the bowel of the premature baby is especially prone to distention and can rapidly undergo necrosis and rupture.

The output of hydrochloric acid by the stomach is strikingly high for a short period after birth, but within a few days falls to low levels. This temporary high production of hydrochloric acid may be an etiologic factor contributing to the formation of perforating peptic ulcer in the newborn, although brain damage (birth injury) acting through vagal pathways or hormonal mechanisms possibly contributes to ischemia of the gastric or duodenal wall, making these more subject to local autolysis.

Enzymes adequate for the digestion of all simple foods, excluding starches, are present at birth although fat is usually tolerated rather poorly by premature infants.

While the full-term infant has sufficient liver development for adequate function, the intensity and duration of *icterus neonatorum* in the premature has been thought to indicate a relative but temporary insufficiency in the organ for clearing the blood stream of pigments.

Levine, Gordon, and Marples[2] have shown that otherwise incomplete metabolisms of certain amino acids in premature infants may be corrected by the addition of vitamin C to the diet.

Urinary System

At birth the kidneys of premature infants, and even those of some full-term babies, are immature; anatomically this is shown by the fetal lobulations which have persisted and by the lack of full glomerular development. Physiologic immaturity is shown by the limited power of concentrating urine, by low clearance levels of urea, sodium, and chloride, and also by frequent albuminuria.

While the hydrogen ion concentration of the blood is essentially normal, averaging 7.4, this is maintained only by compensating for a mild metabolic acidosis. Thus, if any dehydration appears because of abnormal fluid losses (such as from diarrhea, vomiting, or escape from an ileostomy), the premature infant is particularly liable to develop serious acidosis.

Adrenal Glands

The adrenals of the premature baby are usually sufficient to meet most stresses of neonatal life, but under some strains, such as those resulting from chronic infection, major surgery, or the like, poor adrenal response has been observed, as is shown by high eosinophil counts. Adrenal insufficiencies not only can appear from exhaustion of otherwise normal glands but they are particularly apt to follow damage to the organs by hemorrhages which are so common during and following delivery. Adrenal failure may produce temporary collapse or even fatality; this can be warded off in some degree by injection of ACTH, cortisone, or preferably adrenocortical extract. (Upjohn Co., 3 to 5 cc. every eight hours.)

PRINCIPLES OF SURGICAL CARE FOR PREMATURE BABIES

While the premature baby undergoing major surgery for correction of an anatomical abnormality requires all the thought and care necessitated by such procedures in larger subjects, there are additional specific principles and practical considerations which are of utmost importance and which can be listed and summarized as follows.

Preoperative Care

It is not desirable to examine the blood of all these patients to detect those with hypoprothrombinemia; it is disturbing to the baby to collect the blood and it is unnecessary to incur the laboratory expense. It is better and easier to give all premature infants vitamin K (Hykinone, Abbott Laboratories) 2.5 mg. subcutaneously daily before and after operation. Admittedly, this implies giving the material to some babies who do not require it, but as a routine program it is cheap, easy to administer, and is very effective in preventing those tragedies which might otherwise occur from hemorrhages in the brain, lungs, adrenals, or elsewhere. As a routine, penicillin should be used prophylactically to guard against infections. Atropine (0.065 mg.) is given subcutaneously about one hour prior to operation, but no sedative is used. Ideally, the premature infant should be transported from the ward to the operating room in an incubator, but this is usually impossible because of the incubator's electrical and oxygen attachments. Infants can be moved in a warmed bassinet which is covered by a Plexiglas dome, oxygen being supplied from a small portable tank which is attached to and carried along in the bassinet.

Everything in the operating room should be in readiness, so that the baby is not kept unduly exposed to an atmosphere which is dry or of an undesirable temperature. The extremities are wrapped in cotton sheet wadding to minimize loss of body heat. Except for the less complicated procedures such as pyloromyotomy, a cannula or small plastic tubing is inserted by a "cut-down" into a vein so that fluids can be given with ease during or after operation. This can be done under local anesthesia. For most major procedures involving the thorax or abdomen the median ankle vein is employed, but with certain operations such as those for an imperforate anus or removal or a sacrococcygeal teratoma, an antecubital vein of the arm is better.

Anesthesia

For the smallest of babies, under $3\frac{1}{2}$ pounds, we have tended in most cases to employ local procaine (1 or 2 per cent) infiltration of the operative field. To prevent or minimize restlessness or struggling, sedation can be obtained by giving the child brandy (1 part brandy to three parts 10 per cent glucose), either allowing this material to be sucked from a cotton-stuffed nipple or better still by inserting a gastric tube (No. 8 urethral catheter) and instilling a few cubic centimeters of the fluid directly into the stomach. We do not believe that procaine infiltration of the abdominal wall seriously hampers the processes of healing.

Local anesthesia is sometimes unsatisfactory if extensive intra-abdominal manipulations must be carried out. We are convinced that ether anesthesia should be avoided for premature babies because of the chilling which it produces and because of the profound depression which it so often brings about in the immediate postoperative period. Increasingly we have turned to general anesthesia with cyclopropane with a closed system and have found this exceedingly satisfactory when given by a competent anesthesiologist who has had adequate experience in this field. Cyclopropane is the agent of choice because it gives easy and quick induction, satisfactory relaxation, rapid recovery, and permits the continuous administration of oxygen in high concentration.

An intratracheal tube should never be used except in an emergency, because its use is so apt to be followed by postoperative laryngeal edema, respiratory obstruction, and complications which are very difficult to combat and might even lead to fatality. A tightly fitting face mask permits positive-pressure inflation of the lungs when this is required, and it is not accompanied by the dangers of laryngeal trauma and subsequent edema. Even for intrathoracic operations this method of anesthetic administration is quite satisfactory. It is important to remember that the premature infant's lungs are extremely friable and can be easily damaged if an enthusiastic anesthetist overly distends the pulmonary alveoli by giving too much pressure through a tightly fitting system and a laryngeal tube. These serious complications can be rather well prevented by using a face mask (without an intralaryngeal tube) because this almost certainly has some slight leaks which prevent the transmission of excessive pressures to the lung bed.

Operative Technique

The shorter the length of time the premature infant is subjected to anesthesia and operative trauma, the better are his chances for survival. Thus the surgeon must act quickly; the procedure must be technically as simple and as gentle as possible. Unnec-

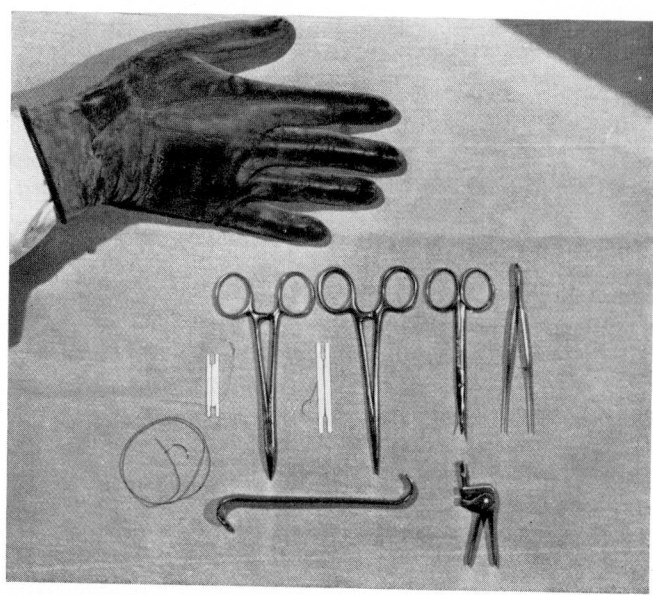

Fig. 19. Small instruments and materials used for surgery in premature babies. The hemostats are "mosquito" clamps. The scissors are vein scissors. For retractors, small S-shaped forms are desirable. On the two card-board loops are 00000 Deknatel silk on atraumatic needles. At the lower left is 0000 Deknatel silk on a French needle. At the right lower corner is a crushing clamp for cutting down spurs of a Mikulicz ileostomy.

essary manipulations or exposures of lung, intestines or other viscera should be avoided assiduously. There is, however, no excuse for haste or for abandonment of sound surgical principles. It is much better to subject the child to an operation which is an hour or two in length, which has the greatest delicacy and which adequately repairs the anatomical defect, than it is to rush quickly through a procedure which is rough, highly traumatic, and possibly insufficient for correcting the abnormality.

For abdominal wounds there is no place for through-and-through sutures which are brutal, ineffective, and not nearly so satisfactory as a closure, layer by layer. For the abdomen, we employ 0000 chromic catgut to the peritoneum and interrupted silks to all of the remaining layers, preferably using 00000 Deknatel silks for the repair (Fig. 19).

Abdominal incisions should never be muscle-splitting; a far stronger postoperative wound is obtained following the lateral retraction of the rectus belly. Needless to say, the wound must be handled with the most meticulous care because any unnecessary or heavy-handed pinching of structures with forceps or hemostats will give rise to post-operative reactions which are unnecessary and inexcusable.

Wound Dressings

Any dressing to the thorax or abdomen should be loosely applied; any compression or restriction around the wound area may seriously hamper the respiratory movements to a dangerous degree. Because of its yielding character, Elastoplast (manufactured by Duke Laboratories, Inc., Stamford, Conn.) makes a most satisfactory covering; its ability to stretch allows some resiliency and gives greater ease to the respiratory movements. Any drainage tubes, such as a thoracotomy catheter or a gastrostomy tube, must be thoroughly anchored with adhesive tape in a satisfactory manner because the premature infant, in spite of his apparent weakness, has often demonstrated his ability to disturb or pull out tubes which have not been appropriately anchored.

General Postoperative Care

One often forgets that these small infants suffer pain which can seriously hinder respiratory movements and can prevent much-needed rest. It must also be remembered that sometimes the infant is so exhausted that he cannot cry to warn of his plight. Morphine or preferably phenobarbital in small doses at appropriate intervals abolishes restlessness and induces sleep which is so beneficial.

Following an operation of any magnitude, complications can occur so quickly in these small patients that it is essential to provide constant nursing care for some days, until the physician can be sure that the baby is stable and is out of danger. The most frequent complications are predominantly respiratory in nature; suction apparatus must be constantly available at the bedside and it is well to have an infant's laryngoscope with suitable intratracheal tubes close at hand in case any aspiration requires their use.

Some very small premature babies have such an unstable respiratory system, evidenced by prolonged periods of apnea or irregular respiration, that it has seemed desirable for a day or two after surgery to stimulate them routinely with Coramine (Ciba Pharmaceutical Products, Inc.) every three or four hours. We cannot prove that this has been of value, but under some circumstances have felt that this central stimulation has been beneficial.

Antibiotics should almost routinely be given before and after surgery. Penicillin (30,000 units per 24 hours) and streptomycin (10 mg. per pound per 24 hours) are the agents of choice, because of their effectiveness, low toxicity, and availability for parenteral administration. Other antibiotics such as aureomycin or terramycin may be effectively given by mouth late in the postoperative period, but because of their tendency to produce venous thrombosis, their intravenous use should be avoided whenever possible. One complication of antibiotic therapy peculiar to infants is the development of thrush; most antibiotics enhance the growth of monilia and their administration should be stopped if thrush appears. In this event, and if bacterial infection must still be combated, the sulfonamides are of considerable value. We prefer sulfadiazine ($\frac{1}{4}$ grain per pound per 24 hours, divided into six-hourly doses) but its administration must be carefully watched and controlled because of possible damage to the kidneys.

Environment of Constant Temperature and Constant Humidity

All premature babies with a surgical condition should be placed in an incubator, the temperature of which is high, until the child's body temperature rises to 98° F. The incubator temperature is then cut back to around 85° F. and the baby allowed to establish his own temperature level. The temperature of the incubator may have to be raised or lowered slightly to a point which allows the baby to establish his own body temperature at a reasonable level. The incubator which we have found most efficient is the Isolette (Fig. 20) (manufactured by Air-Shields, Inc., Hatboro, Pa.), since in addition

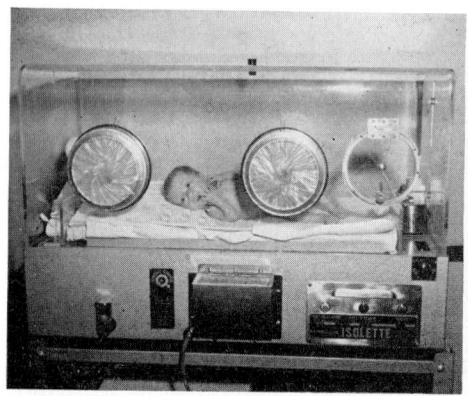 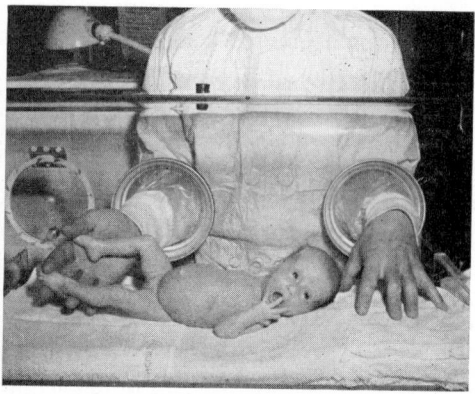

Fig. 20. Incubator unit (Isolette) which is very useful for premature babies. By automatic controls, the atmosphere within the unit can be kept at a constant temperature and humidity. Oxygen can be introduced into the Plexiglas enclosure. The side ports allow introduction of nurse's or doctor's hands for handling the baby.

to its constant temperature and humidity controls, it affords excellent visibility of the child within it, ease of handling the patient, and has adequate provision for the entrance of intravenous and suction tubes as well as ports for the passage inward of the examiner's hands. The atmosphere within the incubator should be of high humidity, approaching saturation. For those children who have had intrathoracic operations, we prefer to have the atmosphere supersaturated, a state which can be easily produced by the use of an apparatus through which air, or preferably oxygen, is passed in such a way that water within the instrument is finely nebulized and sprayed into the enclosure. For this purpose a most useful Mistogen instrument (Fig. 17) has been devised by Denton and Smith[1] (manufactured by the Production Foundry Co., 2700 Magnolia Ave., Oakland, California).

Concentrated Oxygen Atmosphere

Since most premature infants with surgical problems have a condition which directly or indirectly diminishes the respiratory reserve, it is essential that the respiratory system be given every means of assistance by the administration of oxygen in rather high concentration. It is therefore routine for some days following surgery to blow oxygen directly into the Isolette, passing this whenever desirable through a Mistogen apparatus to simultaneously put nebulized moisture into the atmosphere.

Isolation

The premature baby has been acclimatized to the cushioned existence of an intrauterine life, and the less he is disturbed, the better are his chances for survival. By placing the baby in an Isolette where he can be under full vision, there is little need to disturb him and he can be protected from respiratory infections which might be lurking in the doctors and nurses who are in attendance. The baby should be handled as little as possible. Only the most essential diagnostic and therapeutic procedures should be done. No clothing is kept on the child; diapers are simply laid under the buttocks and are replaced as required. The baby should not be given a water bath, but the skin can be cleansed with oil as may be necessary. Temperature-taking, weighing, injections, and various other manipulations should always be restricted to the barest needs.

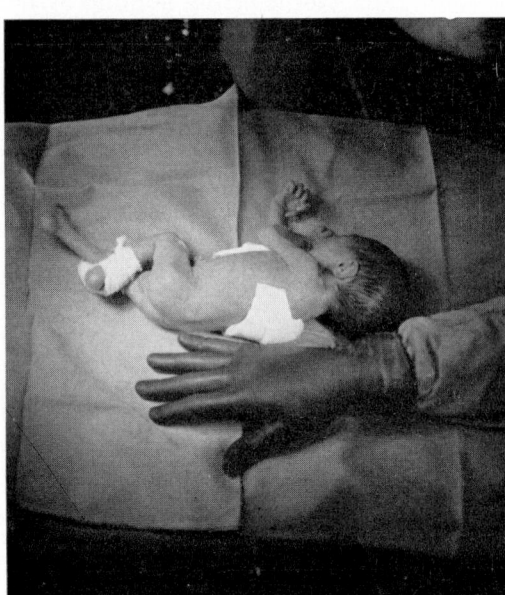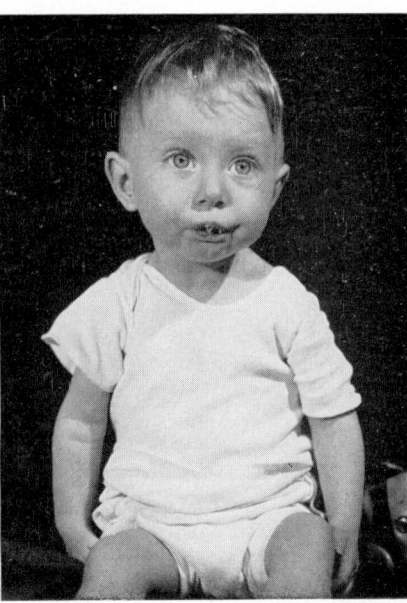

Fig. 21. Premature baby operated upon for esophageal atresia and tracheo-esophageal fistula. *Left*, Photograph of child at the completion of operation. The baby weighed 2 lbs., 15 oz. The esophagus was repaired by end-to-end anastomosis. *Right*, Photograph of this child fifteen months later. There is no difficulty in swallowing.

Gastric Aspiration by Intermittent Methods

In those premature babies who are operated upon for intestinal obstruction there is necessity for decompression of the alimentary tract before and after surgery. Gastric intubation should never be carried out with the use of an oral or nasal tube which is constantly left in place because this is too apt to give rise to irritative swelling in the hypopharynx or epiglottis, leading to laryngeal obstruction of serious or even fata degree. To accomplish gastric decompression, the stomach should be aspirated every three or four hours, passing a No. 8 urethral catheter through the nose or the mouth down into the stomach, lavaging the same, and then immediately withdrawing the tube. Such intermittent aspiration must be continued until that time when the gastric fluid no longer contains bile.

Preset Twenty-four Hour Limitation on Parenteral Fluids

Because of the premature infant's diminished cardiac reserve, his easy tendency toward development of edema, and his inability to excrete concentrated or large amounts of urine, he is particularly susceptible to the dangers of overhydration. In the postoperative period, *we have lost more premature babies from overhydration than from any other single cause.* It is all too easy to give excess amounts of fluid and to bring about a flooding of tissues, particularly the myocardium or the central nervous system, which can be irreversible and can rapidly lead to fatality. While we have seen dozens of premature babies die from overhydration, we have never seen one expire from being too dry! Therefore, from a practical standpoint, we have come to feel that it is essential for four or five days after surgery to keep premature babies distinctly on the "dry" side. It is highly important at the beginning of each day to set a numerical limit on the total amount of fluid which will be given during the next twenty-four hour period. The total, of parenteral fluids of all types, in a premature baby who is taking nothing by mouth

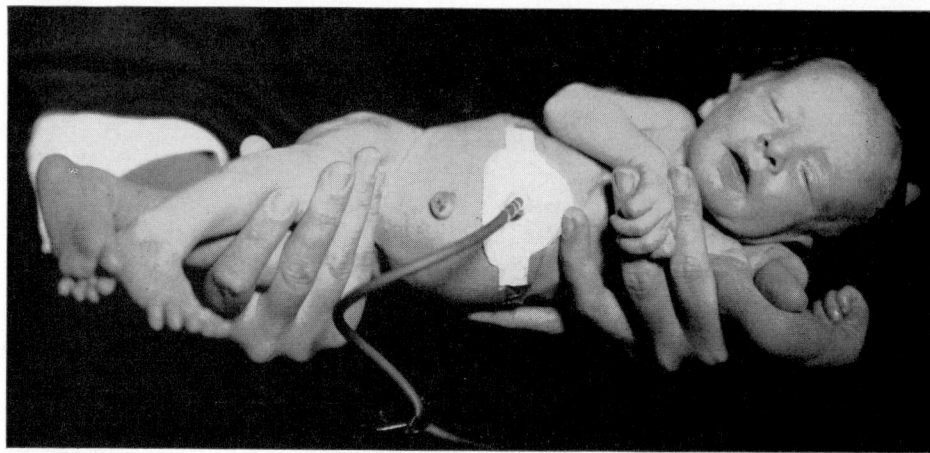

Fig. 22. Photograph of baby weighing 4 lbs., 3 oz. who had esophageal atresia and tracheo-esophageal fistula. The child was treated by primary esophageal anastomosis and by establishment of a temporary gastrostomy. The patient is in excellent health two years later.

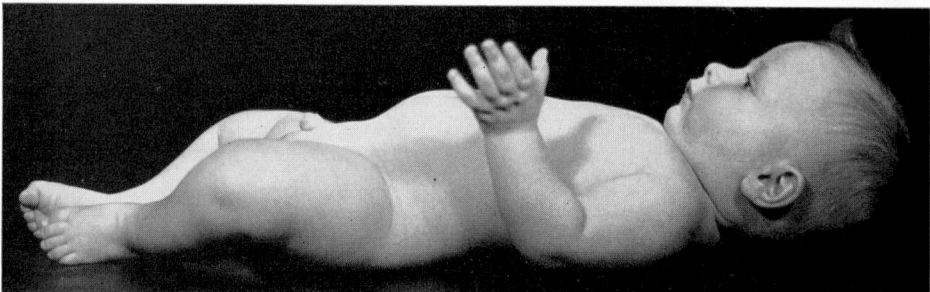

Fig. 23. Baby who weighed 4 lbs., 4 oz. at the time of operation for treatment of esophageal atresia and tracheo-esophageal fistula. Therapy by division of fistula and primary anastomosis of esophageal ends. Photograph six months later. The child is in excellent health seven years later.

should not exceed 30 cc. per pound per twenty-four hours. This total amount, of course, must not all be given at once but should be divided into two doses twelve hours apart, or preferably three doses eight hours apart. To provide fluids and some calories, we have preferred to use 10 per cent dextrose in water intravenously. The fluids can also include *plasma*, or *concentrated albumin* (as described in Chapter 2), or *blood* (if there is a count below 4 million). These amounts are admittedly deficient and are below those required to keep a baby in an ideal state of fluid and electrolyte balance, but experience has shown that attempts to keep these babies in ideal balance are all too apt to be followed by a lapse into a state of overhydration from which the child cannot be retrieved; conversely, if the baby is kept mildly or moderately dehydrated for some days, it is then possible gradually to give more fluid, particularly when this can be given more safely by mouth, to get the baby into an optimum state. After the initial period of dehydration has been purposely maintained for four to six days, the most reliable clinical

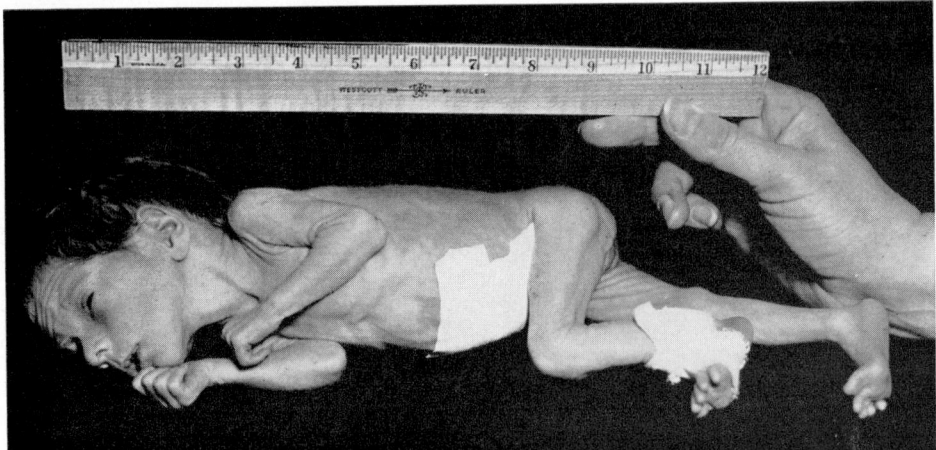

Fig. 24. Child who weighed 2 lbs., 6 oz. at the time of operation for duodenal atresia. Treated by duodenojejunostomy. The entire abdomen is only 2.5 inches in length. The child is in excellent health two years later

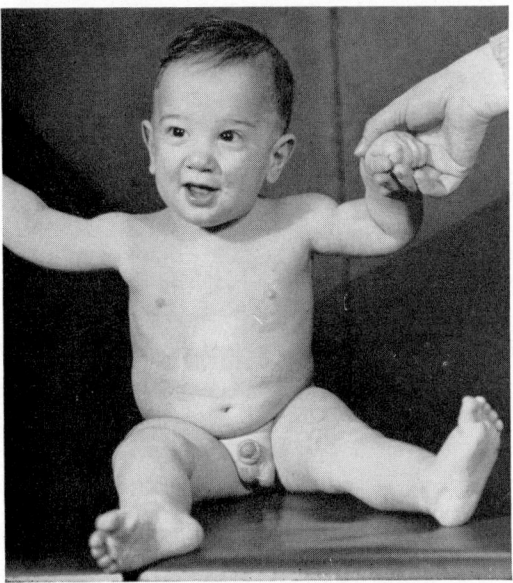

Fig. 25. Child who weighed 2 lbs., 15 oz. at the time of operation for a duodenal atresia. Treated by duodenojejunostomy. Photograph one year later showing excellent condition.

guides by which subsequent fluid requirements can be assessed are skin turgor, tension of the anterior fontanelle, weight gain or loss, number of urinations, and so forth.

Avoidance of Intravenous Saline Solutions

The kidneys of premature babies cannot excrete excess amounts of sodium chloride which may be given to the child in parenteral fluids. While it is true that some premature babies have definite sodium or chloride deficiencies because of gastric or intestinal ab-normalities and the losses produced thereby, it is virtually impossible to give limited amounts of saline without overstepping these requirements and flooding the baby with salt which he is unable to excrete. As a practical approach to the problem, we have found it far better to ignore mild or moderate electrolyte deficiencies for many days and to make a firm rule that *the premature surgical patient shall not be given parenteral saline at any time*. This rule, which has been broken on only the rarest of occasions, has without doubt kept us out of much trouble. As soon as fluids and milk can be ingested by the gastro-intestinal tract, the infant usually rapidly corrects any chemical imbalance himself.

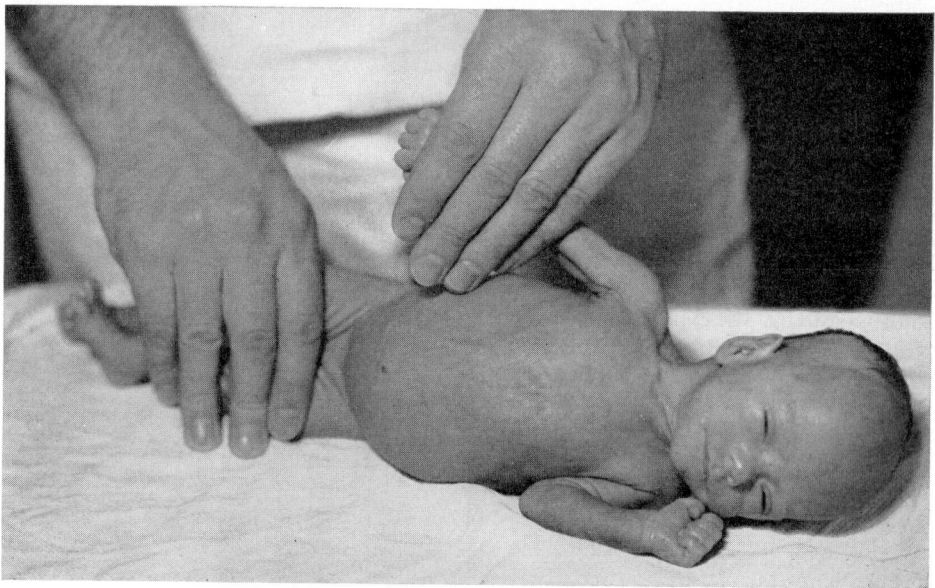

Fig. 26. Child who weighed 2 lbs., 14 oz. at the time of operation for intestinal obstruction. Was found to have multiple ileal atresias and gangrene of a portion of the intestine. Treated by resection of the gangrenous area and side-to-side anastomosis. Photograph two months after operation. Wound is well healed. The child is in excellent health four years later.

Minimal Laboratory Studies

Premature babies need to be protected from the overenthusiasm of interns and house staff who have a high degree of curiosity and want to secure a number of bio-chemical determinations which, of course, are interesting but which are often of little practical value in guiding the care of the child. Premature babies are like the proverbial turnip and very little blood can be gotten out of them. Efforts to withdraw blood often lead to a mauling which does the baby much harm. Furthermore, these small infants are subject to such rapid change that by the time the data are received from the labora-tory, the figures no longer represent the state of affairs in the patient. In premature babies one seldom finds a long drawn-out battle such as the surgeon occasionally en-counters in older children and adults in whom there can be shifts and imbalances of varying sorts, with life hanging by a thread, for protracted periods of time. In the pre-mature baby either the battle will be lost and the baby dead, or else rather promptly the child is on the road to recovery. Therefore, the electrolyte shifts, which certainly exist, do not need to be studied so closely. As a practical matter, we find it possible to

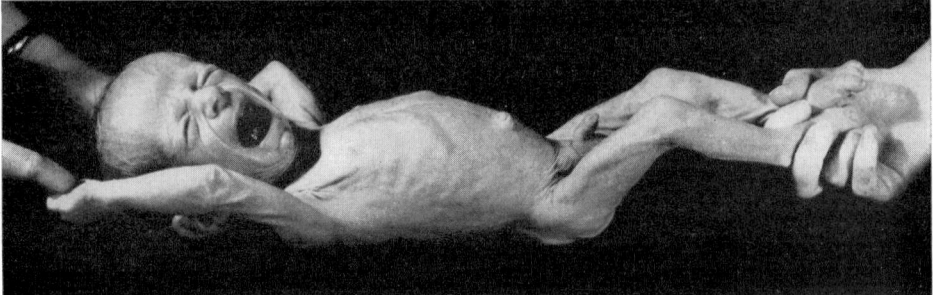

Fig. 27. Child who weighed 4 lbs., 10 oz. at the time of operation for hypertrophic pyloric stenosis.

pull more babies through the postoperative course by relying on "clinical" judgment rather than employing a host of laboratory aids. Under only the most unusual circumstances do we feel that it is justifiable or desirable to perform those tests which require the withdrawal of venous blood.

Daily Use of Intravenous Plasma, Albumin, or Blood

Because of the tendency of premature babies to have low levels of serum protein, a state which is aggravated in most surgical subjects by some degree of starvation, and because of the tendency to the formation of edema (especially dangerous in the myocardium and brain), every effort should be made to keep the plasma protein at a satisfactory level for six or seven days following any major surgical undertaking. From a practical point of view, it is not necessary to study repeatedly the serum protein to actually determine its level; one can usually assume with a fair degree of probability that some deficiency exists. To combat this defect, it has been our policy to administer once each day a small infusion of plasma, not over 10 cc. per pound, or preferably to infuse human serum albumin (of a salt-free or salt-poor variety). This is generally given in concentrated form, three or four times normal, about 2 cc. per pound of body weight. If the blood count is below 4,000,000 cells per cubic millimeter, blood instead of plasma or concentrated albumin can be given for that day.

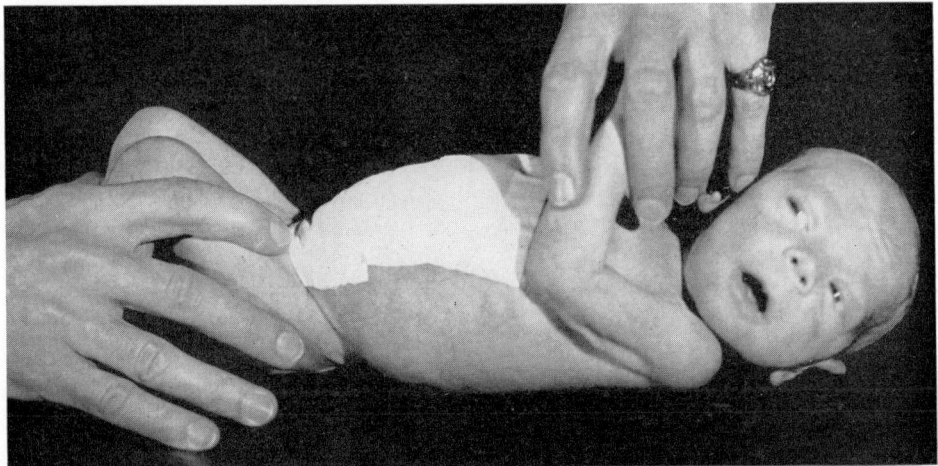

Fig. 28. Child who weighed 4 lbs., 15 oz. at the time of operation for intestinal obstruction. Was found to have ileal stenosis which was treated by side-to-side anastomosis. Photograph ten days later.

Gavage Feedings

When the time comes for resumption of feedings by way of the gastro-intestinal tract, these small surgical patients should be fed in exactly the same way that normal premature babies are given food. The premature infant generally has a poor sucking reflex or may tire himself out unduly by the act of feeding. It is therefore generally better to give the formula by gavage, calculating the fluid and caloric requirements to satisfy the metabolic demands. Because of the premature infant's intolerance to fat, we customarily employ a high protein feeding or breast milk. By gavage, a No. 8 or 10 catheter can be passed down the nose or mouth into the stomach, all fluid and air aspirated therefrom to guard against overdistention, and then the formula slowly instilled, following which the tube is withdrawn. In this way the child is tired very little by the process of feeding and can immediately fall off to sleep.

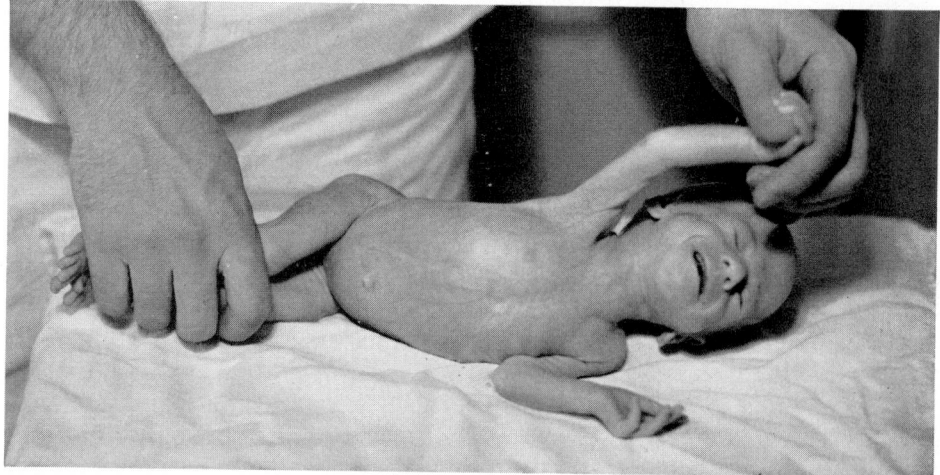

Fig. 29. Child who weighed 3 lbs., 7 oz. at the time of operation for duodenal obstruction and was found to have an annular pancreas which was treated by duodenojejunostomy. Photograph two months later. Wound is well healed. The child is in excellent health four years later.

Length of Hospitalization

In general, the premature baby is ultimately going to survive if he lives twelve to fourteen days after a surgical undertaking; beyond this there are generally but few problems of surgical importance. However, the child is still premature and unable to cope with life in the environment of a home. Therefore, he should be treated like any premature baby without a surgical condition and should be kept in a hospital under ideal surroundings until he is at least 5 pounds in weight. By this time the child is generally stabilized in a reasonably satisfactory way, can be discharged, and can be cared for at home by his physician.

MATERIAL AND RESULTS OF SURGERY IN PREMATURE BABIES

During the sixteen years ending December 31, 1951, 159 premature infants have been operated upon by members of the attending and resident staffs of the general surgical service of the Children's Hospital in Boston. At the time of surgery all these infants weighed 5 pounds or less. The pathologic states for which operations were undertaken and the over-all results obtained are summarized in Table 3. Of all the premature babies operated upon, 88 survived and were discharged from the hospital, a survival rate of 55 per cent. Figures 21 through 33 are photographs of some of the patients; all these babies survived their surgery. It is of interest that in the entire series only one death occurred on the operating table. Some pertinent data regarding each of the survivors are listed in Table 4. In the last year of this study (1951) there were 18 patients with survival of 15, a salvage of 83 per cent.

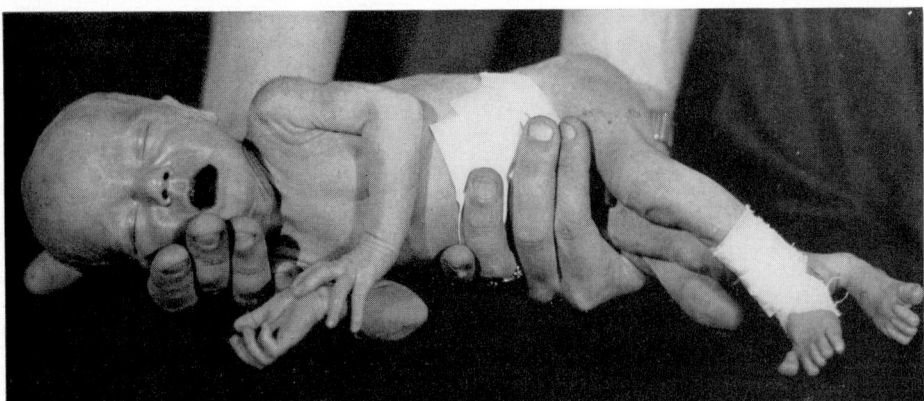

Fig. 30. Photograph of baby who weighed 3 lbs., 12 oz. at the time of operation for duodenal obstruction. Was found to have an annular pancreas and was treated by duodeno-jejunostomy. The child is in excellent health two years later.

In the group of premature babies operated upon there were 10 who weighed less then 3 pounds at the time of operation; 7 of these survived. Some information concerning this group of particularly small babies is shown in Table 5.

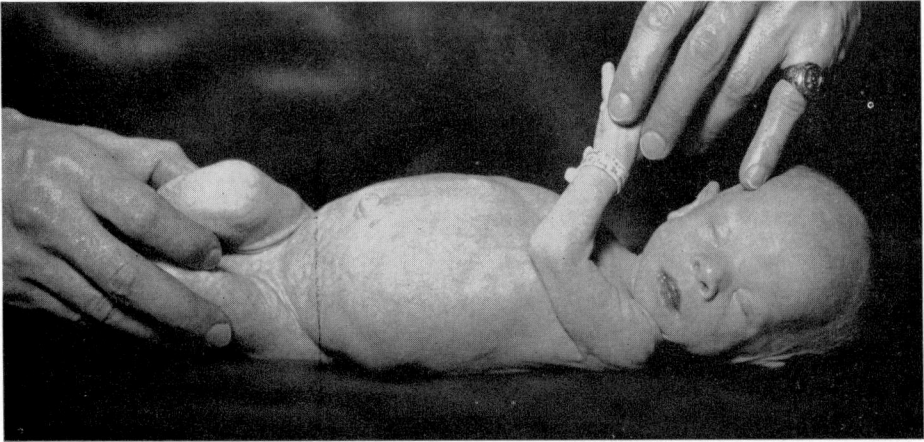

Fig. 31. Child who weighed 4 lbs. at the time of operation and was found to have duodenal obstruction from an annular pancreas and also perforation of the stomach. Treated by closure of the gastric perforation and by duodenojejunostomy. Photograph one month later. The wound is well healed. The child is in excellent health one year later.

The vast majority of subjects in this series of premature surgical patients were operated upon in the first few days of life. However, those with hypertrophic pyloric stenosis and some with other incomplete forms of intestinal obstruction were operated upon at later ages, generally between the second and fourth weeks of life. At the time

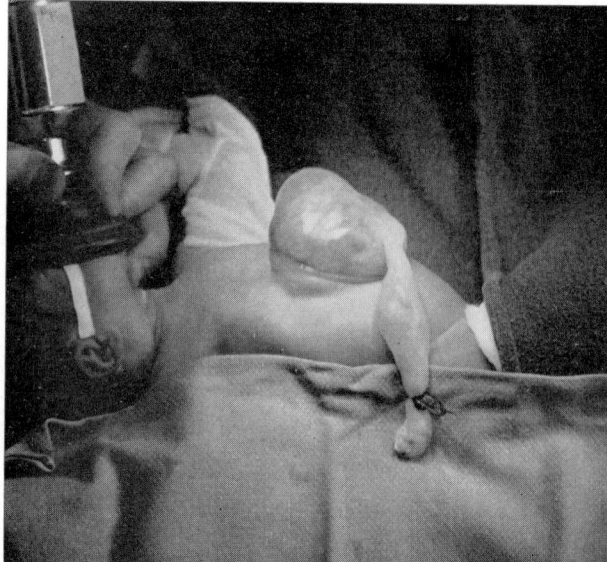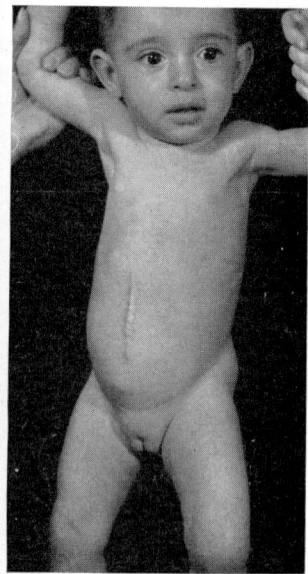

Fig. 32. Premature baby who was treated for a moderate-sized omphalocele by two-stage repair. *Left*, Child weighing 4 lbs. before operation was undertaken. *Right*, Photograph one year later showing the satisfactory repair of the abdominal wall.

of operation the average weight for the entire series of patients was 4 pounds, 3 ounces.

Various types of anesthetic were used as follows: Avertin plus local procaine infiltration, 1 per cent; ether, 14 per cent; local procaine infiltration, 31 per cent; cyclopropane, 54 per cent. While these figures show the use of the different agents throughout the sixteen-year period, within the past few years we have turned almost entirely to cyclopropane anesthesia for these tiny subjects.

Of the 88 infants who were discharged well from the hospital, 10 are known to have died subsequently from causes which were related or unrelated to their primary operation or abnormality. Of the 78 who are surviving, 3 are known to be Mongols,

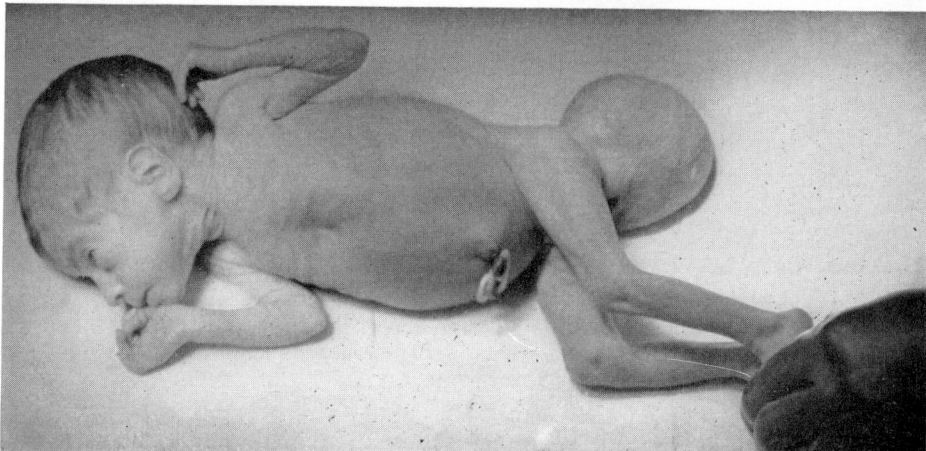

Fig. 33. Premature baby who had a malignant sacrococcygeal teratoma. With the tumor, the child weighed 3 lbs., 4 oz. Following operative removal of the tumor the child weighed 2 lbs., 10 oz. The girl is in excellent health three years later, without evidence of recurrence.

one is mentally retarded and has cerebral palsy, while another has retrolental fibroplasia. The final statistics therefore indicate that of the 159 babies operated upon, 55 per cent survived their operation and were discharged from the hospital apparently well. Ten of these have subsequently died from various causes, leaving 78 who are alive. In the living group 6 have serious defects while 72 children (45 per cent of those originally operated upon) appear to be entirely normal individuals. While the mortality rates are quite high, these figures show that a reasonable percentage of premature babies with serious anatomical malformations can be operated upon for correction of deformities and nearly half of them can be salvaged as children who are sound in mind and body.

Table 3

Pathology and Results of Therapy in 159 Premature Infants
(5 Pounds or Less) Undergoing Surgery

January 1, 1936 through December 31, 1951

Diagnosis	Number of Cases	Survived and Discharged from Hospital
Atresias:		
Esophageal	51	18
Duodenal	11	6
Jejunal	6	3
Ileal	7	3
Imperforate Anus	11	7
Stenoses:		
Pyloric (hypertrophic)	25	23
Duodenal	4	4
Jejunal	1	1
Ileal	2	1
Annular pancreas	7	6
Obstruction for malrotation	5	1
Obstruction of jejunum by bands	1	1
Exploration for ? obstruction	3	3
Intussusception	1	1
Meconium ileus	6	0
Perforated duodenal ulcer	1	0
Omphalocele	6	5
Ruptured omphalocele	4	0
Diaphragmatic hernia	3	1
Strangulated inguinal hernia	2	2
Sacrococcygeal teratoma	2	2
Totals	159	88

Survival Rate—55%

Table 4

List of 88 Premature Infants Who Have Survived Surgical Procedures*

Case	Diagnosis	Weight at Operation		Operation
		lb.	oz.	
1	Esophageal atresia	3	12	Partial repair of anomaly†
2	"	3	12	"
3	"	4	8	"
4	"	4	11	"
5	"	4	11	"
6	"	4	13	"
7	"	2	15	Esophageal anastomosis
8	"	4	3	"
9	"	4	4	"
10	"	4	7	"
11	"	4	8	"
12	"	4	8	"
13	"	4	12	"
14	"	5	0	"
15	"	5	0	"
16	"	5	0	"
17	"	5	0	"
18	"	5	0	"
19	Duodenal atresia	4	1	Gastrojejunostomy
20	"	2	6	Duodenojejunostomy
21	"	2	15	"
22	"	3	3	"
23	"	4	8	"
24	"	4	14	"
25	Jejunal atresia	3	9	Jejuno-ileostomy
26	"	4	3	"
27	"	4	7	"
28	Ileal atresia	2	14	Resection. Ileo-ileostomy
29	"	4	0	Mikulicz anastomosis
30	"	4	4	Ileocolostomy
31	Imperforate anus	2	9	Colostomy‡
32	"	3	5	"
33	"	3	6	"
34	"	4	1	Proctoplasty
35	"	4	10	"
36	"	4	12	"
37	"	4	15	"
38	Pyloric stenosis	3	3	Pyloromyotomy
39	"	3	10	"
40	"	3	14	"
41	"	4	3	"
42	"	4	4	"
43	"	4	4	"
44	"	4	6	"
45	"	4	8	"
46	"	4	9	"
47	"	4	10	"
48	"	4	10	"
49	"	4	10	"

Table 4 (*Continued*)

Case	Diagnosis	Weight at Operation		Operation
		lb.	oz.	
50	Pyloric stenosis	4	12	Pyloromyotomy
51	"	4	12	"
52	"	4	12	"
53	"	4	12	"
54	"	4	13	"
55	"	4	15	"
56	"	4	14	"
57	"	4	14	"
58		4	14	"
59		4	14	"
60	"	5	0	"
61	Duodenal stenosis	3	2	Duodenojejunostomy
62	"	4	5	"
63	"	4	10	"
64	"	4	15	"
65	Jejunal stenosis	4	13	Jejunojejunostomy
66	Ileal stenosis	4	15	Ileo-ileostomy
67	Annular pancreas	3	6	Duodenojejunostomy
68	"	3	7	"
69	"	3	12	"
70	"	4	0	"
71	"	4	7	"
72	"	5	0	"
73	Malrotation	4	8	Ladd's operation
74	Obstruction from jejunal bands	4	12	Release of bands
75	? Obstruction	2	8	Abdominal exploration
76	"	4	11	"
77	"	4	13	"
78	Intussusception	4	9	Reduction
79	Omphalocele	3	6	Repair
80	"	4	0	"
81	"	4	4	"
82	"	4	12	"
83	"	5	0	"
84	Diaphragmatic hernia	4	13	"
85	Strangulated inguinal hernia	4	0	"
86	"	4	4	"
87	Sacrococcygeal teratoma	3	4	Removal of tumor
88	"	3	7	"

* Ten of these babies died subsequent to their hospital discharge. In some, the death was related to the original surgical condition; in others it was not.

† In newborn period, operations consisted of closure of tracheo-esophageal fistula, marsupialization of upper esophageal pouch in neck, and gastrostomy. These children were rehospitalized at subsequent times for intrathoracic or extrathoracic reconstruction of the esophagus.

‡ Repair of anus deferred for subsequent hospital admission.

Table 5

Data from Patients under Three Pounds Requiring Surgical Procedures*

Patient	Weight at Operation		Diagnosis	Operation	Result
	lb.	oz.			
BBP	2	0	Ruptured omphalocele	Repair	Died one day later
DD	2	6	Duodenal atresia	Duodenojejunostomy	Excellent recovery
RB	2	9	Imperforate anus	Colostomy	Discharged well. Sudden death 6 mo. later
BGS	2	8	? Intestinal obstruction	Exploration	Excellent recovery
BT	2	10	Sacrococcygeal teratoma	Excision†	Excellent recovery
NB	2	14	Intestinal atresias	Anastomosis	Excellent recovery
SB	2	14	Intestinal volvulus	Resection	Died one day later
BBD	2	15	Duodenal atresia	Duodenojejunostomy	Died six days later
TP	2	15	Esophageal atresia	Primary anastomosis	Excellent recovery
BBK	2	15	Duodenal atresia	Duodenojejunostomy	Excellent recovery

* All patients in this table are included in the statistics of Table 3. The seven on this table who survived operation are all included on Table 4.

† The baby and tumor weighed 3 pounds, 4 ounces. After excision of the tumor, the baby weighed 2 pounds, 10 ounces.

REFERENCES

1. Denton, R. and Smith, R. M.: Portable Humidifying Unit. II. Large-Capacity Metal Nebulizer. Am. J. Dis. Child., 82:433, 1951.
2. Levine, S. Z., Gordon, H. H. and Marples, E.: A Defect in the Metabolism of Tyrosine and Phenylalanine in Premature Infants: II. Spontaneous Occurrence and Eradication by Vitamin C. J. Clin. Investigation, 20:209, 1941.
3. Smith, C. A.: The Physiology of the Newborn Infant. 2nd Edition. Charles C Thomas, Springfield, Ill., 1951.

CHAPTER 6

Atresia of the Esophagus

In recent years there has been no more dramatic advance in surgery than that which has taken place in the treatment of congenital atresia of the esophagus. In spite of innumerable attempts by many surgeons to correct the malformation by operative means, the abnormality was uniformly fatal throughout the world prior to 1939. In the decade following this, improvements in the surgical handling of babies with this anomaly have been so remarkable that in many centers a high proportion of these children now can be saved and can be provided with a satisfactory pathway for the transport of food to the stomach.

Material for Study

Our experiences in this field were indeed most dismal through the 1930's, when almost every conceivable method of attack on the problem was tried, promising in a few instances a successful outcome, but ending uniformly with fatality. This material, comprising 32 patients treated by various means from 1929 to early 1940, was summarized by Lanman.[10] While there was no cure in any patient, regardless of the surgical attack employed, much of value was learned concerning the handling of newborn babies who required intrathoracic surgical procedures. This fundamental knowledge, gathered from a long series of heartbreaking experiences, forms a substantial foundation upon which rests the modern surgical therapy for correction of esophageal abnormalities.

From 1929 through 1952, there were 259 cases of esophageal atresia admitted to the surgical service of the Children's Hospital of Boston. Because of a moribund state at the time of hospitalization or because of coexisting serious cardiac abnormality, 11 of these were not operated upon. In 248 some form of operation, or combination of procedures, was undertaken. A brief summary of the material *since 1939* is included in Table 7. As seen, we now have 109 children, with ages varying up to fourteen years, who are living following surgical correction of the anatomic abnormality. This total experience in the handling of patients with esophageal atresia forms the basis for discussing the subject in this chapter. Too much credit cannot be given to Ladd, to Leven, to Haight and others for outstanding contributions to the field, bringing it from one of complete disappointment and failure into the realm of successful modern surgical therapy.

TYPES OF ESOPHAGEAL MALFORMATION

Several types of malformation of the esophagus have been encountered. First, the esophagus may have no disruption of its continuity, but can have a *stenosis*, generally in its middle third, and usually involving a rather short segment (Fig. 34, F). The obstruction is sometimes of fairly marked degree and gives symptoms in the early weeks or months of life, but more commonly the block is only of moderate variety and is not detected until the child begins to eat semisolid or solid food. We have encountered 38 such congenital stenoses (see Chapter 7). Second, there may be a *fistula* between the esophagus and trachea, the esophagus having no obstruction (Fig. 34, E). These youngsters have coughing and varying degrees of respiratory distress, particularly during periods when fluid is being swallowed and there is some spillover into the respiratory

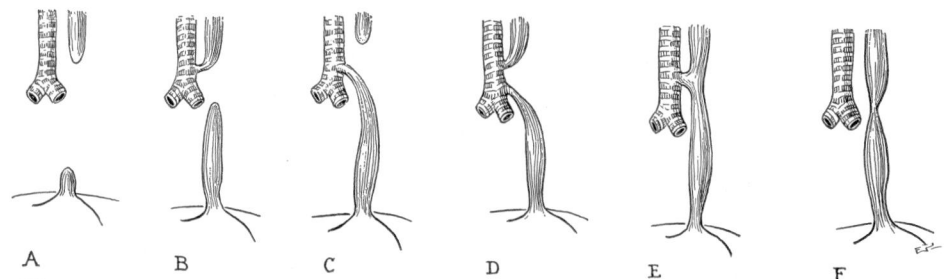

Fig. 34. Types of congenital abnormalities of the esophagus. A, Esophageal atresia. No esophageal communication with the trachea. Under such circumstances the lower esophageal end is very apt to be quite short. B, Esophageal atresia, the upper segment communicating with the trachea. C, Esophageal atresia, the lower segment communicating with the back of the trachea. Over 90 per cent of all esophageal malformations fall into this group. D, Esophageal atresia, both segments communicating with the trachea. E, Esophagus has no disruption of its continuity, but has a tracheo-esophageal fistula. F, Esophageal stenosis.

tract. We have encountered 4 of these abnormalities during the time that we have seen 259 babies with esophageal atresia. For data concerning detection and therapy of tracheo-esophageal fistula (without esophageal atresia), the reader is referred to the excellent articles by Haight[6] and also by Ferguson.[1] Third, there may be an *atresia* of the esophagus.

Atresia of the esophagus is a relatively common abnormality. In well over 90 per cent of cases the configuration is that shown in Figure 34, C; the upper esophageal

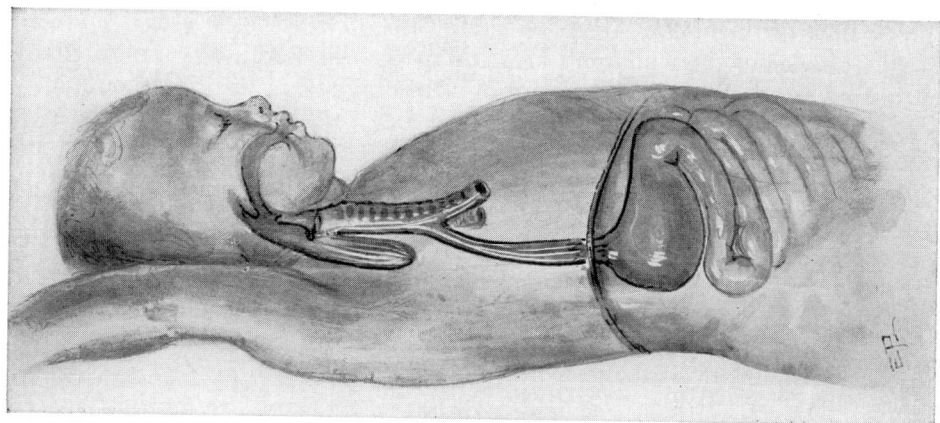

Fig. 35. The common type of esophageal malformation. There is esophageal atresia. The upper pouch ends blindly. The lower pouch communicates with the back of the trachea, just at or slightly above its bifurcation.

pouch ends blindly and has no communication with the trachea, whereas the lower pouch has a tracheo-esophageal fistula. The esophageal ends are separated a variable distance; in some babies they may be quite close to each other, whereas in others the two may be many centimeters apart. In a minority of cases of esophageal atresia, probably less than 10 per cent of any large series, there are variations from this common pattern. In very rare instances there may be a fistula from the upper esophageal pouch to the trachea. Somewhat more commonly the lower esophageal segment has no communication with the trachea, and when this is found the lower esophageal segment is apt to be very short and barely protruding above the diaphragm. Prior to operation it is possible by very simple roentgenographic examinations to obtain rather accurate knowledge regarding the type of abnormality which exists.

CLINICAL PICTURE AND ROENTGENOLOGIC FINDINGS

Symptoms

Esophageal atresia can be suspected and identified in the early hours of life. Certainly the vast majority of the malformations can be detected within the first day or two. One of the commonest findings is that of "excess salivation." A great deal of saliva continually exudes from the child's mouth and one gains the impression that an excessive amount of fluid is being formed. Actually, the total amount of oral secretion is not increased, but since the swallowing mechanism is blocked, this material constantly rolls out of the mouth. Whenever there are attempts at feeding, the hungry child will eagerly take the breast or bottle, but swallowing is accompanied by *gagging, coughing,* and possibly temporary *cyanosis.* After the airway is cleared out, the child's general condition is apparently good, but all subsequent attempts at feeding are similarly followed by the *respiratory distress,* which is obviously produced by a spillover of saliva and milk into the tracheo-bronchial tree. Whenever excess *salivation* or *dysphagia* is encountered in a newly born baby, the patency of the esophagus should be investigated. Important information can be gained quickly and cheaply by gently attempting to pass a No. 10 or 12 urethral catheter down the mouth into the stomach; in the presence of an atresia, the catheter will be stopped by the esophageal obstruction.

Roentgenographic Findings

To gain positive proof of the anatomic abnormality which is present, a few simple roentgenographic studies are very helpful. Through a small urethral catheter which can be introduced through the nose or mouth down into the upper end of the esophagus, 1 or 2 cc. of iodized oil (Lipiodol) can be introduced. This will clearly demarcate the end of the blind upper esophageal pouch (Fig. 36). It is important to view this sac from its lateral aspect, so that any fistula extending forward into the trachea can be detected. Films of the abdomen show the presence, or absence, of gas in the stomach or intestines, thereby giving some information regarding the lower esophageal segment. In the vast majority of cases there is a fistula from the trachea to the lower esophageal segment, which allows air to accumulate in the stomach and intestines. In a small minority of cases no such fistula exists from the trachea to the lower esophageal segment, and no air will be seen below the diaphragm.

Any visualization of the upper esophageal pouch by contrast medium should be made with iodized oil, and not with barium mixture, because the latter is so apt to cause severe reaction in the lungs if it should flow over into the respiratory tract. There is sometimes poor correlation between the appearance of x-ray films of the upper esophageal pouch and the actual position and availability of this pouch when exposed at subsequent thoracic exploration. In some babies the films would seem to indicate an upper segment which extends down to the third or fourth vertebral body, whereas operation shows the pouch to be quite high and difficult to reach and mobilize. Conversely, in a few babies the pouch might seem to be extremely high on films, but at operation it can be reached and freed without too much trouble. Regardless of the picture presented by roentgenograms, we have never seen a pouch so high that it was impossible to expose and manipulate it by thoracic exploration; however, it is true that in some babies it is necessary to carry the mediastinal dissection above the inlet of the thorax to reach the pouch.

Film studies give an idea of the extent and distribution of any pneumonitis which is present, a complication which is found in the vast majority of these babies.

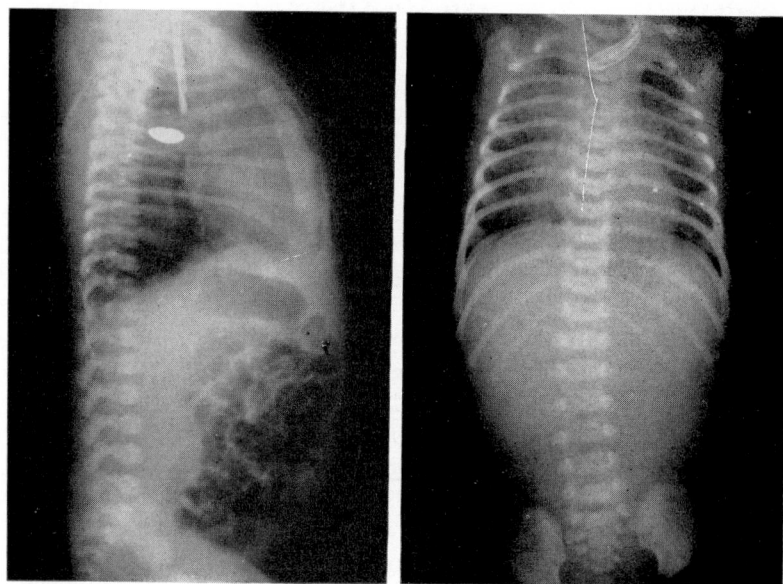

Fig. 36. Roentgenologic findings in cases of esophageal atresia. *Left*, A catheter has been passed down a nostril into the blind upper esophageal pouch. Through it 1 or 2 cc. of Lipiodol has been introduced, which indicates the lowermost point of the blind upper esophageal pouch. None of the Lipiodol has run into the trachea, indicating that there is no opening between the upper esophageal pouch and the trachea. Gas in the stomach and intestines indicates that there is a fistula from the trachea to the lower esophageal segment. *Right*, Findings in another baby in whom there were blind upper and lower esophageal segments. The absence of gas in the abdomen indicates that there is no communication between the trachea and the lower esophageal segment.

Pulmonary Complications

If an esophageal atresia goes unrecognized and untreated, several serious complications appear which portend a downhill course for the baby, eventually leading to death. First, there is starvation and inanition because of the esophageal obstruction. Second, widespread and overwhelming pneumonia follows the spillover of milk and saliva into the tracheo-bronchial tree, literally drowning the baby, and secondarily setting up reactions to the bacteria and lipids which flood the pulmonary tissue. Third, there is very apt to be a reflux of gastric juice from the stomach up the lower esophageal segment and through a fistula into the tracheo-bronchial tree; these acid juices are highly irritating to the respiratory membranes and set up a chemical reaction which augments that already started by the aspiration of milk and saliva from above. These insults rapidly overwhelm the baby; they lead to fatality in a matter of days and are seldom compatible with life for more than a week or two.

Prematurity

There seems to be an extraordinarily high percentage of prematurity in babies with esophageal atresia. Fifty-two of our patients weighed 5 pounds or less at birth. This association of prematurity is distinctly higher than we have seen with other malformations elsewhere in the body.

Associated Abnormalities

While most babies with esophageal atresia and associated tracheo-esophageal fistula have no other important abnormality, it is well to bear in mind that a considerable group of them do have anomalies elsewhere in the body which are a serious threat to health or life. Congenital heart disease, duodenal obstruction and imperforate anus are particularly prominent on the list. Some of these conditions may require surgical relief prior to or at the time of surgical correction of the esophageal obstruction; certainly their existence should be recognized and cognizance taken of them when planning the therapeutic attack in any particular case. Of the 233 patients listed in Table 7, 156 had no other defects, while 77 subjects had the various anomalies shown in Table 6. Some of the babies had several anomalies. The first 9 of the conditions caused death of the subject or were a serious threat to life. For 21 babies another major operation was necessary at the time of, or shortly after, treatment of the esophageal obstruction; these operations were mostly for imperforate anus, intestinal atresia or stenosis, pyloric stenosis, obstruction from malrotation of the intestines, or rupture of the stomach.

Table 6

Other Abnormalities Found in 233 Babies Who Had Esophageal Atresia

Congenital heart disease	24
Malformation of anus or rectum	23
Atresia or stenosis of small intestine	7
Malrotation of colon and intestines	4
Coarctation of aorta	4
Annular pancreas	2
Mongolism	2
Pyloric stenosis	2
Duplication of stomach	2
Meckel's diverticulum	10
Vertebral anomalies	4
Stenosis of ureter	4
Absence of kidney	2
Horseshoe kidney	2
Hypoplasia of kidneys	1
Diaphragmatic hernia	1
Harelip and cleft palate	2
Agenesis of lung	1
Stenosis of bronchi	1
Hypospadias	2
Septate vagina and bicornate uterus	1
Pseudohermaphroditism	1
Club foot	1
Various minor anomalies	7

Early Recognition of Esophageal Atresia

There can be no doubt that the early recognition of esophageal atresia by the pediatrician or general practitioner gives the surgeon better material to work upon; the baby who has little wasting and little or no pneumonia is a much better candidate for surgery than one who is exhausted and has an overwhelming infection.

PREOPERATIVE CARE

Operation Not an Emergency Procedure

Some years ago it was our feeling that all babies with esophageal atresia presented emergency problems requiring immediate operation. Numerous fatalities have now convinced us that it is seldom wise to operate upon these children as soon as they arrive in the hospital. They are starved, they have pneumonitis, and generally they are poor operative risks. Much can be gained by an appropriate period of preparation to get the child into better condition; many hours can be spent profitably in this manner. It is currently our custom to defer operation for twelve or eighteen hours to allow for this preparation, and in some instances this period has been extended to as long as twenty-four or thirty-six hours if pneumonitis appears to be extensive.

Specific Measures Employed

Position of Baby. Whenever there is a fistula from the trachea to the lower esophageal segment, as is found in the vast majority of these subjects, it is advisable to keep the child in a semi-sitting position to minimize the tendency for gastric juice to run up into the tracheo-bronchial tree.

Esophageal Suction. To prevent or to minimize aspiration of saliva, a No. 8 urethral catheter, with several holes cut in its lower end, is threaded through the nose and down as far as it will go into the upper part of the esophagus. Constant suction is applied to this tube so that any saliva which gets down into the blind esophageal pouch will be immediately sucked away.

Chemotherapy. Intensive chemotherapy is started at once, generally employing an intramuscular combination of penicillin (30,000 units each eight hours) and streptomycin (10 mg. per pound each eight hours).

Parenteral Fluid. To supply calories and to combat any existing ketosis, 10 per cent glucose in water is given intravenously, not exceeding 10 cc. per pound each twelve hours.

Oxygen Tent. To alleviate respiratory distress, the child should be placed in an oxygen tent.

Nursing Care. It is highly important to have a nurse with the baby almost continually, paying particular attention to the maintenance of a clear respiratory pathway. If any secretions accumulate in the mouth or throat, the pharyngeal suction tube must be changed or adjusted to make sure that all saliva or mucus is sucked away, in this way minimizing contamination of the trachea.

Intravenous Cannula. Prior to undertaking surgery, a cannula or a fine polyethylene tube should be inserted into an ankle vein through a cut-down incision to allow the administration of blood during operation. As soon as operation is begun, a slow drip of blood is started, so that this can be continued throughout the surgical undertaking, giving a total of about 10 cc. per pound; this has been a most helpful way of supporting these children through a difficult procedure and having them end the operation in a satisfactory state. The cannula can be left in place for the intravenous administration of fluids for twenty-four or thirty-six hours after operation. To leave a cannula in place for longer periods incurs the risk of producing phlebitis.

SURGICAL PROCEDURES

Anesthesia

We have been fortunate in having anesthetists who have had a great deal of experience in the administration of cyclopropane to small babies, which for us has seemed to be the anesthesia of choice in esophageal atresia. The use of an intratracheal tube is purposely avoided whenever possible. It is too apt to set up postoperative irritation in the larynx or the trachea, which adds one more complication during the postoperative course. Furthermore, with such a tube in place it is all too easy for the anesthetist to impart a high pressure to the pulmonary alveoli, overdistend them, and then have pulmonary edema develop within the next twelve to thirty-six hours which may be very troublesome or indeed fatal. We have found that it is best to administer the cyclopropane-oxygen mixture through a tightly-fitting face mask. This generally allows sufficient inflation of the lungs from time to time as may be required. Only under extraordinary circumstances do we resort to the use of an intralaryngeal tube.

Multiple-Stage Operations for Building Antethoracic Esophagus

After stumbling through many dismal experiences and failures, a new ray of light dawned when in 1939 Ladd in Boston and simultaneously Leven in St. Paul, the activity of each being unknown to the other, developed a multiple-stage attack for treatment of esophageal atresia which consisted essentially of: (1) A retropleural exposure and closure of the tracheo-esophageal fistula, to prevent gastric juice regurgitating into the lungs. (2) Establishment of a gastrostomy for purposes of feeding. (3) Marsupialization of the upper blind esophageal pouch on the left side of the neck to allow escape of saliva and thereby prevent spillage into the lungs. These operations could all be completed within the first week or two of life; they protected the lungs from the insults to which they had been subjected, they provided an escape for the salivary juices, and they gave an avenue through which the child could be fed. This general state was now compatible with life, having in mind the construction of an antethoracic esophagus some months or years later when the child was larger and some appropriate tube could be built to join the esophageal opening in the neck with the gastrostomy opening on the abdominal wall. With these multiple-stage repairs, children having esophageal atresia could be made to live, a feat which before had never been accomplished.

The subsequent construction of an antethoracic esophagus brought enormous problems and technical difficulties, requiring infinite patience on the part of the surgeon and patient, necessitating tremendous financial outlay for hospitalization and special treatment, and requiring total periods of hospitalization running into many months or even into several years. While the successes attending the use of multiple-stage attack on the problem, and the formation of an antethoracic esophagus, were remarkable advances in their time, the first successful primary anastomosis of the esophagus for esophageal atresia by Haight in 1941 quickly focused attention on the reconstruction of the esophagus within the mediastinum as a preferable method of therapy. We now feel strongly that multiple-stage construction of an antethoracic esophagus is obsolete therapy; it is greatly inferior to esophageal anastomosis in the mediastinum (or primary esophago-gastrostomy within the mediastinum) as a one-stage repair of the esophageal malformation.

While multiple-stage attacks on esophageal atresia and tracheo-esophageal fistula, with subsequent construction of an antethoracic esophagus, are no longer used by us, it might be well to summarize here some of the experiences gained from the 12 patients who have survived such procedures in this clinic. This brief résumé in no way indicates the innumerable tribulations and infinite patience of Ladd in eventually getting these youngsters through the many complicated steps in the construction of antethoracic subcutaneous tubes. Furthermore, it does not summarize the numerous cases in which there was failure or fatality. However, the résumé does indicate the methods which were employed for each of the children who ultimately survived.

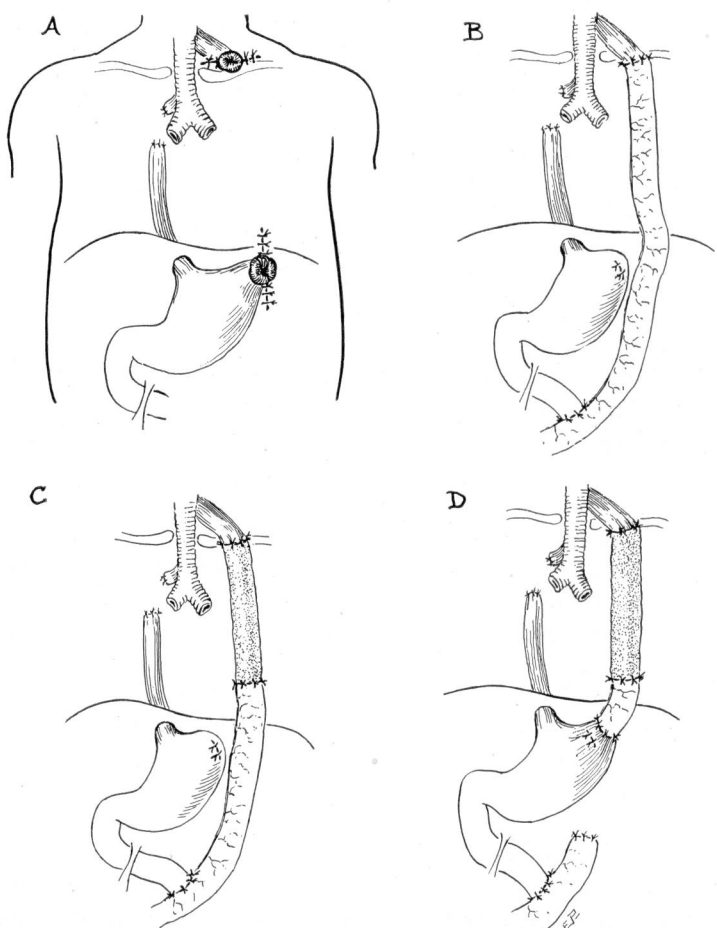

Fig. 37. Types of multiple-stage construction of antethoracic esophagus employed in the early part of the Children's Hospital series for treatment of esophageal atresia, ending with surviving patients. A, Tracheo-esophageal fistula divided; gastrostomy for feeding; upper esophageal pouch exteriorized at base of neck. Esophagus in front of chest not yet made. Two survivors. B, Same as A, but with division of jejunum, bringing up a limb to join the upper esophageal pouch in front of thorax. Three survivors. C, Same as A, with upper portion of antethoracic esophagus made by skin tube, joining the lower end of this to a limb of jejunum. Six survivors. D, Same as C, but because of inanition (the stomach being out of the circuit) the jejunum was cut off and run into the stomach so that all food now passed through the stomach. One survivor.

Types of Antethoracic Reconstruction. In the Children's Hospital material most of the patients in the early 1940's were treated by multiple-stage attack. Twelve of these are surviving at the time of the present review in 1952. The programs of treatment of the esophageal abnormality in these are summarized in Figure 37. Sketch A of Figure

37 shows what was accomplished in the first week or ten days of life: namely, surgical closure of the esophago-tracheal fistula, establishment of a gastrostomy, and marsupialization of the upper esophageal segment in the neck. For different reasons, 2 patients have been left in this situation and an antethoracic esophagus has not yet been constructed. Sketches B, C, and D of Figure 37 indicate the types of construction of an antethoracic esophagus which have been made.

These antethoracic esophaguses, once they have been completed, have been reasonably satisfactory. They can carry fluids and solid food in a fairly efficient way. At times they have developed mild strictures at one or several of their anastomotic lines, requiring surgical dilation, a feat which is sometimes difficult because of the devious course of the pathway. It has become quite clear that any such antethoracic esophagus should not by-pass the stomach and empty directly into the intestine; the failure to pass food

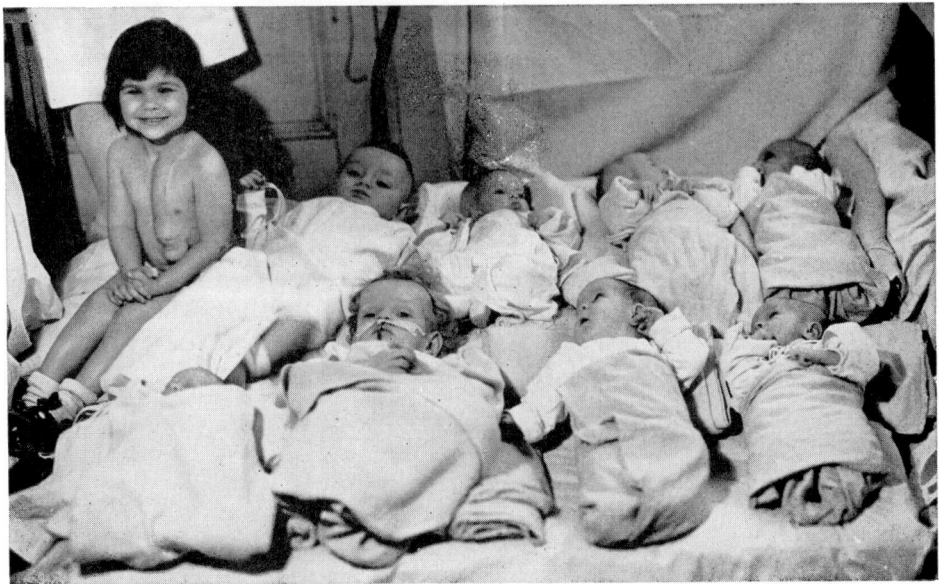

Fig. 38. Photograph of 9 children who were simultaneously in the hospital for treatment of esophageal atresia.

through the stomach leads to a marked retardation of physical growth. This point was made quite evident by one boy, whose stomach had been by-passed, and who was found at the age of seven years to weigh but 27 pounds (Fig. 40). While he took large amounts of food, it was felt that the exclusion of the stomach from his digestive mechanism might in some way be responsible for the physical handicap which was so evident. Therefore, at the age of seven years, five years after the completion of his esophago-skin tube-jejunal pathway, the abdomen was reentered and the jejunum severed from the intestinal tract and turned into the greater curvature of the stomach so that all food now entered the gastric lumen. This boy gained 10 pounds in the subsequent three months! This experience certainly suggests that the stomach plays an irreplaceable role in the digestive functions and that it is quite necessary during the period of growth of an individual. It further suggests that the other children of our series (Fig. 37, B and C) who have exclusion of the stomach will probably require an additional operation to deliver food into the stomach.

Initial Plan for Building Antethoracic Esophagus Changed to Anastomosis of Esophagus in Mediastinum

During the early 1940's when children were being kept alive by the triple procedure of closure of the tracheo-esophageal fistula, gastrostomy, and marsupialization of the upper esophageal pouch, we were carrying along some of these patients with the idea of constructing an antethoracic esophagus in later years. Under Dr. Swenson's able management it was believed that it might be possible to avoid the tribulations of building an antethoracic esophagus and instead provide a distinctly better anatomic arrangement

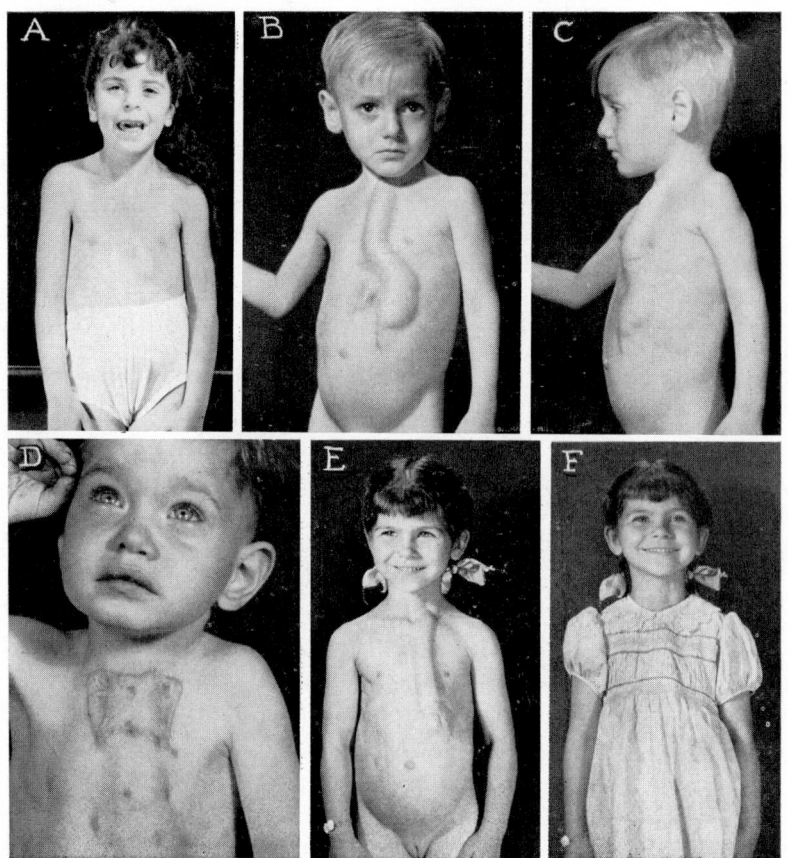

Fig. 39. Children who were treated for esophageal atresia by multiple-stage construction of an antethoracic esophagus. A, Girl treated by Yudin procedure (Fig. 37, B). B and C, Boy with upper part of the antethoracic esophagus made from a skin tube and lower part of it constructed from jejunum (Fig. 37, C). D, Child with same reconstruction (Fig. 37, C). E and F, Girl with same reconstruction (Fig. 37, C).

by attempting to reconstruct the esophageal tube in the posterior mediastinum. In short, the previously marsupialized upper esophageal pouch was threaded back into the base of the neck and down into the posterior mediastinum. By a right retropleural mediastinotomy it was possible to pick up this liberated upper end of esophagus and anastomose it to the lower esophageal segment which has been residing in the mediastinum. Needless to say, this posed many technical difficulties, but it was possible in 5 patients to make such a reconstruction and to establish an esophageal pathway through which the patient has been able to swallow food with considerable satisfaction. In a sixth case (in which there was only a rudimentary lower esophageal segment) reconstruction was done through the left pleural cavity, bringing up about one-quarter of the stomach into the thorax so that this could be joined with the upper esophageal segment (which had been replaced in the chest). These 6 patients represent salvage of a reasonably satisfactory sort; the original decisions to commit the children to multiple-stage construction of an antethoracic esophagus have been changed so that an esophageal (or esophageal-gastric pathway) has been made in the posterior mediastinum.

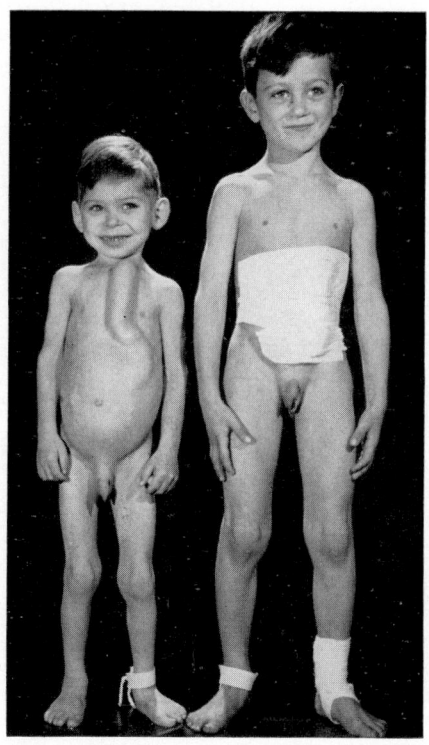

Fig. 40. Example of stunting of nutrition and growth which can occur from exclusion of the stomach from the digestive circuit. *Right*, Normal seven-year old boy (who had appendicitis) for comparison. *Left*, Boy of same age who had been treated for esophageal atresia by type of construction shown in Fig. 37, C. He weighed but 27 pounds. (After the time of this photograph, the jejunal tube was divided and joined to the stomach (Fig. 37, D) so that all food then entered the stomach. He gained ten pounds in three months!)

Disadvantages of Multiple-Stage Repairs

All of these multiple-stage operations for construction of an antethoracic esophagus (or for subsequent replacement of the esophagus into the mediastinum) require an enormous financial outlay, exceedingly long periods of hospitalization, and very complicated surgical and nursing care. For these reasons we believe that all of them are now antiquated and should be completely replaced by attempts at one-stage primary anastomosis of the esophagus in the posterior mediastinum of the newly born baby. It is now possible in all patients (unless there is other existing serious disease such as congenital abnormality of the heart, intestinal obstruction, or the like) to make such a primary repair in the small baby either by bringing together the ends of the esophagus or in an occasional case by bringing the stomach up into the chest, thereby permitting union of the esophageal ends.

Primary Esophageal Anastomosis

Since 1945 we have entirely given up the treatment of esophageal atresia by multiple-stage procedures (construction of an antethoracic esophagus). Since that time we have in all cases attempted a one-stage repair by union (within the mediastinum) of the esophageal ends.

Exposure. To expose the esophagus in the mediastinum of a newborn baby, a right-sided approach is far superior to one on the left. Whether the exposure should be retropleural or transpleural is possibly open to debate. In the early part of this work it was felt by most surgeons that the opening of a pleural cavity in a small baby would be disastrous either because of temporary embarrassment of the lung or because of subse-

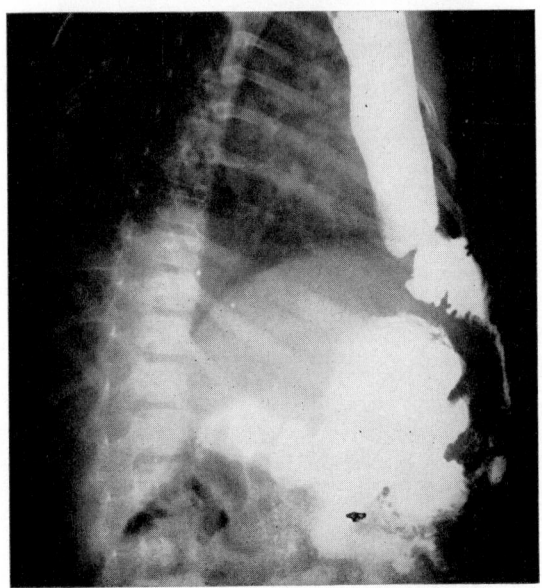

Fig. 41. Roentgenogram of a child treated for esophageal atresia by multiple-stage construction of an antethoracic esophagus (Fig. 37, D). Barium enters the stomach by way of the anterior passage which had been made from a skin tube and a piece of jejunum.

quent contamination of the pleural sac. Hence, a retropleural exposure was generally advocated. The field obtained by this avenue is small; the opening is narrow and deep. It is possible, but difficult, to dissect up into the thoracic apex or down as far as the diaphragm when such extensive explorations are necessary. It is possible to mobilize the esophageal ends and make a reasonably satisfactory esophageal anastomosis. One of the biggest safety factors of this approach behind the pleura was that it permitted an extravasation to the exterior if there should be any postoperative leakage from the anastomosis, a complication which was not uncommon.

More recent experience has made us feel quite conclusively that the retropleural approach, while possessing certain advantages, is distinctly inferior to a transpleural opening, temporarily collapsing the lung away, but reexpanding it immediately at the termination of operation. The *transpleural exposure* is very easy to make. It cuts a great deal off of the operating time. It gives an excellent view from the top to the very bottom of the chest and it allows the widest possible dissection of the esophagus. It permits opening of the diaphragm and mobilization of the stomach when these are required. While it would seem to have the disadvantage of allowing any postoperative leakage from the anastomosis to escape directly into the pleural cavity and thereby be trouble-some or even fatal, it has been our experience that the wider exposure permits us to make a superior anastomosis so that postoperative leakage is now very rare. Therefore, in the last three years *we have used the right transpleural approach for all cases,* regard-less of the size of the baby, the condition of the lung, or the positions of the esophageal ends.

Operative Technique. With the child on the table and his right side uppermost, the right arm is drawn upward out of the way (Fig. 42). A long incision is made just above the midportion of the chest, running from just beneath the tip of the scapula forward beneath the breast. After transecting the external muscles of the chest, an intercostal space is entered, generally the fourth or fifth, this being opened throughout its entire length. It is seldom necessary to divide a rib posteriorly or a costal cartilage anteriorly. The ribs are soft and bend easily, allowing a wide exposure with a spreading instrument, for which a self-retaining thyroid retractor serves admirably. The lung is held forward. Rather than compress this by an overlying pack, it is generally better to grasp the pos-terior portion of it delicately with a half-length clamp so that the lung can be pulled forward, in this way allowing partial expansion of the lung during operation. The azygos vein is doubly ligated and divided as it enters the superior vena cava. With great care a leaf of mediastinal pleura is cut and dissected backward as a flap, preserving this so that it can be sewn back into place over the esophagus at the end of operation.

Attention is now directed to the upper esophageal segment, dissecting upward in the mediastinum until it is encountered, then grasping its tip with several silk sutures which act as traction stitches, rather than crushing the pouch with a clamp. Sharp and blunt dissection is then carried around the sides and the posterior aspect of this blind sac. Finally, the liberation must be carried to the most dangerous part, separating the esophageal pouch from the back of the trachea. It is very easy to make a hole accidentally in the back of the trachea when the latter becomes tented up by virtue of its attachments to the esophagus. Therefore, the dissection should be carried well toward the esophagus itself, to protect the tracheal tube from injury. If a hole is inadvertently made in the trachea, it must be immediately closed by appropriate suture. While making traction on the esophageal pouch, dissection is carried up to the very apex of the chest and even be-yond into the base of the neck, a point of considerable importance in getting adequate mobility of the esophagus and thereby facilitating the subsequent anastomosis. We have never seen any interference with the blood supply of the upper end of the esophagus, no matter how high the dissection has been carried into the base of the neck.

Directing attention downward, the lower esophageal segment is now identified and raised from its bed, a step which should be carried out with two precautions in mind. The vagi and their major branches should not be interfered with or severed (for fear of setting up postoperative gastric atony or pyloric spasm). Furthermore, the dissection around the left side of the esophagus must be done with great care so that the left pleural sac is not broken into, an accident which greatly increases the anesthetist's troubles. We have found it best to start the freeing at about the midpoint of the lower esophageal segment, to dissect around its entire periphery, and then pass a linen tape around the esophagus for traction purposes, which facilitates lifting the esophagus from its bed. Just how far the esophageal dissection must be carried downward will depend on the length of the gap which exists between the two esophageal ends. The dissection should be extensive enough to insure that the esophageal ends will later come together without tension; the lower segment should not be liberated more than this, for fear of diminishing its already poor blood supply. However, when it is necessary to do so, there should be

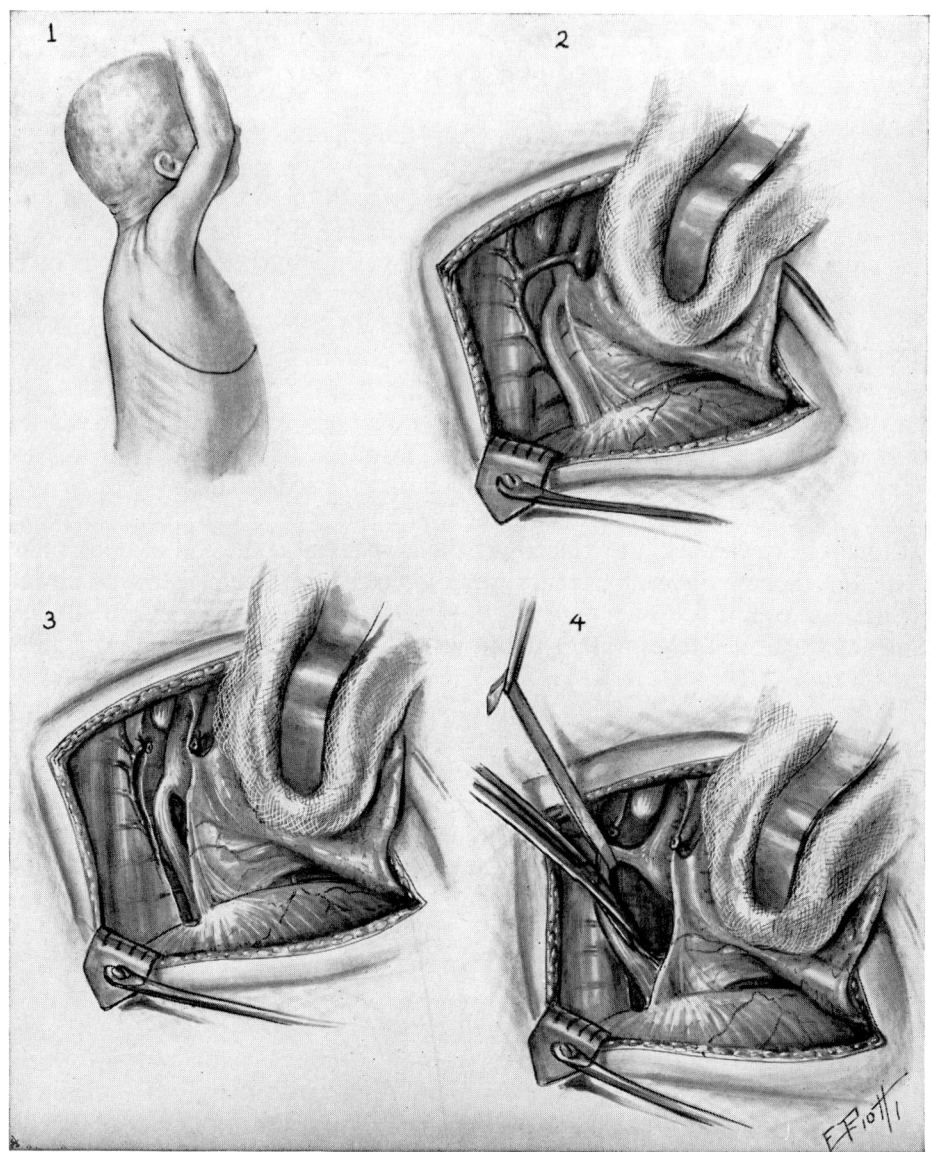

Fig. 42. One-stage primary anastomosis for esophageal atresia. 1. Position of baby with right side of chest uppermost, arm drawn above. Position of incision indicated. 2. Transpleural approach, through fifth interspace, spreading of ribs. The azygos vein can be seen coursing over to the superior vena cava. Above this is the upper blind end of the esophagus. Below it is the lower esophageal segment which communicates with the back of the trachea. 3. Azygos vein divided. Pleural covering of medi-astinum is carefully opened, (preserving the pleural edges so that these flaps can be brought together at the end of operation). The two portions of esophagus are now clearly seen. 4. The upper esophageal pouch has been freed up to the base of the neck. Tape passed around lower esophageal segment, which is being mobilized from its bed.

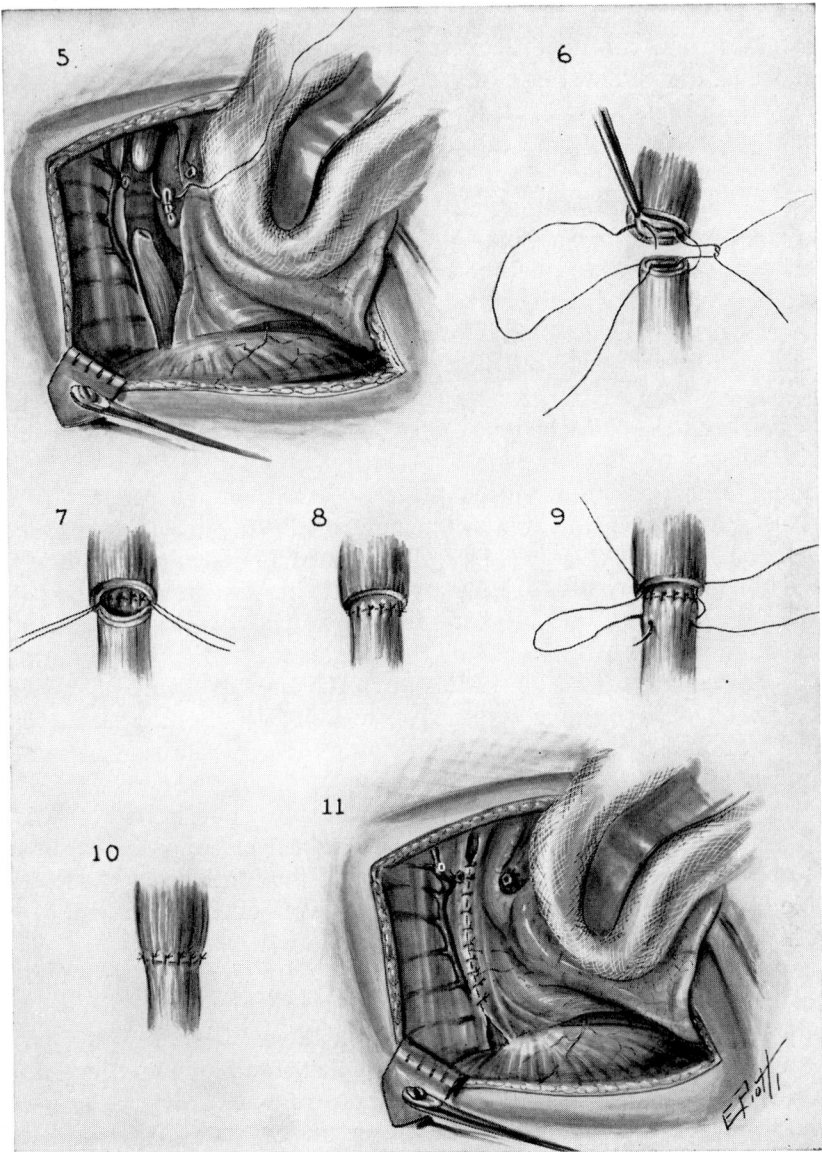

Fig. 42 (*continued*). 5. Lower esophageal segment cut off from trachea. Trachea being closed with interrupted sutures (00000 Deknatel silk), being careful not to constrict the trachea. 6. Details of anastomosis of esophageal ends. The upper pouch has been opened; the lower one has been slightly dilated by passing a hemostat or half-length clamp into it. Union by the method of Haight. The stitch includes the entire thickness of the lower segment, but only the mucosa of the upper segment, knots to lie on inside of lumen. 7. Back row of sutures placed and tied. 8. Inner layer of stitches completed. 9. Second layer of silk sutures, grasping the muscularis of the upper pouch and then the lower esophageal wall below the initial suture line. This second layer of sutures will pull down a cuff of the upper muscular wall to cover the inner union. 10. Outer layer of sutures completed around entire periphery of esophagus, pulling down the outer tissues of the upper segment to cover and seal over the inner reconstruction. 11. After completion of the anastomosis, the pleural edges are carefully brought together to seal off the anastomosis. Small opening left at upper and lower ends so that serum or other fluid will not be trapped in mediastinum, but can escape into the right pleural cavity (which will be drained postoperatively by a catheter).

no hesitation in carrying the mobilization of the esophagus all the way down to the diaphragm.

The fistulous connection between the lower esophageal segment and the trachea is now severed and the tracheal opening closed with interrupted 00000 Deknatel silk stitches. Over this primary line of closure it is generally possible to bring a second layer of adventitial substance, but great care should be taken not to constrict the trachea in any way.

The open end of the lower esophageal segment generally appears rather small for making an anastomosis; we customarily dilate it somewhat, finding that it is possible to increase its diameter to two or three times its preexisting size. In some instances it is necessary to trim off a little of the end to get back to thicker substance and to a larger lumen. The upper esophageal pouch is now opened and for 3 or 4 mm. its mucous membrane is separated from the surrounding muscular coats.

For anastomosis we have tried many methods of union but in general we rely most on that which was described by Haight, feeling that it gives the best sealing of the anastomotic line. The first step in this union is to grasp the *entire thickness* of the lower segment (including muscularis and mucosa) and to join this to the *mucosa* of the upper segment. This is completed by a row of interrupted silk stitches of 00000 Deknatel silk. We have generally found it best to place all of the back row of sutures and then draw the two ends of the esophagus together by a pull which is simultaneously distributed through all of the silks, after which the individual stitches can be snugged up and tied. After this back row is finished, a No. 8 urethral catheter is fed downward into the stomach and the other end is passed upward through the esophagus and pharynx out either the mouth or nose. With this tube in place, the remaining half of the sutures can then be easily taken, without having any fear of grasping the opposite side of the esophagus with the needle. After the inner row has been completed, *a cuff of muscularis* of the upper segment can now be drawn as a *sleeve* over the inner suture line, anchoring this muscular sleeve with a row of interrupted silk stitches around the entire periphery of the esophagus. This sleeve extends down 3 to 5 mm. beyond the inner layer of sutures; it gives considerable strength to the anastomosis and it gives effective sealing of any small aperture which might exist in the inner union.

The flap of mediastinal pleura is now carefully sewed back into place, making a covering over the anastomosis and providing a layer which can quickly become adherent to the esophagus and help seal it over. A small vent is left at the superior and at the inferior end of this pleural reconstruction, so that serum or blood will not accumulate in the mediastinum (and raise the flap of pleura away from the esophagus); the openings allow escape of any fluid into the pleural sac.

A No. 10 or 12 catheter, fitted with several holes, is led out the sixth interspace in the mid-axillary line for postoperative pleural drainage. The chest wound is closed with pericostal sutures of 0000 chromic catgut and the great muscles of the chest wall are repaired with continuous stitches of the same material. A similar approximation is taken in the subcutaneous tissues. The skin is closed with continuous fine silk. Through the intercostal catheter, the pleural cavity can now be lavaged and then all fluid and air sucked away, giving immediate, complete expansion of the lung.

The more one has experience with the treatment of esophageal atresia, the more it becomes obvious that in the vast majority of subjects it is possible to perform a primary anastomosis of the esophageal ends, a feat which is dependent upon wide mobilization of the esophageal segments. However, there are occasional patients in whom there is no lower esophageal end, or else the lower segment is exceedingly short; either condition makes it impossible to perform a primary esophageal anastomosis. It becomes necessary to draw a portion of the stomach up into the chest (Fig. 43). The lower nubbin of esophagus can be grasped and pulled upward so that the pleural and peritoneal reflections around the esophageal hiatus are brought into prominence. These are then opened anteriorly and the scissors swept around the entire circumference of pleura and peritoneum at the esophago-gastric junction to allow the stomach to be pulled up into the chest. In no case have we found it necessary to split the diaphragm to enlarge the hiatus. Furthermore, the hiatus has been big enough to accommodate that portion of the stomach which subsequently passes up through it. Great care must be taken with the left gastric artery as the stomach is drawn upward; this vessel must be identified, doubly ligated, and divided as it comes into view. If this precaution is not taken, the delicate vessel might be ruptured and its proximal portion sink back into the abdomen and produce serious bleeding. As much of the stomach as necessary can be pulled up into the thorax quite readily, but one should bring up only enough to permit the ends of the esophagus to be joined without tension. It is highly important to anchor the stomach around the entire periphery of the diaphragmatic hiatus with interrupted silk stitches, a step which is often difficult to accomplish but which must be done to prevent subsequent herniation of intestines through this area. When the stomach has been drawn up into the chest it is still possible to cover over the esophageal anastomosis with a flap of pleura but it is impossible to obtain enough of a pleural flap to cover the stomach itself.

Gastrostomy. Following primary esophageal anastomosis, many of the babies can be fed by mouth soon after operation without complications of any sort. Indeed, we have used this regimen on several occasions and have been agreeably surprised by the exceedingly smooth course of the patient and the ability to discharge him from the hospital within ten days or two weeks. On several occasions we have also fed these children through a No. 8 urethral catheter which had been led through the nose, down through the esophagus and into the stomach, leaving this in place for ten days and introducing all feedings through it. More recently, a small polyethylene tube has been used for this purpose.

However, we are completely convinced that it is generally much safer to immediately establish a temporary gastrostomy, an adjunct which in our hands has produced almost no complications and which would seem to provide the best possible chance for healing of the esophageal anastomosis. It has been our feeling that the use of inlying rubber or polyethylene tubes through the nose or mouth might not always provide decompression of the stomach and might allow injurious vomiting if the feedings are not well tolerated. Furthermore, one never knows when there may be edema and temporary obstruction of the esophagus in the subsequent few weeks; the presence of a gastrostomy is a tremendous help for putting the esophagus at rest and yet permitting adequate feeding. Therefore, we have generally established a gastrostomy, which in all cases during the last three years has been made immediately after completion of the thoracic procedure. The abdomen having been prepared and draped at the same time that the chest was prepared, there is little disturbance in slightly turning the baby so that a left upper rectus muscle-splitting incision can be made, drawing the greater curvature of the stomach out through the wound and establishing a Stamm gastrostomy, placing a self-retaining catheter in the stomach (Fig. 75). Closure of this wound requires but a few sutures. The establishment of the gastrostomy seldom adds more than fifteen or twenty minutes to the time of the thoracic operation.

In those rare cases when the stomach has been drawn up into the chest, we have not

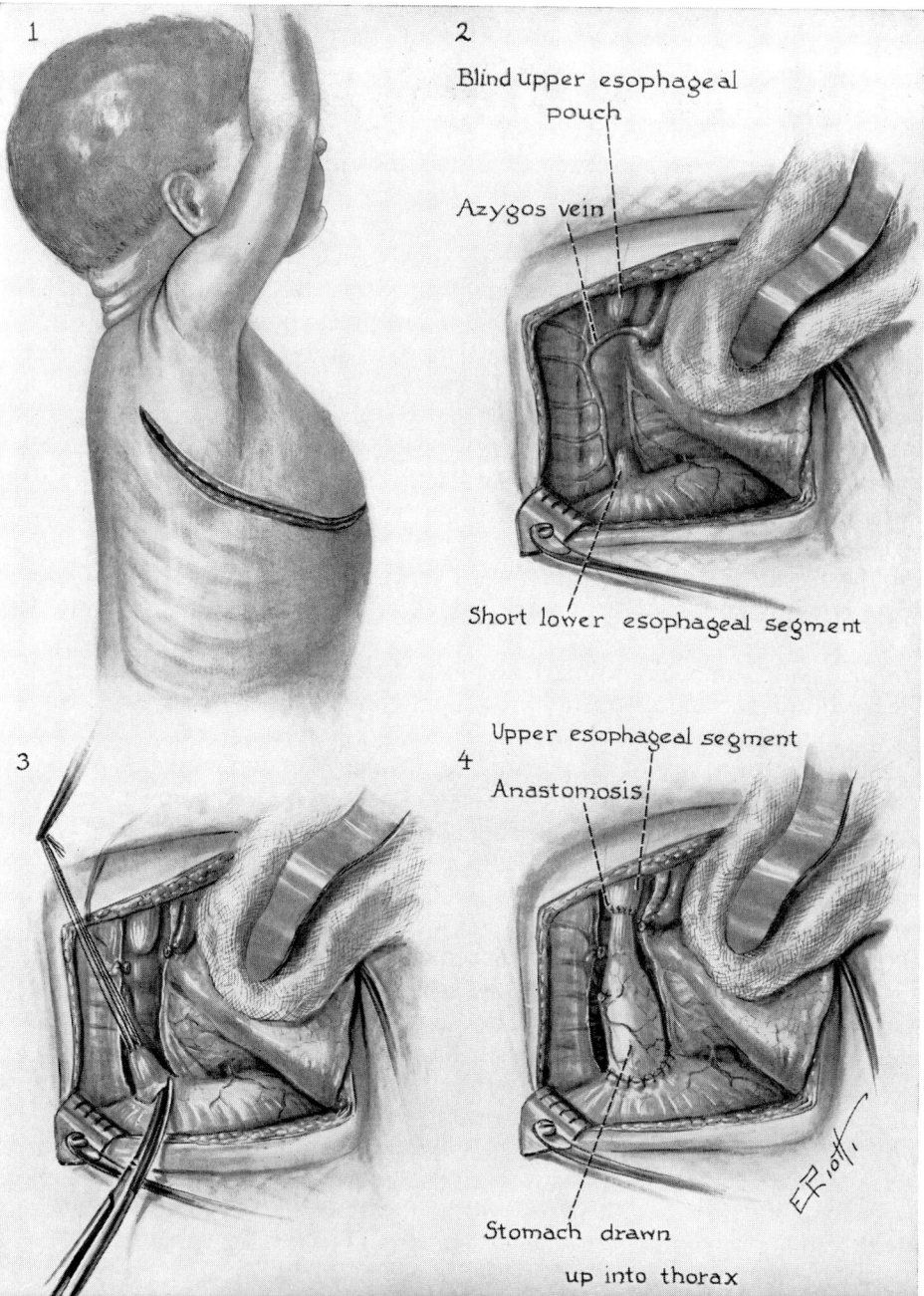

Fig. 43. Type of one-stage reconstruction used for esophageal atresia when where is only a rudimentary lower end of the esophagus. 1. Right transpleural approach. 2. Chest open, showing widely separated esophageal ends. 3. Azygos vein divided. Mediastinal pleura opened from top to bottom of thorax. Upper esophageal pouch has been well liberated from its bed. Lower esophageal nubbin grasped with several traction stitches. Incision being made in pleura (and peritoneum) around esophageal hiatus of diaphragm. 4. Stomach drawn up into thorax, permitting esophageal anastomosis without tension. Stomach carefully anchored around periphery of diaphragmatic hiatus to prevent subsequent herniation here.

established a gastrostomy because so little stomach has remained below the diaphragm that it would be difficult or impossible to make a gastrostomy. Furthermore, in such cases we prefer not to introduce milk into the stomach in the early postoperative period, for fear that it would immediately run up into the thoracic portion of the stomach and thereby soil the esophageal anastomotic line. When the stomach has been drawn up into the chest for an anastomosis, we like to leave the gastro-intestinal tract at complete rest for five or six days and to supply all feeding by parenteral routes.

POSTOPERATIVE CARE

Oxygen, Wet Atmosphere, Antibiotics, Suction

Following surgery, these babies should be placed immediately in some sort of an enclosure, such as an Isolette.* In a plastic enclosure the baby can be seen at all times, can be given a high concentration of oxygen, and furthermore can be provided with a supersaturated atmosphere which can be obtained by blowing oxygen through a Mistogen† apparatus which nebulizes water into the atmosphere. This excess moisture is highly desirable for some days in alleviating the irritations in the nose, mouth, trachea, and lungs which have been brought about by the various insults. Parenteral chemotherapy in the form of penicillin and streptomycin should be continued until it is certain that the pulmonary infection is completely under control. Some suction apparatus should be constantly at hand so that if any saliva accumulates in the mouth or pharynx, it can be sucked away. Generally, within a day or two the saliva will be swallowed in a satisfactory manner.

Gastrostomy Feedings

The gastrostomy tube is left open for twenty-four to thirty-six hours, the stomach being kept deflated during this time. On the second or third day, feedings can be started through the gastrostomy tube, beginning these with caution, generally using an ounce or two of 10 per cent glucose in water every four hours. If this is tolerated well, a milk formula can be given, started in small amounts, never giving enough to distend the stomach fully, thereby preventing regurgitation up into the esophagus. It has been found quite satisfactory to allow such feedings to drip in slowly over a period of twenty or thirty minutes (Fig. 44). The gravity feeding apparatus is provided with a glass segment containing an escape hole so that if there should be any increase in pressure within the stomach during coughing or straining, the milk will not pass up into the esophagus but instead will reflux up into the apparatus and be discharged in a safe manner.

Oral Feedings

If the child is apparently swallowing saliva, the lungs are relatively clear, and the general condition of the patient is satisfactory, it is generally possible and safe to begin oral feedings on the eighth or tenth postoperative day. A few drams of water or glucose solution can be offered, and if these are apparently swallowed without gagging or coughing, small amounts of milk formula can be subsequently offered on a regular schedule. The amounts of milk which are offered can be gradually increased so that it is usually possible to have these children taking full feedings by mouth at the end of two or three weeks after operation. If at any time apprehension develops concerning deglutition, it is well to reduce the oral feedings or to abandon them temporarily and to return

---

* Manufactured by Air-Shields, Inc., Hatboro, Pa.

† Manufactured by Production Foundry Co., 2700 Magnolia Ave., Oakland, Cal.

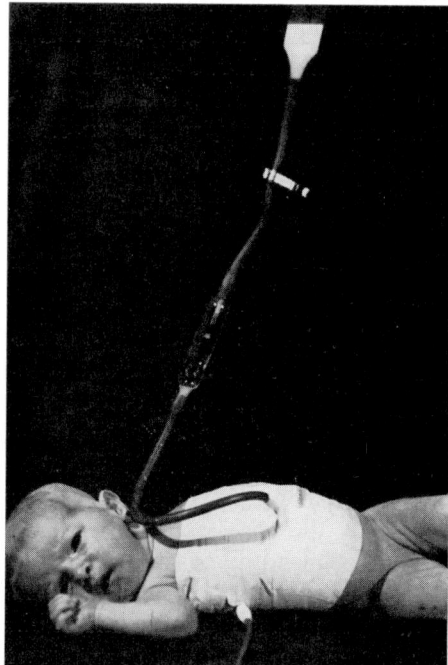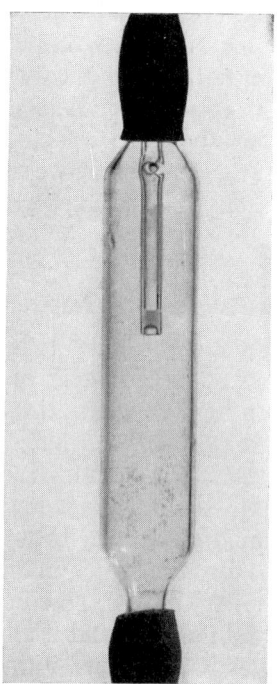

Fig. 44. Method of feeding through a gastrostomy tube. *Left,* Formula is placed in an open tube glass portion of an Asepto syringe). This is connected by tubing to a glass Murphy drip apparatus, which then is joined to the gastrostomy tube. *Right,* The glass Murphy drip appliance. Milk enters by way of the central small tube. The outer glass shell has a tiny opening in its upper end to allow escape of gas or of milk from the stomach if the child should strain or cry and thereby increase the intra-abdominal pressure.

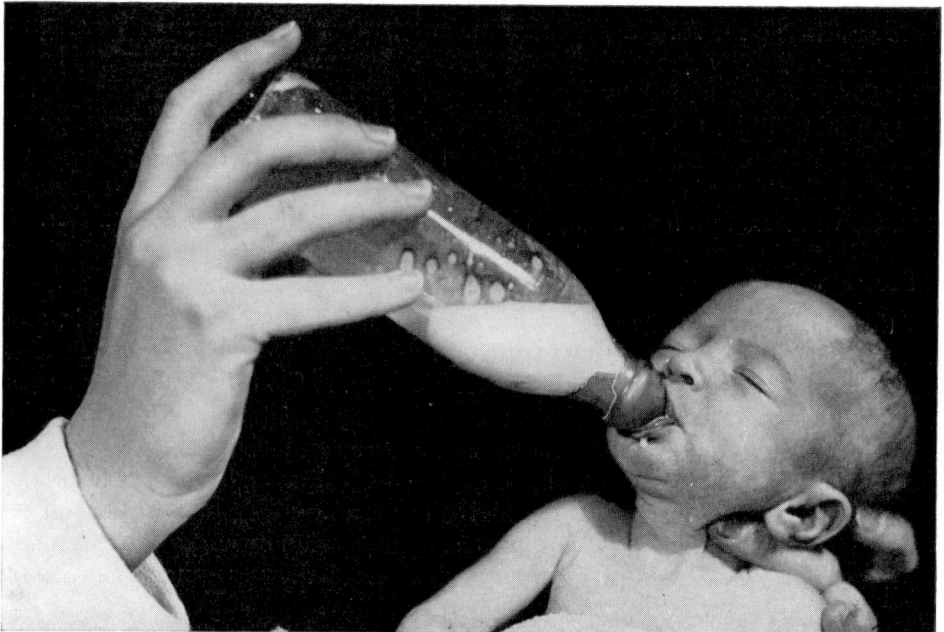

Fig. 45. Child being fed formula by mouth, thirteen days after primary esophageal anastomosis.

for a short time to gastrostomy feeding. It is for such situations that the gastrostomy tube should be left in place, even though it has been clamped off and temporarily not used. Generally, if all is going well, it is possible to discharge these babies from the hospital in about three weeks. Our shortest hospital stay was eight days. If by the end of five or six weeks it is apparent that all feedings can be taken quite well by mouth, the gastrostomy tube is withdrawn and the gastric opening is allowed to close spontaneously.

Complications

In occasional subjects, many sorts of complications appear. These are principally in the form of recurrent pneumonitis, severe coughing, difficulties in swallowing; they may require extended periods of hospitalization. While such troubles and complications tend to plague this field of surgery, it is now possible to avoid most of them and get 75 per cent or 80 per cent of the surviving babies out of the hospital in two or three weeks after operation.

Stenosis at Anastomotic Site

It is very difficult to predict which subjects are going to develop a stenosis at the anastomosis and require subsequent dilation during ensuing months or years. In general, if a good anastomosis has been made, with the establishment of a large lumen and without tension at the suture line, one can feel reasonably certain that important obstruction will not subsequently develop at the anastomotic site. Conversely, whenever an esophageal anastomosis is made under great tension or the union has been a poor one, the stage is set for subsequent reaction and scar-tissue formation which will often require close and extensive supervision and may even require dilation on one or more occasions. Esophageal dilation should not be performed merely because of x-ray appearance (narrowing at one point and dilatation above this). Dilations should be made only when there is clinical evidence of inadequacy of the swallowing mechanism. It is difficult to lay down any rules concerning the management of obstructive complications; they must be managed according to the specific indications in each particular case. In general, if narrowing and stricture at the anastomotic site are going to give difficulties, these will be manifest during the first five or six months of life. After that age, the general growth of the esophagus permits sufficient enlargement of the anastomotic ring so that dysphagia becomes less troublesome or disappears entirely. The subject of postoperative strictures is discussed more fully in Chapter 7.

RESULTS OF THERAPY

General Statistics

From the beginning of 1939 through 1952, 233 patients with esophageal atresia were seen on the surgical service of the Children's Hospital. Nine of these babies were not operated upon because they entered the hospital in extremis, had Mongolism, or possessed serious cardiovascular abnormalities. The remaining 224 subjects were operated upon by various procedures. A year-by-year summary of the material is shown in Table 7. As can be seen, multiple-stage construction of an antethoracic esophagus brought our first living patient in 1940; this method of therapy was in vogue up through 1945, but has been abandoned thereafter. While many attempts at primary anastomosis had been made before, our first success with this came in August, 1943. This child is in excellent general health nine years later and has an esophageal tube which carries solid food very satisfactorily. From 1943 through 1945 attention gradually turned from mul-

Table 7

Data from 233 Cases of Esophageal Atresia, 1939 through 1952

(This list includes all patients coming into the hospital, including those operated upon and 9 who were not)

Year	Total No. of Cases	Number Dead	Number Living	Living After Multiple Stage Construction of Antethoracic Esophagus	Living with Esophageal Anastomosis (or Esophago-Gastrostomy) in Mediastinum	Per Cent Survival
1939	4	4	0	0	0	0
1940	4	3	1	1	0	25
1941	8	8	0	0	0	0
1942	9	8	1	1	0	11
1943	17	11	6	3	3	35
1944	13	5	8	4	4	61
1945	17	12	5	3	2	29
1946	34	15	19	0	19	55
1947	23	6	17	0	17	73
1948	23	13	10	0	10	43
1949	18	10	8	0	8	44
1950	25	15	10	0	10	40
1951	17	7	10	0	10	58
1952	21	7	14	0	14	67
Totals:	233	124	109	12†	97*	

* Six of these started out as multiple stage construction of an antethoracic esophagus, but ended up with esophageal anastomosis (or esophago-gastrostomy) in the mediastinum. One of these cases was in 1943, three in 1944, and two in 1946.

† Two of these not completed yet.

tiple-stage attack to primary anastomosis of the esophagus. An attempt at primary esophageal repair has been made in all subjects since 1945. Today (1953) there are 12 subjects living with multiple-stage construction of an antethoracic esophagus (2 of these not yet entirely completed) and there are 97 patients living and in excellent condition with esophageal anastomosis (5 of these with stomach drawn up into the chest).

Condition of Patient Prior to Surgery in Relation to Survival

There seems to be little doubt that the over-all outlook for a patient with esophageal atresia is related somewhat to the rapidity with which the diagnosis has been made by the attending physician. The longer a child is subjected to pulmonary inflammation, the less are the chances of surviving a surgical correction of the esophageal abnormality. Within recent years the vast majority of babies in our series have been referred in the first day or two of life, which is a good indication of the alertness of the physicians who have attended them and made the diagnosis.

Effect of Prematurity

Without doubt, the outlook for survival in any series of babies with esophageal atresia will depend somewhat upon the frequency of occurrence of prematurity. Esophageal atresia seems to be associated with a very high incidence of prematurity, nearly 25 per cent in our series. Babies weighing less than 4 pounds have little possibility of surviving the surgical correction, whereas the larger subjects have an excellent chance of recovery. In our series, there were 52 babies who weighed less than 5 pounds at birth; 17 of these have survived. Our smallest surviving subject weighed 2 pounds, 15 ounces at the time of operation for primary anastomosis of the esophageal ends; the child is in excellent condition two years later. In short, prematurity decreases the chances of successful issue from corrective surgery, but does not necessarily imply that the baby will not survive such an undertaking.

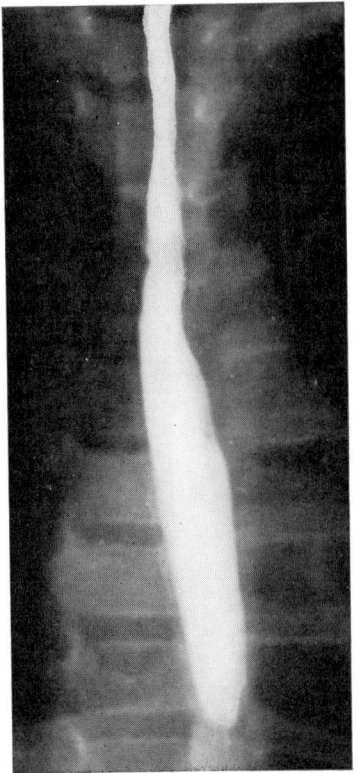

Fig. 46. Roentgenogram of esophagus, two years after primary anastomosis for treatment of esophageal atresia.

Effect of Associated Malformations

For babies with esophageal atresia and other coexisting abnormalities of the heart, intestine, anus, et cetera, the therapy of the esophageal abnormality and the other anomalies may require literally months of hospitalization and involve the treatment of numerous complications before the youngster can eventually be discharged. Obviously, secondary operations for duodenal atresia, malrotation of intestines, correction of an imperforate anus, and so on, all tend to raise fatality rates, but a considerable number of babies have survived such corrections in addition to the treatment of an esophageal atresia.

Average Care Required

The vast majority of children with esophageal atresia can be given a primary anastomosis of the esophageal ends, can be discharged from the hospital within two or three weeks, and are usually taking all feedings by mouth at this time. If a gastrostomy has been established, it is generally our policy to leave this open for an additional few weeks

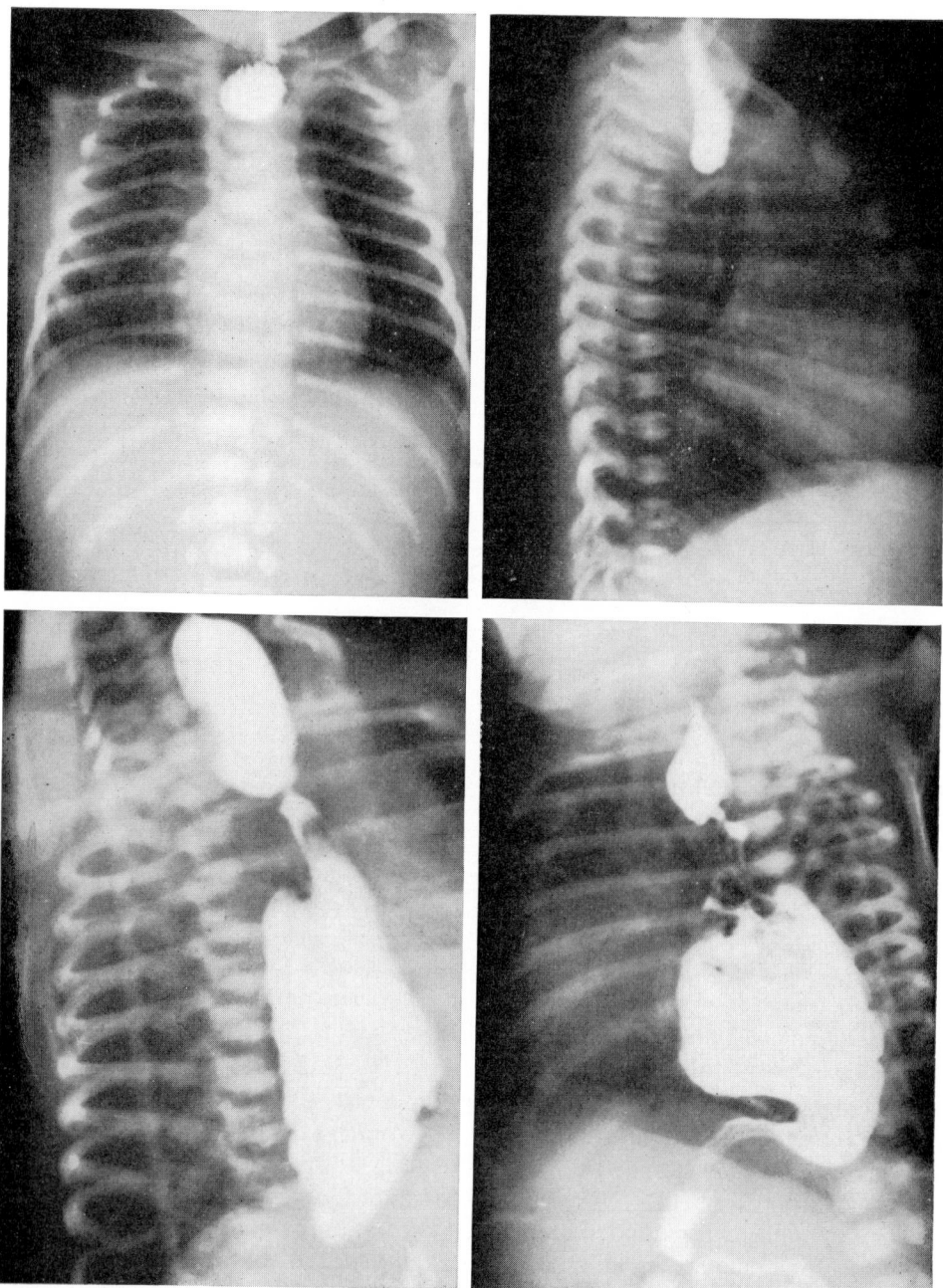

Fig. 47. Roentgenogram from a child with esophageal atresia, having a rudimentary lower esophageal end; treatment by drawing stomach into thorax to permit esophageal union (Fig. 43). *Above,* Films before operation, showing high upper pouch and the absence of gas in the abdomen. *Below,* Films several months after operation. The entire stomach is above the diaphragm.

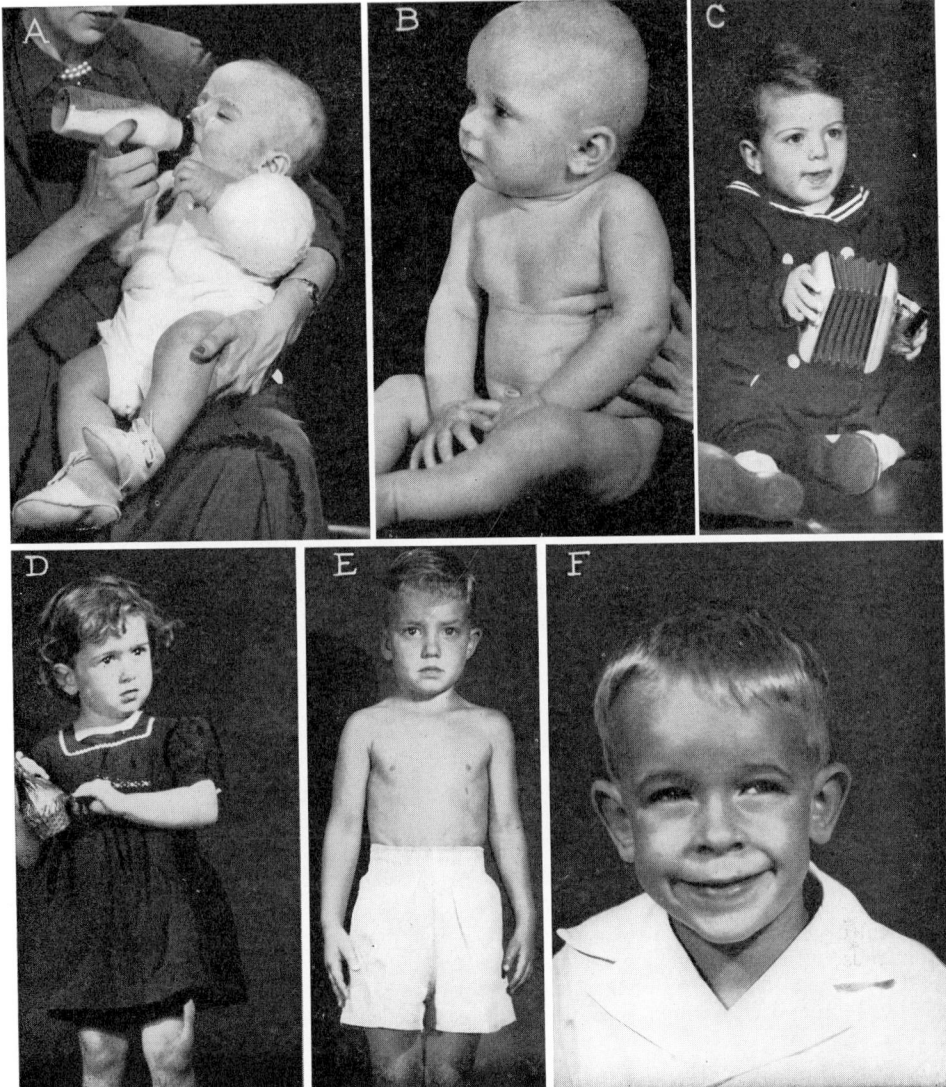

Fig. 48. Photographs of children who have been treated for esophageal atresia by one-stage esophageal anastomosis in the mediastinum. A, Baby five months after operation. B, Boy six months after operation, showing the excellent nutrition. C, Boy sixteen months of age. D, Girl three years old. E, Boy five years after operation. F, Child nine years after operation.

so that it might be available if any emergency might require its use. If all is going well and the child is continuing to take feedings satisfactorily by mouth, the gastrostomy tube can be withdrawn at six or seven weeks of age, and the opening allowed to close spontaneously. It is seldom necessary to close the opening surgically.

Necessity for Esophageal Dilations

In some patients it has been necessary to dilate the esophageal anastomosis at subsequent times. A full consideration of the problem of stricture following esophageal anastomosis is given in Chapter 7. Of the 97 patients who are living with an anastomosis of the esophagus, we have never performed dilation in 63 of them. For the other

34 subjects it has been necessary from time to time to dilate a stricture which appeared at the operative site. A half dozen of these have required only one or two dilations, the majority have needed three or four dilations over a period of two or three years, and the remainder have required a considerable number of dilations extending over a period of several years. In general, narrowing at the point of anastomosis has been most troublesome within the first year of life; it has generally been found that beyond this period the

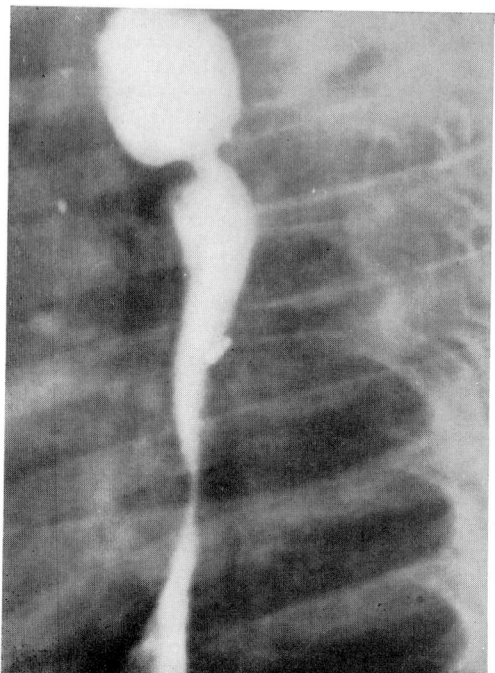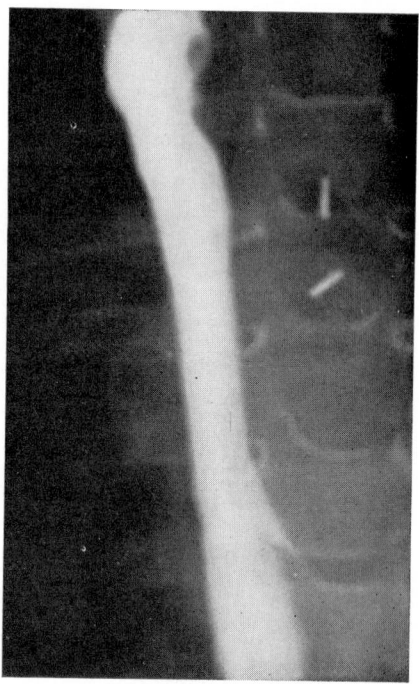

Fig. 49. Roentgenograms from a child who developed severe stenosis at anastomotic site, following treatment of an esophageal atresia by primary anastomosis. The stricture was unyielding, even after numerous dilations. Secondary operation was undertaken, at two years of age, to cut out the strictured zone and bring fresh esophageal ends together. *Left,* Preoperative film showing the narrowed zone. *Right,* Film two weeks after operation showing excellent pathway. When attempted in a few cases, these secondary operations have been very worthwhile and have been carried out without fatality.

esophagus and the anastomotic area grow rather well along with the development of the child so that the need for subsequent dilation becomes less and less as the child gets older. While x-ray visualization of the esophagus and the anastomotic site by the use of contrast media gives an excellent view and record of the esophageal lumen, we have relied decreasingly upon this examination for determination of the necessity for dilation. We have leaned more and more upon the history of the manner in which solid or fluid materials have been swallowed to judge the need for esophageal dilation.

Secondary Resection of Esophageal Stricture

Dilation of any stricture in the esophagus can usually accomplish all that is required in the way of therapy, but there is an occasional case in which a more radical attack is necessary. In 4 subjects we have had considerable contraction at the operative site, which failed to yield satisfactorily to repeated dilation, and have performed secondary operations at one or two years of age for secondary removal of the scar tissue

with very satisfactory results in all cases (see Chapter 7). At these times there was sufficient elasticity in the esophageal tube to permit mobilization, resection, and a clean
anastomosis.

Postoperative Cough

Some of these children have had a dry unproductive cough for many months following the intrathoracic operations, a complication which is probably due to the original
pulmonary infection and also to scarring along the posterior aspect of the trachea with
fixation of tissues in the posterior mediastinum. As the child becomes older, it is generally found that such coughing will eventually disappear without any specific therapy
tor it. However, it is important to point out that persistent respiratory symptoms might
have a basis in some recurring defect which requires a surgical correction. An increasing
stenosis at the operative site might cause impediment of swallowing or spillage of saliva
or other material into the larynx with constant irritation of the trachea. Furthermore,
one should always be mindful of the possibility of recurrence of a fistula between the
trachea and the esophagus. If there is any suspicion of this latter complication, careful
visualization with the use of contrast media should be made, and if any fistula is found,
immediate surgical closure of it should be undertaken. In two children we have had
such a fistula recur after primary esophageal anastomosis; secondary operation for
closure of the fistula has abolished the coughing in each case.

Summary

Without doubt, the surgical correction of esophageal atresia by surgical closure ot
the tracheo-esophageal fistula and by primary anastomosis of the esophageal ends (or
esophago-gastrostomy) represents one of the greatest advances of surgery in modern
times. These abnormalities can be recognized quickly and with great accuracy. The
surgical correction is attended with a high degree of success and these patients can be
transformed to subjects who are functionally normal and whose health is excellent
(Fig. 48).

Our most recent statistics are as follows: During the year 1952, 21 babies with esophageal atresia have been operated upon, all by direct anastomosis, all through a right
transpleural approach. Fourteen of these babies survived, an over-all recovery rate of
67 per cent. In the entire group of 21 babies there were 7 who were premature (under 5
pounds in weight) or who had other serious abnormalities. There were 14 babies who
weighed more than 5 pounds and had no other serious malformation; out of these 14
infants, 12 survived their primary anastomosis of the esophagus—a recovery rate of
85 per cent.

REFERENCES

1. Ferguson, C. F.: Congenital Tracheoesophageal Fistula Not Associated with Atresia
   of the Esophagus. Laryngoscope, 61:718,
   1951.
2. Garrison, R. F. and Mayer, J. H.: Congenital
   Tracheo-Esophageal Fistula—Nasogastric
   Polyethylene Tube in Lieu of Gastrostomy.
   American Surgeon, 18:131, 1952.
3. Gross, R. E. and Scott, H. W., Jr.: Correction of Esophageal Atresia and Tracheo-
   esophageal Fistula by Closure of Fistula
   and Oblique Anastomosis of Esophageal

Segments. Surg., Gynec. & Obst., 82:518,
1946.
4. Haight, C. and Towsley, H. A.: Congenital
   Atresia of the Esophagus with Tracheo-
   esophageal Fistula. Surg., Gynec. & Obst.,
   76:672, 1943.
5. Haight, C.: Congenital Atresia of the Esophagus with Tracheoesophageal Fistula. Reconstruction of Esophageal Continuity by
   Primary Anastomosis. Ann. Surg., 120:623,
   1944.
6. Haight, C.: Congenital Tracheoesophageal

Fistula without Esophageal Atresia. J. Thoracic Surg., *17*:600, 1948.

7. Holt, J. F., Haight, C. and Hodges, F. J.: Congenital Atresia of the Esophagus and Tracheo-Esophageal Fistula. Radiology, *47*:457, 1946.

8. Ladd, W. E.: The Surgical Treatment of Esophageal Atresia and Tracheoesophageal Fistula. New England J. Med., *230*:625, 1944.

9. Ladd, W. E. and Swenson, O.: Esophageal Atresia and Tracheo-Esophageal Fistula. Ann. Surg., *125*:23, 1947.

10. Lanman, T. H.: Congenital Atresia of the Esophagus. A Study of Thirty-Two Cases. Arch. Surg., *41*:1060, 1940.

11. Leven, N. L.: Congenital Atresia of the Esophagus with Tracheoesophageal Fistula. J. Thoracic Surg., *10*:648, 1941.

12. Leven, N. L., Varco, R. L., Lannin, B. G. and Torgen, L. A.: Surgical Management of Congenital Atresia of the Esophagus and Tracheo-Esophageal Fistula. Ann. Surg. In press.

13. Longmire, W. P., Jr.: Antethoracic Jejunal Transplantation for Congenital Esophageal Atresia with Hypoplasia of the Lower Esophageal Segment. Surg., Gynec. & Obst., *93*:310, 1951.

14. Swenson, O.: End-to-end Anastomosis of the Esophagus for Esophageal Atresia. Surgery, *22*:324, 1947.

CHAPTER 7

Esophageal Stenosis or Stricture

Whereas esophageal atresia (Chapter 6) is an abnormality with complete obstruction and demanding surgical therapy within the first few days of life, stenoses or strictures are conditions with only partial blockage of the esophageal pathway and hence present problems which are met later in infancy or in childhood.

Strictures may be long, short, or multiple; they can appear in any part of the esophagus, and they can produce obstruction varying from mild to very marked. There may be different etiologic types, including: (1) Congenital; (2) postoperative; (3) following peptic esophagitis; (4) due to chemical burns. Because of great differences in treatment of these four forms of obstruction, it is best to consider them separately. Our material includes 95 patients, with representatives of the various groups.

CONGENITAL ESOPHAGEAL STENOSIS

Clinical Picture

Children with congenital esophageal stenosis generally have symptoms which begin very early in life (Fig. 50). Most of the malformations are discovered within the first year or two; even those which are not detected until later in childhood have given symptoms dating back to infancy. Males and females are affected with the same frequency.

Symptoms. The dominant symptoms are regurgitation of part of each feeding and a failure to gain weight properly. While spitting-up may be severe in the first weeks or months of life, more often the complaints appear initially when the baby is started on semi-solid or solid food. As would be expected, the more marked the stenosis, the sooner the onset of symptoms. It is rare to have any forceful vomiting; the material merely rolls out of the mouth in an indolent manner. What is brought up can be recognized as frothy saliva or undigested milk and food; it does not smell sour. In some of the older children, the esophagus above the level of obstruction attains such enormous size that it becomes a great sac filled with food; it presses against the trachea and bronchi, and produces wheezing. It is not uncommon to have choking spells during or after feeding; these might be accompanied by temporary cyanosis. There may be repeated bouts of bronchitis, or even bronchopneumonia, which undoubtedly are sequelae of tracheal aspiration.

Physical Findings. Physical examination usually shows but little, except possibly for malnutrition in some cases. Often the nutritional status is excellent if the parent has avoided solid food and has supplied plenty of milk or other nourishing fluids. Laboratory studies often reveal a moderate anemia.

Other Abnormalities. Of our 38 patients with congenital esophageal stricture, three were known to have some other abnormality of the alimentary tract; in one there was an imperforate anus and duodenal atresia, in another duodenal stenosis, and in a third there was a very small tracheo-esophageal fistula just above the area of esophageal narrowing.

Roentgenographic visualization of the esophagus during a swallow of barium fluid or mixture shows the lesion very well. The narrowed area can be identified easily; it persists during fluoroscopic observation or through a series of film exposures. The obstruction is almost always short; it appears as a diaphragm or veil, with an opening located either centrally or eccentrically. Oftentimes it is impossible to differentiate between a firm, unyielding fibrous plate and a mass of heaped-up, extra muscle which is bulging into the esophageal lumen; generally, the pathology would show a combination of the two elements. The esophageal segments above and below this area are usually in straight alignment (Figs. 58, 60, 61) but in some instances there can be an offset in

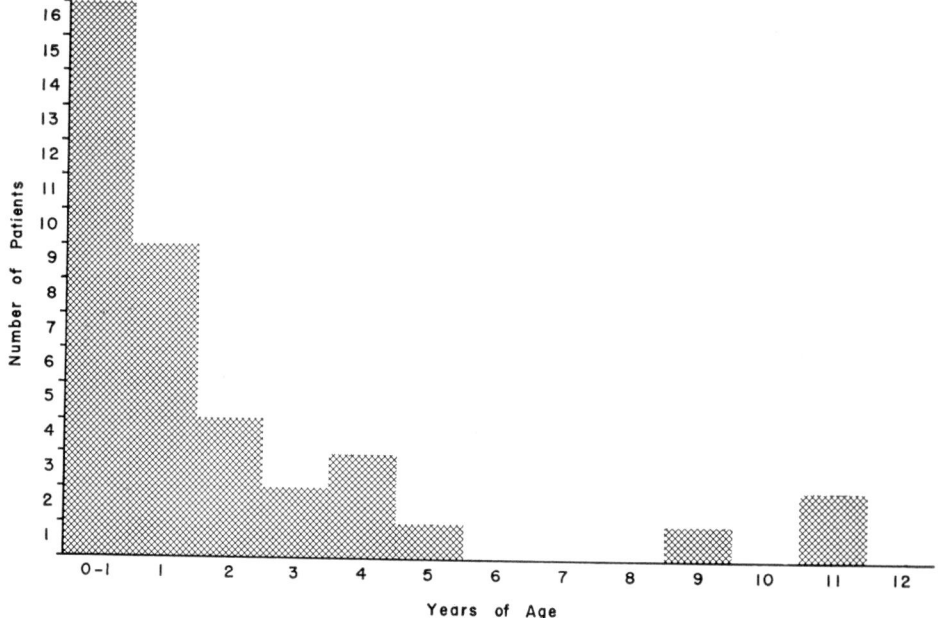

Fig. 50. Chart showing ages of patients at time diagnosis of congenital esophageal stricture was made. Most of these children had had symptoms dating back to early infancy.

relation of one to the other (Fig. 59). Above an obstruction the esophagus is dilated; below it is normal or collapsed. Occasionally (4 of our patients) a foreign body was seen lodged at the narrowed point, the ingestion and stoppage of this object in the esophagus being the factor which first called attention to the underlying abnormality.

Congenital obstructions are found anywhere in the esophagus, but about half of them appear in the middle third. In the quarter which we have seen in the lower third of the esophagus, it was not always entirely clear whether the narrowing was one which had existed since birth or whether it represented scarring and cicatricial contraction after peptic ulceration and esophagitis (from regurgitation of gastric juice into the lower esophagus or from aberrant gastric mucosa in the esophagus itself). When there is obstruction at the cardia, it is sometimes difficult to differentiate between achalasia (incoordination, with a strong and overactive muscle) and fibrosis at this level; generally there is some element of both mechanisms.

Esophagoscopy, which should always be done under general anesthesia in babies and children, is helpful in confirming the diagnosis, in determining the yielding or unyielding character of tissue at the site of obstruction, and in appraising the state of preservation of the mucous membrane at and above the stenosis.

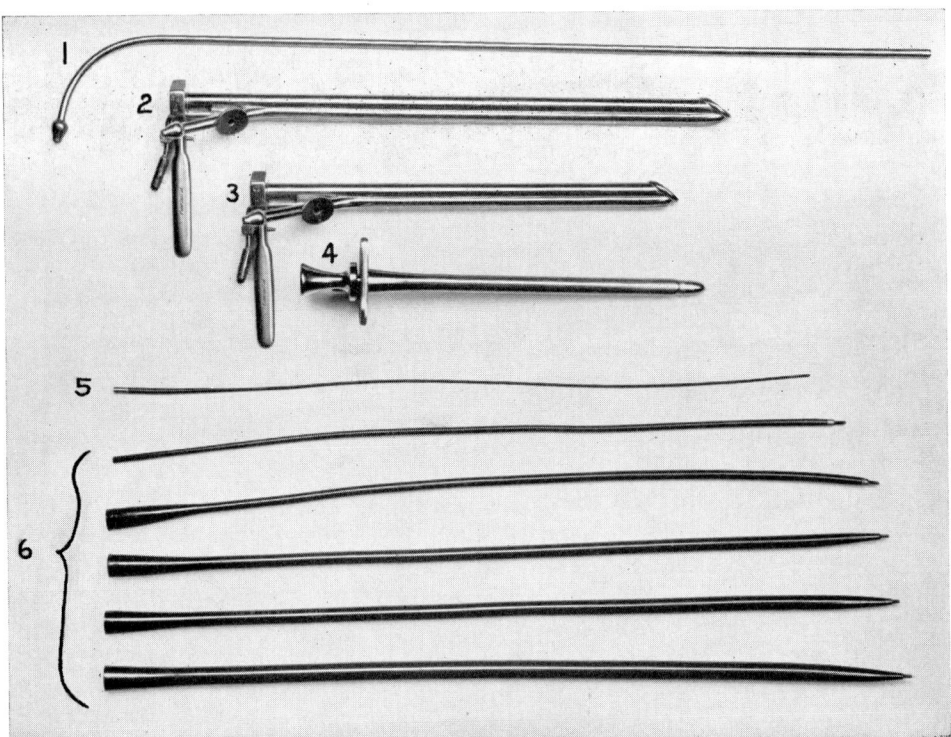

Fig. 51. Instruments for dilation of esophageal stricture in babies and small children, particularly useful for treatment of congenital or postoperative strictures. 1. Sucker tube. 2. Esophagoscope, 7 x 25 mm. 3. Esophagoscope, 7 x 19 mm. 4. Urethral endoscope, very helpful in tiny babies. 5. Filiform leader, with screw-socket at its larger end. 6. A few of the elastic dilators which can be screwed onto the filiform leader; these are available up through No. 40.

Treatment

Dilation. In the vast majority of cases, congenital esophageal stenosis can be treated satisfactorily and safely by dilation. We perform all of these under general anesthesia. For babies under a year or two, a filiform leader (Fig. 51) can generally be directed through the stenotic opening, while visualizing it through an esophagoscope. With the filiform properly in place, the scope can be withdrawn over it, and then a small gum-webbing dilator screwed onto the filiform leader. The well oiled dilator is then passed

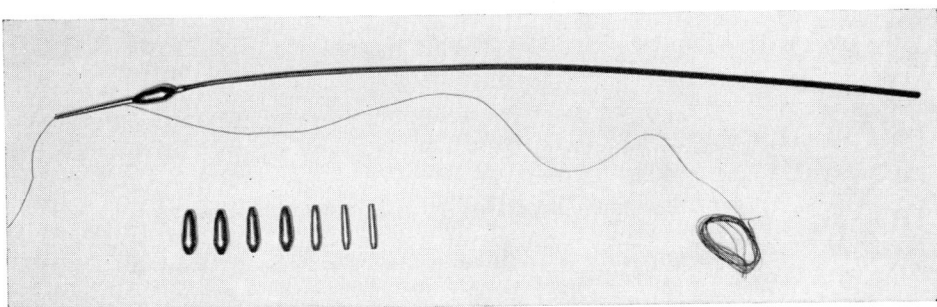

Fig. 52. Mixter type of dilator which can be pushed down the esophagus, employing a string guide. The leading part of the instrument can be fitted with metal dilators of different sizes, some of which are shown below.

down the esophagus. After withdrawing the dilator, it is unscrewed from the leader, so that larger ones of appropriate size can be attached and directed downward to stretch the esophagus progressively. For children beyond a few years of age, the most difficult portion of a dilation can be done in this manner, after which gum-webbed elastic dilators (without leaders, Fig. 53) can be passed.

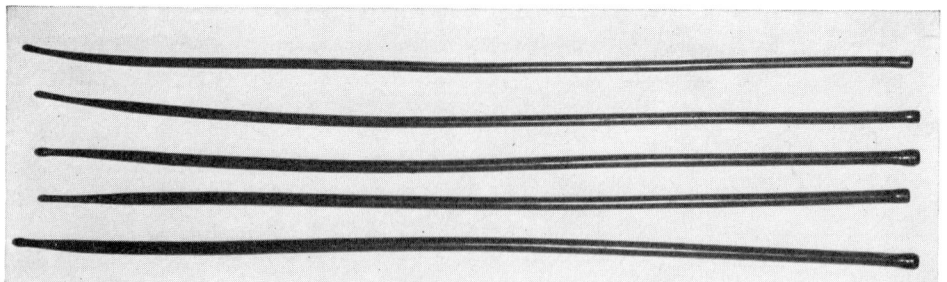

Fig. 53. Gum-webbing dilators, 30 inches long, which can be used for dilating the esophagus of a larger child, especially useful when the orifice is not very narrow. Various sizes are available.

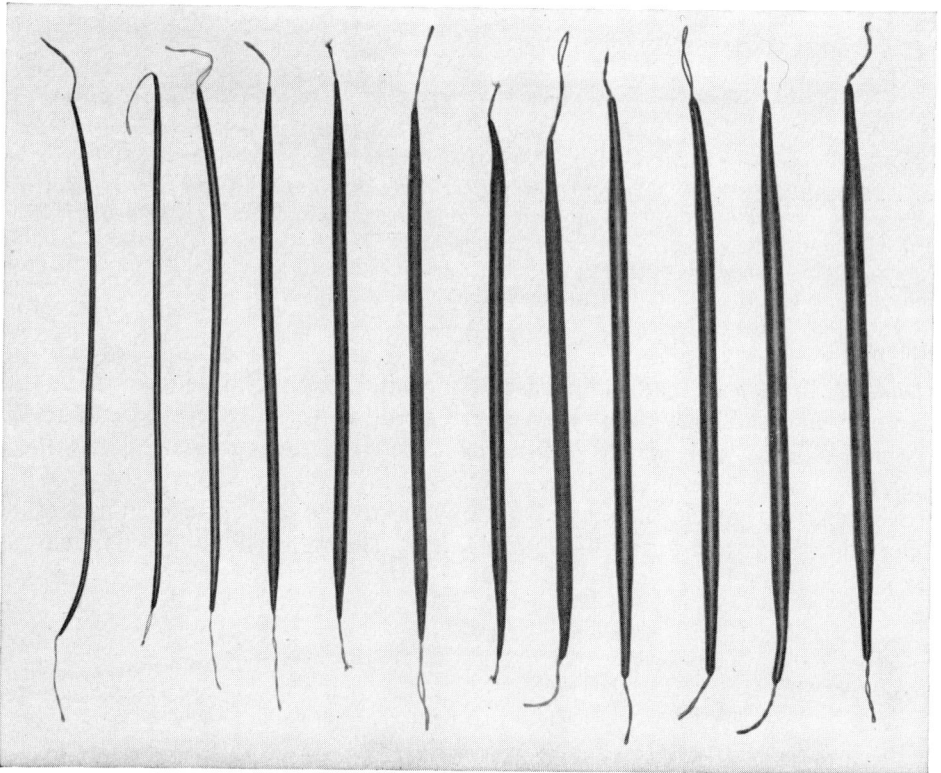

Fig. 54. Tucker soft rubber dilators, for retrograde dilation of the esophagus.

Gastrostomy. When nutrition is poor and ample nourishment cannot be supplied through the strictured esophagus, the establishment of a gastrostomy gives immediately an avenue for feeding and it also provides a means for dilation by retrograde methods. For such a gastrostomy, we always employ the Stamm method (Chapter 10). Just before a dilation is to be done, the child is made to swallow a thread or string; when under anesthesia this can be fished out of the gastrostomy with a blunt hook. One then attaches to the lower end of the string a series of solid (but soft) rubber Tucker dilators (Fig. 54) arranged in tandem in increasing sizes. By pulling on the string in the pharynx, the dilators are drawn upward through the esophagus, carrying the dilation to a point which seems to be effective in stretching it but yet not enough to do damage thereto. While it is

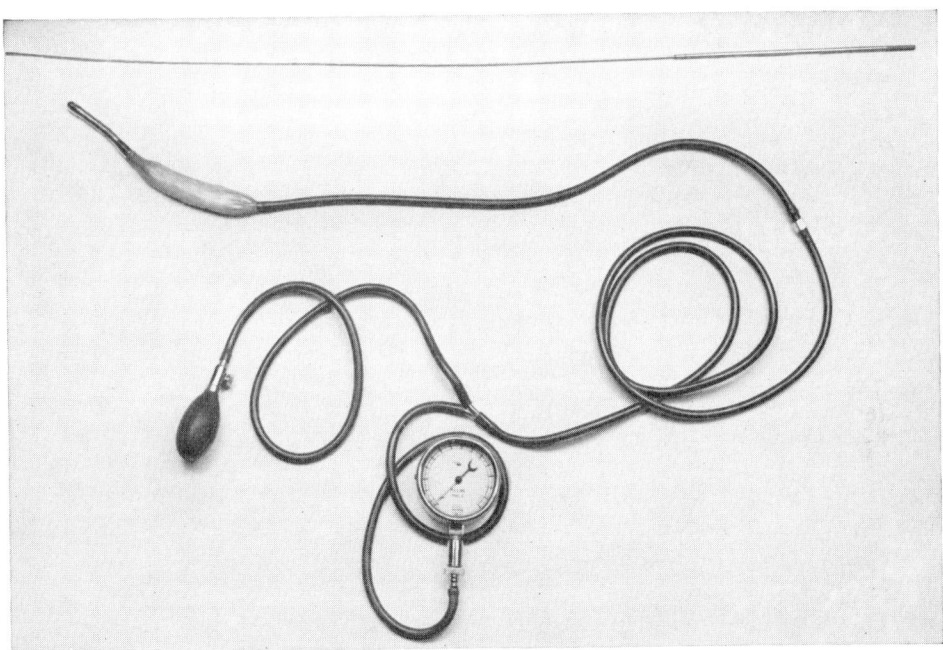

Fig. 55. Mosher pneumatic esophageal dilator which is very effective in stretching the esophago-gastric junction in cases of achalasia of the cardia. The wall of the balloon is made with a barium-impregnated fabric so that it can be identified while being maneuvered under fluoroscope control (see Fig. 56).

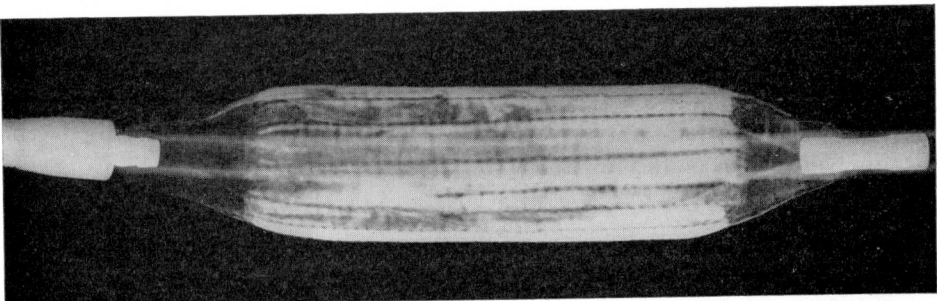

Fig. 56. Roentgenogram of the inflatable balloon of a Mosher dilator. The opaqueness of the bag is a desirable feature which helps to position the instrument under fluoroscopic guidance.

possible to perform these retrograde dilations without anesthesia, we generally prefer to do them under general narcosis.

Treatment of Spasm or Stricture at the Cardia. For those rare patients with obstruction at the cardia itself, we have had very satisfactory results by introduction of a Mosher dilator (Figs. 55 and 56) (under general anesthesia and under fluoroscopic control), pushing this down the esophagus to a point where the dilating mechanism lies at the

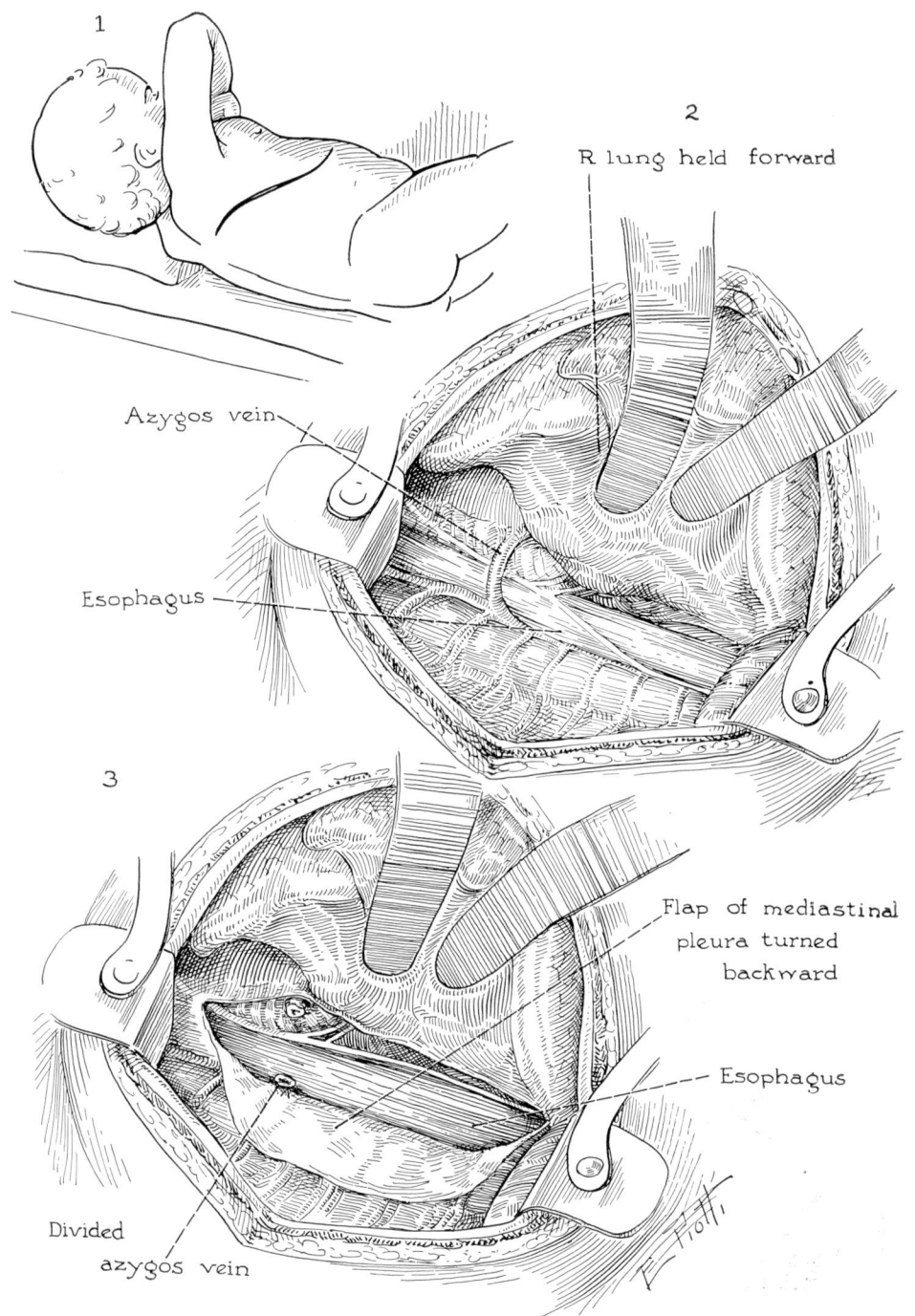

Fig. 57. Method of resection for removal of a short stricture of the esophagus, with repair by end-to-end anastomosis. 1. Position of thoracic wound. 2. Exposure through sixth interspace, and transpleural approach to the mediastinum. 3. Exposure of the esophagus. Flap of mediastinal pleura carefully reflected and saved. It is generally impossible to determine the exact level of the stricture by external inspection of the esophagus.

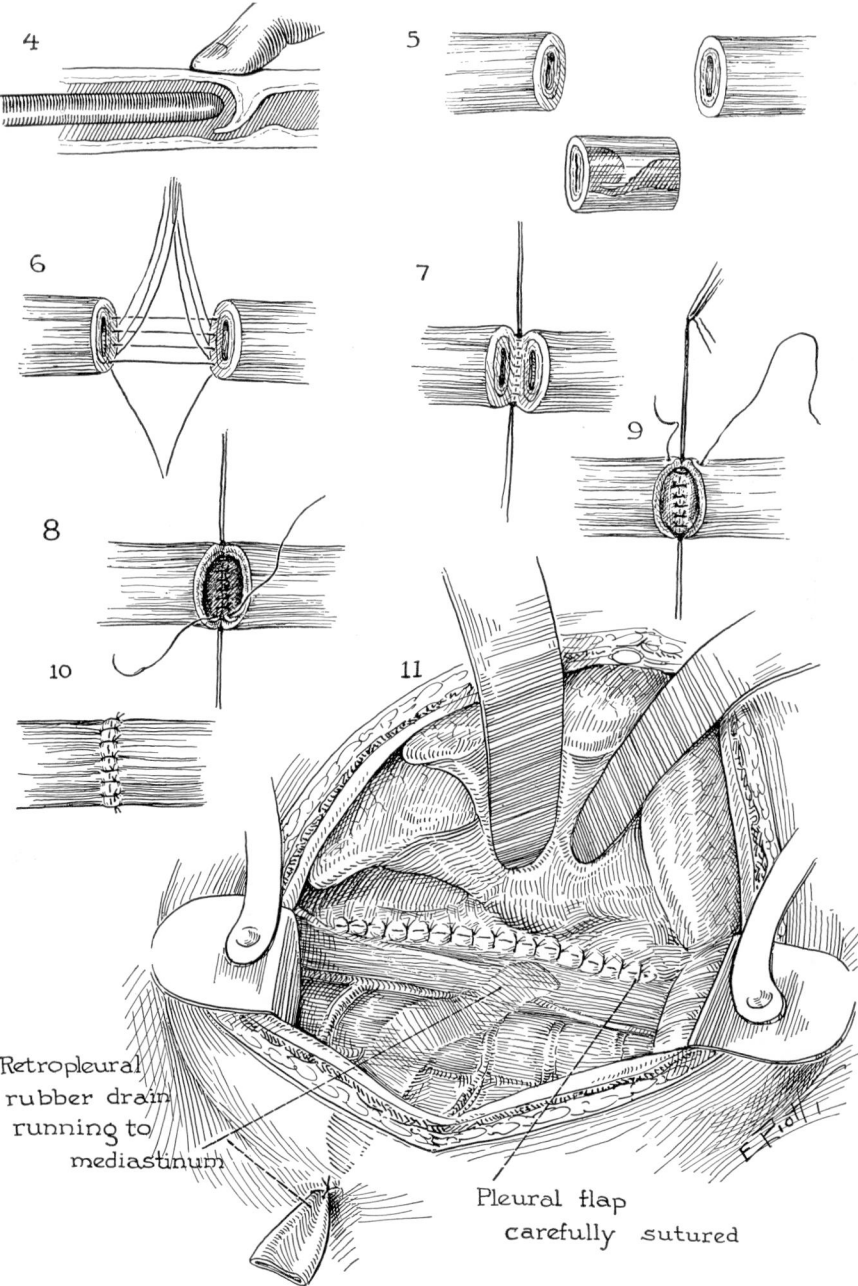

Fig. 57 (*continued*). 4. Portion of esophagus mobilized from its bed, carefully saving the vagus nerves. Bougie or stiff catheter passed down the esophagus, so that finger palpation can find exact level of the obstruction. 5. Stenosed segment excised. 6. Placement of posterior row of interrupted silk sutures through muscularis and submucosa (about a dozen sutures should be used in this posterior row). Placing all the sutures *first* allows them to be drawn up together, thus distributing the pull as the esophageal ends are later approximated. 7. Posterior stitches drawn up and tied. 8. Mucosa being closed with interrupted fine silk sutures, the knots presenting in the lumen of the esophagus. 9. Mucosa entirely closed. External row of sutures being completed in the muscularis-submucosal tissues. 10. Anastomosis completed. 11. Extrapleural drain led from back into mediastinum. Pleural covering of mediastinum closed tightly. (In most cases we have preferred to omit the retropleural drain, and instead leave a small opening at the end of the pleural closure to allow escape of any mediastinal fluid into the pleural cavity which is always drained by an intercostal catheter.)

cardia, and then inflating the expansile bag to 10 or 12 pounds pressure, maintaining this for five to ten minutes. Generally, two or three such treatments are all that are required to give relief.

Esophageal Resection. In an occasional case, it is preferable to attack surgically the stenotic area of an esophagus and either to remove it entirely (followed by an end-to-end union of the remaining esophageal ends) (Fig. 57), or to open the esophagus longitudinally at the stenotic area and then close it transversely. When the latter is done, it is sometimes possible, while the esophagus is open, to cut away part of the presenting internal diaphragm.

Results of Therapy

We have treated 38 patients with congenital stenosis of the esophagus, including 3 in whom the lesion was at the cardia.

Of those with lesions above the cardia, the following regimens of dilation have been carried out (5 of this group subsequently came to surgical resection or revision of the stenotic area):

2 patients had no dilation.
8 patients have been dilated once.
4 patients have been dilated twice.
10 patients have been dilated less than 6 times.
11 patients had 7, 8, 9, 10, 11, 16, 20, 34, 55, 58, and 91 dilations respectively.

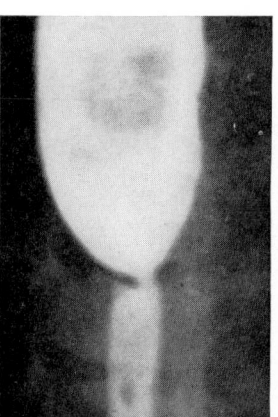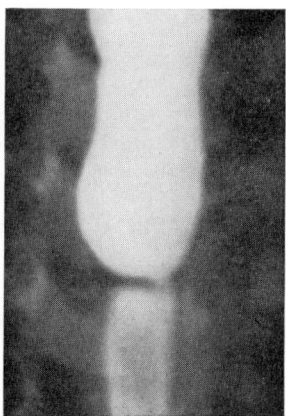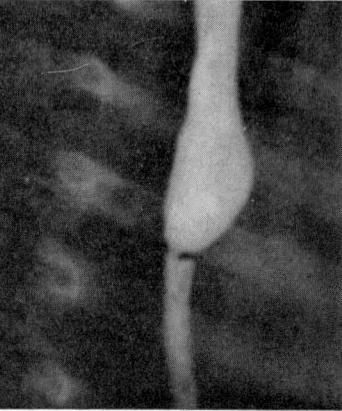

Fig. 58. Congenital stricture of the esophagus in a fifteen-month old boy who had severe difficulties in swallowing since two months of age, being able to take only fluid diet. Three views showing the lesion. Effectively treated by four esophageal dilations. Complete relief of symptoms thereafter, and ability to take solid food without hesitation.

No fixed course of therapy could be prescribed or predicted. The management of cases has had to be on an individual basis, some strictures yielding easily to dilation and others being most obstinate. In about two-thirds of the cases, six dilations or less, over a span of months or several years, have been followed by complete and apparently permanent relief of symptoms. About a third of cases have presented most vexing problems and have required an excessive number of dilations over a period of many years. Some of these children will obviously need further therapy, but in general there seems to come a time beyond which treatment is no longer necessary or is only occasionally required. An outstanding example of this is a boy who, during the first eight years of

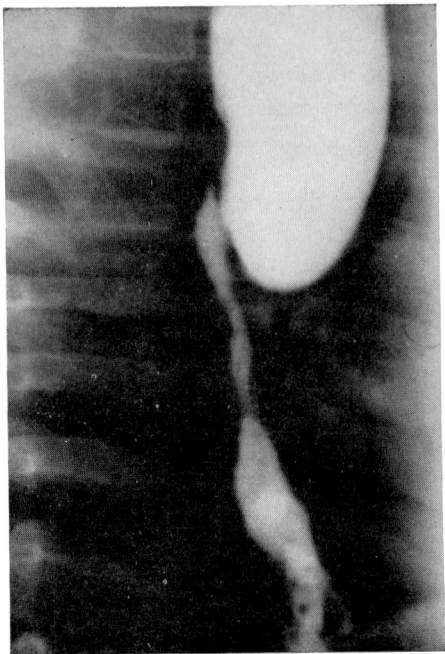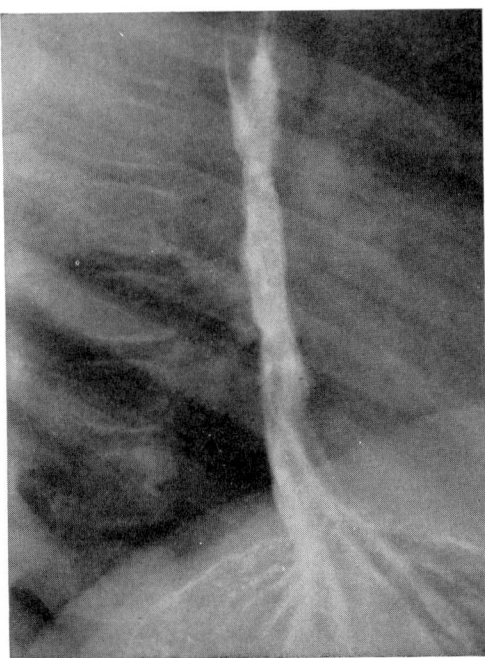

Fig. 59. Congenital stricture of the esophagus in an eleven-month old boy who had had intermittent vomiting since birth. *Left,* Roentgenogram showing the constriction and the off-set alignment of the esophageal lumina. *Right,* Two years following resection of the stenotic area and reconstruction of the esophagus by end-to-end anastomosis (Fig. 57).

life, was given 91 dilations (the expense and the tribulations of hospitalization attendant to these were enormous!); since then he has had excellent health and satisfactory swallowing during the fourteen years he has been followed.

All of the children with congenital esophageal stricture have survived to date (excepting one who died of acute leukemia). A program of esophageal dilations has generally sufficed to give eventually a satisfactory result in adolescent and adult life, but certainly in some instances there has been a long and desperate battle.

Six patients in the group had gastrostomies followed by retrograde dilations (these

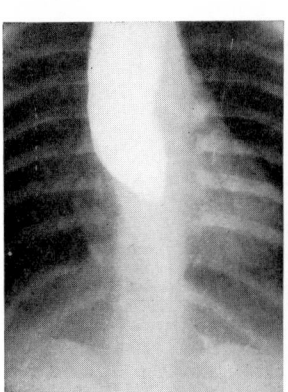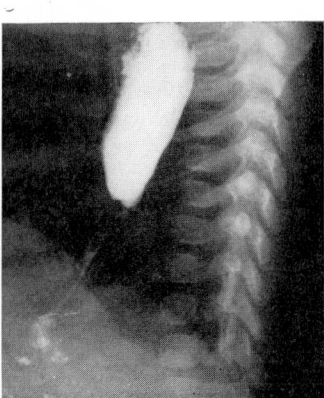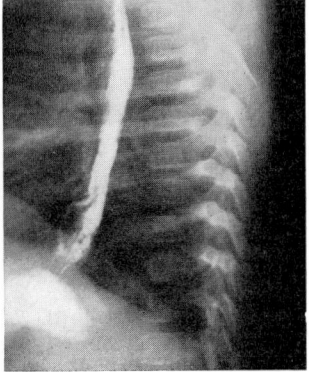

Fig. 60. Congenital esophageal stricture in a three-month old baby treated by resection and end-to-end anastomosis of the esophagus. *Left* and *middle,* Roentgenograms before surgery, showing the obstruction. *Right,* Appearance of esophageal pathway following surgical reconstruction.

all being included in the above enumeration of dilation procedures); some needed only 3 or 4 such dilations, while one required 91.

During dilations, one esophagus was perforated. This was recognized within a few hours by air in the left pleural cavity. It was treated by immediate tube drainage of the pleural cavity, administration of antibiotics, and restriction of intake of fluids by mouth. The child survived.

In recent years, we have elected to treat by resection 5 of the patients with congenital esophageal stenosis. At the time of operation they were 3 months, 10 months, 16 months, 10 years, and 11 years of age respectively. In the first 4, the lesion was excised and the esophagus was reconstructed by end-to-end anastomosis of the remaining segments (Fig. 57). In the last patient, the lesion was quite close to the diaphragm; it was ap-

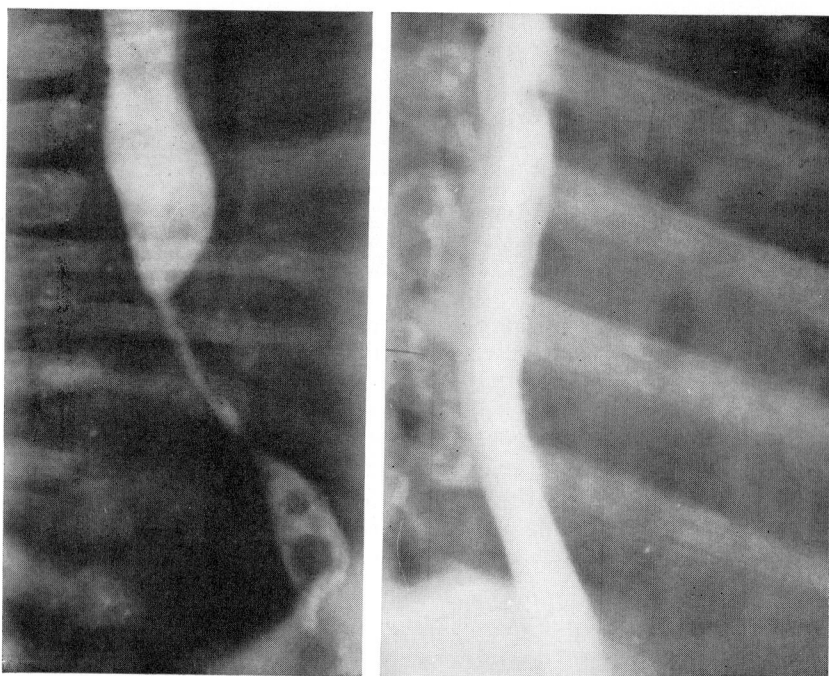

Fig. 61. Congenital esophageal stricture over a rather long segment. Regurgitation of feedings since fifth day of life. *Left*, Appearance of esophagus at five weeks of age. Treated by gastrostomy, retrograde dilations and then segmental resection of esophagus at ten months of age. *Right*, Appearance three and a half years after esophageal resection.

proached through the left pleural cavity. It was feared that mobilization of the esophagus (for resection and anastomosis) might interrupt the vagus nerves and give troublesome complications; therefore the esophagus was not raised out of its bed, but was opened longitudinally, some of the diaphragm was cut out, and then the esophagus was closed transversely. The boy ate meat within two weeks! All of these surgically treated patients have survived, have done well, and have had very gratifying results; 2 of them had to have a few dilations shortly after surgery, but have been well thereafter. The results have been so gratifying that we believe that any congenital esophageal stenosis which does not seem to be yielding after a half dozen attempts at dilation should be strongly considered for surgical resection or revision of the strictured area.

Of the 3 children who had obstruction at the cardia, it has been impossible to say whether the narrowing was due to "spasm" of an overactive sphincter or due to a fibrotic ring; probably there was some element of both mechanisms. In each case we have had extremely satisfactory results with the use of a Mosher dilator. With only a few treatments, relief of obstruction has been attained very quickly and apparently permanently. In no instance has it been necessary to resort to the Heller operation or one of the anastomotic procedures of esophago-gastrostomy for treatment of obstruction at the cardia in childhood.

POSTOPERATIVE ESOPHAGEAL STRICTURE

Clinical Picture

In this group, we are concerned with the development of stricture at the site of a previous esophageal anastomosis, a consideration which has to do entirely with the late results following surgery for esophageal atresia.

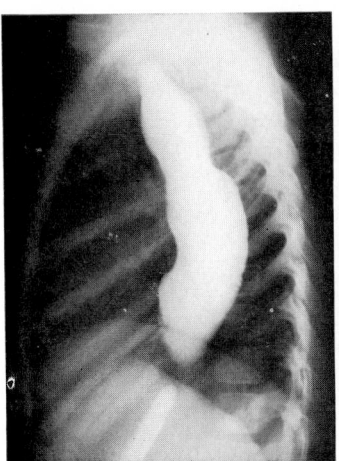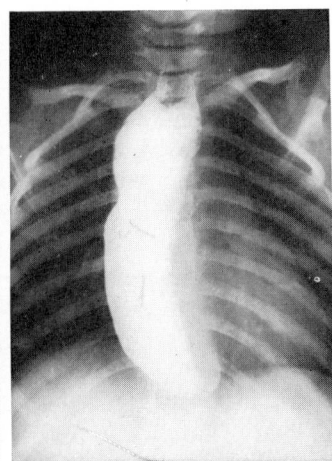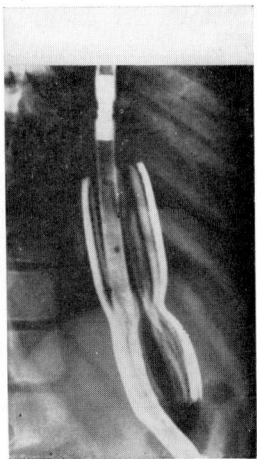

Fig. 62. Achalasia of the cardia, with marked obstruction at lower end of esophagus and great distention above this (which gave wheezing and respiratory distress). Film on right, shows Mosher dilator in place. Patient completely relieved of all symptoms after a few dilations with this instrument.

During the past decade we have turned to the routine use of primary anastomosis for all newborn infants who have atresia of the esophagus (whether or not it is combined with a tracheo-esophageal fistula, and regardless of the positions of the esophageal stumps). In the vast majority of cases, sufficient esophageal tissue is available to permit union of the esophageal ends in the posterior mediastinum. Only in a few cases has the lower end been quite short, treatment requiring drawing a portion of the stomach into the right side of the chest so that the esophageal ends could be united. The routine treatment of all cases of esophageal atresia by primary anastomosis has, on the whole, been quite successful (Chapter 6). Of 97 patients who are living with an anastomosis of the esophagus, we have never performed dilation in 63 of them. For the other 34 it has been necessary from time to time to dilate a stricture which appeared at the operative site. A half dozen of these have had only one or two stretches, the majority have needed 3 or 4 dilations during the first two or three years of life, and the remainder have required a considerable number of dilations extending over a period of several years. It is the group of 34 patients that we would like to consider in detail in this chapter.

These 34 patients could be divided into three, rather easily defined groups, depending upon the time of onset of dysphagia:

Dysphagia appearing *early* (within a few weeks after the esophageal anastomosis)   9 cases
Dysphagia *delayed* in appearance from 1 to 5 months   15 cases
Dysphagia *late* in appearance, coming on after 10 or 11 months   10 cases

There are very good reasons for separating cases into these categories, because the problems of therapy and the prognosis are quite different in each. Almost always, those babies who exhibit symptoms of obstruction *early* (within a few weeks) after establishment of an esophageal anastomosis (for esophageal atresia) are those with the most perplexing problems. In these babies, it is usually known that the anastomotic unions have been technically poor, or else there had been some postoperative leakage, which has since closed off spontaneously but which has left a great deal of regional scarring. Such strictures are the most troublesome to treat because the esophageal substance is unyielding, and indeed the esophageal tube is generally encased in a fibrous mass which limits its distensibility. In these very young babies, the inability to swallow correctly and the marked debility which accompanies a series of harassing complications often leads to a spillover of milk or saliva into the trachea; such aspiration is a great hazard and the superimposed recurrent or chronic pneumonia can enormously increase the problems of caring for the youngster. This whole picture generally suggests that a long siege of therapy will be required. Conversely, those dysphagias which are *delayed* or *late* in onset usually come from an esophageal tube which is quite elastic and yielding, but which is accompanied by a short zone of fibrous ring or an excessive "turn-in" at the anastomotic site which begins to give symptoms only when solid food is offered; such constrictions yield readily to a few dilations.

Methods of Therapy

The decision to start instrumental therapy should not be based on a roentgenographic picture alone. Some children show by x-ray an area of esophageal narrowing, even with some dilatation above it, and yet get along reasonably well. We believe it is best to use roentgenographic study as only one part of the evaluation. Specific therapy should not be undertaken unless there are sufficient clinical symptoms to warrant such a step.

Early Symptom Group. It is well to bear in mind that a portion of the symptoms may be due to residual or recrudescent inflammation in the operative area of the esophagus. Much of this swelling and edema can subside if the esophagus is put at rest for a short time. Certainly, all semi-solid food should be stopped at once, and only milk (or formula) offered; adequate nourishment can be given with this alone. It is best to withhold completely orange juice, which has an irritative effect. If milk or formula is not tolerated, all feedings by mouth should be discontinued for several days. Such a period of rest often permits an esophagus to regain reasonably good function. During these few days, the child will have to be fed by parenteral routes, or if a gastrostomy is still open (we usually leave it open until four to six weeks of age) it is easy to supply full feedings by this route.

There should be considerable hesitation about attempting esophageal dilation too soon after an esophageal anastomosis has been established, for fear of disrupting the suture line and making matters worse. Generally, a very young baby can be tided over on supportive measures, and it is not necessary to stretch the esophagus in the first month or six weeks of life. When the time comes for dilation, two methods have been used. *First*, if a gastrostomy is still open, the safest approach is to use small retrograde Tucker dilators. Under anesthesia, a filiform leader can be passed down the esophagus into the stomach, fishing out the lower tip of this through the gastrostomy opening. A string is now tied to the tip; the filiform leader and its attached string are drawn up out of the mouth. By means of the string, retrograde dilators are pulled up through the esophagus. *Second,* if no gastrostomy is available, esophageal dilation can be done

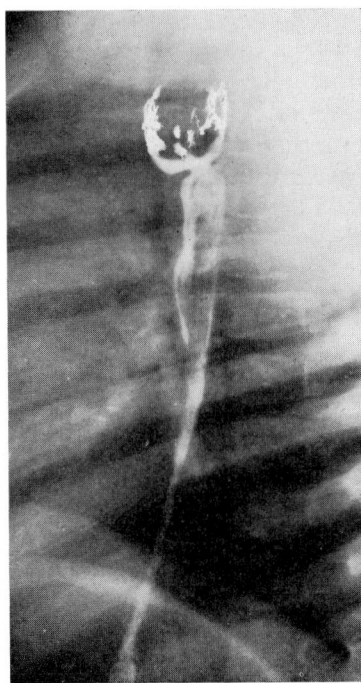 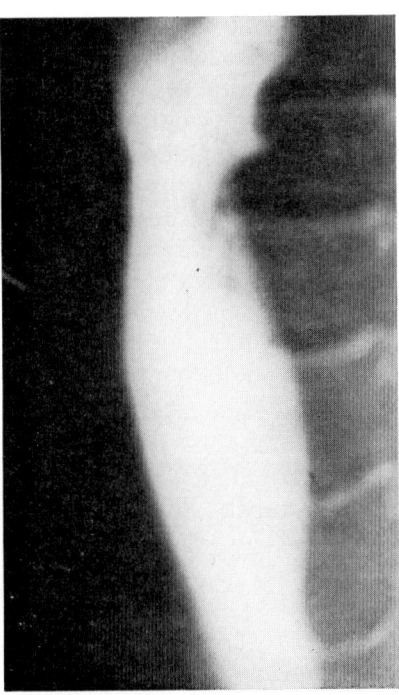

Fig. 63. Esophageal stricture following anastomosis of the esophagus for esophageal atresia. The child required three dilations in the first four months of life. *Left,* Appearance at ten months of age, considerable constriction and obstruction remaining. No subsequent therapy. *Right,* Appearance at three years of age. Excellent esophageal pathway; the child could swallow food very well. This case demonstrates what frequently happens; the esophagus begins to open up after the first year of life.

(under anesthesia) by passing a small scope to the point of stricture, directing a filiform leader down through the narrowed zone, withdrawing the scope while leaving the leader in place. Appropriate gum-webbing dilators can then be screwed on to the filiform leader and passed down the esophagus.

Just how often, and over how long a period of time, the esophagus will have to be dilated varies from case to case. In general, one should be very guarded in making any statements about the extent of therapy which will be required. Some of these babies can (if the child is carried along for six to nine months) eventually improve greatly, the esophagus then attaining accelerated growth along with the development of the child (Fig. 63). In contrast, other youngsters have such high degree of regional scarring that a large number of dilations are required, or secondary operative attack on the lesion is necessary at a later time. In our 9 cases with dysphagia appearing at an *early* date, the number of dilations given was 30, 14, 11, 9, 9, 8, 7, 6, and 5 respectively (an average of 11). These extended over periods varying from one month to five years; in half of the cases they were completed in seven months. Of the 9 patients, 5 eventually did well on dilations alone, and now in late childhood seem to be in a very satisfactory state; the other 4, because of very persistent or repeated troubles, were subjected to secondary resection of the strictured zone.

While a conservative attitude is desirable in handling by dilation those patients in whom there has been early onset of symptoms of esophageal stricture, it is possible to treat the more difficult cases by a second operation for revision or removal of the strictured area. This should not be done until one is convinced that a program of dilations will not produce the desired result. Furthermore, in a second operation which is performed too soon one would probably encounter extensive reactions and adhesions in the posterior mediastinum whereas at older ages these difficulties would tend to be somewhat less. The 4 patients on whom we performed secondary operations were 7, 10, 22, and 24 months of age respectively. While there was considerable fibrosis in the mediastinum of these, in each it was possible to free the esophagus (and also spare the vagus nerves) without too much trouble. They were all operated upon by right trans-

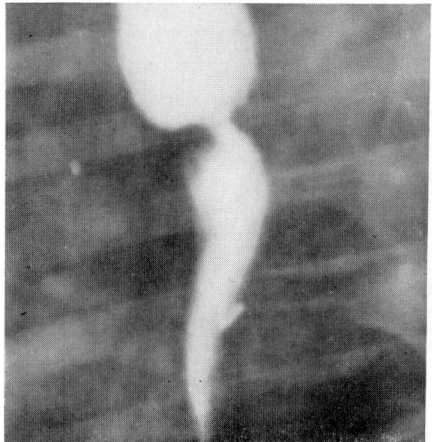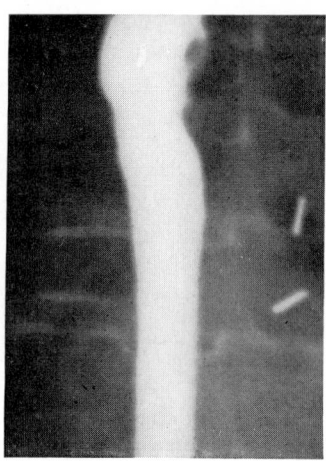

Fig. 64. Local resection of esophageal stricture. Two-year-old child who previously had had a primary anastomosis for esophageal atresia; poor union obtained. There was much scarring subsequently, requiring a large number of dilations through the first two years of life, without gaining much headway on the problem. *Left,* Film at two years of age, showing the high degree of stricture. *Right,* Esophagus following resection and re-anastomosis. The child has been completely relieved of dysphagia.

pleural approaches, being careful to save a mediastinal pleural flap which could be sewed back later to cover the esophageal suture line. In the first case, the esophagus was opened longitudinally in the strictured area and was closed transversely. In the other three, the entire strictured area was cut out and discarded, bringing together the remaining rather normal-appearing esophageal ends for a clean anastomosis. There was no postoperative leak from the suture line in any of these four cases. The first child required several dilations following the surgery, but after six months was taking solid food by mouth; the other 3 have had no postoperative dilations and have been taking solid food since a few weeks after operation (Fig. 64). We are strongly inclined to believe that the complete excision and re-anastomosis gives results which are superior to those of any "plastic" revision of a strictured area.

Delayed Symptom Group. The 15 patients in this group seldom presented any serious problems from the therapeutic angle. Dilations have been done (under anesthesia) by introducing a filiform leader, to which gum-webbing dilators of increasing size were attached and then passed into the esophagus from above. The program was seldom burdensome; the patients were handled as follows:

1 had 6 dilations
3 had 5 dilations
2 had 3 dilations
4 had 2 dilations
5 had 1 dilation

The average was 2.6 dilations per case. After these series had been completed, there was almost always ability to partake of a normal diet.

Late Symptom Group. These youngsters, who had symptoms of dysphagia coming on toward the end of the first year of life or after that time, presented only minor problems which could be treated very quickly, easily, and effectively. We were impressed in this group by several children who were getting along quite well until they swallowed some foreign body which became lodged at the slightly narrowed part of the esophagus.

Dilations were done (under anesthesia) by use of a filiform leader carrying gum-webbing dilators. After these had been used up to a maximum size available, we have in some cases used the long gum-webbing dilators (without leaders, Fig. 53). For the 10 patients in the group, the treatments were as follows:

1 had 5 dilations
1 had 3 dilations
3 had 2 dilations
5 had 1 dilation

The average number was 1.7 dilations per case.

Results of Therapy

For the entire group of 34 patients with stricture following a previous esophageal anastomosis for treatment of esophageal atresia, the following general statements can be made.

The seriousness, or benignity, of the situation depends greatly upon the *time* when the symptoms of dysphagia first appear. In those children who had *late* or *delayed* onset of symptoms, the condition was always one which could be handled easily and effectively by a few dilations of the strictured zone. In contrast, for those babies who had *early* onset of dysphagia or inability to swallow, the outlook was almost always a serious one since the esophageal scarring was extensive and the situation was generally accompanied by aspiration, pulmonary complications, and marked debility. Slightly more than half of these patients eventually (after a year or two) developed a good esophageal pathway and are now eating normal diets; almost half came to more radical therapy by secondary operation for plastic revision or complete excision of the strictured area. Of these two secondary types of operation we believe that resection is much to be preferred. These secondary operations have proved to be safe, and the results following them are exceedingly good.

There have been no perforations of the esophagus during any of the dilation procedures. There was no esophageal leakage nor was there any death in the patients subjected to secondary resection.

ESOPHAGEAL STRICTURE FOLLOWING PEPTIC ESOPHAGITIS

Clinical Picture

The esophagus is highly vulnerable to the ravages of peptic ulceration; it is probably more susceptible to such injury than is the duodenum or jejunum. Hydrochloric acid and pepsin can invade the esophagus: (1) When there is relaxation of the cardia and reflux of gastric juices. (2) When there is a hiatus hernia, a lack of the pinch-cock shut-off of the cardia, and a portion of the gastric cardia residing above the level of the diaphragm. (3) When there is aberrant gastric mucosa in the esophageal lining. In any of these situations, peptic erosion can set up an extensive and very intense inflammatory reaction in the esophagus, throwing it into spasm (Fig. 65), and eventually leading to fibrosis and cicatricial contraction. The stages of spasm (from esophagitis) merge im-

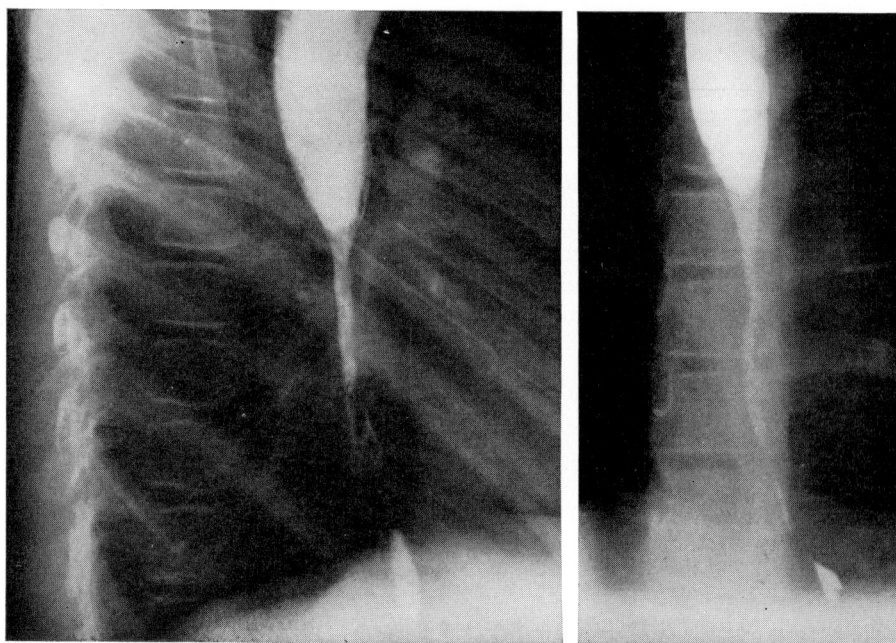

Fig. 65. Peptic esophagitis in a twelve-year-old boy. The films suggest a long stricture; esophagoscopy showed the esophagus diffusely inflamed, but distensible. (The x-ray appearance is therefore due to marked spasm.) The child was completely relieved of dysphagia by anti-acid medical therapy.

perceptibly into those of stricture (from scarring). In either, or both, there are symptoms of esophageal obstruction which include dysphagia, regurgitation, vomiting, weight loss (or failure to gain), bleeding into the alimentary tract, and possibly spillover of food into the trachea giving pulmonary infection, a complication which is particularly apt to be seen in babies.

Esophagitis can appear in newborn infants. Indeed, it is our impression that if peptic esophagitis is ever going to arise, symptoms are usually manifested from the earliest months of life. Such obstruction (spasm) can be so severe in infancy that gastrostomy may be necessary as a lifesaving measure. The length of time required for transition from stages of spasm to those of stricture is important in outlining the course of the therapy which is required. Apparently the development to a cicatricial form is very slow; it is seldom seen in childhood, and is largely a problem of adult life. Therefore, it is rarely necessary in childhood to employ those measures which have been undertaken for adults, namely, excision of the strictured area (which is very apt to be followed by peptic ulceration in remaining parts of the esophagus) or extensive gastric resection to reduce acid-producing tissue (this in a child would almost certainly lead to retardation of growth).

Therapy

While esophageal stricture (from peptic inflammation) is seldom of serious degree in childhood years, its forerunner (peptic esophagitis) can be most extensive and can be very stubborn to treat in the young. We have seen very little in the way of beneficial effects from Banthine, and little help from belladonna. Still much can be accomplished by an anti-acid regimen. The child is offered a normal diet at regular meal hours; such food will neutralize the free acid for a period of possibly two hours. Then, two hours *after* each meal a moderate-sized drink of milk *or* a swallow of other acid-neutralizing substance such as Creamalin is given. No water or other fluid should be taken to wash these down, thus allowing them to linger in the esophagus as long as possible. This

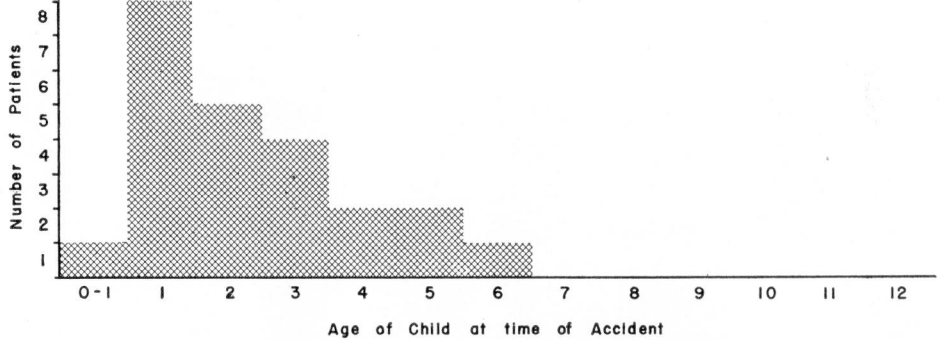

Fig. 66. Ages of patients with lye strictures of the esophagus.

regimen supplies the child with a neutralizing substance in the middle of the morning, the middle of the afternoon, and at bedtime. If the child wakens during the night, a drink of warm milk is beneficial. We have seen this simple regimen work wonders with cases in which the esophagus presented a raw-looking, granular, and bleeding surface (when viewed through an esophagoscope) and was in marked spasm, producing a high degree of obstruction. Generally, within weeks or a few months, the condition has been markedly ameliorated and the child's health greatly improved. Certainly, such conservative measures should always have a very thorough trial; we believe that by their use, surgical resection can always be avoided in the childhood ages.

ESOPHAGEAL STRICTURE FROM LYE BURNS

Clinical Picture

Of the various injurious chemicals which children can swallow and which give rise to esophageal damage, lye is the worst and the most frequent offender. This substance, raw or in various commercial products, containing high concentrations of sodium hydroxide, is commonly used in the home for cleaning of toilets, drains, or floors. In a solid or powdered form it is rarely ingested, but if put into solution and left standing about, the colorless or pale whitish fluid is apt to be taken by a thirsty and unsuspecting child, thinking it is water or milk. Commonly a youngster swallows the caustic solution because it has been left in a container customarily used for food or drink, such as a cup, a glass, or a soda pop bottle. The accidents are almost wholly confined to children in the first few years of life (Fig. 66); our youngest patient was six weeks and the oldest six years at the time.

Lye solutions make disastrous burns rapidly around the lips, in the mouth, and particularly in the esophagus. That part of the fluid which is in the oral cavity is spit out almost instantly; the mucosal lesions here can be extensive and terrifying at first, but they are not very deep and they almost always heal rather promptly and completely. Any material which reaches the stomach is quickly diluted and neutralized by the hydrochloric acid of the gastric juice; burns of the stomach are rare. The chemical has its longest and most damaging contact with the esophageal lining; the burns can be extensive, deep, and devastating.

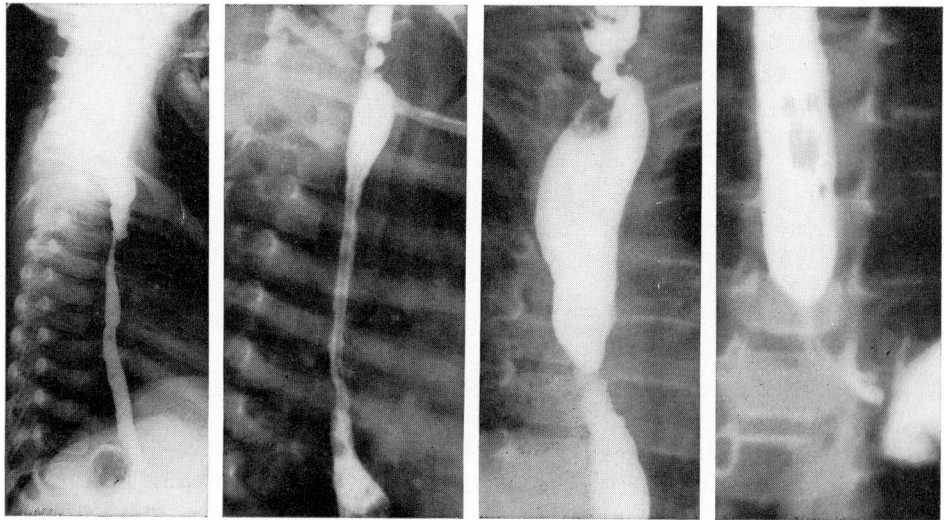

Fig. 67. Lye strictures of the esophagus in four children, showing varying extents and positions in which the esophagus can be burned and obstructed.

In a review of our 23 cases of lye burns of the esophagus, the following locations and extents of lesions were found:

Upper third of esophagus................................. 5 cases
Middle third... 6 cases
Lower third.. 7 cases
Multiple... 3 cases
Just below cricopharyngeus............................... 1 case
Entire esophagus... 1 case

Therapy

Acidic Solutions. Theoretically, the immediate use of a mild solution such as lemon juice, orange juice, or weak vinegar to rinse the mouth and to swallow might have some beneficial neutralizing effects, but as a practical measure this is almost valueless. In the atmosphere of excitement at the time of the accident, such materials can seldom be obtained quickly enough to do any real good.

General Measures. With a child excited and in pain from a fresh lye burn, sedation should be given in generous doses and continued as long as the patient must be made comfortable. In one of our patients, some of the caustic material had spilled into the larynx; a tracheotomy was required. Sipping a teaspoonful of olive oil every half hour for the first twelve hours, and then every hour for twenty-four hours, will help to soothe the painful membranes of the lips and mouth. At first, all food or drink will be refused. After some days, water will usually be taken, and if this can be swallowed, milk should be offered for its nourishing value and for its soothing effect on the necrotic membranes.

After soreness of the mouth has subsided somewhat, roentgenographic visualization is in order while a thin barium fluid is being swallowed, so that the presence or absence of esophageal burn can be determined, and if present, its position and extent can be ascertained. Not all lye burns of the mouth are accompanied by esophageal lesions; sometimes the fluid has been ejected quickly and has not reached the esophagus.

The problems of care can be summarized as follows: In the *acute cases*, treatment is directed toward preserving life, supporting the general state of health so that the lesion can heal, maintaining a patent esophageal lumen, and restoring the lumen to a size compatible with relatively normal esophageal function. In patients with *chronic stricture*, the first three steps have been accomplished already and the problem is one of providing an esophageal pathway which will be satisfactory for the passage of food. Little more than relatively good function can be expected, since a perfectly normal tube can never be provided and the patient must be continually observed throughout life for the possibility of recurring stricture.

Early Dilation. In some quarters *early* dilations of the esophagus have been advocated; by beginning within a few days after the injury, passing a mercury-filled rubber-bag bougie daily, it is believed that subsequent scarring and contraction can be minimized. To this view we take strong objection. The program seems to be completely opposed to all sound principles of treating damaged tissues; it is hard to believe that early instrumentation does not increase the trauma. That additional damage actually does take place is commonly indicated by the fact that bougienage during acute stages of the burn is accompanied by a flare-up of fever, pain, and bleeding. This "preventive" treatment must be carried out daily (or at very frequent intervals) for a period of months. While the method has many advocates, we have not used it.

Gastrostomy. For some cases of esophageal stricture it is possible to maintain fairly good nutrition and also to dilate the esophagus from above, but in many instances the esophageal pathway is so tiny that a gastrostomy becomes necessary for purposes of feeding and also to allow for a better method of treating the esophagus by retrograde dilation. For all such gastrostomies, we prefer the Stamm method (Chapter 10). Once a gastrostomy has been made, it will usually have to be left open many months, or possibly several years. With this opening, nutrition can be rapidly improved; usually it is not long until a high caloric diet can be given by mouth, at least in the form of liquids or possibly pureed foods. Once a gastrostomy has been made, the advantages and superiority of retrograde methods of dilation generally make one reluctant to close the gastrostomy until it is quite clear that little more in the way of esophageal dilation will be required. Of our 23 patients with lye strictures, a gastrostomy was made in 16 of them (69 per cent).

Dilations. While a few esophageal burns are of minimal extent and do not give rise to severe stricture, the vast majority of them do produce marked scarring, contracture, and obstruction which will require instrumental dilation. We prefer to defer starting this until most of the active, inflammatory phase is past; it is generally possible to put off this therapy for a month or six weeks. Dilations, particularly the first ones, must be exceedingly gentle so that esophageal rupture will not occur. To prevent perforation, dilations should either be made in a retrograde manner (with Tucker dilators) or else made from above *always* employing a string guide. A silk thread (such as Champion surgeon's silk, No. 12 white braided) is passed through the nose or through the mouth into the oropharynx and its tip then allowed to proceed down the esophagus. Aves et al.[1] have employed a small mercury-laden rubber sac to expedite passage of the guide string. A roll of reserve string is kept strapped to the side of the face. From time to time as the child swallows, more string from the reserve can be released so it is pulled down through the stomach and into the intestine. Usually 3 or 4 yards are necessary to anchor it sufficiently, the process of getting the string down usually requiring one or two days. Hubbard and Leven[6] have pointed out that the use of a swallowed string is contraindicated whenever there is an anatomic loop (such as gastroenterostomy or entero-enterostomy) at any level in the alimentary tract, for fear that the string might cut the loop or ulcerate the mucosa.

When the string is in place, general anesthesia is given, the string is fished out of the mouth, is pulled up tautly, and is used as a guide over which Mixter dilators (Fig. 52) can be run down through the strictured zone. Only gentle pressure should be used. Too much stretching should not be done at one sitting, since it is apt to tear the esophageal wall and make matters worse. Little or no blood should be seen on the dilators which are withdrawn.

It is impossible to predict what course of therapy will be necessary for any given case. The number and the frequency of dilations are factors which vary tremendously from case to case; treatments must be used as indications present themselves. In general, the intervals between dilations should be as long as possible. While it is sometimes necessary to perform them a few weeks apart, it is usually possible to lengthen the intervals to five to six weeks, sometimes longer. After some reasonable headway has been made, it is often possible to increase the intervals to several months or more. The necessity for dilations can best be judged by observing how soon dysphagia returns and the intake of food diminishes. Most patients will require long courses of dilation, extending over a span of many years.

In our 23 patients with lye stricture who have had courses of therapy completed, or who are currently under treatment, there have been the following number of dilations.

        6 had   1 to   6 dilations
        9 had   6 to 13 dilations
        3 had 14 to 20 dilations
        5 had 30, 36, 52, 52, and 59 dilations respectively.

In no instance have we had esophageal perforation. For about half of these patients the course of dilations has apparently ended, though it is possible that they may require an occasional stretching in adult life; for the remaining patients, the end is yet nowhere in sight and it is obvious that a much longer program of therapy will be necessary.

Resection. There are few conditions which require more prolonged treatment and more patience on the part of the child and doctor than some of the severe lye strictures of the esophagus; they are most vexatious problems to deal with. When faced with a long series of dilations, it is very tempting to think of excision of the damaged portion of esophagus to attain permanent relief of obstruction.

A radical attack on the problem of impermeable stricture of the esophagus has been made by the establishment of some form of antethoracic esophagus. Such undertakings have had great impetus from the work of Yudin,[15] who reported the surgical treatment of 80 patients by stage operations which consisted of division of the jejunum, bringing up the distal loop of jejunum in front of the thoracic cage for anastomosis with the esophagus in the neck above the stricture, and reestablishment of the continuity of the intestinal tract by anastomosing the proximal end of the divided jejunum to the lower jejunum or to the upper ileum. Yudin's mortality rates have been amazingly low and the end results have been satisfactory from the standpoint of function. Yudin's method has the disadvantage of completely sidetracking the stomach, duodenum, and upper jejunum; these are thrown out of function except for their activity in producing alimentary juices. It is important to point out that most of Yudin's subjects were adults; for children, the Yudin operation has certain adverse features. In our clinic, attempts at similar antethoracic jejunal transplantation in children (for treatment of esophageal atresia) have been troublesome, or have failed, because of the shortness of the loop which can be brought up onto the chest or because of insufficient blood supply (and sloughing) of this limb. Furthermore, the failure to deliver food into the stomach has been followed by a marked stunting of growth. In two cases, Harrison[4] has made a reconstruction by transplanting a segment of jejunum into the posterior mediastinum to connect the upper portion of esophagus to the stomach.

While the methods of Yudin and of Harrison represent tremendous advances in surgical thinking, they will probably be relegated to a position of historical interest because of the more logical and the safer procedures developed by Sweet[12] and others, whereby subtotal resection of the esophagus (left-sided approach) is combined with a high intrathoracic esophago-gastric anastomosis. Paine[10] prefers to carry out these steps by a combination of simultaneous abdominal and right thoracic approaches. Variable proportions of the stomach will have to be displaced upward into the thorax, depending upon how much of the esophagus must be sacrificed. Sweet has clearly described the operative procedure and has recorded 3 cases in which it was performed successfully for treatment of extensive esophageal stricture; Paine has written of 2 others. Because of the length of lye strictures which are generally encountered, it is very doubtful if they can often be treated by resection and end-to-end anastomosis of the esophagus, leaving the stomach in the abdomen.

In 1951 Paine found that there had been only 18 patients reported in the American literature with lye strictures of the esophagus from whom the stricture had been removed and the continuity of the gastro-intestinal tract restored. In these there was one fatality; in all the surviving patients the result was described as excellent or satisfactory, though some of the follow-up studies were only brief ones.

Our one attempt at resection was in a three-year-old Negro girl (Fig. 68) who had an impermeable stricture of the entire esophagus; the lumen was completely blocked off. A gastrostomy had been established for purposes of feeding. A subtotal resection of the esophagus was performed, bringing the fundus of the stomach up to the very apex of the left pleural cavity where it was anastomosed to the stump of esophagus. This child had a very stormy convalescence requiring several months of hospitalization. There were profound disturbances of intestinal motility and diarrhea which at first were exceedingly difficult to control; we assumed that these were due to disruption of the vagi which had to be sacrificed in the dense peri-esophageal scar tissue. Furthermore, there was loss of a sphincteric mechanism between the pharynx and the stomach. During inspiratory movements of the chest, air rushed into the stomach, so that it was constantly a great wind-filled sac, making the patient very uncomfortable and largely putting the left lung out of commission by compression. Enormous accumulations of air gathered

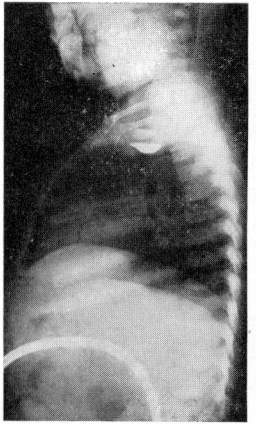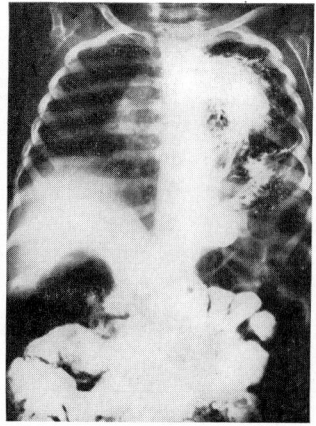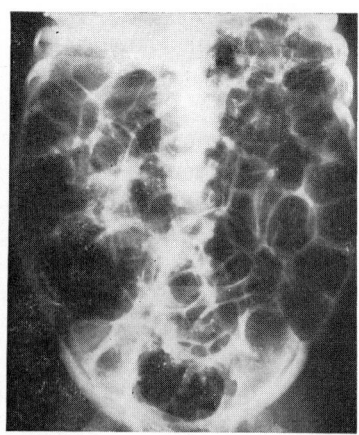

Fig. 68. Three-year-old colored girl with impermeable stricture of the esophagus, after swallowing lye. *Left*, Showing the complete obstruction. *Middle*, Postoperative film, after removal of esophagus and bringing stomach up to the apex of the chest for anastomosis to the esophageal stump. *Right*, Film one month after surgery. This child had severe intestinal disturbances for several months. Excessive amounts of air were gulped into the stomach during inspiration, the pharyngeal constrictor mechanism being interfered with. Furthermore, there was a great deal of diarrhea, presumably because the vagi had been transected in the chest (involved in peri-esophageal scar tissue). Esophagogastrostomy can be followed by troublesome complications.

in the intestines. The child could swallow and could eat; her nourishment became reasonably good, but the over-all result certainly left much to be desired. This case has dampened our enthusiasm for undertaking resection in other cases of lye stricture, though it cannot be denied that under some circumstances this radical approach might be employed with greater satisfaction. Conservative treatment (if dilations can be termed such) has in no case led to fatality in our series; this fact makes us somewhat hesitant to employ resection which (while it is apparently attended by low risk to life) is apt to introduce complications of a troublesome nature.

REFERENCES

1. Aves, F. H., Desforges, G. and Strieder, J. W.: Mercury-Bag Bolus to Expedite Passage of Esophageal Dilator Guide String. J. Thoracic Surg., *24:*34, 1952.
2. Bosher, L. H., Jr., Burford, T. H. and Ackerman, L.: The Pathology of Experimentally Produced Lye Burns and Strictures of the Esophagus. J. Thoracic Surg., *21:*483, 1951.
3. Gross, R. E.: Treatment of Short Stricture of the Esophagus by Partial Esophagectomy and End-to-End Esophageal Reconstruction. Surgery, *23:*735, 1948.
4. Harrison, A. W.: Transthoracic Small Bowel Substitution in High Stricture of the Esophagus. J. Thoracic Surg., *18:*316, 1949.
5. Holinger, P. H., Johnston, K. C., and Greengard, J.: Congenital Anomalies of the Esophagus Related to Esophageal Foreign Bodies. Am. J. Dis. Child., *78:*467, 1949.
6. Hubbard, T. B., Jr., and Leven, N. L.: Esophageal Dilatation: A Contraindication to the Swallowed Thread, and an Alternative Method. Surgery, *27:*126, 1950.
7. Kernodle, G. W., Taylor, G., and Davison, W. C.: Lye Poisoning in Children. Am. J. Dis. Child., *75:*135, 1948.
8. Lisa, J. R. and Taylor, H. M.: Congenital Malformation of the Esophagus without Tracheoesophageal Fistula. N. Y. State J. Med., *48:*1622, 1948.
9. Mixter, S. J.: Symposium on the Surgery of the Esophagus From the Standpoint of the General Surgeon. Tr. Am. Laryng. A., *31:*342, 1909.
10. Paine, J. R.: Excision of Extensive Lye Stricture of the Esophagus. N. Y. State J. Med., *51:*2628, 1951.
11. Salzer, H.: Early Treatment of Corrosive

Esophagitis. Wien. klin. Wchnschr., *33:* 307, 1920.

12. Sweet, R. H.: Subtotal Esophagectomy with High Intrathoracic Esophago-Gastric Anastomosis in the Treatment of Extensive Cicatricial Obliteration of the Esophagus. Surg., Gynec., & Obst., *83:*417, 1946.

13. Tuttle, W. M. and Day, J. C.: The Treatment of Short Esophageal Strictures by Resection and End-to-End Anastomosis. J. Thoracic Surg., *19:*534, 1950.

14. van den Wildenberg: Contribution a l'étude des rétrécissements congénitaux de l'oesophage et des diverticules de l'oesophage. Ann. d'oto-laryng., *65:*390, 1948.

15. Yudin, S. S.: The Surgical Construction of 80 Cases of Artificial Esophagus. Surg., Gynec., & Obst., *78:*561, 1944.

CHAPTER 8

Cardio-Esophageal Chalasia

Vomiting in newborn babies generally indicates the existence of some form of obstruction in the alimentary tract. There are many anomalies which produce partial or complete blockage and which require surgical intervention for their relief. Among babies who vomit, there is also a small group with a neuromuscular disturbance in the esophagus and cardia, who might at first be regarded as having a clinical picture suggesting obstruction, but who on further investigation are found to have a condition which can be treated entirely by medical means. Relaxation of the gastric cardia is not a surgical problem, but it is well to include here a short consideration of the lesion, since surgeons are apt to be called to see these patients during their initial study. Some young babies, who are otherwise completely normal, have a persistent laxity of the lower portion of the esophagus and a failure of the gastric cardia to assume its usual sphincteric action; Neuhauser and Berenberg[4] have termed the lesion "chalasia" of the esophagus and cardia.

ETIOLOGY

Little is known about the etiology of chalasia. Normally, the esophageal hiatus relaxes during the act of swallowing, but is otherwise kept closed. According to Jackson,[3] this constriction is produced by the "pinchcock-like" action of the diaphragm. Hurst and Stewart[2] have demonstrated special diaphragmatic muscle bundles which surround the lower esophagus, and which by their action open and close the cardia. It has been postulated that absence of these bundles, improper development of them, or alterations in their neural control might bring about the abnormal physiology. Since also the esophagus of these patients is usually atonic and has a diminished peristalsis, it would appear likely that there is a widespread neuromuscular defect in the intrinsic musculature of the esophagus and the cardia.

CLINICAL PICTURE

Chalasia occurs with equal frequency in males and females. The history, the clinical findings, and the course of the illness in infants afflicted with this syndrome are rather uniform. Usually pregnancy and delivery have been uneventful, and the newborn baby at first shows no evidence of being abnormal. However, within a week after birth the baby starts to vomit. This becomes progressively more frequent, and soon appears during or immediately after each feeding. Otherwise, the infant appears well, active, and hungry. The vomiting seems to be effortless and is rarely forceful or projectile; it is more of a regurgitation. The vomitus is usually not bile-stained, but may contain gastric juice and therefore is curdled and sour-smelling. Although vomiting may occur during a feeding, it more commonly comes during eructations and especially when the baby is placed back in his crib in a supine position. Frequently the mother volunteers the information that there is no vomiting as long as the baby is held upright. Untreated, the infant continues to vomit, lose weight, or gain poorly. In some, aspiration gives rise to a pulmonary infection. Physical examination is generally negative except for varying degrees of dehydration and malnutrition; occasionally there is an associated pneumonia.

DIAGNOSIS

Chalasia may be suspected from the history, but can only be confirmed by elimination of other causes of vomiting and by radiologic detection of the persistent cardio-esophageal relaxation. At fluoroscopy the barium-filled esophagus appears larger than usual, and gives the impression of being atonic and flaccid. Esophageal peristaltic waves are diminished in frequency and strength. There is great laxity of the cardia and there is an absence or weakness of the diaphragmatic sphincteric shut-off; following deglutition the cardia remains open and widely patulous (Fig. 69). Together, the esophagus and

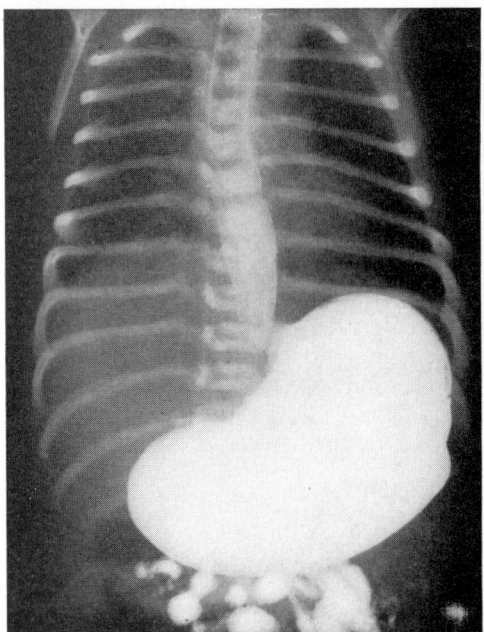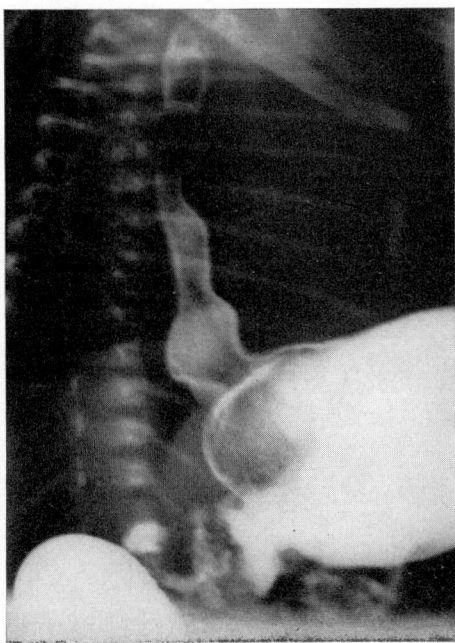

Fig. 69. Roentgenograms from two babies with relaxation of the esophagus and cardia. Barium freely flowed from the stomach back up through the patulous cardia into the hypotonic esophagus.

stomach appear as a toneless sac; barium flows freely back and forth from one part to the other, entirely dependent upon the position of the baby. When the patient is supine, any slight pressure upon the abdominal wall causes retrograde filling of the esophagus with air or barium from the stomach. Crying or struggling raises the intra-abdominal pressure and produces a similar result. If the patient is held erect, regurgitation is not observed, although it is apparent that the esophageal hiatus still remains open. Occasionally, reflux into the pharynx elicits a gag reflex, and forceful vomiting occurs. The stomach and the pylorus usually appear otherwise normal.

TREATMENT

Relief from vomiting is obtained by feeding the baby in a sitting position, and by keeping him so for thirty minutes to an hour after each meal. The infant may be strapped into a small, padded chair (Fig. 70), or be bolstered up in his crib by pillows. This upright posture is maintained day and night; it is continued for several weeks or months until vomiting no longer occurs. Babies easily get accustomed to the continuous erect position; they are peaceful, they sleep well, and they do not object to being propped up in this manner. Thickening the feedings by adding an ounce of cereal to each 15 ounces of formula may help to prevent regurgitation, but drugs—such as atropine—are of no value unless there is an associated pylorospasm.

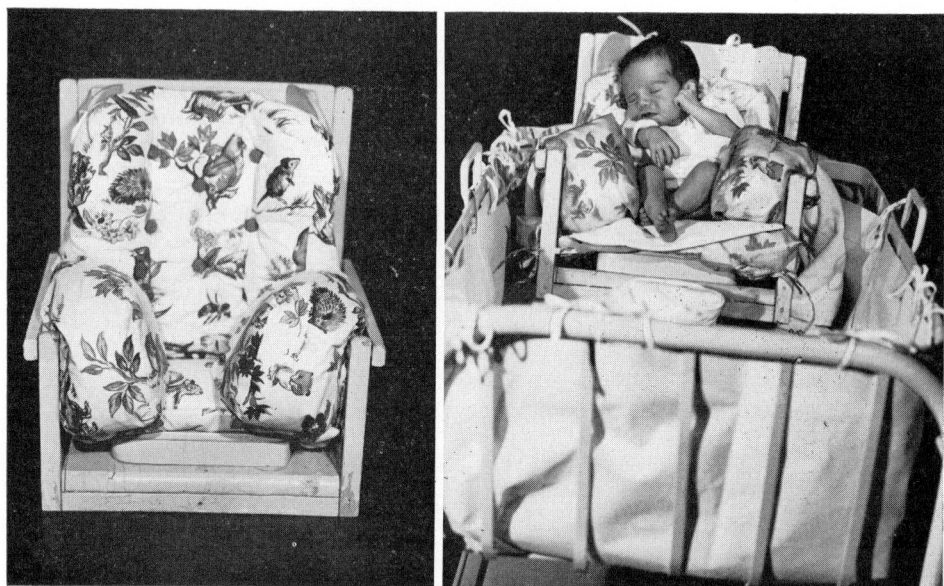

Fig. 70. *Left*, A small padded chair into which a baby with chalasia can be strapped. *Right*, Child with chalasia being kept in the upright position by holding him in a padded chair.

After this regimen is employed, the babies immediately start to gain weight, and to develop normally. Usually after two to three months a barium swallow shows no abnormality in the esophagus or cardia; they have acquired a normal tone and function.

RESULTS OF TREATMENT

The chalasia syndrome has been recognized only within recent years. In many instances, the symptoms are so mild that the infant is not fluoroscoped, and the diagnosis not made. Thus it is difficult to ascertain accurately the true incidence of chalasia. At the Children's Hospital, during the seven-year period from 1944 through 1950, there were 30 infants with troubles serious enough to warrant roentgenologic investigation and for whom a diagnosis of chalasia was established. Studies were carried out in all cases to exclude other possible causes of vomiting. All infants were treated by thickened feedings and by the use of the upright position, both while in the hospital and later at home. In most instances, therapy could be discontinued after three to four weeks, at which time repeat roentgenographic studies revealed markedly improved or normal function of the esophagus and cardia. Some patients required several months of therapy before the esophageal functions returned to normal.

One infant was slow to respond, and one failed to improve under the treatment; both of these were found later to have cerebral defects and mental retardation. One child still has mild chalasia as shown by x-ray examination, although vomiting and regurgitation have disappeared. One infant had an extremely severe degree of esophageal involvement; the entire structure was flaccid, with no peristaltic activity whatsoever.

While lying down the child had difficulty even swallowing her saliva; sitting up she could handle her saliva, but still could not take feedings. Because of the severity of the condition, a feeding gastrostomy was established; with this, in addition to the upright position, the baby began to gain weight and to improve. In two months all feedings could be taken by mouth and retained; after an additional month the gastrostomy tube was removed and the gastrostomy was allowed to close. The child has since done extremely well

REFERENCES

1. Berenberg, W. and Neuhauser, E. B. D.: Cardio-Esophageal Relaxation (Chalasia) as a Cause of Vomiting in Infants. Pediatrics, 5:414, 1950.
2. Hurst, A. F. and Stewart, M. J.: Gastric and Duodenal Ulcer. Oxford University Press, New York, 1929.
3. Jackson, C.: The Diaphragmatic Pinchcock in So-called "Cardiospasm." Laryngoscope, 32:139, 1922.
4. Neuhauser, E. B. D. and Berenberg, W.: Cardio-Esophageal Relaxation as a Cause of Vomiting in Infants. Radiology, 48:480, 1947.

CHAPTER 9

Congenital Hypertrophic Pyloric Stenosis

Hypertrophic stenosis of the pylorus is the most common condition requiring surgical therapy in infancy. In this abnormality the pylorus has a marked increase in size of its circular musculature, compression of its mucosa, and obstruction of its lumen. Clinical findings include all of the cardinal symptoms and signs of mechanical blockage at the outlet of the stomach.

Operative attack on congenital pyloric stenosis is one of the greatest advances in abdominal surgery in the last few decades. Prior to 1912, when the technique of pyloromyotomy was introduced, the mortality in this condition varied from 50 to 75 per cent or more; today proper surgical management, combined with adequate preoperative and postoperative care, carries fatality rates less than 1 per cent. Experience gained from the operative treatment of 1787 patients up to December 31, 1952, forms the basis of the following presentation.

PATHOLOGY

Gross Pathology

There is hypertrophy of and increase in the number of smooth muscle fibers of the pylorus. Such enlargement gives a bulbous or fusiform mass. The *dimensions* of this swelling vary somewhat with the age of the baby and with the degree of hypertrophy which is present. In an average case, the swollen pylorus is about $\frac{3}{4}$ inch in length and about $\frac{5}{8}$ inch in diameter.

The pylorus is quite firm and rubbery in consistency. Its external surface is smoothly covered by serosa. A longitudinal hemisection shows the *musculature* to be of such thickness that it pushes the mucosa inward and thereby greatly diminishes the lumen of the stomach at this point. The great bulk of muscular tissue is unyielding and it impedes the passage of curds from the stomach into the duodenum. When the thickened musculature is examined in cross section, it is found to be yellowish gray, quite firm, and of a gristly consistency.

A longitudinal section of the hypertrophied pylorus shows important anatomic differences in the configuration of the mucosa at the gastric and duodenal ends. As shown in Figure 71, the lumen of the stomach is gradually reduced in size as one approaches the pylorus, but *the duodenum assumes its full size at once*, because of the abrupt termination of the pyloric sphincter at its distal end. It is important to remember this during operation, for there is great danger of sweeping a scalpel into the duodenal lumen at the point where it balloons out just beyond the pylorus.

Microscopic Pathology

Sections of specimens which have been found at autopsy (without surgical intervention) do not show any increase in nerves, nor is there any other neurologic abnormality to suggest that muscular hypertrophy is brought about by a neurologic disturbance. In specimens obtained from infants under a week or ten days of age, the mucosa and submucosa are essentially normal. After this time, the forcing of curds through the small opening produces *edema of the mucosa* and a slight increase of *leukocytes* in this layer. The mechanical irritation brings about a thickening of the mucosa which further reduces the size of the pyloric opening. Presumably, it is for this reason that infants do not exhibit signs of obstruction until they are one or two weeks of age, in spite of the fact that the hypertrophied muscle has been present since birth (or before birth?).

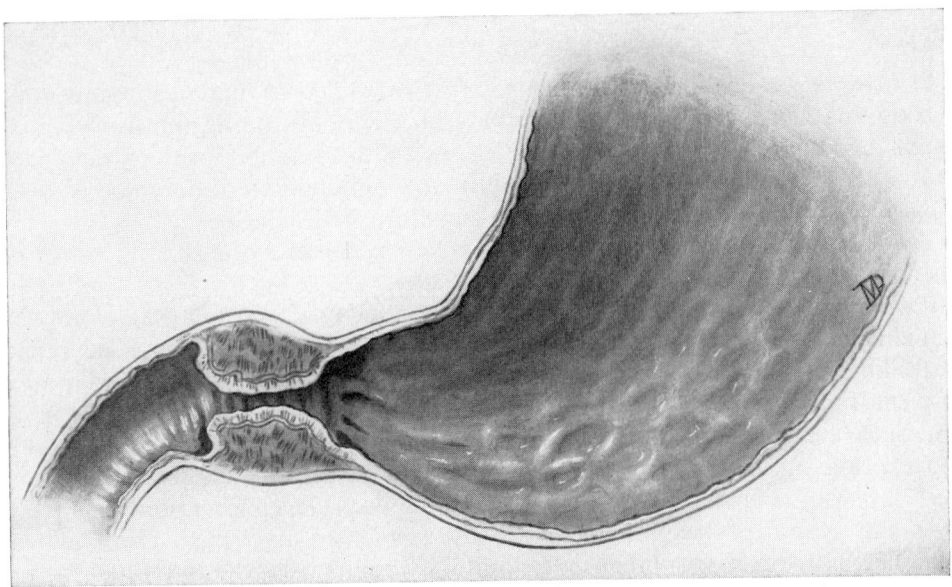

Fig. 71. Longitudinal section from a case of pyloric stenosis, showing hypertrophy of musculature at outlet of the stomach. The thickened muscle tapers off gradually on its gastric side but stops abruptly on the duodenal end.

Dependent upon the obstruction of the pylorus, there are secondary changes of lesser importance in the wall of the gastric antrum and fundus, such as mild hypertrophy of the muscular coats of the stomach and an increase in prominence of the mucosal rugae. These reactions are similar to those which are found in any portion of the gastro-intestinal tract above a lesion which has caused longstanding mechanical obstruction.

ETIOLOGY

There is no satisfactory explanation for the etiology of congenital hypertrophic stenosis of the pylorus. Some writers have propounded the theory that *injury to the central nervous system* during birth might be an etiologic factor, but the absence of other signs of cerebral damage in the great majority of cases tends to refute this view. It has also been suggested that the disease might be analogous to conditions such as megaloureter or Hirschsprung's disease of the colon, in which there is some local neurologic abnormality, imbalance, or failure of development; we have no reason to condemn this theory, nor do we know of any evidence to support it.

Some pediatricians regard pyloric stenosis as the end result of a *preexisting pyloric spasm*. In other words, the muscle, which has been overactive for long periods of time, now becomes hypertrophied. Such muscular spasm could have been originally brought about by abnormal reflex disturbances which are occasionally seen in other parts of the gastro-intestinal tract, for example, at the gastric cardia. While this theory might be attractive, it does not appear to be entirely plausible, because pyloric hypertrophy can be found so early in life that spasm could not have preexisted for any appreciable length of time.

There is no racial predisposition to the condition.

In short, we are at a loss to explain hypertrophy of the pylorus, and regard this problem as one of only academic interest which is far overshadowed by practical considerations of the surgical treatment.

SYMPTOMS

Pyloric stenosis is more apt to occur in *first-born children* than in subsequent ones. The condition can *recur in families;* a study of this point during the five years 1946 through 1950 (490 cases) shows that in 12 cases another member of the family (sibling or parent) had had the condition. In one instance four children of the same parents all had pyloric stenosis and had been operated upon for it.

The symptoms are all indicative of *a high obstruction* and of a serious loss of body fluids and electrolytes, especially hydrochloric acid.

Vomiting seldom occurs before the ninth or tenth day of life, and usually not before the child is two weeks of age. At first, vomiting may be little more than a regurgitation after feeding, but soon it becomes more forceful and projectile; at the start it may be infrequent, but later it appears after most of the feedings and is the outstanding complaint. Since the obstruction is above the duodenum, the vomitus does not contain bile. The child is continually hungry, because little food passes into the intestine to be absorbed. He will therefore eagerly nurse or take the bottle, even after vomiting.

As the pyloric obstruction increases, the *stools become less frequent* and more scanty. The bulk diminishes because less and less food reaches the intestine.

With continued *starvation, failure to gain weight* or the *loss of weight* is always seen. There is a loss of subcutaneous fat. Marked *dehydration* is evidenced by wrinkling of the face, neck, and extremities. If vomiting has been long continued and severe, *alkalosis* may give hyperpnea or other respiratory disturbance.

PHYSICAL EXAMINATION

Inasmuch as four-fifths of the patients with pyloric stenosis are males, the *sex* of the patient is of some importance. The majority of subjects are from four to six weeks of *age* (Fig. 72).

The general *physical appearance* of patients who are brought to the physician early may show little variation from normal. However, signs of weight loss, wrinkling of skin, sunken appearance of the eyes, and a decrease of subcutaneous fat are more characteristic of advanced stages. Practically all patients have evidence of dehydration, which is best determined by the pliability of the skin. In a normal infant, when the skin of the chest, abdomen, or extremity is picked up by the fingers and then released, it will immediately sink back into its normal position. In contrast, a dehydrated baby has skin of thinner texture which falls back into its flattened contour very slowly.

Examination of the abdomen is of great importance. If there is any distention, it is confined to the epigastrium. During or after feeding, inspection shows gastric waves passing from left to right. Palpation may show a distended stomach if the child has recently been fed. Of greatest interest and value is the palpation of the right upper quadrant with the tip of one finger tip in the attempt to feel the hypertrophied pylorus. In well over 95 per cent of cases, the pyloric "tumor" can be felt through the abdominal wall; in occasional cases it can be felt only after repeated examinations. If the tumor cannot be detected, feedings of some fluid material such as milk formula, saline and glucose, or dilute orange juice will relax the abdominal wall and make possible satisfactory examination. If the enlarged pylorus cannot be felt, the feeding should be kept up until the baby vomits, because this is followed by a momentary period of great relaxation during which the abdominal viscera can be best palpated. The vomitus, of course, does not contain bile, a fact which clearly indicates that the obstruction is above the ampulla of Vater.

Palpation for a pyloric "tumor" requires *gentleness and patience;* a physician who expects to feel the mass by poking quickly will probably find that the baby becomes

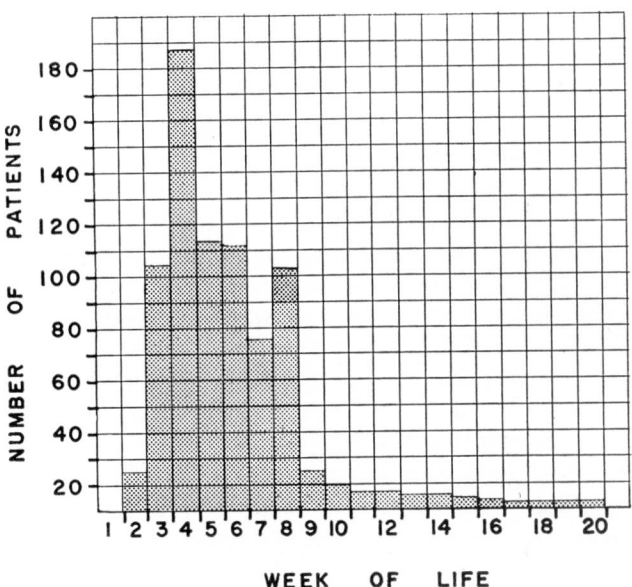

WEEK   OF   LIFE

Fig. 72. Study from a series of cases, showing age of patients at time of admission to the hospital for treatment of pyloric stenosis.

rigid, so that little is learned. Conversely, if the examiner rests his fingers gently on the infant's abdomen and takes sufficient time to feel around slowly in the right upper quadrant, he will be rewarded in the vast majority of cases by identifying the enlarged pylorus and thereby establishing the correct diagnosis.

If the child has been untreated for a long time, the recurring loss of hydrochloric acid brings about *alkalosis,* so that hypertonicity or respiratory disturbances may be found.

It is surprising to find that starvation over long periods does not produce nutritional *eaema.* In only one case have we observed marked edema—the serum protein level was 4.9 mg. per cent—which could be ascribed solely to starvation. This explanation was further supported by the fact that there was no reappearance of edema subsequent to operative relief of pyloric obstruction.

DIFFERENTIAL DIAGNOSIS

Pylorospasm must be differentiated from pyloric stenosis. Babies with this condition are apt to have generalized muscular hypertonicity of the trunk and extremities. The vomiting tends to appear in spells; that is, the child will vomit for two or three days and then be relieved spontaneously for several days before vomiting reappears. No pyloric tumor can be felt by abdominal palpation. The symptoms vary from day to day, whereas with pyloric stenosis they become progressively more frequent and more severe. Symptoms arising from pylorospasm can be relieved by using atropine derivatives, particularly when they are employed in conjunction with sedatives such as phenobarbital; these drugs do not ameliorate symptoms when they arise from pyloric stenosis.

Intracranial Injury or hemorrhage which is derived from birth trauma or hemorrhagic disease is a frequent cause of vomiting and may have to be considered in the differential diagnosis. In children so afflicted, the vomiting is not apt to be as forceful as that seen with mechanical obstruction. Furthermore, the vomiting is more likely to be in small amounts and to be unrelated to the ingestion of food. Vomiting may be the only symptom or sign of intracranial pathology, but one is more likely to find other evidence of neurologic disorder, such as convulsions, spasticity, hypotonicity, bulging fontanelle, or possibly bloody fluid by spinal or subdural taps.

Other Types of Intrinsic Intestinal Obstruction must be considered in the differential diagnosis. It is important to remember that atresia (or marked stenosis) of the esophagus, duodenum, or intestine produces vomiting within the first day or two of life. This is in sharp contrast to the vomiting which occurs in pyloric stenosis, which seldom begins in the first week. Furthermore, these other forms of congenital obstruction are apt to show findings which are not encountered in obstruction at the pylorus. With atresia of the esophagus, there may be a communication between the esophagus and the trachea, or else there is a spilling over of saliva into the larynx; in either situation respiratory difficulties are common. If an atresia exists in the lower duodenum or other portion of the intestinal tract, the vomitus will contain bile or fecal material, which clearly indicates that the obstruction is beyond the pylorus.

Chalasia. Recently we have begun to recognize a new symptom-complex which may be described as a chalasia of the cardia (see Chapter 8). These babies vomit persistently but lack other signs of pyloric stenosis. The condition may be differentiated from pyloric stenosis by roentgenologic examination; this shows that the gastric cardia is continually relaxed and that there is frequent regurgitation of barium from the stomach up into the esophagus. Babies with this condition respond promptly to a therapeutic regimen during which they are given thickened feedings and are propped up in Fowler's position. After a few months, the cardia regains tone and regurgitation disappears.

Extrinsic Forms of Congenital Obstruction, brought about by *incomplete rotation* of the alimentary tract, can give signs within the first few weeks of life. When the intestine is improperly turned or anchored, peritoneal folds come to lie across and compress the lower duodenum; there is vomiting of material which generally contains bile. No pyloric tumor can be felt. Roentgenologic studies are very helpful in differentiating such anomalies from those in which there is pyloric obstruction.

Poor Feeding Regimens for babies can induce vomiting, with clinical findings which can often simulate those of pyloric stenosis. Unduly *prolonged* feedings at breast, or the use of *too concentrated* or *too bulky* formulas can be disturbing to a child. Whenever one must care for a baby who has been vomiting, it is important to review the feeding history in detail, to eliminate the possibility of unreasonable amounts or types of food as a basis for the complaints. Not infrequently, patients are admitted to the hospital with a presumptive diagnosis of pyloric stenosis, only to find that adoption of a sensible feeding regimen completely eliminates the vomiting.

ROENTGENOLOGIC EXAMINATION

Since the symptoms and signs of pyloric stenosis are sufficient to establish definitely the proper diagnosis, roentgenologic examination is not necessary in average cases. There are, however, some instances in which the history is atypical, or the physical findings are inconclusive. Under such circumstances the diagnosis is in doubt and it is best to obtain additional information by x-ray study. We find that roentgen examination is necessary in only one out of 18 or 20 cases.

Methods and Findings

Two methods of examination are available. A *film* of the abdomen without contrast medium will often show a large, dilated, gas-filled stomach, with relatively little gas in the intestine beyond the pylorus. If the stomach is not thus outlined by entrapped air, a gastro-intestinal examination may be done with *the use of contrasting barium*, which is added to a formula feeding.

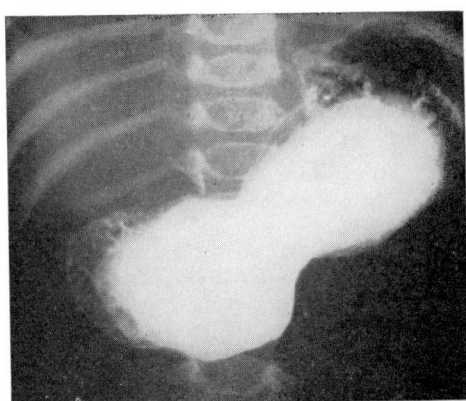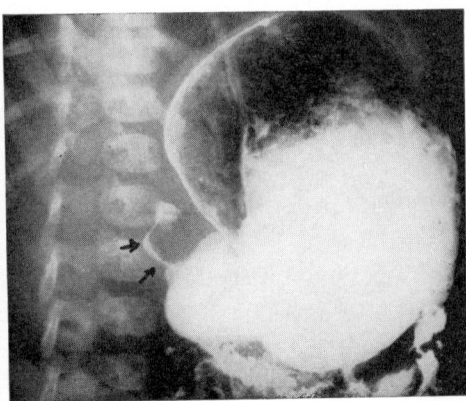

Fig. 73. Roentgenograms from a baby with pyloric stenosis. *Left*, Showing gastric distention and marked peristaltic waves. *Right*, Visualization of outlet of stomach. The pyloric canal (arrows) is greatly attenuated and narrowed. Only small amounts of barium escape into the duodenum.

Fluoroscopic and film findings may be listed as: (1) An enlarged stomach (Fig. 73) with a rounded end (due to ballooning and a curving of the antrum). (2) Greatly increased gastric peristalsis. (3) Passage of the barium to the pylorus but escape of only tiny amounts of it into the duodenum. (4) An elongated and greatly narrowed, thread-like lumen to the pylorus. (5) Abnormal retention of barium in the stomach. Normally, a baby's stomach is completely empty in three hours; the presence of a large part of the barium after this time (when combined with vigorous peristalsis) is indicative of pyloric obstruction.

PREOPERATIVE CARE

To obtain good surgical results and low mortality rates it is essential to give pre-operative support to babies who are dehydrated or are in poor electrolyte balance. Attention must be directed toward treatment of ketosis and replacement of body fluids, electrolytes, and carbohydrate stores.

Administration of Parenteral Fluids

The giving of parenteral fluids is the greatest factor in improving the general condition of these youngsters. A day or two can be well spent in thus strengthening the child; indeed, in extreme cases a longer period may be required to get the baby into optimum condition.

Appropriate fluids should be administered morning and night of each preoperative day. If dehydration is marked, at each of these times an intravenous injection is given, and this is immediately followed by a hypodermoclysis. For *intravenous* therapy, 10 per cent glucose in sterile water is given, in the proportion of 10 cc. per pound of the baby's body weight. For the *hypoaermoclysis*, physiologic saline is used, in amounts equalling 15 cc. per pound of body weight. In average cases in which dehydration is only moderate, we are inclined to give morning and night only the intravenous injections of glucose.

The combination of intravenous and subcutaneous fluids appears to be superior to the administration of fluids solely by the subcutaneous route. However, in general practice or in many general hospitals, where comparatively little infant work is being done, there may be difficulty in giving intravenous infusions. Under such circumstances, all of the parenteral administrations may be given by *subcutaneous routes* if the sites of injection are frequently changed from the pectoral region to the back and to the thighs. If desired, these can be facilitated by the addition of hyaluronidase. When the subcutaneous route is the only one employed, we are inclined to use a mixture (1 part of physiologic saline to 1 part of 5 per cent glucose in water), the total amount of fluid not exceeding 15 or 20 cc. per pound of body weight at any one administration; this can generally be done twice in a twenty-four-hour period.

Transfusion

Transfusion is occasionally of considerable help in preparing an undernourished child for operation, if the blood count is below 4 million. There may be a lowered level of plasma protein which augurs for poor wound healing after operation; hence it is wise to raise the protein level by infusion of blood or plasma from a suitable donor. Blood should never be given in amounts exceeding 10 cc. per pound of body weight at any one time. Transfusions are but rarely needed in cases of pyloric stenosis but are sometimes helpful for the poorer-risk type of patient.

Feedings

While the child is being thus prepared for operation, it is well to continue the oral feedings. The infant may vomit most of this material, but some of it does go through the pylorus and is absorbed from the intestinal tract. The feeding may be milk formula or thickened with small amounts of cooked cereal in the proportion of one part of cereal to 15 or 20 of formula.

More recently, we have omitted entirely the use of milk feedings during the preoperative period, and have offered only saline and glucose solution every three or four hours, feeling that vomiting is possibly reduced thereby and that more liquid gets through the pylorus.

Drugs

When there is some doubt whether a baby has pylorospasm or pyloric stenosis, the use of *atropine*, either by the subcutaneous route or incorporated in the feeding, may be of some value. If the child is fussy and hypertonic, phenobarbital every eight or twelve hours will have a quieting and beneficial effect. These drugs have a rather limited usefulness in typical cases of pyloric stenosis.

Vitamins

Administration of *vitamin C* has been routinely adopted in all of our cases in recent years; this is done in an effort to promote better healing of the wound after operation. If the child is vomiting most of its feedings, 25 mg. of ascorbic acid can be incorporated daily in the parenteral fluids.

OPERATIVE PROCEDURES

Before 1912 gastro-jejunostomy was the surgical treatment for congenital pyloric stenosis; the mortality was usually well above 50 per cent. In 1908 Fredet introduced an operation which consisted of splitting the hypertrophied pyloric muscle in a longitudinal fashion, without opening the mucosa, and then suturing the muscle in a transverse direction. This had the great advantage of being an aseptic technique, and the results were definitely better than were the previous ones with gastro-jejunostomy. In 1912 Ramstedt described the operation which is now universally employed in treatment of pyloric stenosis in babies. It consists of splitting the hypertrophied circular muscle longitudinally, but not incising the mucosa. The mucosa is allowed to pout out into the slit in the muscle. No attempt is made to cover over the muscular defect. The obstruction is quickly and completely relieved.

Anesthesia

Morphine should not be given preoperatively, because of its depressant effect on the respiratory system. Atropine should be given, 0.06 mg. subcutaneously. The anesthesia of choice is *ether*, administered by the drop and open-mask method. We have employed this in 99 per cent of our cases, and have found it extremely satisfactory. In no case has there been a death which could possibly be attributed to the anesthetic. We are not unmindful of the fact, however, that the anesthetic care of our cases has been by nurses or doctors whose work is confined wholly to childhood and infancy. It would be unwise to use ether universally for these operations in those communities where anesthetists have not had experience in dealing with babies.

Instead of a general anesthesia, some clinics have routinely employed local *procaine* infiltration of the abdominal wall, possibly combining this with use of a whiskey-and-sugar nipple. In institutions where competent anesthetists are not available, this method is without doubt the preferable one. We have not chosen to adopt it, because the infiltration of the abdominal wall prolongs the operative procedure unnecessarily, the baby might struggle while the abdomen is open, and there is also a slight risk of interfering with the healing of the wound in thin and undernourished subjects.

In a few babies, because of current respiratory disease, we have employed *Avertin* (100 mg. per kilogram of weight) in conjunction with procaine infiltration of the abdominal wall, and the anesthesia was most satisfactory. In a few cases *cyclopropane* anesthesia has been used; it is quite satisfactory, but the explosive hazards make us feel that its use is justified only if the baby has a respiratory infection.

Preparation for Operation

Conservation of body heat during operation, so important for infants, may be accomplished by wrapping the arms and legs with several layers of sheet wadding. At the wrists and ankles this sheet wadding may be pinned down to the operating table so that the extremities will not move into the operative field. A hot-water bottle slipped under the baby's back serves the dual purpose of arching it forward to give a better operative exposure, and also of supplying heat to the patient during operation.

For *gastric deflation*, a No. 10 or 12 French urethral catheter should be passed through the nose or mouth down the esophagus and into the stomach just before operation, so that all fluid and air can be withdrawn. The catheter is left in place during the entire operation so that any gas which appears in the stomach can be aspirated by the anesthetist.

Operative Technique

The *abdominal incision* can take a variety of forms: (1) Formerly it was our custom to use a right rectus, muscle-splitting incision. It gave unexcelled exposure, but was followed by an appreciable number of wound disruptions. It has therefore been completely abandoned. (2) Some operators prefer a longitudinal incision in the anterior rectus fascia, withdrawing the muscle belly laterally, and making a transverse incision in the posterior rectus sheath and peritoneum. (3) It is rather satisfactory to make a longitudinal incision, retracting the muscle belly laterally, and longitudinally opening the posterior sheath and peritoneum. In those rare cases in which some lesion in addition to a pyloric stenosis is suspected, we prefer this approach because it can be made to give a wide exposure and a fairly strong repair. (4) For all routine pyloric cases we have, for more than a decade, employed a right upper quadrant gridiron incision, described by Robertson. It gives an adequate exposure when pyloromyotomy alone is performed; its repair gives a very strong abdominal wall. Our wound problems have completely disappeared since adopting it.

For a *gridiron incision*, an opening about 3 cm. long is made in the skin extending outward from the lateral border of the right rectus muscle and 1 cm. below and parallel to the costal border (Fig. 74). The external oblique muscle is divided in the direction of its fibers, exposing the internal oblique. The fibers of this latter muscle are in turn separated, and the peritoneum and transversalis are opened while keeping them together as a single layer. The thickened pylorus is now drawn up through the wound and can be held just outside the abdominal wall by the assistant's left hand. Examination of the hypertrophied pylorus will now show it to be of firm consistency. Its main *blood supply* swings around from its inferior border; one finds the *superior anterior surface* to be the least vascular part of the entire pyloric ring. It is in this zone of least vascularity that the constricting muscle is to be incised.

The operator can now press the tip of his left index finger up against the duodenal end of the pylorus; this stabilizes the pylorus and it also clearly demarcates the distal extent of the pyloric mass. With a small scalpel (No. 15 Bard-Parker blade), a *longitudinal cut* 10 or 12 mm. in length is made, passing through the serosa and superficial bits of the musculature. From this stage onward the remainder of the muscle may be cut with the scalpel if desired, but it is better to use a blunt instrument because this will readily divide all the gristly and friable fibers of the muscular coat, but will not sever the submucosa. This precaution minimizes the danger of entering the lumen of the gut. Ordinarily, we use the point of a closed hemostat to scrape along and divide the deeper portion of the muscle; the hemostat can then be opened and the points expanded between the edges of the muscle, thus stretching and widening the gap to 4 or 5 mm. If this has been done properly, the muscle will be opened so that a large V-shaped defect presents, but at the same time there will be no tear of the underlying submucosa. Spreading of the muscular ends is continued until the mucosa pouts up to the level of the serosa. It is quite necessary to have the mucosa thus protrude up into the muscular defect to insure an adequate lumen for the pylorus and also to prevent the severed ends of the muscle from reuniting. No attempt is made to cover the pyloric defect with serosa or omental fat.

This procedure is practically bloodless. If there is any oozing from the cut serosa or muscular ends, it can usually be controlled by the application of a warm saline pack for a few minutes. If *bleeding* still persists, it may be necessary to ligate one or two small vessels with fine silk or catgut. In the vast majority of cases no ligatures are necessary. When the operator has satisfied himself that hemostasis is complete, the pylorus is dropped back into the abdomen.

Complications. The outstanding danger in this operative procedure is the possibility of *perforating the mucosa*—an accident which is most likely to occur at the duodenal end of the pylorus. This is due to the fact that the lumen of the gut gradually diminishes in size on the gastric end of the pylorus, but balloons out quite rapidly as it expands into the duodenum (Fig. 71). If the operator hopes to sever all of the muscle in one or two sweeps of a scalpel, he may easily cut into the duodenum where the musculature ends abruptly. Hence, great care must be exercised when working in the duodenal end of the incision. If a duodenum has been accidentally opened, prompt recognition of the error is highly important, because an unchecked escape of duodenal contents will lead to *peritonitis*, whereas immediate closure of the opening will avoid such a catastrophe. Any small opening can be closed with one or two sutures to *invert* the pouting mucosa and possibly to bring serosa over this area; before tying any such stitches, it is well to bring up and include in the sutures a wad of omentum which will help to seal any leak. Whenever a duodenum has been accidentally opened, it is our custom to keep the baby on constant gastric suction for twenty-four hours after operation before starting any feedings.

Closing the Abdomen. The abdomen must be closed with care, if subsequent troubles with the wound are to be avoided. The abdominal wall in most of these patients is only $\frac{1}{8}$ or $\frac{1}{16}$ inch thick, and hence fine sutures are necessary and delicate grasps of tissue must be taken. Routinely, we close the peritoneum and each of the muscle layers with continuous catgut, never larger than 000 chromic. The subcutaneous tissues are approximated with fine interrupted sutures of 000000 Deknatel silk. The skin is not sutured; if a small sterile pad is placed over the wound and adhesive straps are applied, so that the skin is wrinkled up in the wound region, the edges of the skin wound will fall together and be held there in a most satisfactory manner. This dressing should not be taken off or disturbed at the time of hospital discharge (three or four days later); it is left on until the baby is seen on about the tenth day for a check-up. Thus it is not necessary to place or to remove skin sutures; the wound heals nicely.

POSTOPERATIVE CARE

Standard Feeding Regimen

Considerable variation is possible in the treatment after operation. It apparently does not make a great deal of difference what *kind* of fluid or formula is offered for the first day or two; it is very important that the *amounts* which are given should be reasonably small. If large quantities are taken, the baby is all too apt to start a bout of vomiting which merely prolongs convalescence.

In an institution where pyloric cases are frequently seen, it is best to adopt a standard form of postoperative feeding in order that house staff, nurses, and ward attendants may know what is expected in the after-care. For feeding of postoperative pyloric patients it is, of course, possible to use a wide variety of formulas. For the sake of standardization,

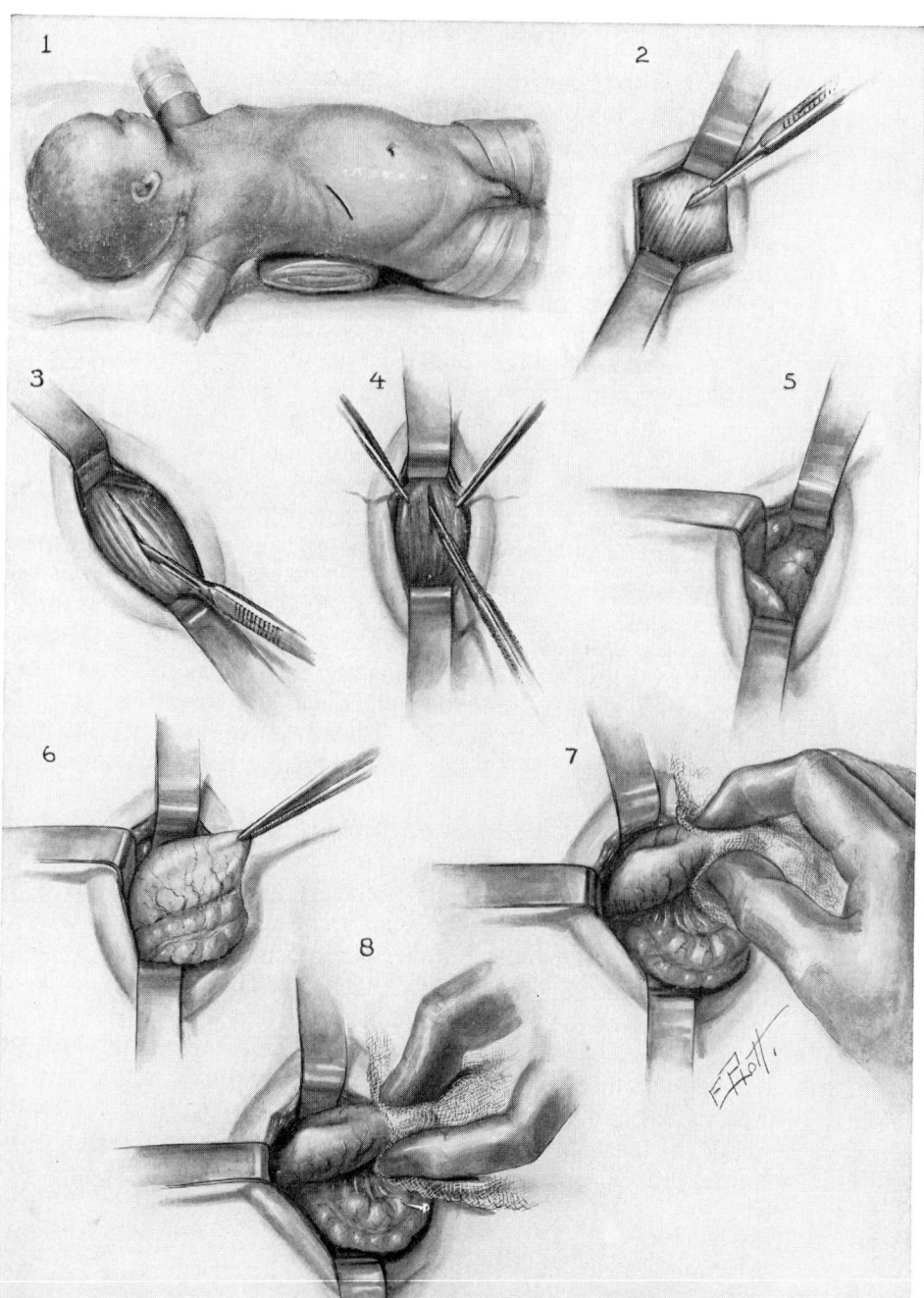

Fig. 74. Ramstedt pyloromyotomy, employing a gridiron incision. 1. To lessen heat loss, arms and legs are wrapped in sheet wadding. Position of oblique skin incision below costal margin. 2. Two retractors (1 cm. wide and 1 cm. deep) in place. Splitting external oblique muscle along direction of its fibers. 3. Retractors shifted. Division of internal oblique muscle (or fascia). 4. Retractors shifted to a transverse direction. Transversalis muscle and peritoneum being opened simultaneously. 5. Retractors placed within abdomen. A third retractor holds the liver edge upward. 6. Antrum of stomach being grasped and withdrawn. 7. Pylorus pulled out through the abdominal wound. 8. Gastric antrum given to assistant, who holds it with his left thumb and forefinger. (*See facing page 141 for illustration of 9.*) 9. Tip of surgeons left forefinger presses against duodenal end of pylorus to stabilize the same and also to point out clearly its termination.

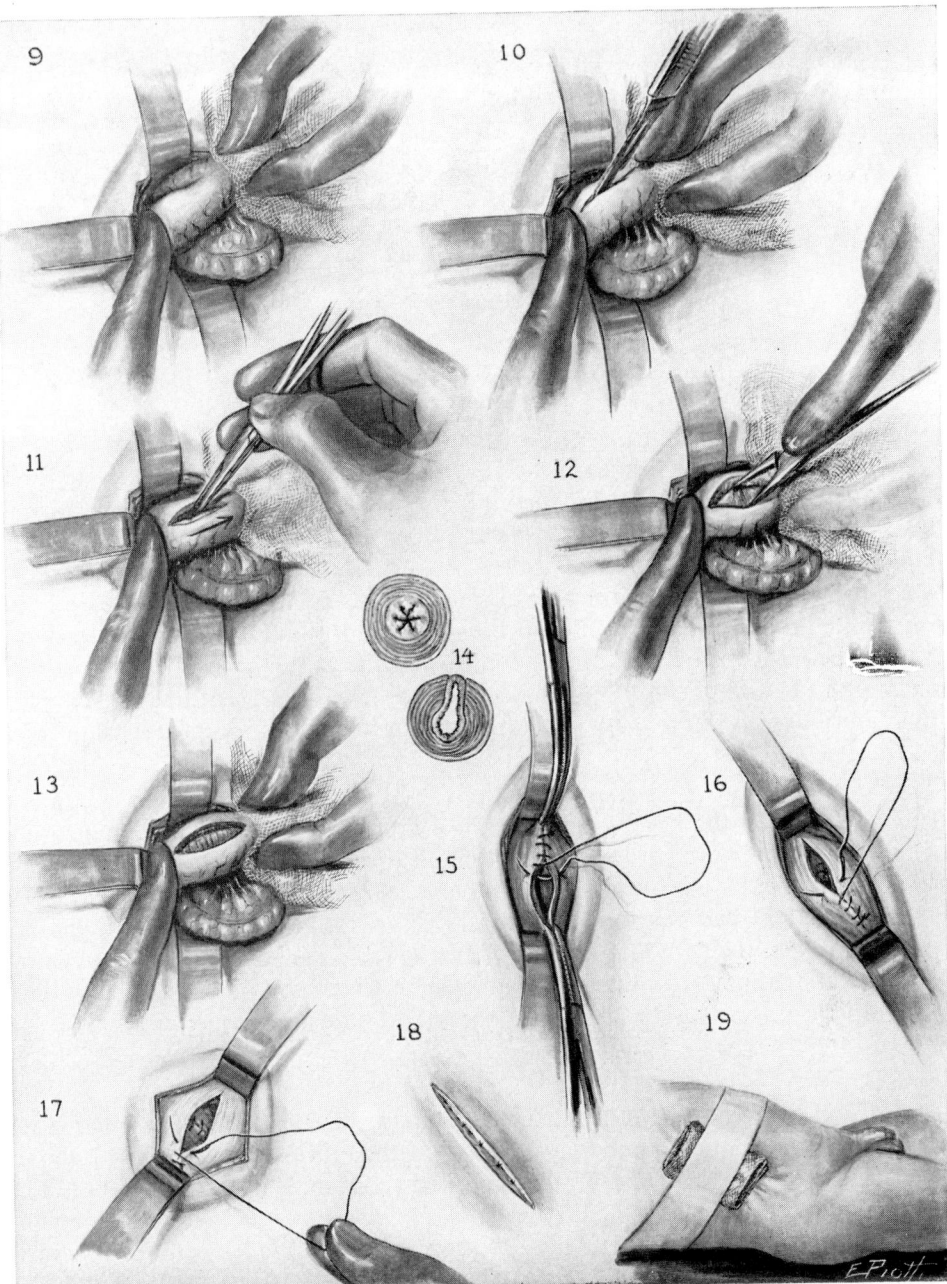

Fig. 74 (*continued—See previous page 140 for description of 9*). 10. Incision being made on *anterior-superior* surface, where the vascularity is minimal. The cut is made only through the serosa and the outer part of the thickened muscle. 11. The point of a closed hemostat scraped along the remaining deep portion of the muscle will sever it, but will not cut the underlying mucosa. 12. Tips of hemostat inserted between severed edges of the muscle; opening the instrument will spread the muscle. 13. Pyloromyotomy completed; the submucosa bulges up between the edges of muscle. 14. Cross-section of a hypertrophied pylorus before operation (*above*) and after operation (*below*); after splitting the muscle the mucosa pouts up through the muscular defect, providing an adequate lumen. 15. Closure of abdominal wall begun; the peritoneum and transversalis muscle are sutured as one layer. 16. Closure of the internal oblique muscle. 17. Closure of the external oblique muscle. 18. Interrupted 000000 silk sutures to the subcutaneous tissues. (No cutaneous sutures will be employed.) The skin edges gape slightly. 19. Adhesive dressing being applied. (By tightening the adhesive tape until the skin is well wrinkled, the cutaneous edges of the wound are brought into apposition.) The upper and lower ends of the gauze will now be covered with additional adhesive.

ease of preparation in the diet kitchen, and reduction of costs, we routinely use an evaporated milk modification* and the following feeding regimen:

BEGINNING 4 HOURS AFTER OPERATION:

1 oz.	5% glucose	every 2 hrs.	3 feedings
1 oz.	formula	every 2 hrs.	till 8 P.M. day after op.
$1\frac{1}{4}$ oz.	formula	every 2 hrs.	6 feedings

BEGINNING SECOND MORNING AFTER OPERATION:

2 oz.	formula	every 3 hrs.	8 feedings

BEGINNING THIRD MORNING AFTER OPERATION:

$3\frac{3}{4}$ oz.	formula	every 4 hrs.	6 feedings

This schedule runs till the morning of the fourth day after operation. Beyond this, orders can be given which take cognizance of the fluid and caloric requirements of the individual baby. The child can generally be discharged from the hospital on the fourth or fifth day.

For a few days after operation there may be occasional vomiting; generally, the feeding schedule should be continued, since it will usually be found that soon all vomiting or regurgitation ceases. In only occasional cases is it necessary to reduce the oral intake to more limited amounts or to build up the intake more gradually. The postoperative feedings are better tolerated for the first few days if the bottle is given while the child is still reclining in bed. After the feeding has been taken, the baby can be picked up and held in an upright position to allow eructation of gas which has collected in the stomach.

Parenteral Fluids

It is obvious that the feeding schedule above outlined gives an inadequate amount of fluid for the first thirty-six or forty-eight hours. Hence, it is usually advisable to supplement the oral intake by use of parenteral fluids. Customarily two intravenous infusions are given on the first and possibly the second postoperative day. Such fluids should be continued as long as the baby shows signs of any dehydration, but generally they may be discontinued after thirty-six hours. For babies who have been in fairly good condition prior to surgery, it is not essential to give parenteral fluids after operation.

RESULTS OF THERAPY

Advance in the treatment of hypertrophic pyloric stenosis can be appreciated when one recalls that at about the time of World War I the *mortality* often ranged above 50 per cent, whereas today there are several published series in which fatalities are less than 1 per cent. There are few other fields of surgical endeavor in which the improvement of results has been so striking. Table 8 lists our mortality rates with operations in various periods from 1915 through 1952.

These operations have been performed by the senior and junior staffs; more recently the vast majority have been done by residents and assistant residents. In the series of 1787 cases there have been 4 infants in whom division of the pyloric muscle was incomplete and a secondary operation had to be resorted to.

Patients who have recovered from the operative procedures have had excellent and lasting relief of symptoms. Our average postoperative period of hospitalization has been reduced to four or five days. Some of these individuals have been followed for as long

---

* Evaporated milk.............. 6 parts
50% Karo (red label type)........ 1 part
Water....................... 8 parts

Table 8

Summary of Results in 1787 Cases of Pyloric Stenosis

Years (Inclusive)	Number of Cases	Deaths	Mortality, Per Cent
1915–1922	125	13	10.4
1923–1928	150	11	7.3
1929–1931	151	3	2.0
1932–1935	162	8	4.9
1936–1939	177	1	0.6
1940–1945	380	4	1.0
1946–1950	490	4	0.8
1951–1952	152	1*	0.6

* This death was in a premature baby who also had been treated for esophageal atresia.

as thirty-five years, and none is known to have any detrimental effect from having the pyloric muscle divided.

A critical review of all cases in the seven-year period 1946 through 1952 discloses the following facts: 642 cases have been treated. There were 5 deaths, giving 0.7 per cent mortality from all causes, including other congenital abnormalities. These 5 died of: peritonitis following omphalocele repair, diarrhea and pneumonia, diarrhea, prematurity and diarrhea, prematurity and complications from esophageal atresia. For babies who had only pyloric stenosis, the mortality rate was 0.3 per cent. In short, over 99 per cent of babies with pyloric stenosis (even when accompanied by other abnormalities or by prematurity) have survived operation and have been completely and promptly relieved of their symptoms.

REFERENCES

1. Akin, J. T., Jr., and Forbes, G. B.: Congenital Hypertrophic Pyloric Stenosis. Surgery, *21*:512, 1947.
2. Baker, R. P. and Sager, W. W.: Congenital Hypertrophic Pyloric Stenosis. A Review of 329 Cases. Clin. Proc. Child. Hosp., *7*:95, 1951.
3. Donovan, E. J.: Congenital Hypertrophic Pyloric Stenosis. Am. J. Surg., *39*:377, 1938.
4. Flynn, J. G.: Hypertrophic Pyloric Stenosis in Infants: A Result of Birth Injury. Texas State J. Med., *37*:367, 1941.
5. Horgan, E.: The Use of a Transverse Abdominal Incision in, and Comments on, the Surgical Treatment of Infantile Pyloric Stenosis. Surgery, *18*:339, 1945.
6. Jacoby, N. M.: Pyloric Stenosis. Selective Medical and Surgical Treatment. Lancet, *247*:748, 1944.
7. Lamson, O. F.: Congenital Hypertrophic Pyloric Stenosis. Treatment of Accidental Perforation of Mucosa during Rammstedt Operation. Surg., Gynec. & Obst., *57*:398, 1933.
8. Maizels, M. and McArthur, C. B.: Cell and Plasma Chloride in the Pyloric Stenosis of Infants. Am. J. Dis. Child., *41*:35, 1931.
9. Schnohr, E.: Chemical Changes in Blood and Tissues in Congenital Hypertrophic Pyloric Stenosis. Acta Paediat., *14*:49, 1932.
10. Wyatt, O. S.: Hypertrophic Pyloric Stenosis; A Review of 100 Cases. Journal-Lancet, *59*:233, 1939.

CHAPTER 10

Peptic Ulcer.   Gastrostomy

PEPTIC ULCER

Incidence

Ulcers of the stomach and duodenum, while admittedly rare, are occasionally the cause of serious or even fatal illness in some children. They can appear at any age and they have been described in stillborn or even premature infants. In a three-week-old baby who died from another condition, we have found a duodenal ulcer which by histologic examination showed evidence of chronicity suggesting that it had been present before birth. Guthrie reported 9 cases of peptic ulcer in children found among 6059 autopsies at the Glasgow Royal Hospital for Sick Children. In 1941 Bird, Limper and Mayer collected 243 cases from the literature, and it is estimated that well over 350 cases of ulcer in childhood have now been recorded. In most of the reported cases, the ulcer was discovered only at autopsy; this would suggest that there is room for improvement in recognizing the condition during life.

Peptic ulcers appear to be somewhat more numerous in infancy than in childhood. As a whole they tend to run a more acute course than they do in adult life, presumably because the more bland diet and the more active regenerative processes of children promote faster healing.

Types of Ulcer

Two types of ulcer are likely to be met: a "primary" type in which the ulcer and its effects comprise the main clinical and pathologic picture, and a "secondary" form in which localized or diffuse ulceration develops (generally as a terminal event) in a child already seriously ill from infection, burn, or intracranial disease. In the latter group are Cushing-Rokitansky and Curling ulcers; they need not concern us here.

Symptoms

An ulcer is relatively asymptomatic in a high percentage of cases, and frequently the lesion is unsuspected until the time of autopsy. It is barely possible that some of the vague abdominal pains and the recurrent alimentary disturbances which are so frequent in childhood may be due to ulcer more often than is now believed. While a "silent" clinical course is the general rule in infancy, the symptoms after the first year or two are usually quite similar to those observed in adult life. *Epigastric distress* which is relieved by eating should suggest the correct diagnosis. *Pain* during the night is particularly common. *Pain* and *vomiting* which appear an hour or two after ingestion of food can result from pylorospasm or from actual mechanical block from scar formation. Peptic ulcers in the young may give rise to: (1) malnutrition and repeated gastric upsets; (2) exsanguinating and even fatal hemorrhage; (3) perforation into the general abdominal cavity; and (4) mechanical obstruction from cicatricial tissue near the pylorus.

In general, severe bleeding or perforation is more common in the infant while obstructive symptoms (from either pylorospasm or scar) are more apt to appear in oldre children. In the *very young*, we have seen perforation in a premature infant only one day of age, and intra-uterine perforation has been described (Lee). Usually the infant has vomited or refused feedings, but it is only when the abdomen is distended and tense that serious abdominal disease is suspected. An x-ray film of the upright abdomen reveals free air under the diaphragm. In two infants we have undertaken laparotomy for control of exsanguinating hemorrhage from a peptic ulcer. In *older children* the disease is more apt to take on a more chronic recurring form resembling that seen in adults.

Medical Treatment

When there are no complications, a cure can be effected in most cases by rest, a modified ulcer regimen with bland diet, antacids, frequent small feedings, and tincture of belladonna with or just before meals. Banthine in appropriate dosage may prove to be of considerable value.

Hemorrhage is apt to be tolerated poorly, and while *transfusions* should not be given too frequently or in too large amounts, the reports of fatalities from bleeding would imply that blood should be administered sooner and more liberally than is the custom with adults.

Surgical Treatment

Perforation carries a very high risk of mortality, and the one hope for survival rests in *surgical closure* of the hole. Plication or excision of the ulcer should never be done because these procedures are almost certain to constrict and obstruct the gut and require a gastroenterostomy—a combination which is productive of great shock in an already seriously ill child. It is better, and it is sufficient, to take three or four sutures which grasp opposite margins of the perforation and then lay a piece of omental fat (free or attached) over the opening. This fat is held in place by the sutures, which are now tied over it. This operation can be quickly completed; it does not constrict the duodenum (or stomach); and it effectively and permanently plugs the hole.

Mechanical obstruction is best treated by a *posterior gastrojejunostomy*. The surgeon should not be tempted to perform any type of resection, for while these have a definite place in the treatment of some adult cases, they are unnecessary in the young. On two occasions we have established gastro-enterostomies for obstructing duodenal ulcer in children. These were both followed by alleviation of pain, by termination of vomiting, and by very satisfactory gains in weight.

Table 9

Form of Ulcer in Various Age Groups
(From Bird, Limper, and Mayer[2])

Age Years	Bleeding	Perforating	Stenosing	Persistently Painful	Totals
0–2	45	33	9	7	94
2–7	10	3	2	5	20
7–12	8	15	18	16	57
12–15	3	26	31	12	72
Totals	66	77	60	40	243

Table 10

Indication for Operation in Infants and Children with Peptic Ulcer
(From Bird, Limper, and Mayer[2])

Age Years	Perforation	Hemorrhage	Obstruction	Persistent Pain	No. of Patients Operated Upon
0–2	8	3	4	—	15
2–7	3	4	1	—	8
7–12	7	2	18	4	31
12–15	25	3	30	7	65
Totals	43	12	53	11	119

Results of Treatment

In the Children's Hospital material 4 children were known positively to have peptic ulcer, and were treated medically. Some data concerning these are listed in Table 11.

Concerning the surgical therapy for peptic ulcer in infants and children, Bird, Limper, and Mayer[2] have made an excellent summary of the literature; this included a study of 119 patients in whom some operative procedure had been carried out. In the cases treated in the first two years of life, the mortality rate was 70 per cent—a figure dependent not only upon the very young age of the patients, but also upon the more serious form of the complications. In children beyond the second year, the total mortality following operation was 5 per cent. Bird, Limper, and Mayer reported the youngest case with successful operation—a $34\frac{1}{2}$-hour old baby with perforation of a duodenal ulcer. At the Boston Children's Hospital there have been (between 1930 and 1952) 8 patients treated surgically for primary peptic ulcer; data concerning these are shown in Table 12.

GASTROSTOMY

Indications

Gastrostomy is an operation which must occasionally be performed on infants and children, the indications usually being some form of mechanical obstruction above the cardia of the stomach.

It is frequent practice to establish a temporary gastrostomy during an operative repair of an *abnormality of the esophagus*. While primary anastomosis is a very satisfactory treatment for esophageal atresia, and can be performed in many instances without establishment of a gastrostomy, it is our general policy to establish a temporary gastrostomy for feeding for some weeks to allow the most perfect healing of the esophageal union. Although such a gastrostomy can be done a day or two after the esophageal operation, we now usually establish it at the same time since it seldom requires more than an additional fifteen or twenty minutes.

A common esophageal obstruction in childhood is that resulting from *lye burns*. The great majority of these can be adequately treated by dilation from above, the dilator being passed along a string guide (see Chapter 7). In the more severe burns, the esophageal scarring interferes greatly with the child's nutrition and the lumen of the esophagus may be so small that dilation cannot be safely performed when one is working solely through the mouth. In such instances a gastrostomy has a definite place in the thera-

Table 11

Cases of Peptic Ulcer at Children's Hospital Treated Medically

Case	Age	Sex	Chief Symptoms	Ulcer Site	Result
1	1 day	M	Hematemesis Melena	Duodenum	Excellent
2	26 days	M	Vomiting Marasmus	Duodenum	Died. Autopsy: Chronic duodenal ulcer
3	2½ mos.	F	Vomiting Marasmus Melena	Stomach	Died. Autopsy: Perforated gastric ulcer
4	9 yrs.	M	Hemorrhage	Duodenum	Excellent

peutic regimen: first, to provide a route by which food can be given; second, to establish an avenue for retrograde dilation of the esophagus.

Operative Technique

A number of methods for constructing a gastrostomy have been described. We have now completely abandoned the Janeway procedure, the Witzel technique, and all other methods in favor of the Stamm gastrostomy.

By the *Stamm technique* an opening is made in the anterior surface of the stomach and a catheter is thrust into it, which is then held in place by a circular silk suture which

Table 12

Peptic Ulcer at Children's Hospital Treated Surgically

Case	Age	Sex	Indication for Surgery	Operation	Ulcer Site	Result
1	2 days (premature)	M	Perforation and hemorrhage	Suture of Perforation	Duodenum	Died 3rd postop. day
2	5 wks.	M	Hemorrhage	Laparotomy	Duodenum	Died 2nd postop. day
3	9 mos.	M	Stenosis	Gastro-jejunostomy	Duodenum	Good
4	14 mos.	M	Hemorrhage	Transduodenal suture of bleeder	Duodenum	Excellent
5	15 mos.	M	Hemorrhage	Laparotomy	Duodenum	Excellent
6	17 mos.	M	Perforation	Suture of perforation	Duodenum	Excellent
7	9 yrs.	M	Hemorrhage	Laparotomy	Duodenum	Excellent
8	11 yrs.	M	Stenosis	Gastro-jejunostomy	Duodenum	Excellent

infolds the gastric wall (Fig. 75). When this suture has been tightened, another is taken to turn the wall in farther. The stomach should always be anchored to the anterior abdominal wall. For babies, a No. 12 or 14 French catheter is amply large. For older

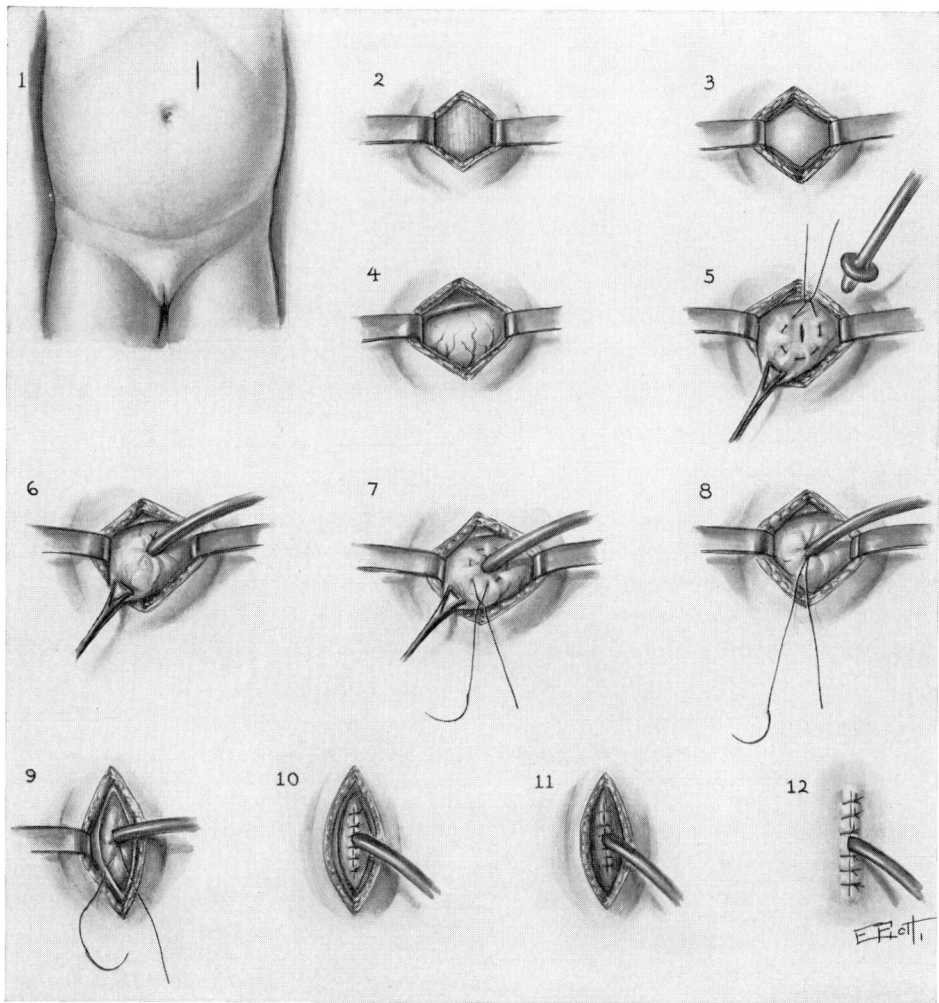

Fig. 75. Method of establishment of a Stamm gastrostomy. 1. Position of the short incision, midway between the medial and lateral borders of the rectus muscle. 2. Anterior rectus fascia exposed. 3. Anterior rectus fascia opened and rectus muscle split, exposing posterior rectus sheath. 4. Peritoneum opening, exposing liver edge and greater curvature of stomach. 5. Stomach pulled out through wound with Babcock clamp. Purse-string suture of silk placed. Stomach punctured. Mushroom catheter about to be inserted. 6. Catheter in stomach, purse-string suture tied up. 7. Second purse-string of silk placed. 8. Second purse-string tied up. 9. End of the purse-string stitch carried through parietal peritoneum, for anchoring stomach to the anterior abdominal wall. 10. Peritoneum closed around catheter. 11. Rectus muscle closed. 12. Skin approximated.

children, larger tubes are generally required. If the opening in the abdominal wall is kept very short, it will be necessary to place but a few stitches in it; for newborn babies, the incision need not be more than 1.5 cm. long. Keeping the wound very short virtually abolishes the complications of wound disruption and evisceration.

After-care

A small dry dressing should be placed around the gastrostomy tube to absorb any moisture and to keep the skin from macerating. If the tube has been placed snugly enough in the stomach, there will be no leakage around it. If a gastrostomy has been correctly performed and if the dressings have been adequate, there is rarely any erosion of the abdominal skin.

When it is desired to close such a gastrostomy, the tube can be withdrawn and the sinus tract will generally close spontaneously. Certainly in those where the tube has not been unduly large and the opening has been present for only a month or two, the opening will close promptly by itself. When a catheter of very large size has been used, and in some patients in whom the gastrostomy has been of such long standing that gastric mucosa has grown out through the tract, it might be necessary to stitch the opening to gain permanent closure.

REFERENCES

1. Beattie, J. W. and Bohan, K. E.: Perforation of Gastric Ulcer in Premature Newborn with Operation and Survival. American Surgeon, *18*:1146, 1952.
2. Bird, C. E., Limper, M. A. and Mayer, J. M.: Surgery in Peptic Ulceration of Stomach and Duodenum in Infants and Children. Ann. Surg., *114*:526, 1941.
3. Bloch, L. and Serby, A. M.: Peptic Ulcer in Children: Follow-Up Study of Cases Reported Previously and Report of Additional Cases. Am. J. Digest. Dis. *4*:15, 1937.
4. Brockington, C. F. and Lightwood, R.: Duodenal Ulceration in Infants. An Account of Two Cases. Lancet, *2*:1209, 1932.
5. Clyne, D. G. W. and Rabinowitch, J.: Four Cases of Duodenal Ulceration in Children Simulating Appendicitis. Arch. Dis. Child., *17*:102, 1942.
6. Fisher, J. H.: Duodenal Ulcers in Infants. Am. J. Dis. Child., *79*:50, 1950.
7. Guthrie, N. J.: Peptic Ulcer in Infancy and Childhood with a Review of the Literature. Arch. Dis. Child., *17*:82, 1942.
8. Hunter, W. and Dryerre, H. W.: Duodenal Ulceration in Newborn. Brit. M. J., *2*:15, 1939.
9. Kunstadter, R. H. and Gettelman, E.: Gastric Ulcer with Fatal Hemorrhage in Newborn. J.A.M.A., *106*:207, 1936.
10. Miller, R. A.: Observations on the Gastric Acidity During the First Year of Life. Arch. Dis. Child., *17*:198, 1942.
11. Palmer, D. W.: Duodenal Ulcer in Infancy. Ann. Surg., *73*:545, 1921.
12. Tashiro K. and Kobayashi, N.: Duodenal Ulcer in Infancy and Childhood. Am. J. Surg., *29*:379, 1935.
13. Theile, P.: Beitrag zur Kenntnis der Gerschwürsbildungen des Magens und Duodenum im Kindesalter. Deutsche Ztschr. f. Chir., *150*:275, 1919.

CHAPTER 11

Congenital Atresia of the Intestine and Colon

Congenital atresia of the intestine and colon is an uncommon malformation in which there is complete obstruction of the alimentary tract. It rapidly produces vomiting, severe dehydration, starvation, and possibly rupture of the blind intestine. If no surgical relief is given, death supervenes in most cases in the first week of life, but a few patients have lived to the age of ten or twelve days. Surgical therapy is followed by high mortality, but an increasing number of successfully treated cases are appearing in the literature. Prompt recognition of the obstruction and immediate operation give the only hope of survival.

It is incorrect to speak of "partial atresia" or "complete atresia" because the term *atresia* itself means a complete block. To describe constriction with narrowing of a lumen, the term *stenosis* is appropriate.

The first successful surgical treatment for an intestinal atresia was by Fockens in 1911. The following chapter is based almost entirely on experiences from the surgical management of 140 cases at the Boston Children's Hospital. Portions of this material have been published on several previous occasions.

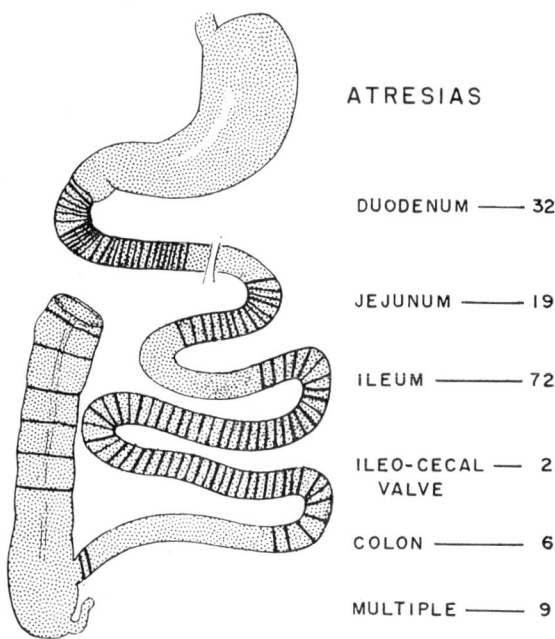

ATRESIAS

DUODENUM ——— 32

JEJUNUM ——— 19

ILEUM ——— 72

ILEO-CECAL — 2
VALVE

COLON ——— 6

MULTIPLE ——— 9

Fig. 76. Diagram showing position of atresias in 140 cases.

Page 150

EMBRYOLOGY

Most of the relevant embryologic events take place between the fifth and tenth weeks of fetal life. Prior to the fifth week the intestine presents a well defined lumen lined with epithelium. Soon after this the epithelium rapidly proliferates, and the lumen of the intestine from the pylorus to the ileo-cecal valve becomes obliterated by epithelial concrescences. Thus, the formerly patent intestine now passes through a *solid stage* for a short period. Later, vacuoles appear among these epithelial cells and a coalescence of the cystic spaces reestablishes the intestinal lumen by the twelfth week. It is well known that such a solid stage normally exists in the human intestine, but there is some question concerning the presence, extent, and duration of a solid stage in the colon.

An arrest in development during the second or third month of fetal life results in either *atresia* or *stenosis* of the intestine. A stenosis arises if the hollow tube is reformed, but fails to attain a normal diameter. An atresia occurs if there is a persistence of one of the septa. If, during its solid stage, the intestine becomes pinched off, an atresia results in which there is discontinuity of the two intestinal limbs.

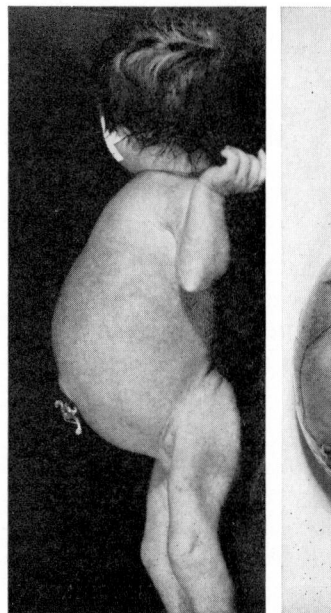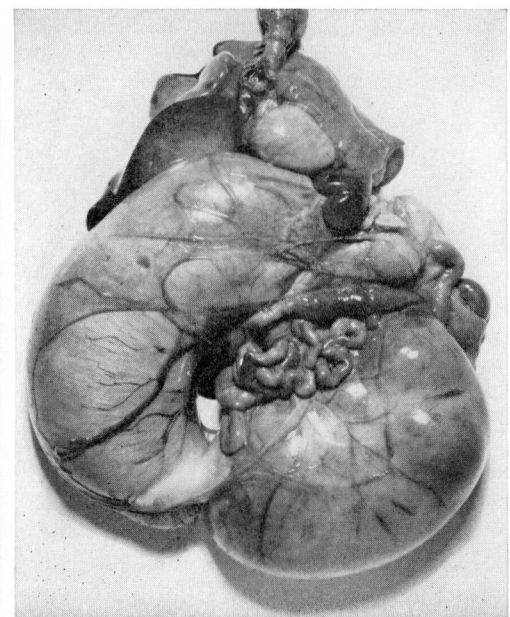

Fig. 77. Seven-day old child who entered hospital in extremis and was found to have atresia of distal duodenum. *Left,* Showing the marked distention, which came solely from the stomach and duodenum. *Right,* Autopsy specimen. Above and to the left is a greatly dilated stomach. Below and to the right is a huge duodenum. In center of specimen, note the tiny, collapsed intestines.

PATHOLOGY

Intestinal atresia may be found in two forms. In the first variety, there is an internal *diaphragm* or *veil* which completely blocks the lumen (Fig. 83). In the other, the intestine ends as a *blind sac* and there is a discontinuity of the bowel (Fig. 78); the distended proximal segment may be detached from the collapsed distal loop, or else the two may be joined by a thread-like fibrous band. In some cases there may be several atresias; the isolated, blind segments of intestine—joined to one another by tiny threads—give the appearance of a miniature string of sausages.

Proximal to the obstruction, the intestine is tensely dilated and the obstructed loops

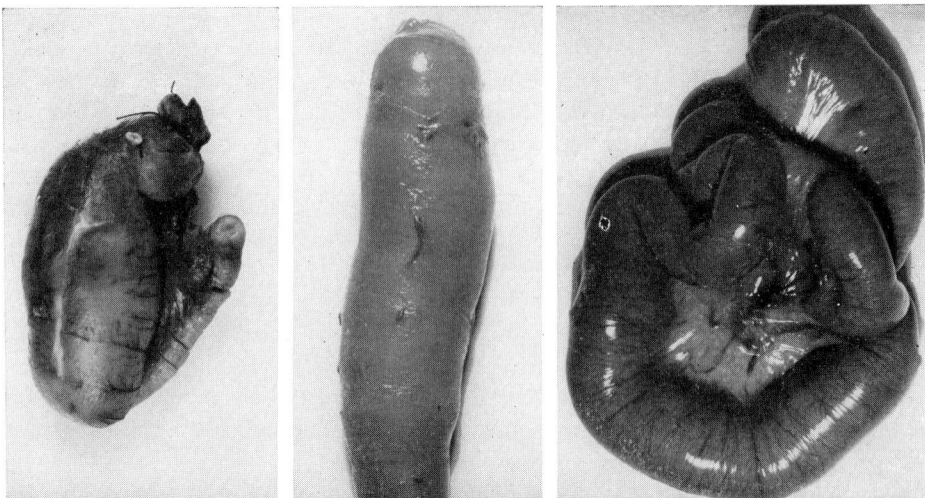

Fig. 78. Three specimens from babies with intestinal atresia. The blind end of gut is at upper part of each photograph. *Left*, Jejunal atresia, 6-day old baby. *Middle*, Atresia of mid-ileum, 3-day old boy. *Right*, Atresia of terminal ileum, 4-day old girl.

may be 3 or 4 cm. in diameter. This degree of distention in a newly born baby greatly thins the intestinal wall and leads to local ischemia. Necrosis and perforation of the bowel are therefore imminent dangers in any baby with intestinal atresia which has not been relieved by the third day of life.

Distal to the obstruction, the intestine is very small, contains no gas, and has within its lumen only small amounts of mucus and cellular detritus which have been cast off from the lower intestinal mucosa. This collapsed intestine usually measures no more than 4 to 6 mm. in diameter and a collapsed colon is not much larger.

The Meconium in Intestinal Atresia

The meconium stool from a normal child is composed of: (1) Dead cells from the intestinal lining; (2) various secretions from the stomach, intestine, liver, and pancreas; (3) material from the amniotic fluid which is swallowed by the baby *in utero*. One of the constituents of amniotic fluid, noted as long ago as 1861 by Jacobi, is the *vernix caseosa*— squamous epithelium desquamated from the fetus's skin. The meconium of a normal baby, therefore, contains many of these cornified cells which have passed through its intestinal tract. It is obvious that an atresia of the intestine or colon will not allow them to pass beyond the obstructed point.

Farber's Test. Farber called attention to the above facts and devised a simple test whereby the meconium of a baby can be quickly examined and the presence or absence of swallowed vernix cells can be rapidly determined. A specimen of meconium is obtained, care being taken that it comes from the center of the stool, and is smeared on a glass slide. This is covered for about one minute with Sterling's gentian violet. It is washed with running water and decolorized with acid alcohol. This decoloration removes dye from all of the specimen except the cornified epithelial cells. In any newly born child with intestinal obstruction, the absence of cornified epithelial cells in the meconium is presumptive evidence that an intestinal or colonic atresia exists, whereas the finding of such cells in appreciable numbers suggests that the obstruction is only partial (intestinal stenosis, or else obstruction from extrinsic pressure). False positive tests can easily occur by contaminating the stool with material scraped from the skin of the peri-anal area. If care is used to insure that the specimen studied comes from a representative (central) portion of the stool, this test is of considerable aid in establishing the correct preoperative diagnosis.

CLINICAL FINDINGS

Babies with intestinal or colonic atresia have symptoms on the first day of life. During or after nursing there is *vomiting* which becomes progressively more frequent and more intense as subsequent feedings are taken. Intestinal atresia above the papilla of Vater is very rare; hence the vomitus from most patients with atresia almost always contains bile. The character of the vomitus will depend somewhat upon the level of the obstruction; if it is high, the material will be curdled milk or thin yellowish fluid, whereas a low obstruction will produce vomitus which is malodorous and which is fecal in appearance. Any baby who continues to vomit during the first day or two of life while being fed a normal amount of breast milk or a reasonable formula should be investigated by roentgenographic means, searching for intestinal obstruction.

The character and size of the *stools* are of some importance in making the diagnosis of intestinal atresia in a newborn child, but they can be misleading. Usually the stools are smaller in amount, drier in consistency, and grayish green in color rather than having the tarry appearance of normal meconium. However, in some instances the stools may resemble normal meconium very closely in gross appearance. The failure to find cornified epithelial cells in the first forty-eight hours of life (or the failure to find milk curds at a later date) is of great significance.

Abdominal distention may or may not be present, depending upon the level of the atresia and the length of time the patient has gone untreated. If the obstruction is duodenal, distention will be limited to the epigastrium or indeed may be absent if the stomach has been emptied by repeated vomiting. If the atresia is in the jejunum or at a lower level, abdominal distention may be marked and generalized. The time at which distention appears is variable. In some cases it has been noticed by the obstetrician at birth, the baby presumably having swallowed enough amniotic fluid to dilate the intestine down to the point of obstruction. In other cases the distention does not appear until the child is twenty-four to forty-eight hours old, depending upon how much milk has been ingested and how effective vomiting has been in emptying the alimentary tract. In some babies, particularly those beyond three or four days of age, the abdomen may be enormously distended because the stomach or intestine has ruptured and has allowed air or fluid to escape into the peritoneal cavity.

When there is duodenal blockage, *peristaltic* (gastric) *waves* may be seen crossing the epigastrium from left to right or (duodenal) they may course downward in the right upper quadrant. If the obstruction is jejunal, ileal, or colonic, intestinal patterning may be seen over any portion of the abdominal wall.

Fever is a not uncommon finding. Some degree of it can be caused by dehydration alone. If the temperature is above 102° or 103° F., the possibility of intestinal rupture and peritonitis must be thought of.

ROENTGENOLOGIC EXAMINATION

If these babies are carefully observed during the first twenty-four to forty-eight hours of life, the clinical findings are usually sufficient to make the correct diagnosis, or certainly to suggest it. However, roentgenologic studies will give confirmatory evidence of obstruction, and in some cases will help to localize the site of the lesion. *Films of the* abdomen, without the use of contrast media, will give all the important information in most cases. Markedly dilated duodenum or distended loops of small intestine are usually sufficient to make a correct diagnosis. One does not see the speckled or granular-appearing material which is so apt to be found in babies with meconium ileus. If the clinical course and the x-ray findings together suggest strongly an obstruction, operation should be undertaken without further attempt to localize the actual level of the block.

Use of Barium

The administration of barium to these babies is not without some risk, because the material can become inspissated and clog the intestinal tract; furthermore, there is always the possibility of aspirating any barium which might be vomited. If barium is given,

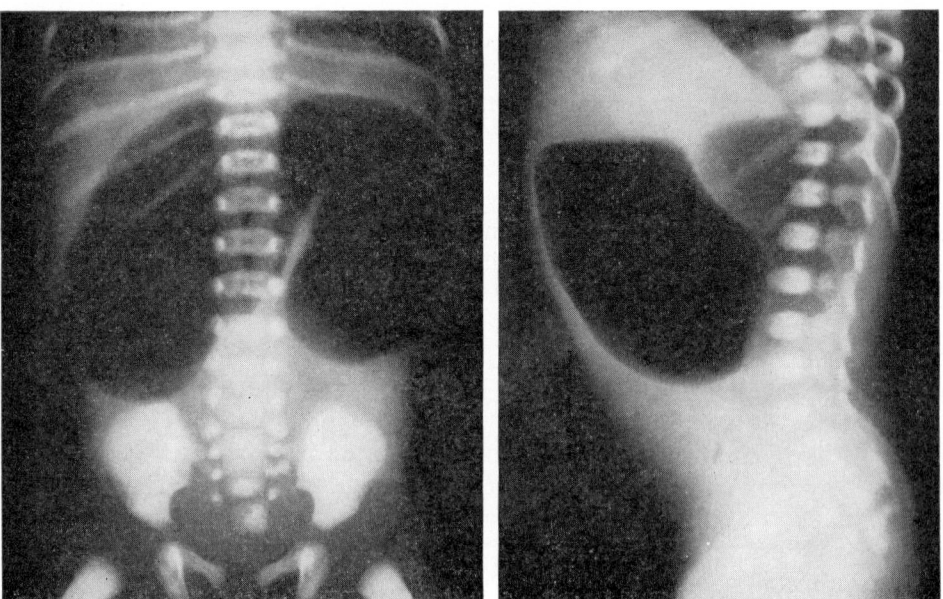

Fig. 79. Roentgenograms of a newborn baby with atresia of the duodenum. Tremendous gaseous distention of the stomach and duodenum; no gas in intestine beyond this.

only a thin mixture should be employed. Furthermore, after completion of the examination, a gastric tube (small urethral catheter) should be inserted into the stomach and as much barium as possible be removed by gastric lavage.

In Figure 80 the findings are well illustrated from a case of atresia in the *third portion of the duodenum*. The ballooned-out duodenum is almost as large as the stomach and no barium or gas bubbles are seen in the intestines beyond. With obstructions lower in the *jejunum*, two or three loops of distended bowel are seen. With atresia of the *ileum*, multiple loops are distended with gas or fluid. It is generally impossible to differentiate between a low ileal and a colonic obstruction by x-ray films.

Because of the marked distention in most of these subjects (examples of which appear in Figs. 81 and 82), the use of a barium enema to determine the *patency of the colon* only adds to the great discomfort and distress of the baby. Even if an obstruction in the colon were demonstrated by this means, it would not alter the operative exposure in any way, hence this examination should seldom be employed when abdominal distention is present.

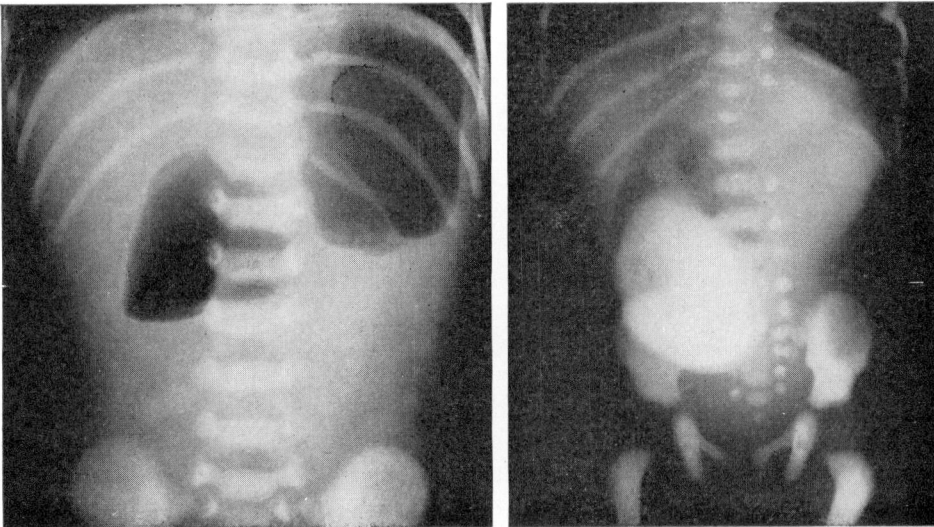

Fig. 80. Roentgenograms from a five-day old baby with atresia of the duodenum. *Left*, Plain film, upright position. *Right*, Film after ingestion of barium. There is no gas or barium beyond the duodenum.

If a child has already been treated with ileostomy for temporary relief of obstruction, and decompression has thus been accomplished, a *barium enema* examination may give valuable information in determining the size and continuity of the colon. If the lower bowel is thus found to be patent but small, the ileostomy may be closed and an anastomotic procedure established with a feeling of certainty that the bowel below the anastomosis can function.

The *presence of fluid* within the abdominal cavity can be suspected from x-ray films in some individuals, when there are opaque areas between adjacent loops of bowel. Such findings do not necessarily mean perforation and peritonitis; a large amount of fluid can be poured out from serous surfaces of obstructed intestine.

When there has been rupture of the intestine before birth, and a sealing over of the same, the sterile peritonitis thus set up can sometimes be recognized by the small, calcified deposits which are scattered throughout the abdomen.

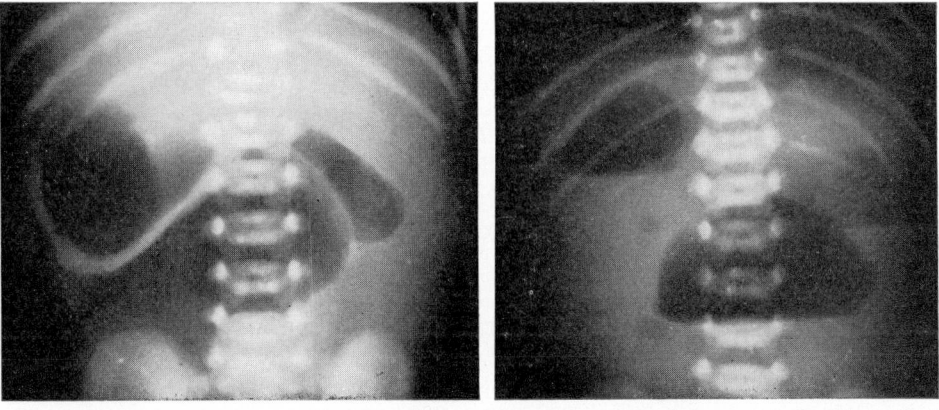

Fig. 81. Roentgenograms from a newborn baby with atresia of the jejunum. *Left*, Film with baby lying down. *Right*, Film with child in upright position.

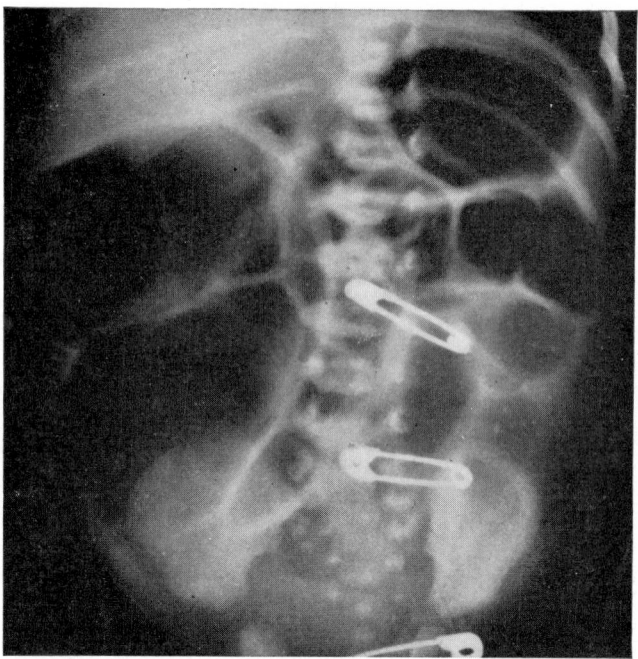

Fig. 82. Film from four-day old baby with atresia of mid-ileum, showing extensive and marked gaseous distention.

TREATMENT

Babies with atresia of the intestinal tract will die if left untreated; they seldom survive for more than a week without surgical relief. Usually perforation and fatal peritonitis will supervene if the intestine is not decompressed in some manner by the third or fourth day. However, some infants who are not operated upon until the sixth or seventh day will have only impending necrosis, without actual disruption of the intestine.

The mortality for operative procedures is extremely high, and successfully treated cases are still rarities in the medical literature. However, it is becoming evident that earlier recognition of the anomaly and properly performed surgical therapy are giving an increasing number of survivors. Surgery should always be undertaken, no matter how desperate the condition of the child might seem. Appropriate preoperative measures can increase the chances of successful issue.

Preoperative Measures

Prior to operation, an *inlying gastric tube* should be inserted to deflate the stomach. A No. 8 F or 10 F soft rubber urethral catheter, with extra holes cut in it, makes a satisfactory tube. Gastric suction or lavage will prevent vomiting and pulmonary aspiration, an important consideration; chest complications are frequently the cause of death in these babies.

Preoperative treatment includes liberal administration of *parenteral fluids* which may be given as 10 per cent glucose intravenously (10 cc. per pound of body weight) and as physiologic saline subcutaneously (15 cc. per pound of body weight). If preferred, the fluids can all be given through a cannula or plastic tube inserted by "cut-down" into an ankle vein. Vitamin K should be given to avoid the possibility of bleeding due to hemorrhagic disease of the newborn.

When placed on the operating table, the baby's arms and legs should be wrapped with sheet wadding to *conserve body heat*, and a hot-water bottle should be placed under the back to supply heat and reduce shock.

Anesthesia

We have routinely used drop *ether* with an open mask, feeling that this gives better relaxation and exposure. *Cyclopropane*, with a closed system, has been very satisfactory when there has been available an anesthetist who had experience in giving this to small babies. When dealing with very small infants (under 5 pounds) we have sometimes preferred local anesthesia, infiltrating the appropriate portion of the abdominal wall with 2 per cent procaine. The baby can be made somewhat stuporous by the ingestion of brandy, using a mixture of one part brandy and three parts 10 per cent glucose. Ten or 15 cc. of this mixture can be introduced into the inlying gastric tube; if necessary this can be repeated in twenty to twenty-five minutes.

Exposure

A long right rectus incision, 3 or 4 inches in length, with its midpoint opposite the umbilicus, retracting the muscle laterally, will give exposure to any part of the intestinal tract. On opening the abdomen there is always some free peritoneal fluid. As much as

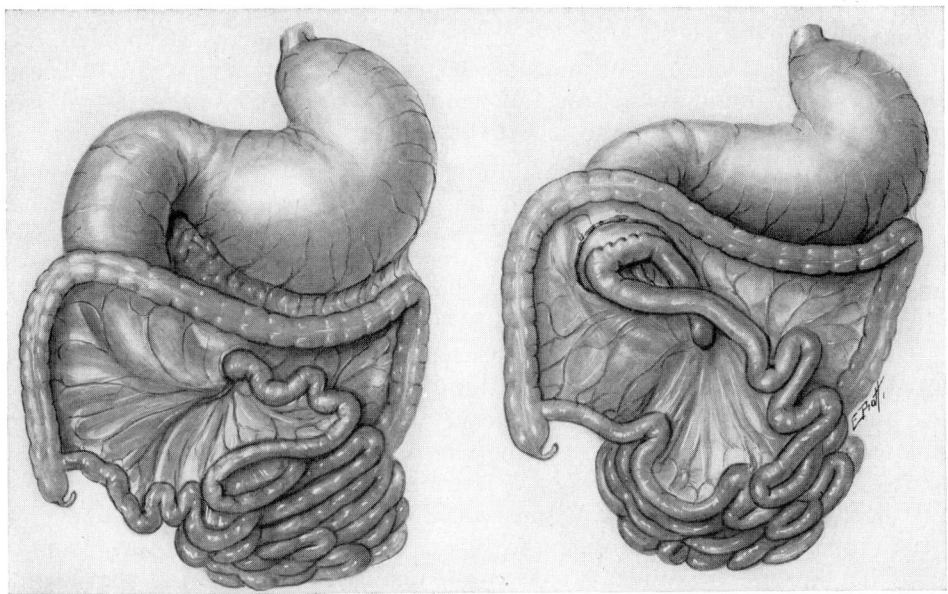

Fig. 83. Operative findings and treatment in a case of *atresia of the third part of the duodenum.* *Left*, Marked distention of the stomach and duodenum. *Right*, Treatment by retrocolic duodeno-iejunostomy.

several hundred cubic centimeters of this clear, yellowish material can be found. If the fluid is cloudy or malodorous, a perforation of the gut must at once be suspected and sought for.

Intestines proximal to the point of obstruction will be found greatly dilated and will usually extrude themselves through the abdominal wound. These loops may be as much as 3 or 4 cm. in diameter; they are very tense and they must be carefully handled for fear of rupture. The intestines below the obstruction are collapsed, and are generally not more than 3 to 5 mm. in diameter. They contain no gas and by the time operation is performed usually little or no meconium can be palpated within their lumina.

Multiple Atresias

The finding of one atresia, above which the intestine is distended, should never be accepted as representing *all* of the pathologic abnormality present in the abdomen. Multiple atresias occur in a small but important percentage of cases so that a search should always be made with this possibility in mind. This need not be disturbing to the child and it does not require more than a few moments. The intestine can be rapidly inspected from the known atresia down to the ileo-cecal valve; only in this way can the operator be sure that the alimentary tube can be functional below any anastomosis which is made. Statistically, it is exceedingly rare for an atresia to appear in the colon if one exists in the small intestine, hence it is our practice to avoid extensive inspection and manipulation of the colon, except in its most accessible parts. Whenever several atresias are found in the small intestine, a point for the anastomosis must be selected in the distal loop which is beyond the lowermost block. If there are several isolated, collapsed, sausage-like bits of bowel, these may be resected, but if the child is in a precarious state, it is sometimes better to leave them in place and to remove them subsequently if they give trouble (in the way of cyst formation).

Other Types of Abnormalities

It is well to make a cursory inspection for other abnormalities which might require correction, such as a defect of the mesentery or an error of intestinal rotation. The latter is not infrequently found as an associated anomaly (6 per cent of our cases); it *must* be corrected at the same operation to relieve the baby of all obstruction.

Selection of Type of Operation

We are firmly convinced that it is unwise to make a direct attack on those atresias which have the form of a single veil or diaphragm obstructing the alimentary tube. It is very tempting to believe that the intestine can be opened above or below this block, that the diaphragm can be cut out, and that the obstruction can thereby be relieved. A few cases have been treated successfully in this manner, but one usually finds these local attacks unsatisfactory because it is impossible to cut away all the obstructing membrane or else the intestinal wall at the circumference of the diaphragm is fibrous and nondistensible. Much valuable time is lost in these local endeavors which usually end up unsatisfactorily or disastrously. *Therefore, it is always better judgment to leave the atresia strictly alone and to circumvent it by some appropriate anastomotic procedure.*

For the higher atresias—those in the duodenum or jejunum—there can be no question but that direct anastomosis, by side-to-side union of a structure just above with one just below the block, gives the best chance of survival. When dealing with atresias of the ileum, ileo-cecal valve, or colon there is room for debate regarding the best method of approach to the problem. In the early work of Ladd in this field, some enterostomies were made, were allowed to remain open for protracted periods, and led to such disastrous consequences in the way of fluid and electrolyte loss, inanition, etc. that he developed a feeling they should never be used in the treatment of atresias; he believed that primary anastomosis was the treatment of choice regardless of the level of the atresia. In recent years we have developed a viewpoint which differs from this; statistics show that primary anastomoses have been quite successful in treatment of the high blocks (duodenum or jejunum), but that they have been followed by exorbitant mortality rates when used for ileal atresias. We have therefore been exploring the possibility of treating ileal or colonic atresia by a Mikulicz type of exteriorization of the two blind ends, leaving the enterostomy open only a week or two before closing it. While adequate statistics are not yet available to prove, or disprove, the merits of this procedure, the results to date have been encouraging and have been better than we have been able to obtain by direct anastomoses.

When treating duodenal or jejunal atresias, *gastro-enterostomies should be avoided* whenever possible. In his early work, Ladd employed some of these but often found that some food would pass the pylorus and churn back and forth in the blind duodenum. This produced anorexia, nausea, and abdominal discomfort, which could be relieved only by secondary operations in which duodeno-jejunostomies were established. The two situations demanding a gastrojejunostomy are: (1) Those very rare lesions in which the atresia is in the first part of the duodenum. (2) For those babies who are quite premature and have such small parts that the performance of a duodeno-jejunostomy is

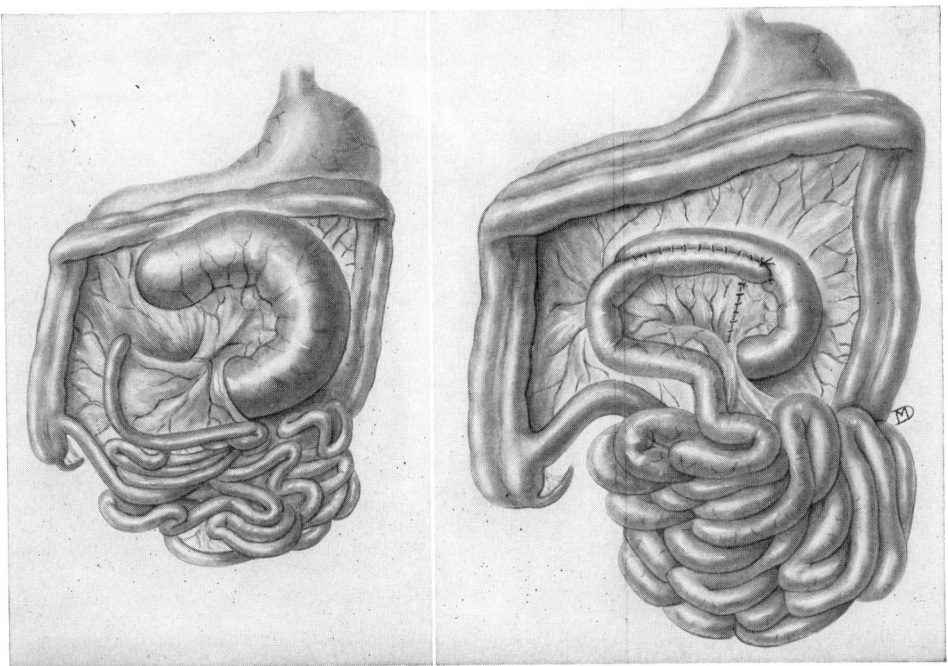

Fig. 84. Operative findings and treatment in a case with *jejunal atresia. Left,* Anatomic data The jejunum ends blindly and is not connected with the lower segment of bowel. Jejunum greatly distended; ileum and colon collapsed. *Right,* Surgical treatment by side-to-side isoperistaltic jejuno-ileostomy. Ileal loops and colon enlarge in a few days after establishment of such an anastomosis.

exceedingly difficult. (From 1940 through 1952, in 40 cases of atresias of the duodenum or jejunum, we have performed gastrojejunostomy but once.) In short, *isoperistaltic duodeno-jejunostomy is the treatment of choice for atresias of the duodenum or high jejunum.*

Establishment of a Side-to-Side Anastomosis

The great disparity in size of loops which are to be joined presents one of the most difficult features of operation. It is well to inflate the collapsed distal bowel by injection into it of 3 to 5 cc. of mineral oil and several cubic centimeters of air. This material will not only distend the segment which is to be used for the anastomosis, but will percolate down through the tiny lower intestine and begin to open it up. If the proximal loop is very distended, it is best to collapse it by aspiration. The use of aseptic types of anastomoses, such as the Parker-Kerr technique, is not practical with intestines so small. Since the suture of intestines of diminutive size cannot be completed satisfactorily by end-to-end union, a side-to-side anastomosis should always be used in these small infants.

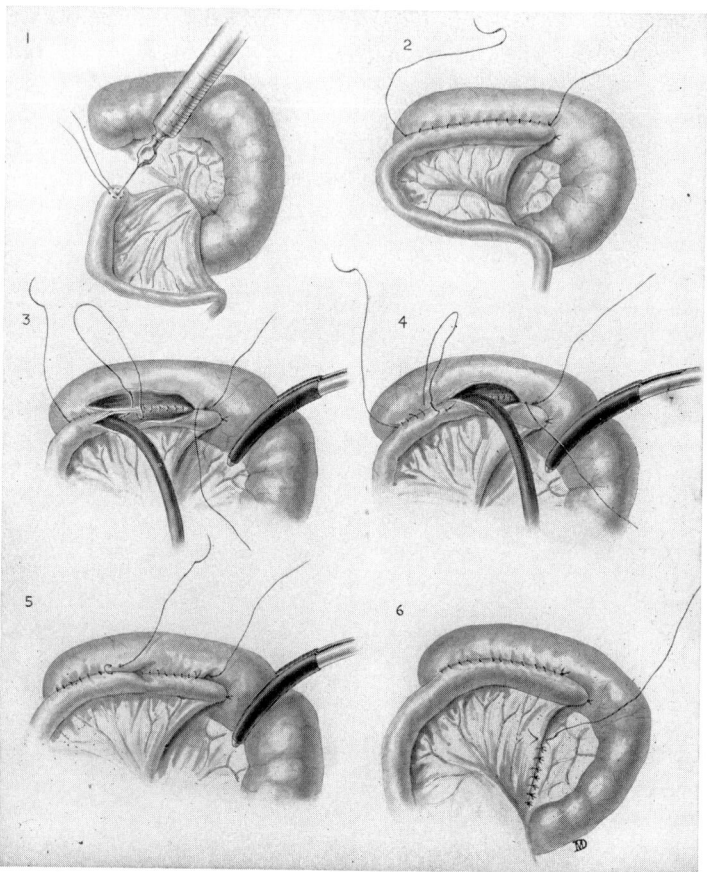

Fig. 85. Details of operative steps in side-to-side anastomosis for atresia of *jejunum* or *upper ileum*. 1. Dilated proximal and collapsed distal loops end blindly. The latter is being distended with mineral oil and air. 2. First line of suture with 00000 silk on an atraumatic needle (such as an eye suture or blood vessel suture). 3. Rubber-covered clamp on proximal loop to prevent peristaltic rushes. Loops opened. Continuous over-and-over stitch of fine atraumatic silk or chromic catgut (0000). Catheter in distal loop to help define the edge and to prevent constriction of tiny intestine when corner is rounded with inner layer of suture. 4. Inner suture being continued anteriorly as a Connell stitch. 5. Inner row complete. Outer continuous row being placed. Anastomosis completed. Mesenteric defect being closed.

A lateral anastomosis can always be made in two layers (Fig. 85); a continuous *00000 silk* suture on a small atraumatic needle is best suited for the external layer. The inner layer may be performed with a *0000 chromic catgut* on an atraumatic needle, the type used for ureteral sutures serving well for this purpose. The inner catgut layer is taken as an over-and-over stitch on the posterior row, and is continued anteriorly as a *Connell* stitch. Great delicacy must be used in the suture of such intestines, because the distal loop is extremely small and the proximal loop is apt to be thin and friable. Very small forceps must be used; a small hemostat serves best for a needle-holder. No clamp need be applied across the distal intestine; it is unnecessary and is too apt to injure the bowel. If the proximal loop is free (as in the ileum or the lower jejunum), an intestinal clamp can be used on it to minimize soiling during the open phase of the anastomosis.

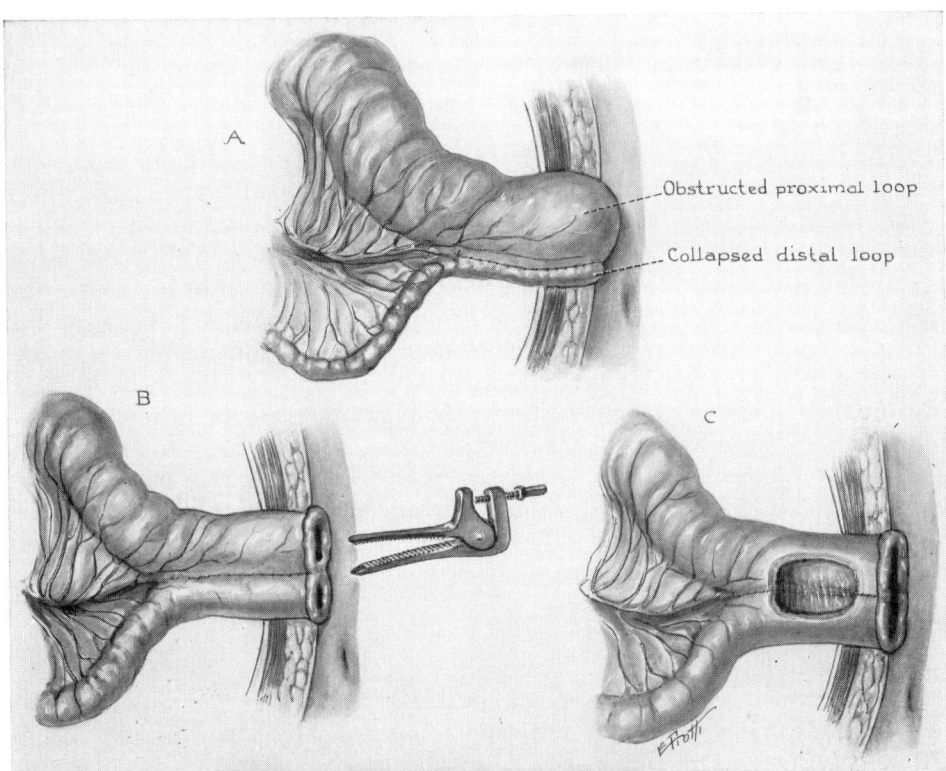

Fig. 86. Aseptic treatment of atresia in distal half of ileum by the exteriorization method. A, The two blind loops are sewed together and brought out through the abdominal wall. Both limbs will be opened as soon as the abdominal wound is closed. B, The upper and lower loops have been opened. This decompresses the proximal intestine. Intermittent introduction of fluids into the distal loop distends it. After four or five days, the small crushing clamp (manufactured by Codman and Shurtleff, Inc.) can be inserted, as indicated, to crush down the septum between the two limbs. C, The septum has been cut down and the single stoma is now ready for closure (extraperitoneally) within one or two weeks.

Exteriorization Operation

From a theoretical point of view, exteriorization of the blind ends, after sewing the proximal and distal loops together, has certain advantages: (1) It is a completely aseptic procedure. (2) It diminishes the length of the operation. (3) It gives quicker relief of the intestinal obstruction. (4) It permits the gradual introduction of material into the distal loop so that it can be properly distended before turning a fecal stream into it. (5) It avoids the danger of leakage which sometimes follows primary anastomoses in tiny intestines.

In the treatment of atresias by the exteriorization method, the two limbs must be sewed together so that no other loop of intestine can get between them before the crushing clamp is applied. This union should be made with fine silk stitches, preferably but not necessarily interrupted. It is usually not possible to insert two parallel rows of sutures (to make a broad surface on which a crushing clamp can later be placed); the distal loop is so small that only a single row of stitches can be inserted. As the loops are drawn out through the abdominal wall wound, they should be anchored around their periphery to the peritoneal edges by interrupted black silk sutures; at the time of subsequent closure of the enterostomy the dissection can be carried down *to* these sutures and the peritoneal cavity need not be entered. After the abdominal wound is completely closed, the proximal loop can be opened and the intestine decompressed at once. The distal loop can be opened and from time to time fluids injected into it so that it will assume a normal caliber.

Exteriorization procedures have certain disadvantages, but these can be minimized. The child should not be allowed to languish and lose intestinal fluid indefinitely. Within a few days after operation, a small crushing clamp can be applied in the two spurs so that they can be made into a common lumen. Care must be taken to cut down the spurs sufficiently far. The depth of the septum between the two limbs must be accurately estimated before attempting to close the enterostomy; if the septum is not low enough, it must be cut down further by another application of the crushing clamp. It is usually possible to close the stoma in a week or two.

At the time of closing the enterostomy, the presenting portion of intestine is freed down to the peritoneal level, and the intestinal end then turned in in an appropriate fashion. It is not difficult to do this if the stoma has been present for more than two or three weeks. If closure is attempted within a week or ten days after the initial operation, the two limbs are apt to be only lightly stuck together and hence must be handled very carefully for fear of tearing them apart.

Postoperative Treatment

Treatment following operation demands a great deal of patience, attention, and supportive care. The *stomach* should be repeatedly washed out or should be *aspirated* by constant suction as long as any bile-stained material is recovered from it. The *colon* should be *dilated* with saline or soap suds enemas two or three times per day. *Chemotherapy* is important in most cases for combating pneumonitis which these patients commonly have. *Feedings* must not be started until there is reasonable assurance that they will not induce vomiting. They should be in very small amounts ($\frac{1}{2}$ ounce every three to four hours), and not stepped up until it is known that these trial amounts are well tolerated. It is impossible to set schedules which will be applicable to all patients; the feeding regimens must be individualized, carefully supervised, and slowly built up. *Parenteral fluids* two or three times per twenty-four hours must be given for some days to maintain the fluid balance. A *transfusion* of citrated blood will be required immediately during or after operation to prevent shock. Thereafter, transfusions of blood or plasma should be given as often as is necessary to maintain the red blood count and the plasma protein at normal levels.

RESULTS OF THERAPY

To review the results of operative treatment for intestinal atresia is discouraging because the failures have been numerous. However, it is necessary to study the results of various forms of therapy to evaluate the different methods and to lay the basis for improving the results in the future. Data from the Children's Hospital surgical cases are summarized in Table 13. The fatalities did not all occur in the hospital; several of them followed one to several months later, but the nature of the child's course or the terminal

Table 13

Results of Operative Treatment in 140 Cases of Intestinal or Colonic Atresia

Site of Atresia	Up to 1940		1940 through 1952	
	Alive	Dead	Alive	Dead
Duodenum.....................	1	4	15*	12
Jejunum........................	3	3	5	8
Ileum..........................	3	31	21	17
Ileo-cecal Valve.................	0	2	0	0
Colon..........................	0	2	2	2
Multiple Atresias.................	0	3	4	2
Totals.........................	7	45	47†	41

* Two of these are Mongols.
† From 1940 through 1952, recoveries were 53 per cent. (In 1952 there were 17 cases of atresia at all levels; 12 survived, a recovery of 70 per cent.)

illness suggested that the intestinal tract was not functioning normally and that this disturbance was largely responsible for the death. Therefore these have all been listed as deaths from atresia.

Site of Atresia

The level of an atresia has little bearing on the prognosis. A review of our material (Table 13), especially in the 1940 to 1952 series, shows about the same proportion of survivals and fatalities in atresias at various levels of the alimentary tract. However, in the survivors there does seem to be an important difference in the postoperative course which bears some relation to the level at which there had been an atresia. Those who had an atresia in the duodenum or jejunum usually recovered from operation quite promptly and had a smooth course thereafter. In contrast, a few of those who had atresia in the lower intestinal tract had long-continued disturbances, such as poor nutrition, feeding difficulties, and bouts of partial obstruction, which have almost certainly been related to intestinal adhesions. Presumably, operations for the lower atresias are more prone, for a variety of reasons, to be followed by the development of adhesions. Before chemotherapy and antibiotics were available, these adhesions were generally ascribed to bacterial contamination of the peritoneal cavity during open operations, but we doubt if the incidence of adhesions has been reduced appreciably since the introduction of antibiotics. Furthermore, we have been troubled by adhesions—in spite of the greatest care in trying to prevent them—in some of the patients who had completely aseptic operations by the Mikulicz method of anastomosis.

Causes of Death

In a small minority of our cases, fatality was caused by some other important anomaly such as congenital heart disease. In a few cases there was peritonitis from rup-

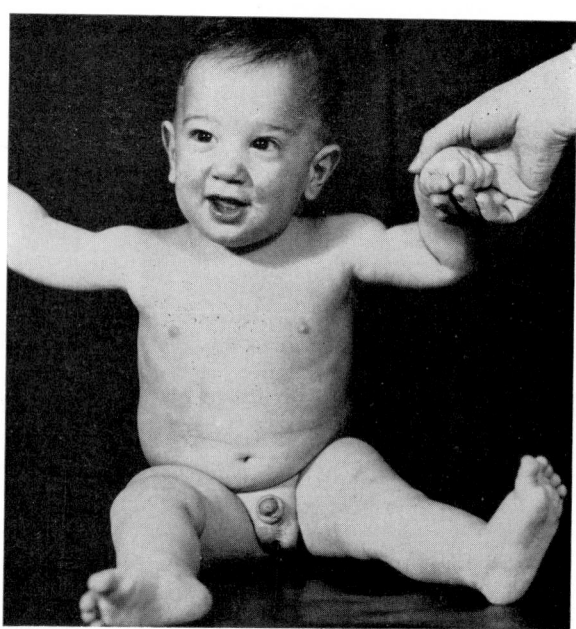

Fig. 87. Photograph of child one year after treatment of a duodenal atresia by duodeno-jejunostomy.
(The baby weighed 2 pounds, 15 ounces at the time of operation.)

ture of intestine prior to hospitalization, which progressed in spite of surgical closure of the leak and administration of supportive chemotherapy. A few of the earlier deaths were in patients treated by ileostomies which were left open for extended times; death came from dehydration, inanition, and gradual wasting. In more recent years, enterostomies have not been followed by these disastrous complications because the electrolytic and fluid balances have been better controlled and the openings have been closed within a week or two. The chief cause of fatality after treatment of intestinal atresia is obstruction from peritoneal adhesions; this complication has been responsible for about three-fourths of our failures.

Mongolism

Atresias of the colon or lower intestine do not seem to be accompanied by central nervous system disturbances; the survivors have had good mental development. However, a significant percentage of subjects with duodenal atresia have survived operation and it has later been found that they are Mongols. Presumably, there was in fetal life some arrest which simultaneously interfered with the normal development of the duodenum and also of the brain. Two of our survivors are Mongols. This disappointing fact makes it apparent that all babies with duodenal atresia should be carefully evaluated before undertaking any surgery.

Over-all Results

The Boston Children's Hospital material is summarized in Table 13. From 1940 through 1952 there were 88 cases, with 47 babies relieved of obstruction and with reconstruction of the continuity of the alimentary tract; this is a recovery rate of 53 per cent.

In the period 1940 through 1952, the ileal atresias treated by Mikulicz double enterostomy (or entero-colostomy) showed 14 survivals and 6 deaths, while those treated by primary anastomosis gave 7 survivals and 11 deaths. These figures would seem to be distinctly in favor of the exteriorizing procedures for the ileal obstructions. The soundness of this principle is made all the more evident by picking out the figures for 1952 (which are included in the above statistics). There were 7 cases of ileal atresia, all treated by exteriorizing procedures; there were 6 survivors and 1 death. (The death occurred in a child who also had an omphalocele, which greatly complicated the therapy.)

In 1952 we treated 17 babies with atresia, at all levels of the intestine; 12 of them survived, a recovery rate of 70 per cent.

END RESULTS IN INTRINSIC CONGENITAL INTESTINAL OBSTRUCTION (ATRESIA AND STENOSIS)

In subjects with obstruction of the jejunum, ileum, or colon, there is usually no difficulty in determining at the operating table whether the blockage is partial or complete. Should the intestine below the obstruction contain any gas, the lesion obviously must be a stenosis. But a stenosis of the duodenum or intestine may have a pin-point opening; the gut beyond may be quite collapsed and the operator led to believe that the obstruction has been a complete one. We have made this mistake on several occasions, and have found at subsequent autopsy that a small opening actually existed. Therefore, there is some justification for not making too sharp a line of demarcation between the atresias and the stenoses. For some discussions, it is probably better to group the two conditions together as *intrinsic obstruction* of the intestine. Table 14 lists the end results in our 211 cases of intrinsic obstruction, which includes the atresias considered in this chapter and the stenoses discussed in the following chapter.

Table 14

Operative Results in 211 Cases of Intrinsic Obstruction (Atresia or Stenosis) of the Intestine or Colon

Site of Atresia or Stenosis	Up to 1940		1940 through 1952	
	Alive	Dead	Alive	Dead
Duodenum......................	8	8	36*	19
Jejunum........................	4	4	6	10
Ileum..........................	5	36	29	21
Ileo-cecal Valve.................	0	3	1	4
Colon..........................	0	3	2	2
Multiple........................	0	3	4	3
Totals.........................	17	57	78†	59

* Seven of these are Mongols.

† From 1940 through 1952, recoveries were 57 per cent. (In 1952 there were 19 cases of atresia or stenosis with 13 recoveries, 68 per cent.)

REFERENCES

1. Bolling, R. W.: Complete Congenital Obstruction of the Duodenum, Duodenoiejunostomy at Nine Days. Ann. Surg., *83:*543, 1926.
2. Demmer, F.: Atresia Ilei. Resectio ileocoecalis Heilung. Arch. f. klin. Chir., *147:*471, 1927.
3. Donovan, E. J.: Congenital Atresia of the Duodenum in the Newborn. Ann. Surg., *103:*455, 1936.
4. Ernst, N. P.: A Case of Congenital Atresia of the Duodenum Treated Successfully by Operation. Brit. M. J., *1:*644, 1916.
5. Evans, C. H.: Surgery in the Newborn. J. M. Soc. New Jersey, *45:*471, 1948.
6. Evans, C. H.: Atresias of the Gastrointestinal Tract. Internat. Abstr. Surg., *92:*1, 1951.
7. Farber, S.: Congenital Atresia of the Alimentary Tract: Diagnosis by Microscopic Examination of Meconium. J.A.M.A., *100:*1753, 1933.
8. Fockens, P.: Ein operativ geheilter Fall von kongenitaler Dünndarmatresie. Zentralbl. f. Chir., *38:*532, 1911.
9. Glover, D. M. and Barry, F. McA.: Intestinal Obstruction in the Newborn. Ann. Surg., *130:*480, 1949.
10. Ladd, W. E.: Congenital Obstruction of the Duodenum in Children. New England J. Med., *206:*277, 1932.
11. Ladd, W. E.: Congenital Obstruction of the Small Intestine. J.A.M.A., *101:*1453, 1933.
12. Ladd, W. E.: Surgical Diseases of the Alimentary Tract in Infants. New England J. Med., *215:*705, 1936.
13. Ladd, W. E.: Congenital Duodenal Obstruction. Surgery, *1:*878, 1937.
14. McConahay, H. A.: Congenital Micro-colon Associated with Multiple Small Intestine Stenoses and Atresias. Nebraska M. J., *30:*237, 1945.
15. McIntosh, R. and Donovan, E. J.: Disturbances of Rotation of the Intestinal Tract; Clinical Picture Based on Observations in 20 Cases. Am. J. Dis. Child., *57:*116, 1939.
16. Miller, E. M.: Bowel Obstruction in the New Born. Ann. Surg., *110:*587, 1939.
17. Morton, J. J. and Jones, T. B.: Obstructions about the Mesentery in Infants. Ann. Surg., *104:*864, 1936.
18. Neuhauser, E. B. D.: The Roentgen Diagnosis of Fetal Meconium Peritonitis. Am. J. Roentgen., *51:*421, 1944.
19. Sweet, G. B. and Robertson, C.: A Case of Congenital Atresia of the Jejunum (with Recovery). Arch. Dis. Childhood, *2:*186, 1927.
20. Webb, C. H. and Wangensteen, O. H.: Congenital Intestinal Atresia. Am. J. Dis. Child., *41:*262, 1931.
21. Weeks, A. and Delprat, G. D.: Congenital Intestinal Obstruction: Atresia of Jejunum. Report of Two Cases. S. Clin. North America, *7:*1193, 1927.

CHAPTER 12

Congenital Stenosis of the Intestine and Colon

Congenital stenosis of the intestinal tract presumably arises in the same manner as does an atresia, the process of local obliteration being less complete. From some points of view it can be grouped with and discussed with the atresias, classifying them both as "intrinsic obstructions," but it seems wiser to set them apart because of very real differences in prognosis. Many reports in the literature give rise to confusion because authors have not carefully differentiated between intestinal atresia and intestinal stenosis. A close scrutiny of some published cases of "successfully treated atresia" makes plain the fact that what is listed as atresia often is actually a stenosis.

Marked stenoses give symptoms and demand treatment in the first week or two of life; fatality rates are apt to be high. Less marked constrictions do not show up until later infancy or even childhood years; surgical correction carries an excellent outlook. Our material includes 71 patients who have been operated upon for treatment of a stenosis.

EMBRYOLOGY

In the preceding chapter on atresias of the intestine it was noted that the intestinal tube passed through a *solid stage* at one time during its embryologic development. The epithelial concrescences which give rise to this solid form subsequently disappear in the normal embryo. If, however, there is an *incomplete reduction* from the solid stage, a diaphragm of tissue remains which may be perforated in only one small point. Such an obstructing lesion may appear at any level from the pylorus to the rectum.

PATHOLOGY

Stenoses are much more common in the duodenum than elsewhere; about half of our patients had a duodenal obstruction while one-quarter of them had an ileal lesion (Fig. 88).

At the *narrowed zone* the intestinal lumen is of variable size. In many cases the opening is little more than 2 or 3 mm. in diameter, and will barely admit a probe. The aperture may be larger, and in a few specimens there is only a slight constriction of the bowel. (A small proportion of duodenal stenoses are accompanied by an annular pancreas, which surrounds the duodenum at the stenotic area, as described more fully in Chapter 15.) *Microscopic examination* of the narrowed zone shows heaped-up mucosa and submucosal tissues which may be supported by accessory smooth muscle and irregularly distributed, excess connective tissue in all layers. In those stenoses with only a slight narrowing of the intestine, microscopic examination of a longitudinal section may show little more than increased fibrous tissue in the submucosa or muscularis.

Page 167

Above the obstruction the intestinal tube is always dilated to some degree. If the stenosed area has a very small diameter, the proximal intestine is markedly distended (Figs. 89 and 90). When the stenosis is in the second or third part of the duodenum, the duodenum above may be almost as large as the stomach, and the pylorus is apt to be

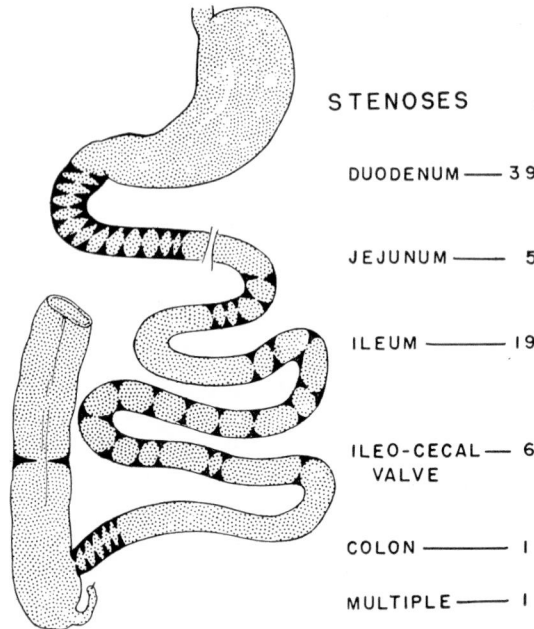

STENOSES

DUODENUM —— 39

JEJUNUM —— 5

ILEUM ———— 19

ILEO-CECAL — 6
VALVE

COLON ———— I

MULTIPLE —— I

Fig. 88. Sketch showing positions of stenoses of intestinal tract in 71 patients.

quite patulous. While the distention in some of these cases may be marked, we have never encountered rupture of the gut such as is seen occasionally in cases of atresia. In only one patient have we encountered multiple stenoses.

SYMPTOMS AND SIGNS

Age Incidence

The ages at which our patients were hospitalized are as follows:

First week of life	31 cases
Second week	12 "
Third week	7 "
One month to one year	13 "
One year to nine years	8 "
Total	71 cases

Symptoms in Young Babies

About half of the patients, being only a week or two of age, have clinical findings which are difficult or impossible to distinguish from those of intestinal atresia. The most marked complaint is *persistent vomiting*. Since the obstruction is generally below the ampulla of Vater, the vomitus contains bile. *Abdominal distention* is present if the obstruction is low, but it is limited to the epigastrium when the obstruction is in the jejunum or duodenum. Generally the *stools* are diminished in number and size. In some individuals the stools contain milk curds, indicating an incomplete type of obstruction. *Loss of weight* or failure to gain is common.

Symptoms in Late Cases

While symptoms in the above-described group are severe enough to bring babies to the hospital in the first week or two of life, the remaining half of patients with intestinal stenosis do not appear until a later age. A small group are first seen in the third or fourth week, and in these the frequency of *vomiting* and the degree of *dehydration* are not as great as in those babies who are hospitalized earlier. The *stools* in these babies may be scanty, and of course they do contain some milk curds; the infants are apt to be brought in to a medical service for "regulation of feeding," or for other study to determine the nature of their trouble, which is seldom apparent at first examination.

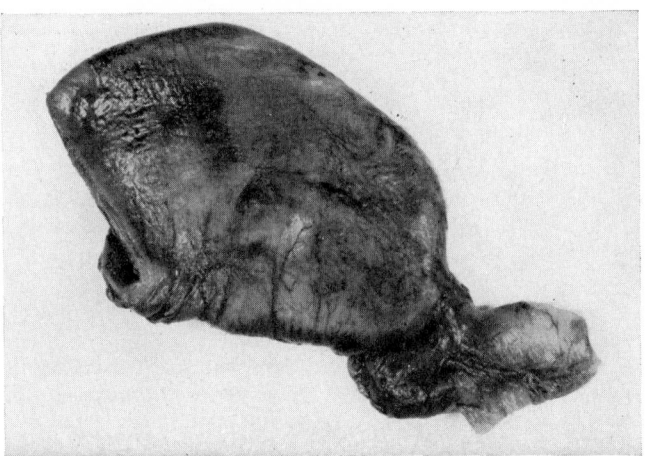

Fig. 89. Segment resected from mid-ileum of two-day old girl, showing stenosis which had produced high degree of obstruction.

About a third of our patients with stenosis were initially hospitalized after the first month of life. The symptoms were so mild that some patients had gone for months or even years with only occasional vomiting, intermittent abdominal pain, or retarded gain in weight. These older subjects are apt to have symptoms which are vague and hence are often treated for long periods by change of diets, administration of laxatives, or by use of atropine compounds before it is evident that an organic abnormality is present.

Physical Findings

The physical findings vary with the age of the individual and with the degree of constriction. If the obstruction is at a high level, *distention* of the epigastrium or of the right upper quadrant may be obvious, and a dilated duodenum can usually be palpated if it has not been deflated by repeated vomiting. *Peristaltic* waves may pass downward in the right upper quadrant. When the obstruction is in the lower jejunum or ileum, large dilated loops may give rather general distention and visible peristalsis in any part of the abdomen. In babies coming to the physician's attention in the first week of life, the obstructions are usually of a severe grade, the physical findings are striking, and dehydration is advanced. This is in contrast to those patients who have their initial symptoms in later months or years and in whom the physical findings are apt to be minimal.

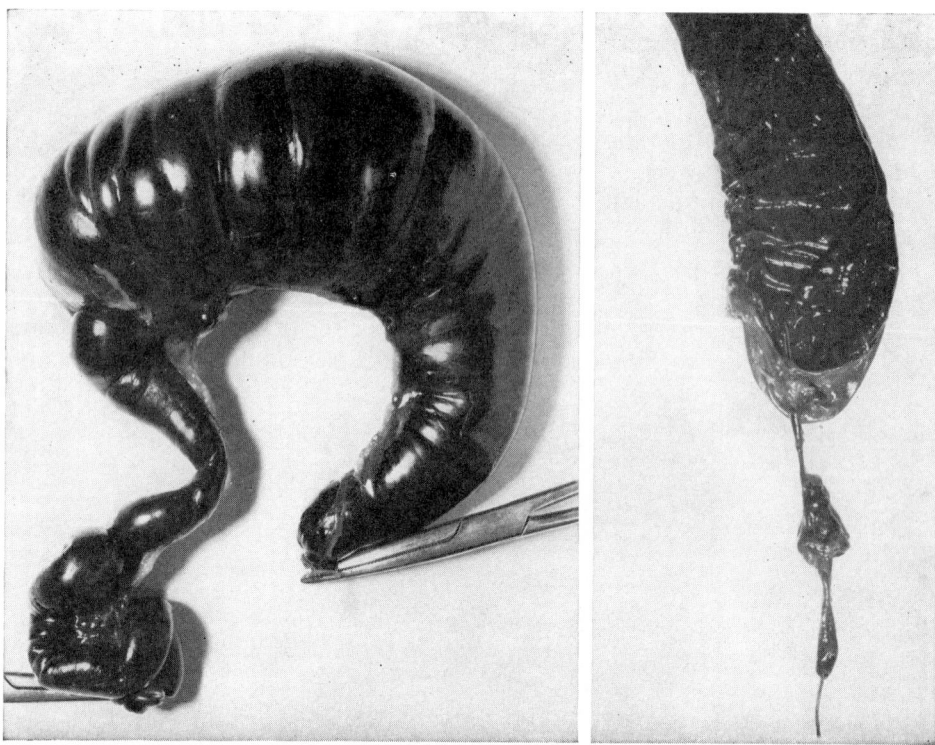

Fig. 90. Segment resected from a three-day old boy; stenosis of distal ileum. The entire segment was gangrenous because it had prolapsed through a hole in the mesentery. *Left*, Exterior view of the specimen. *Right*, Specimen opened, to show the narrowed zone which would barely admit a hairpin.

ROENTGENOLOGIC EXAMINATION

In all cases there is roentgenologic evidence of dilated intestine above the point of obstruction. A *film* of the abdomen without the use of contrast media may give all the information which is required. Proximal to the block, the duodenum or other portion of intestine is greatly dilated. If such observations are made, no further roentgenologic examination need be done and operation can be resorted to at once.

Use of Barium

If there is any question about the presence of obstruction, a thin barium mixture should be fed. Typical findings are illustrated in Figures 91 and 92; the duodenum or intestine is greatly distended and only a few flecks of barium pass into the intestine beyond. The ingestion of barium is not without danger, and one of our patients suddenly died twelve hours after such an examination. Postmortem examination showed no demonstrable cause of death; there was no evidence of aspiration. Presumably, a greatly dilated stomach and duodenum either pressed on the inferior vena cava, or else set up reflex mechanisms which in some way disturbed the cardiovascular apparatus. If barium is given and an obstruction demonstrated, as much barium as possible should be retrieved from the stomach by gastric lavage.

TREATMENT

Dehydration and ketosis should be combated adequately before operation is started.

The upper intestinal tract should be deflated to facilitate the operative procedure and to prevent vomiting and aspiration.

Operative Technique

Exposure of the Intestine. For all of these cases a right rectus, muscle-retracting incision is preferable. It gives adequate exposure, and it can be extended upward or downward without difficulty if conditions require it.

Dilation or Plastic Reconstruction of the Stenotic Region. Often it is very tempting to try dilation of the stenotic area, or else to cut longitudinally across it and sew up this defect in a transverse manner. While some of these local attacks are successful, generally they are ineffectual and disappointing. It is best to avoid them completely.

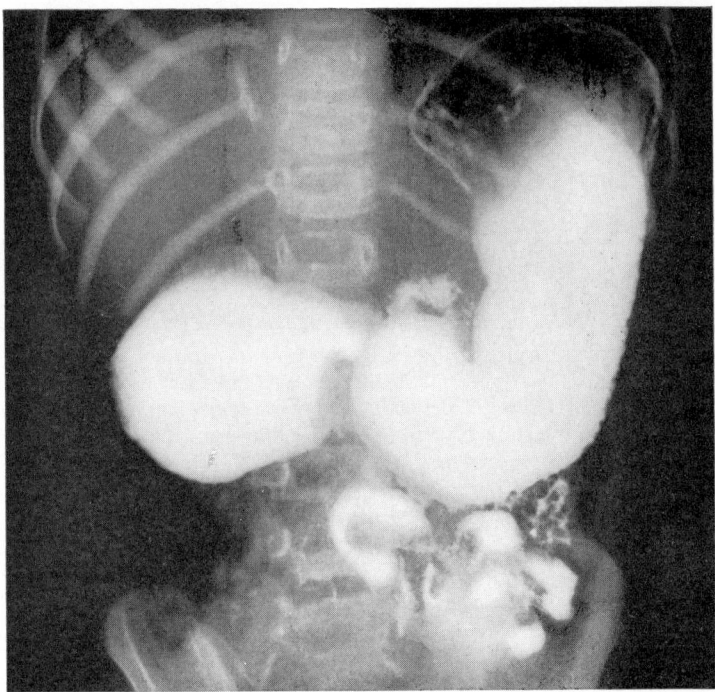

Fig. 91. Barium study from a two-year old child who had gained weight poorly and had vomited intermittently. The pylorus is quite patulous, the duodenum is greatly distended. At operation stenosis was found in second part of the duodenum.

High Obstruction. If there is a duodenal obstruction above the papilla of Vater (which is very rare), a *gastro-jejunostomy* must be made, but for all other duodenal or upper jejunal obstructions, a *duodeno-jejunostomy* gives better drainage of the duodenal loop. A duodeno-jejunostomy can be made behind the colon by piercing the transverse mesocolon; if for any technical reason an *antecolic* union seems easier, it is an acceptable procedure. When short-circuiting anastomoses are done, they should be made in an isoperistaltic manner.

Side-to-side anastomoses for intestinal stenosis usually offer little in the way of technical difficulties; the distal bowel, while somewhat collapsed, is always large enough to work on with ease. Therefore, two layers of sutures can always be placed. It has been our practice to employ an external continuous layer of 00000 silk and an internal layer of continuous 0000 chromic catgut suture with an over-and-over stitch posteriorly and a Connell stitch anteriorly.

Lower Obstruction. For those obstructions which appear in the lower jejunum or anywhere in the intestine beyond, two methods of treatment are available. First, if the child is in precarious condition, it is quickest and safest merely to perform a side-to-side isoperistaltic union of those loops which are just above and just below the block. If the child is in satisfactory condition it is oftentimes more satisfying—but by no means essen-

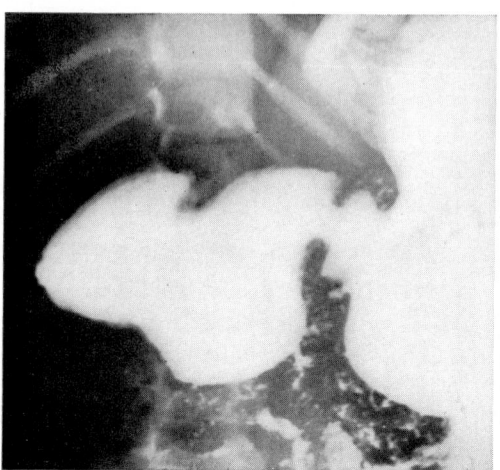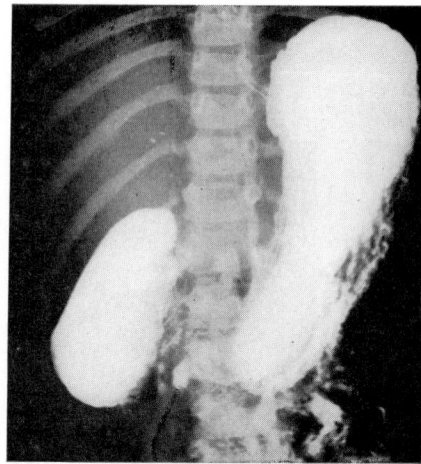

Fig. 92. Roentgenograms from two patients who had intermittent vomiting and poor gain in weight. Both were found to have duodenal stenosis. *Left*, Film from a three-year old girl, showing marked dilatation of duodenum, marked peristaltic activity in this sector, and with only small amounts of barium escaping into the intestine beyond. *Right*, Findings in a nine-year old boy, with marked dilatation of the duodenum.

tial—to excise the narrowed segment and join appropriately the remaining ends by end-to-end suture. This latter procedure is particularly useful for children beyond a year of age.

Postoperative Treatment

Postoperative care includes an immediate *transfusion* if much blood has been lost during the operative procedure. For several days the stomach and duodenum should be kept *deflated by an inlying tube* to diminish the tension on the suture line and to reduce peristaltic activity. *Feedings* should be withheld for three or four days to permit healing of the anastomosis. *Fluid and caloric requirements* can be met by parenteral routes. Intensive antibiotic and chemotherapy should be maintained after operation until all risk of infection has passed.

RESULTS OF TREATMENT

Statistics from 71 patients treated at the Boston Children's Hospital are summarized in Table 15. In the first portion of the series several patients were treated by temporary enterostomy or colostomy, which we have now completely abandoned for treatment of intestinal stenosis. Since 1940 only anastomoses (or for the lower stenoses, excision of the stenosis combined with primary anastomosis) have been used. The immediate restoration of the intestinal tract continuity has given a marked improvement in the survival rates.

Table 15

Results of Operative Treatment in 71 Cases of Intestinal or Colonic Stenosis

Site of Stenosis	Up to 1940		1940 through 1952	
	Alive	Dead	Alive	Dead
Duodenum......................	7	4	21*	7
Jejunum.........................	1	1	1	2
Ileum...........................	2	5	8	4
Ileo-cecal valve....................	0	1	1	4
Colon...........................	0	1	0	0
Multiple stenoses	0	0	0	1
Totals...........................	10	12	31†	18

* Five of these are Mongols.
† From 1940 through 1952, recoveries were 63 per cent.

While it was previously our feeling that the high obstructions provided better outlooks, this no longer seems to be true. There does not appear to be any good correlation between the level of obstruction and the prognosis.

As in babies with atresia of the duodenum, it has been found that a few of the subjects with duodenal stenosis are Mongols. This association has not been found with obstruction at other levels. It should be emphasized again that any baby with intrinsic duodenal obstruction should be carefully examined for the possibility of Mongolism.

The over-all picture in the treatment of intestinal stenosis is becoming increasingly satisfactory. During the period from 1940 through 1952, 63 per cent of our patients have been relieved of their obstruction.

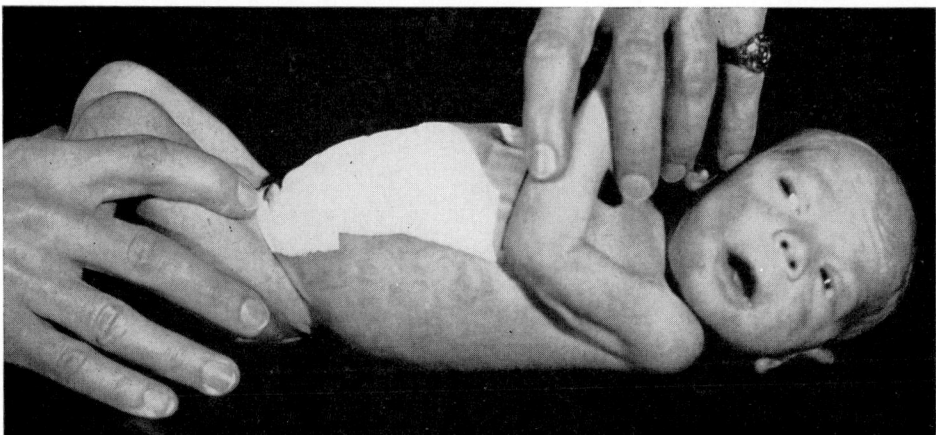

Fig. 93. Photograph eleven days after operation. Baby weighing 4 pounds, 15 ounces, operated upon for jejunal stenosis, and successfully treated by side-to-side jejuno-ileostomy.

REFERENCES

1. Cannon, P. R. and Halpert, B.: Congenital Stenosis of the Third Portion of the Duodenum with Acute Occlusion and Rupture of the Stomach. Arch. Path., *8:*611, 1929.
2. Cautley, E. Duodenal Stenosis. Brit. J. Child. Dis., *16:*65, 1919.
3. Evans, C. H.: Atresias of the Gastrointestinal Tract. Internat. Abstr. Surg., *92:*1, 1951.
4. Garvin, J. A.: Congenital Occlusion of the Duodenum. Am. J. Dis. Child., *35:*109, 1928.
5. Glover, D. M. and Barry, F. M.: Intestinal Obstruction in the Newborn. Ann. Surg., *130:*480, 1949.
6. Kuliga, P.: Zur Genese der congenitalen Dünndarmstenosen und Atresien. Beitr. z. path. Anat. u. z. allg. Path., *33:*481, 1903.
7. Ladd, W. E.: Congenital Obstruction of the Small Intestine. J.A.M.A., *101:*1453, 1933.
8. Ladd, W. E.: Congenital Duodenal Obstruction. Surgery, *1:*878, 1937.
9. Webb, C. H. and Wangensteen, O. H.: Congenital Intestinal Atresia. Am. J. Dis. Child., *41:*262, 1931.

CHAPTER 13

Intestinal Obstruction in the Newborn Resulting from Meconium Ileus

Intestinal obstruction of the newborn arising from impacted meconium is one of the most difficult conditions to treat in early life. While meconium ileus has been well recognized as a pathologic and clinical entity for several decades, the condition was almost uniformly fatal (at least in its severe degrees) until the middle forties, in spite of the fact that numerous attempts had been made by various procedures in a number of clinics to treat surgically this form of obstruction. The lesion used to carry an exceedingly gloomy and almost uniformly fatal prognosis, but today this picture is quite changed. A considerable number of these infants can now be relieved of their intestinal obstruction and a reasonably high proportion of them can subsequently be prevented from having a chronic nutritional disturbance or a serious pulmonary infection, which is so apt to descend upon the child who began life with a meconium ileus.

In the handling of these patients, it is highly important to recognize that we are faced not only with a disagreeable form of intestinal obstruction in a newborn baby, but also with an individual who has a generalized disease in which there is marked reduction in formation of exocrine pancreatic enzymes and a widespread disturbance in the mucus-secreting glands of the alimentary and respiratory tracts. Throughout the body, all mucus is extremely thick and viscid, and the patient is very apt to develop a serious or even fatal nutritional disturbance or chronic pulmonary infection. The care of these children can therefore be divided into two separate categories. First, there is the surgical problem of relieving intestinal obstruction in the early days of life. Second, there is the medical problem of subsequently supervising the nutritional state for many years by proper control of the diet and feeding of enzymes, and also the prevention or control of respiratory infections by the use of antibiotics and other supportive measures.

PATHOLOGIC DATA

The pathologic findings have long been clearly defined. As early as 1905, Landsteiner[10] focused upon the association of intestinal obstruction and a thickened, inspissated meconium, found in conjunction with lesions of the pancreas. The classical works of Andersen[1, 2] and of Farber[7, 8] have clarified our knowledge and have emphasized the widespread nature of the disturbance. The essential features of the picture are: (1) A profound change in the pancreas, appropriately called "fibrocystic disease of the pancreas" in which the acini are atrophied and apparently inactive. The ducts are greatly dilated, filled with an esinophilic staining material; the lining cells are flattened. The interacinar and interlobular structures have a great increase in connective tissue. Grossly, the pancreas is contracted and has a great increase in firmness. No diminution in islet activity or formation of insulin has been demonstrated, but there have been many measurements to show that the discharge of pancreatic juice into the duodenum is profoundly altered. This fluid is greatly reduced in amount and in enzyme content. (2) The mucus-secreting glands of the alimentary tract, and also those of the respiratory system, show widespread change; they exhibit but slight goblet formation and the secretion produced is diminished in amount, is exceedingly thick, and is very sticky.

The secondary effects are threefold: First, the meconium in the lower intestinal tract of the newly born child, because of its putty-like consistency, produces intestinal obstruction. Second, (if the child survives the obstruction of the newborn period) there is a greatly altered absorption from the intestine. The diminution in certain pancreatic enzymes can lead to abdominal distention, severe wasting of the body, and other features of a chronically disturbed nutritional state. Third, the altered physiology in the respiratory tract membranes makes the child particularly prone to recurring infections which are debilitating and indeed are often fatal. The sticky fluid on the surfaces of the bronchi greatly impairs the efficiency of the cleansing ciliary movements, so that material accumulates in the smaller passages of the lung and either induces infection or complicates that which is already present. Whether the change from cuboidal and columnar epithelium to a more flattened or even a squamous form is dependent upon vitamin A deficiency (which indeed many of these children have because of poor fat absorption), or whether it is secondary to severe inflammation, is open to debate, but without doubt the onset of these changes is accompanied by a reduction in local resistance to bacterial invasion.

The fundamental disturbance leading to altered pancreatic physiology and pathologic anatomy and also to the widespread mucoviscidosis needs further study. The experiments of Farber, wherein the pancreatic lesions were simulated in animals by administration of large doses of parasympathomimetic drugs, strongly suggest that the whole picture can be produced by an overactivity of the vagal mechanism. Baggenstoss et al.[4] have believed that "vagal juice" of the pancreas is thick and viscid, whereas "secretin juice" of the pancreas is watery and has both a diluting and a flushing effect. The dual stimulation of the pancreas by these two mechanisms, vagal impulse on the one hand and secretin hormone on the other, would imply that a normal production of normal pancreatic juice results from a balanced combination of these two influences. Theoretically, then, a diminution or an absence of the secretin factor would give a pancreatic discharge which is diminished in amount and greatly increased in viscosity. Whether fibrocystic disease of the pancreas in humans is caused by underactivity of the secretin factor or overactivity of the vagus nerves is unknown.

In *meconium ileus* the obstruction is one of purely mechanical blockage by the unusual material which is present in the lumen of the intestine. In the mid-ileum the contents are rather fluid, but below this there is meconium which is dark, very thick, exceedingly sticky, putty-like, and which adheres with great persistence to the intestinal wall or to anything with which it comes in contact. It is gummy and sticks to instruments used to try to scrape it away. It clings tenaciously to the gloves of the surgeon who tries to remove it at the operating table, or to the gloves of the pathologist who tries to clean it out of the bowel at autopsy examination. This thick substance may be found in a segment of variable extent in the lower ileum. It may fill only a short loop, but more commonly it is found plugging the last 10, 20 or even 30 cm. of ileum. The obstructed ileum is considerably dilated and is greatly thickened. The ileo-cecal valve and the colon are apt to be normal or subnormal in diameter; they contain very hard, dry, pellet-like nubbins of meconium concretions.

Not infrequently, an enlarged and distended loop of mid- or lower ileum becomes twisted upon itself, turns gangrenous, and then adheres to surrounding structures. Occasionally, a distended intestine will perforate, either in the presence of or in the absence of volvulus. Such a disruption is apt to appear in the lower ileum, but we have seen it in the cecum, and indeed in the sigmoid. Perforations can occur before birth, in which instance there is a widespread sterile peritonitis, development of adhesions, and generally a sealing off of the perforation. The escape of sterile intestinal contents into the peritoneal cavity gives scattered, minute, foreign-body reactions, in which there is

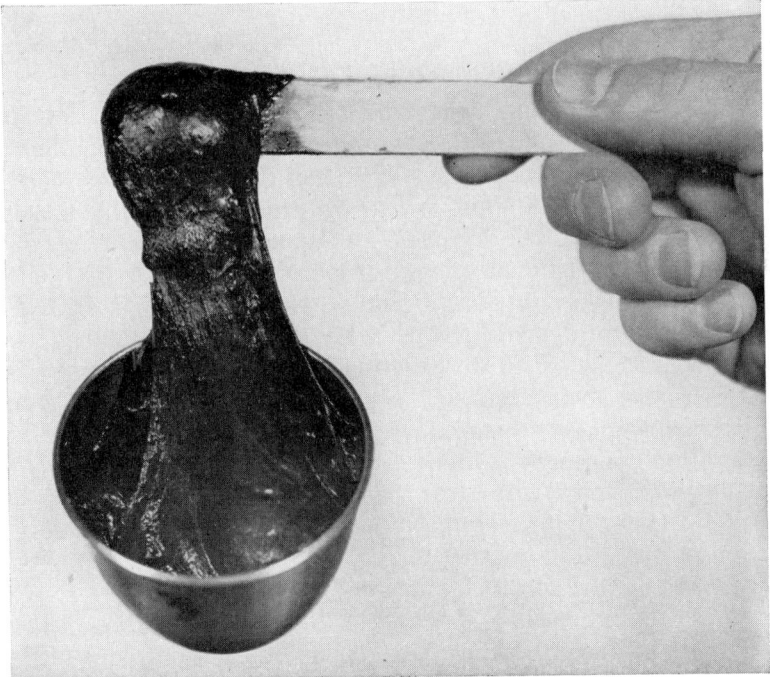

Fig. 94. Very thick and tenacious material removed from intestine of a baby with meconium ileus. With a stick dipped into the material, the metal cup can be lifted!

calcification and which can later be identified in x-ray films of the abdomen. If rupture of intestine occurs after birth, the peritoneal cavity is flooded with material which is high in bacterial count and which gives rise to an overwhelming peritonitis.

CLINICAL PICTURE

The clinical picture of meconium ileus can strongly simulate several other forms of intestinal obstruction in the newborn. Within the first day or two of life the baby begins to vomit, the vomiting becoming progressively more frequent and more copious, the material ejected being first clear, and then subsequently more dark and murky in appearance. The abdomen is moderately or markedly distended, and the pattern of intestinal loops can frequently be seen and felt through the abdominal wall. In not all cases, but certainly in a rather high percentage of them, palpation of the abdomen will reveal not only generalized distention, but also firm masses within the intestinal loops—a fact which should strongly suggest the proper diagnosis. When intestinal concretions are felt, they are most apt to be found within the lower abdomen and particularly toward its right side. Generally, very little is learned from examination of the stools or from a history concerning the bowel functions. There may have been no passage of meconium per rectum, but in some instances several bowel movements have appeared and are usually reported as being essentially normal in appearance for meconium of a newborn child. Almost never do the stools become light in color, nor do they contain curds, even though the child may have been fed on a milk formula for some days.

While no definite reason has yet been discovered why a mother should produce babies who have pancreatic insufficiency and generalized mucoviscidosis, the fact remains that these conditions are very apt to appear in multiple siblings of a family, even though other normal children may be brought forth before, between, or after children who have pancreatic deficiencies and mucoviscidosis.

ROENTGENOLOGIC EXAMINATION

Roentgenologic examination of the abdomen should include anteroposterior films with the patient in the supine and also in the upright position. Lateral films are of some value in occasional cases. At once it is evident that there is rather extensive intestinal distention, the gas and fluid-filled loops appearing throughout the abdomen, particularly in its upper half or two-thirds. The degree of distention of loops leaves no doubt concerning the presence of an obstruction in the mid or lower intestine. Of importance is the fact that loops of intestine *vary greatly in size;* some are enormously ballooned out, others are only moderately enlarged, some may be rather normal in size, and a few might seem to be even somewhat smaller than the expected normal. This great range in the size of various loops is usually in contrast to the picture found when there is an intestinal stenosis or atresia, wherein the visualized loops are all apt to be quite large, and one does not see in association with them any loops of normal or subnormal size.

Of particular importance is the fact that inspissated *meconium gives a mottled or granular appearance* (Fig. 95) in those areas where it is in great concentration. This spotty substance is almost never seen in other forms of intestinal obstruction in the newborn period.

In some cases flecks of calcium may appear throughout the abdomen (scattered on parietal or visceral peritoneum), indicative of a burned-out peritonitis of fetal life. In a few patients there may be frank evidence of postnatal disruption of the bowel, with marked ballooning of the abdominal parietes, collection of fluid between intestinal loops, and entrapment of free air within the peritoneal cavity.

In some subjects it is not possible by physical examination or even by roentgenologic study to differentiate meconium ileus from other forms of intestinal obstruction in the newborn baby. However, in 70 to 80 per cent of cases, one can, by feeling the hard abdominal masses on palpation, and by study of carefully exposed films, recognize meconium ileus prior to operation.

TREATMENT

Meconium ileus may occur in various degrees of severity. Occasionally, one encounters a baby in whom signs of obstruction are mild and the intestinal tract can be relieved of all evidence of obstruction by enemas, by gastric lavage, and by feeding pancreatic enzymes which can percolate down the intestinal tract and thereby dissolve the inspissated material. It is tempting to think that all babies with meconium ileus could be treated by such simple techniques, thereby avoiding abdominal operation. However, such does not prove to be the case. In 1941 a child was seen at the Children's Hospital

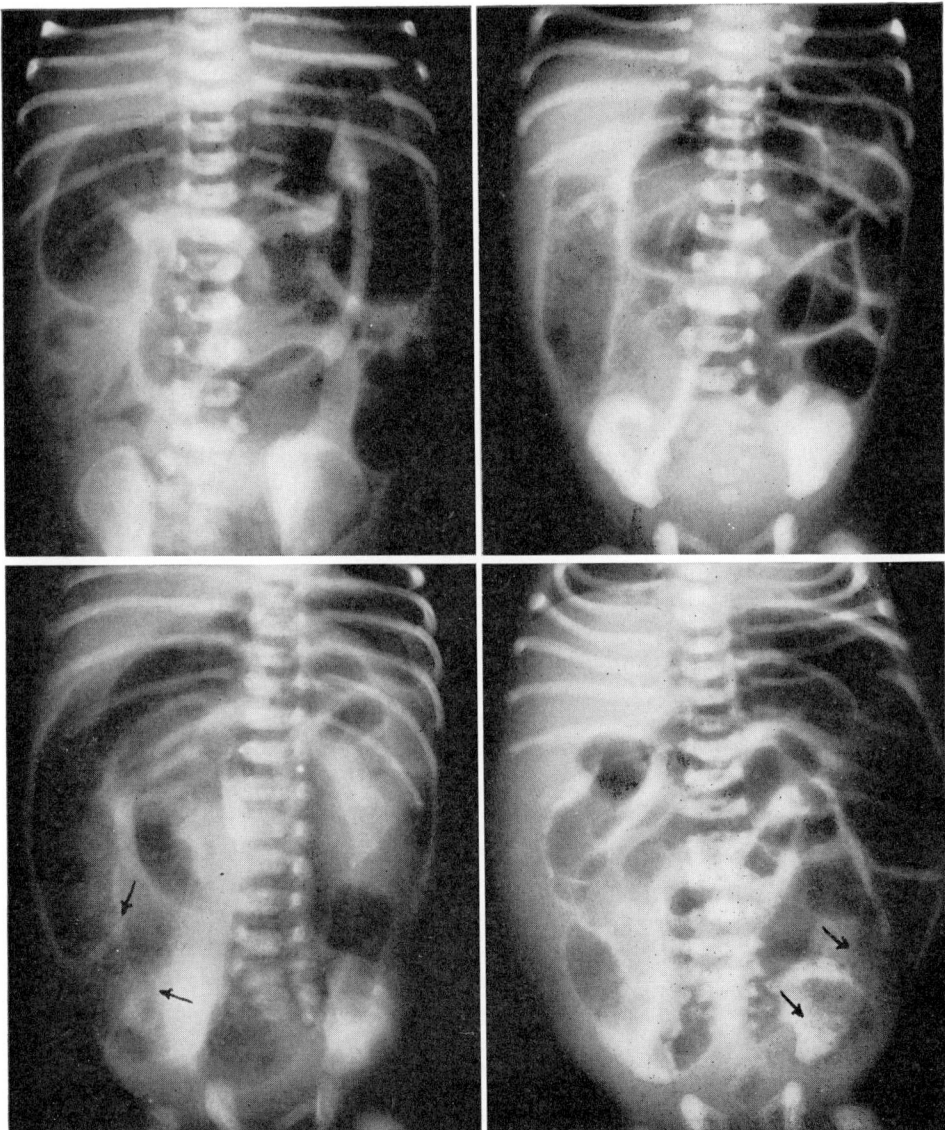

Fig. 95. Roentgenograms from four babies who had intestinal obstruction from inspissated meconium. Each case shows great variation in the size of intestinal loops, seen particularly well in the eft upper film. Granular, inspissated meconium can be seen (arrows) in both lower films.

with a moderate degree of intestinal obstruction in the newborn period and the alimentary tract was completely cleared by our medical confreres with conservative therapy. In 1947 a newly born baby with a high degree of intestinal obstruction was entered on the Surgical Service and operative relief was thought to be almost certainly necessary, but the periodic deflation of the stomach with a tube and the instillation of pancreatic material into the upper intestine eventually completely deflated the entire alimentary tract in a very satisfactory way. Both of these children have been carried along to the present time (1952), and though they have had definite evidence of pancreatic insufficiency by examination of the duodenal juices, they are in excellent health because of the replacement therapy and the antibiotics which have been given. In short, an occasional patient can have the alimentary tract cleared by conservative measures, but the vast majority of babies with well defined evidence of intestinal obstruction will demand some operative relief.

From 1920 to 1940, various members of our staff operated upon a considerable number of babies with meconium ileus, these undertakings carrying an exceedingly poor and almost hopeless outlook, regardless of the method of surgical therapy which had been used. In a few instances, the intestinal tract could be deflated and cleared (generally by the use of a Witzel enterostomy and instillation of proteolytic enzymes through this tube), only to have the child die a week or two later of overwhelming pulmonary infection. These bitter experiences led to the belief that there was little use in relieving these babies of obstruction because almost certainly they would die thereafter from pneumonitis. This attitude of hopelessness has now been changed, because there is adequate proof that if the surgeon can relieve the baby of obstruction, the medical man can usually keep the child in good nutritional status by dietary measures and can often prevent or control respiratory infections by the use of appropriate antibiotics.

From 1940 onward, 63 cases of meconium ileus have been observed and treated on the Surgical Service of the Children's Hospital. The types of operation and the results therefrom are listed in Table 16. The distribution of cases by years is shown in Table 17.

Table 16

Results of Surgical Attempts in Treatment of Meconium Ileus
Boston Children's Hospital Series, 1940 through 1952

	Died	Cured of Obstruction
No operation (child in extremis)................	1	0
Exploratory laparotomy only...................	5	0
Lysis of adhesions...........................	1	0
Gastrostomy and intubation of intestine.........	1	0
Resection of plugged terminal ileum, end-to-end anastomosis.................................	2	0
Sigmoidostomy (for perforated sigmoid).........	0	1
Ileostomy and cecostomy.....................	1	0
Witzel enterostomy...........................	15	1
Mikulicz resection, ileo-colostomy..............	4	2
Mikulicz ileo-colostomy, plus Witzel ileostomy....	2	0
Mikulicz resection and double ileostomy.........	9	18
Total.................................	41	22

Of the 63 patients, 41 died on the Surgical Service and 22 were relieved of their obstruction; of the 22 survivors 8 subsequently died from a chronic nutritional disturbance or from pulmonary infection.

The methods of surgical therapy employed for the 63 babies listed in Table 16 can be described and commented upon as follows:

No operation was performed for one baby who was obviously in extremis and who died within a few hours after hospital admission.

Exploratory laparotomy only was carried out in 5 instances, in each of which a rather hopeless situation was encountered. There was old or recent perforation, widespread peritonitis, extensive gangrene of the intestines or some such condition which made it impossible to accomplish anything by surgical means.

Lysis of adhesions was performed in one child, the intestines being bound together as the result of an old fetal peritonitis. The inspissated material within the gut seemed to be of only moderate dryness, and it was hoped that freeing of the intestines would allow peristaltic activity to be improved and the intestine to be cleared—a forlorn hope.

Gastrostomy and intubation of intestine was carried out once. Attempts had been made before operation to feed a small catheter through the nose and stomach into the intestinal tract, but this was unsuccessful. It was felt that, rather than extensively handling distended and damaged intestine, it might be simpler to open the anterior wall of the stomach and to feed a long tube directly through the duodenum and down into the upper intestine (bringing the tube out through the anterior abdominal wall). It was hoped that through this accessory passage some of the gummy, semi-fluid material in the upper intestine could be withdrawn and that proteolytic enzymes could be introduced which might get down into the lower intestine and dissolve the inspissated meconium. There was great difficulty in feeding the tube around the duodenal bend. The whole undertaking was a disappointing one.

Resection of Plugged Terminal Ileum, End-to-End Anastomosis. Attempts were made to open the lower intestine, milk down some of the thickened meconium, or to flush it out. Short portions of the terminal ileum, containing material which could not be dislodged, were resected and the remaining ends of intestine joined by end-to-end union. We were impressed by the fact that extensive massaging of the intestines or flushing of them (while the abdomen is open) is too traumatizing and too productive of fatal shock. Furthermore, a primary intestinal anastomosis is too hazardous in a small baby in whom there is still a question about the functional status of the bowel beyond it; the line of anastomosis is subjected to great strain and is apt to rupture.

In connection with these two cases, it is important to refer to the work of Hiatt,[9] who was the first to bring forth any important progress in the treatment of meconium ileus. His therapy consisted of exposure of the involved intestinal loops by laparotomy, the insertion of a sizable catheter into the gut, and the repeated lavage with saline until the inspissated material had been washed out. He emphasized that the use of enzyme solution for this lavage (while the abdomen was open) was quite dangerous because any spillage into the peritoneal cavity would produce a serious reaction there. We concur with this observation. We are amazed at the apparent ease with which Hiatt has been able to wash out the intestines with saline. We had tried this in many cases at the operating table (prior to 1940) and became convinced that it is almost impossible to soften, dilute, or wash away inspissated meconium with water or saline.

Sigmoidostomy was performed in one child who had a high degree of obstruction, who likewise had a colon filled with putty-like material, and who had a perforation of the sigmoid. The perforated area was exteriorized; subsequently the gut could be washed out with pancreatic enzymes and cleared. Later, the sigmoidostomy was closed and the child has been cured of the obstruction.

Ileostomy and cecostomy were performed for one baby, the ileostomy being established at a rather high level, where the trapped material was semi-fluid in nature. The cecostomy was beyond the putty-like substance in the terminal ileum but was proximal to the hard, stony material in the colon. It was our hope that these two vents would give avenues by which the alimentary tube could be decompressed and could be flushed out with various enzymes, but the outcome was fatal.

Witzel enterostomy has certainly had a thorough trial. It was extensively used by us during the 1930's with almost uniform failure. In addition, it has been performed 16 times in that portion of our series summarized in Tables 16 and 17. A No. 10 or 12 urethral catheter was inserted into the bowel wall in an oblique fashion, placing the tube at that level in which the content of the ileum was semi-fluid (above that portion where the contents were putty-like). In some cases the tube was directed upward, and in others it was pointed downward. It was the hope that this rather simple procedure, performed under local or general anesthesia, would allow aspiration of that part of the intestinal material which was fluid and would also give an opening through which "pancreatic" or other proteolytic enzyme could be introduced into the ileum and allowed to run down and dissolve the putty-like material distal to the enterostomy. In the

Table 17

Meconium Ileus Obstruction—Results of Therapy
Boston Children's Hospital Series

Year	Dead	Relieved of Obstruction	Relieved of Obstruction, but Subsequently Died of Nutritional Disturbance or Pulmonary Infection
1940	1	0	– –
1941	3	0	– –
1942	7	0	– –
1943	4	0	– –
1944	1	0	– –
1945	1	1	1
1946	4	0	– –
1947	7	2	1
1948	6	2	1
1949	3	4	2
1950	3	3	1
1951	0	4	1
1952	1	6	1
	41	22	8

series (since 1940) one child has been cured of intestinal obstruction by this means. The other 15 came to a fatal termination rather promptly. While there might be theoretical factors in favor of a Witzel enterostomy as a form of treatment for meconium ileus, our long and sad experience has caused us to completely abandon the procedure. In an intestine so small, the infolding of a portion of its wall often completely blocks the lumen of the gut. Furthermore, instillation of a highly potent pancreatic or other proteolytic enzyme through such a channel is very apt to give dissolution of the gut wall at the line of suture, thus causing leakage into the peritoneal cavity. Furthermore, in a few instances the inlying catheter, even though apparently soft and not particularly rigid, eroded the opposite intestinal wall against which it lay, leading to disruption and fatal peritonitis. We are quite sure that Witzel enterostomy for this type of case is almost worthless.

Mikulicz resection, with ileo-colostomy, has been adopted in a small number of cases in which it was necessary to remove a segment of the terminal ileum and first portion of the colon because of perforation of the same, or because they contained exceedingly solid material. It seemed wise to exteriorize and remove this portion of gut.

In some of these, the alimentary tube was entered while the abdomen was still open; it was necessary to deflate the mid-intestine to a point where it could be put back into the abdomen. It is obvious that such an opening of the gut (while the abdomen is open) introduces the possibility of peritoneal soilage; this should certainly be avoided if possible. A review of our 6 patients in whom a Mikulicz ileo-colostomy was performed leaves us with the impression that it is sometimes necessary to use this form of operation when the cecum or colon has been perforated, but that it should never be used for any other circumstance. The procedure necessitates mobilizing the cecum, ascending colon, or right half of the colon; this is too extensive an undertaking in a child who is extremely ill to begin with.

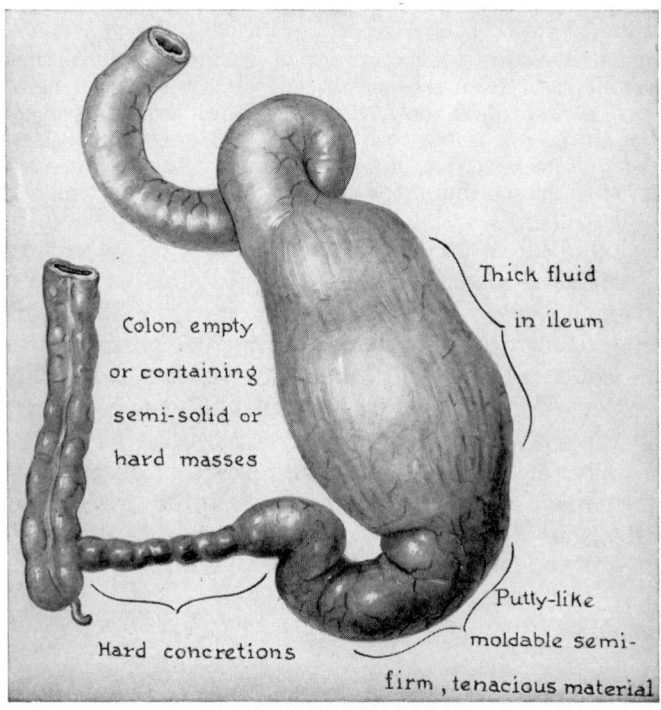

Fig. 96. Findings in typical case of intestinal obstruction of the meconium ileus type. For therapy, we have had the best success by removing (with an aseptic Mikulicz procedure) that dilated portion of gut which contains the moldable, semi-firm, tenacious material.

Mikulicz Ileo-colostomy plus Witzel Ileostomy. In two patients the Mikulicz removal of terminal ileum and some portion of the right side of the colon were necessary, but a considerable amount of putty-like meconium still remained above in the ileum; we wondered whether this would be evacuated spontaneously after operation. To give an additional vent to the intestines, a Witzel ileostomy was established just above the upper level of the putty-like mass. Both children died. This combination of procedures does not seem to be warranted.

Mikulicz Resection and Double Ileostomy

We have come to believe that this type of attack is by far the best procedure which is now available for treatment of meconium ileus. It has several advantages. In an aseptic manner, it allows one to exteriorize (and subsequently remove after the abdomen

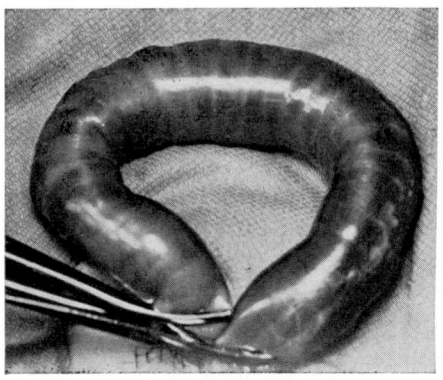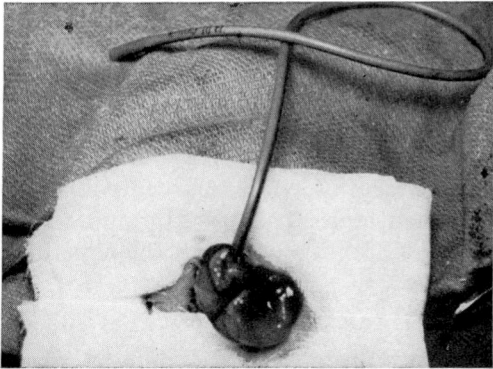

Fig. 97. Photograph immediately at termination of operation for treatment of meconium ileus obstruction. The loop of distal ileum showing the greatest distention has been exteriorized. *Left*, The abdominal wound is closed; here shown is the loop which has been brought out and will now be cut off. *Right*, The distended loop has been cut away. The proximal opening of the ileum is left open for decompression of the same. The distal limb has a small catheter tied into it, so proteolytic e nzymes can be instilled in the subsequent few days for cleaning out the terminal ileum and colon.

is closed) that portion of the distal ileum which is greatly distended and which contains a large mass of inspissated material. It provides a double vent, the proximal one of which is used for immediate decompression of the intestine above, and the distal one of which will allow instillation of enzymes during the postoperative period so the terminal ileum and colon can be flushed out. Since we have had a much higher success with this operation than with any other we have used, this has now become our standard form of treatment for meconium ileus. Twenty-seven cases have been treated in this manner; 9 subjects have died and 18 have been relieved of obstruction.

Among the 27 patients who were treated by Mikulicz resection and double ileostomy, our over-all results are apparently improving within the last four years, pre-

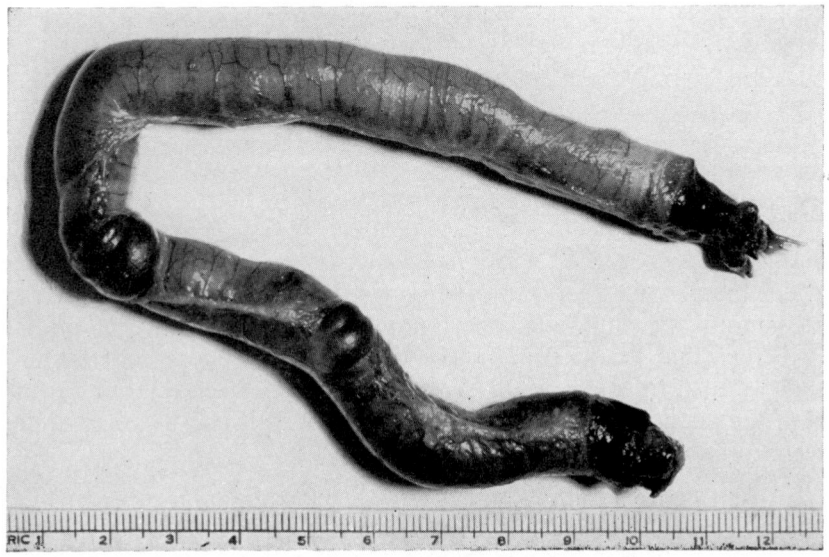

Fig. 98. Photograph of portion of ileum which has been cut out during an exteriorizing operation (see Fig. 97). Note that the segment stays distended; the material within it is so thick that it will *not run out*.

sumably because greater attention is paid to handling of the bowel at operation and to the support of the child after operation. Prior to 1949, 8 babies were treated by this method; 5 died and 3 were relieved of their obstruction. Since 1949, 19 have been treated by this method; 4 died and 15 have been relieved of their obstruction, a survival of 79 per cent.

While there might be some features which make it undesirable to establish a double ileostomy by the Mikulicz technique, certain comments are in order. There is practically no erosion of the abdominal wall in the presence of such an ileostomy, because the child's intestinal fluids are markedly deficient in enzymes. Hence, there is not the disturbing factor of cutaneous irritation which so frequently is a serious complication when an ileostomy is established for other conditions (such as for ulcerative colitis). Second, while fluid and electrolyte loss might cause one to hesitate to open the intestine externally in a small child, we have not found it difficult to combat this loss with intake by mouth and by parenteral routes. Third, one does not need to permit a baby with an ileostomy to languish in this state for a protracted period of time. A crushing clamp can be applied to the two limbs within a few days so that some intestinal juice seeps down into the lower bowel rather soon. While some of our ileostomies have been left open for many months, it is now our common practice to close them within two or three weeks. (Both of the operations are done under cyclopropane anesthesia, in the attempt to reduce the risks of pulmonary infection.)

Examination of Pancreatic Juice

Because of the critical condition of the baby, it is not practical to examine the duodenal juice prior to operative relief of obstruction from impacted meconium. However, it is important to carry out such examination in all patients who survive surgical relief of the condition, for only in this way will information be available to guide appropriately the subsequent dietary management. The marked deviation from normal which can be observed in the enzymatic activity of the duodenal fluid has been recorded by Maddock, Farber, and Schwachman,[11] and is indicated in Table 18.

Table 18

Units of Enzyme Activity in Duodenal Juice for One Hour before and for One Hour after Stimulation by Intravenous Secretin

(From Maddock, Farber, and Schwachman[11])

	Trypsin		Lipase		Amylase	
	Before	After	Before	After	Before	After
5 normal infants and children........	4325	6720	1573	2682	3293	5780
7 patients with pancreatic fibrosis.....	21	26	13	9	216	137

Supportive and Medical Therapy

When a baby has been relieved of obstruction of the meconium ileus type, its surgical problem has been solved, but the youngster must have adequate and long-continued medical supervision thereafter. Chronic nutritional disturbance (from pancreatic insufficiency) and progressive pulmonary disease (from the mucoviscidosis) are very apt to bring about profound changes or even fatal complications. From the earliest moments appropriate measures must be taken to combat these; it is far more effective to ward them off than it is to treat them after they have become established.

For long-term care the following items are of importance: (1) The deficiency of protein disintegration and assimilation by the intestinal tract must be corrected by either giving a diet of amino acids and polypeptides or else giving a normal diet and adding to it enzymes (in the form of Viokase). For the former choice materials are now commercially available, such as Nutramigen, which is a fortified casein hydrolysate. If tolerated by the infant (without vomiting or diarrhea), it is the best substitute which is available at this writing; if it causes too much gastro-intestinal disturbance, some other hydrolysate without the additional fat can be tried. We much prefer to employ a normal diet for babies (such as an evaporated milk formula) and add accessory enzymes in the form of $\frac{1}{8}$ teaspoonful of Viokase to each bottle. (This material cannot be added while preparing the formula; it is destroyed by heat.) This regimen is simple to conduct, gives the child good nourishment and weight gain, and is inexpensive.

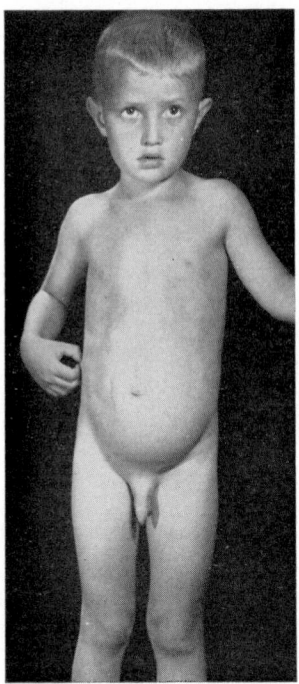

Fig. 99. Case 3, Table 19. Child treated in newborn period for meconium ileus. Photograph at four and one-half years, showing excellent general health.

(2) The total caloric value of the diet should be greatly increased—as much as 40 to 50 per cent above that offered a normal baby of the same age. (3) Vitamin K should be given, 5 mg. per day for several weeks, and later two or three times per week, to prevent the bleeding which has been occasionally seen in some of the children. (4) There should be a high intake of vitamins *which are of a water-miscible variety*. Twice a day 0.6 cc. of preparation is given, each oral dose containing at least: Vitamin A, 5000 units, vitamin D, 1000 units, thiamine chloride 1.0 mg., riboflavin 0.4 mg., nicotinic acid 2.0 mg., and ascorbic acid 50 mg. (5) In older children, when solid food is taken, proteolytic enzymes are given by mouth with each of the meals ($\frac{1}{4}$ teaspoonful of Viokase for a one-year old child, larger doses for older patients). (6) Daily oral antibiotics should be given to stave

off pulmonary infection. For this purpose terramycin has been most useful, in doses of 50 mg. twice a day, maintaining this indefinitely for months or years. If there are episodes with flare-up of respiratory infection, the basic maintenance dose of terramycin can be increased as the conditions demand, or other drugs can be employed which might be more suitable, using parenteral routes if they seem to be indicated in more serious infections.

RESULTS OF THERAPY

In the not-too-distant past the surgical treatment for meconium ileus was a most disappointing undertaking. Children died with a high degree of regularity following the many types of operation which were tried. In a few instances the alimentary tract was relieved of obstruction, only to find that the child quickly succumbed thereafter from a

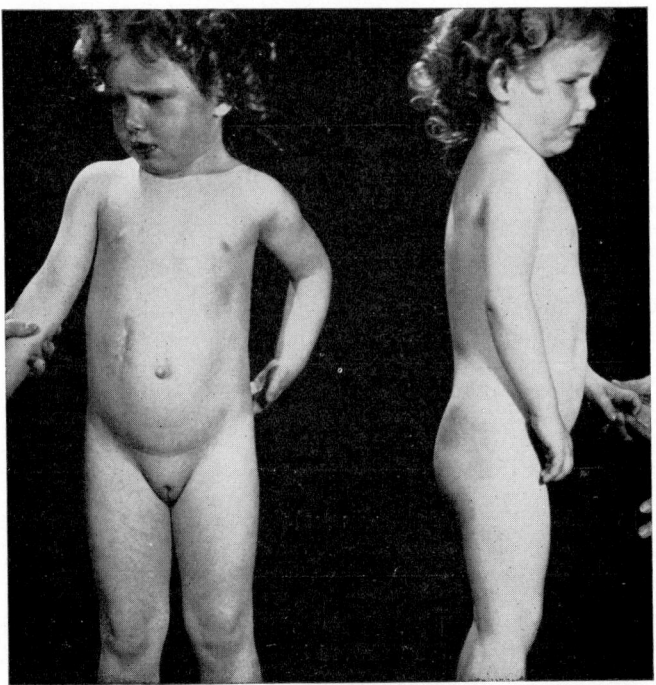

Fig. 100. Case 4, Table 19. Girl treated at three days of age for intestinal obstruction from inspissated meconium. Treatment by Mikulicz resection of plugged terminal ileum. Photograph at three and one-half years, showing excellent health.

severe nutritional disturbance or a progressive pulmonary infection. This exceedingly poor prognosis has changed since the middle of the 1940's, because it has now become evident that it is possible by certain surgical maneuvers to free the ileum and colon of the obstructive material, and furthermore, medical treatment has been able to prevent or to combat successfully the ravages of pancreatic insufficiency and pulmonary infection.

A variety of operative procedures which we have tried are discussed in the foregoing pages. While some of them have theoretical or practical value under certain circumstances, most of them have fallen into disuse and should not be employed any more.

From our own experience, we have felt that it is generally impossible to wash out the intestines in the manner described by Hiatt, and we have preferred to perform a Mikulicz resection of the terminal portion of the ileum which contains the firm meco-

Table 19

Children's Hospital Cases of Meconium Ileus Relieved of Obstruction

Case	Sex	Age at Operation	Operative Procedure	Remarks
1. 296160	M	1 day	Volvulus with gangrene, intestinal perforation, and peritonitis. Mikulicz resection of gangrenous volvulus 7/16/45. Closure of ileostomy 8/3/45.	Discharged 8/16/45. Developed celiac nutritional disturbance and pulmonary infection. Died 12/9/45.
2. 318415	M	2 days	Witzel ileostomy 5/20/47.	Bowel washed out with pancreatin. Relieved of obstruction. Developed chronic pulmonary infection. Died 7/3/47.
3. 313663	M	2 days	Mikulicz ileo-transverse colostomy 1/23/47. Closure of ileo-colostomy 12/31/47.	Excellent condition Oct. 1951.
4. 329113	F	3 days	Mikulicz ileo-ileostomy 2/13/48. Closure of ileostomy 2/28/48.	Completely relieved of obstruction. Excellent condition Oct. 1951.
5. 332365	M	2 days	Mikulicz ileo-ileostomy 6/17/48. Closed 11/15/48.	Died at 6 months of pulmonary infection.
6. 343872	F	3 days	58 cm. impacted ileum removed by Mikulicz ileo-ileostomy 4/15/49.	Completely relieved of obstruction. Died of pulmonary infection 5/15/49.
7. 345766	F	1 day	Also had multiple atresias of ileum. 23 cm. of ileum removed by Mikulicz ileo-ileostomy 5/22/49.	Relieved of obstruction. Died of nutritional disturbance and pulmonary infection 6/23/49.
8. 346556	M	1 day	Mikulicz ileo-ileostomy (high) 6/4/49. Closure of ileostomy 6/25/49.	Completely relieved of obstruction. Excellent health 5/17/51.
9. 348650	M	3 days	Peritonitis from sigmoid perforation. Exteriorization of perforated sigmoid 7/31/49. Closure of sigmoid-ostomy 2/15/50.	In excellent health. Sept. 1951.
10. 356771	F	2 days	Mikulicz ileo-ileostomy 2/26/50. Ileostomy closed 3/13/50.	Excellent condition 8/16/51.
11. 366293	M	5 days	Ileo-ileostomy (Mikulicz) 11/15/50. Closed 12/9/50.	Died Jan. 1951 of pulmonary disease.

Table 19 (Continued)

Case	Sex	Age at Operation	Operative Procedure	Remarks
12. 369902	M	4 days	Ileo-ileostomy Mikulicz 2/12/51. Ileostomy closed 2/28/51.	Very good condition Oct. 1951.
13. 372074	F	3 days	Perforation of cecum. Mikulicz resection of cecum and terminal ileum 5/12/51. Drainage of abdominal abscess 6/12/51. Closure of ileo-colostomy 7/2/51.	Chronic nutritional problem and pulmonary infection. Died 8/12/51.
14. 376244	F	4 days	Mikulicz ileo-ileostomy 7/29/51. Closure of ileostomy 8/13/51.	Satisfactory condition. Some pulmonary infection Oct. 1951.
15. 375792	F	2 days	Ileo-ileostomy (Mikulicz) 7/22/51. Ileostomy closed 7/31/51.	Severe pulmonary infection Oct. 1951.
16. 378380	M	5 days	Mikulicz ileo-ileostomy 9/17/51. Closed on 10/4/51.	Good condition Oct. 1951.
17. 387289	M	3 days	Mikulicz ileo-ileostomy 6/12/52. Closure of ileostomy 9/29/52.	Good condition 12/31/52.
18. 389216	F	2 days	Mikulicz ileo-ileostomy 7/2/52. Closure of ileostomy 7/26/52.	Good condition 12/31/52.
19. 392736	F	1 day	Mikulicz ileo-ileostomy 10/14/52. Closure of ileostomy 12/5/52.	Good condition 12/31/52.
20. 392948	M	3 days	Mikulicz ileo-ileostomy 10/18/52. Closure of ileostomy 10/29/52.	Died 11/20/52 of pulmonary disease.
21. 395612	M	2 days	Mikulicz ileo-ileostomy 12/16/52.	Well 12/31/52.
22. 395671	F	6 days	Mikulicz ileo-ileostomy 12/21/52.	Well 12/31/52.

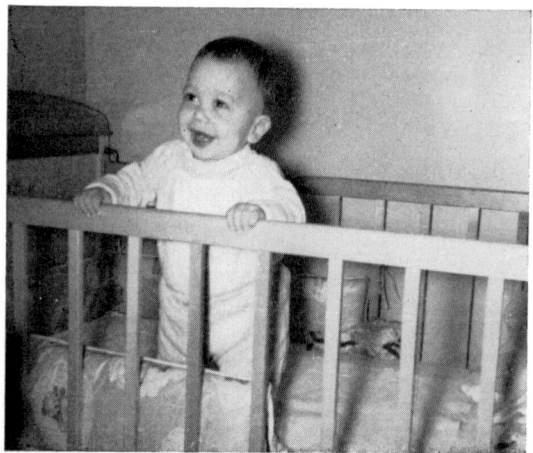

Fig. 101. Case 8, Table 19. Child who was treated by Mikulicz resection of meconium-plugged terminal ileum. Photograph at eight months, showing excellent status.

nium mass, making this exteriorization in an aseptic manner, cutting off the exteriorized loop after the abdominal wall has been closed. The upper and lower loops can usually be flushed out with proteolytic enzymes and made to function satisfactorily within a few days. A crushing clamp can be put on between the two spurs shortly thereafter. The ileostomy can be closed within two or three weeks after the initial operation.

Adequate medical supervision is of great importance in bringing these children through subsequent years and giving them reasonable health and vitality. The costs of

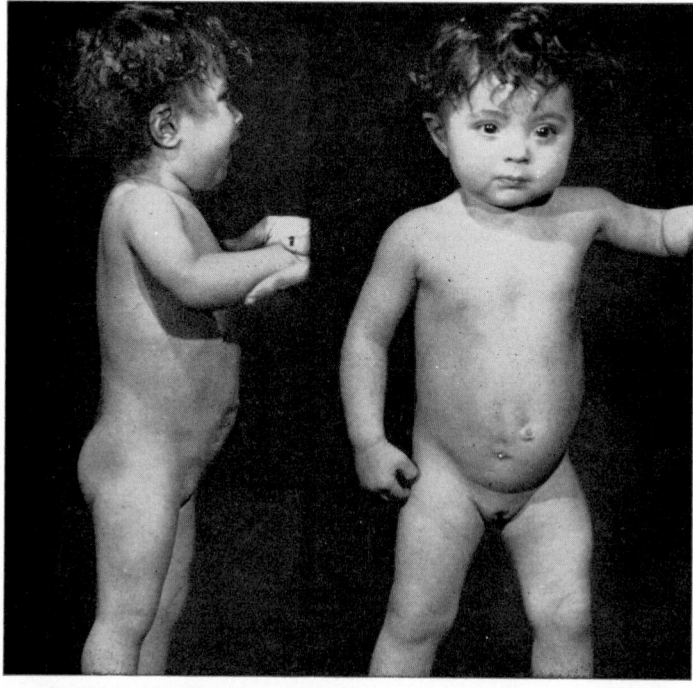

Fig. 102. Case 10, Table 19. Child who had obstruction of the meconium ileus type. Treated by Mikulicz resection of the obstructed terminal ileum. Ileostomy closed two weeks later. Photograph at one year of age, indicating excellent general health.

this are low, the program is one which is not usually difficult to follow, and the over-all results are extremely satisfactory in a very high percentage of cases, as is evidenced by the fact that a small group of these children have been followed for periods up to five years of age and are in a very satistactory state of health. In Table 19 are listed 22 patients who have been surgically cured of meconium ileus; some pertinent data are given for each case. Of these 22 patients, 8 have subsequently died (within one to six months) of severe nutritional disturbance from a pancreatic insufficiency or from overwhelming pulmonary infection; the remaining 14 are in very good health and state of nutrition. The impression is gained that if a child does not succumb from pulmonary disease within the first six months, pneumonic infections become less of a threat thereafter.

REFERENCES

1. Andersen, D. H.: Celiac Syndrome. II. Fecal Excretion in Congenital Pancreatic Deficiency at Various Ages and with Various Diets, with Discussion of the Optimal Diet. Am. J. Dis. Child., *69*:221, 1945.
2. Andersen, D. H.: Celiac Syndrome. III. Dietary Therapy for Congenital Pancreatic Deficiency. Am. J. Dis. Child., *70*:100, 1945.
3. Ayers, W. B., Stowens, D. and Ochsner, A.: Fibrocystic Disease of the Pancreas. Treatment by Sympathetic Denervation of the Pancreas and Presentation of a Theory of Neuroeffector Mechanisms: Preliminary Report of Five Cases. J.A.M.A., *142*:7, 1950.
4. Baggenstoss, A. H., Power, M. H. and Grindlay, J. H.: The Relationship of Fibrocystic Disease of the Pancreas to a Deficiency of Secretin. Pediatrics, *2*:435, 1948.
5. Dodd, K.: Intestinal Obstruction due to Meconium Ileus in a Newborn Infant. J. Pediat., *9*:486, 1936.
6. Ehrenpreis, T.: Meconium Ileus and Hirschsprung's Disease. Acta paediat., *40*:227, 1951.
7. Farber, S.: Pancreatic Function and Disease in Early Life. V. Pathologic Changes Associated with Pancreatic Insufficiency in Early Life. Arch. Path., *37*:238, 1944.
8. Farber, S.: The Relation of Pancreatic Achylia to Meconium Ileus. J. Pediat., *24*:387, 1944.
9. Hiatt, R. B. and Wilson, P. E.: Celiac Syndrome. VII. Therapy of Meconium Ileus; Report of Eight Cases with a Review of the Literature. Surg., Gynec., & Obst., *87*:317, 1948.
10. Landsteiner, K.: Darmverschluss durch eingedicktes Meconium. Pankreatitis. Centralbl. f. allg. Path. u. path. Anat., *16*:903, 1905.
11. Maddock, C. L., Farber, S. and Schwachman, H.: Pancreatic Function and Disease in Early Life. II. Effect of Secretin on Pancreatic Function of Infants and Children. Am. J. Dis. Child., *66*:370, 1943.
12. Schwachman, H., Crocker, A. C., Foley, G. E. and Patterson, P. R.: Aureomycin Therapy in the Pulmonary Involvement of Pancreatic Fibrosis (Mucoviscidosis). New England J. Med., *241*:185, 1949.

CHAPTER 14

Malrotation of the
Intestines and Colon

Of particular interest to the surgeon who must deal with abdominal surgery in children is the condition of incomplete rotation of the intestine. Malrotation (which is almost always an incomplete rotation) produces high intestinal obstruction because of external pressure on the second or third portion of the duodenum.

There have been literally hundreds of reports in the literature describing this condition. Many of these are of autopsy findings and quite a few of them represent post-mortem studies following unsuccessful abdominal explorations. Until the late twenties our own experience with these anomalies was most disappointing, fatality usually occurring because of use of procedures which incompletely alleviated the obstruction or which, by some open anastomotic procedure in a very ill child, gave rise to a fatal peritonitis. After a number of deaths following such surgery, studies at the autopsy table showed that an apparently complicated lesion could be treated by rather simple means. Within the last fifteen years several excellent reviews have been published regarding the condition and its surgical correction. Outstanding among these are the contributions of Ladd in his aseptic method of relieving the obstruction. With the institution of this form of therapy a striking improvement in results has been obtained.

If the surgeon has not familiarized himself with this condition, he will be confused on opening the abdomen of a newly born baby with such an anomaly. Conversely, if he recognizes the abnormality immediately he can easily institute measures which give high promise of successful issue.

The following discussions are based almost entirely on experience at the Children's Hospital up to January 1, 1951, during which time 156 babies and young children have been operated upon by modern methods.

EMBRYOLOGY

The pathologic condition described in this chapter is wholly concerned with the development and position of the *midgut*, which includes that portion of the alimentary tube from the duodenum to the midpart of the transverse colon. This is the segment supplied by the superior mesenteric artery.

Normal Rotations and Attachments of Intestinal Tract

From the sixth to the tenth weeks of embryonic life, the alimentary tube grows at a faster rate than does the celomic cavity, and a portion of the midgut normally protrudes out into the base of the umbilical cord (Fig. 103). At about the tenth week the peritoneal cavity grows at an accelerated rate and the midgut is withdrawn into it. As this recedes into the abdomen, it *rotates* in a counterclockwise direction (as one faces the fetus).

The lower portion of the midgut (including the terminal ileum, cecum, ascending colon, and transverse colon) lies wholly in the left side of the abdomen. The anticlockwise rotation continues until the cecum comes to reach the superior part of the abdomen. Thus, in the eleventh week the cecum and first portion of the colon are in the epigastrium. As the rotation subsequently progresses, the cecum passes into the right upper quadrant and finally ends its migration in the right lower quadrant.

After this rotation is completed, the ascending mesocolon and the descending mesocolon both fuse to the back wall of the abdomen, which in effect anchors the base of the mesentery posteriorly, from the ligament of Treitz obliquely downward toward the cecal area. Thereby the normal developmental sequence of events becomes completed.

Malrotations

Most of the clinical findings in malrotations of the intestinal tract can be understood if this normal embryology is borne in mind. *Arrests of development* during the tenth or eleventh week of fetal life will give rise to anomalies which are characterized by: (1) A lack of attachment of the mesentery along the posterior abdominal wall; (2) an incompletely rotated cecum; or (3) a completely rotated cecum which is mobile and unattached.

PATHOLOGY

Obstruction of the Descending Duodenum

With incomplete rotation of the cecum, one commonly finds this viscus just below the distal half of the stomach; bands of reflected peritoneum run from it (or the ascending colon) to the right posterolateral part of the abdominal wall (Fig. 105). These bands or folds lie directly across the descending portion of the duodenum and partly obstruct it by external pressure. In some cases the cecum itself lies on the duodenum where it is held by the parietal peritoneum; anchored in this manner, it presses against and obstructs the duodenum.

Volvulus of Midgut

In association with these abnormal positions of the cecum, the mesentery of the small intestine lacks a normal posterior fixation; it has only a rudimentary attachment near the origin of the superior mesenteric artery. Hence the intestine, from the duodeno-jejunal junction to the mid-transverse colon, is supported by an incompletely anchored mesentery. Obviously, this entire mass can twist. Such a volvulus of the midgut generally takes place in a clockwise direction; the twist can be for one or two complete turns. When volvulus takes place, a coil of intestine wraps itself around the base of the mesentery (and at first glance might give the impression that there is a herniation of bowel through a hole in the mesentery). This is an illusion, because untwisting the volvulus shows that there is no hole in the mesentery. Of all the cases which have come to surgery because of duodenal obstruction from an incompletely rotated cecum, *approximately one-half also have had a volvulus of the midgut.*

On two occasions we have seen incomplete rotation of the intestines and a midgut volvulus in a patient who had complete *situs inversus* of the abdominal viscera.

Effects of Volvulus. When a volvulus occurs, two serious conditions are at once established. First, the twisting of structures around the rudimentary attachment of the mesentery angulates and obstructs the alimentary tube at both the duodeno-jejunal junction and the transverse colon. Second, the torsion partially or completely occludes the superior mesenteric vessels. Hence *infarction* of the entire midgut may supervene.

From the above descriptions, it is obvious that there are really two separate but

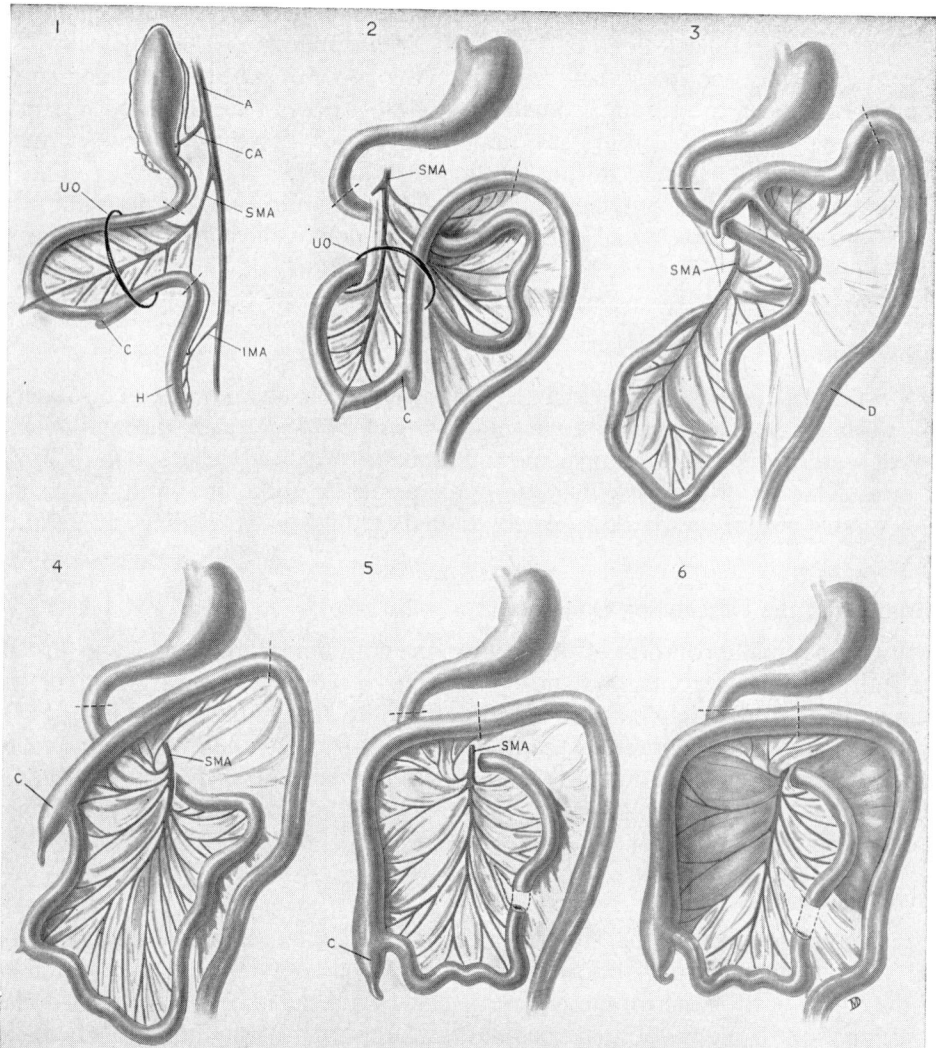

Fig. 103. Schematic drawing of normal development, rotation, and attachment of the midgut. The midgut in each sketch is that part included between the dotted lines and represents that portion of the alimentary tract from duodenum to midtransverse colon which is supplied by the superior mesenteric artery.

A, Aorta	H, Hindgut
C, Cecum	IMA, Inferior Mesenteric Artery
CA, Celiac Axis	SMA, Superior Mesenteric Artery
D, Descending Colon	UO, Umbilical Orifice

1. Fifth week of fetal life—lateral view. The foregut, midgut, and hindgut with their respective blood supplies are indicated. Most of the midgut is extruded into the base of the umbilical cord where it normally resides from about the fifth to the tenth week. 2. Tenth week of fetal life. The intestine is elongating and the hindgut is displaced to the left side of the abdomen. The developing, intra-abdominal intestines come to lie behind the superior mesenteric artery. A portion of the midgut still protrudes through the umbilical orifice into the base of the cord. 3. Eleventh week of fetal life. All of the alimentary tract is withdrawn into the abdomen. The cecum lies in the epigastrium, beneath the stomach. 4. Late in eleventh week of fetal life. The colon is rotating; the cecum lies in the right upper quadrant of the abdomen. 5. Rotation of the colon is complete, and the cecum lies in final position. There is a common mesentery—the mesocolon of the ascending colon being continuous with the mesentery of the

related lesions in these cases. One is concerned with the *obstruction of the descending duodenum* by an overlying cecum or peritoneal band. The other is concerned with the *volvulus of the midgut*. It is important to appreciate the fact that these two conditions can coexist, because many operators have merely reduced the volvulus and have subsequently had the patient die from unrelieved duodenal obstruction (caused by the transduodenal bands).

One may deduce that obstructions from these abnormalities will bring about dilatation of certain portions of the gastro-intestinal tract. In the usual case, the duodenum is considerably dilated in its proximal half (Fig. 104). If there is a volvulus of the midgut, the jejunum and ileum may be quite collapsed at first, because duodenal contents cannot enter this obstructed segment. However, if the volvulus is present for some time, gas accumulates in this isolated midgut segment because of local bacterial growth. Hence, the jejunum, ileum, and ascending colon may become greatly distended.

Recognition at Operation. On opening the abdomen one is presented with small intestinal loops without seeing the ascending or transverse colon (Fig. 105). Hence, when the right half of the colon is hidden from immediate view (particularly if presenting loops are bluish or are congested), the operator should suspect at once that he is dealing with an improperly attached mesentery and a volvulus of the midgut.

Normally Placed, Mobile Cecum

The majority of children who have come to our attention because of anomalous rotation of the alimentary tract have had an incomplete rotation of the cecum and also a lack of normal attachment of the mesentery to the posterior abdominal wall, but in a few cases there have been minor degrees of these malformations. One can find: (1) a normally placed, unattached cecum with an unattached mesentery of the small intestine; or (2) a normally placed, unattached cecum with a partially attached ileal mesentery. Either one of these gives intermittent symptoms if there is momentary twisting of the cecum or of the cecum and terminal ileum.

Partly Attached Great Omentum

An additional finding in some cases, which has little clinical significance, is related to the attachment of the great omentum. Normally, this structure arises from the stomach and later overlies the transverse colon to which it becomes fused. In some patients with incomplete rotation of the colon, the stomach and colon are not connected with each other, and the omentum hangs only from the stomach.

SYMPTOMS AND SIGNS

The majority of humans with anomalies of malrotation have complaints which bring them to the physician's attention in the neonatal period. A few have symptoms appearing at a later time; some do not have trouble until late childhood or even adult life. A rare individual can have the anomalous rotation and peculiar mesenteric attachments without ever showing symptoms therefrom. Of our 156 patients coming to operation for treatment of obstruction from malrotation, 87 were in the first month of life, 40 were from one to twelve months of age, and 29 were from one to fifteen years of age

---

ileum. There is no posterior attachment of this common mesentery except at the origin of the superior mesenteric artery. 6. Final stage in attachment of the mesenteries. The ascending and the descending mesocolons become fused to the posterior abdominal wall; thereby the mesentery of the jejunum and ileum gain a posterior attachment from the origin of the superior mesenteric artery obliquely downward to the cecum.

(with a rather even distribution of these latter through the childhood years). In babies, the symptoms were generally those of high grades of obstruction demanding immediate surgery. In the group of older children, the symptoms, on the whole, had been less striking, were generally of an intermittent nature, and in some had been recurring for months or years.

Clinical Picture in Infancy

Obstruction of the duodenum causes *vomiting*, and this is the outstanding complaint. Since the obstruction is low in the duodenum, the vomitus usually contains bile, but the peritoneal bands are on rare occasions above the papilla of Vater and the vomitus is not greenish. Vomiting is usually persistent and occurs after most of the feedings. Inasmuch as the obstruction is usually partial, there may be passage of some curd-containing stools.

Abdominal distention usually follows, but at first it is limited to the epigastrium, because only the stomach and duodenum are dilated. Careful inspection may show peristaltic waves passing downward in the right side of the epigastrium. *Dehydration* and *electrolyte depletion* of severe degrees can occur rapidly because there is loss of pancreatic juice, bile, and gastric secretions in copious amounts. If dehydration is marked, a *fever* of moderate or high degree may be encountered.

If the patient is untreated for some days, the abdominal distention may become generalized if there is an associated midgut volvulus which entraps gas in the jejunum and ileum. The temperature may reach 105° F. or more, such fever arising either from dehydration or from volvulus and infarction of a large part of the intestinal tract. In cases with generalized abdominal distention the *stools* are usually scanty and there are poor returns from enemas, because a volvulus of the midgut has obstructed not only the duodenum but also the colon.

Of the various patients we have treated surgically for malrotation obstruction, 39 were under one week of age. In this group, the clinical picture might easily be confused with—and possibly indistinguishable from—that arising from *intestinal atresia* or *stenosis*. It is not really important to determine exactly which of these three conditions exists, for all of them demand immediate exploration and operative relief.

Laboratory data will usually show concentration of urine and there may be an elevation in the red blood count. Hemoconcentration may also give rise to a slightly elevated white blood count, but a marked *leukocytosis* should immediately arouse suspicion of intestinal gangrene.

Clinical Picture in Older Children

When malrotation is found in older children, there has usually been a history of long-continued or recurring attacks of *abdominal pain, nausea,* and *vomiting.* These children may have only recurring minor abdominal complaints for which study is undertaken, or else they may have a single alarming episode which requires prompt surgical treatment.

Patients with Celiac Syndrome

Of some interest is a small group of children with a clinical picture simulating celiac disease. These have persistent or recurrent abdominal distention with or without pain, poor absorption of food, intolerance to certain substances, and either constipation or diarrhea. The complaints are presumably brought about by twisting of the midgut in such a way that the terminal ileum is temporarily obstructed, or else mesenteric compression gives congestion and edema of the intestinal wall. It is therefore important to examine roentgenologically (by barium enema) all individuals with a celiac syndrome to detect any unrotated cecum or mobile cecum, because surgical correction of such abnormality can at times completely relieve the patient's symptoms.

ROENTGENOLOGIC EXAMINATION

History and physical findings will often suggest the correct diagnosis, but this should be confirmed by roentgenologic investigation (Fig. 104). A film of the abdomen without the use of contrast media may show a gas-filled, dilated stomach and duodenum, but in some cases vomiting has been so effective that the duodenum and stomach are empty and no evidence of high intestinal obstruction is gained from this simple study. If a baby is seen in the first week of life, there may be only a few small bubbles of air in the intestinal tract below the level of the duodenum. In marked contrast, there may be an enormous distention of the entire jejunum and ileum.

Visualization of the duodenum or the colon with contrasting barium almost always gives significant information. There is no set rule regarding which should be studied first. In general, if the patient has rather acute symptoms suggesting high obstruction, it is probably best to give a few swallows of barium for this can quickly supply the data on which the diagnosis of duodenal blockage is made. If one is studying a patient who has had recurrent symptoms, and there is nothing urgent at the moment, it is probably better to start with a barium enema. Any anomalies of position or mobility of the cecum can be detected thereby; the barium can be evacuated before beginning a gastro-intestinal series. In many cases it is not necessary to examine the patient with contrast media by mouth and also by enema; either one can give all the information which is necessary. In other instances, examination by both routes is very desirable.

When examined from above, the stomach is usually larger than normal and the first part of the duodenum is distinctly dilated. Barium can be seen passing down to the point of obstruction, and *fluoroscopically* may be observed to churn up and down in the enlarged duodenum. Only a small amount of the material will pass beyond this region.

A *barium enema* will show the cecum in the epigastrium or right upper quadrant, and in an incompletely rotated position. In a few cases the transverse colon appears in a normal position as far proximal as the hepatic flexure, but then the ascending colon and cecum are sharply angulated and tucked up underneath this transverse colon.

It is well to bear in mind that abnormal positions of the cecum and ascending colon may be the only roentgenologic findings, and no evidence of intestinal obstruction may be forthcoming if the patient is not currently having an attack.

TREATMENT

In recent years the great improvement in therapeutic results can be attributed to better preoperative care, adoption of an operation which completely relieves obstruction in an aseptic manner, and proper supportive management during the early post-operative days.

Preoperative Preparation

The majority of these patients present acute surgical emergencies, are dehydrated, and are in rather poor general condition. Fluids and electrolytes should be restored by parenteral administration of both *physiologic saline* and *glucose*. A small catheter should be introduced through one nostril, and led down into the stomach for aspiration of fluid and gas which has collected there. In small infants a No. 8 or 10 soft-rubber urethral

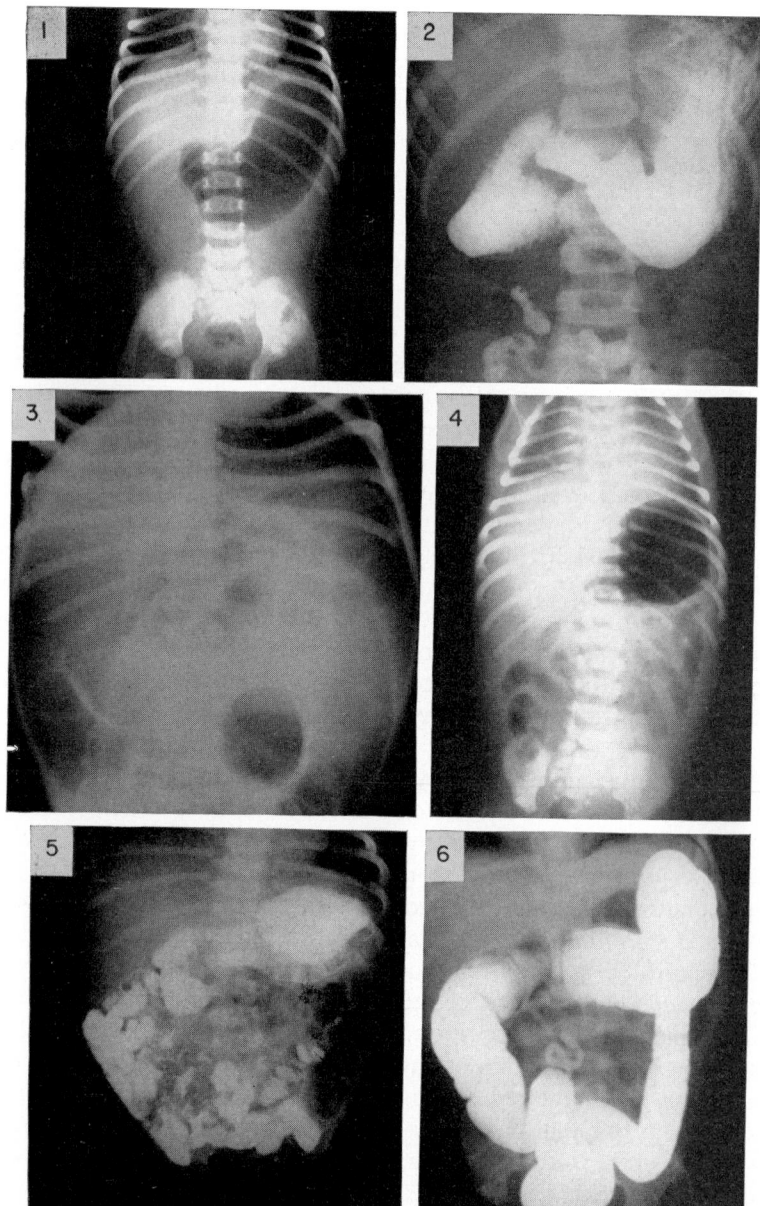

Fig. 104. Films from 6 babies with malrotation, to show some of the roentgenographic pictures which can be obtained. 1. Two-day old child with duodenal obstruction. Large amount of gas in the stomach; very little gas in intestines beyond duodenum. 2. Three-year old boy with intermittent vomiting since birth. Barium shows considerable dilatation of duodenum, with blockage in its terminal portion, only little barium escaping into the intestines. 3. Three-month old baby with symptoms and signs of acute intestinal obstruction for thirty-six hours. Abdomen greatly distended. Intestinal loops diffusely dilated in the film. Findings at operation—unattached cecum and mesentery, with a volvulus of the entire midgut. Gas has entered and become trapped in the twisted midgut. 4. From a child with volvulus of the intestines. There is some gas collecting in the intestines, and a great deal of fluid pouring out between loops (interference with venous return by a twist of the mesenteric base). 5. Barium series in a child who had had intermittent duodenal obstruction (from transduodenal peritoneal bands). The duodenum is moderately dilated and obstructed. There are many coils of intestine in an anomalous position on the (patient's) right side of the abdomen. 6. Barium enema from a child who had intermittent duodenal obstruction. The cecum and appendix can be seen shifted to a medial position; (under the fluoroscope, the cecum and ascending colon were seen to be quite mobile).

catheter serves admirably for this purpose, if several holes are cut in the end which lies in the stomach. *Deflation of the stomach* is important for two reasons. First, the danger of vomiting and aspiration will be lessened. Second, the intra-abdominal manipulations at operation will be greatly facilitated.

Operative Technique

Anesthesia. The anesthesia in all of these cases should be general narcosis, preferably with *ether.* Great relaxation of the abdominal wall will be necessary to explore the abdomen completely and to deliver the loops of intestine as subsequently described. It is essential to have an anesthetic which will completely abolish pain when the intestines are delivered and the mesentery is pulled upon. Therefore, local anesthesia is rarely satisfactory.

Exposure of the Intestine. In exploring one of these patients it is necessary to have a generous exposure. A *long right rectus incision* running from the xiphoid process downward well below the umbilicus will be found essential. The rectus muscle is retracted laterally. Some peritoneal fluid is always encountered which can be rapidly sucked away. On inspection of the abdominal viscera one of two conditions is found: (1) *The ascending and transverse colon lie in the right upper quadrant, and there is no intestinal volvulus.* The duodenum is obstructed by pressure from the overlying cecum, or from peritoneal bands which cross over to the colon and cecum. This duodenal compression is relieved by a comparatively simple operation devised by Ladd. The posterior parietal peritoneum is incised just to the right of the cecum, which permits clearing of the anterior surface of the duodenum until the latter is exposed throughout its whole length. In doing this the cecum is displaced to the patient's left and all pressure is taken off the duodenum. It is sometimes necessary to divide a few nondescript folds or bands near the duodenal-jejunal junction to completely bring the duodenum out into clear view and to insure that it lies in an unobstructed way. No attempt is made to restore the normal anatomic position of the cecum, which is not only unimportant, but is apt to be unrelated to relief of the patient's symptoms. This operation is aseptic, affords lasting relief, and is far superior to any short-circuiting anastomosis.

(2) *The entire small intestine is twisted (midgut volvulus).* If, on opening the abdomen, the surgeon sees only the small intestinal mass (which may be discolored) and cannot view the right half of the colon, he should at once suspect a midgut volvulus (Fig. 105). To one who is unfamiliar with this picture, it may be extremely puzzling; it often appears that loops of ileum are herniating through some part of the mesentery. If the surgeon attempts to evaluate the findings without delivering all the intestines outside the abdomen, he will become hopelessly confused, will waste valuable time, and usually not find out what he is dealing with. *The whole midgut must be pulled out onto the abdominal wall.* This can be done readily and with little shock in these patients, who have only a rudimentary attachment of the mesentery to the posterior abdominal wall. After the intestines have been delivered, the volvulus can be recognized. It has usually taken place in a clockwise direction and may go through an arc of 360 degrees, or, as in one of our patients, through four complete turns. The volvulus is reduced by unwinding the mass in the appropriate direction. When this is done, a normal color returns to the intestines and the surgeon might be led to believe that everything necessary has been done. *This is a grave error which generally leads to fatality. The cecum and ascending colon, which now lie in the right upper quadrant, must be freed and transferred to the left.* This can be accomplished rapidly by merely incising the peritoneum to the right of the ascending colon or high cecum. When this fold has been slit and the right half of the colon dis-

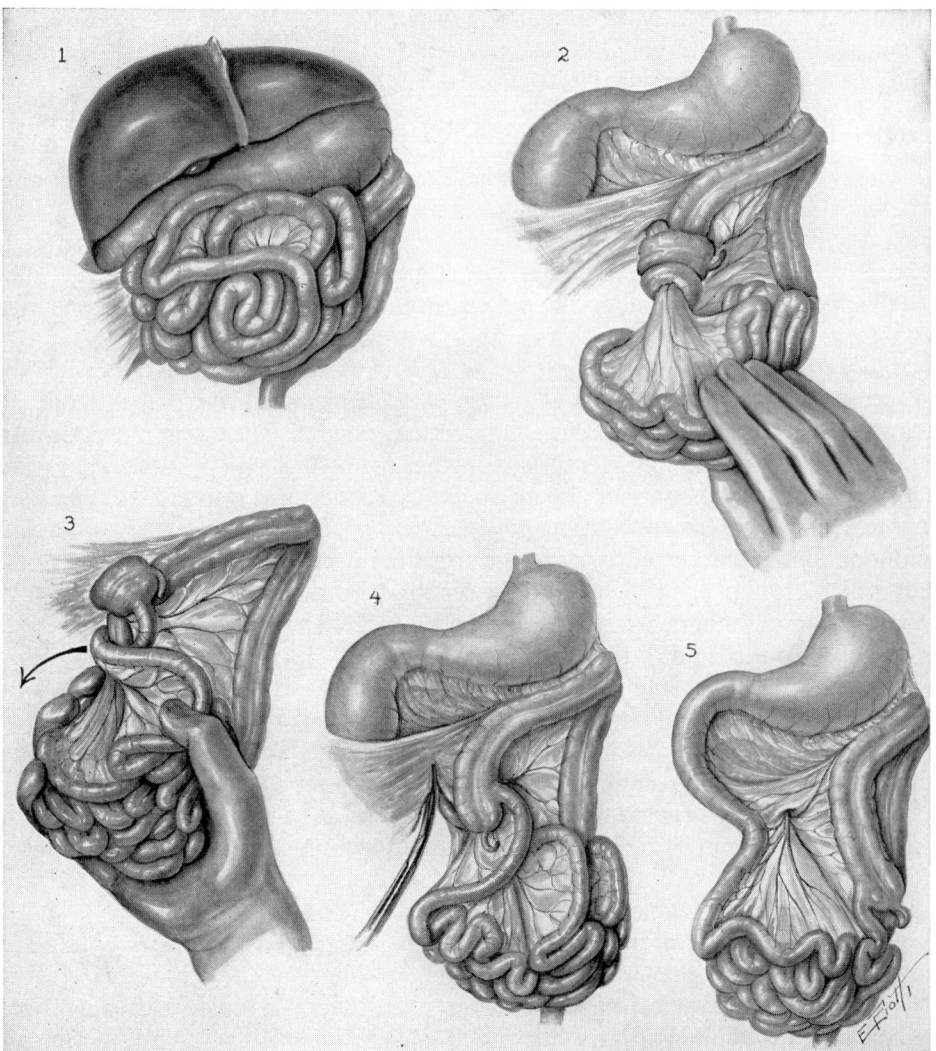

Fig. 105. Operative treatment of acute intestinal obstruction arising from incompletely rotated cecum associated with volvulus of the midgut. 1. Appearance of viscera on opening abdominal cavity. The small intestines are seen at once and appear to hide the right half of the colon. 2. The intestinal mass is delivered out of the wound and pulled downward, showing the base of the mesentery. Coils of intestine or ascending colon are wrapped around the root of an incompletely anchored mesentery. The volvulus has taken place in a clockwise direction. The descending duodenum is dilated because of extrinsic pressure from the peritoneal folds which cross it and run to the colon. 3. The volvulus is reduced by taking the entire intestinal mass in the hand and rotating it in an anticlockwise direction (in most cases). 4. The volvulus is now completely reduced and the cecum lies in the right side of the abdomen. The peritoneal folds from the cecum can now be seen as they press on the duodenum; the duodenum is still obstructed by these folds. The folds are now being severed; they do not carry any blood supply to the intestine or colon. 5. Appearance of the intestines and ascending colon at end of the operative procedure. The duodenum descends in the right paravertebral gutter to join the jejunum. The small intestines lie on the right side of the abdomen, while the cecum and ascending colon slide to the midline or left side of the abdomen. All obstruction is relieved by this procedure. The superior mesenteric artery and its branches are left exposed as shown.

placed from the right upper quadrant, the duodenum will be seen coursing downward in the right paravertebral gutter to join the jejunum. The entire colon will reside in the left side of the abdomen.

Removal of Appendix

It is generally inadvisable to remove the appendix incidentally in these operations. Most of these patients have been extremely ill before operation; the surgical procedure opens up wide raw areas within the abdomen and requires much handling and manipulation of the intestines. Under these circumstances, the contamination of the peritoneal cavity with any organisms may end disastrously. Removal of the appendix is justifiable only in older subjects and those who have been in reasonably good general condition prior to the time of operation.

Symptomless Cases

All children who are found to have an incompletely rotated colon need not necessarily be candidates for surgery. We have followed a few individuals who are known to have a partially displaced cecum but who have never had symptoms therefrom. This group is relatively small when compared to the number of persons who do have complaints from an abnormally located colon.

Mobile Cecum

Occasionally one sees a child who has no duodenal obstruction but who has symptoms from a mobile cecum which can twist or angulate upon itself. Treatment may be in one of two ways: (1) If the mesentery has a rather normal attachment to the posterior abdominal wall, the mobile cecum can be tacked down posteriorly with suitably placed silk sutures. (2) If the mesentery has very little posterior attachment, it is easier, safer, and quicker to carry out the Ladd technique and slit the peritoneum at the right of the hepatic flexure, so that the entire right half of the colon can shift over into the left side of the abdomen.

Postoperative Therapy

All of the various measures which are desirable for the care of patients after extensive abdominal surgery should be carried out; it is particularly important to use constant gastric suction. The extensive intra-abdominal manipulations almost invariably produce profound disturbances of intestinal motility for several days. To combat abdominal distention and to prevent the dangers of vomiting and aspiration, the stomach should be kept deflated as long as green material comes up the tube. This period generally lasts for one or two days; sometimes it is longer.

RESULTS OF TREATMENT

On perusing the literature one often finds that the treatment of these abnormalities is followed by *mortality figures* which are unwarrantably high. A summary of our own material gives a most encouraging picture of the prognosis, provided the condition is not associated with some other serious malformation.

Statistical Data

A considerable number of these patients, particularly those seen in the first few weeks of life, have some other serious malformation in the abdomen which greatly complicates the surgical care and which contributes heavily to mortality rates. To gain a more clear picture of our material, it is analyzed here by dividing it into: (1) Those subjects who were treated for malrotation alone, and (2) those who were treated for a malrotation and also required additional surgery for some other serious intra-abdominal or alimentary tract anomaly. The data are listed in Table 20. In the group of children who had only a malrotation to be operated upon, there were 85 per cent survivors. In the group requiring surgery for malrotation and also for some other condition, there were 43 per cent survivors.

Relief of Celiac Syndrome

There have been some gratifying results in a few older children who had clinical pictures suggestive of celiac disease and who had roentgenologic findings of an incompletely rotated cecum. In these cases a release of the cecum toward the left side of the abdomen, and freeing of the base of the mesentery, has produced clinical improvement. Presumably there had been some interference with the venous return of the small intestine which altered its absorptive function. It is evident that all subjects with symptoms suggestive of celiac disease should be roentgenologically examined by barium enema to detect any unusual position or mobility of the cecum and ascending colon which might be corrected by surgery.

Recurrence of Volvulus

In one patient there has been subsequent appearance of intestinal volvulus. The fact that this does not occur more often is probably dependent on the postoperative development of a few abdominal adhesions which prevent the intestines from swinging again.

Subsequent Appendicitis

Since it has been our policy in most of these operations to leave the appendix, there is the risk that these subjects might subsequently develop appendicitis with unusual physical findings. One child is known to have developed appendicitis some years later;

Table 20

Statistics on the Treatment of 156 Malrotations by Ladd's Operation
(to January 1, 1951)

Patients Treated Only for Malrotation		Patients Treated for Malrotation and Also for Some Other Abnormality	
Living—108	Dead—20	Living—12	Dead—16
Causes of Death:		These also had:	These also had:
Preoperative perforation or gangrene of intestine 5		Pyloric stenosis..... 4	Pyloric stenosis..... 1
Recurrence of volvulus................... 1		Duodenal stenosis... 3	Duodenal stenosis or
Evisceration......................... 2		Biliary obstruction.. 3	atresia.......... 8
Subsequent adhesions and obstruction....... 5		Annular pancreas... 1	Omphalocele....... 2
Inanition............................ 1		Intestinal duplication 1	Annular pancreas... 1
Thrombosis of mesenteric vessels........... 1			G.U. anomalies 1
Uncontrollable diarrhea.................. 1			Esophageal atresia.. 3
Congenital heart disease................. 3			
Pneumonia........................... 1			
Per Cent Survivors.....................85		Per Cent Survivors.....................43	

the pain and tenderness were in the left side of the epigastrium, and it was from this region that the appendix was removed.

Relief of Duodenal Obstruction

A long experience in treating malrotation of the colon has given ample evidence of the effectiveness of the Ladd operation in completely and permanently curing duodenal obstruction. In all of the patients listed as survivors in Table 20, there has been lasting and very gratifying relief of obstructive symptoms.

REFERENCES

1. Brown, R. B. and Ross, D.: Congenital Abnormalities of Intestinal Rotation and Mesenteric Attachment—a Cause of Intestinal Obstruction in the Adult. Ann. Surg., *134:* 88, 1951.
2. Dott, N. M.: Anomalies of Intestinal Rotation: Their Embryology and Surgical Aspects, with Report of Five Cases. Brit. J. Surg., *11:*251, 1923.
3. Frazer, J. E. and Robbins, R. H.: On the Factors Concerned in Causing Rotation of the Intestine in Man. J. Anat. & Physiol., *50:*75, 1915.
4 Gardner, C. E., Jr., and Hart, D.: Anomalies of Intestinal Rotation as a Cause of Intestinal Obstruction; Report of Two Personal Observations; Review of One Hundred and Three Reported Cases. Arch. Surg., *29:*942, 1934.
5. Raymond, H. E. and Dragstedt, L. R.: Anomalies of Intestinal Rotation: A Review of the Literature with Report of Two Cases. Surg., Gynec. & Obst., *53:*316, 1931.
6 Hecker, P., Grunwald, E. and Kuhlmann, C. J.: Les anomalies congénitales de forme et de position du gros intestin et leur importance chirurgicale. Rev. de chir., *64:*661, 1926.
7. Jones, T. B. and Morton, J. J.: Congenital Malformations of the Intestine in Children. Am. J. Surg., *39:*382, 1938.
8. King, E. S. J.: Two Uncommon Forms of Intestinal Obstruction Occurring Consecutively; Compound Volvulus and Retroposition of the Transverse Colon. Brit. J. Surg., *24:*817, 1937.
9. Koszler, V.: Zur Klinik des Mesenterium commune. Arch. f. Kinderh., *110:*166, 1937.
10. Ladd, W. E.: Congenital Obstruction of the Small Intestine. J.A.M.A., *101:*1453, 1933.
11. Ladd, W. E.: Surgical Diseases of the Alimentary Tract in Infants. New England J. Med., *215:*705, 1936.
12. McIntosh, R. and Donovan, E. J.: Disturbances of Rotation of the Intestinal Tract; Clinical Picture Based on Observations in Twenty Cases. Am. J. Dis. Child., *57:*116, 1939.
13. Miller, R. and Gage, H. C.: Gastromegaly and Chronic Duodenal Ileus in Children. Arch. Dis. Childhood, *5:*83, 1930.
14. Mole, R. H.: Congenital Non-Rotation of the Intestine. Brit. J. Surg., *17:*670, 1930.
15. Morton, J. J. and Jones, T. B.: Obstructions About the Mesentery in Infants. Ann. Surg., *104:*864, 1936.
16. Reisman, H. A.: Congenital Obstruction of the Alimentary Tract. J. Pediat., *10:*622, 1937.
17. Rubin, E. L.: Radiological Aspects of Anomalies of Intestinal Rotation. Lancet, *2:*1222, 1935.
18. Silverman, F. N. and Caffey, J.: Congenital Obstructions of the Alimentary Tract in Infants and Children: Errors of Rotation of the Midgut. Radiology, *53:*781, 1949.
19. Wakefield, E. G. and Mayo, C. W.: Intestinal Obstruction Produced by Mesenteric Bands in Association with Failure of Intestinal Rotation. Arch. Surg., *33:*47, 1936.
20. Wangensteen, O. H.: New Operative Techniques in the Management of Bowel Obstruction. Surg., Gynec. & Obst., *75:*675, 1942.
21. Waugh, G. E.: Congenital Malformations of the Mesentery: A Clinical Entity. Brit. J. Surg., *15:*438, 1928.

CHAPTER 15

Annular Pancreas Producing Duodenal Obstruction

An uncommon but interesting form of obstruction is that which arises from an annular pancreas, in which there is a ring of pancreatic substance surrounding and constricting the second portion of the duodenum. The degree of obstruction varies from case to case. In those cases in which the constriction is mild, there may be no symptoms or there may be related difficulties only in adult life. In those cases in which obstruction is marked, there is striking evidence of duodenal blockage early in life, even in the neonatal period. The obstruction is one which can be corrected by surgical means with a high degree of success.

PATHOLOGY

In this malformation the head of the pancreas lies in its customary position in the bend of the duodenum. From this head, two arms of pancreatic tissue extend around the second part of the duodenum, one anteriorly and one posteriorly; these usually fuse and form a complete encircling mass. In some subjects there is a gap between the two ends; if this occurs it is apt to appear anteriorly. Such a ring of pancreatic tissue almost invariably produces, or is accompanied by, some degree of compression and stenosis of the duodenum. In rare instances, there is an atresia of the duodenum at the level of the pancreatic ring.

The annular portion has all of the histologic characteristics of normal pancreas. It contains islet as well as acinar tissue. The ducts for the external secretions have been the subject of considerable investigation. They may be rudimentary and may run from the anterior part of the ring toward the left to join the main pancreatic duct. However, it is more common for the annular part of the pancreas to be traversed by a major duct which begins anteriorly, runs to the right, and then curves around laterally and posteriorly, finally, to join either the common bile duct or the main pancreatic duct. In some cases the lower segment of the common duct passes through the posterior portion of the annular pancreas and is obstructed either by constriction or angulation.

The pathologic data can be divided into four general categories: (1) The changes which occur in the pancreatic substance itself. (2) The secondary effects upon the alimentary system. (3) The derangements which are sometimes found in the lower biliary passages. (4) The associated congenital abnormalities in other portions of the body.

Numerous writers have commented upon the finding of some form of pancreatitis, either acute and hemorrhagic in nature, or chronic and cicatricial in type. Such changes may involve the main body of the pancreas, only the annular portion, or the entire organ. Severe pancreatitis is not infrequently the illness which brings the patient to the operating table or to autopsy. The relatively high incidence of inflammatory lesions in patients

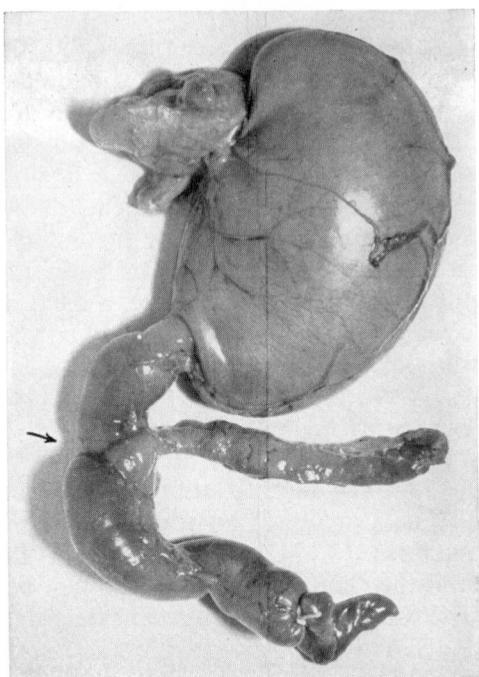

Fig. 106. Annular pancreas from an eight-day-old baby who died of congenital heart disease and obstruction. A ring of pancreatic tissue surrounds and obstructs the duodenum.

with annular pancreas suggests an origin related to abnormal form of the ducts. Certainly, it is conceivable that an attenuated or angulated ductal system could produce stasis and back pressure. Similarly, a direct communication with the biliary system, associated with compression of the lower portion of the common duct, might lead to reflux of bile into the pancreatic tissue and thereby activate the pancreatic enzymes.

The secondary changes in the intestinal tract are obvious. Dilatation and thickening of the first part of the duodenum are in direct proportion to the degree of obstruction which has been produced by the pancreatic ring. Gastric or duodenal ulceration has been frequently reported. This may be dependent upon stasis of gastric or duodenal material or it might be secondary to a reduced flow of pancreatic juice.

Any disturbances in the biliary system, if they occur, are purely those brought about by partial blockage of the common duct as it traverses pancreatic tissue. Dilatation of the extrahepatic ducts, stasis of bile within the liver, and evidence of icterus throughout the body may be of mild or marked degree. Biliary obstruction generally does not appear in patients who have an annular pancreas, but if it is going to appear it is apt to be manifest in infancy or early childhood.

Like any congenital malformation in the human, an annular pancreas may be associated with a considerable incidence of other anatomic abnormalities in neighboring or distant parts of the body. Some of these are of only academic interest and do not necessarily disturb the patient's health. However, many of them are of considerable importance, have given rise to serious symptoms, or even have brought fatality. Of the 10 patients we have operated upon for duodenal obstruction, 9 had some other abnormality, and in 3 of them it was serious enough to require operative correction, was a menace to well being (Mongolism), or was a threat to life (congenital heart disease). Some data regarding these cases are listed in Table 21.

EMBRYOLOGY

Embryology of the annular pancreas has been thoroughly discussed by McNaught[10] and others. Theoretic explanations for development of the anomaly are mainly in one of two categories. Lerat[9] and others contend that the annular arrangement is merely the result of hyperplasia—that is, overgrowth of pancreatic substance—dissecting in such a way beneath the serosal coat of the duodenum that it finally surrounds this part of the alimentary tube. They suggest that the enlargement follows fetal peritonitis as a regenerative process. Most workers, however, favor the theory that the malformation results from the failure of the tip of the ventral pancreatic anlage to rotate with the duodenum—as does its ductal outlet. In consequence, a band of elongated, pancreatic tissue becomes wrapped around the duodenum in a napkin-ring fashion, and the duct from the ventral anlage sweeps around the entire duodenum to enter the duct of Wirsung.

CLINICAL DATA

In 1933, McNaught[10] reviewed the literature and collected 40 cases of annular pancreas. In 1935, he and Cox[11] presented an additional case and cited three others, which had been already recorded. In 1942, Lehman[8] brought this total up to 48 cases, and particularly emphasized the clinical problem which can be produced by the congenital abnormality. In 1943, Chapman and Mossman[3] described the findings in a dissection room subject. Ravitch and Woods[12] listed 3 cases treated by surgery. In 1952 Shapiro, Dzurik, and Gerrish[13] presented 4 cases with obstruction in the neonatal period. In all, about 85 cases have been published; only a minority of these have been in infancy and childhood.

It is evident that duodenal obstruction can be complete or nearly complete so that there is duodenal obstruction in the first few days of life; conversely, the degree of blockage may be so slight that no complaints are referable to it until subsequent years or even adult life.

When an annular pancreas produces symptoms, it usually manifests itself in the form of acute or chronic duodenal obstruction. There may be epigastric pain, nausea, vomiting, and possibly malnutrition. The vomitus may or may not contain bile, depending upon the anatomic relationship of the common duct to the narrowed portion of duodenum.

Roentgenologic examination by a barium series gives rather conclusive proof of a partial block, with dilatation of the first part of the duodenum compared to a more collapsed third part of the organ. The mid-duodenum is notched or constricted. Such filling defects, and associated delay in emptying of the stomach and first part of the duodenum, may be indistinguishable from the picture produced by a healed duodenal ulcer which has given marked duodenal deformity. However, in a subject of childhood years, such roentgenologic findings are more suggestive of a congenital duodenal stenosis or annular pancreas than of a cicatrizing peptic ulcer.

While evidence of pancreatitis is a complication which has been seen in adults, we have not detected it in any of our childhood cases.

In rare instances, usually in infants dying within the first few months of life, *jaundice* has been a presenting complaint. It may be mild or marked. The stool contains much or little bile pigment—depending upon the degree of obstruction of the biliary passage. In one specimen studied by Dr. Sidney Farber in our pathology laboratory the common duct was completely blocked; the baby had had acholic stools and a very high icteric index prior to its death at five months.

TREATMENT

Aside from the consideration of any biliary obstruction which might exist, the necessity for operation will depend upon the degree of duodenal obstruction which accompanies the lesion. Under rare circumstances the duodenum may be atretic and surgical relief is imperative in the first few days of life. Similarly, those babies who have only a tiny, pinhole opening in the duodenum require early operative intervention. In some cases one finds that a fluid or even solid diet can be tolerated for many years before symptoms of high intestinal obstruction manifest themselves and demand surgical therapy.

The alleviation of duodenal obstruction can be conceivably effected in three different ways, and each type of operation has been supported by various proponents:

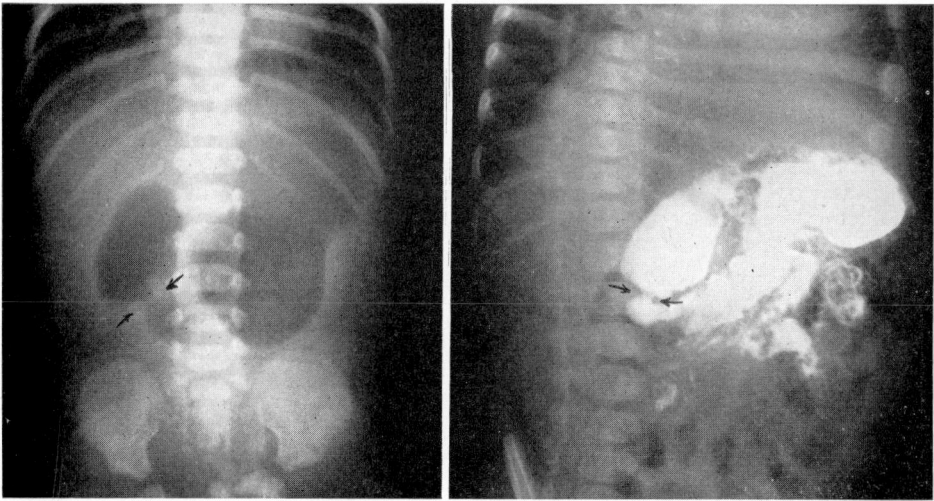

Fig. 107. Roentgenograms from patients with duodenal obstruction from an annular pancreas. *Left*, Plain film from a three-day-old baby. Gas in the stomach and dilated first portion of the duodenum. No gas seen in remainder of abdomen. *Right*, Barium meal examination of a five-day-old child, showing the marked constriction of the duodenum (at the arrows).

1. *Division of the ring of pancreatic tissue*, or a resection of part of the same, has been performed by Lerat,[9] Howard,[7] Lehman[8] and others. Zech followed this procedure by a Heineke-Mikulicz type of plastic enlargement of the constricted duodenal wall. Many of these patients survived, but not infrequently they developed a pancreatic fistula which gave some concern during the postoperative course. Such leakage is a distinct hazard in this type of therapy. Since the pancreatic ducts may exhibit considerable variation in their distribution, the operator can never be certain when a major duct will be severed if the pancreatic ring is divided. Furthermore, simple section (or partial resection) of the ring will not always insure a complete release of the duodenum, since the latter may be constricted by fibrous tissue within the wall itself. A review of cases which have been treated by these methods shows that incomplete relief of obstruction has oftentimes required a second operation. *There is no doubt that direct attack on the pancreatic ring or constricted portion of duodenum is inferior to a short-circuiting type of operation.*

2. *A posterior gastro-enterostomy* has been established by some operators. Relief of the duodenal obstruction by such a measure will probably have the largest number of adherents, since this operation is one which is well standardized and which will un-

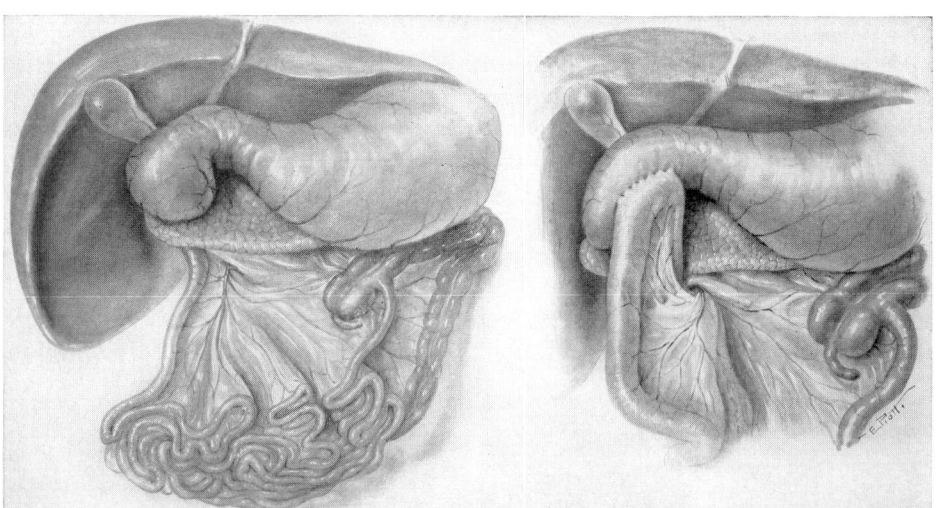

Fig. 108. Abnormality and treatment in patient 1, Table 21. *Left,* Findings at operation. There was an incomplete rotation of the colon and intestines. Continuous with the body and head of the pancreas was a ring of pancreatic substance which completely surrounded and obstructed the duo-denum. First portion of duodenum was dilated; beyond the obstruction, the intestine and colon were collapsed. *Right,* Method of surgical alleviation of duodenal obstruction by establishment of an isoperistaltic duodeno-jejunostomy.

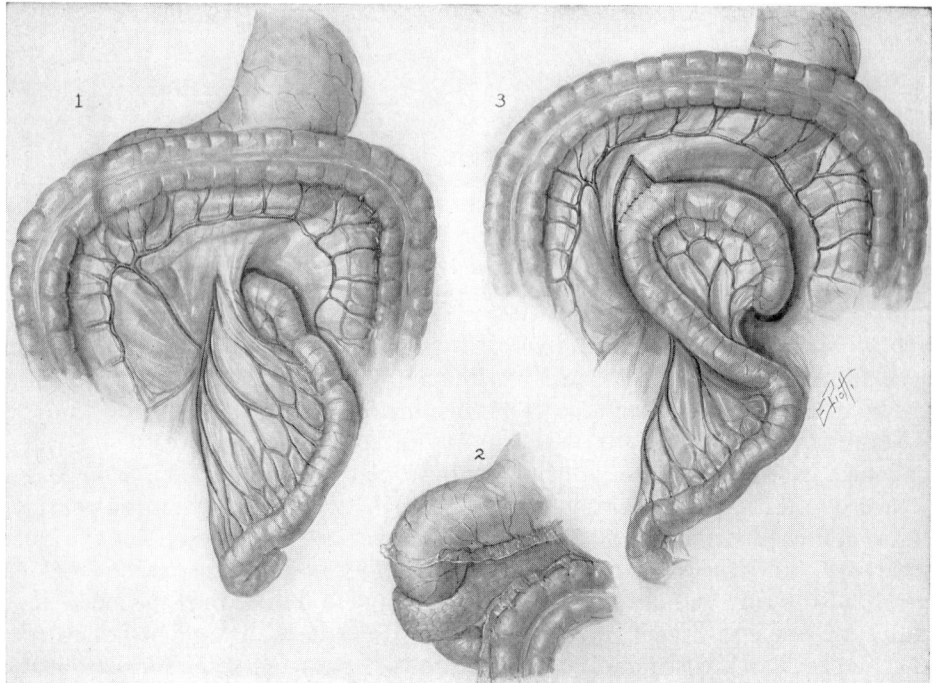

Fig. 109. Usual findings in cases with annular pancreas; recommended method of therapy. 1. An-nular pancreas, producing high degree of duodenal obstruction. 2. Hepatic flexure of colon reflected to show better the duodenum. 3. Operative treatment by retrocolic isoperistaltic duodeno-jejunostomy. The transverse mesocolon has been opened to expose the first part of the duodenum. The jejunum has been brought over against this for an anastomosis. For the two-layered union in babies, the outer stitch has been made with continuous 00000 Deknatel silk on an atraumatic needle and the inner layer has been made with 00000 chromic catgut.

doubtedly relieve symptoms in the majority of cases. However, in some patients it will not effectively drain the proximal duodenum, hence we believe that it is inferior to a duodeno-jejunostomy.

3. *Duodeno-jejunostomy* was first proposed and used by us[6] in 1942 for the treatment of obstruction arising from annular pancreas. We believe this to be the ideal type of surgical correction, because it completely relieves the duodenal stasis, does not interfere in any way with the gastric functions, and does not possess any of the hazards of cutting the pancreatic ring with its attendant danger of fistula. In spite of the diminutive size of the distal collapsed loop of intestine, it is possible to perform an isoperistaltic duodeno-jejunostomy in a small baby. In one of our cases (Fig. 108) this was greatly facilitated by an incomplete rotation of the colon (which made the duodenum more approachable). When the colon is situated in its normal position, the mesocolon can be pierced, bring-

Table 21

Data from Cases of Annular Pancreas Cases
(Through 1950)

Case	Age Sex	Year	Duration of Symptoms	Operation	Other Congenital Anomalies	Result
1	3 days F	1942	Since birth	Duodeno-jejunostomy	Malrotation	Cured
2	5 mos. F	1946	Since birth	Duodeno-jejunostomy	Ectopic kidney Meckel's diverticulum Accessory spleen	Died 14 hours post-operatively
3	2 days F	1948	Since birth	Duodeno-jejunostomy	Malrotation	Died after 7 days. Subdural hemorrhage
4	1 day F	1948	Since birth	Duodeno-jejunostomy	Meckel's diverticulum	Cured
5	5 days F	1948	Since birth	Duodeno-jejunostomy	. . . . . .	Cured
6	5 days F	1949	Since birth	Duodeno-jejunostomy	? Mongol	Cured
7	1 day M	1949	Since birth	Duodeno-jejunostomy	Esophageal atresia (op. for it). Congenital heart disease	Died after 8 days
8	5 days M	1950	Since birth	Duodeno-jejunostomy	Malrotation. (Ladd's op. for it)	Cured
9	1 day M	1950	Since birth	Duodeno-jejunostomy	Esophageal atresia (op. for it). Imperforate anus (colostomy for it). Congenital heart disease	Died at 3 months (cardiac)
10	2 days M	1950	Since birth	Duodeno-jejunostomy	? Mongol	Cured

ing into view the dilated proximal portion of duodenum which can then be anastomosed to the jejunum which is brought over against it (Fig. 109).

RESULTS OF TREATMENT

In the Children's Hospital material there have been 5 babies, from eight days to five months of age, who died from various causes and were found at autopsy to have also an annular pancreas. In only one of these did duodenal obstruction contribute to the exitus (Fig. 106). In addition there have been 10 patients who came to our Service because of duodenal obstruction and were operated upon for this. Data concerning them are listed in Table 21. Six patients are alive, well, and completely cured of their obstruction. In the 4 who died, death was primarily related to esophageal atresia in one, cardiac malformation in one, subdural hemorrhage in one, and shock in one.

In summary, if the duodenal obstruction is accompanied by other serious malformation or malady, the outlook is grave, but if it exists as the sole lesion giving rise to the child's complaints, the patient can be cured in the vast majority of cases by establishment of a duodeno-jejunostomy.

REFERENCES

1. Brines, O. A.: Annular Pancreas, Involved in Acute Hemorrhagic Pancreatitis. Ann. Surg., *92:*241, 1930.
2. Brines, O. A.: Annular Pancreas Associated with Peptic Ulcer. Am. J. Surg., *12:*483, 1931.
3. Chapman, J. L. and Mossman, H. W.: Annular Pancreas: Accompanied by an Aberrant Pancreatic Nodule in the Duodenum. Am. J. Surg., *60:*286, 1943.
4. Cunningham, G. J.: Annular Pancreas. Brit. J. Surg., *27:*678, 1939–40.
5. dos Santos, R.: Deux lésions rare du duodenum. XV Congrés International de Medicine, Lisbon, *9:*419, 1906.
6. Gross, R. E. and Chisholm, T. C.: Annular Pancreas Producing Duodenal Obstruction. Ann. Surg., *119:*759, 1944.
7. Howard, N. J.: Annular Pancreas. Surg., Gynec., & Obst., *50:*533, 1930.
8. Lehman, E. P.: Annular Pancreas as a Clinical Problem. Ann. Surg., *115:*574, 1942.
9. Lerat, P.: Contribution chirurgicale a l'Étude du pancréas annulaire. Bull. Acad. roy. de méd. de Belgique, 4th Series, *24:*290, 1910.
10. McNaught, J. B.: Annular Pancreas. A Compilation of 40 Cases, with a Report of a New Case. Am. J. M. Sc., *185:*249, 1933.
11. McNaught, J. B. and Cox, A. J., Jr.: Annular Pancreas. Report of a Case, with a Simple Method for Visualizing the Duct System. Am. J. Path., *11:*179, 1935.
12. Ravitch, M. M. and Woods, A. C., Jr.: Annular Pancreas. Ann. Surg., *132:*1116, 1950.
13. Shapiro, D. J., Dzurik, F. J. and Gerrish, E. W.: Obstruction of Duodenum in the Newborn Infant Due to Annular Pancreas. Pediatrics, *9:*764, 1952.
14. Silvis, R. S.: Annular Pancreas. Ann. Surg., *135:*278, 1952.

CHAPTER 16

Meckel's Diverticulum

Meckel's diverticulum is said to occur in 2 or 3 per cent of all cases coming to autopsy examination. This outpocketing from the ileum does not often give rise to important pathologic abnormalities, but when it does so the resulting lesion may be a serious one. The vagaries of Meckel's diverticulum are well known to surgeons who have had any breadth of experience in abdominal surgery, particularly if they have done much children's work. Our material includes 149 patients (up through 1950) for whom a diverticulectomy was performed.

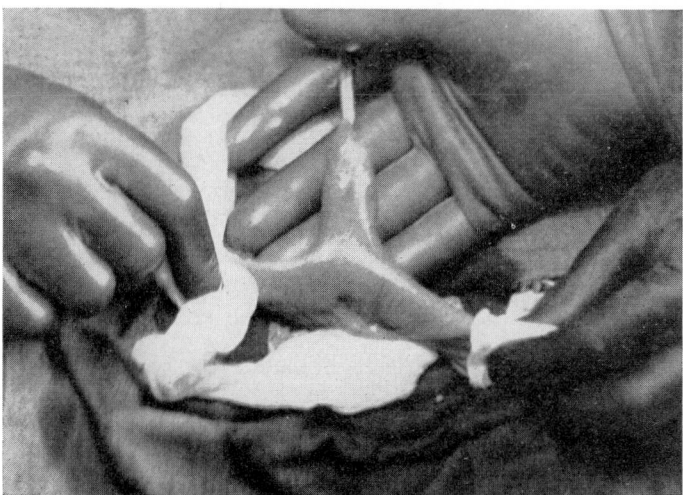

Fig. 110. Photograph of Meckel's diverticulum taken at the operating table. (From Hudson, the New England Journal of Medicine.)

EMBRYOLOGY

During early embryonic life the intestine has a wide anterior communication with the yolk sac. This opening is gradually narrowed to form the tube-like vitello-intestinal duct. The yolk sac remains within the cord and the vitelline duct becomes reduced to the long, slender yolk stalk which then loses its connection with the intestine at about the 7 mm. stage.

Meckel's diverticulum represents that portion of the vitelline duct which had opened into the ileum. This small pouch is usually disconnected from the umbilicus, but a cord of tissue, the remnant of the primitive yolk stalk, may join the terminal ileum to the inner aspect of the umbilicus. If a longer portion of the vitelline duct remains patent, the intestine may retain an external opening at the navel.

PATHOLOGY

Meckel's diverticulum arises from the ileum 18 inches to 3 feet above the ileo-cecal valve. It opens on the antimesenteric side of the intestine, but may curve around and lie against the side of the gut, to which it becomes adherent. Rarely the diverticulum swings over against the mesentery and acquires a filmy covering which gives it the appearance of having an intramesenteric position.

The diverticulum is a finger-like outpocketing, which usually has a diameter somewhat less than that of the adjacent bowel and a length varying from $\frac{1}{2}$ inch up to 2 or 3 inches. One of our specimens was a large orange-sized cyst which had only a small communication with the intestine. Several writers have described examples of "jejunum duplex," "ileum duplex," or "giant diverticula," which are tube-like structures a foot or more long, lying on the mesenteric border of the bowel. These have been thought to originate from Meckel's diverticula, but we do not agree with this view. Accumulated evidence favors classifying these with the "duplications" (Chapter 17), which can occur anywhere along the alimentary tract from the tongue to the anus.

The *lining* of a Meckel's diverticulum does not necessarily correspond to that of the ileum, to which it is attached. In 130 diverticula in which there was histologic examination, the mucosae were as follows:

Gastric and ileal.. 53 cases
Gastric... 14 cases
Gastric and colonic...................................... 2 cases
Gastric, ileal, and colonic.............................. 1 case
Pancreatic tissue and ileal.............................. 7 cases
Ileal only.. 45 cases
Duodenal and ileal....................................... 4 cases
Colonic and ileal.. 4 cases

Important *pathologic complications* can arise from a Meckel's diverticulum in many ways (Fig. 112). In 149 patients we have removed this structure because of the following conditions.

Ulcer and hemorrhage.................................... 50 cases
Abdominal pain.. 29 cases
Leading point of intussusception........................ 28 cases
Inflammation, with or without perforation................ 18 cases
Umbilical fistula....................................... 11 cases
Formation of cyst inside of umbilicus.................... 1 case
Obstruction from band (to umbilicus or to mesentery)......... 8 cases
Volvulus and infarction of diverticulum.................. 4 cases

Hemorrhage from a diverticulum almost invariably arises from a small peptic ulcer at the neck of the pouch or in the near-by intestine, which is presumably due to local digestion of the mucous membrane by the action of hydrochloric acid and pepsin which are secreted from aberrant gastric mucosa which lines the diverticulum.

It is not uncommon for a diverticulum, particularly if it is broad and short, to become inverted; and when it does so it may be the starting point of an *intussusception*. When once this process has started, the intussusceptum will be progressively dragged along into the terminal ileum or colon.

Inflammation of a diverticulum can be found in a small proportion of cases. Whether this appears from bacterial invasion or from chemical and enzymatic digestion is unknown; probably both contribute to the reaction. While microscopic examination shows significant bacterial growth and inflammation, the finding of gastric mucosa in some specimens suggests the possibility that digestive ferments have initiated the erosion. Once started, the disease is very apt to progress to actual *rupture* and contamination of the abdominal cavity by intestinal contents. This condition is particularly dangerous, because the migratory nature of the diverticulum and the absence of a protecting omentum in young children make free perforation a rapidly spreading and often fatal type of infection.

A vestigial band connecting a diverticulum to the inner side of the umbilicus may produce *intestinal obstruction* if a loop of gut is pulled tightly over it. If the tip of a diverticulum becomes adherent to near-by intestine or mesentery, a pocket is formed through which coils of gut can prolapse and become obstructed.

Tuberculosis and *neoplasms* in Meckel's diverticula have been described, but we have not encountered either of these in our series.

Meckel's diverticula appear to be more common in males than in females, the proportion being 75 per cent and 25 per cent, respectively, in our patients.

CLINICAL FINDINGS

Meckel's diverticulum may manifest itself at any age. If, however, complications do arise, they are more apt to do so early in life (Fig. 111). Approximately half (45 per cent) of all patients came to the hospital within the first two years of life. The youngest was five hours of age; the oldest was fourteen years.

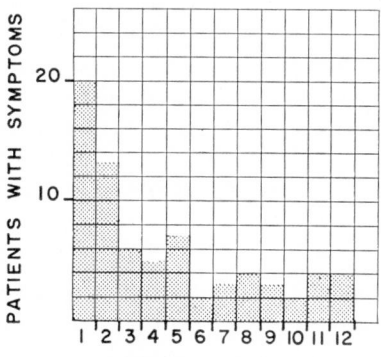

YEAR   OF   LIFE

Fig. 111. Chart showing age at which patients developed symptoms from a Meckel's diverticulum or its complications.

Hemorrhage

Massive hemorrhage was the chief symptom in 50 children, 80 per cent of whom were under two years of age. The principal and alarming symptom is usually the sudden passage of a *bloody stool* by a young child in whom there have been no previous symptoms. This bleeding is apt to be copious, and while the first stool might be dark or black in color, subsequent ones are almost invariably bright red. The extent of bleeding may be judged from the fact that the red count sometimes drops to 1,500,000 or 2,000,000. The massiveness of the bleeding is in contrast to the spotting of blood which occurs with anal fissures or rectal polyps. Bleeding from a Meckel's diverticulum is unattended by pain, or else there is only mild discomfort, which is in sharp contrast to the agonizing pain which accompanies the bleeding of intussusception. Though several of our patients had one to three previous episodes of melena, it is more common to have a single attack of bleeding which is severe enough to bring the child quickly to a physician's attention. With such hemorrhage, *lethargy, collapse, pallor,* and *increased pulse rate* are frequently concomitant findings.

Vague Symptoms without Demonstrable Pathology

In a small number of children, abdominal pain of a vague and nagging sort can apparently originate from a Meckel's diverticulum. The pain may be periumbilical or poorly localized; it is usually unattended by vomiting; and it may recur at irregular intervals. Physical examination reveals no abdominal abnormality. When the diverticulum is exposed at operation there may be no inflammation, kinking, or intestinal obstruction, and it is not clear just why the structure should give rise to symptoms. It is possible that there is some interference with the proper peristaltic activity of the intestine when the diverticulum is present. In most of these cases the concurrent removal of the appendix makes it difficult to tell which of the two caused the pain. However, relief has been obtained from diverticulectomy alone in a sufficient number of cases to prove that symptoms can originate from a diverticulum which on pathologic examination shows nothing remarkable.

Intussusception

When intussusception is started by a diverticulum, there are no features to distinguish it from the idiopathic type of intussusception which is common in childhood and in which no anatomic abnormality can be found. The clinical picture is one of *intermittent abdominal pain* which recurs at intervals of fifteen to twenty minutes. In the early hours of the illness the child will double over, cry out in distress, turn pale, and vomit during the momentary paroxysms of pain. Between seizures he will be relaxed, comparatively comfortable, and even playful. As the condition progresses he will give evidence of *shock and collapse* in the interims. Abdominal pain and symptoms of intestinal obstruction may exist for many hours before blood appears in the stools.

Appendicitis Simulated

The clinical course of a Meckel's diverticulitis may simulate that of acute appendicitis and indeed may be indistinguishable from it. The sequence of periumbilical pain, nausea, vomiting, fever, and leukocytosis is common to both conditions. If appendicitis is of some hours' standing, there may be shift of pain and maximal tenderness to the right lower quadrant. In diverticulitis, however, there is no such shift, or else the shift is to some other part of the abdomen in which the diverticulum happens to lie for the moment. Frequently the child is too young to analyze the position of his pains.

Umbilical Sinus

An umbilical sinus from which there is a repeated discharge of mucus or other fluid should at once arouse suspicion of a Meckel's diverticulum communicating with the navel. Insertion of a small catheter into the fistula, instillation of a bit of Lipiodol, and roentgenologic study may give important information concerning a communication with the intestine and thus rule out a patent urachus, which would connect with the urinary bladder. If *fecal material* exudes from the umbilicus—and there has been no previous operative procedure or disease of the abdomen to cause an intestinal fistula—one can make the proper diagnosis quickly and with great certainty. In one of our patients a

mucoid discharge was found to contain both hydrochloric acid and pepsin; examination of the subsequently removed diverticulum showed it to contain gastric mucosa.

Obstruction

Constrictions of intestinal loops which are caught over an omphalomesenteric cord have no symptoms to distinguish them from other forms of acute intestinal obstruction.

ROENTGENOLOGIC EXAMINATION

Roentgenologic examinations are practically useless in attempting to visualize a Meckel's diverticulum. We have conducted many gastro-intestinal series with contrast media in patients who were subsequently found to have a diverticulum at operation. In

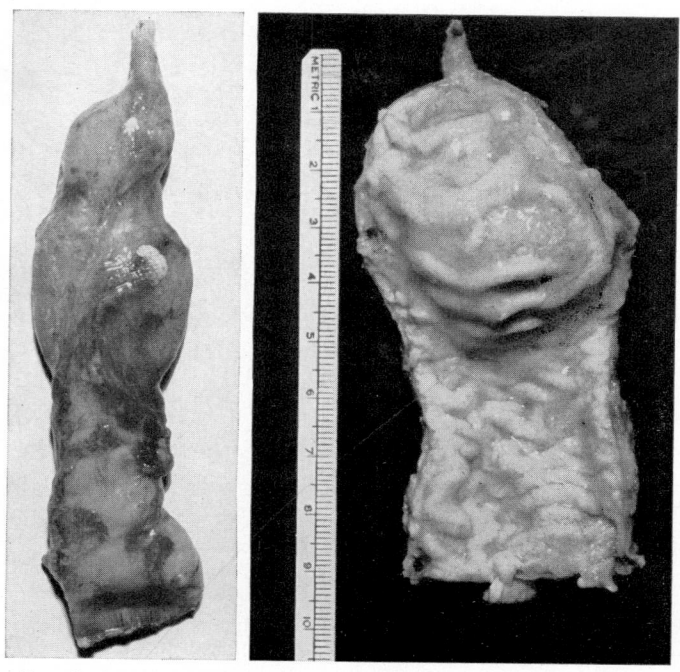

Fig. 114. Meckel's diverticulum from a nine-month-old child who had severe melena. The distal half of the pouch (upper part of photograph) was lined by gastric mucosa.

only two children did some of the barium collect in a small area which presumably represented the pouch. Our disappointing experiences have led us to abandon roentgenography as a means of searching for this congenital anomaly.

TREATMENT

Diverticulectomy

Excision and Suture. Some practical points in the treatment of Meckel's diverticula might be suggested. After removing one of them, the remaining stump should not be turned in with a purse-string suture for fear of unduly constricting the gut. Removal of the pouch should be done by first placing two clamps (half-lengths or Kocher clamps) obliquely across its base to prevent spillage, and then cutting between these with the actual *cautery* (Fig. 115). The bowel can be closed in several ways, but it is sufficient to use a single row of silk Halsted stitches. This method of diverticulectomy is practically aseptic and is superior to the operation in which the intestine is opened longitudinally and sutured transversely. If an oblique line of resection and intestinal suture has been made, the closure will not obstruct the gut.

Diverticulum with Thickened Base. Most diverticula have a thin enough base so that the above-described method of removal can be carried out. In some cases, however, the base of the diverticulum is thickened because of edematous gastric mucosa, aberrant pancreatic tissue, or inflammatory disease. In such cases it is impossible to get a satisfactory turn-in of the intestinal coats, and it is preferable to make a large, *wedge-shaped excision* of the diverticular base followed by suitable repair of the intestine. In some cases there is such extensive thickening around the base of the diverticulum that it is

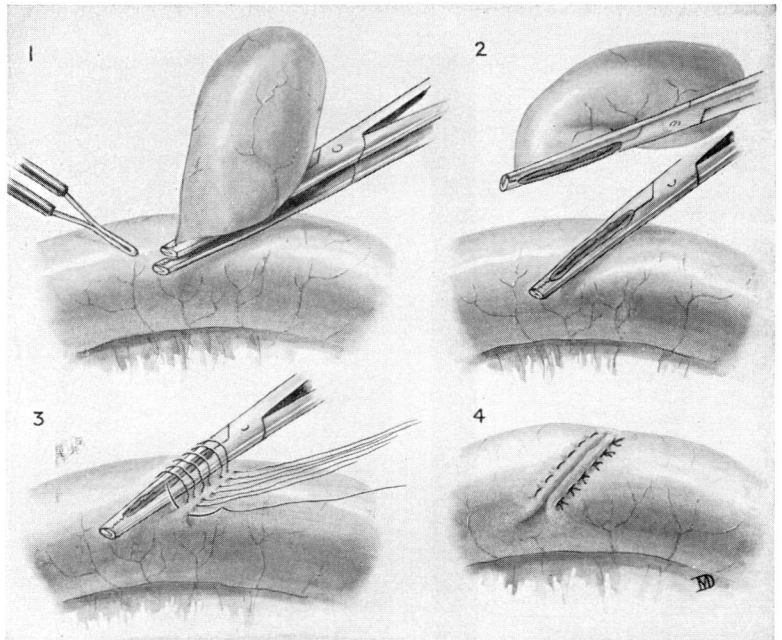

Fig. 115. Recommended method of removal of a Meckel's diverticulum: 1. Cautery cutting away diverticulum between Kocher clamps. 2. Diverticulum has been cut away. Position of the remaining clamp is shown. 3. Placement of silk Halsted sutures. 4. Clamp removed; sutures snugged up.

necessary to resect it with a short piece of bowel, reconstructing the continuity of the intestine by direct anastomosis, or (if the child is very ill) by a Mikulicz exteriorization.

Diverticulum Which Is Leading Point of Intussusception. When a diverticulum has been the leading point of an intussusception, the intussusception should be reduced (if possible) and the diverticulum everted. If the child is in satisfactory condition, the diverticulum can be removed; in some instances the child is so ill that it is much better judgment to leave the diverticulum (if it is not gangrenous) for removal at a second operation a week or two later. Whenever there is considerable damage to the diverticular or intestinal wall, this must, of course, be removed at once.

Symptomless Cases. A diverticulum which has not given rise to symptoms, but which is discovered during the course of laparotomy for some other lesion, should be excised if the condition of the patient is satisfactory. A Meckel's diverticulum is always a potential source of future trouble and should be eliminated if it is possible to do so without appreciable risk.

RESULTS OF THERAPY

Employing the above-outlined methods of treatment in 149 patients, the mortality figures given in Table 22 have obtained.

Table 22

Results of Operative Treatment in 149 Cases of Meckel's Diverticulum

Presenting Complication of Meckel's Diverticulum	Recovered	Died
Hemorrhage	48	2
Abdominal pain	28	1
Leading point of intussusception	19	9
Inflammation, with or without perforation	10	8
Umbilical fistula or cyst	11	1
Obstruction from band	8	0
Twist and infarction of diverticulum	4	0
Totals	128	21

Of the 149 patients, 128 survived and 21 died. When broken down into statistics from the early and the more recent parts of the series, the following figures are found:

	Recovered	Died
Prior to 1940	57	16
1940 through 1950	71	5

Reviewing our material with the intent of finding ways in which the operative mortality can be reduced, we come to the following conclusions:

1. In those patients with *massive hemorrhage*, transfusion and operation should be performed immediately to prevent death from exsanguination.

2. When resection must be employed for a *gangrenous diverticulum* or intestine following an *intussusception*, it is preferable to use aseptic methods because of the great danger of a spreading peritonitis. This is best executed by the Mikulicz procedure, which exteriorizes the bowel and closes the abdominal wall before cutting off the damaged intestine.

3. When *inflammatory conditions* of the diverticulum are suspected, operation should be performed immediately, to prevent tree perforation into the general peritoneal cavity and its attendant high mortality rate.

REFERENCES

1. Christine, A.: Meckel's Diverticulum. A Pathologic Study of Sixty-three Cases. Am. J. Dis. Child., *42:*544, 1931.
2. Collins, D. C., Collins, F. K. and Andrews, V. L.: Ulcerating Carcinoid Tumor of Meckel's Diverticulum. Am. J. Surg., *40:* 454, 1938.
3. Faust, L. S. and Walters, W.: Fibrosarcoma of Meckel's Diverticulum Producing Intestinal Hemorrhage. Minnesota Med., *14:* 233, 1931.
4. Gray, H. K. and Kernohan, J. W.: Meckel's Diverticulum Associated with Intussusception and Adenocarcinoma of Ectopic Gastric Mucosa; Report of Case. J.A.M.A., *108:*1480, 1937.
5. Halstead, A. E.: Intestinal Obstruction from Meckel's Diverticulum. Ann. Surg., *35:*471, 1902.
6. Hudson, H. W., Jr.: Meckel's Diverticulum in Children; Second Clinical and Pathological Study with a Report of Thirteen

Additional Cases. New England J. Med., *208:*525, 1933.

7. Kittle, C. F., Jenkins, H. P. and Dragstedt, L. R.: Patent Omphalomesenteric Duct and Its Relation to the Diverticulum of Meckel. Arch. Surg., *54:*10, 1947.

8. Lindau, A. and Wulff, H.: The Peptic Genesis of Gastric and Duodenal Ulcer, Especially in the Light of Ulcers of Meckel's Diverticulum and Postoperative Ulcers in Jejunum. Surg., Gynec., & Obst., *53:*621, 1931.

9. Michael, P.: Tuberculosis of Meckel's Diverticulum. Arch. Surg., *25:*1152, 1932.

10. Poate, H. R. G.: Volvulus of Meckel's Diverticulum. Australian & New Zealand J. Surg., *7:*351, 1938.

11. Skinner, I. C. and Walters, W.: Leiomyosarcoma of Meckel's Diverticulum, with Roentgenologic Demonstration of Diverticulum. Proc. Staff Meet., Mayo Clinic, *14:*102, 1939.

12. Womack, N. A. and Siegert, R. B.: Surgical Aspects of Lesions of Meckel's Diverticulum. Ann. Surg., *108:*221, 1938.

CHAPTER 17

Duplications of the Alimentary Tract

Duplications are spherical or elongated hollow structures which (1) possess a coat of smooth muscle; (2) are lined by a mucous membrane similar to some part of the alimentary canal; and (3) are intimately attached to some portion of the alimentary tube. They may appear at any level from the base of the tongue to the anus. They are more commonly found in relation to the small intestine than to any other part of the gastrointestinal tract.

Terminology

These malformations have been described in the literature under various names, including "enterogenous cysts," "enteric cysts," "ileum duplex," "giant diverticula," "inclusion cysts," "gastric thoracic cysts," and a number of other terms which are quite descriptive of the individual specimens, but do not call attention to the fact that they all have a common embryologic derivation and should therefore be grouped together as similar anomalies. Some names as "enteric cyst" and "enterogenous cyst" indicate a close relationship to the intestine, but they can hardly be applied to the long tubular structures which course through the mesentery alongside of the gut. Likewise, "giant diverticula" adequately describe some specimens which have free connections with the enteric tube, but such an opening is lacking in many others. "Ileum duplex" has been used to designate some of the anomalies, but does not properly describe those which are seen in the jejunum, duodenum, stomach, or colon. "Inclusion cysts" conveys the idea that the structure is largely embedded within the intestinal wall; while this is true in a few cases, it certainly is not characteristic of the group as a whole. It is more fitting to employ an all-inclusive name for these malformations which have appeared in divers locations and which have many shapes, sizes, and varying characteristics. We have therefore chosen to group them as *duplications of the alimentary tract*, because each is similar to some portion of the alimentary tract, though not necessarily to that portion to which it is contiguous.

PATHOLOGY

A number of these lesions have been described in the literature, but the following summary has been largely based upon studies of 68 of them from surgical or autopsy material by Dr. Sidney Farber at the Boston Children's Hospital. Duplications present a great variety of gross findings, some of which are portrayed in the figures of this chapter.

Sites of Occurrence

The sites at which duplications have been observed in our series of 68 lesions (in 67 patients) were as follows: base of the tongue, 1; within the thorax and arising from the esophagus, 13; long tubular diverticula within the thorax arising from the duodenum or jejunum, 3; stomach, 2; duodenum, 4; jejunum, 4; ileum, 19; at ileo-cecal valve, 8; cecum, 3; near terminal ileum or colon, but having a separate mesentery, 2; sigmoid, 2; rectum, 3; double-lumened colon or rectum, 4. Figures 116 and 117 graphically indicate the locations of these anomalies, while Table 23 summarizes some of the pertinent data from the individual cases.

Firm Union with Intestine

The adherence of a duplication to esophagus, stomach, intestine, or colon is an important point in most instances in recognizing or dealing with these lesions at the operating table. While a few of them are long side-arms directed away from the alimentary tract, and in rare instances (Cases 47 and 56 in Table 23) the lesion has a separate "mesentery" from which it hangs, the vast majority of duplications are intimately attached to (or are an integral part of) the digestive tube. There might be a slight furrow between the duplication and the alimentary tube, but attempts to dissect away the lesion will show that there is a firm union, made by the coalescence of the muscular layers of the two where they lie together. This feature is best appreciated by a microscopic study, which shows that the muscular coats really fuse into a common wall. The cystic structure may or may not communicate with the lumen of the nearby alimentary tube; in 13 there was such a communication, but in the remaining 80 per cent there was no such opening.

Nature of the Outer Coats

A feature common to all duplications, regardless of size, origin, or attachment, is the possession of a well developed coat of *smooth muscle*, which may consist of one, two, or three layers, with fibers running in the same or in varying directions. This characteristic gives a wall several millimeters in thickness which can be recognized grossly; it quickly serves to differentiate the anomaly from lymphatic or chylous cysts which have walls considerably thinner.

Types of Epithelial Lining

The epithelium which lines a duplication always resembles that of some part of the alimentary tract, but it does not necessarily correspond to the mucosa of that level at which the duplication is found. Thus, a cyst of the base of the tongue can have its interior coated by colonic mucosa, or a cyst of the rectum can be partially lined by gastric epithelium, and so forth. In some of the specimens two or even three types of alimentary tract mucosa are found. For the most part, the lining is well preserved and can be readily identified by microscopic study, but in occasional specimens it is partially destroyed by pressure necrosis, or by enzymatic digestion from the fluid which the structure contains. The thickness of a duplication lining usually helps to differentiate it grossly from the very thin membrane possessed by cysts of lymphatic origin.

Types of Fluid

The nature of the fluid within a duplication depends upon several factors. Commonly, it is a *clear, colorless, mucoid substance* which has been secreted by its own membrane. In occasional specimens the secreted and entrapped fluid is under such high pressure that there is necrosis and sloughing of the lining membrane; the fluid may then become *hemorrhagic or murky*. If a duplication is one which possesses a communication from the alimentary tract, succus entericus or fecal material and gas can regurgitate

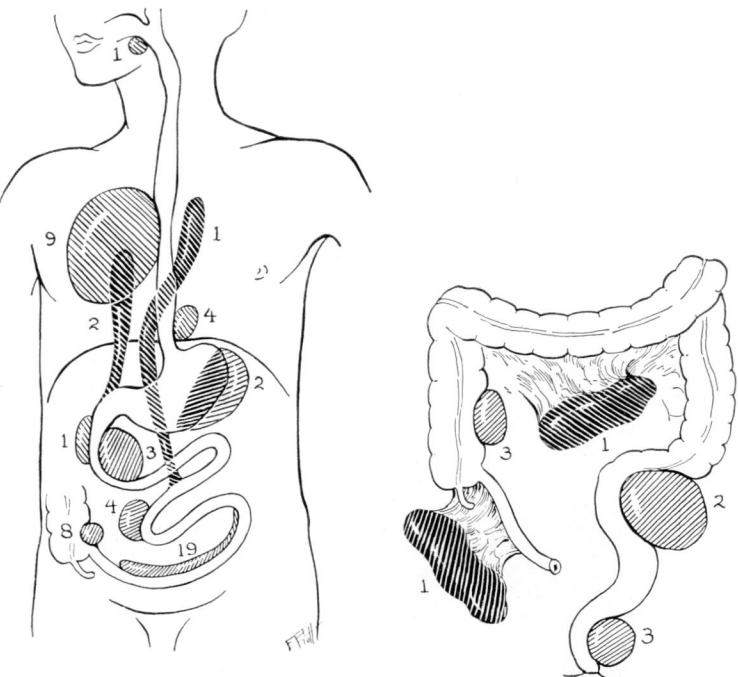

Fig. 116. Sketch showing distribution of duplications of the alimentary tract. The figure beside each lesion indicates the number of malformations found in the area.

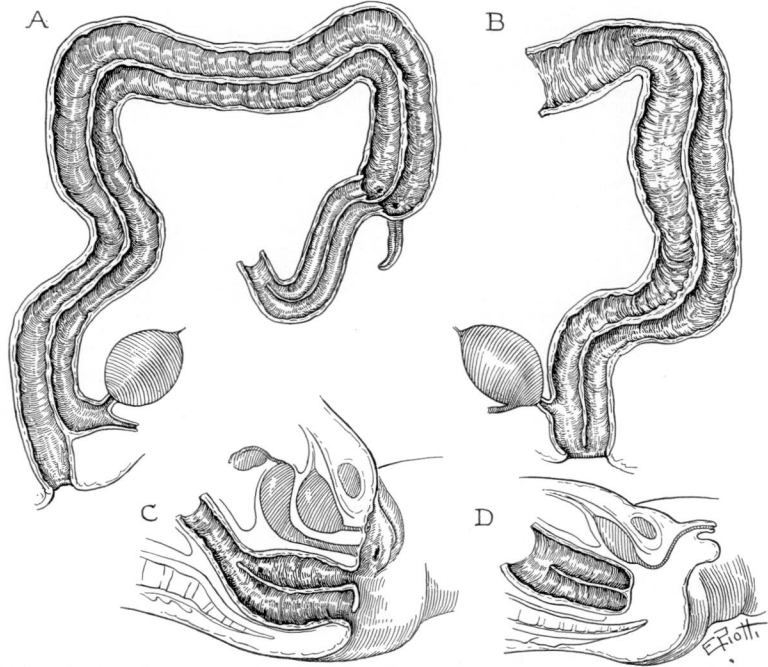

Fig. 117. Sketch showing general extent and form of abnormalities in which there was a double colon or rectum. A. Extensive duplication, combined with recto-urethral fistula, Case 66. B. Duplication of entire descending colon, with recto-urethral fistula, Case 67. C. Duplication of rectum, with two anal openings. Genital tract in two separate halves, each with a separate external opening, one side of which is shown here, Case 68. D. Duplication of rectum, with imperforate anus, Case 65.

into it. Since the large majority of duplications are closed structures, it is possible to sample some of its contained fluid to study the type of material elaborated by the cyst wall. If there is a combination of gastric and other types of lining, the retained fluid may have a pH and an enzymatic activity of widely varying range. If it is only intestinal or colonic in nature, the fluid is quite basic and contains mucus. If, on the other hand, the lining membrane is entirely or largely gastric in nature, the fluid contains hydrochloric acid and pepsin, and has a very low pH (1 to 3).

Variations in Shape and Size

Duplications vary tremendously in shape: (1) A few are diverticular structures branching out from a side of the intestine, running for a distance of several to 40 or 50 cm.; these can lie within the mesentery, extend off into unexpected places, or stretch from the abdomen up into the chest. (2) Somewhat similar are those which are long tubular affairs communicating at one end with the intestine or colon, and running

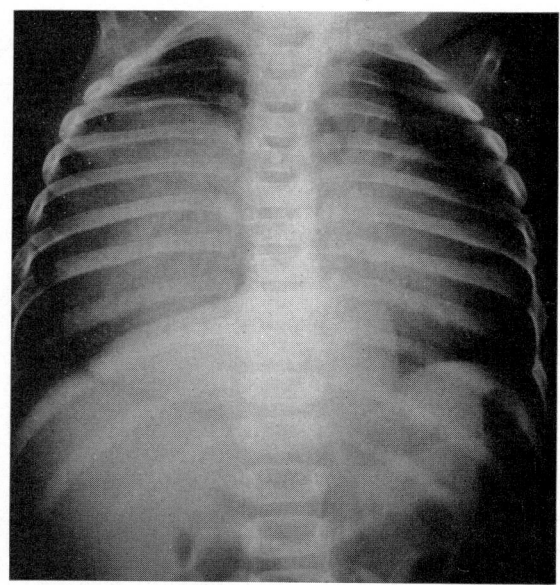

Fig. 118. Roentgenogram of baby with a large duplication in the right side of the thorax, compressing pulmonary tissue and pushing mediastinum and heart to patient's left, Case 4.

alongside of the same, giving a double-barreled appearance. These are apt to be of great length. (3) A few are elongated sacs, generally lying within the leaves of the mesentery, contiguous to and firmly attached to the intestine, usually not communicating with the intestine. (4) Most common of all are the spherical or ovoid hollow structures, arising from some part of the alimentary tube, occasionally communicating with it, but generally not.

Duplications also vary greatly in size. The tubular ones tend to be about the same diameter as intestine or colon; they can be anywhere from a few centimeters to more than half a meter in length. The rounded lesions may be as small as a centimeter or two in diameter; the larger ones can be the size of a grapefruit or even bigger. Some representative specimens are displayed in the accompanying figures.

Differentiation from Mesenteric Cysts

It is highly important for the surgeon to recognize the pathologic difference between duplications (of the spherical variety) and mesenteric cysts. The latter are lymphatic in origin, have a thin wall, and can be readily peeled away from adjacent viscera. In contrast to these findings, a duplication has a thicker, muscular wall which can rarely be dissected away from the intestine without opening the duplication or the intestine. It is therefore evident that the mesenteric cyst can usually be removed without disturbing the intestine, but that in removing a duplication a portion of the intestine usually has to be resected along with it.

EMBRYOLOGY

Several theories have been put forth to explain the origin of duplications. Those arising from some part of the ileum were previously thought to represent aberrations in development of a Meckel's diverticulum. For several reasons this theory is scarcely tenable, and in any event it does not explain the origin of duplications in other portions of the alimentary tract. *Sequestration,* or a pinching off of a group of cells from the

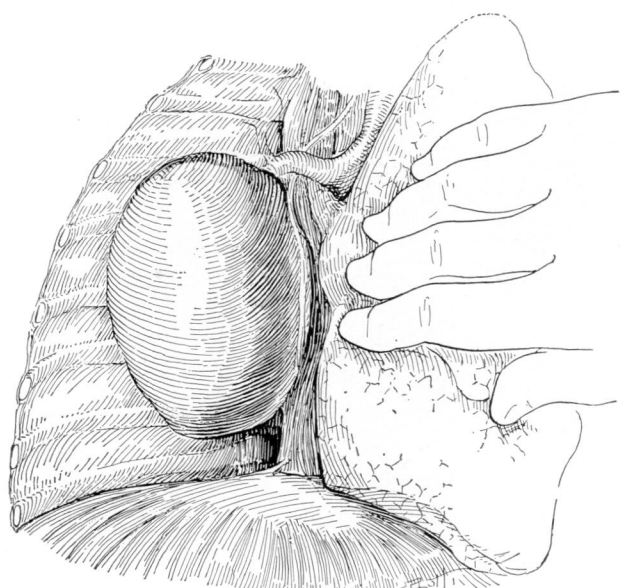

Fig. 119. Sketch of a right-sided thoracic duplication, arising from and attached to the esophagus, bulging into the pleural cavity behind the lung.

primordial intestinal tube, could easily account for the development of nearby cysts which attain all of the histologic elements of an alimentary tract wall, and which are attached to the intestine or are hanging from a separate mesentery.

A most plausible theory is that advanced by Lewis and Thyng,[9] who frequently found *diverticula* in various portions of fetal alimentary tracts of pigs, rabbits, cats, sheep, and humans. These outpocketings are most often seen in the ileum, a fact which corresponds to the greater frequency of duplications in the ileum. These small outpocketings in the intestinal wall—which are not related to the omphalomesenteric duct (Meckel's diverticulum)—normally regress, but if one of them is pinched off the structure could easily give rise to an adjacent duplication.

Bremer[2] has pointed out that development of the alimentary tube after the solid stage (which is normal) can give rise to hollow structures which do or do not communicate with the alimentary canal. During the late stage of the solid phase, multiple vacuoles appear within the cell mass. These are linearly arranged; they later coalesce and intercommunicate so that a single hollow tube is formed. It is not improbable that some of these cystic spaces can fail to join up with the main, epithelial-lined tube which is forming. The isolated unit could thereby form a hollow (rounded or tubular) duplication which has in its wall all of the histologic elements of some part of the alimentary tract and furthermore is attached to the otherwise normal alimentary system.

CLINICAL SYMPTOMS AND SIGNS

Age

Duplications are usually found in infancy or childhood, but they may be discovered at any period of life. The lesions are such that they attract attention in early years. Our youngest patient was one day of age; the oldest was thirteen years. In our series of 68 lesions, 65 per cent were found in the first year of life, 9 per cent in the second year, 8 per cent in the third year, and only a scattering of cases thereafter.

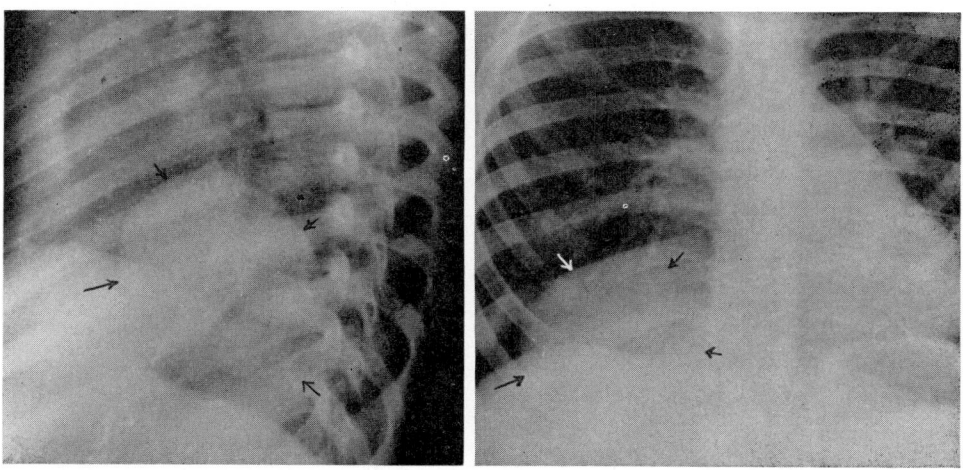

Fig. 120. Films from a child with duplication cf the esophagus, in lower part of the right-hemithorax, Case 14.

Symptoms

The various symptoms produced by these abnormalities may be roughly grouped under four categories: (1) The cyst or tube-like structure becomes so dilated that it encroaches upon the adjacent intestine and partially *obstructs* it. (2) The lining membrane produces such a large amount of fluid that internal pressure is high and *pain* is produced by distention of the structure. (3) The duplication, lying as it often does within the leaves of the mesentery, may press upon mesenteric blood vessels and produce *necrosis, sloughing,* and *bleeding* of the adjacent intestine. (4) The duplication may be lined by gastric mucosa, liberating hydrochloric acid and pepsin, the erosive action of which extends through the wall (in the closed variety of duplication) or produces an ulcer in the nearby intestine (in the communicating type); *hemorrhage* results. With these general statements in mind, more specific remarks can be made regarding the special complaints or complications produced by particular varieties of duplications as they appear in different parts of the body.

Duplications Arising in the Thorax

Only one of our 13 duplications which originated in the thorax had a communication with the esophagus. They therefore accumulate fluid and become sizable masses, usually making themselves evident by *pulmonary compression and respiratory symptoms.* They may fill half or two-thirds of a pleural cavity (Fig. 118). While these cysts may reside entirely within the mediastinum, they are much more apt to lie along one side of the esophagus and balloon out into a pleural cavity, pushing the lung forward. They are more than twice as common on the right than the left. Those on the right tend to attain a larger size than those on the left.

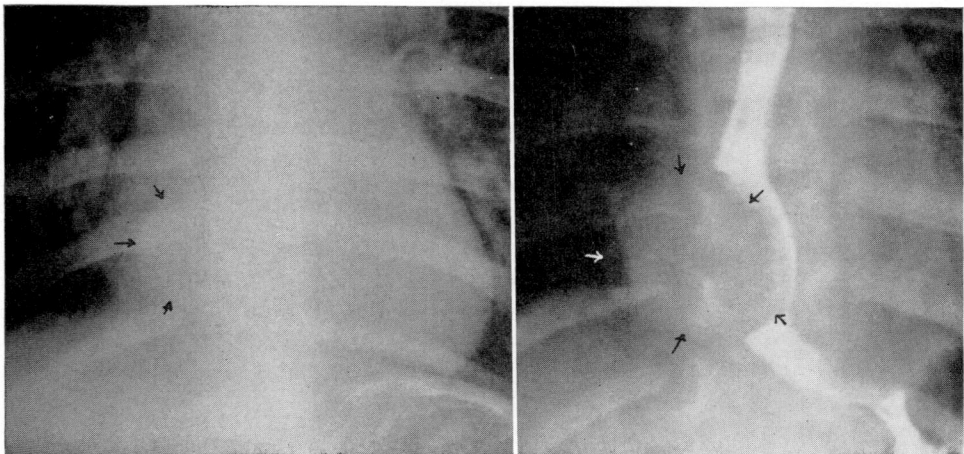

Fig. 121. Roentgenograms of a small duplication in lower part of right side of chest. With barium in the esophagus, the deformity of the latter is readily apparent, Case 10.

There is a marked tendency for duplications of this group to be lined by gastric mucosa, a fact which has frequently led to their description in the literature as "gastric thoracic cysts," "mediastinal cysts of gastric origin," etc. The fluid entrapped within them contains rennin, pepsin, and hydrochloric acid in very high concentration; the pH has been measured as being very low. This unneutralized fluid is very apt to bring about autodigestion of the cyst wall, setting up an exceedingly intense inflammatory reaction. The greatly vascularized wall becomes densely adherent to the lung or the esophagus, from either of which bleeding occurs. *Repeated hemoptysis or hematemesis can be a major symptom.* In Case 9 (Table 23) the reaction was so severe that there was erosion into the left upper lobe, with development of a fistula into the same, giving such marked destruction that the lobe had to be removed along with the cyst. Physical signs may be minimal or absent in the smaller lesions, but with larger ones there are diminished breath sounds, dullness or flatness, and changes indicative of pulmonary compression, or of accumulation of pleural fluid.

Duplications in the Thorax, but Arising from Intestine

These lesions are very rare, but are a fascinating group. We[5] have seen but three of them (Cases 15, 16, and 17, Table 23); Fischer[3] has described another. They are long diverticula, originating from the duodenum or jejunum, which course upward, pierce the diaphragm and enter the thorax, where they may extend well toward the apex of the chest (Figs. 124 and 125). These tubular outpocketings give rise to symptoms in two ways. First, intestinal gas and fluid may back up into them, distend the intrathoracic portion, lead to compression of the heart or lung, and hence produce *cardio-respiratory symptoms* of an intermittent nature. Second, the tube may be partially or completely lined by gastric mucosa, liberating gastric juice which produces an ulcer in its wall or in the intestine and leads to *exsanguinating hemorrhage, melena,* and *anemia.*

Duplications of the Stomach

In a very large duplication of the stomach (Case 18, Table 23) there was no mechanical obstruction; the complaints were those of epigastric fullness and discomfort; the large mass could be palpated in the epigastrium.

Duplications of the Intestine

Since these have a wide variety of sizes, shapes, and locations, some communicating with the intestine while most of them do not, there is a tremendous range of symptoms and signs related to them. The duodenal ones are generally situated along the inner curve of the same, compress the duodenum and give findings of *high intestinal obstruction;* in some instances the duodenal mass is large enough to palpate. The majority of duplications of the jejunum and ileum produce partial intestinal obstruction with *colicky pain, vomiting, visible peristalsis,* and possibly signs of *dehydration.* The long tubular duplications of the ileum are apt to give severe, painless, and repeated *hemorrhage* from the intestinal tract, because of sloughing and ulceration of the ileal mucosa. Many of the jejunal and ileal duplications are of considerable size, and a rather mobile and nontender mass can be felt by palpation. In contrast, the long, narrow tubular formations can seldom be felt through the abdominal wall. The cysts near the ileo-cecal valve do *not* attain a large size, because very early they obstruct the ileo-cecal valve or else become the leading point of an intussusception.

Duplications of the Colon and Rectum

It is rather uncommon to find a cystic duplication along the colon or sigmoid (Cases 57–61, Table 23); they gradually compress and partly block the bowel and produce palpable masses. Those behind the rectum (Cases 62–64) all appeared in babies; in the narrow pelvic canal, rather small lesions give early compression of the rectum, obstipation, and abdominal distention; by digital examination the mass can easily be felt in the hollow of the sacrum. A rather special group (Fig. 117) consists of 4 youngsters (Cases 65–68) in whom long segments of the rectum or colon (and in one case, the terminal ileum) possessed a double lumen, each of which carried a fecal stream; in each instance the peculiarity of the lower end of the duplication produced the symptoms for which medical relief was sought. In one there was an imperforate anus. In another, a female, there was an accessory perineal opening which discharged fecal material. In the other two, males, the secondary colonic tube emptied into the urethra, with a discharge of fecal material into the same.

ROENTGENOLOGIC DATA

Roentgenographic investigation generally gives important data in the various forms of duplication, indicating the general size, position and space relationships of the

Table 23

Data from 68 Duplications of the Alimentary Tract

Case	Age	Location of Cyst Relevant Figures	Size of Duplication Type of Mucous Membrane	Treatment	Result
1	. . . . . .	Base of tongue	1 cm. in diameter. Colonic	Excision	Recovered
2	7 wks.	Right plural cavity (middle)	5 cm. in diameter. Gastric	Excision	Recovered
3	2 yrs.	Right pleural cavity	10 x 6 x 5 cm. Gastric	Excision	Recovered
4	7 mos.	Right pleural cavity (Fig. 118)	8 x 5 x 4 cm. Gastric	Multiple marsupializations	Died
5	22 mos.	Para-esophageal left (lower) (Fig. 123)	8 x 5 x 4 cm. Pseudo-columnar	Excision	Recovered
6	3 wks.	Lower esophagus, left	1.5 cm. in diameter. Gastric	Marsupialization and curettage	Recovered
7	6 wks.	Lower esophagus, right	5 cm. in diameter	Marsupialization and curettage	Recovered
8	20 mos.	Esophagus, right	3 x 2 x 0.5 cm. Pseudo-columnar	Excision	Recovered
9	6 wks.	Esophageal, with fistula to left upper lobe	2.5 x 2 cm. Gastric	Excision of duplication and left upper lobectomy	Recovered
10	5½ yrs.	Lower esophagus, right (Fig. 121)	12 x 8 x 8 cm. Pseudo-columnar	Excision	Recovered
11	1 yr.	Mid-esophagus, right	. . . . . . Gastric	Marsupialization	Recovered
12	5 wks.	Upper esophagus, right	5.5 x 3.5 x 3 cm. Small intestine	Excision	Recovered
13	1 mo.	Lower esophagus, left (Fig. 122)	6 x 2.5 cm. Colonic	No therapy. Found at autopsy	Same patient as No. 28
14	3½ yrs.	Right pleural cavity (attached to diaphragm) (Fig. 120)	5 x 6 cm.	Excision	Recovered
15	4½ yrs.	From duodenum, entering right chest) (Fig. 124, *left*)	20 x 2.5 cm. Gastric	Excision of supradiaphragmatic portion	Recovered

Table 23 (continued)

Case	Age	Location of Cyst Relevant Figures	Sign of Duplication Type of Mucous Membrane	Treatment	Result
16	4 mos.	From jejunum, entering right chest (Fig. 124, *right*)	27 x 2.5 cm. Small intestinal	1 stage complete resection and anastomosis of jejunum	Recovered
17	3½ mos.	From jejunum, entering right chest and into left chest	30 x 2 cm. Colon, ileum, pesudocolumnar	Multiple stage removal of supra-diaphragmatic portions	Recovered
18	7 yrs.	Along stomach	Large as stomach. Necrotic mucosa	Partial excision and marsupialization	Recovered
19	3 days	Greater curvature of stomach	4 cm. in diameter. Gastric	Excision duplication and gastrostomy	Died
20	5 wks.	Duodenum (Fig. 126)	4.5 x 3.5 x 3.5 cm. Duodenal	Resection. Gastrojejunostomy	Recovered
21	8½ yrs.	Duodenum	3 x 4 cm. Small intestinal	Window cut into duodenum	Recovered
22	1½ yrs.	Duodenum	5 cm. in diameter	Window cut into duodenum	Recovered
23	2 yrs.	Right side of duodenum	2.5 x 2.5 cm. Gastric	Excision	Recovered
24	6 mos.	Jejunum	22 x 6 x 6 cm. Gastric	Mikulicz resection	Died
25	2 wks.	Jejunum	4 cm. in diameter. Jejunal	Resection and anastomosis	Recovered
26	3 days	Jejunum	4 x 3 x 3 cm. Small intestinal	Resection and anastomosis	Died
27	13 yrs.	Jejunum (Fig. 127)	30 x 5–10 cm. Gastric	Resection and anastomosis	Recovered
28	1 mo.	Jejunum and ileum (Figs. 129 and 130)	65 cm. long. Small intestine	(Perforated). Resection and anastomosis	Died
29	1 day	Upper ileum	23 x 9 cm. Pyloric	Resection and anastomosis*	Recovered
30	10½ mos.	High ileum	1.5 x 1.5 cm. Ileal	Reduction intussusception Resection of duplication	Recovered
31	3 yrs.	Upper ileum	6 cm. diameter. Small intetine	Excision*	Recovered

* Also had Ladd procedure for malrotation.

Table 23 (continued)

Case	Age	Location of Cyst Relevant Figures	Size of Duplication Type of Mucous Membrane	Treatment	Result
32	4 mos.	Detached from high ileum	52 cm. long. Gastric	Anastomosis distal end duplication to ileum*	Recovered
33	3 mos.	Ileum	7 x 4 x 4 cm. Gastric	None	Died
34	1 day	Ileum	5.5 x 4.5 x 2.5 cm. Necrotic	Resection and anastomosis	Recovered
35	9 days	Ileum	3.5 x 2 cm. Small intestine	Resection and anastomosis	Recovered
36	6 yrs.	Ileum	3 cm. diameter. Ileal	Resection and anastomosis	Recovered
37	2 yrs.	Ileum (Fig. 131)	38 cm x 2 cm. Gastric	Resection and anastomosis	Died
38	4 mos.	Ileum	1 x 1 cm. Gastric	Resection and anastomosis	Recovered
39	9 days	Mid ileum	30 x 5 cm. Pyloric and colonic	Resection and Mikulicz ileostomy	Recovered
40	1 day	Low ileum (Fig. 132)	44 x 1 cm. Small intestine	Excision	Died
41	12 days	Terminal ileum	1.5 cm. diameter. Ileal	Resection and anastomosis	Recovered
42	2 mos.	Terminal ileum	2 cm. diameter. Ileal	Resection and anastomosis	Recovered
43	2 yrs.	Terminal ileum	3.8 x 3.2 cm. Gastric	Resection and anastomosis	Recovered
44	10 days	Lower ileum	3.5 x 2 cm. Pyloric	Resection and Mikulicz ileostomy	Recovered
45	18 mos.	Terminal ileum	3 x 2 x 1.6 cm. Gastric, ileal, colonic	Excision	Recovered
46	3 wks.	Terminal ileum	3 x 1.5 cm. Ileal	No therapy. Found at autopsy	Died
47	19 mos.	Detached from terminal ileum	15.5 x 4 x 5 cm. Columnar	Excision	Recovered
48	3 mos.	Ileo-cecal junction	3 x 2 x 2 cm. Small intestine	Resection and ileocolostomy	Recovered

Table 23 (continued)

Case	Age	Location of Cyst Relevant Figures	Size of Duplication Type of Mucous Membrane	Treatment	Result
49	3 days	Ileo-cecal junction	3 cm. diameter. Small intestine	Mikulicz resection gangrenous ileum and cecum*	Died
50	1 wk.	Ileo-cecal junction	5.5 x 3 cm. Small intestine	Resection and ileocolostomy	Recovered
51	10 mos.	Ileo-cecal junction (Fig. 134)	5 x 4 x 3.5 cm.	Resection and Mikulicz ileocolostomy	Recovered
52	10 mos.	Ileo-cecal junction	2.5 cm. diameter. Low cuboidal	Resection and Mikulicz ileocolostomy	Recovered
53	13 mos.	Ileo-cecal junction	5 x 4 cm. Ileal	Reduction intussusception. Resection and ileocolostomy	Recovered
54	3½ yrs.	Ileo-cecal junction	3 x 3.5 cm. Small intestinal	Resection and ileocolostomy	Recovered
55	8 mos.	Ileo-cecal junction	6 x 3.5 x 3.5 cm. Columnar epithelium	Resection and ileocolostomy	Recovered
56	5 days	Detached from transverse colon	3.5 x 2.5 cm.	Excision	Recovered
57	8 mos.	Cecum	2 cm. diameter. Colonic	Reduction intussusception. Resection and ileocolostomy	Recovered
58	3 mos.	Cecum	4 cm. diameter. Colonic	Reduction intussusception. Resection and anastomosis	Died
59	3 wks.	Cecum	5 cm. diameter. Colonic	Resection and ileocolostomy	Recovered
60	2 wks.	Sigmoid	12 x 10 x 8 cm. Ileal and colonic	No therapy. Found at autopsy	Died
61	2 yrs.	Sigmoid	2.5 x 0.6 cm. Large intestinal	Resection and anastomosis	Recovered
62	6 mos.	Posterior to rectum (Fig. 135)	5 x 2.5 x 2.5 cm. Mixed	Excision. Rectum repaired	Recovered
63	1 yr.	Posterior to rectum	4 cm. diameter. Mucosa ulcerated	Excision	Recovered

Table 23 (continued)

Case	Age	Location of Cyst Relevant Figures	Size of Duplication Type of Mucous Membrane	Treatment	Result
64	2 mos.	Posterior to rectum	2.4 cm. diameter. Intestinal	Excision	Recovered
65	14 days	Double lumen rectum. Imperforate anus. (Fig. 117, D)	5 x 0.5 cm. Rectal	No therapy. Found at autopsy	Died
66	4 mos.	Double lumen terminal ileum, appendix, transverse and descending colon (situs transversus) (Fig. 117, A)	Terminal ileum to rectum. Colonic	Closure recto-urethral fistula. Resection descending colon. Two rectal lumina made into 1 (3 operations)	Recovered
67	6 wks.	Double lumen, descending colon to anus (Fig. 117, B, and 137)	15 x 5 cm. Colonic	Closure recto-urethral fistula. Resection descending colon. Two rectal lumina made into 1 (3 operations)	Recovered
68	12 yrs.	Double lumen, colon and rectum (Fig. 117, C)	18 x 2 cm.	Accessory anal opening closed. Two rectal lumina made into 1	Recovered

anomaly, often permitting positive identification of the lesion, but in other instances providing insufficient information for making an accurate diagnosis.

Duplications Arising within the Thorax

Esophageal duplications give roentgen changes suggestive of posterior mediastinal tumors or pleural cysts. Details of the duplication's outline may be obscured by secondary changes in the lung or by pleural fluid. Most of the cysts have a spherical form, a homogeneous density, and a continuity with the mediastinal shadow (Fig. 118). The heart and mediastinal structures are apt to be displaced to the opposite side. There may be erosion of vertebral bodies or of overlying ribs.

Lipiodol bronchograms usually show pulmonary compression from the retropleural duplication, and aid in differentiating the latter from bronchogenic cysts and other anomalies. Examination of the esophagus with contrast media rarely shows a fistulous connection to the lesion; the esophagus is usually indented, displaced, or angulated by the adjacent mass.

Duplications in the Thorax, but Arising from the Intestine

Films without contrast media show a widening of the mediastinal shadow, particularly on the right side, because of the elongated mass lying in either one of the paravertebral gutters (Fig. 124). Films taken with the patient in an erect position might show some gas in this shadow, suggesting a diaphragmatic hernia—a point which might be further suggested by regurgitation of barium up into the area after ingestion of a barium meal. Indeed, differentiation from a congenital hernia might be virtually im-

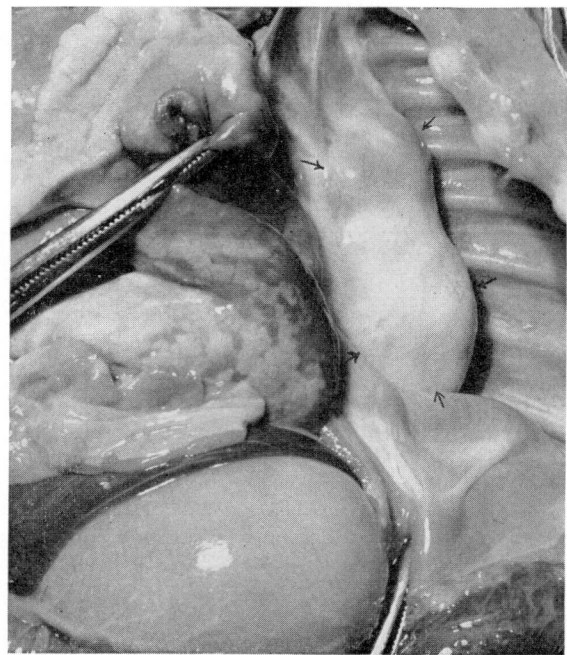

Fig. 122. A small, asymptomatic duplication in left side of chest, found at autopsy, Case 13.

possible. If, however, the gas-filled shadow is quite close to the mediastinum (not spread out laterally in the chest) and if the patient is known to have had melena, a diagnosis of *duplication* is more plausible than hernia.

Duplications of the Stomach

Roentgen studies aid in showing the size of the lesion and help in determining its position with relation to other abdominal viscera. A gastro-intestinal series indicates the mass to be behind or below the stomach, with a smooth bulge into the gastric lumen along the greater curvature; a barium enema visualizes the transverse colon displaced downward and not obstructed.

Duplications of the Intestine

Duodenal cysts compress the first and second portion of the duodenum and exhibit evidence of duodenal obstruction when studies are performed with a barium series. Dilated intestine is found above some but not all of the jejunal and ileal lesions. Not infrequently, as much can be learned from films in the postero-anterior and lateral directions without contrast media as can be determined with the use of a barium series. Distention of intestinal loops, particularly if localized to one part of the abdomen, indicates obstruction and often gives some idea of the level at which the lesion exists. In a few instances, when there is a communication, barium will flow into and will outline the duplication (Fig. 127). In the presence of a duplication which does not communicate with the intestine, a space-filling shadow can be seen in the films with displacement of gas shadows away from this.

Duplications of the Colon

For the cystic variety of anomaly occurring along some part of the colon or behind

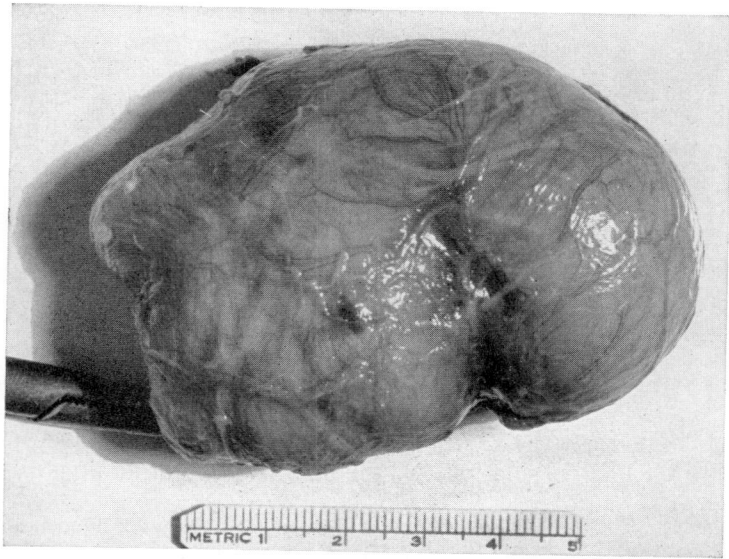

Fig. 123. Duplication, excised from left side of esophagus without opening esophagus, Case 5.

the rectum, examination by barium enema gives considerable information regarding the size, position, and attachments of the lesion. In those forms of duplication which can be best described as a double-lumen colon, barium (which has been fed for a gastrointestinal series) might outline the two parallel and contiguous colonic tracts (Fig. 136). In some cases it is possible to inject barium in a retrograde manner through the anus and also simultaneously through some other orifice (as a perineal sinus, the urethra in

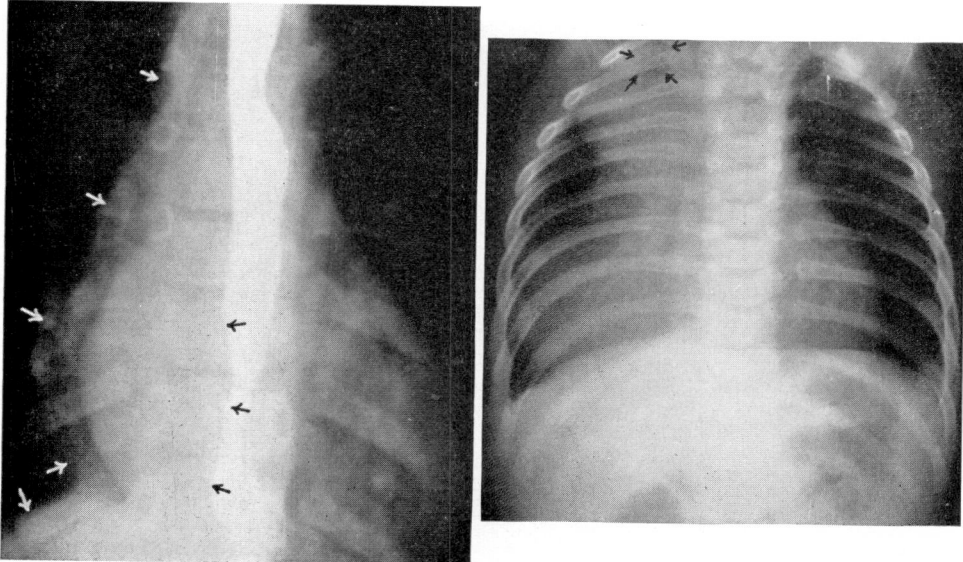

Fig. 124. Roentgenograms from two cases with long diverticula originating from intestine and extending up into chest. *Left*, Case 15, mass running up along right side of mediastinum. Compare Figure 125, A. *Right*, Case 16, mass projecting out from right side of mediastinum. Arrows indicate gas bubble in the structure. Compare Figure 125, B.

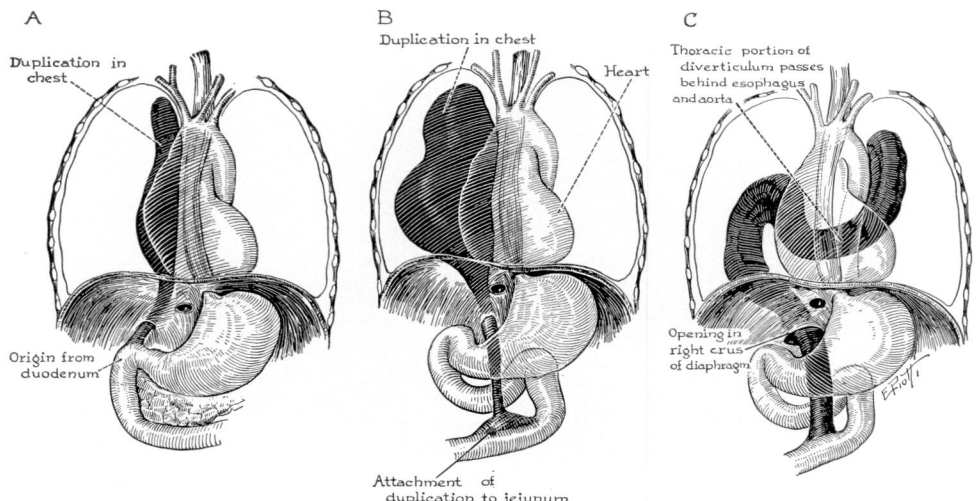

Fig. 125. Sketches of three very long diverticula which arose from the duodenum or jejunum and extended up into the thorax. In A and B, the duplication was lined by gastric mucosa and gave rise to severe melena. In C, the duplication filled with intestinal gas and fluid, giving rise to cardio-respiratory distress. A, Case 15. B, Case 16. C, Case 17.

the male, etc.) so that the two parallel rectal or colonic tubes can be filled and their relationships visualized. In two of our patients we were not aware that a double-lumen colon existed until a loop sigmoidostomy was established (preparatory to treatment of a perineal or urethral anomaly); cutting open the sigmoid loop presented four lumina instead of the expected two! Injection of barium into these four ostia gave excellent delineation of the double rectum and colon.

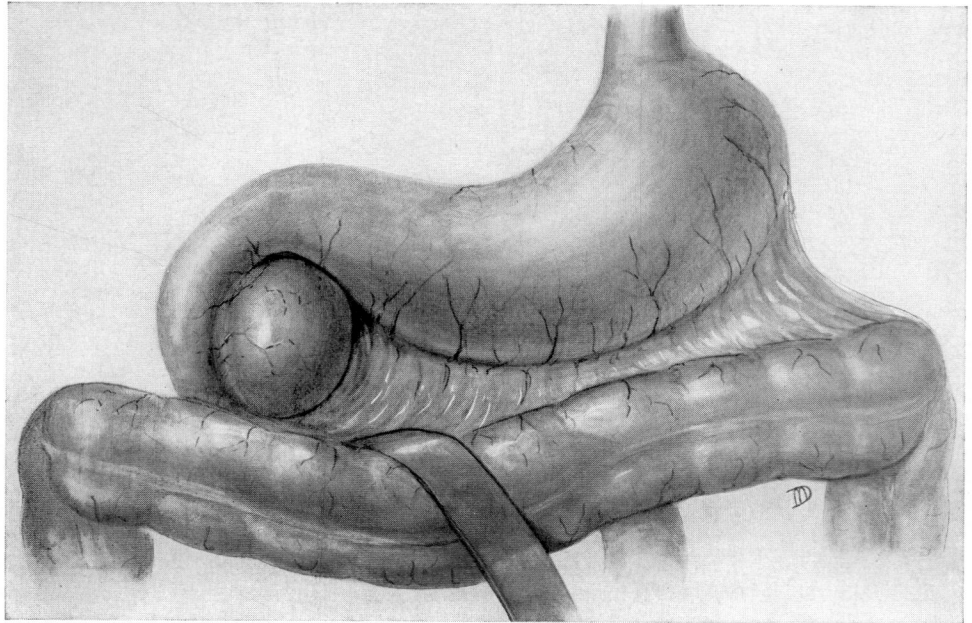

Fig. 126. Duplication of first and second parts of duodenum in a five-week-old baby. Case 20.

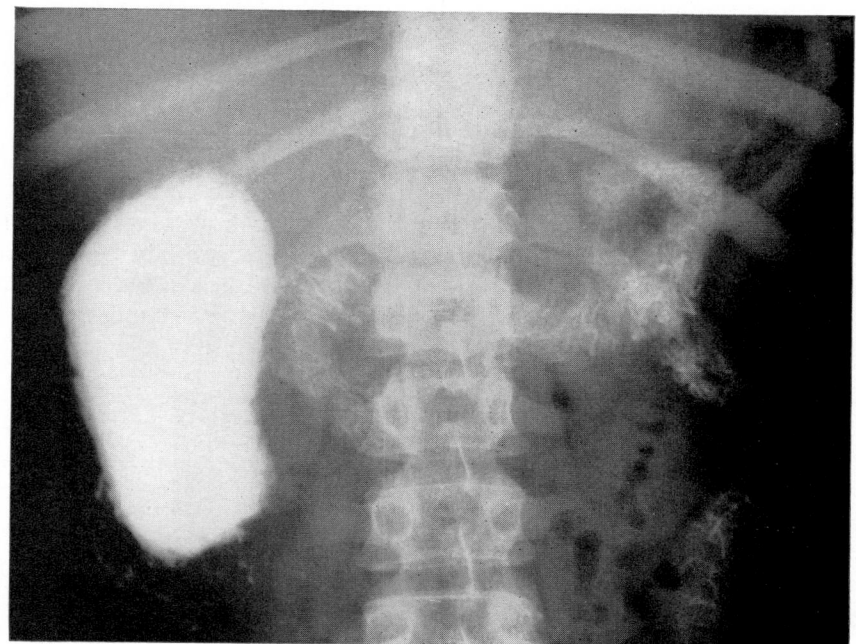

Fig. 127. Roentgenogram from a thirteen-year-old girl with a large duplication which communicated with the jejunum and which filled with barium. Case 27.

TREATMENT
Pathologic Considerations

These malformations cannot be treated by any means other than surgical attack. Two points must be borne in mind which stress the importance of pathologic anatomy in relation to operative procedure. First, the cystic structure and alimentary tube have a common wall (in 64 of our 68 specimens) and as a general rule it is quite difficult or impossible to separate one from the other without injuring the bowel. Second, arteries

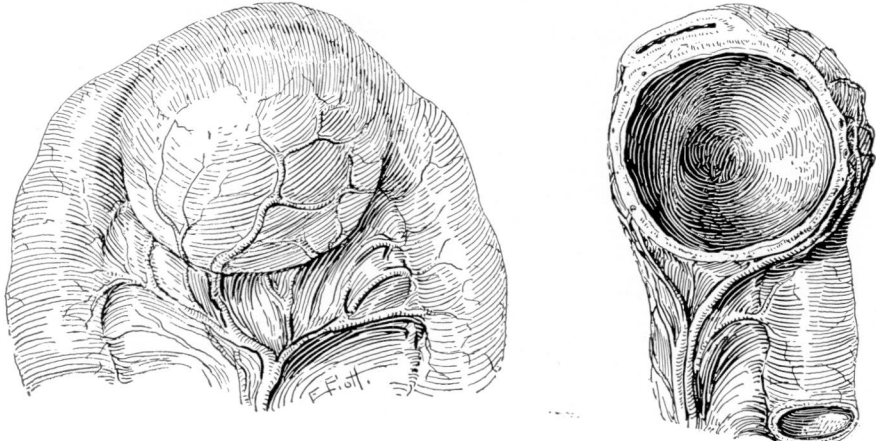

Fig. 128. Sketch of a rather typical duplication of the small intestine, indicating the manner in which it lies within the leaves of the mesentery, against the intestine, and the course of blood vessels over both of its exposed surfaces.

and veins of the contiguous portions of the alimentary tract usually course over the surface of the cyst (especially true of the intestine and colon); any attempts to resect the cyst alone may so interrupt these vessels that there is an impairment of the blood supply.

Operative Technique

In the majority of cases the treatment of choice is *resection* of the duplication and its adjacent gut, followed by reestablishment of intestinal or colonic continuity by a *primary anastomosis*. When dealing with some lesions (such as those at the ileo-cecal valve), or when operating upon a seriously debilitated child, it might be more desirable to perform a quicker and aseptic removal by exteriorization, using the Mikulicz technique. While these general statements are applicable in many instances, there are certain locations which prohibit such forms of treatment because of the anatomic peculi-

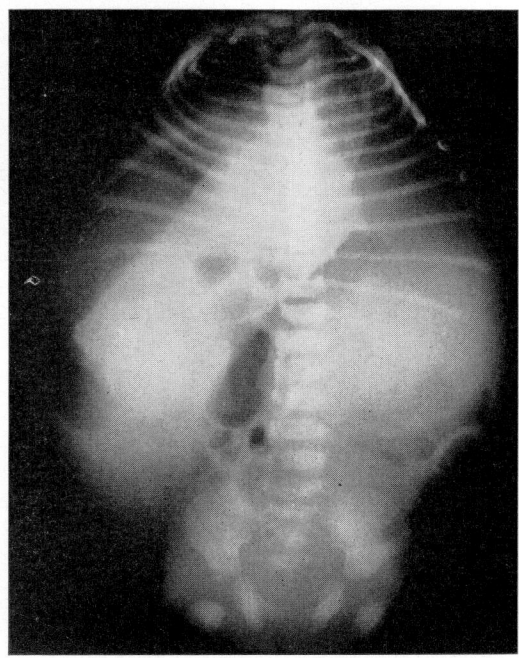

Fig. 129. Roentgenogram from a one-month-old baby with enormous abdominal distention from a huge duplication. (See Fig. 130.) Case 28.

arities of the region; hence special considerations are necessary under these circumstances. Examples of these problems might be mentioned in more detail as follows:

Duplications Arising in the Thorax. It was the original contention of Ladd[8] that these anomalies in the thorax are best treated by marsupialization and by subsequent attempts to destroy the lining membrane by repeated curettage, injection of cauterizing fluids, or pressure packing. Such procedures are very apt to be followed by recurrence of the cyst because it is sometimes impossible to destroy *all* of the lining membrane; some tiny remnant of it remains and is a nidus from which a new lining regenerates. The necessity for multiple-stage operations—which beyond the first stage can be exceedingly difficult—greatly condemns this operative attack. We now feel that marsupialization of the thoracic lesions is obsolete. It is far better to expose the cyst widely by a transpleural approach and remove it. This method can be made safe by several precautionary measures: (1)

As the cyst is approached, a pleural coat should be stripped back off of it, so that this can be saved for subsequent buttressing and closing over of the esophagus. (2) The cyst can usually be peeled away from most adjacent structures without too much difficulty, but as the esophagus is approached the dissection must be meticulous and slow. In some cases it is possible to dissect the cyst away from the esophagus without entering either. If this does not appear to be feasible, the cyst can be freed down to its neck, and cut off at this level—leaving a small remnant of its muscular wall and lining membrane attached to the esophagus. Under direct vision, this remnant of membrane can be cut off, leaving any muscular coat attached to the esophagus. (3) If perchance an opening is made into the esophagus, this can be closed in an appropriate fashion with inverting silk stitches, followed by transpleural, or preferably retro-pleural, mediastinal post-operative drainage.

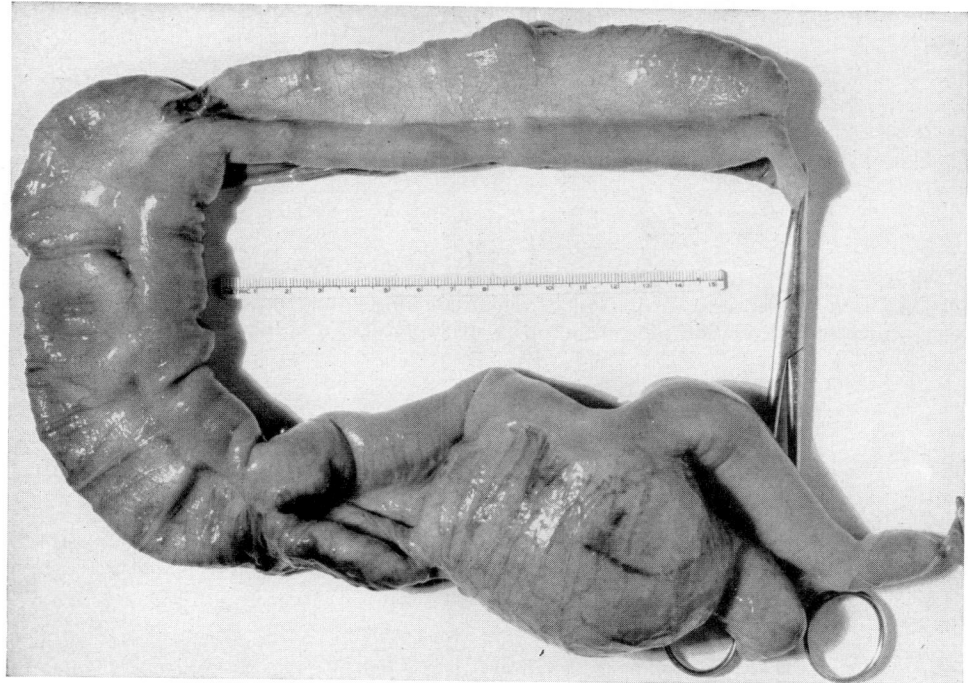

Fig. 130. Extensive duplication of the ileum. The scale is 15 cm. long. The intestine lies along the interior of the specimen, and the duplication is around the periphery. Case 28.

Duplications in the Thorax Arising from Intestine. Because they traverse two body cavities, these anomalies may require extensive or multiple-stage procedures to effect a cure.[3, 5] Just how much has to be done in an operative way depends somewhat upon the type of symptoms which are present and the character of the membrane which lines the tube. If the lining is intestinal or colonic in nature and the symptoms have been only those related to *distention* of the intrathoracic portion, it is sufficient to remove only that part which lies above the diaphragm, leaving in place the segment of diverticulum which resides below the diaphragm (Case 17, Table 23). Conversely, if the long diverticulum is lined by gastric mucosa and the symptoms have been those of bleeding from the intestinal tract, it is important to remove *all* of the anomalous structure. This might require separate thoracic and abdominal undertakings, depending upon the extent of

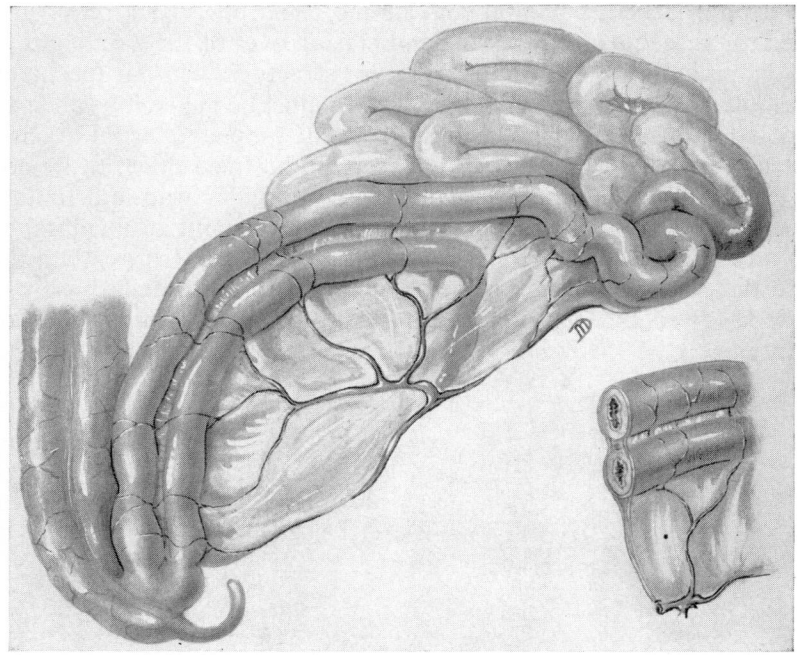

Fig. 131. Drawing of a long tubular duplication of the lower ileum, which communicated with the intestine near the ileocecal valve. Duplication 38 cm. long. Insert shows cross-section of the double-barreled structure and relation of duplication to the mesentery and the intestine. Case 37.

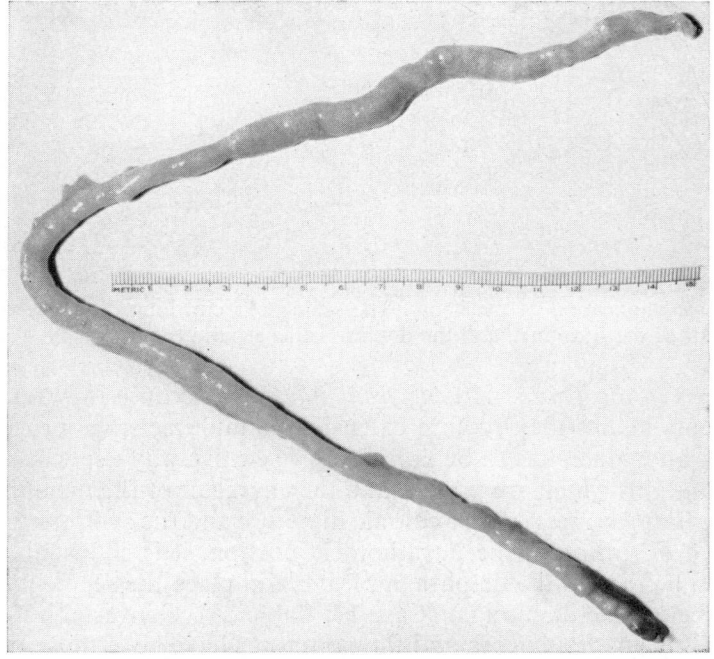

Fig. 132. Extremely long duplication removed from the ileum in a day-old baby. The structure is 44 cm. long. Fatal termination. Case 40.

the lesion, condition of the child, and the like. In Case 16 we were able to accomplish a complete excision in one stage by a right thoracotomy and a simultaneous right upper quadrant laparotomy, removing the entire diverticulum and a portion of the jejunum from which it arose, reestablishing the continuity of the jejunum by end-to-end suture.

Duplications of the Stomach. In a small lesion, such as in Case 19, the entire duplication can be excised. However, in extensive ones, such as Case 18, the therapy might be total gastrectomy and establishment of an esophago-jejunostomy; this undertaking appears to be rather hazardous. As an alternative, the cyst can be opened, a portion of

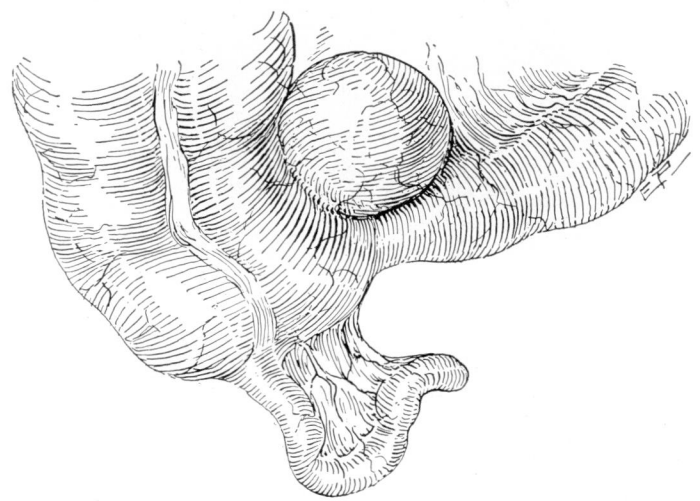

Fig. 133. Sketch of a duplication arising near ileocecal valve, Cases 48–55.

it resected, and the remainder marsupialized to the anterior abdominal wall so that it can be tightly packed with gauze to destroy its lining. Withdrawing the packing some days after operation allows the cyst walls to fall together and coalesce, an attack which was successful in our Case 18.

Duplications of the Duodenum. Because of special anatomic considerations, these deserve particular comment. One cystic duplication of the duodenum was treated by *excision of the mass* and the first part of the duodenum, combined with a *posterior gastro-jejunostomy*. The postoperative result was quite satisfactory, but this form of therapy is not to be recommended since it is fraught with danger of injury to the common bile duct, head of the pancreas, and regional blood vessels. As an alternate and superior method, Gardner and Hart[4] cut a *window* between the cyst and adjacent duodenum, with success. We have since been pleased with the employment of this approach in two cases, traversing the cyst and creating an opening between it and the duodenum. It would seem to be of importance to make this window toward the *distal* end of the duplication, and to make the stoma of *ample size*, both of which factors would tend to prevent the entrapment of duodenal contents in the side pouch.

Duplications of the Intestine. For the vast majority of duplications of the jejunum, ileum, and the ileo-cecal valve region there seems to be little if any justification for attempts to peel them away from the adjacent gut since these efforts are so apt to be followed by injury to the latter. It is far preferable—in these areas where there is a mesentery—to excise the lesion along with the attached segment of alimentary tube,

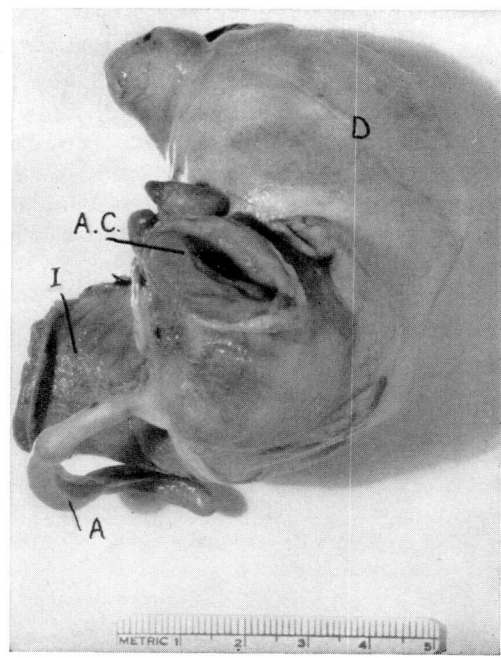

Fig. 134. Surgical specimen of duplication removed from ileocecal region (viewed from behind). A appendix. AC, ascending colon. D, duplication. I, ileum. Case 51.

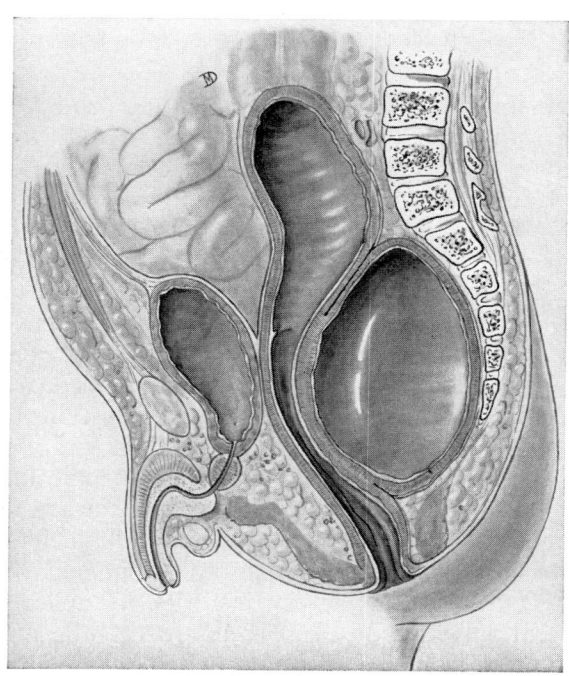

Fig. 135. Reconstruction drawing showing duplication anterior to the sacrum producing partial obstruction of the rectum. Case 62.

and to reestablish the continuity of the tract by direct anastomosis or by a Mikulicz procedure.

Duplications of the Colon and Rectum. When occurring in the free portion of the colon, such as the transverse and sigmoidal areas, the same principles apply as those used for small intestinal anomalies, namely, excision along with the adjacent bowel. For those occurring behind the rectum, the baby can be placed in a face-down position (the abdomen raised over a sandbag and the legs hanging) so that an incision behind the anus allows dissection up into the hollow of the sacrum. There is a good plane of cleavage between the pelvis and the cyst, but the latter may be difficult or impossible to peel away from the rectum. In two of our cases the rectum was not entered, but in a third it was torn into; the rent in the rectum could be satisfactorily closed by inverting sutures of catgut, reinforced with silk.

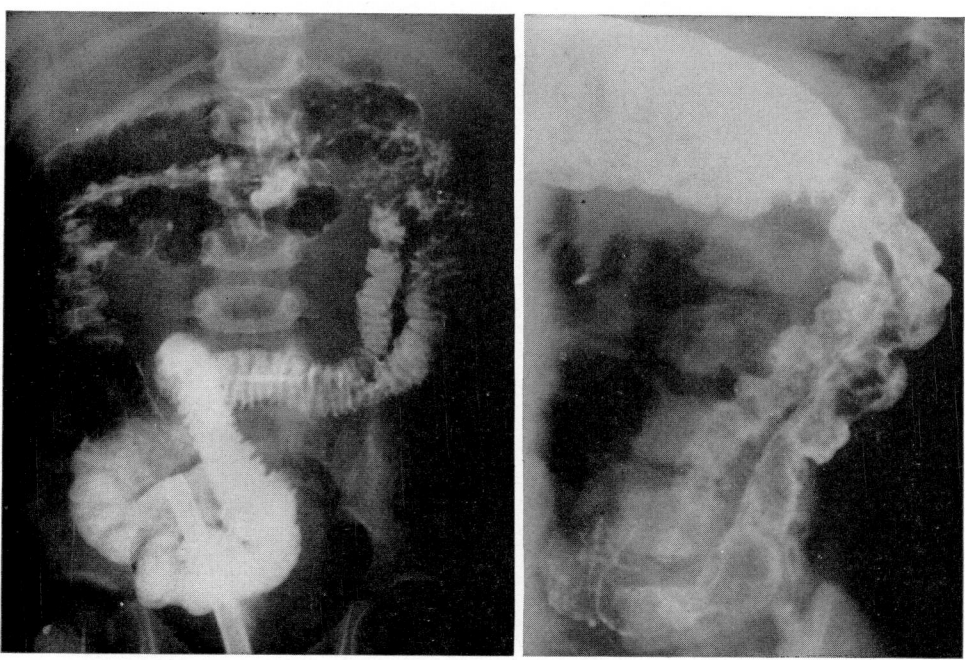

Fig. 136. *Left,* Roentgenogram from Case 66, shows the double lumen in the transverse colon and terminal ileum (patient has situs transversus). Compare Figure 117, A. *Right,* Roentgenogram from Case 67, showing a double, descending colon. Compare Figure 117, B.

For the long double-barreled lesions of the colon it is important to point out that it may *not* be necessary to treat the entire anomaly; it is usually sufficient to direct therapeutic attempts toward its lower end. In each of the four instances (Cases 65–68) the upper ends of both colonic tubes were open to the fecal stream and each tube seemed to have propulsive activity. Therefore, as a general principle, it would seem necessary to correct only the disturbances which exist at the lower end of the anomaly. In Case 65 this would have involved correction of an imperforate anus. In Case 68 an extra opening to the exterior had to be closed off and the two rectal lumina converted into a single cavity. In Cases 66 and 67 a fistula to the urethra had to be closed off and the two rectal tubes converted into one lumen, so that all fecal material is now discharged through the anus. To cut down the walls between such parallel tubes, we have found it

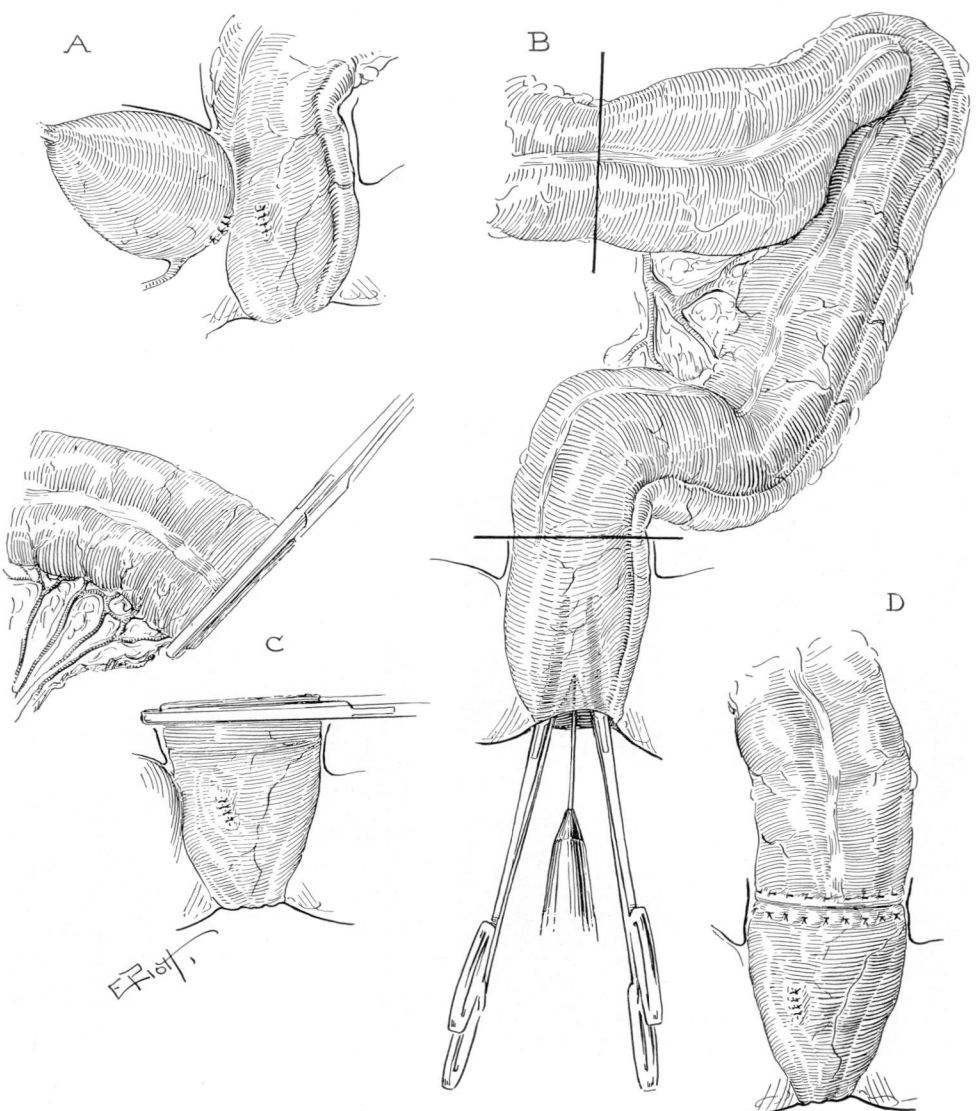

Fig. 137. Operative procedure used in Case 67. **A,** The recto-urethral fistula is closed off. **B,** The septum within the rectum is cut by endothermy, between Kocher clamps. The entire descending colon, between the lines, will be removed. **C,** Transverse colon brought down to upper part of rectum. **D,** Anastomosis completed.

satisfactory to apply two Kocher clamps lengthwise along the septum and cut between these with an endothermy knife. When one such cut has been made, the clamps can be inserted on the septum at a higher level, for another cut, carrying out such progressive divisions as far as is necessary. (While we resected portions of the descending colon in patients 66 and 67, we now believe that this additional step might have been unnecessary.)

RESULTS OF TREATMENT

The increasing awareness of the problems presented by these congenital anomalies, the application of newer concepts of chemotherapy and electrolyte balance, and the improvement in techniques of bowel surgery have substantially reduced the mortality or duplication patients in spite of the fact that some of them present most fo rmidable undertakings. From 1928 through 1940, 15 patients were operated upon with4 deaths, a mortality rate of 27 per cent. During the ten years since 1940, 48 patients have received surgical treatment for this condition at the Children's Medical Center; there have been 4 deaths in this group, a mortality rate of 8 per cent. It is significant that in the last 20 patients there have been no fatalities. For individual consideration of the various cases, some material is given on each of them in Table 23, so that the results of various forms of therapy can be studied.

REFERENCES

1. Black, R. A. and Benjamin, E. L.: Enterogenous Abnormalities: Cysts and Diverticula. Am. J. Dis. Child., *51*:1126, 1936.
2. Bremer, J. L.: Diverticula and Duplications of the Intestinal Tract. Arch. Path., *38*:132, 1944.
3. Fisher, H. C.: Duplications of the Intestinal Tract in Infants. Arch. Surg., *61*:957, 1950.
4. Gardner, C. C., Jr., and Hart, D.: Enterogenous Cysts of the Duodenum: Report of a Case and Review of the Literature. J.A.M.A., *104*:1809, 1935.
5. Gross, R. E., Neuhauser, E. B. C. and Longino, L. A.: Thoracic Diverticula Which Originate from the Intestine. Ann. Surg., *131*:363, 1950.
6. Ladd, W. E. and Chisholm, T. C.: Double Uterus, Vagina and Rectum. Am. J. Dis. Child., *66*:629, 1943.
7. Ladd, W. E. and Gross, R. E.: Surgical Treatment of Duplications of the Alimentary Tract: Enterogenous Cysts, Enteric Cysts, or Ileum Duplex. Surg., Gynec., & Obst., *70*:295, 1940.
8. Ladd, W. E. and Scott, H. W., Jr.: Esophageal Duplications or Mediastinal Cysts of Enteric Origin. Surgery, *16*:815, 1944.
9. Lewis, F. T. and Thyng, F. W.: The Regular Occurrence of Intestinal Diverticula in Embryos of the Pig, Rabbit and Man. Am. J. Anat., *7*:505, 1907.
10. McLanahan, S. and Stone, H. B.: Enterogenous Cysts. Surg., Gynec., & Obst., *58*:1027, 1934.
11. Mixter, C. G. and Clifford, S. H.: Congenital Mediastinal Cysts of Gastrogenic and Bronchogenic Origin. Ann. Surg., *90*:714, 1929.
12. Pachman, D. J.: Enterogenous Intramural Cysts of the Intestines. Am. J. Dis. Child., *58*:485, 1939.
13. Poncher, H. G. and Milles, G.: Cysts and Diverticula of Intestinal Origin. Am. J. Dis. Child., *45*:1064, 1933.
14. Slomovitz, Z., Cash, I. I. and Enzer, N.: Duplication of the Ileum. Gastroenterology, *11*:528, 1948.

CHAPTER 18

Foreign Bodies in the Alimentary Tract

Infants and children are prone to put into their mouths non-digestible materials which are not infrequently swallowed. A wide variety of objects may enter the alimentary canal, ranging from sharp pins or nails to smooth coins or buttons and from small finger rings to moderate-sized toys of all sorts. It is almost inconceivable how some of these pointed or sharp objects can move along the alimentary tube without injuring its mucous membrane or causing important difficulties. Indeed, it is difficult to understand how some of the larger bodies pass through the esophagus, the pylorus, or the ileo-cecal valve at all. The great majority of them start on their way with little more than a gulp or a short fit of coughing. In fact, many are swallowed without the slightest difficulty and the accident is suspected only because of the disappearance of an object with which a child had been playing.

Foreign bodies which stop in the hypopharynx or esophagus can be troublesome, at times can be difficult to treat, and occasionally can lead to serious complications. Those which reach the stomach will, in the vast majority of instances, pass through the remainder of the intestinal tract; in only a small minority of cases is their operative removal required.

Objects Recovered

In a series of patients at the Children's Hospital, the foreign bodies listed in Table 24 were retrieved from the alimentary tract.

Age Incidence

The majority of these children with foreign bodies in the esophagus or gastro-intestinal tract were from six months to four years of age. The youngest was one month and the oldest was fifteen years. The distributions were as follows:

Under 1 year	85
1 year	131
2 years	178
3 years	124
4 years	87
5 years	56
6 years	29
7 to 15 years	76

Trichobezoar

The formation of a hair-ball is apt to be followed by poor health over a long period of time, because the gastric lumen becomes largely occluded by a dense mass which

Table 24

766 Foreign Bodies Swallowed by Babies and Children

(The figures in parentheses indicate the numbers of objects which stuck in the esophagus and had to be removed therefrom.)

Item	Count	Item	Count	Item	Count
Penny	154 (30)	Metal toy parts	4 (3)	Dice	1
Open safety pin	88 (32)	Bead	3	Moth ball	1
Nickel coin	61 (13)	Metal cap	3 (1)	Book fastener	1
Closed safety pin	60	Paper clip	3	Thermometer bulb	1
Bobby pin	56 (1)	Piece of wire	3 (2)	Toy watch	1
Straight pin	33 (2)	Shoe buckle	3	Rubber balloon	1
Quarter (coin)	23 (12)	Phone slugs	3	Key ring	1
Tack	21 (4)	Staples	3	Lead soldier	1
Nail	20	Jackstone	3 (2)	Toy train car	1
Screw	14	Bone	3 (2)	Toy scissors	1
Ring	13	Steel nut	2	Comb teeth	1
Marble	13	Pen point	2	Wooden splinters	1
Button	12 (5)	Wooden ball	2	Razor blade	1
Impacted food	12 (12)	Toy horn	2	Steel wool	1
Piece of glass	10	Locket	2	Spring	1
Toy whistle	10 (3)	Collar button	2 (1)	Hatpin	1
Campaign button	9 (1)	Ball bearing	2	Sea shell	1
Needle	7	Plastic toys	2	Flashlight bulb	1
Key	7 (3)	Stone	2 (1)	Rubber nozzle	1
Bolt	5	Plastic disc	2 (1)	Toy shoe	1
Religious medal	5 (1)	Ear ring	2 (2)	Chain	1
Piece of lead pencil	5	Toy pipe	1	Medicine dropper	1
Piece of steel	5 (1)	Dental brace	1	Rubber nipple	1 (1)
Toy coins	5 (2)	Toy spoon	1	Cellophane	1 (1)
Doll eye	4	Rattle handle	1	Metal washer	1 (1)
Small bell	4 (2)	Tooth	1	Cup hook	1 (1)
Hair ball	7	Lead type	1	Egg shell	1 (1)
Dime coin	4 (1)	Metal plug	1 (1)	Small crucifix	1 (1)
Fruit stones	4 (1)	Jewelry pin	1 (1)	Metal disc	1 (1)
Barrettes	4 (1)	Rivet	1		

interferes with the ingestion and digestion of food. The habit of plucking and chewing hair would appear to be an innocuous one, but the gradually enlarging and matted bolus finally produces partial gastric obstruction and malfunction. A history of hair-eating, poor appetite, occasional vomiting, eructations of malodorous gas, and failure to gain weight properly are highly suggestive of a trichobezoar, particularly if a mass can be palpated in the epigastrium. The diagnosis can be proved by roentgen examination after a swallow of barium.

SYMPTOMS

About one-quarter of all foreign bodies lodge in the esophagus and may give rise to spells of choking, inability to swallow, and vague feelings of discomfort. If they have remained in place very long, they may cause reaction in adjacent structures including the larynx and trachea. In rare instances, sharp objects can perforate the esophagus and puncture the aorta, pericardium, or parietal pleura. About three-quarters of objects which are swallowed pass directly into the stomach, and once they have done so it is uncommon for them to give rise to symptoms. Of those reaching the stomach, well over 90 per cent progress through the alimentary tract without discomfort of any sort and their elimination may not be recognized unless the stools are carefully searched. If the bodies are unusually large in relation to the size of the patient, there may be occasional mild *abdominal cramps* and rarely *vomiting*. Jagged or irregular objects may scratch the anus and initiate minor *bleeding*. The appetite is rarely interfered with. *Perforation* of the intestine is exceedingly rare, and even if it does take place it occurs so slowly that omentum, liver, or other viscus becomes adherent to the intestine at this point to prevent escape of the sharp object or infected material into the general peritoneal cavity. Therefore, perforation is usually not attended by pain, tenderness, spasm, or fever.

ROENTGENOLOGIC STUDY

Fortunately, most foreign bodies which are swallowed are opaque to x-rays. Roentgenologic examinations are of value in determining that a missing object actually resides in the alimentary tract, and also in watching its progress or lack of progress. Fluoroscopic observation, or a plain film, will usually give all the information which is desired, but the use of a contrast medium is occasionally of value.

In one of our patients the position of a stationary needle was not clear. Studies with a barium gastro-intestinal series and a barium enema gave the impression that it was outside of the alimentary tract. This was confirmed at laparotomy, when it was found to have escaped completely from the stomach or intestine (site of perforation could not be located) and was wrapped in a wad of omentum.

TREATMENT

The treatment of foreign bodies in the alimentary tract cannot be dogmatically stated, for it will necessarily depend upon the exigencies of the individual case. Approximately a quarter of them lodge in the esophagus and require operative endoscopic removal, particularly if the object lies in the hypopharynx where it is apt to give rise to respiratory difficulties. For the three-quarters which slip through into the stomach, conservative treatment is all that is required in most instances. Without doubt, many laparotomies can be avoided if several days' delay and patience are exercised. Of our 615 patients with gastro-intestinal foreign bodies, the foreign material was eliminated in the stool of 572, while operation was deemed advisable in only 43.

Esophageal Foreign Bodies

Some foreign bodies, because of their large size, irregularity, or sharpness, lodge in the esophagus and must be removed promptly. Urgency for doing this is greater if the object sticks at a high level, where there is the possibility of giving rise to respiratory complications. When a foreign body lodges in the esophagus, it is well to bear in mind that there might be some previously existing intrinsic esophageal pathology (such as an old lye stricture, a congenital narrowing, etc.). Such was the case in about 10 per cent of our patients from whom an esophageal foreign body had to be extracted. Of all the foreign bodies listed in Table 24, those marked by parentheses (totaling 151) had to be removed from the esophagus in the ten-year period ending December 31, 1950. All of these patients recovered rapidly, excepting 9 in whom convalescence was delayed by a tracheitis (1), pneumonitis (1), peri-esophageal inflammation (1), esophageal perforation (2), pyopneumothorax (2), cervical abscess (1), or pericarditis (1). There was eventual recovery in all of these excepting the last, in whom an open safety pin had entered the pericardium, giving rise to suppuration which could not be controlled by surgical drainage or by chemotherapy.

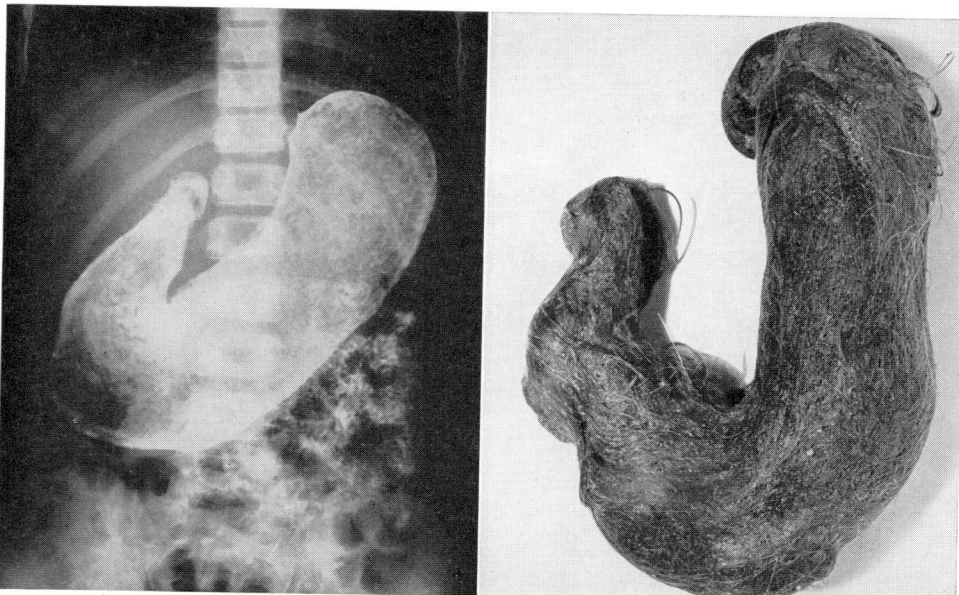

Fig. 138. Trichobezoar in the stomach of a seven-year-old girl who had a habit of pulling and eating strands of her hair. *Left,* Roentgenogram. The barium surrounds a large matted and fibrillar mass (hair-ball) which fills the gastric lumen. *Right,* The hair-ball which was removed from the stomach

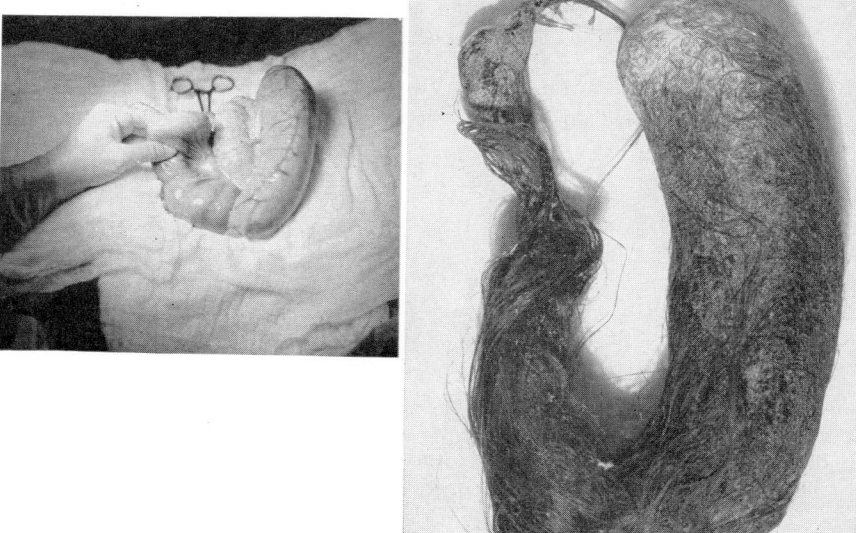

Fig. 139. Findings in a child with a hair-ball which filled the stomach and a large part of the duodenum. *Left,* Operative photograph, showing the mass in the stomach and in the duodenum. *Right,* The specimen which was removed by gastrotomy; the duodenal portion could be pulled back through the pylorus.

Gastro-intestinal Foreign Bodies

Since it is known that most objects which reach the stomach will pass spontaneously, there is seldom any need for advising early operation for those which have passed the esophagus. Unless there is some symptom to suggest perforation of the bowel, which is rarely the case, conservative management should be given a thorough trial.

Table 25

List of All Babies under Twenty-four Months of Age with Gastro-intestinal Foreign Bodies

Spontaneous Passage in Stool (138 Patients)

Age in Months	Object	Age in Months	Object
23, 22, 22, 20, 19, 16, 15, 15, 14, 14, 14, 12, 12, 11, 11, 11, 11, 11, 10, 10, 9, 9, 9, 9, 8, 8, 8, 7, 7, 6, 5	Open safety pin	19, 9	Button
		13, 11	Toy coin
		17	Moth ball
23, 22, 22, 22, 22, 22, 22, 21, 21, 20, 20, 20, 19, 19, 18, 18, 17, 16, 14, 1	Penny	14	Rivet
		15	Screen wire
20, 20, 20, 19, 19, 19, 16, 15, 11, 11, 10. 8, 6, 4	Closed safety pin	11	Rattle handle
		22	Collar button
20, 17, 16, 12, 11, 5, 5, 3	Straight pin	10	Piece of lead pencil
22, 20, 18, 18, 17, 6, 4	Bobby pin	16	Comb teeth
21, 20, 14, 10, 10, 7, 6	Tack	1	Wood splinter
22, 14, 12, 12, 11, 11	Piece of glass	11	Broken razor blade
22, 20, 15, 12	Nickel coin	21	Steel wool
21, 16, 14, 14	Ring	22	Metal ball
18, 9, 9, 5	Screw	21	Quarter
18, 18, 16	Marble	20	Piece of light bulb
17, 16, 11	Stove bolt	4	Rubber tip
19, 10	Religious charm	6	Small chain
18, 14	Key	21	Paper clip
11, 9	Toy eye	16	Medicine dropper

Surgical Removal (14 Patients)

Age in Months	Object
17, 15, 15, 13, 11, 11, 10, 10, 9, 6, 5, 5	Open safety pin
14	Barrette
21	Penny

Conservative Therapy. With conservative therapy, the child should be kept on its *normal diet.* Large amounts of bread or porridge (with the idea of forming a protecting bolus around an open safety pin or needle) have little to recommend them. Active *catharsis* should certainly be avoided for fear of increasing the intestinal peristalsis and enhancing the possibility of intestinal irritation or perforation. If constipation has been present, small amounts of *mineral oil* may be prescribed with impunity. All of the *stools* should be collected in a suitable container so that they can be examined until the foreign body is identified. In general, there need be no haste about discontinuing a conservative regimen in favor of operative treatment. Most of these objects will be eliminated within a few days, but occasionally one will require several weeks. The mere size of an object is not often a deterrent factor in its passing through the intestine, for almost any solid and rigid object which can get into the stomach (no matter how small the patient) will

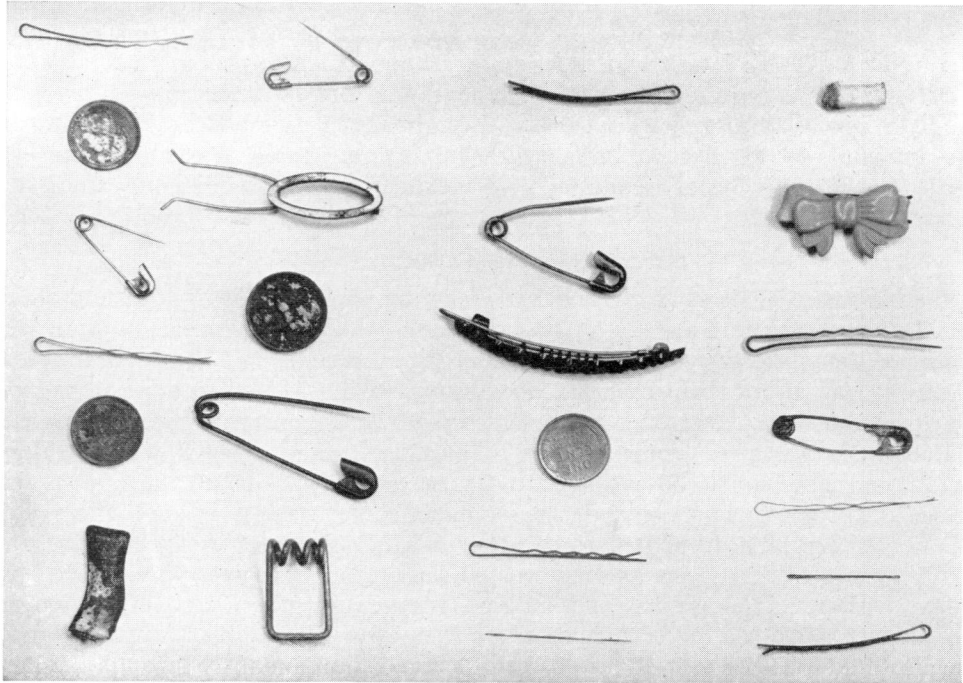

Fig. 140. Some foreign bodies which failed to pass spontaneously and had to be removed by laparotomy, mostly from the stomach and duodenum.

be eliminated eventually and spontaneously in the stool. *Smooth materials,* such as buttons, coins and toy whistles, may be left unoperated upon for as long as *three or four weeks* or more without danger, and indeed we have never had to remove one of these rounded or relatively smooth bodies by operative means, if the intestine was normal to begin with. Sharp objects, such as straight pins, open safety pins, needles, broken glass, and nails, must be regarded with some concern. Most of these can be spontaneously passed in the majority of instances, but frequent checks with x-ray films are desirable to make sure that progress is being made. If a sharp object remains in one place for more than three or four days, it is well to consider surgical removal.

Operative Treatment. The indications for operation in our cases were: (1) Failure of progress of a needle, open safety pin, or hairpin, in 16. (2) Failure of progress of a nickel coin which had stopped at a congenital stenosis of the jejunum, in one. (3) Failure of progression of blunt objects (barrettes, bobby pins, coin, metal spring, et cetera, in 15. (4) Suspected perforation by a nonprogressing pointed object, in 4. (5) For removal of a gastric hair-ball, in 7. (6) Appendectomy (signs of acute appendicitis) when foreign body lodged in appendix, 3.

The chances for a spontaneous passage of foreign substances through the intestinal tract of an infant or older child would presumably depend somewhat on the *size* of the object in relation to the size of the individual. In order to point out what the alimentary tract is capable of eliminating, Table 25 lists all infants under two years of age, the objects which entered the gastro-intestinal canal, and whether there was spontaneous passage or surgical removal. This summary indicates that any object which can be swallowed by a baby will pass about as readily as it would in an older child, and that operation need not be urged merely because a patient is small or young.

Operative withdrawal of a foreign body from the gastro-intestinal tract is almost always an upper abdominal procedure. In the present series the pylorus, duodenal curves, and jejunal angulation were the main anatomic structures which arrested progress in such a way as to require operation. Whenever the foreign object passed beyond the jejunum, there was almost always a subsequent unimpeded course through the remainder of the alimentary tract (except for one girl with a coin caught at a congenital jejunal stenosis, 3 in whom objects lodged in the appendix, and 2 in whom they stuck in the sigmoid).

SUMMARY AND CONCLUSIONS

The treatment of most foreign bodies which are swallowed by infants and children should be conservative. In a series of 766 babies and children who ingested a wide variety of objects it was necessary to remove 151 from the esophagus by endoscopic means and 43 from the gastro-intestinal tract by laparotomy. When lodged in the esophagus, all sharp objects and any large ones which failed to progress promptly were removed immediately by endoscopic means. Of the manifold substances which were swallowed, about 20 per cent had to be extracted from the esophagus. Of all the objects which traversed the esophagus and reached the stomach, some concern was felt when straight pins, open safety pins, bobby pins, needles, or other sharp objects were being dealt with. While the vast majority of these passed safely, their progress was checked every few days with roentgenograms, and surgical intervention considered if lodgment occurred in one place for more than three or four days. If an object once entered the stomach, it had a 93 per cent chance of being passed spontaneously through the bowel; surgical removal was necessary for only 7 per cent of them.

In a series of 766 foreign bodies in the alimentary tract there was a death from one which punctured the esophagus and entered the pericardium; there was no death in that group in which the object had entered the stomach.

REFERENCES

1. Best, R. R.: Management of Sharp Pointed Foreign Bodies in the Gastrointestinal Tract. Am J. Surg., 72:545, 1946.
2. DeBakey, M. and Ochsner, A.: Bezoars and Concretions: Comprehensive Review of the Literature with Analysis of 303 Collected Cases and Presentation of 8 Additional Cases. Surgery, 4:934, 1938.
3. Delaney, C. J.: Foreign Bodies Swallowed by Children. N. Y. State J. Med., 40:1024, 1940.
4. Donovan, E. J.: Meckel's Diverticulum Perforated by Foreign Body. Ann. Surg., 106: 953, 1937.
5. Forbes, R. P.: Bezoar Causing Intestinal Obstruction. J. Pediat., 24:574, 1944.
6. Jackson, C. and Jackson, C. L.: Foreign Bodies in Intestines. M. Rec., 140:285, 1934.
7. Johnson, C. I. and Ferguson, C. F.: Foreign Bodies in the Air and Food Passages. New England J. Med., 215:1054, 1936.
8. Lyons, C. G. and Cody, G. L.: Bezoar. Radiology, 31:225, 1938.
9. McEnery, E. T. and Fox, P. F.: Foreign Bodies of Duodenum Causing Urinary Disturbance. J. Pediat., 29:226, 19 6.
10. Silber, S., Kaplan, C. and Epstein, B.: The Use of a Permanent (Alnico) Magnet in the Peroral Removal of a Metallic Foreign Body (Padlock) from the Stomach. Ann. Otol., Rhin., & Laryng., 53:589, 1944.
11. Storck, A., Rothschild, J. E. and Ochsner, A.: Intestinal Obstruction Due to Intraluminal Foreign Bodies. Ann. Surg., 109: 844, 1939.

CHAPTER 19

Appendicitis

Appendicitis is the most common lesion requiring intra-abdominal surgery in childhood. It is still a highly important problem because of the great frequency of the condition, and because it continues to be responsible for deaths which should be preventable. Although the mortality rates in first-class hospitals have been gradually improving, this does not necessarily reflect the state of affairs in all institutions, particularly those in some smaller communities.

The following considerations, opinions, and data are based upon generally accepted knowledge of the disease and upon information gathered from the treatment of 2070 children with appendicitis up to January 1, 1951, at the Boston Children's Hospital.

Differences in Appendicitis in Children and in Adults

While appendicitis is the same disease in the adult and the child, the reactions and the complications can be quite different in these two age groups. The physician who tries to employ the same details of treatment for both will often invite, and will frequently meet, disaster. To obtain reasonably good results in handling appendicitis in young subjects it is essential to recognize that the criteria for establishment of a diagnosis are different, that the untreated disease runs a more rapid and deadlier course, and that a somewhat different therapeutic attack must be used in combating the condition.

PATHOLOGY

Inflammation of the appendix begins in the mucosa or submucosa with bacterial invasion, leukocytic infiltration, vascular engorgement, edema, and hemorrhage. This is followed by ulceration of the mucosa and accumulation of purulent exudate within the appendiceal lumen. It is characteristic for the process to spread outward and to involve the muscularis and serosa. Distention of the appendix or thrombosis of its vessels diminishes the blood supply to the organ so that gangrene and rupture may follow. In the course of the disease, fibrin is formed on the serosal surface, making the organ adhere to nearby structures, particularly to the omentum if this is long enough to reach to the iliac fossa. This defense mechanism for localizing the infection is efficient in older children and adults, but it is poor in infants and younger subjects in whom the omentum is notoriously short, thin, and almost devoid of fat.

Fluid is poured into the peritoneal cavity when the appendiceal veins are thrombosed, or when the appendiceal lumen is blocked by exudate, fecalith, or a swollen mucosa. For a few hours this is clear, but soon fibrin and leukocytes accumulate and make it a thin, cloudy, odorless but sterile *exudate*. Bacteria may then invade such a medium by rupture of the appendix, or by traversing a highly inflamed but still intact appendiceal wall.

In the natural course of the disease, checking of the inflammation will depend upon the immunity of the individual and upon the availability of mobile structures for *walling off* the process. The complete encirclement and enclosure of an appendix in a protective omental sheath takes place in some fortunate cases. A less effective mode of defense is that in which loops of intestines, mesentery, cecal wall, or parietal peritoneum become adherent to one another to form a pocket which encases the distending and rupturing appendix, giving a regional abscess. If these walling-off reactions have not appeared in time, rupture of an appendix *contaminates the general peritoneal cavity*. Once this has occurred, spread of infection is very rapid. While a generalized peritonitis is a supreme menace to the life of the individual, a final defense is still possible by a gathering of the exudate into one or more regions of the abdomen to form *localized abscesses* in the pelvis, between intestinal loops, under the liver, below the diaphragm, etc.

Much has been said about the *danger of purgatives* in patients with acute appendicitis. There is overwhelming statistical evidence to show that the ingestion of castor oil or other active laxatives will greatly increase intestinal and appendiceal peristalsis so that perforation and dissemination of infection are more likely to occur.

The *bacteriology* in cases with abscess or peritonitis is variable. In many peritoneal cultures there are doubtless important organisms which are lost sight of because of a luxuriant overgrowth of colon bacillus. In a series of 336 peritoneal cultures which showed growth, the following identifications were made:

Colon bacillus	202
Enterococcus	4
Streptococcus hemolyticus	5
Streptococcus nonhemolyticus	1
Staphylococcus aureus	3
Pneumococcus	4
Mixed (intestinal)	95
Other organisms	22

ETIOLOGY

Not much is known about the etiology of acute appendicitis. The greater frequency of the disease at certain periods of the year when respiratory infections are common suggests that the organisms responsible for the respiratory diseases also have a predilection for invasion of the vermiform appendix, but there is little statistical evidence to support such a hypothesis. While a head cold, pharyngitis, or bronchitis not uncommonly precedes the onset of acute appendicitis, actually this combination is found in only a minority of cases. The fact that early stages of appendicitis do not show uniform involvement of all layers of the organ is rather against the theory of a hematogenous origin of the lesion. Most frequently, the disease probably starts by bacterial invasion from the highly infective material which resides in the appendiceal lumen.

The frequency with which inflammation originates in the *inner coats* of the appendix tends to support the thesis that *obstruction to its lumen* is an important etiologic factor in appendicitis. Wangensteen and his colleagues exteriorized and artificially obstructed appendices in humans (adults) and then demonstrated that there was sufficient formation of mucus to raise the intra-appendiceal pressure to figures approaching the systolic blood pressure. This mounting tension of entrapped secretory products is certainly sufficient to bring about ischemia and necrosis of the appendiceal walls. Therefore, it is reasonable to believe that a *fecalith* or *inspissated material* which obstructs an appendiceal lumen plays an important part in the onset of inflammatory disease. The frequency with which fecaliths are found in gangrenous or ruptured appendices lends strong support to this view. That this is not a universal factor is suggested by those cases in which no fecalith, foreign body, hyperplastic lymphoid tissue, or other form of obstruction can be demonstrated.

There is a widespread impression (difficult to prove statistically) that an appendix which once has been acutely inflamed is very apt to have another infection at a subsequent time. Presumably, this is true because *scar tissue* forms in a place where it blocks the drainage of the organ. This marked tendency to recurrent infection is the basis for the belief that appendicitis (with rupture) which has been treated by drainage of an abscess (or peritoneal cavity) should always be followed some months later by surgical removal of the appendix to prevent a recurrent bout of the disease.

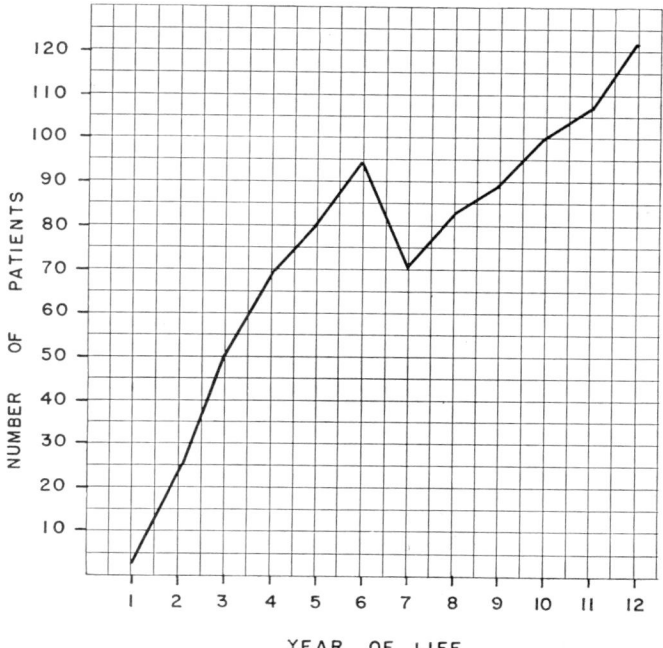

YEAR OF LIFE

Fig. 141. Graph showing age incidence of acute appendicitis in children. The condition is rare in the first year and is uncommon in the second year of life.

SYMPTOMS AND SIGNS

Difficulty in recognition of acute appendicitis in young children has been emphasized often, but the more skill one has in managing patients of this age, the rarer will be the errors in diagnosis. Certainly it is possible in most instances to identify the condition before rupture has taken place. To do this in the less clear-cut instances requires careful examination by an experienced physician or surgeon.

The triad of *abdominal pain*, *vomiting*, and *slight fever* must be considered as indicative of appendicitis until proved otherwise. If any or all of these are accompanied by important abdominal tenderness, appendicitis should be the diagnosis which is given greatest consideration.

Age and Sex Incidence

The youngest individual in the Children's Hospital series with acute appendicitis was six months of age, but younger ones have been reported. Appendicitis is quite rare in the first year of life, is infrequently found in the second year, but from then on it becomes common. More cases are seen in the period from six to twelve years than in the period from one to six years. The disease is slightly more frequent in males than in females, 55 per cent against 45 per cent in our series. This ratio is slightly higher than the predominance of males over females in the general population.

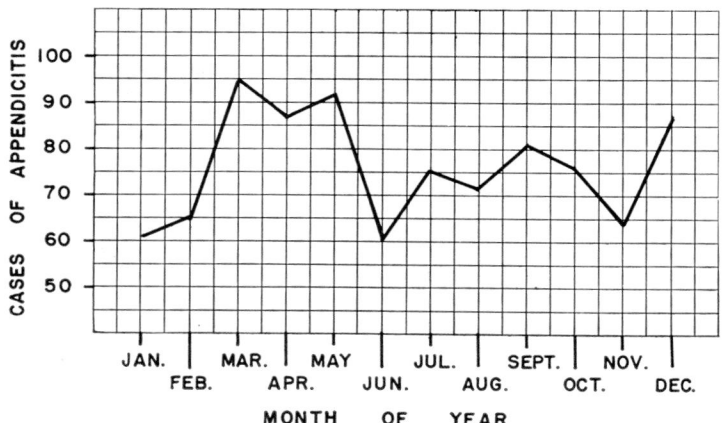

Fig. 142. Incidence of acute appendicitis by months of the year. The greater frequency of the disease during March, April, and May might possibly be related to the prevalence of respiratory infections during these spring months.

Symptoms

Pain. The usual history is one of acute abdominal pain, followed by nausea and vomiting. Pain is apt to begin around the umbilicus or in the epigastrium, but often children are vague and inaccurate about describing their complaints and it may be impossible to elicit a story of early periumbilical discomfort. After a variable number of hours, the pain is most intense in the *right lower quadrant.* When a child is seen in this stage, the severity of his current troubles may make him forget and even deny that he previously had any peri-umbilical symptoms. Pain of appendiceal origin can be maximal in the *right upper quadrant,* if the cecum is incompletely rotated and lies—with the appendix—in a very high position. If inflammation advances to a spreading involvement of the peritoneum, pain will become diffuse and severe. Appendiceal pain is apt to be constant, but occasionally it is colicky because of obstruction of the *appendiceal lumen*

Table 26

Relationship between Age of Patient and Extent of Appendicitis
(Statistics from 2070 Cases)

Patient's Age	Cases with Acute Unruptured Appendicitis	Cases with Ruptured Appendicitis	Per Cent with Rupture
Less than 1 year	1	6	85
1 to 2 years	7	65	90
2 to 4 years	78	261	77
4 to 6 years	164	206	55
6 to 12 years	781	400	34
12 to 16 years	91	10	9

Table 27

Relation between Duration of Symptoms and Extent of Appendicitis
(in 1399 Cases)

Duration of Symptoms	Acute Unruptured Appendicitis	Acute Ruptured Appendicitis	Per Cent with Perforation
0 to 12 hours..................................	143	18	11
12 to 24 hours.................................	289	58	13
24 to 36 hours.................................	135	72	34
36 to 48 hours.................................	55	92	64
2 to 3 days....................................	61	120	67
Over 3 days...................................	80	276	78

(by fecalith, swollen mucosa, or a kinking of the organ) or because of disturbed peristalsis of nearby intestinal loops.

Vomiting. This is an almost universal finding in acute appendicitis; rarely is it absent. Vomiting may occur only once or twice, but it is apt to be repeated and persistent.

Fever of 100° to 101° F. is the rule, but the temperature may be normal, particularly if the child has been exposed on a cold day while being brought to the physician or hospital. A *temperature* above 102° F. is rare unless there is peritonitis, in which case it may reach 103° F. or more.

The bowel movements may be normal, but *constipation* is common. An inflamed appendix which lies against the lower sigmoid, or a spreading peritonitis which irritates the intestinal tract, can produce a diarrhea. Urinary symptoms are usually absent, but frequency or dysuria can be brought about by an inflamed appendix which lies against the right ureter or the urinary bladder.

A history of recent *upper respiratory infection* is obtained in about one-fifth of the cases. This may be only incidental, but occasionally one gains the impression that the respiratory disease was a forerunner of the abdominal infection. Intestinal disorders, principally *acute enteritis*, are found in some cases and any important changes for the worse in a patient with gastroenteritis should arouse the physician's suspicions of a superimposed appendicitis. Appendicitis may occur at any time during the *acute exanthemata* of childhood, particularly measles. The onset of abdominal symptoms during one of these infections should make one mindful of this possibility.

Technique of Physical Examination

Everything which can be learned by *inspection* should be noted first. The general appearance of the child, the luster or sunkenness of the eyes, the dryness or perspiration of the skin, the position of the legs, the manifestations of pain and the rate of respiration will frequently give considerable information regarding the seat of pathology, the extent of the lesion, and the degree of toxicity.

If the physician is mindful of a few details, he will be able to gain the maximum information from his examination. An approach which is hurried and rough will only agitate the child and produce a crying, alarmed, and uncooperative patient. The common routine of starting with the head, gagging the youngster with a throat stick, upsetting him with a cold stethoscope, and then suddenly palpating the abdomen with a heavy hand is almost certain to give an unreliable impression of the presence or absence

of abdominal inflammation. The findings under such circumstances are apt to be misleading and the resulting diagnosis is often incorrect. It is essential to gain the child's
confidence before proceeding with abdominal palpation, in spite of the fact that this
may actually take as long or longer than the examination itself. A great deal of patience
is often required to accomplish this, but the time is well spent.

Very gentle superficial *palpation* must precede deep palpation and will usually give
more valuable information than the latter, which may throw the whole abdominal
musculature into spasm. If one portion of the abdomen appears to be tender, this

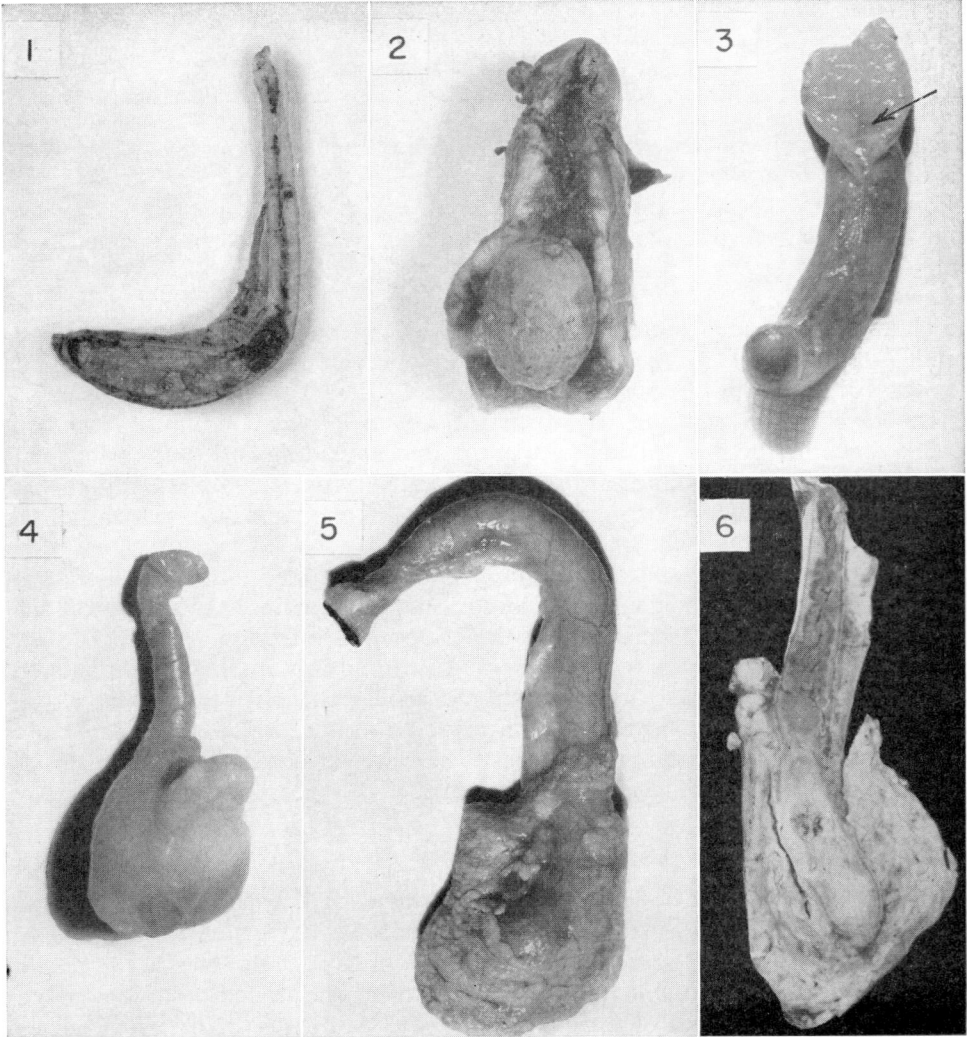

Fig. 143. Photographs of six specimens which were removed because of acute appendicitis. The
base of the appendix is up in each picture. 1. Appendix, diffusely inflamed, and gangrenous in its distal
half. 2. Opened appendix, diffusely inflamed, containing a fecalith. 3. Result of old and recent appendicitis. There is a complete block of the lumen (arrow) from an old process. Organ beyond this tensely
swollen with exudate. 4. Acutely inflamed appendix with marked swelling and edema. 5. Appendix
with inflammation limited to its bulbous tip. 6. Longitudinal section of a gangrenous appendix and a
protective mass of omentum which encased the distal half of it.

should be avoided until all other parts are examined. A warm hand which is applied slowly and gently and kept on a tender area without moving will often give more information and upset the child less than will a palpating hand which is hastily and heavily moved from one region to another. If pneumonia or pleuritis is the basis of the patient's complaints, abdominal spasm will gradually disappear if the observer's hand takes over the function of splinting the lower chest wall. Spasm which remains in spite of continued manual pressure on the abdomen is an indication of peritoneal irritation. Palpation should always include bimanual examination of the kidney regions to rule out renal disease.

Tenderness. The appendix of the child is larger in relation to the size of the abdominal cavity than is that of the adult, and the meso-appendix is correspondingly longer and less well fixed. Therefore, the *point of maximal tenderness* may vary more in location than it does in the adult. It may appear near the midline, well down in the pelvis, or even out in the right flank. If tenderness is accompanied by involuntary muscle spasm, this is evidence of inflammatory involvement of the parietal peritoneum. A low-lying pelvic appendix may give exquisite tenderness by rectal examination which is not too apparent by abdominal palpation. Rebound tenderness is difficult to elicit except in older and more cooperative children. If generalized peritonitis complicates the picture, tenderness is widespread and marked. If the disease has been present for four or five days or more, a tender walled-off abscess may be felt by rectal or abdominal palpation. *Tenderness is the most important single finding upon which the diagnosis of appendicitis is based.* It must be heeded above all other symptoms, signs, or laboratory data. If it is indubitably present, well marked tenderness demands laparotomy.

A *positive psoas* or *obturator sign* may be difficult to detect. Irritation of the psoas muscle by an abscess or inflamed appendix is most apt to be recognized by noting what position the child assumes when left undisturbed, for there will be a tendency to lie with the right thigh partially flexed.

Abdominal *auscultation* may reveal increased peristalsis if there is a spreading peritonitis, or a diminished activity if paralytic ileus has set in.

The cardinal points of a complete general physical examination should follow the abdominal inspection and palpation. *Digital rectal examination* should be left until the last.

Hospitalization for Observation

When seen for the first time in the home or office, a child with abdominal complaints may present a very puzzling picture from which no definite conclusions can be drawn. The youngster is frightened or will not relax; the observations from abdominal examination are inconclusive. It is important that such a child be seen a time or two again, for only by repeated examinations can one be sure whether the abdominal complaints are indicative of some minor ailment or whether appendicitis actually exists. If the physician can see the patient again several times at home, this provides adequate coverage of the case. In some instances *when it is impossible to make such repeated visits, it is highly important to hospitalize the child for a period of twenty-four or even forty-eight hours* so that a close contact can be kept and a conviction can be formed whether the abdominal findings are decreasing or increasing. Such a period of observation does not require extensive or expensive laboratory investigation. It is seldom necessary to have more than a urine examination and one or two white blood counts. Such hospitalization provides coverage mainly in the form of making it easy for someone to see the youngster frequently and to examine the abdomen repeatedly. If the symptoms and signs subside quickly, the child can be discharged without delay; if the findings progressively indicate that appendicitis is present, appropriate therapy can be undertaken. It is much better to handle the situation this way than to allow the child to languish at home and have an appendicitis progress to peritonitis, a disastrous state of affairs which has occurred all too often.

LABORATORY DATA

Leukocytosis to levels of 12,000 or above is common; counts above 18,000 to 20,000 are apt to imply that a local or generalized peritonitis exists. The polymorphonuclear ratio is commonly increased to 85 or 95 per cent. While leukocytosis of some degree generally accompanies acute appendicitis, gangrene or even spreading peritonitis is occasionally found without a striking rise in the white count.

Urine examination usually shows acetone or other ketone bodies. The sediment should be examined to rule out infection of the urinary tract, but it is to be remembered that irritation of the ureter by adjacent appendicitis can make a few white or red blood cells appear in the urine.

Roentgenologic study has been used in some clinics, seeking for free gas in the peritoneal cavity to differentiate ruptured from nonruptured appendicitis; this procedure is unwarranted and has little practical importance. X-ray studies of the chest have great value in cases of suspected appendicitis when there is any question of detecting and ruling out a central pneumonia.

DIFFERENTIAL DIAGNOSIS

Bronchopneumonia

This may be suspected by a higher fever, a higher leukocytosis, a cough, and an increased respiratory rate. In early stages of the disease, or if the pneumonia is central in location, auscultation and percussion of the chest may give rather normal findings. More commonly auscultatory changes are evident. Abdominal spasm may accompany pneumonia, but will gradually disappear if a supporting hand is laid on the abdomen and maintained there steadily for a few minutes. When this differential diagnosis is in question, a roentgenogram of the chest should be obtained.

Pyelitis

Pyelitis can usually be differentiated by a higher fever, white cells in the urinary sediment, and tenderness which is maximal over one of the kidneys.

Idiopathic Primary Peritonitis

When peritoneal infection comes from streptococcal or pneumococcal organisms, it almost always produces a high fever (104° to 105° F.), generalized tenderness, and a doughy abdomen in infants or a spastic one in older children. As a rule this condition is more common in the first year or two of life, but when it does occur in older children, the history may indicate that the pain was generalized at its onset and did not begin around the umbilicus or in the right lower quadrant as would be the case with appendicitis. Leukocytosis is usually higher in primary than in secondary peritonitis. In pneumonia, pyelitis, or idiopathic peritonitis the illness may be ushered in by nausea, vomiting, and abdominal pain, but the temperature is apt to be 103° to 105° F.; whereas in appendicitis the temperature is rarely over 101° F. and is usually not above 103° F. even when complicated by early peritonitis.

While primary peritonitis used to be common, it is now an exceedingly rare condition (presumably because of the widespread use of antibiotics). In past years it was necessary to bear it in mind constantly; now it is not so important in the differential diagnosis.

Acute (Nontuberculous) Mesenteric Adenitis

This is the most common condition which must be differentiated from acute appendicitis. It almost invariably accompanies a respiratory infection, so that examination of the pharynx, nose, and chest is important. Abdominal pain may be generalized or may be localized to any region where the swollen lymph nodes are located. They are larger and more numerous in the mesentery of the terminal ileum, hence the abdominal pain and tenderness are more marked in the right lower quadrant. Nausea and vomiting seldom accompany the condition. Fever is low grade or absent. Tenderness is only slight and is usually not as marked or as localized as that found in acute appendicitis. The white blood count is rarely above 10,000.

When mesenteric adenitis is suspected, observation of the child for several hours is usually sufficient to indicate that the process is stationary or subsiding, and hence is not typical of acute appendicitis. Thus, a course which is characterized by (1) no vomiting, (2) minimal tenderness on repeated examinations of the abdomen, (3) normal or only slightly elevated temperature, and (4) white counts which are not appreciably elevated, generally is sufficient to convince a conscientious physician that there is no pathologic lesion within the abdomen requiring surgery. Several hours' delay in making such observations will usually do no harm, even if appendicitis is present, and a number of useless laparotomies can be avoided thereby. However, if any reasonable suspicion persists about the possibility of appendicitis, laparotomy should be undertaken.

Constipation

Constipation can cause abdominal pain, nausea, and even vomiting, which may be confused with appendicitis. A normal temperature and white blood count are the rule but either can be slightly elevated. There might be slight tenderness in the right lower quadrant (from the distended cecum). If the bowels have not been moving well, or if fecal concretions can be felt within the rectum or along the sigmoid, a warm soapsuds enema should be given and the child examined again within an hour or two. If constipation is the cause of the complaints, this treatment will almost certainly bring relief; unnecessary operation can be avoided. If acute appendicitis really exists, little or no harm has been done by evacuating the bowel.

Gastro-enteritis

This may be confused with appendicitis. A history of a similar condition in other members of the family, or a diarrhea without significant abdominal tenderness, tends to rule out appendicitis. Gastro-enteritis and vomiting may give mild or diffuse abdominal tenderness by retching and straining of the abdominal wall, but there is little or no localization of it such as is the case with appendicitis. (If diarrhea is a manifestation of an inflamed pelvic appendix or a spreading peritonitis, these should be readily detected by marked tenderness on rectal or abdominal palpation.)

Anomalies of the Right Ureter

A right kidney which is blocked by a stricture at the uretero-pelvic junction, by an aberrant blood vessel crossing the ureter, or by a ureteral stone, may give fever, nausea, vomiting, and abdominal pain, but the pain and tenderness are maximal in the flank. The urine may or may not contain white cells, according to the presence or absence of superimposed infection. If the abdominal complaints have been recurrent or if there is a reasonable possibility of urinary tract pathology, it is highly desirable to obtain intravenous pyelograms. A considerable number of patients come to the attention of urologists for complaints which persist after an appendectomy, and adequate studies then make it evident that the ureter or kidney has actually been the seat of the important abnormality all of the time.

Chronic Cicatrizing Enteritis

This is a longstanding inflammatory condition which has been described under many names, including "regional ileitis," "nontuberculous granuloma of the intestine," "Crohn's disease," etc. It may involve the colon or small intestine, particularly the latter, and is most common in the terminal ileum. Ulcerations, the etiology of which is poorly understood, appear in the mucosa and inflammatory cell infiltration and fibrosis may involve all layers of the intestinal wall so that it is narrowed, stiffened, and tube-like. A pannus of edematous or fibrotic mesenteric fat appears around the sides of the intestine. Tubercle-like lesions develop on the serosal surfaces. In late stages the intestinal lumen is markedly diminished in caliber and becomes obstructed.

While much more common in adult life, this condition can occur in childhood. It manifests itself by symptoms of great chronicity, chiefly characterized by recurring bouts of abdominal pain, possibly vomiting, and especially diarrhea. X-ray examination is often negative, but there may be evidence of partial obstruction. Barium studies (gastro-intestinal series or enema) may visualize the segment (or segments) of narrowed intestine. The inflammatory reaction has been known to disappear spontaneously; recurrence has often been observed even after surgical resection. Surgery is indicated only for treatment of obstructive symptoms.

TREATMENT

Immediate Appendectomy

When a diagnosis of acute appendicitis (unruptured) has been made, there should be no question about the form of treatment, for *immediate appendectomy* carries very little risk and is followed by a short convalescence.

Dangers of Expectant Treatment in Advanced Cases. When the inflammatory process has spread beyond the appendix and a generalized peritonitis has developed, there is some divergence of opinion concerning when to operate, how to operate, whether to drain, and what the after-care should be. There has been a recent tendency to return to treatment by the "Ochsner method," that is, delaying of operation for some days or weeks in the hope that a localized abscess will be formed which can then be drained and the appendix removed. This expectant treatment, while desirable under some circumstances for adults, if used in childhood will often result in death of the patient from overwhelming infection before any abscess develops! In the child, an appendix which is ruptured and is seeding the abdominal cavity with infected material is a constant menace, and if it can be quickly and gently removed the individual has an improved chance for combating the peritonitis which already exists.

In cases of abscess or of generalized peritonitis of appendiceal origin, we are firmly opposed to extended delay (beyond a few hours) in performing operation. We are strongly of the opinion that most cases of abscess or of generalized peritonitis run a smoother course, have a better chance of recovery, and have a shorter hospitalization, *if the appendix is removed and appropriate supportive measures are employed.* This course of attack is necessarily one which requires constant supervision by a competent staff. It implies that appendectomy must be performed with a minimum of trauma, with little or no disturbance of other intraperitoneal structures, and with as short an operating time as is consistent with gentleness and safety. The preoperative preparation and the postoperative supportive care are extremely important and may actually require greater skill and judgment than the operation itself.

In some clinics a definite *symptom duration,* such as thirty-six hours, is used to decide the question of immediate operation versus delayed operation (some weeks later). In childhood, we do not agree with this arbitrary method of determining forms of treatment, because some patients may still be in good general condition forty-eight or more hours after the onset of appendicitis symptoms, whereas others will have a ruptured appendix and spreading peritoneal infection in less than twelve. *Each case should therefore be considered individually and should be treated according to the conditions which are found to be present.*

Treatment of Seriously Ill Peritonitis Patients

While we are strongly opposed to the "deferred" or non-operative treatment of children with peritonitis of appendiceal origin, it must be emphasized that immediate operation in some of these cases can be disastrous and that conversely a short period of preparation is highly important in the care of the desperately ill subject.

There can be no doubt that immediate operation on a child who is in a toxic state from an overwhelming peritonitis adds an insult from which he might not recover. This should not be taken to imply that surgery should be deferred indefinitely or avoided entirely. The optimum choice lies somewhere between these extremes. *Operation should always be undertaken, but it is of utmost importance to prepare the patient aaequately for some hours before this is done.* While the less ill subjects can be spared most of this delay, the very ill ones must be given every attention in this regard if they are to survive. This raises the question of how to choose those who can be operated upon rather promptly and those who must receive preparation in every detail. To make this separation of cases, we have found an ill defined but practical dividing line by picking out for supportive therapy all subjects whose pulse is above 140, or whose temperature is above 103°, or whose facies and general appearance suggest great toxicity.

For preoperative preparation, the following measures are instituted: (1) Full sedation with morphine, to give comfort and rest. (2) Constant gastric suction through a nasal tube, to deflate the stomach and reduce the hazards of vomiting. (3) Insertion of a cannula or a plastic tubing into an arm or leg vein for constant intravenous infusion of appropriate fluids. (4) Intravenous administration of 5 per cent glucose in physiologic saline to combat starvation, ketosis, and electrolyte depletion (ranges of 150 to 250 cc. for subjects two to four years of age, 250 to 500 for those four to ten years of age). (5) Intravenous injection of 150 to 250 cc. of plasma (in the exceedingly ill patients) to provide protein and to combat shock or impending collapse. (6) Intravenous injection of penicillin (250,000 to 750,000 units per twenty-four hours) and sodium sulfadiazine ($\frac{1}{4}$ to $\frac{1}{2}$ grain per pound per twenty-four hours). These twenty-four hour doses are divided into four parts, and one is given each six hours. (In some instances we have preferred to administer the penicillin and sodium sulfadiazine by intramuscular injection. The latter can be given in a 5 per cent solution in distilled water.) (7) Placement of the child in a semi-sitting position to allow peritoneal exudate to gravitate toward the lower part of the abdomen and also to facilitate breathing.

Just how long such measures should be continued will vary from case to case. It is desirable to improve the hydration and general appearance of the child, to bring the

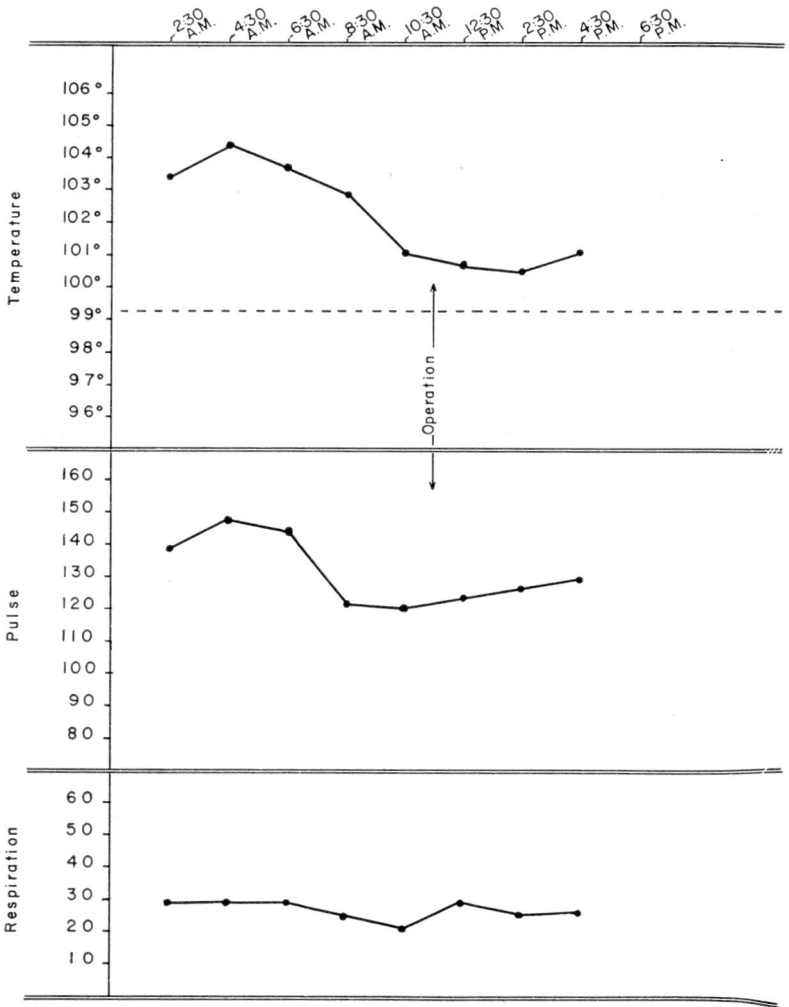

Fig. 144. Chart from a seven-year-old girl with acute appendicitis and generalized peritonitis. Because of the extreme illness of the patient at the time of hospital admission, operation was deferred for nine hours, during which supportive therapy was given in the form of sedation, gastric suction, intravenous administration of glucose and saline, injection of penicillin and sodium sulfadiazine. During this nine-hour period there is a marked lowering of the temperature and pulse; at the end of the period operation could be carried out safely.

pulse below 130, and the temperature below 103° F. These can usually be accomplished in four to eight hours; in rare cases ten to twelve hours may be required. There is seldom any justification for putting off operation beyond twelve hours, because there are diminishing returns in terms of improvement, and indeed beyond this time the situation is apt to deteriorate and the patient become more ill. Figure 144 illustrates the favorable changes which can be produced by the measures outlined above; after such support, operation can be carried out, the appendix removed, and the abdomen drained.

Treatment of Appendiceal Abscess

If an appendiceal abscess has formed during the time prior to hospitalization, this is an indication that the individual's powers of resistance are good and that intestinal loops, omentum, or other viscera have become adherent to one another to limit the spread of infection. The outlook in such cases is always excellent. After existing dehydration or ketosis has been properly combated, appendectomy and drainage are in order.

Incision should be made directly over the presenting mass. If the abdominal cavity should be traversed before the abscess mass is come upon, it is sometimes better to close this wound and make a more lateral one which will enter the abscess directly from the side by a retroperitoneal approach and thus avoid soiling of the general peritoneal cavity. If an abscess is in a position which necessitates opening it across the abdominal cavity, this does relatively little harm if an aspirator is available for immediate removal of purulent material as soon as it appears. If the appendix presents itself and can be readily excised, it is best to do so. If it is surrounded by vascular *granulation tissue* or by dense *adhesions*, it is sometimes wiser merely to insert a drain, and defer appendectomy until four to six months later when it can be performed with greater ease and safety. (We find it is possible to remove the appendix in 98 per cent of cases at the initial operation.)

Anesthesia for Appendectomy

Anesthesia is preferably *ether* or *nitrous oxide-oxygen* with ether. These may be advantageously combined with a basal dose of Avertin (90 mg. per kilogram of body weight, without morphine) if there is a concurrent respiratory infection. If available, *cyclopropane* has proved to be satisfactory for those who are very ill; when so used, it appears to be a little less debilitating than does ether. *Spinal* anesthesia has no place in childhood cases and *local* anesthesia is only satisfactory when it is proposed to make a small opening solely for inserting a drain into an abscess.

Type of Incision

It was formerly our practice to employ almost routinely a right rectus incision, but in recent years we have turned to the use of a McBurney incision in most cases. However, it is well to recognize that in some children the cecum and appendix are very high and would be difficult to expose them adequately through a McBurney opening.

A McBurney incision is good for drainage of a palpable abscess or for the removal of an appendix which can be accurately localized because of tenderness limited to this region, but its habitual use in childhood will at times lead the surgeon into operative difficulties. This small opening, with the forceful and brutal retraction which might be required to get exposure, can lead to a stormy convalescence which could be avoided by a wider opening through a rectus incision which permits wider exposure and therefore gentleness in treatment of the tissues.

Whenever there is doubt about the diagnosis, or when an inflamed appendix is believed to be in a very high position, a right rectus incision will be preferable because of the ease with which it can be extended. Splitting of a rectus muscle is poor, because of the weakening of the abdominal wall and the danger of postoperative dehiscence. Medial retraction of the rectus is advantageous for some cases but we never use it because of the limited exposure which is obtained, and because of the danger to nerve supply if it

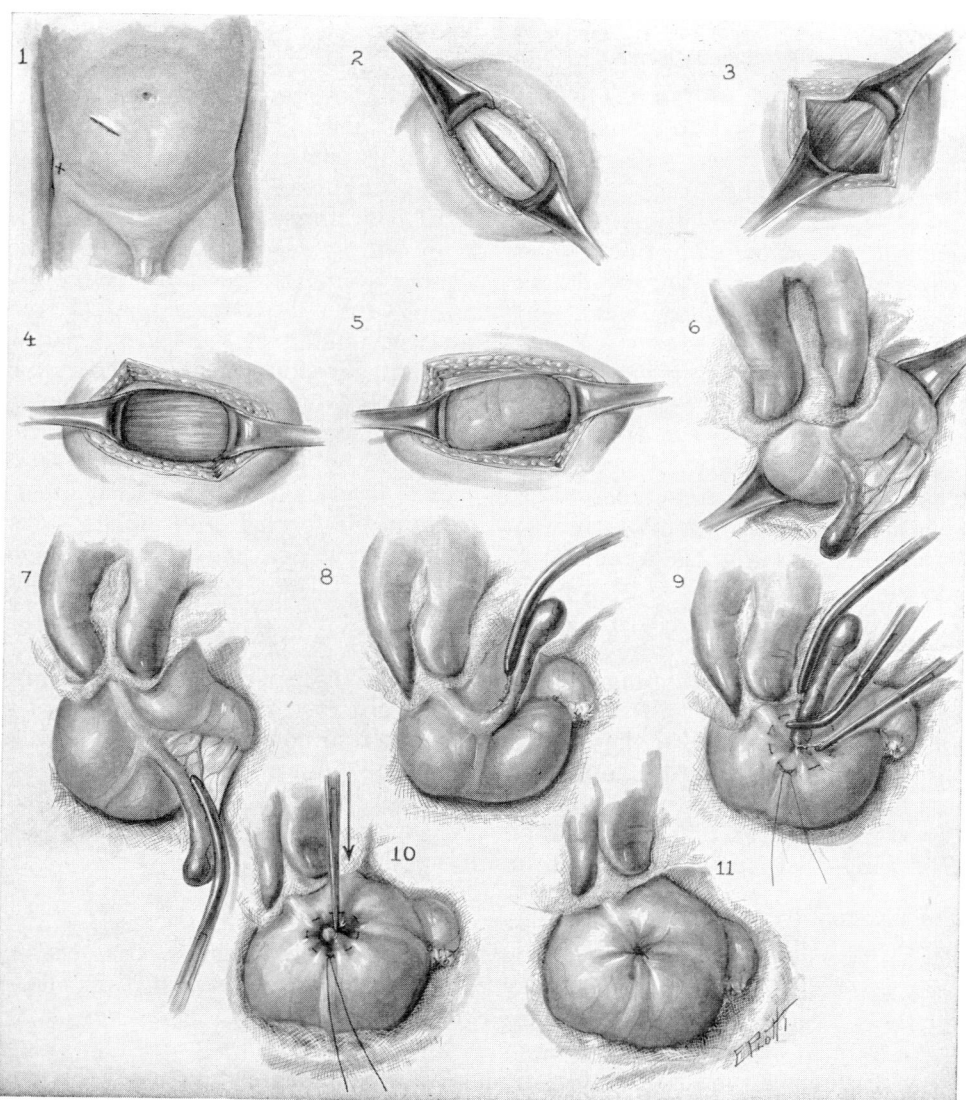

Fig. 145. Operation for acute appendicitis. 1. Position of McBurney incision, made a little higher than is customary in adults. 2. External oblique fascia slit open, McBurney retractors always put in direction of incision in each layer. 3. Internal oblique muscle split open. 4. Transversalis muscle exposed. It will be cut simultaneously with the peritoneum. 5. Peritoneum opened, exposing the cecum. 6. Cecum pulled out of abdomen and rolled up onto abdominal wall by left fingers of surgeon. 7. Cecum transferred to right hand of assistant, who should hold it steady throughout the remainder of the procedure. 8. Appendix grasped along its mesentery with a half-length clamp. Meso-appendix divided. 9. Right-angle clamp on appendix, near its base. Base of appendix ligated with catgut, which is then held with a hemostat. Silk purse-string stitch placed around cecal wall. 10. Appendix cut off. As the circular silk stitch is tightened, the appendiceal stump is pushed in. 11. Stump closed.

is extended. If a rectus incision is to be employed, it is far better to retract the muscle belly laterally; this is followed by maximum strength in the postoperative wound.

Excision of the Appendix

The actual removal of an appendix presents no special problems in most cases, but the dislodging of a high retrocecal, deeply embedded, inflamed appendix may be a most difficult surgical task. Not infrequently it is easier to sever the appendix at its base before dividing the mesoappendix. Great care must be exercised to avoid rupturing an acutely inflamed, edematous, and friable organ. If an appendix is surrounded by a wad of *adherent omentum* (Fig. 143, 6) this fatty protecting sheath should not be dissected off because it probably encloses a gangrenous organ, the exposure of which would contaminate the operative field. Such adherent omentum should always be left attached to the appendix and should be excised with it.

When removing a ruptured appendix, care should be taken to remove from the abdominal cavity (or abscess cavity) any fecalith which might have escaped from the organ. Leaving this nidus within the abdomen is very apt to leave residual infection or provide the focus for a late abscess.

Whenever possible, it is best to *invert the cecum* with a purse-string silk suture, since this probably reduces the chances of establishing a fecal fistula. In the occasional case in which the caput of the cecum is diffusely inflamed, thickened, and edematous, it is folly to attempt inversion of the stump, for the suture will pull out, undue bleeding will occur, and considerable damage may be inflicted on the cecal wall.

Drainage

The peritoneal fluid which may accompany an acutely inflamed but unruptured appendix does not necessarily contain bacteria. If it is odorless or if an immediate smear shows no organisms, all of the obtainable fluid should be sucked away and the abdomen closed without drainage. If, however, there is any question about the presence of bacteria in this fluid, the operator will be wise to insert a single cigarette drain down into the pelvis; this may be withdrawn in twenty-four or forty-eight hours if the peritoneal cultures subsequently show no growth.

Drainage for *generalized peritonitis* is a debatable question. In recent years many surgeons have inclined toward the closure of such abdomens without drainage, but with this view we are distinctly in disagreement. While we agree that this choice is satisfactory in many cases, we have the distinct impression that some patients, so treated, have an unduly long or complicated convalescence which probably could have been avoided or minimized if a drain had been used. While a drain is admittedly ineffective in evacuating the general abdominal cavity after a few days' time, there seems to be little doubt that individuals with generalized peritonitis of appendiceal origin convalesce better and quicker if the abdomen is allowed to evacuate itself early through a drain-hole. Such an avenue allows escape of pus which would otherwise have to be absorbed by the general circulation. Furthermore, any collections of pus which might subsequently form in the iliac fossa or pelvis can break into this drainage tract and easily discharge themselves to the exterior.

Stiff rubber tubing as a drain should be decried because of the danger of pressure erosion of nearby intestines. A thin, pliable, rubber wick with a center core of loose gauze (a *Penrose* drain) will not erode or damage surrounding structures. Drains should not be indiscriminately placed among coils of intestines, but should be laid along the lateral wall of the abdomen and thereby led down into the pelvis. To avoid the formation of a fecal fistula, a drain should be placed so that it does not rest against the appendiceal stump.

Sulfonamides in Abdomen

We have never had any enthusiasm for the introduction of sulfonamide compounds in an abscess cavity or in the peritoneal cavity in cases of generalized peritonitis. It is far better to saturate the patient with the appropriate drugs by intravenous or subcutaneous routes, accomplishing this before operation is begun.

Type of Operation Employed

In our series of cases of acute appendicitis the types of operation employed are listed in Table 28. It is obvious that with progression through the years there has been a much greater tendency to remove the appendix whenever possible in cases of generalized peritonitis. The continued use of drains in cases of generalized peritonitis is in direct contrast to the current practice of many surgeons and clinics.

Table 28
Types of Operation Employed

Operation	Jan. 1, 1929 to Dec. 31, 1938	Jan. 1, 1939 to June 31, 1944	July 1, 1944 to Jan. 1, 1951
Appendicitis without rupture:			
Appendectomy	365	253	373
Appendectomy with drainage	101	19	11
Appendicitis with peritonitis or abscess:			
Appendectomy	...	12	39
Appendectomy with drainage	331	185	300
Drainage of peritoneum or abscess	41	34	6
Totals	838	503	729

POSTOPERATIVE CARE FOLLOWING SIMPLE APPENDICITIS

Following simple appendectomy for acute, unruptured appendicitis, little in the way of special treatment is necessary during the postoperative course. Vomiting may be troublesome for twenty-four or thirty-six hours, during which time the oral intake should be very limited. In the average case, fluids can be taken as desired after the first day and soft solids after the second day. Because of the rapidity of wound healing in the young patient, the individual may safely be allowed out of bed in a few days. Our average hospital stay has been 6.7 days.

POSTOPERATIVE CARE FOLLOWING APPENDICITIS WITH RUPTURE

Gastric and Duodenal Aspiration

Following operation for an appendiceal abscess or generalized peritonitis, the postoperative period requires utmost vigilance. The intestinal tract should be put at rest by withholding all oral feedings until there is clinical evidence that the infection has subsided and the gastro-intestinal tract is beginning to function properly. Abdominal distention is combated or prevented by the use of an *inlying gastric aspiration tube;* constant suction is applied to it by some suitable apparatus. In only the most serious cases is it necessary to pass a Miller-Abbott or Cantor tube into the small intestine for decompression.

Since it is much easier to avoid distention than to treat it after it has appeared, we have routinely inserted an inlying gastric tube in all cases with peritoneal infection. After it is in place and is known to be functioning properly, the patient should be permitted to drink water or clear fluids as desired (and the liquid allowed to suck back through the tube). These fluids keep the oral and esophageal mucous membranes moistened, irrigate the stomach, and cleanse the suction tubing as they wash back through it. It is very inconsiderate to withhold oral fluids merely because the physician wishes to prevent washing out of gastric electrolytes; it is much easier on the patient to let him drink all the clear fluid he desires and then to replace parenterally any electrolytes which are lost.

The length of time during which it is necessary to continue gastric (or intestinal) suction will vary from case to case. The tube should not be removed at a set time limit. It should be left in place until the (gastric) returns are free of bile-stained material, until the patient is passing gas per rectum, and until auscultation reveals a return of intestinal peristalsis. In some patients these events take place within twenty-four or thirty-six hours, in others they do not appear for six to seven days. In average cases the tube must remain in place for three or four days.

Fowler's Position

An erect position of the patient in bed is believed to aid in keeping peritoneal exudate away from the upper part of the abdomen. Some observers deny this, but we are strongly in favor of maintaining Fowler's position (Fig. 146) when peritoneal infection

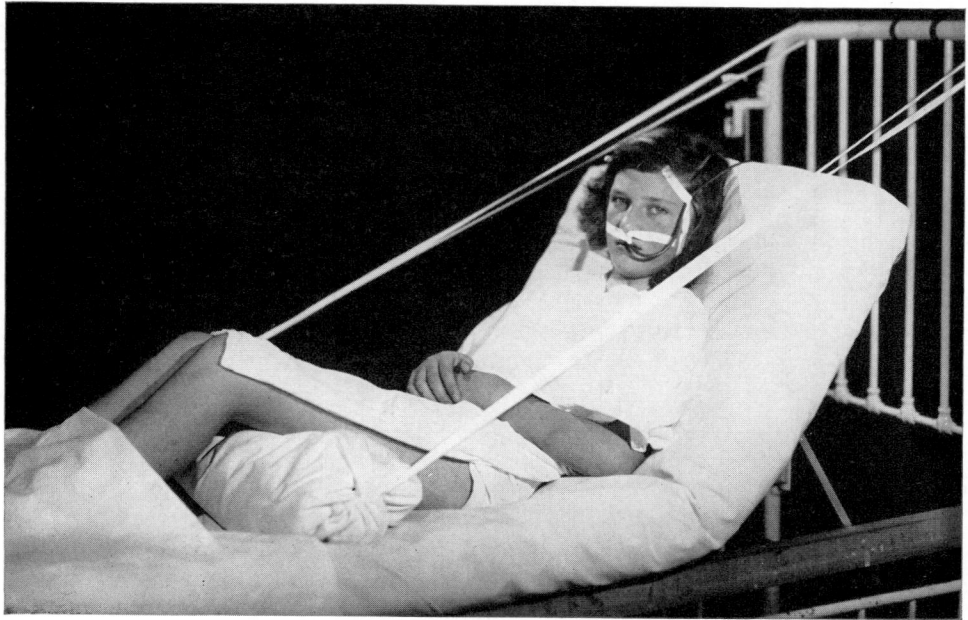

Fig. 146. Method of holding a child up in Fowler's position with a knee roll.

is known to exist. Under this regimen, subdiaphragmatic abscesses are extremely rare and localization of infection to the pelvis appears to be better than when the individual is allowed to lie in a horizontal position. Furthermore, the sitting position allows the patient to breathe more easily; it probably helps to reduce the incidence of pulmonary complications. While in adults a semi-sitting position might favor the production of vein thrombosis in the pelvis and legs, in a child there is little such risk.

Oxygen Tent

A valuable adjunct in combating abdominal distention is a tent which contains 90 to 95 per cent of oxygen (Fig. 147). Fine and his co-workers have demonstrated that trapped, inert intestinal nitrogen (from swallowed room air) can be removed rather

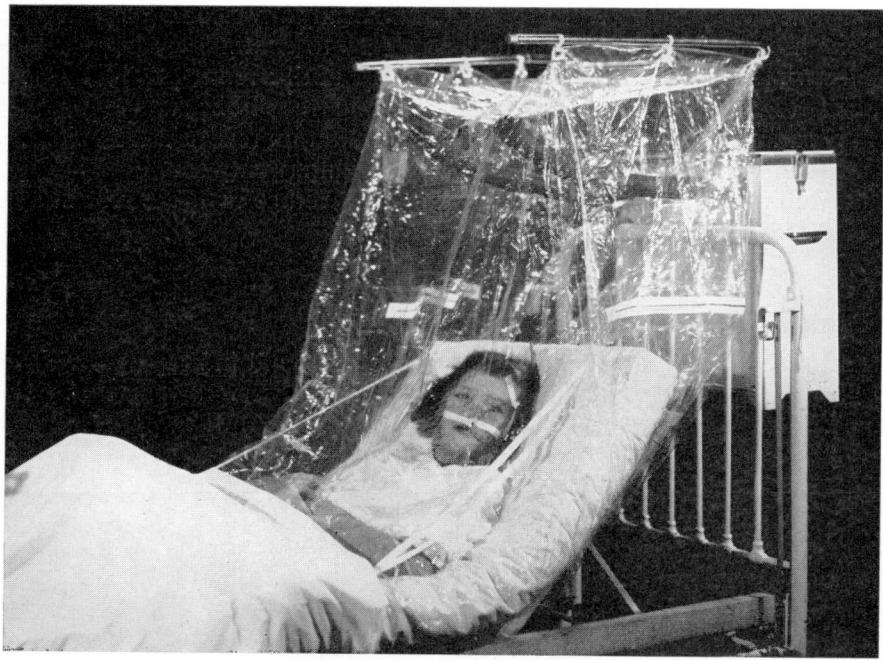

Fig. 147. A satisfactory type of oxygen tent for administration of high-concentration (90%) oxygen. Gastric suction is currently employed. Because of the continuous flow of oxygen, a cooling apparatus is seldom necessary. When this is required, the oxygen can be passed through a wide-mouthed stoppered bottle containing ice. For large children, an icing unit can be suspended in the tent.

effectively if the patient is placed in an atmosphere where the concentration of oxygen is high and that of nitrogen is low. It is helpful in all cases in which gaseous distention is present. To gain effective results, the tent must be employed for twelve to twenty-four hours; we have yet to observe any deleterious effects on the lungs when continued as long as four or five days. While this form of treatment may be expensive, troublesome, and often disappointing for the adult patient, it is much more satisfactory for the child. The amount of oxygen required depends upon the individual's consumption, leakage from the apparatus, number of times the tent is opened, and other factors, but with good equipment the oxygen cost is not excessive. While a patient is in such a tent, constant gastric suction should be simultaneously employed to remove any fluid which accumulates in the upper part of the alimentary tract.

Heat to Abdomen

Heat applied to the abdomen at two- or three-hour intervals has a soothing effect, possibly aids in reducing abdominal distention, and certainly helps in resolving any inflammation which might develop in the surgical wound.

Morphine

This drug has an important place in the postoperative care. In the uncomplicated case it may be given every three or four hours, as needed to control pain and restlessness. When peritonitis exists, morphine should be given by the clock at four-hour intervals for the first day or two so the patient is kept in a somewhat stuporous condition. Adequate sedation permits rest which is so beneficial. Treatments are much facilitated if the child is relaxed and quiet. After the first forty-eight or seventy-two hours, discomfort can be controlled with smaller and less frequent injections of morphine.

Parenteral Fluids

In recent years when so much stress has been laid upon the administration of parenteral fluids, this aspect of the treatment need hardly be emphasized. Fluids by *subcutaneous* or preferably by the *intravenous* route, two or three times per twenty-four-hour period, are usually sufficient to maintain positive fluid balance, normal electrolyte levels, and a fair caloric intake. If intravenous therapy is difficult to administer, a constant *venoclysis* may be employed, a procedure which we now routinely employ for all seriously ill patients. When this is used, the cannula or plastic tubing should not be left in any one vein for more than twenty-four or thirty-six hours because thrombosis or peri-phlebitis may become very troublesome.

The *amount of solution* administered will depend upon the exigencies of the case. Rough estimates of the degree of hydration can be gained by the frequency and the amount of urinary voidings. For a patient who is critically ill, who has fever and extensive infection, who has constant gastric suction, and who at the same time is having fluids administered by parenteral routes, it is essential to keep a written balance sheet of the fluids which are given and those which are excreted or sucked away. Such a tabulation enables the physician to evaluate quickly the fluid status of the patient at any time.

If suction is maintained or if parenteral fluids are administered for more than two days, the level of *blood chlorides* and *serum protein* must be checked at appropriate intervals. If the chloride level is low, more saline solution should be given. If the serum protein begins to fall below 6 grams per 100 cc. of plasma, a transfusion or plasma infusion (depending upon the red blood count) is indicated. In most of the routine cases it is not necessary to study the plasma potassium levels, but in the particularly ill patient who has been depleted in many ways, it is certainly advisable to determine the potassium concentration and to correct any existing deficiency by appropriate parenteral administration of potassium-containing fluid.

Removal of Drains

If drains have been used, they should be loosened slightly from their bed in thirty-six to forty-eight hours and should be withdrawn a little each succeeding day so that they are completely removed by the fifth or sixth day after operation.

Chemotherapy

There can be no question about the fact that modern chemotherapy has enormously altered the outlook for patients with peritonitis of appendiceal origin. However, these drugs should not glibly be given credit for low fatality rates which in reality could be approached without them. It has long been known that appendicitis is a more serious disease and is accompanied by higher mortality rates in children than in adults, and yet our total mortality rate from 1928 through 1939 (before chemotherapy was available) was 3.1 per cent. In more recent years the reduction of this figure to nearly zero can be largely attributed to the various antibiotics. While these drugs have slightly reduced the number of fatalities, one of the most impressive features attending their usage has been the amazing reduction in toxicity of patients, reduction of the incidence of complications, and the shortening of convalescence. In peritonitis cases, the entire recovery period is much less stormy that it was in the years before these drugs were available.

We have long disagreed with the advice that penicillin, in massive dosage, is the drug of choice in treating peritonitis of appendiceal origin. Regardless of what other organisms might be present, the exudate almost invariably contains large numbers of colon bacilli, against which penicillin has very little action. It is our belief that penicillin, while destructive of any gram-positive organisms which are present, should never be given alone. If it is employed at all, it should always be combined with some other drug which has bactericidal activity against a wider spectrum of organisms, particularly those in the gram-negative series.

Streptomycin, while particularly potent against colon bacilli, has proved to be somewhat disappointing in the practical results which are obtained. When first it was available, we welcomed it as a substance which might be particularly useful for peritonitis cases, but clinical trial has shown that it is inferior to other substances. We have come to rely on it less and less; we lean much more heavily to other drugs, particularly sulfadiazine.

Aureomycin and terramycin are excellent for the mixed flora in peritonitis of appendiceal origin, but from a practical viewpoint they have a limited usefulness. It is difficult or painful to administer them through the small veins of children. While highly effective when given by the oral route, this method of administration is not possible during the first few days of therapy when the alimentary tract is disturbed and constant suction is being employed. These drugs are particularly useful after three or four days whenever there is some residual peritoneal infection to combat and when the patient can maintain an oral intake.

By far, we have come to rely most on sulfadiazine. It has a high potency against a very wide range of gram-positive and gram-negative organisms, it is cheap, and it can be given easily by parenteral or later by oral routes. For children two to four years of age the dosage is about $\frac{1}{4}$ grain per pound of body weight per day, divided into four doses, six hours apart. For children four to twelve years, this needs to be increased to about $\frac{1}{2}$ grain per pound per day. If given subcutaneously or intravenously, the sodium salt should not be given in concentrations greater than 5 per cent (in distilled water). It cannot be combined with penicillin in a common mixture for subcutaneous injection. If given intravenously, it can be added to the glucose or saline which is being given to maintain fluid and electrolyte balance. Adequate drug levels lie between 9 and 10 mg. per 100 cc. of plasma.

COMPLICATIONS

Paralytic Ileus

Ileus may result from a spreading peritoneal infection, from undue trauma to the intestines during operation, or from low levels of blood chloride and protein. Recognition of the early stages of a dynamic ileus is important because it is easier to ward off distention than it is to treat it after it has become established. While neostigmine,

Pituitrin, and other such drugs can increase intestinal tone and peristalsis, their use is contraindicated when there lurks in the background the possibility of hidden peritoneal infection or a mechanical form of obstruction. Constant gastric suction, high-concentration oxygen tent, hot abdominal poultices, and rectal tubes are effective in most cases. If these more simple measures are not sufficient to combat a paralytic ileus, the use of a Miller-Abbott or Cantor tube will almost certainly progressively deflate intestinal loops as its tip descends; the various loops are decompressed and they will regain their peristaltic activity. (Enterostomy has little or nothing to offer for treatment of paralytic ileus because it usually deflates only the one loop which is opened.)

Intestinal Obstruction

Mechanical intestinal obstruction may occur at two periods after appendicitis operations; it appears much more frequently in patients who have had appendiceal rupture and peritonitis. *Early* obstruction may appear from a few days to two weeks, when intestines are matted together and are adherent to one another by plastic, fibrinous exudate. *Late* obstruction occurs after several months or years, when a firm fibrous band compresses or strangulates an intestinal loop. Early and late obstructions require entirely different forms of therapy.

In the *early* form of obstruction no attempt should be made to explore the abdomen, for doing so involves a high risk of spreading infection which nature is doing its best to wall off. Conservative treatment by *constant suction* of the stomach or intestine will tide most patients over the critical period. With the intestines thus deflated, the fibrinous peritoneal exudate will usually liquefy and disappear within four or five days so that the intestines become released. (While a Witzel enterostomy used to be a common method of treating early mechanical obstruction, this has now been replaced almost entirely by nasal intestinal intubation.) From July 1, 1944 to January 1, 1951, in a series of 729 cases of acute appendicitis (384 unruptured and 345 ruptured) there were 30 instances of early intestinal obstruction. Data from these are summarized in Table 29.

In the *late* form of obstruction—coming on months or years after the appendiceal inflammation and operation—the peritoneal bands causing obstruction are tough and fibrous; there is a high probability that ischemia and gangrene of an incarcerated loop will supervene if prompt and adequate relief is not given. A few of these patients can be decompressed and tided over their difficulties by adequate intestinal intubation and deflation, but it is our belief that—since it is sometimes exceedingly difficult to determine whether intestinal gangrene is present—the vast majority of these patients should be explored so that adhesions can be severed, intestinal loops released, and, whenever necessary, gangrenous loops can be excised.

Generalized Peritonitis Followed by Abscess Formation

A localized abscess occasionally forms after subsidence of a generalized peritonitis. Our experience with this complication (from July 1, 1944 to January 1, 1951) is summarized in Table 30. When pain, tenderness, and swelling show that an abscess is forming in the lower abdomen or in the pelvis, a gentle daily examination will indicate whether it is resolving itself or whether it is accumulating more exudate which must be evacuated. Considerable judgment is required to determine the optimum time for instituting drainage. If fever is maintained or is climbing, if there is increasing local pain, or if there is increasing intestinal obstruction (from a loop which is involved in the inflammatory mass) *incision and drainage* should be resorted to. In general, there is no need for haste in opening one of these abscesses; what often appears to be an abscess

Table 29

Time of Onset and Treatment of Early Intestinal Obstruction
(Successful Results in All Cases)

Patient	Year	Type of Appendicitis	Onset of Obstruction, Postoperatively	Treatment
1	1944	Ruptured, general peritonitis	32 days	Lysis of adhesions
2	1944	Ruptured, general peritonitis	26 days	Lysis of adhesions
3	1944	Ruptured, general peritonitis	3 days	Witzel enterostomy
4	1945	Ruptured, general peritonitis	34 days	Lysis of adhesions
5	1945	Ruptured, general peritonitis	1 day	Gastric suction (10 days)
6	1945	Ruptured, general peritonitis	9 days	Gastric suction (5 days)
7	1945	Ruptured, abscess formation	On admission	Miller-Abbott suction (7 days)
8	1946	Ruptured, general peritonitis	14 days	Miller-Abbott suction (5 days)
9	1946	Ruptured, abscess formation	16 days	Miller-Abbott suction (2 days)
10	1946	Ruptured, abscess formation	1 day	Miller-Abbott suction (5 days)
11	1947	Ruptured, general peritonitis	On admission	Miller-Abbott suction (7 days)
12	1947	Ruptured, general peritonitis	1 day	Gastric suction (5 days)
13	1947	Ruptured, general peritonitis	1 day	Miller-Abbott suction (4 days)
14	1947	Ruptured, general peritonitis	13 days	Miller-Abbott suction (3 days)
15	1947	Ruptured, abscess formation	2 days	Miller-Abbott suction (4 days)
16	1947	Ruptured, general peritonitis	18 days	Miller-Abbott suction (2 days)
17	1947	Ruptured, abscess formation	20 days	Miller-Abbott suction (3 days)
18	1948	Ruptured, local peritonitis	1 day	Miller-Abbott suction (5 days)
19	1948	Unruptured, without fluid	7 days	Miller-Abbott suction (4 days)
20	1948	Ruptured, abscess formation	6 days	Miller-Abbott suction (2 days)
21	1948	Ruptured, general peritonitis	On admission	Miller-Abbott suction (14 days)
22	1948	Ruptured, abscess formation	5 days	Miller-Abbott suction (5 days)
23	1949	Ruptured, abscess formation	6 days	Miller-Abbott suction (7 days)
24	1948	Ruptured, general peritonitis	7 days	Miller-Abbott suction (7 days)
25	1949	Ruptured, local peritonitis	3 days	Miller-Abbott suction (6 days)
26	1949	Ruptured, abscess formation	2 days	Miller-Abbott suction (4 days)
27	1949	Ruptured, local peritonitis	4 days	Miller-Abbott suction (6 days)
28	1950	Unruptured, without fluid	2 days	Miller-Abbott suction (4 days)
29	1950	Ruptured, local peritonitis	5 days	Miller-Abbott suction (5 days)
30	1950	Ruptured, abscess formation	3 days	Miller-Abbott suction (4 days)

will spontaneously subside. It is then evident that the swelling consisted mainly of edematous, matted intestinal loops without an actual accumulation of pus. Watchful waiting will tide over many of these patients with an abdominal mass; what was thought to be an abscess will often prove to have been only a localized, non-suppurative inflammatory swelling.

If an abscess appears in the pelvis, no attempt should be made to open it through the rectum until definite fluctuation is detected by digital examination, and until the mass is large enough to impinge upon the adjacent pelvic nerves and paralyze the anal sphincters. A low-lying collection of pus often spontaneously ruptures into the vagina or rectum or it can be satisfactorily evacuated through the rectum; the resulting wound heals with remarkable rapidity. It is well to remember that a rounded, soft mass presenting against the rectum may prove to be a loop of intestine which is stuck in the pelvis! The surgeon should be confident of the nature of any mass before plunging a knife into it. In a child it is almost always better to drain a pelvic abscess by a transabdominal route.

Avoidance of Complications

Without doubt, many children with generalized peritonitis or abscess formation can be treated by supportive measures and chemotherapy, avoiding operation for some weeks or months at which time the appendix is removed. We are firmly convinced that such a method of therapy, while possibly not more hazardous as far as risk of life is concerned, is certainly more stormy, is more productive of complications, and requires a much longer period of hospitalization. We have always believed that immediate operation (with preoperative preparation never longer than six to twelve hours) gives the best chance to recover with a less hectic convalescence and the shortest possible length of hospitalization. During the four years ending January 1, 1951, we find the following length of hospitalizations: In patients treated for unruptured appendicitis it averaged 6.7 days. In those treated for appendicitis with local or generalized peritonitis it averaged 12.02 days. In those treated for appendicitis with abscess formation it averaged 13.4 days.

Summary of Postoperative Complications and of Secondary Operations

Intra-abdominal abscess, paralytic ileus, and intestinal obstruction are the commonest and the most serious postoperative complications which are encountered. These have been individually considered above. Table 31 lists all postoperative complications encountered and all the secondary operations performed during the series of 729 cases of acute appendicitis treated in childhood from July 1, 1944, to January 1, 1951

MORTALITY FACTORS

Extent of Appendicitis

Acute appendicitis, without rupture, has a well standardized method of treatment and is attended by a death rate which is just about nil. Appendicitis with peritonitis, however, is still a major surgical problem, and continues to carry risks which endanger a patient's life. Even with this more extensive form of the disease the results of therapy have been steadily improving and the fatality rates can now be negligible. Table 32

Table 30

Postoperative Abscesses in Relation to Treatment

Operative Procedure	Cases	Pelvic Abscess	Wound Abscess	Sub-hepatic Abscess	Subdia-phragmatic Abscess	Multiple Intra-abdominal Abscesses	Brain Abscess
Appendectomy..........	405	5	8	—	—	—	—
Appendectomy with sulfonamide compounds locally	7	—	—	—	—	—	—
Appendectomy with drain..	277	18	12	2	3	2	—
Appendectomy with drain and sulfonamide compounds locally..........	32	5	11	1	—	1	1
Appendectomy with drain and streptomycin locally.	2	1	—	—	—	1	—
Incision and drainage......	6	—	—	—	—	—	—
Totals..................	729	29	31	3	3	4	1

Table 31

Postoperative Complications Encountered and Secondary Operations Performed
(In 729 Cases of Appendicitis, 7/1/44 to 1/1/51)

Complication	Occurring in Cases of Unruptured Appendicitis	Occurring in Cases of Ruptured Appendicitis	Cases Requiring Secondary Operation
Pelvic abscess	1	28	5
Multiple small intra-abdominal abscesses	0	4	4
Subhepatic abscess	0	3	3
Subphrenic abscess	0	3	3
Brain abscess	0	1	1
Wound abscess	8	23	9
Intestinal obstruction	2	28	4*
Pneumonia	0	4	0
Atelectasis	3	0	0
Fecal fistula	0	1	0
Contagious disease	2	3	0
Hematuria—due to diazine	1	6	0
Purpura—cause unknown	0	1	0
Ether convulsions	1	0	0
Incisional hernia	0	2	1
(Interval appendectomy)	0	6	6

* Lysis of adhesions—3; Witzel enterostomy—1.

summarizes our own statistics. Our last fatality from appendicitis occurred in 1944; there has been no subsequent death up till the time of the present writing (September 1952).

Duration of Symptoms

It is quite evident that the treatment of acute appendicitis before rupture has taken place is followed by a rapid convalescence and carries an excellent prognosis. Conversely, if inflammation has spread through the peritoneal cavity, treatment is followed by a

Table 32

Type of Appendicitis and Related Mortality Rates

Type of Appendicitis	Cases	Deaths	Mortality Percentage
1928 to 1938:			
Acute, unruptured	466	2	0.42
Acute, ruptured with local or diffuse peritonitis	372	24	6.45
1939 to June 30, 1944:			
Acute, unruptured	272	1	0.36
Acute, ruptured with local or diffuse peritonitis	231	7	3.03
July 1, 1944 to Jan. 1, 1951:			
Acute, unruptured	384	0	0.00
Acute, ruptured with local or diffuse peritonitis	345	1	0.02

more stormy course and possibly by a serious threat to the patient's life. Since rupture of the acutely inflamed organ is the dangerous turning point in appendicitis, it is of some interest to know when this takes place in most cases. In 1399 cases in which the duration of symptoms was known, the condition of the appendix as found at operation is summarized in Table 27. These figures show that after twenty-four hours the incidence of rupture rises sharply. It is apparent that great responsibility rests upon the pediatrician or general practitioner to make a diagnosis within the first twenty-four hours if the disease is to be treated while rupture is uncommon and good results can be expected.

While the treatment of acute appendicitis, with or without rupture, has been improved tremendously in recent years, much can yet be accomplished in more prompt recognition of the condition so that it can be treated in its early stages. During recent years (July 1944 to January 1951), of the 729 patients who entered the Children's Hospital of Boston, 345 (47 per cent) had rupture of the organ and either a localized abscess or a diffuse peritonitis!

Age of Patient

The individual's age, *per se*, is not believed to be a factor in mortality rates, for in very young children acute unruptured appendicitis can be treated with as low a mortality as in older subjects. However, the more rapid progression of inflammation to a generalized peritonitis in the young subject, and the greater difficulty in arriving at a correct diagnosis in babies and small children, combine to make appendicitis a much more serious disorder in the first two or three years of life; a much higher percentage of the appendices have ruptured before being referred for treatment. Table 26 gives some figures relevant to this point.

PINWORMS AND APPENDICITIS

Pinworms or their ova have been recognized in about 3 per cent of our surgically removed, acutely inflamed appendices, but only rarely was there histologic evidence of burrowing of worms into the submucosal tissues which might have initiated the inflammatory process.

Symptoms

Pinworms are often found in appendices which show no inflammation despite the fact that the patients have had clinical findings which are highly suggestive of acute appendicitis. Such symptoms include *nausea, vomiting, abdominal pain*, mild right lower-quadrant *tenderness*, a degree or two of *fever*, and a mild or moderate *leukocytosis*. Mechanical obstruction of the appendix by a bolus of the parasites undoubtedly accounts for this syndrome which is often indistinguishable from that of acute appendicitis.

The frequency with which pinworm infestation of the appendix gives rise to symptoms will undoubtedly vary with the prevalence of the disease in the particular community and the stratum of society from which patients are drawn. A survey at the Children's Hospital has revealed that approximately one-fifth of the general ward population harbors these parasites (some of these children had various symptoms which might be attributable to pinworms; most of them were asymptomatic).

Treatment

Given a child with minor abdominal complaints, equivocal findings on abdominal examination, and proved to have pinworms in the stools, a *vermifuge* may be tried, but if there is any lighting up of abdominal signs *appendectomy* should be undertaken forthwith. As a general rule, it is not wise to administer a vermifuge to patients with impressive appendiceal symptoms; it will seldom empty an appendix of worms, and indeed the patient may actually have appendicitis. The safest treatment of well marked appendiceal symptoms due to pinworms is appendectomy.

For the *medical treatment* of pinworms a number of drugs are available. We currently prefer the use of gentian violet. No purgation is necessary before or after the therapy. The drug is administered orally and is available in enteric coated "Enseal" tablets, 0.012 or 0.03 gram each. For children the dose is 0.01 gram per day for each year of age; this total dose is divided and is given in two or three parts through the day, limiting any individual administration to 0.03 gram. The adult dose is 0.18 daily. The drug is best tolerated when taken with meals. Nausea and vomiting may occur but are not contraindications to continuance of treatment. The therapy is maintained for eight days, discontinued for one week, and then repeated. The first period of treatment usually kills all mature worms and the second one kills any larvae hatched from eggs. Little or no permanent good will result from the treatment unless all members of the family are treated in a similar manner. It is extremely important for all members to wash their hands thoroughly after each bowel movement and before each meal. A 90 per cent cure rate can be expected with this therapy.

APPENDECTOMY FOR RECURRENT ABDOMINAL PAIN

Any physician who undertakes the care of children is familiar with the frequency and worrisome character of recurrent and unexplained abdominal pain. These bouts of discomfort may appear alone, may be accompanied by nausea, or even by vomiting. Fever is usually absent or minimal. Relatively little is found on examination of the abdomen. Individual attacks as a rule are not severe, but the nagging and repetitious quality of the symptoms is finally sufficient to arouse the parents' apprehensions. These cases provide considerable anxiety for the practitioner, as well as the surgeon, who wants to avoid unnecessary operation and yet give the patient any benefit which surgical treatment might offer.

Preoperative Study of Patient

A case of this sort requires careful consideration and study before any surgery is contemplated. The possibility of *constipation* as a cause of complaints should be completely eliminated. If there is any question of incomplete evacuation, daily administration of mineral oil over a period of two or three weeks should be tried. *Pinworms* as a source of complaints must be investigated. A history of perianal itching, finding of worms around the anus, or the identification of ova in the stools calls for a course of vermifuge treatment.

Provided constipation and parasitic intestinal infection have been excluded, three investigations should be made: (1) The *stool* should be examined by benzidine or guaiac tests; occult bleeding may turn attention to an unsuspected polyp or Meckel's diverticulum. (2) *Intravenous pyelography* should be performed even though the urine is normal. An unsuspected hydronephrosis or other anomaly in the urinary tract may be uncovered. (3) A *roentgenologic examination* of the colon by barium enema should be made to rule out colonic polyp or incomplete rotation of the colon. These fluoroscopic and film studies of the abdomen will incidentally reveal any calcification which might be present in tuberculous mesenteric lymph nodes. Examination of the upper intestinal tract by roentgenologic means is so seldom productive of positive findings in the childhood ages that such an examination may be omitted in most cases (unless there are specific indications for doing it).

Surgical Treatment

Provided these studies are all negative and the child's symptoms are severe enough, *laparotomy* is justifiable and indeed advisable—providing the operator is willing to perform a thorough exploration. The small intestine from the ligament of Treitz to the ileo-cecal valve should be carefully inspected and palpated to make sure there is no polyp, Meckel's diverticulum, obstructing band, or other abnormality. The gallbladder should be palpated for stones. Any undue mobility of the cecum should be corrected. Finally, after the entire examination has been completed, *appendectomy* can be undertaken. A satisfactory exploration implies that a rectus incision is employed; a McBurney opening gives an entirely inadequate exposure for this undertaking.

The appendix in such a child may give symptoms because it is kinked, scarred, or is obstructed by some solid material within its lumen. Quite often the appendix is disappointingly normal in appearance and yet the individual is subsequently relieved of pain. Children with vague and recurring abdominal pain should not be subjected to hasty and lightly considered appendectomy, but in those patients who have had adequate studies to rule out other pathologic conditions, this operation, while at times disappointing, will bring relief in a majority of instances. Even if the abdominal symptoms continue, something has been gained because the family and the responsible physician can rest assured that a low-grade appendicitis will not flare up and give serious trouble.

REFERENCES

1. Botsford, T. W., Hudson, H. W., Jr., and Chamberlain, J. W.: Pinworms and Appendicitis. New England J. Med., *221:*933, 1939.
2. Bower, J. O.: Acute Appendicitis: A Survey of Its Incidence and Care in Philadelphia. J.A.M.A., *96:*1461, 1931.
3. Caldwell, E. H.: Appendicitis in Childhood. Surg., Gynec. & Obst., *67:*169, 1938.
4. Coller, F. A. and Potter, E. B.: The Treatment of Peritonitis Associated with Appendicitis. J.A.M.A., *103:*1753, 1934.
5. Crile, G., Jr.: Peritonitis of Appendiceal Origin Treated with Massive Doses of Penicillin. Report of 50 Cases. Surg., Gynec. & Obst., *83:*150, 1946.
6. Fine, J., Hermanson, L. and Frehling, S.: Further Clinical Experiences with Ninety-five Per Cent Oxygen for the Absorption of Air from the Body Tissues. Ann. Surg., *107:*1, 1938.
7. Giertz, K. H.: Twenty-five Years' Experience in the Treatment of Peritonitis. Ann. Surg., *104:*712, 1936.
8. Gordon, H.: Appendiceal Oxyuriasis and Appendicitis, Based on Study of 26,051 Appendices. Arch. Path., *16:*177, 1933.
9. Griswold, M. L. and Goodspeed, W. K.: Factors in the Mortality of the Ruptured Appendix. Ann. Surg., *129:*260, 1949.
10. Harris, W. H. and Browne, D. C.: Oxyuris Vermicularis as a Causative Factor in Appendicitis. J.A.M.A., *84:*650, 1925.
11. Hudson, H. W., Jr. and Chamberlain, J. W.: Acute Appendicitis in Childhood. J. Pediat., *15:*408, 1939.
12. Hudson, H. W., Jr., and Krakower, C.: Acute Appendicitis and Measles. New England J. Med., *215:*59, 1936.
13. Kaufman, L. R. and Mersheimer, W. L.: Sulfonamides in Appendicitis. A Review of 412 Consecutive Cases and an Analysis of Fatalities. Am. J. Surg., *65:*393, 1944.
14. Ladd, W. E.: Immediate or Deferred Surgery for General Peritonitis, Associated with Appendicitis in Children. New England J. Med., *219:*329, 1938.
15. McLanahan, S.: Further Reductions in the Mortality in Acute Appendicitis in Children. Ann. Surg., *131:*853, 1950.
16. Miller, E. M., Fell, E. H., Brock, C., and Todd, M. C.: Acute Appendicitis in Children. J.A.M.A., *115:*1239, 1940.
17. Paulson, E. C.: Analysis of 10,000 Appendectomies. Minnesota Med., *33:*46, 1950.
18. Scott, H. W. and Ware, P. F.: Acute Appendicitis in Childhood. Arch. Surg., *50:*258, 1945.
19. Slattery, L. R., Yannitelli, S. A. and Hinton, J. W.: Acute Appendicitis. Evaluation of

Factors Contributing to the Decrease in Mortality in a Municipal Hospital Over a Twenty Year Period. Arch. Surg., *60:*31, 1950.

20. Sperling, L. and Myrick, J. C.: Acute Appendicitis; A Review of 518 Cases in the University of Minnesota Hospitals from 1932 to 1935. Surgery, *1:*255, 1937.

21. Strohl, E. L. and Sarver, F. E.: Acute Appendicitis. An Analysis of 878 Cases at St. Luke's Hospital, Chicago. Arch. Surg., *55:* 530, 1947.

22. Taylor, E. S. and Hodges, R. G.: Acute Appendicitis in Children. Surg., Gynec. & Obst., *73:*288, 1941.

23. Thieme, E. T.: Appendicitis. A Ten Year Survey: 1935 through 1944. Arch. Surg., *59:*514, 1949.

24. Wangensteen, O. H. and Dennis, C.: Experimental Proof of the Obstructive Origin of Appendicitis in Man. Ann. Surg., *110:*629, 1939.

CHAPTER 20

Intussusception

Intussusception is the telescoping of a portion of intestine or colon into a more distal segment of the enteric tube. When an intussusceptum has been drawn into its intussuscipiens, the process is almost invariably a progressive one until death supervenes or therapeutic relief is given.

Intussusception is one of the most important surgical emergencies in infancy and early childhood. The *frequency* with which this condition is encountered may be judged from the fact that 702 cases have been treated at the Children's Hospital. During the past decade, an average of about 20 patients per year have been encountered. Some high mortality rates are still being reported in the literature; they indicate the need for more widespread knowledge of the condition and its treatment. Reduction of these death rates in the future must depend not only upon the surgeon's skill in operative technique, but also upon the recognition of cases by the pediatrician and general practitioner within a period of twenty-four hours, when the prognosis is still excellent.

ETIOLOGY

Intussusception in the adult is usually brought about by some mechanical abnormality, whereas in the childhood and infancy group such factors are found in only a small minority of cases. In our series of 702 patients, demonstrable etiologic agents were found as listed in Table 33; these comprise only 6 per cent of the entire group.

Table 33

Demonstrable Causes of Intussusception in 702 Cases

Meckel's diverticulum	32 cases
Intestinal polyp	5 cases
Lymphoma of bowel	2 cases
Duplication of terminal ileum	3 cases
Hematoma of ileum	1 case
Total	43 cases

In the remaining 659 individuals no definite cause for the intussusception could be found. The fact that intussusception is so apt to occur between the ages of four and ten months strongly suggests that the change from a milk to a more solid *diet* might alter the intestinal peristalsis in such a way that intussusception is initiated. It is well recognized that intussusception occasionally makes its appearance during or shortly after *acute enteritis*, at which time the disturbed intestinal peristaltic movements may set the stage for prolapse of one segment into another. Occasionally *allergic states* may possibly account for altered peristaltic activity; this has been suggested in a few cases of intussusception, but

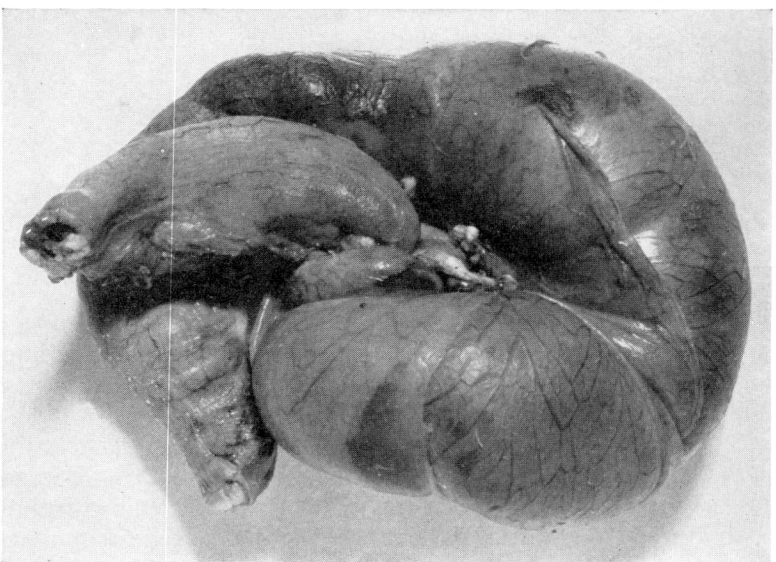

Fig. 148. Irreducible ileo-ileal intussusception removed from a nine-month-old girl.

more extensive investigation of other patients has left us with little evidence regarding the culpability of allergic conditions. In short, the etiologic factor in 90 to 95 per cent of childhood intussusceptions is still unknown.

TYPES OF INTUSSUSCEPTION

Intussusceptions are classified by compound appelations which indicate the part of the intestinal tube (intussusceptum) which telescopes into the intussuscipiens. Thus, the name of the most common form, the *ileo-colic*, implies that the ileum has advanced into the colon. Complex varieties are occasionally seen, for example the *ileo-ileo-colic* (Fig. 151), in which the ileum enters the ileum and this entire mass then prolapses into the colon. The percentage of occurrence of these various types is listed in Table 34.

Table 34

Types of Intussusception in 702 Cases

Type of Intussusception	Per Cent of Series
Jejuno-ileal or ileo-ileal	5
Ileo-colic	77
Ileo-ileo-colic	12
Colo-colic	2
Type not stated	3
Multiple intussusception	1
Retrograde intussusception	0.2

SYMPTOMS AND SIGNS

Intussusception tends to occur within more or less definite age groups. Table 35, Figure 153, and Figure 154 point out the ages of patients in our series. The peak of incidence occurs from the third to the eleventh months. Seventy-five per cent of the

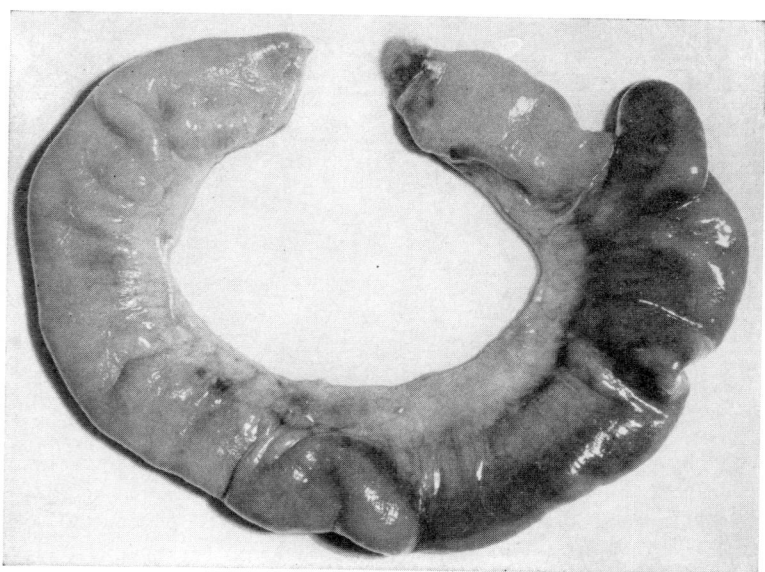

Fig. 149. Specimen removed from a seven-year-old boy; Meckel's diverticulum had been a leading point of intussusception. Reduction of the intussusception could be accomplished, but the intestine was damaged to a degree which made resection desirable. (Intussusception in older children usually has some demonstrable etiologic factor.)

patients are under one year of age; 85 per cent are under two years. Our youngest patient was three days of age; the oldest was fourteen years. Boys are more often affected than girls; the proportion is 65 per cent males and 35 per cent females in our series.

Table 35

Incidence of Intussusception According to Age (702 Cases)

Age	Cases	Age	Cases	Age	Cases	Age	Cases
1 month (or less)	2	10 months	43	19 months	9	5 to 6 years	9
2 months	15	11 months	28	20 months	6	6 to 7 years	6
3 months	21	12 months	7	21 months	3	7 to 8 years	3
4 months	57	13 months	16	22 months	7	8 to 9 years	4
5 months	88	14 months	6	23 months	3	9 to 10 years	1
6 months	83	15 months	3	24 months	4	10 to 11 years	1
7 months	86	16 months	3	2 to 3 years	32	11 to 12 years	0
8 months	54	17 months	3	3 to 4 years	20	over 12 years	2
9 months	46	18 months	9	4 to 5 years	22		

One rarely finds intussusception in a child who is thin, undernourished, and poorly developed. On the contrary, babies with intussusception are usually very well nourished and are generally far above the average in physical development. This *fat and healthy appearance* is apt to mislead the physician if he sees the baby in the early hours of illness. Thus, the first visit may result only in the impression that the parent is overanxious, whereas a return visit the next day shows that the child is desperately ill.

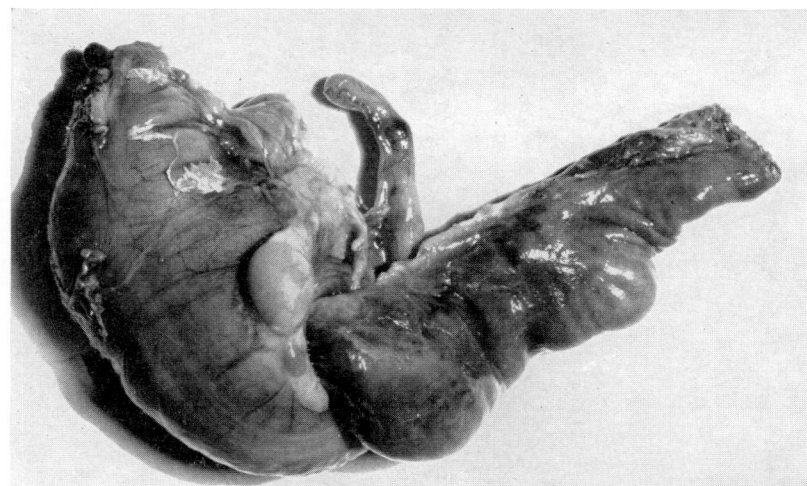

Fig. 150. Irreducible intussusception from a six-month-old baby. Terminal ileum is tightly jammed into the cecum and ascending colon.

Symptoms

The clinical manifestations of intussusception are almost always alarming and should immediately suggest the correct diagnosis. In about 90 per cent of the cases there is recurrent, colicky *abdominal pain*, in a child who was previously well. While these patients are usually so young that they cannot describe their complaints, the parent or attendant notices that the child intermittently becomes pale and either doubles over or draws up his legs in obvious, severe pain. This ten- or fifteen-second paroxysm may be

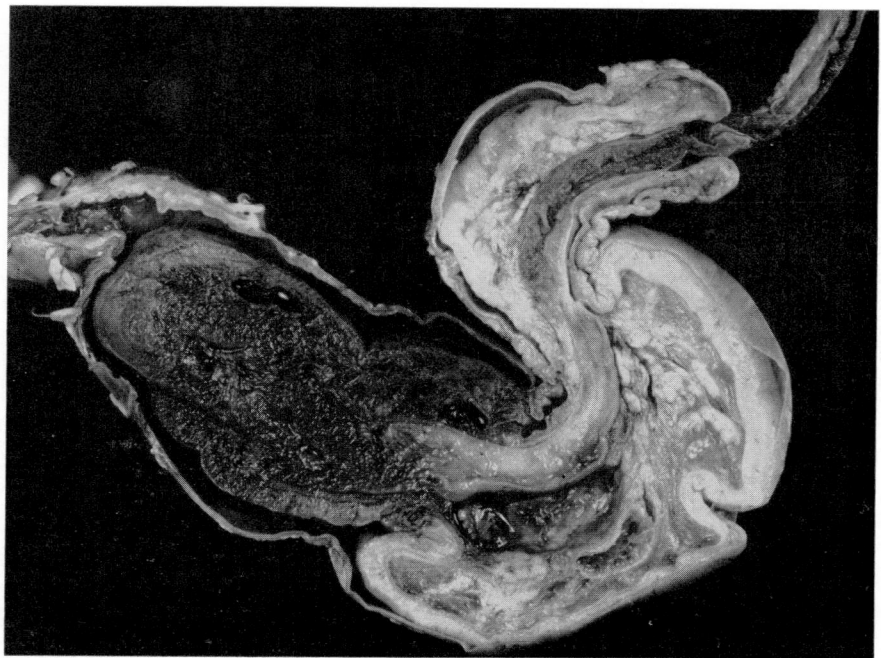

Fig. 151. Irreducible ileo-ileo-colic intussusception from a one-year-old girl.

accompanied by grunting respirations and by a burst of crying. After it is past, the child may resume a playful attitude and appear well, only to have a return of pain five or ten minutes later. *Vomiting* is an early symptom, is repeated and severe, and is seen in about three-quarters of the children.

During the first hours of illness, the intense, recurring pain is the alarming symptom; but as the obstruction continues, *pallor, sweating, dehydration,* and *shock* appear and they increase in severity as time elapses. If the condition is left untreated, the individual becomes moribund at the end of two or three days.

The passage of *bloody stools* occurs in about 85 per cent of the cases, but they may not be found in the first twelve to fourteen hours. After the initiation of symptoms there may be one or more normal bowel movements, but after this, bright red or dark brownish bloody mucoid material is passed. The amount of bleeding varies greatly from case to case. It may only stain the diaper or it may be copious enough to induce severe shock.

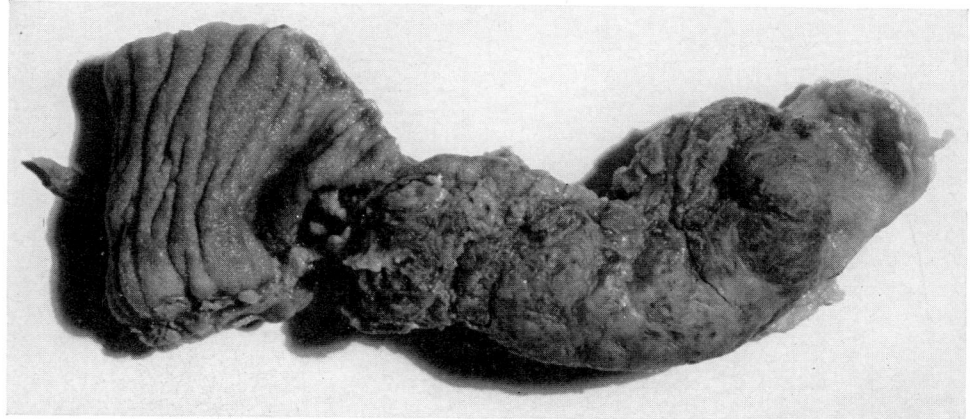

Fig. 152. Gangrenous intussusception from a thirteen-month-old baby.

Physical Findings

The general condition of the baby varies with the duration of symptoms. If obstruction has existed for only a few hours, the child may appear relatively well. If intussusception has been present for a longer period, the baby is listless and extremely ill, the body tissues are dehydrated, and the eyes are sunken and lusterless. Usually the pulse is rapid, the skin pale, and sweating marked. Even though a state of partial collapse exists, there will be momentary periods during which the baby cries out and thrashes around in agony. Fever is absent in early stages of the condition, but it is usually present in those who have had symptoms long enough to become dehydrated.

Careful *palpation* of the abdomen is most important, because a *mass* can be felt in about 85 per cent of the cases. While this may be only an ill defined lump, it is more often described as a sausage-shaped structure. It is rather firm and as a rule is not tender. Occasionally it can be felt to increase in hardness if the baby is examined during a paroxysm of pain. If the intussusception has not progressed far, the mass may be situated under the edge of the liver where it evades detection. The right lower quadrant may appear to be empty when it is palpated (*Dance's sign*) because of dislocation of the cecum up into the colon. If no definite mass can be felt in a very fat or uncooperative child whose history is strongly suggestive of intussusception, it is imperative to examine the colon immediately by roentgenographic visualization during a barium enema.

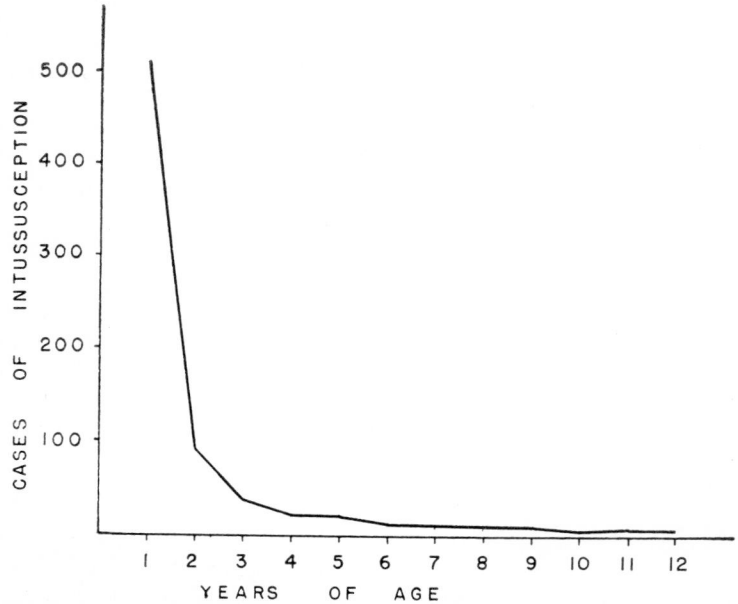

Fig. 153. Age distribution of 702 cases of intussusception; 85 per cent of the patients are less than two years of age.

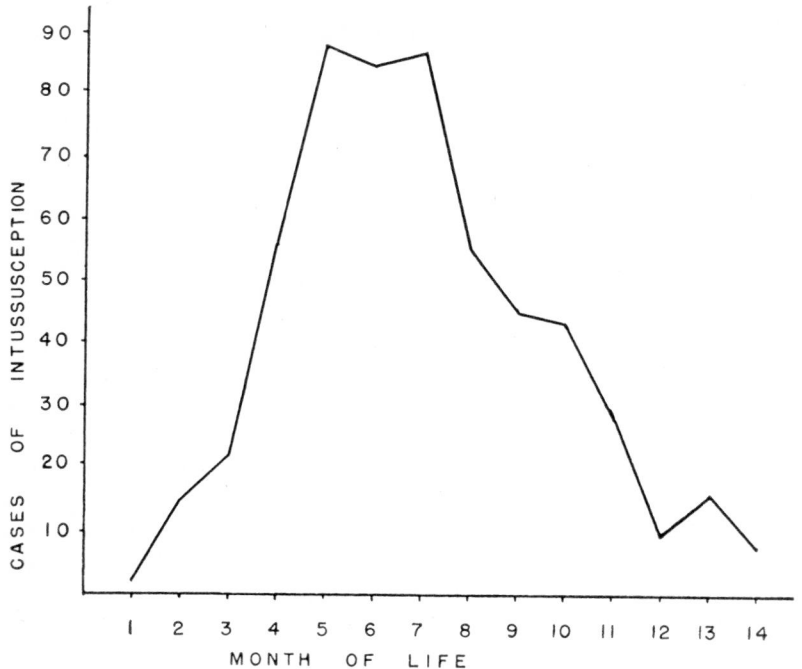

Fig. 154. Age distribution of patients with intussusception which occurred in the first fourteen months of life. The peak incidence is between the fourth and tenth months of life.

By *rectal examination* blood is found in the great majority of patients. The finger may detect an advancing portion of bowel within the rectal lumen. This intussusceptum has the general shape of a uterine cervix. Even though the tip of the advancing bowel cannot be felt within the rectal lumen, bimanual examination may reveal a mass higher up in the peritoneal cavity which might be missed by abdominal palpation alone. In rare cases, the intussusceptum may actually protrude from the anus. The differentiation between intussusception of this type and a *prolapsed rectum* can be readily made by passing a finger into the rectum *between* the intussusceptum and the surrounding anal sphincter; in a prolapse of the rectum there is no such space to admit a finger.

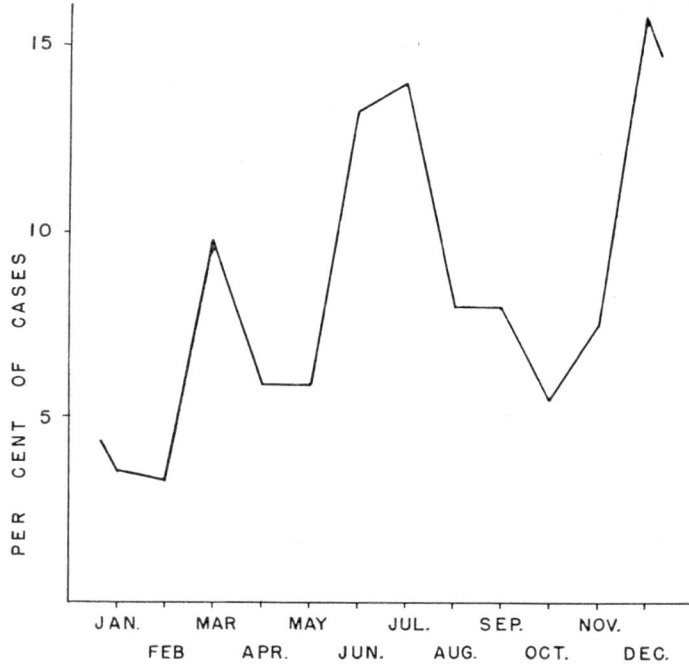

Fig. 155. Incidence of intussusception during various months of the year.

ROENTGENOLOGIC EXAMINATION

In typical cases of acute intussusception, the history and physical findings are sufficient to make a diagnosis, and roentgenologic studies are not necessary. In only about 5 per cent of cases have we found the diagnosis sufficiently in question to require x-ray examination with a barium enema.

In those rare cases of ileo-ileal intussusception, a barium enema is of no aid in gaining information but plain films of the abdomen will almost certainly show evidence of small intestinal obstruction. Inasmuch as the majority of intussusceptions in infancy and childhood progress so that an intussusceptum enters the colon, certain features are found on *barium enema examination*, summarized as follows: (1) Obstruction to the retrograde injection of barium. (2) A cupola effect or cupping in the head of the barium as it meets the intussusceptum. (3) A thin casing of barium surrounding the intussusceptum (and inside the intussuscipiens). (4) A cylindrical shell of barium, surrounding and outlining the intussusceptum, which remains after evacuation of the bowel. (5) In some cases, a partial (or complete) retrogression of the intussusceptum if the barium is injected with sufficient pressure. (6) Gaseous distention of the ileum just proximal to the intussusception.

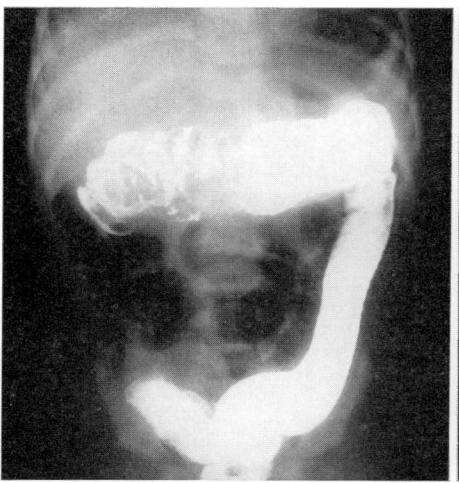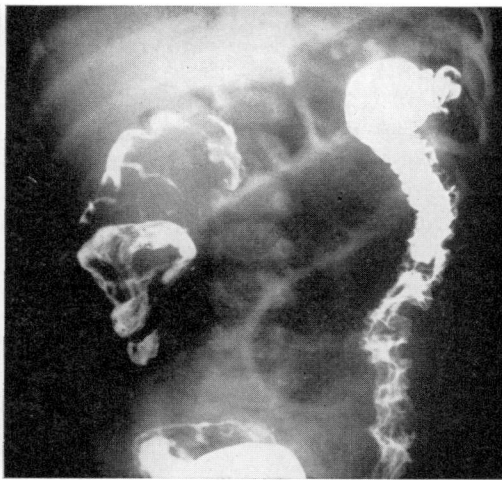

Fig. 156. Typical roentgenographic findings with barium enema in cases of intussusception. *Left,* Filling defects in the column of barium; air-distended intestine proximal to this. *Right,* Post-evacuation film showing a thin sheath of barium around an intussusceptum which lies in the hepatic flexure and proximal half of the transverse colon.

TREATMENT

Non-operative Methods

In 1874 Hutchinson first successfully performed operative reduction of an intussusception, and since that time the treatment of this condition has progressively tended toward surgical intervention. In spite of the almost universal adoption of such treatment, there have been several reports, notably those of Hipsley[7] and Monrad,[13] favoring reduction by *colonic injection of fluids or air.* Arntzen and Helsted,[1] Retan,[18] and Stephens[22] advocated reduction with a barium enema under fluoroscopic control; more recently Ravitch[17] has revived such therapeutic management.

Without doubt, many early ileo-colic intussusceptions can be reduced by these means. However, we are strongly opposed to the routine treatment by colonic inflation for several reasons: (1) A considerable number of patients come to subsequent operation because of irreducibility or because the physician is uncertain that complete reduction has been effected. Operation is therefore delayed and the child has been subjected to a procedure which depletes his narrow margin of reserve. (2) Colonic inflation has a limited effectiveness above the ileo-cecal valve and an ileal portion of an intussusception may be left unreduced. (3) Any existing ileal polyp or Meckel's diverticulum will be completely overlooked, whereas this additional pathologic condition could be recognized if laparotomy had been performed.

During the course of barium enema examination of a few patients we have seen an intussusception slip back—indeed with relatively little pressure—and we have avoided any subsequent operation; this all seemed so simple that it is tempting to adopt it as a routine therapeutic measure. An extensive experience with intussusception convinces us it is probably wise to resist this temptation and resort to surgery when there are proper facilities and personnel for performing this.

Operative Treatment

Short Duration of Symptoms a Factor in Favorable Results. By limiting ourselves to operative treatment, a simplification of therapy has been obtained which has significantly improved our results.

When one studies published surgical mortality rates, which run as high as 45 per cent, the 100 cases treated by Hipsley with hydrostatic pressure, with a mortality of 5 per cent, at first glance appear favorable. However, it is misleading to compare the results of different authors or of different methods without considering the *average duration of symptoms* in each series of cases. It is important to note that quicker hospitalization was obtained in Australia (Clubbe's[4] and Hipsley's[7] series) several decades ago than is accomplished in many centers in the United States today. Thus, Clubbe's cases in 1909 with an average illness of 17 hours may be compared with the following illustrative series in America: Robbins'[19] patients had an average symptom-duration of almost 45 hours; Peterson's and Carter's,[16] 32 hours; our own recent patients, 30 hours.

To the casual observer these differences of a relatively few hours may seem to be trivial, but a glance at Figure 160 shows that the prognosis is excellent in the first 24 hours of the condition, whereas the mortality rises sharply after this time. Inasmuch as the average duration of symptoms in Hipsley's series was only 17 hours, we regard his mortality of 5 per cent as unduly high, because we have had *no* mortality in patients with symptoms of similar duration. It is probable that Hipsley's good results were not due so much to a superior method of treatment as to the rapidity with which patients were referred to him. This early procurement of cases was the fruit of many years' effort on the part of Hipsley and his teacher, Clubbe, in encouraging the pediatrician and practitioner of Australia to recognize the condition and act before it was too late. Too high an estimate cannot be placed upon the educational work of these men.

Preoperative Measures. Since intussusception is regarded as a surgical emergency, it has been our practice to expedite operation as much as possible. An average patient can be admitted, operated upon, and put to bed within an hour. Whenever shock or dehydration is marked, thirty or forty minutes can be profitably spent by administering parenteral *fluids* or giving a *transfusion* before operation. When the general condition of a child is poor, it may be wise to use several hours in supportive and restorative measures. We routinely *deflate the stomach* before operation to reduce to a minimum the dangers from aspirating vomitus. The child's extremities should be wrapped with cotton batting to *prevent loss of heat*, and a hot-water bottle should be placed under the back to supply heat during the surgical procedure.

Anesthesia. Ether by the open-drop method is the anesthesia of choice for routine cases. For those youngsters who are seriously ill, we prefer cyclopropane because it seems to be less debilitating. With gravely ill subjects we have employed only procaine infiltration of the abdominal wall, but in general this has led to such poor relaxation during intra-abdominal manipulations that the method has little to recommend it.

Exposure. Proper placement of the *incision* facilitates the procedure. It should *not* be made over the presenting mass if this appears in the epigastrium or on the left side of the abdomen. It should be made routinely as a right paramedian opening, with its central part opposite the umbilicus, retracting the rectus muscle laterally. Reduction of that part of the intussusception which involves the descending or transverse colon seldom presents much difficulty, but as the region of the ileocecal valve and terminal ileum are approached the operative problems can be great. Hence, an incision on the right side of the abdomen will give the maximum exposure during the most troublesome part of the operation.

Reduction of the Intussusception. In the manipulation of an intussusception the operator must always remember that the incarcerated bowel might be hemorrhagic, friable, or gangrenous. Hence *gentleness* is essential at all times to avoid intestinal disruption and peritonitis. Several fingers are passed into the left side of the abdomen (Fig. 157) to locate the head of the intussusception which is then milked backward along the colon. When it reaches the cecum or ascending colon, the entire remaining intussusception mass can be delivered outside of the abdomen so that it can be more easily inspected and handled. Reduction is continued with a process of milking back or taxis—the gentle compression of the intussuscipiens with the entire hand in such a way that the invaginated part is slowly squeezed out. There may be a temptation to pull out the intussusceptum, but this should be either strictly avoided or else done with the utmost delicacy because it is very apt to jam the entrapped bowel in its intussuscipiens and make matters worse. The dripping-on of warm saline and continued annular pressure of the hand over a swollen intestine tend to keep the bowel in a better state of viability. Slight stretching of the receiving ring with a blunt instrument may help in the reduction. With persistence and patience, 90 to 95 per cent of intussusceptions can be manually reduced.

Small *tears* in the peritoneal coats of the gut are in themselves not particularly dangerous, but they serve as a warning to the operator that the muscularis or mucosa will soon give way if subjected to undue pressure. If peritoneal tears are long, or if they extend into the musculature, a few quickly placed interrupted sutures will suffice to repair them.

Once an intussusception has been completely reduced, the involved portion of gut should be examined to determine its *viability*. There is always some degree of hemorrhage, swelling, edema, and discoloration, but an intestine of questionable viability will often improve in appearance within a few minutes if it is warmed and moistened. If there is peristaltic activity over the involved area, or if it contracts when gently pinched with smooth forceps, the intestine will survive and should not be resected.

Only through experience can an operator know how long to persist in attempts at reduction. Sometimes it is better to spend twenty minutes or half an hour in completing a reduction than it is to resort too soon to resection which is a more complicated operation. On the other hand, long-continued unsuccessful attempts at reduction may so exhaust the child that the operator is eventually forced to resection in spite of the fact that the patient then cannot possibly survive such a formidable procedure; when faced with this dilemma the operator will wish that he had proceeded with resection as an initial step.

Additional Operative Procedures. In conjunction with reduction of an intussusception, additional procedures are sometimes necessary, but *our general policy is to do nothing more than is absolutely necessary during operation for intussusception.* If a Meckel's diverticulum is present and is gangrenous or cannot be everted, obviously it must be removed. If an intestinal polyp is so large that it blocks the lumen of the gut, it should be excised. If the appendix has been injured severely by being included in the intussusception mass, it should be removed. However, mere engorgement and swelling of an appendix is not a sufficient indication for appendectomy. Some authors have advised routine removal of the appendix, believing that irritation from appendicitis produced the invagination and intussusception. Little credence should be placed in this theory. The cautious operator will not remove the appendix unless it is gangrenous or its vessels are thrombosed. *Any procedure which opens the intestinal tract in one of these cases greatly increases the possibility of a peritonitis,* because the injured intestine has a lowered vitality and cannot withstand infection as well as a normal one. Hence, the slightest soiling of the peritoneal cavity might start off a spreading infection with a high proba-

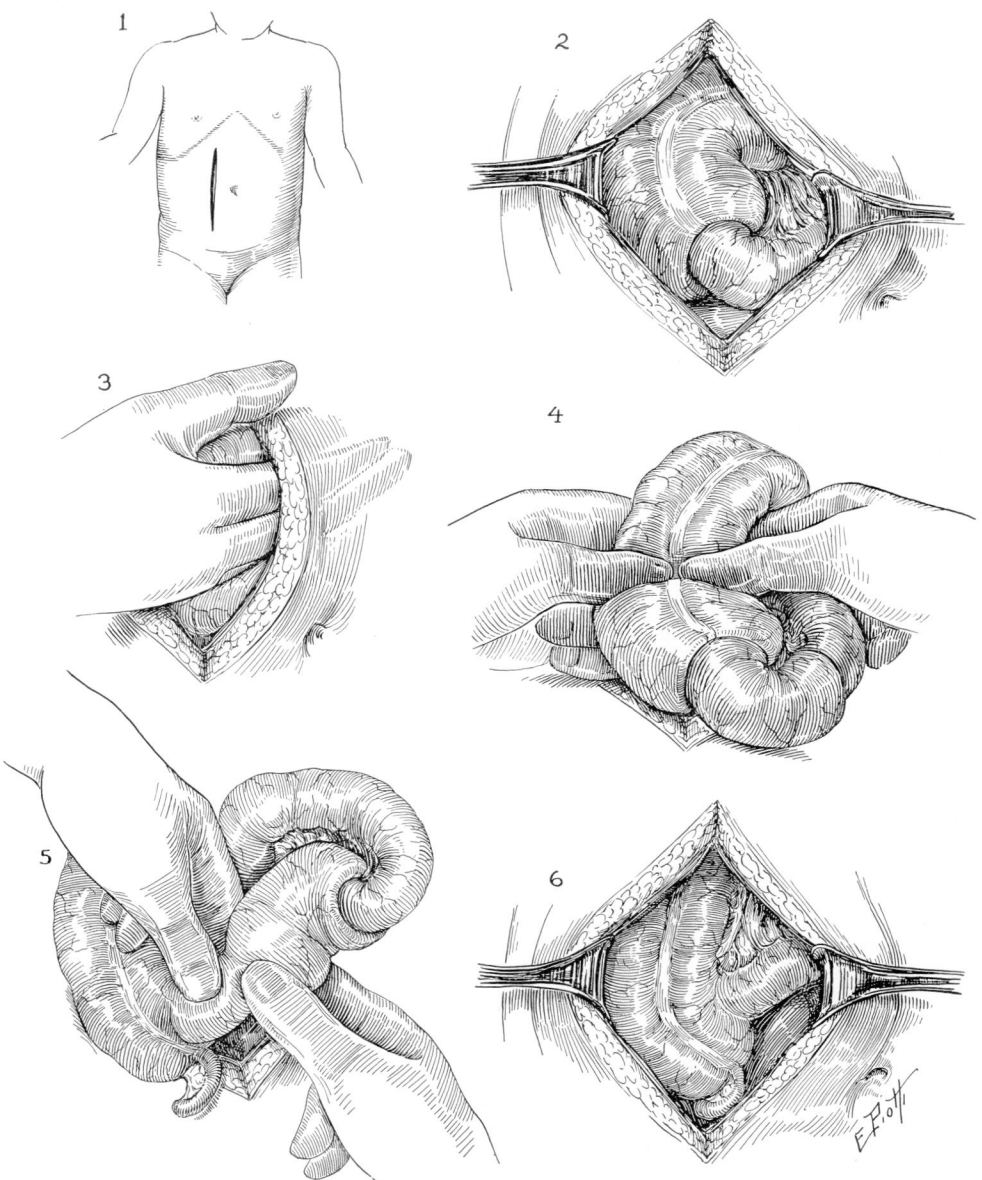

Fig. 157. Method of operative reduction of ileo-colic intussusception. 1. Incision is always made on right side of abdomen, regardless of position of palpable mass. 2. Findings on opening abdomen. Ileum is intussuscepted into ascending colon. Intussusception extends almost to the splenic flexure. 3. Portion of hand passed in to left side of abdomen so the finger tips can push back intussusceptum. 4. Intussusception has been reduced to the ascending colon which is now delivered out of the abdomen. Squeezing over the distal end of the mass is now begun. 5. Cecum and appendix have been delivered. Remaining intussusception in ileum is reduced by continued pressure on the receding mass. 6. Reduction completed and intestines returned to abdomen.

bility of fatal issue. Therefore, whenever possible it is better to defer any opening of the intestinal tract to a *second* procedure (ten days or two weeks later) at which time the circulation of the intestine will have returned to normal and the peritoneal cavity can better withstand the slight soiling which accompanies removal of a polyp, a Meckel's diverticulum, or an intestinal duplication.

In an occasional patient who has had an intussusception for only a short time, who is in good general condition, and whose intussusception reduces easily, it is reasonably safe to remove the appendix as an incidental procedure; recently we have done this in about 20 per cent of cases. This combination of surgical undertakings without fatality does not invalidate the warnings made above regarding limiting the extent of operation for most children with intussusception.

Resection of an Intussusception. In any large series of cases, there will always be some individuals for whom it is necessary to resect an intussusception or damaged intestine. The indications for resection are threefold: (1) When the lesion is irreducible. (2) When the intestine has been irreparably damaged. (3) When a child is critically ill. While the first two categories are obvious, it is important to stress also the last one. When a child is dangerously ill, it might be possible to reduce an intussusception and indeed have a viable intestine, but the disengagement of the bowel releases "toxic" substances into the circulation which are sufficient to produce uncontrollable shock. It is therefore better to avoid reduction (even though this might be feasible technically) and remove quickly the entire mass so that all necrotic material is removed from the body.

When a resection must be performed, the decision must be made whether a primary anastomosis is to be done or whether an exteriorization of the remaining intestinal limbs is preferable. This decision must rest upon the condition of the patient and the technical proficiency of the surgeon. It is very tempting to try primary anastomosis of the bowel and thus reduce the length and complexity of subsequent hospitalization. We have had many fatalities with primary anastomoses but have had 11 survivals following resection and primary anastomosis. Dennis[5] performed 8 resections with primary anastomoses, all patients recovering! In spite of these favorable aspects, we have in recent years (when the house staff performs most of these operations) progressively turned away from primary anastomosis and have almost entirely adopted exteriorizing methods, making certain that the procedure is kept completely aseptic. Without doubt, for the surgeon who is only occasionally dealing with intestinal problems in small subjects, the exteriorization method will give higher recovery rates. By employing it, certain advantages are gained: (1) The operating time is shortened. (2) Shock is minimized. (3) Immediate decompression is accomplished. (4) Asepsis is rigidly preserved. We have not encountered difficulty in maintaining fluid and electrolyte balance during the short time that ileostomies have been open; modern parenteral therapy makes it possible to compensate for juices which are lost from an enterostomy. Furthermore, it is important to emphasize that a crushing clamp can be applied to cut down the septum between the spurs within a few days, and that the enterostomy can be closed within six or seven days after the initial operation.

MIKULICZ RESECTION: TECHNICAL POINTS. If a Mikulicz type of resection is to be done (Fig. 158), it should be performed so that absolutely no soiling of the peritoneal cavity takes place. In other words, the intussuscepted mass or the nonviable gut should be exteriorized and *the abdominal wound completely closed around it before the diseased portion of the intestine is cut away.* A catheter can then be sewed into the upper loop to carry away gas and fluid for twenty-four or forty-eight hours to prevent contamination of the cutaneous wound while it is sealing off. It is best to sew together the distal and proximal spurs before closing the abdomen so that nothing can prolapse between these two loops and be injured when a crushing clamp is subsequently applied. Inasmuch as babies do not tolerate well the loss of succus entericus, the spurs should be cut down with a crushing clamp as soon as it is certain (in two or three days) that the two loops are firmly adherent to the abdominal wall. The child should not be allowed to languish and to lose fluids unnecessarily; we have usually found it possible to close the ileocolostomy (or ileo-ileostomy) in about a week. Of 18 patients treated by these steps and with these precautions, 15 recovered.

Postoperative Treatment and Complications

Administration of Fluids. If no parenteral fluids had been administered before operation, they should certainly be given by intravenous and subcutaneous routes as soon as the surgery is completed. Water, electrolytes, and carbohydrates should be given in this way at least twice a day for two or three days, and in some cases this period must be longer. Ten per cent glucose intravenously and physiologic saline subcutaneously are generally all that are required. Blood or plasma infusions are necessary for the more seriously ill babies.

Deflation of Stomach. It is important to keep the stomach deflated to prevent vomiting and aspiration shortly after operation. Because of the loss of several patients by this regrettable accident, we have adopted routine decompression of the stomach both before and after the operative procedure.

Feeding. For the first postoperative day, or as long as there is return of colored material through the gastric tube, only water in limited amounts should be given by mouth. This keeps the mouth and esophagus moist; it sucks back through the tube immediately, keeping it flushed. After reverse peristalsis has ceased, the gastric tube can be withdrawn and oral ingestion of fluids started cautiously. The full caloric or volume intake for the age and weight should not be offered until the fourth or fifth day. The intestinal tract has been extensively damaged and should not be subjected to its full normal activity until the reparative processes are well under way.

Postoperative Diarrhea. Not infrequently a diarrhea develops during the first week of convalescence, because the traumatized intestine is more susceptible to infection and peristaltic disturbances, particularly in the summer months of the year. It is therefore obvious that strict precautions must be taken to guard against exposure to other patients who have infectious diarrhea or other such disorders. If such a complication develops, the oral intake of food should be reduced, sedatives administered, and appropriate fluids given by parenteral routes.

Postoperative Peritonitis. Shock, dehydration, and toxicity exact a high toll, and fully four-fifths of those who die have these factors listed as the immediate cause of death. Since such conditions cause most of the mortalities, the majority of deaths occur within twenty-four or forty-eight hours after operation. If the intestine has been opened during operation, peritonitis is the greatest hazard. Because of this fact, chemotherapy with a drug with wide range of antibacterial activity (such as sulfadiazine) should be given postoperatively whenever any soiling of the peritoneum has occurred.

Postoperative Fever. Almost universally some rise in temperature is found for several days after operation (Fig. 159). It is not uncommon to find a temperature of 103° or even 104° F. during the immediate postoperative course, but levels above 105° F. carry a grave and usually fatal prognosis. This postoperative pyrexia is presumably due to absorption of foreign proteins through the damaged intestinal wall or to assimilation of products of necrosis liberated by the damaged intestine itself.

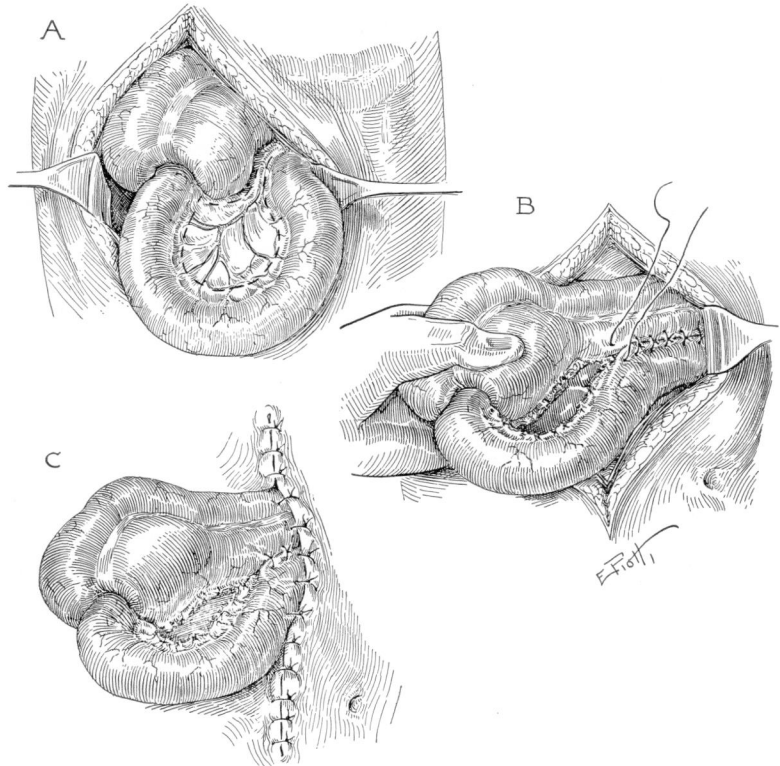

Fig. 158. Method for aseptic resection of an intussusception. A, Right rectus incision. Ileo-colic intussusception. Mesentery and mesocolon will be divided along the dotted line. B, Bowel freed from mesenteric attachments. Limbs of ileum and colon being joined by interrupted fine silk sutures, which must not pierce mucosa. C, Intussusception exteriorized, and abdominal wound closed around the limbs of ileum and colon. The limbs have been sewed to peritoneum and to the skin.

FACTORS IN PROGNOSIS

Early Treatment

The most effective way to reduce the mortality of intussusception is to shorten the period between onset of symptoms and the initiation of treatment. There are few illnesses in which the clinical history and physical findings are more suggestive of the correct diagnosis. One may therefore reasonably expect an intelligent and alert pediatrician or practitioner to recognize this condition within the first twenty-four hours. The direct relationship of the duration of symptoms to corresponding mortality figures is summed up in Table 36. In this study of 202 patients (treated from 1928 through 1939) the over-all mortality was 14 per cent, whereas in the 110 patients who were operated upon within the first twenty-four hours of illness there was no mortality. These relationships are graphically portrayed in Figure 160.

In summary, symptom-durations up to twenty-four hours should carry no mortality, whereas longer symptom-durations show progressively and rapidly mounting fatality rates.

Improvement in Technique

Recent advances in the treatment of intussusception may be attributed to greater effort on the part of both physicians and surgeons. In our material, the physician's

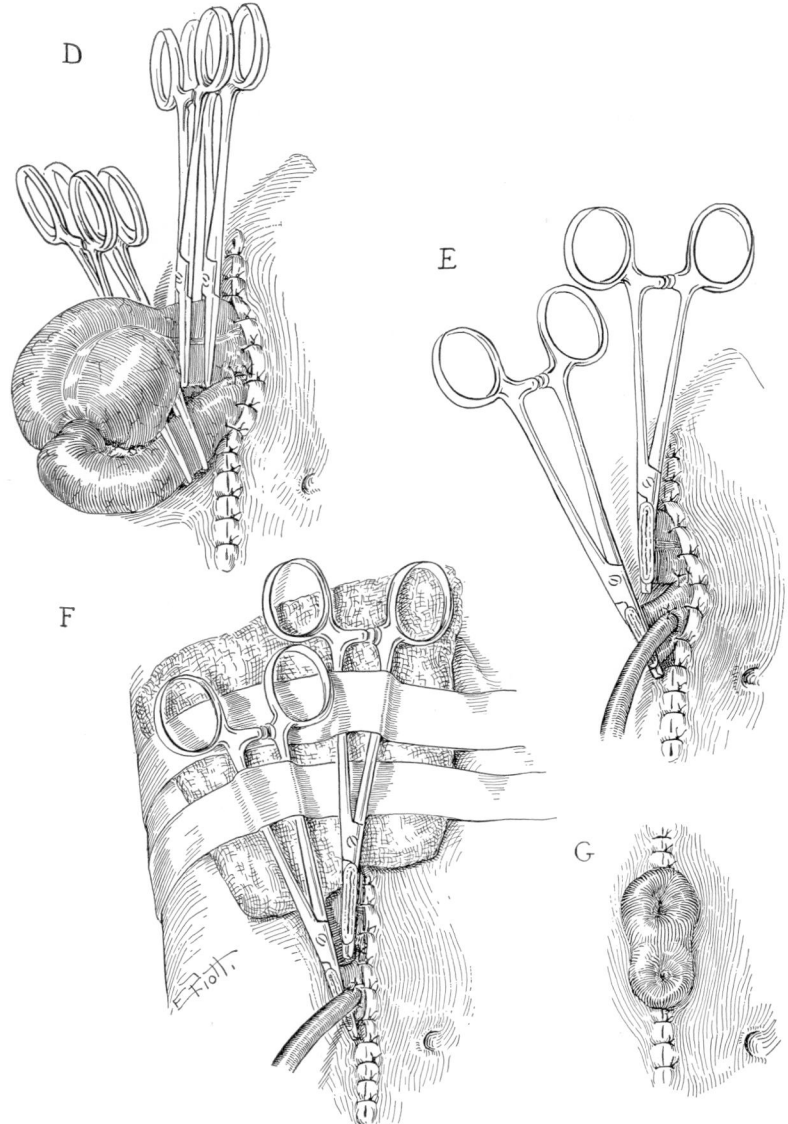

Fig. 158 (*continued*). D, Removal of intussusception deferred until abdominal wound is completely closed. Appropriate clamps applied to the two limbs. E, Intussusception cut away. Catheter inserted into ileum for immediate and continued decompression of the small intestine. F, Two clamps left on limbs to stabilize them for several days until limbs become stuck to abdominal wall. G, Appearance of ileo-colostomy several days following operation, and after removal of clamps. (The septum between the two spurs can now be cut down and the remaining opening of the bowel can be turned in without entering the peritoneal cavity.)

activity may be seen in the drop of the *average symptom-duration* from 38 hours (1908 to 1927) to 30 hours (1928 through 1939). The surgeons' improvement in operative technique and supportive care becomes evident when one compares cases of given symptom-durations which were treated in the earlier period (1908 to 1927) with parallel cases treated in later years. Such a study is shown in Table 37. In each symptom-duration

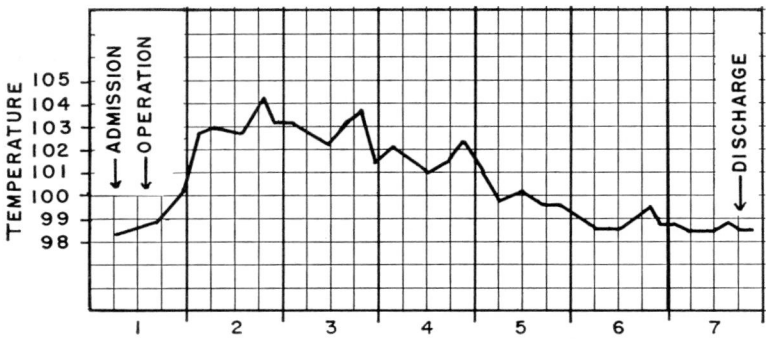

Fig. 159. Typical temperature chart of an infant with intussusception. Patients often have a fever of 103° or 104° F. for two or three days after operation.

group there has been an appreciable reduction in mortality in the second period as compared to that of the first.

Patients in the private ward have usually had a lower mortality rate than those on the charity service. These favorable figures can be partially attributed to the fact that the cases were handled by senior surgeons, but considerable importance is attached to the fact that intussusception is recognized earlier in private patients than in charity ones.

Preoperative Temperatures

The temperature of an intussusception patient prior to operation has considerable prognostic value because it roughly reflects the existing degree of dehydration and toxicity. In general, the higher the temperature, the greater is the likelihood of a subsequent death. As graphically shown in Figure 161, a normal admission temperature is a good sign; a temperature of 100° to 101° F. or more implies a rather poor outlook.

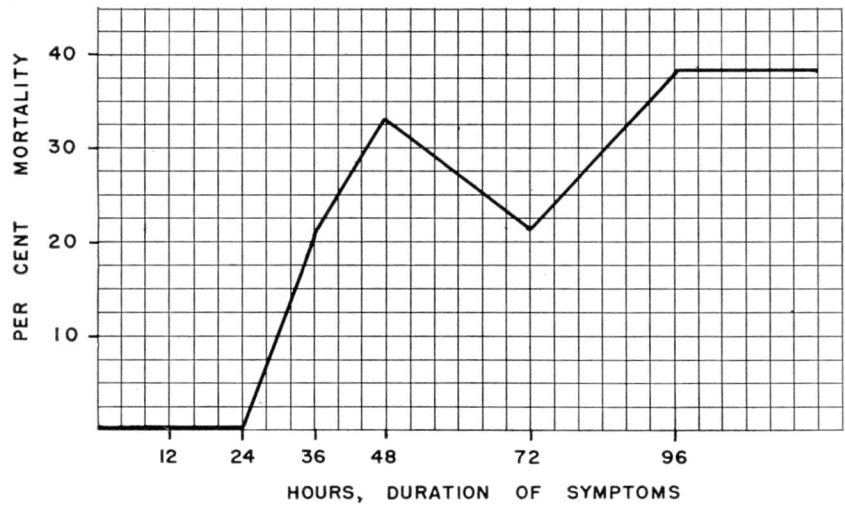

Fig. 160. Graph showing relationship between duration of symptoms and corresponding mortality rates (202 patients with intussusception treated from 1928 through 1939). Operation was performed in 110 patients within the first twenty-four hours of illness without fatality.

Table 36

Duration of Symptoms and Corresponding Mortality Statistics in 202 Patients with Intussusception
(1928 through 1939)

Symptom-Duration	Operative Results		
	Number of Survivals	Number of Deaths	Mortality Percentage
0 to 12 hours.....................	66	0	0
12 to 24 hours.....................	44	0	0
24 to 36 hours.....................	20	6	23
36 to 48 hours.....................	12	6	33
48 to 72 hours.....................	15	4	21
72 to 96 hours.....................	8	5	38
More than 96 hours..............	10	6	38
Totals..........................	175	27	13

Death Rates

The fatality rates over a period of years in 702 cases are charted in Figure 162. Beginning with a mortality of 59 per cent in the 1908 to 1912 period, a gradual decline has taken place. During the three-year period, 1948 through 1950, there were 92 cases without a fatality. This dramatic improvement in results is due to a combination of prompt recognition and better surgical care.

CHRONIC INTUSSUSCEPTION

Subacute or chronic intussusception has been arbitrarily defined as that type in which the symptoms have lasted from five days to two or more weeks. An intussusception which can persist this long without killing the individual must necessarily be of a form which does not completely obstruct the bowel. Indeed, such a patient may have some bowel movements during the illness, and may not appear particularly sick. There may be irregular and intermittent vomiting, moderate abdominal pain, or passage of small amounts of blood in the stool. In short, partial obstruction produces symptoms

Table 37

Comparison from Two Different Periods of Cases with Similar Durations to Show the Improvement in
Surgical Therapy

Symptom-Duration	Mortality Percentage	
	1908 to 1927 Series	1928 to 1939 Series
0 to 12 hours....................	7	0
12 to 24 hours....................	24	0
24 to 36 hours....................	49	23
36 to 48 hours....................	53	33
48 to 72 hours....................	53	21
72 to 96 hours....................	60	38
More than 3 days................	54	38

which are not so pronounced and fulminating as those of acute intussusception, in which the bowel is largely or completely occluded.

Not infrequently the chronic form of intussusception is seen in association with or following *acute enteritis;* accordingly any turn for the worse in a case of enteritis in a young child should arouse one's suspicions of the possibility of intussusception. When chronic intussusception is suspected, a barium enema examination should be the deciding factor in establishing the diagnosis. The prognosis in these individuals is usually rather good, presumably because intestinal obstruction has been only partial and because damage to the intestine and mesentery is minimal.

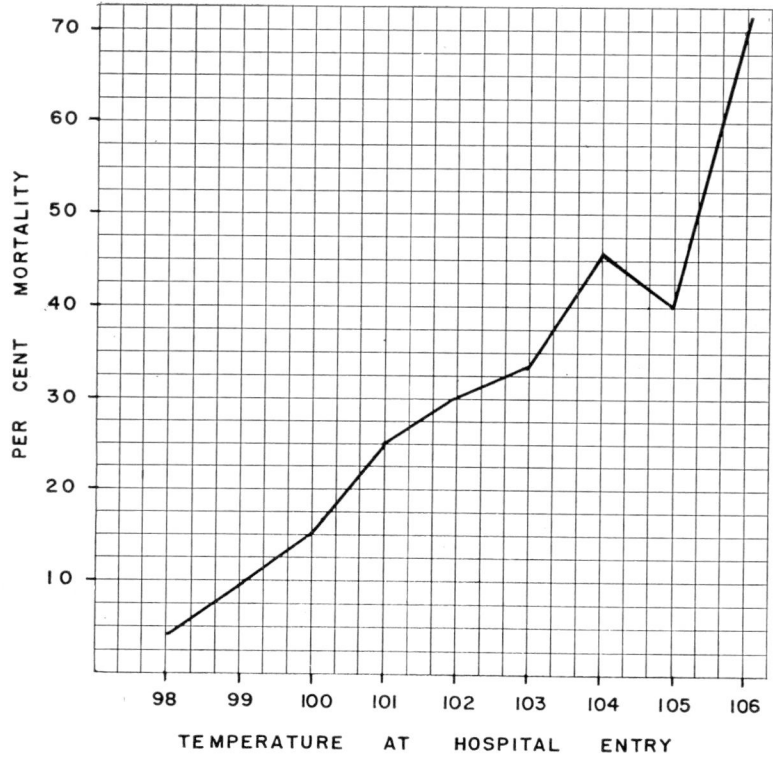

Fig. 161. Graph of relationship between body temperature at time of hospitalization and corresponding mortality rate. Fever at the time of hospitalization implies a poor prognosis, presumably because it indicates severe dehydration or extensive intestinal damage.

RECURRENT INTUSSUSCEPTION

Recurrence of the condition is found in a small percentage of patients with intussusception. The second attack may appear within a few days after the initial episode or it may be delayed for several years. In cases gleaned from the literature the longest interval between attacks was eight years and the shortest was thirty hours. The largest number of recurrences ever reported in one individual was in a child who required four operations. In our series there has been a recurrence rate of about 2 per cent. In one subject there was simple reduction of an intussusception on three separate occasions. In all of our recurrent cases there was survival.

Because of the low incidence of recurrence we believe that *it is not desirable to undertake procedures which are designed to prevent return of intussusception.* The chances of a second attack are so small that there is little justification for performing additional operative steps in a critically ill child. Furthermore, it is questionable whether any of the steps which have been devised to date are effective in preventing subsequent recurrence of the trouble. Another reason for not using "preventive" measures lies in the fact that recurrence does not necessarily take place in the same location as did the original intussusception. The fact that there has been no death in our recurrent cases we attribute primarily to the acuity of the mothers, who invariably recognized the second attack as being similar to the first, and wasted no time in hospitalizing the children within periods when treatment could be given without danger.

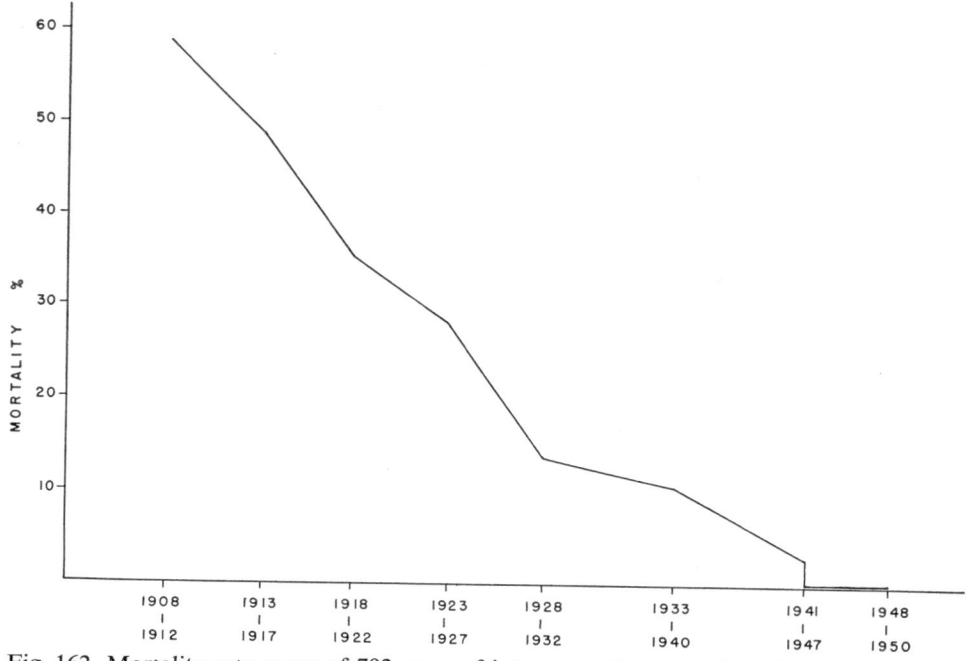

Fig. 162. Mortality rate curve of 702 cases of intussusception treated at the Children's Hospital from 1908 through 1950. There has been a progressive decrease in the death rates throughout this period. There were no deaths in the 92 cases treated from 1948 through 1950.

For those children who have three, four, or five attacks of intussusception, each of which has required therapy, there arises the problem of what to do to prevent these harrowing episodes. Under such conditions, intussusception is generally caused by a very prominent lip of redundant mucosa at the ileo-cecal valve; this projects into the lumen of the cecum and acts as a leading point. Removal of this is very effective in preventing recurrence; this is most easily accomplished by resection of the terminal ileum and cecum. If the child is in good condition, a primary end-to-end anastomosis can be made between the ileum and the colon. If the child is in poor condition, the terminal ileum and cecum can be mobilized rapidly and exteriorized by the Mikulicz technique, subsequently reestablishing continuity of the alimentary tract by crushing down the walls between the two limbs and closing the single stoma.

REFERENCES

1. Arntzen, L. and Helsted, A.: Desinvagination unter Roentgendurchleuchtung bei akuter Darminvagination im Kindesalter. Acta chir. Scandinav., 65:70, 1929.
2. Asbury, H.: Roentgenological Aspects of Intussusception. Am. J. Roentgenol., 18:536, 1927.
3. Beaven, P. W.: The Occurrence of Chronic Intussusception in Young Children. Am. J. Dis. Child., 37:373, 1929.
4. Clubbe, C. P. B.: The Diagnosis and Treatment of Intussusception. Oxford University Press, New York, 1921.
5. Dennis, C.: Resection and Primary Anastomosis in the Treatment of Gangrenous or Non-reducible intussusception in Children. Ann. Surg., 126:788, 1947.
6. Gross, R. E. and Ware, P. F.: Intussusception in Childhood; Experiences from 610 Cases. New England J. Med., 239:645, 1948.
7. Hipsley, P. L.: Intussusception and Its Treatment by Hydrostatic Pressure. M. J. Australia, 2:201, 1926.
8. Hutchinson, J.: A Successful Case of Abdominal Section for Intussusception. Tr. Roy. M. & Chir. Soc., 57:31, 1874.
9. Kirsner, J. B. and Miller, J. F.: Roentgen Diagnosis of Intussusception. Radiology, 31:658, 1938.
10. Lehmann, C.: Ein Fall von Invaginatio ileocecalis im Rontgenbilde. Fortschr. a. d. Geb. d. Rontgenstrahlen, 21:561, 1913.
11. McIver, M. A.: Intussusception of the Small Intestine with Special Reference to Meckel's Diverticulum as a Causative Factor. New England J. Med., 199:453, 1928.
12. Mayo, C. W.: Spontaneous Expulsion of an Intussuscepted Bowel. Proc. Staff Meet., Mayo Clin., 7:345, 1932.
13. Monrad, S.: Acute Invagination of the Intestine in Small Children. Acta paediat., 6:31, 1926.
14. Montgomery, A. H. and Mussil, J. J.: The Treatment of Irreducible Intussusception in Children. Surg., Gynec. & Obst., 51:415, 1930.
15. Perrin, W. S. and Lindsay, E. C.: Intussusception: A Monograph Based on Four Hundred Cases. Brit. J. Surg., 9:46, 1921.
16. Peterson, E. W. and Carter, R. F.: Acute Intussusception in Infancy and Childhood. Ann. Surg., 96:94, 1932.
17. Ravitch, M. M. and McCune, R. M., Jr.: Reduction of Intussusception by Barium Enema; Clinical and Experimental Study. Ann. Surg., 128:904, 1948.
18. Retan, G. M.: Nonoperative Treatment of Intussusception. Am. J. Dis. Child., 33:765, 1927.
19. Robbins, F. R.: Acute Intussusception. Ann. Surg., 95:830, 1932.
20. Schoenfeld, H. H.: Retrograde Intussusception. Virginia M. Monthly, 58:242, 1931.
21. Southern, A. H. and Crawshaw, C. H.: Resection of Intestine for Acute Intussusception. Brit. M. J., 1:266, 1921.
22. Stephens, V. R.: Acute Intussusception: Manipulation Under Fluoroscopic Control. Am. J. Dis. Child., 35:61, 1928.
23. Sussman, M. L.: The Roentgenologic Aspect of Subacute and Chronic Intestinal Intussusception. Am. J. Roentgenol., 27:373, 1932.
24. Thorndike, A.: Acute Recurrent Intussusception in Children. New England J. Med., 207:649, 1923.
25. Wardill, W. E. M.: Polypi in the Bowel Causing Intussusception. Brit. J. Surg., 13:158, 1925.

CHAPTER 21

Polyps of Intestine and Colon

Polyps of the alimentary tract are frequently encountered in childhood. They are found in any portion of the intestine or colon, with predilections for certain areas, and give rise to symptoms which vary according to the position of the lesion. In the vast majority of cases they are single, or else occur as a small group within a short segment of gut, but it is well known that polyps appearing at one site carry a certain implication that additional ones may concurrently exist or subsequently appear at other levels of the intestinal tract. Polyps commonly present rather trifling symptoms and may be easily treated by minor surgical procedures, but in some instances they produce serious illness which requires the most major sort of surgery for adequate therapy.

The following remarks are based largely on material from 203 patients with polyps of the intestine, colon, and rectum who have been treated at the Children's Hospital from January 1931 through December 1950.

PATHOLOGY

Size and Structure

Polyps range from a few millimeters to several centimeters in diameter. The average is 1 cm. or less in maximum cross-dimensions. They are soft and often are friable. At first, the base usually has a sessile attachment to the bowel wall, but later this can become pedunculated as the suspended and enlarging mass is pulled upon by the fecal current. The intestinal or colonic mucosa extends up over the stalk onto the polyp proper, and indeed many polyps appear to be little more than localized redundancies of the regional mucosa and submucosa. However, some of them exhibit definite evidence of neoplastic growth of a benign sort, and goblet, mucus-secreting cells are arranged in irregular adenomatous formations. All polyps show some degree of edema, hemorrhage, and chronic inflammation. Surface ulceration and granulation-tissue formation are common.

Locations

Polyps are most commonly located in the rectum, but they may occur at any point distal to the cardia of the stomach. In a series of 203 cases treated at the Children's Hospital, the lesions were distributed as follows:

In rectum only	144
Sigmoid only	21
Descending colon only	8
Transverse colon only	4
Cecum only	1
Ileum only	2
Scattered through stomach, jejunum, and ileum	1
Scattered in various parts of colon, but none in rectum	4
Scattered in colon and rectum	8
Multiple polyposis of colon	10
Total	203

Approximately two-thirds of our patients had a single polyp, while somewhat less than a third had two to nine polyps. There were 10 with multiple polyposis of the colon. While polyps tend to be single or to be confined to a short segment of gut, they may be scattered diffusely throughout the alimentary tract. An example of this was encountered in an eight-year old girl who at autopsy was found to have four polyps in the stomach, fourteen in the jejunum, and four in the ileum.

"Scattered Polyps" and "Polyposis"

Because the therapeutic approaches are different, it is well to classify polyps into one of three groups, namely: *single, scattered*, or *polyposis*. By "scattered" is meant isolated lesions in the rectum, colon, or ileum, each unit of which can be attacked locally; such scattered lesions may all be detected at one time, or they may appear in stages over a period of years. By "polyposis" is meant the extensive involvement of a segment by so many polyps (Figs. 169 and 170) that the general character of the bowel lining is altered to the point where adequate therapy requires a resection of the entire segment (excepting possibly the rectum). In these patients polyps develop in enormous numbers, particularly in the colon. An example of this was a seven-year-old boy whose colonic wall from cecum to anus was found to have about 400 polyps of different sizes. Some of these were sessile, others were pedunculated; many had an adenomatous structure on microscopic examination. With polyposis of the colon, there are very apt to be other members of the family with the same condition.

CLINICAL FINDINGS

Sequelae

Three important complications can appear from intestinal or colonic polyps: (1) Surface erosion may give *hemorrhage*, particularly if the pedunculated structures are large or multiple. (2) A polyp may act as the leading point of an *intussusception*, a sequence which was found in 5 of our cases. (3) *Malignant degeneration* can occur. This danger is believed to be negligible in the small, isolated polyp such as is found in the rectum, but it is a serious hazard for those individuals with polyposis of the colon, in whom carcinomatous degeneration in later life has been estimated to be as high as 50 per cent. If malignant changes appear, they seldom do so before adult life, but we have seen a twelve-year-old girl with colonic polyposis and with adenocarcinoma of the rectum.

Bleeding

Passage of blood per rectum is the most frequent symptom. Polyps of the small intestine may produce occult blood in the stool which is demonstrable only by chemical tests, or there may be gross amounts of dark red or tarry material intermixed with the excretions. Polyps of the descending colon, sigmoid, or rectum are particularly apt to bleed because they are constantly irritated and ulcerated by the more solid fecal masses which move through these parts of the colon. While isolated polyps in these positions frequently bleed, it is unusual for more than a few cubic centimeters of blood to be passed at any one time; only rarely does massive hemorrhage appear. *Polyposis of the colon* causes almost continuous loss of small amounts of blood, which may induce a state of virtual exhaustion of red cells, hemoglobin, and blood proteins. In one of our children the red count had fallen to 2,500,000 and the serum protein to 2.7 gm. per cent; there was weakness, pallor, orthopnea, leg edema, and clubbing of the fingers.

Abdominal Pain

Aside from bleeding and possible prolapse out through the anus, rectal polyps are usually silent, but lesions higher in the alimentary canal can occasionally produce *abdominal discomfort, cramps*, or even *severe pain*. Abdominal pain which is excruciating, colicky, and possibly associated with vomiting suggests that peristaltic activity has pulled a polyp into the intestine in such a way that an intussusception has been initiated.

Rectal Findings

A polyp of the rectum can usually be felt with the finger and is most commonly attached to the posterior or postero-lateral wall. If it cannot be palpated in this way, it can always be identified by proctoscopy.

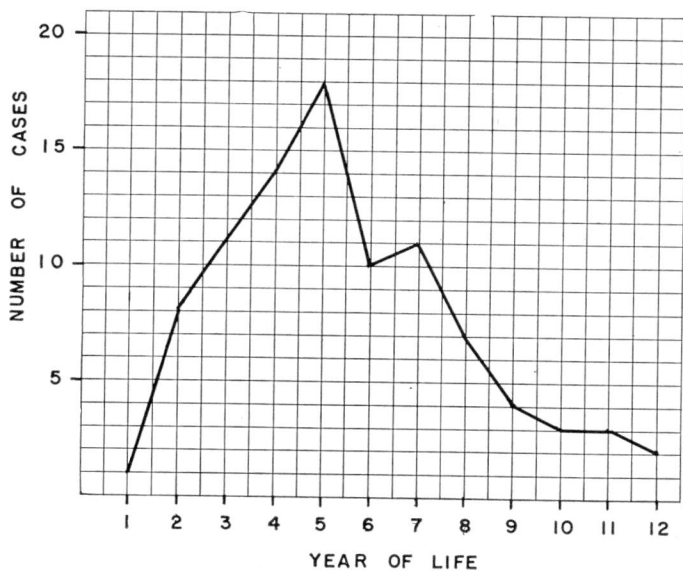

Fig. 163. Age incidence of intestinal or colonic polyps in a study of 92 children.

Age and Sex Incidence

Polyps are rarely discovered in the first year of life. They are most frequently seen from the ages of two to eight years, with a peak of incidence at four or five years. Age distribution studies are set forth in Figure 163. Our youngest subject was fifteen months; the oldest was twelve years.

Males are affected with somewhat greater frequency than females, the proportion being 58 to 42 per cent in our series.

Peri-oral Melanin Spots

Jeghers et al.[12] have described 10 cases with the combination of intestinal polyps and the appearance of melanin spots in the peri-oral skin and in the buccal membranes (Fig. 167).

Familial Tendency

A familial tendency is rarely found when a patient has only one or two polyps, but it is very marked in those cases in which there is polyposis. A striking example of this

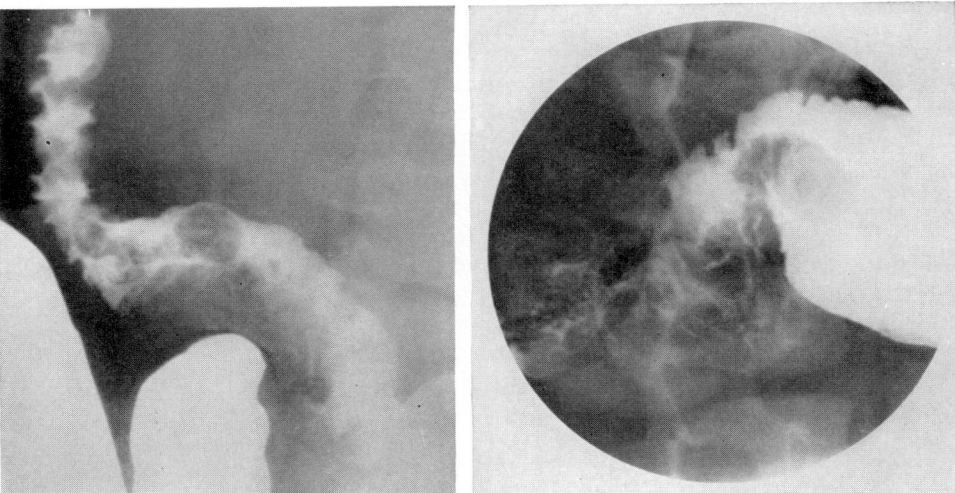

Fig. 164. Roentgenograms from 2 patients; single polyp of the colon.

was exhibited by one family, three of whose children were treated by us; the pertinent facts were:

Patient, nine-year-old boy, polyposis of colon, requiring subtotal colectomy.

Patient, six-year-old girl, polyposis of colon, requiring subtotal colectomy.

Patient, twelve-year-old girl, polyposis of colon and carcinoma of rectum, requiring ileostomy, removal of entire colon, resection of rectum.

A sibling, treated elsewhere, had colonic polyposis.

The mother of these four children had multiple polyposis and died at twenty-nine of carcinoma of the rectum.

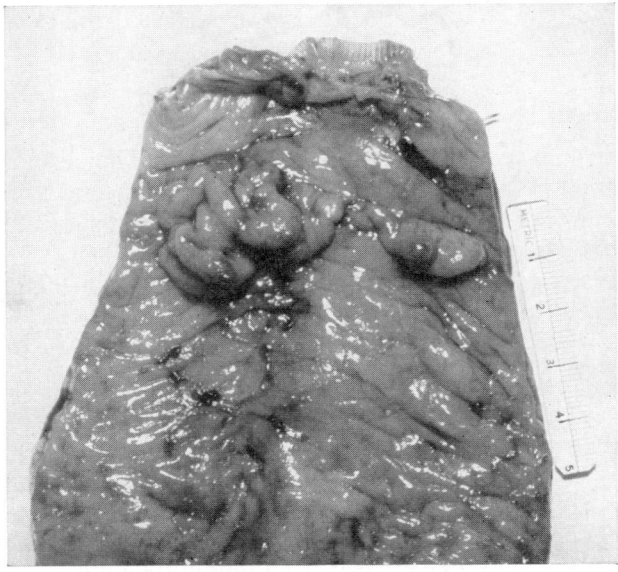

Fig. 165. Segment of sigmoid resected from an eight-month-old baby because of sessile polyps.

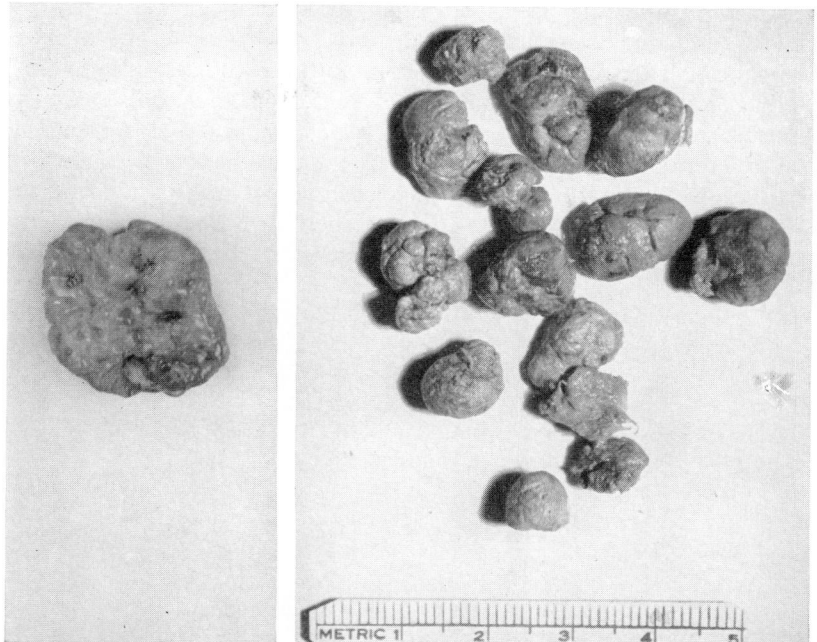

Fig. 166. *Left*, Single polyp removed from cecum. *Right*, Multiple polyps removed from a boy who had polyposis of the colon.

Three maternal uncles died of carcinoma of rectum at ages of twenty-seven, twenty-eight, and thirty-one years.

ROENTGENOLOGIC EXAMINATION

The identification of one or several polyps in the rectum always raises the question of whether more of these lesions are present in other parts of the alimentary tract. While it is true that the vast majority of children who have a polyp of the rectum have no other lesion—and roentgenologic study in such cases will generally be fruitless—it is probably a wise policy to examine the colon by barium enema in all of them.

When there is polyposis of the rectum, the colon should always be visualized by

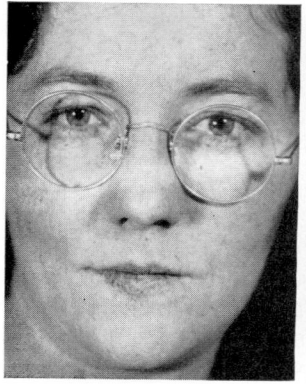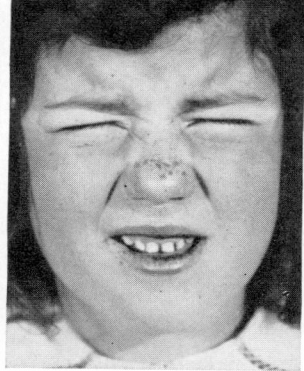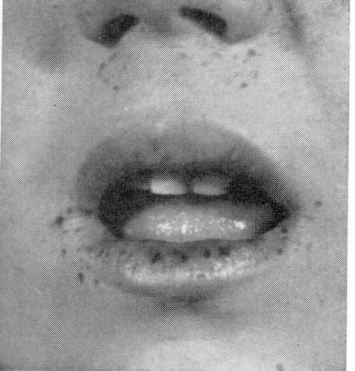

Fig. 167. Photograph of mother (*left*) and patient (*middle* and *right*), both of whom had multiple intestinal polypi and melanin spots about the mouth.

x-ray studies to determine the upper extent of the condition, and a gastro-intestinal series should be conducted to detect any polyps of the stomach or small intestine.

Polyps of the *colon* are found by fluoroscopic or film studies as filling defects during inflation of the colon with a barium mixture (Figs. 164 and 168). In postevacuation films a polypoid mass may retain a thin coating of barium which outlines its borders. Polyps can be differentiated from fecal masses by the fact that they cannot be dislocated by manual palpation during the fluoroscopic examination, and by the fact that a filling defect persists in a given region. Double-contrast enemas (filling the colon with a barium mixture and later inflating it with air) are particularly effective in visualizing polyps.

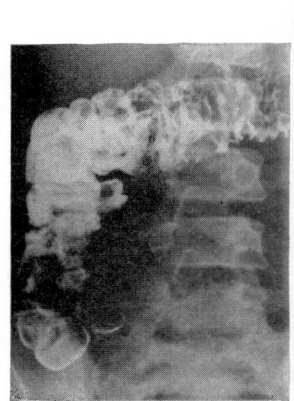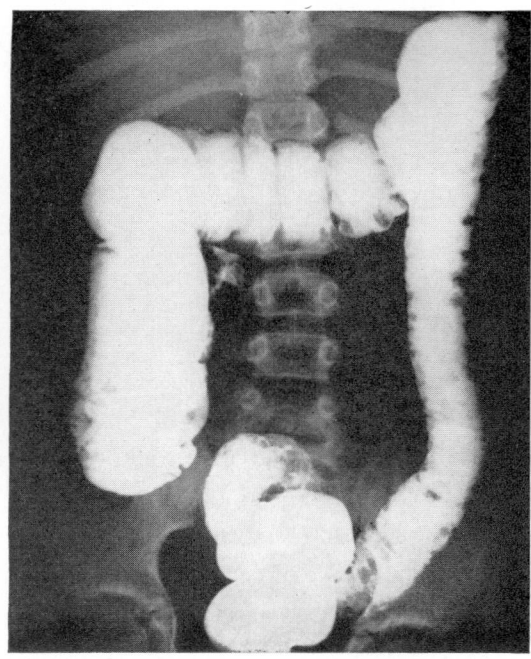

Fig. 168. Barium enema findings in a ten-year-old girl with multiple polyposis of the colon.

DIFFERENTIAL DIAGNOSIS

The passage of blood per rectum by a baby or child is a symptom of variable significance. In the vast majority of cases it indicates a minor ailment, in some it is evidence of an existing lesion which demands surgical relief, and in a few it may be the warning of a condition which threatens the individual's life.

Constipation is probably the most common cause of rectal bleeding in young subjects. Dyschezia and bleeding may come from a small anal fissure if the stools are too hard; these symptoms will be completely alleviated by mild catharsis (mineral oil) for a few days.

A *Meckel's diverticulum* may give rise to bleeding which, when it appears, is usually copious in amount. It is rather typical for the hemorrhage to start suddenly and silently and to terminate abruptly in a few days; in a few subjects it can continue to the point that anemia and exhaustion are evident. The blood which is passed tends to be dark in color; this is in contrast to bleeding found with rectal or colonic lesions where it is apt to be brighter. Severe bleeding may occur on two or three occasions before it leads to laparotomy or exsanguination, but it is unusual for a Meckel's diverticulum to give

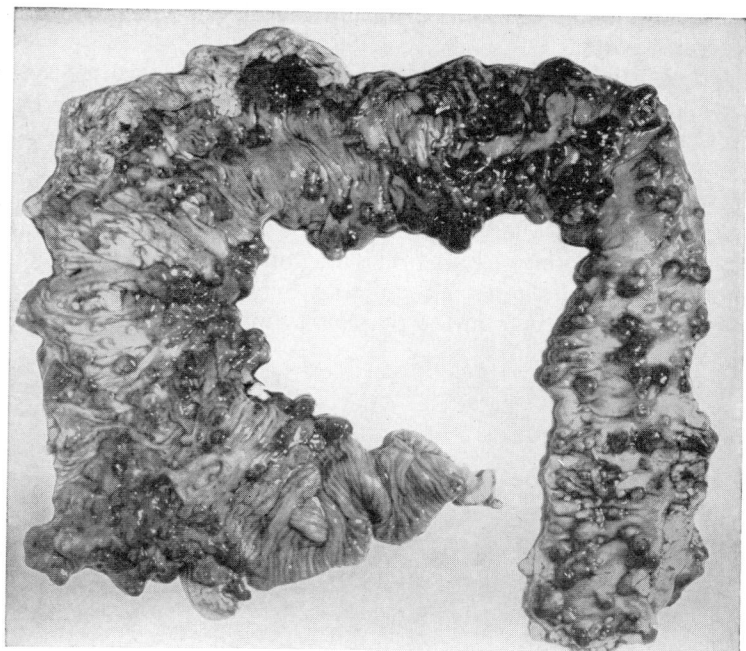

Fig. 169. Colon removed from a six-year-old boy who had multiple polyposis.

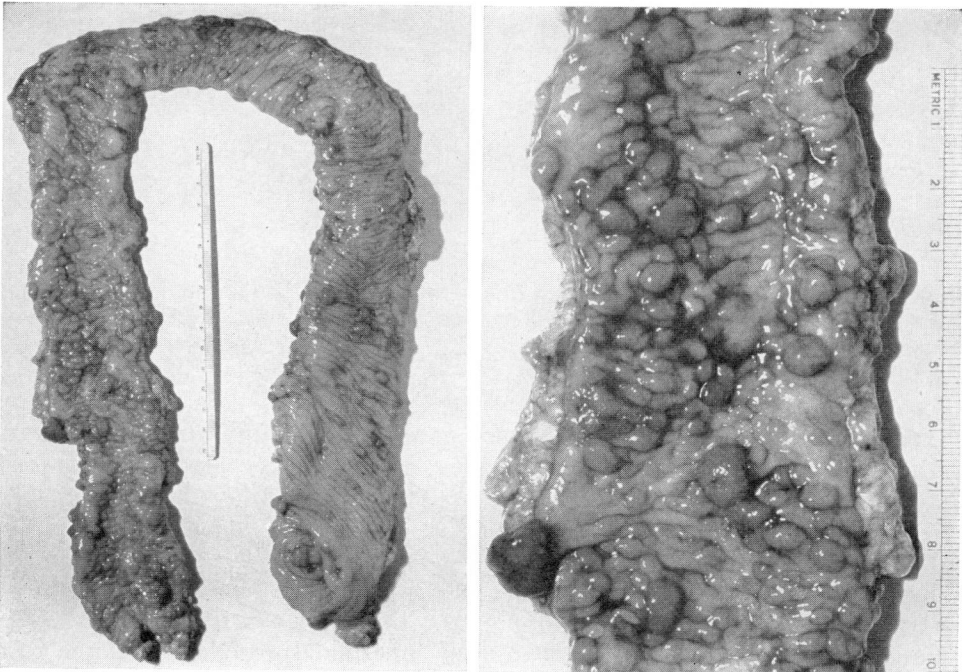

Fig. 170. Colon removed from a six-year-old girl who had familial polyposis of the colon (sibling of patient whose specimen is shown in Fig. 171).

frequent appearance of small amounts of bright red blood, which is more suggestive of anal fissure or rectal polyp.

Intussusception usually has rectal bleeding as one of its cardinal symptoms, but it is almost always accompanied by severe abdominal pain, collapse, and possibly a palpable abdominal mass. This combination of findings, particularly in a chubby baby, is usually sufficient to warrant making a diagnosis of intussusception. It can be proved, or disproved, by barium enema examination.

Scurvy may cause rectal bleeding, but when it does so there is almost always evidence of the disease in the gums or long bones and a history of deficient vitamin C intake.

Blood dyscrasias are usually accompanied by hemorrhagic tendencies in other parts of the body and by some change in the platelet count, clotting time, or bleeding time.

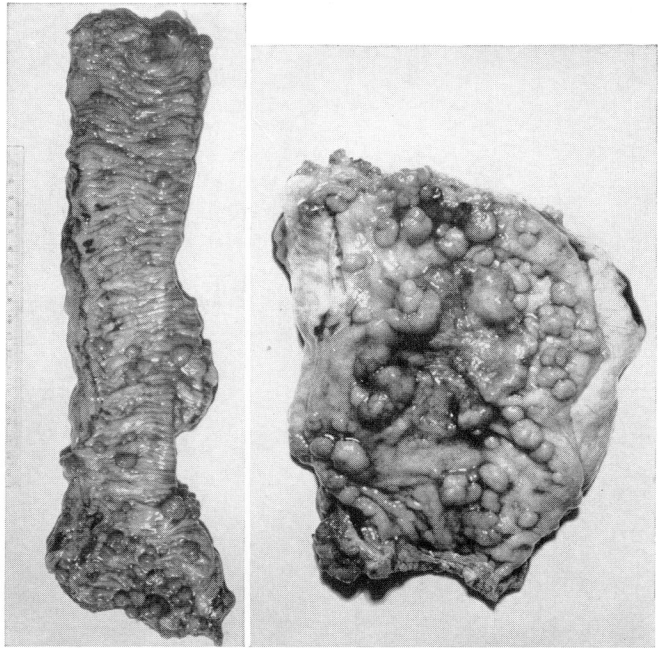

Fig. 171. *Left*, Portion of colon removed from a twelve-year-old girl for multiple polyposis. *Right*, Rectum from the same girl. The central, crater lesion by microscopic examination was a typical adenocarcinoma.

TREATMENT

Treatments for intestinal or colonic polyps are divided into four types of operation, each of which is designed for a particular set of circumstances. Data from some of our more complicated cases are gathered in Table 38.

1. Excision through Proctoscope

Removal of polyps through a proctoscope or sigmoidoscope is the procedure most often used (Fig. 173). By this means all polyps within the lower 10 or 12 inches of bowel can be easily excised. This should always be done under *general anesthesia*, to make certain that the child will not injure himself by moving while the instruments are in place. The *lithotomy* position is preferable to the knee-chest one since it gives the best view of the lesions which commonly arise from the posterior wall of the rectum. The bowel is prepared with a soapsuds enema the evening before operation, and by a second enema about two hours before operation. If fecal material still obscures the view, the rectum can be further irrigated at the operating table, and the fluid then aspirated with a piece of tubing (connected to a suction apparatus) passed in through the proctoscope.

Polyps can often be grasped with an instrument and pulled down to a level where they can be directly handled through a short anoscope possessing a side slit. In this way the base can be transfixed before the pedunculated mass is cut off. This manipula-

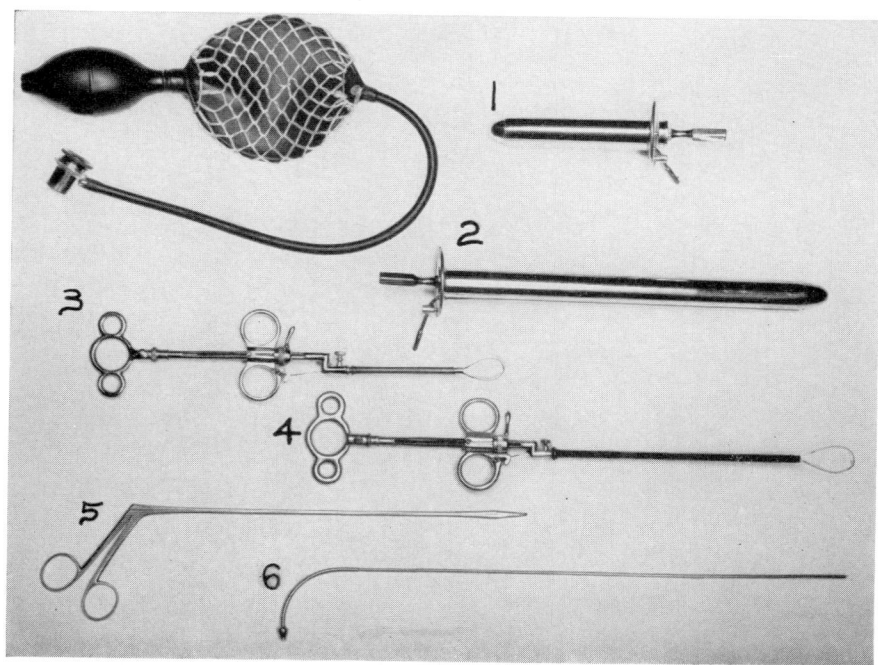

Fig. 172. Instruments for excision of rectal polyps. 1. Short proctoscope, 4 inches long, $\frac{3}{4}$ inch in diameter. 2. Sigmoidoscope, 10 inches long. 3 and 4. Tonsil snares with elongated stems. Thin rubber tubing is drawn over the stems for insulation. 5. Long alligator forceps for grasping and coagulating sessile polyps or bleeding points. 6. Metal suction tube for removing smoke or fecal fluid.

tion is sometimes difficult because polyps tend to tear and bleed, or the rectal wall cannot be easily pulled down into a convenient position. Because of these troubles we have now completely abandoned the ligature method of excising a polyp. It is much preferable to *snare* a polyp with an elongated tonsil snare while simultaneously passing a *coaguiating current* through the instrument. A small polyp with a sessile base is best treated by grasping its central portion with an alligator forceps (through the proctoscope) and then passing a *coagulating (endothermy) current* through it. Coagulation is continued under direct vision until the entire polyp is charred white. Coagulation must be discontinued at this point to avoid perforation of the bowel wall. (We have never had a case of sloughing or perforation of a rectum or colon from endothermy coagulation or snaring of a polyp.)

To facilitate the various manipulations described above, we have revamped a tonsil snare, giving it a long shank (Fig. 172). Furthermore, the shaft is insulated by covering it with a thin rubber tube so that it will not be short-circuited if it touches the interior of the proctoscope.

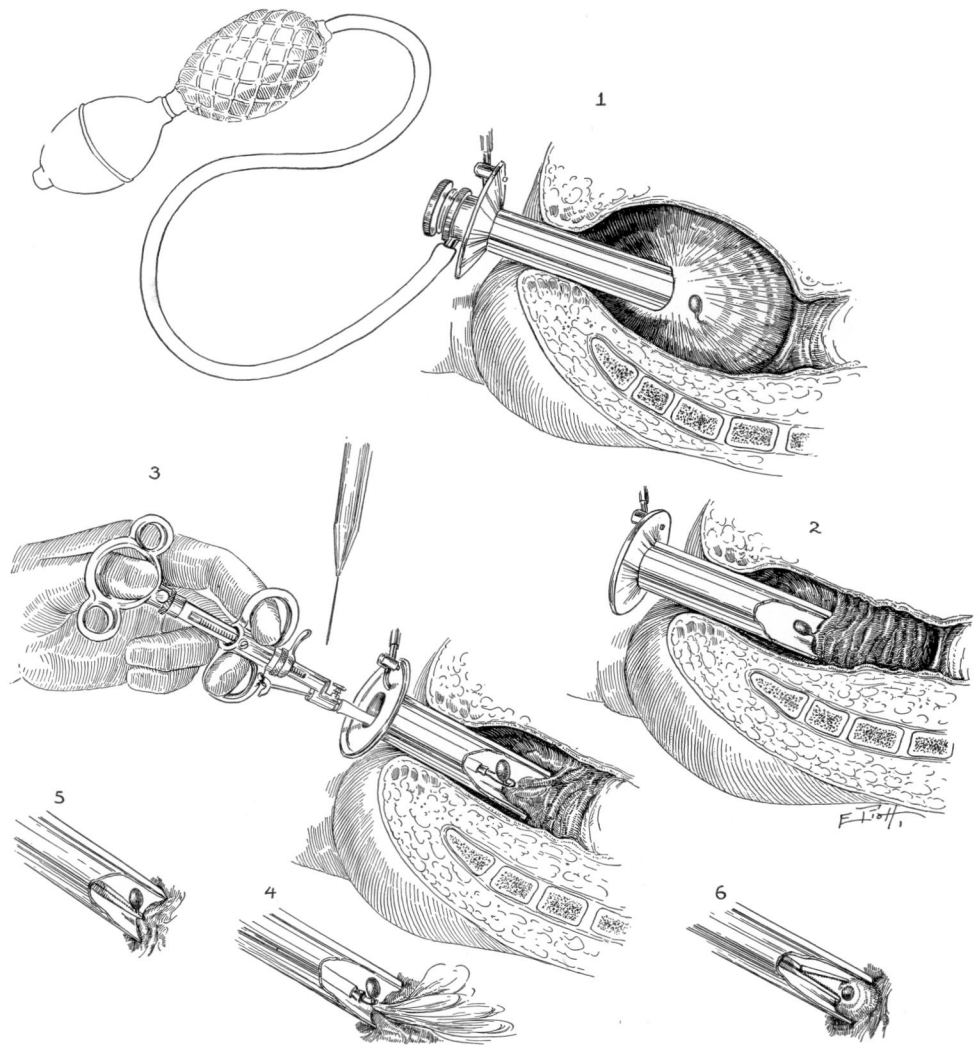

Fig. 173. Method of removal of polyps from rectum or lower sigmoid. 1. Patient in lithotomy position. Bowel inflated through proctoscope. Instrument placed so that its tip lies just distal to polyp. 2. Air pressure released. Polyp prolapses into lumen of proctoscope. 3 and 4. Pedicle of polyp constricted with elongated tonsil snare. Coagulating current passed through snare and pedicle of lesion. 5. Alternate method of removing pedunculated polyp by grasping it with an alligator forceps through which a coagulating current is passed. The friable stalk can be severed by this squeezing and desiccation. 6. Treatment of a sessile polyp by grasping it with an alligator forceps and then passing a coagulating current through it.

2. Abdominal Exploration with Ileotomy or Colotomy

Abdominal exploration with ileotomy or colotomy is employed for those polyps which lie in any part of the tract above the mid-sigmoid. When the abdomen is opened, the entire intestine should be carefully examined to determine accurately how many polyps exist. The segment of the intestine or colon which is to be treated is then drawn up into the wound and packed off carefully to avoid any subsequent soiling of the general peritoneal cavity. Rubber-covered clamps are placed across the proximal and distal ends of the exposed loop to prevent rushes of fecal material. Incision may be made opposite the polyp so that its pedicle can be tied, or an elliptical incision can be made around the base so that the entire mass (with its base) is removed. In either case, the wall is closed with an inverting Connell continuous suture which is reinforced with a row of interrupted stitches, preferably of fine silk.

In dealing with adults, Welch[22] has suggested that colotomy and excision of a polyp should be discarded in favor of segmental resection of any area which bears a polyp. This change in therapy has been proposed because occasionally a polyp will, on microscopic examination, prove to be carcinomatous; a second operation is then required and the chances of curing the patient of cancer may have been lost. In childhood, it is extremely rare that an isolated polyp will show carcinomatous change, hence simple removal of a polyp and its base is all that need be done.

3. Temporary Colostomies

Establishment of one or several temporary colostomies provides avenues of attack on polyps of the colon which are too numerous for multiple colotomies and yet not numerous enough to warrant colectomy. Thus, a sigmoidoscope passed in through a *sigmoidostomy* allows the operator to remove polyps up to the splenic flexure by snare and endothermy coagulation. Similarly, a *transverse colostomy* permits treatment of lesions lying between the hepatic and splenic flexures, and a *cecostomy* gives access to those in the ascending colon. If necessary, all three of these temporary openings can be made, for through them and the anus it is possible to remove scores of polyps from any part of the colon. It is rare that this therapeutic approach via colostomies will be necessary, but we have used it on two subjects with the gratifying result of saving the colon in each. This technique is useful if there are eight, ten, or fifteen polyps scattered through the colon above the lower sigmoid; if a larger number are present, colectomy is to be preferred.

When this plan of treatment is undertaken, the colostomy (or colostomies) should be made in such a way that the fecal stream is not completely diverted out through the abdominal wall. It is necessary to make only a short incision, not over $1\frac{1}{2}$ inches long, in the proper area of the abdominal wall, grasp the sigmoid (or transverse colon, or cecum), and pull the presenting surface of this up to the skin, to which it is stitched. An area of colonic wall about $\frac{1}{2}$ inch in diameter is thus left exposed, at the periphery of which will be the sutures which anchor the bowel to the skin. If the abdominal-wall incision has been kept sufficiently small, it will not be necessary to put any sutures in the peritoneum, muscle, or fascia. This entire procedure is aseptic and the fecal stream of the colon is not diverted or obstructed; after a few days have elapsed, the presenting bowel wall can be punctured. A sigmoidoscope can then be introduced into the colon for removal of polyps. If these openings are suitably small, they contract spontaneously and seldom require secondary surgical closure.

4. Colectomy

Colectomy is mandatory for treatment of *polyposis of the colon*. X-ray irradiation has been tried in some of these, but on the whole it has given disappointing results. Generally, resection of most of the colon can be performed in such a way that the rectum and anal sphincter are preserved. This is done by preliminary removal of polyps from the rectum (possibly requiring several sittings), resection of the colon from cecum to lower sigmoid, and then joining the terminal ileum to the prepared rectum (Cases 7, 8, 9, and 11, Table 38). While some authorities might argue—with considerable justification—that the rectum should always be removed (for fear of carcinomatous change in later life), we feel that sparing the rectum permits a much more normal existence, avoids the disagreeable features of a permanent colostomy, and that the method is justified *provided* the individual remains under the care of a physician or clinic (proctoscopy two or three times per year) so that any recurrent polyps can be excised or if carcinoma develops the rectum can be removed promptly.

A variation of the above colectomy procedure was employed in a seven-year-old boy (Case 7, Table 38) whose colon, including rectum, contained over 400 polyps. This child had such severe and debilitating bleeding that it seemed too hazardous to spend time cleaning out the rectum in the initial stages of treatment. Repeated transfusions raised the blood count to satisfactory levels, but the serum protein remained below the critical level and peripheral edema persisted. The following plan was therefore adopted

Table 38

Data from Complicated Cases of Intestinal or Colonic Polyps

Cases	Sex and Age	Polyps, Distribution, etc.	Treatment	Result
1	F 15 mos.	Numerous polyps descending colon, sigmoid, and rectum.	None.	Mongol. Died of pneumonia and cardiac failure.
2	F* 9 yrs.	20 polyps in stomach, jejunum, ileum, and rectum. Intussusception from jejunal polyp.	Resection of jejunal intussusception.	Death from peritonitis.
3	M 3 yrs.	12 sizable, isolated polyps in left half of colon, during 14 yrs.	Four proctoscopic and two transabdominal removals of polyps during six admissions (through 14 yrs.).	No further polyps now detected.
4	M† 7 yrs.	Extensive polyposis of colon. Colo-colic intussusception.	Colectomy for polyposis and intussusception.	Death from peritonitis.
5	F† 9 yrs.	Innumerable, uncounted, polyps scattered throughout entire colon and rectum.	Fulguration of rectal polyps in stages. Subtotal colectomy, ileosigmoidostomy.	Doing well 11 yrs. later. Symptom-free.
6	M 6 yrs.	Over 400 polyps diffusely scattered throughout colon and rectum.	Ileostomy, multiple-stage colectomy and abdomino-perineal resection of rectum.	Good health 10 yrs. later. Tolerates ileostomy fairly well.
7	M 7 yrs.	Extensive polyposis, colon and rectum.	Temporary ileostomy. Fulguration and removal of more than 75 rectal polyps. Colectomy (319 polyps.) Closure of ileostomy; ileosigmoidostomy.	Excellent general condition in 12 yrs. followed. At semi-annual checks occasional polyp removed from rectum.

Table 38 (continued)

Cases	Sex and Age	Polyps, Distribution, etc.	Treatment	Result
8	M‡ 9 yrs.	Innumerable polyps studding the mucosa of the entire colon and rectum.	Fulguration of rectal polyps. Colectomy, ileosigmoidostomy (Mikulicz method).	Excellent during 5 yrs. followed. At semi-annual checks 2 small polyps fulgurated.
9	F‡ 6 yrs.	At least 100 polyps in colon and rectum.	Rectum cleared by fulguration. Colectomy and ileosigmoidostomy.	Excellent condition in 3 yrs. followed.
10	F‡ 12 yrs.	Innumerable polyps diffusely throughout colon and rectum. Carcinoma of rectum with node metastases.	Abdomino-perineal resection of rectum and multiple-stage total colectomy. Permanent ileostomy.	In good health 6 yrs. followed. Delivered of baby by cesarean section at 17 years of age.
11	F 6 yrs.	Approximately 75 polyps in rectosigmoid with innumerable polyps throughout the entire colon.	Fulguration of rectal polyps. Two-stage subtotal colectomy and ileosigmoidostomy.	Excellent condition in 3 yrs. followed. At semi-annual checks 3 polyps removed from rectosigmoid.

* Patient's mother operated upon previously for intestinal polyp and intussusception.
† Cases 4 and 5 were siblings.
‡ Cases 8, 9, and 10 were siblings.

with successful issue: *First stage*, Transection of lower ileum, establishment of an ileostomy; resection of terminal ileum, cecum, and entire colon down to the lower sigmoid, turning in the lower sigmoid to make a blind rectal pouch about 6 inches long. (In this way the major portion of the bleeding was immediately stopped.) *Second stage*, Removal of all polyps from the rectal pouch by endothermy coagulation and snaring through a proctoscope. This required several procedures. *Third stage*, Taking down the ileum from the ileostomy on the abdominal wall and anastomosing it to the prepared rectal pouch. The boy stood these procedures quite well; with some limitation of fruits and green vegetables in the diet, he has only two or three semi-solid bowel movements a day and has good sphincteric control. He has been followed for twelve years, during which time he has been checked by proctoscopy twice a year and a few additional polyps have been removed from time to time. He has remained in excellent health.

In two children with extensive polyposis of the colon and rectum, the therapy has consisted of removal of all, or most of, the colon, added to an abdomino-perineal resection of the rectum. In one of these polyps were so extensive in the rectum that it was deemed safer to remove it; in the other there was frank carcinoma with lymph node metastases.

RESULTS OF THERAPY

In a series of 203 patients with intestinal, colonic, or rectal polyp (or polyps) two deaths have resulted from polyps or their complications (Cases 2 and 4, Table 38); all others have survived. In the vast majority of cases, therapy was a simple matter, carried out solely by a rectal removal of a polyp; in a few instances a transabdominal operation was required.

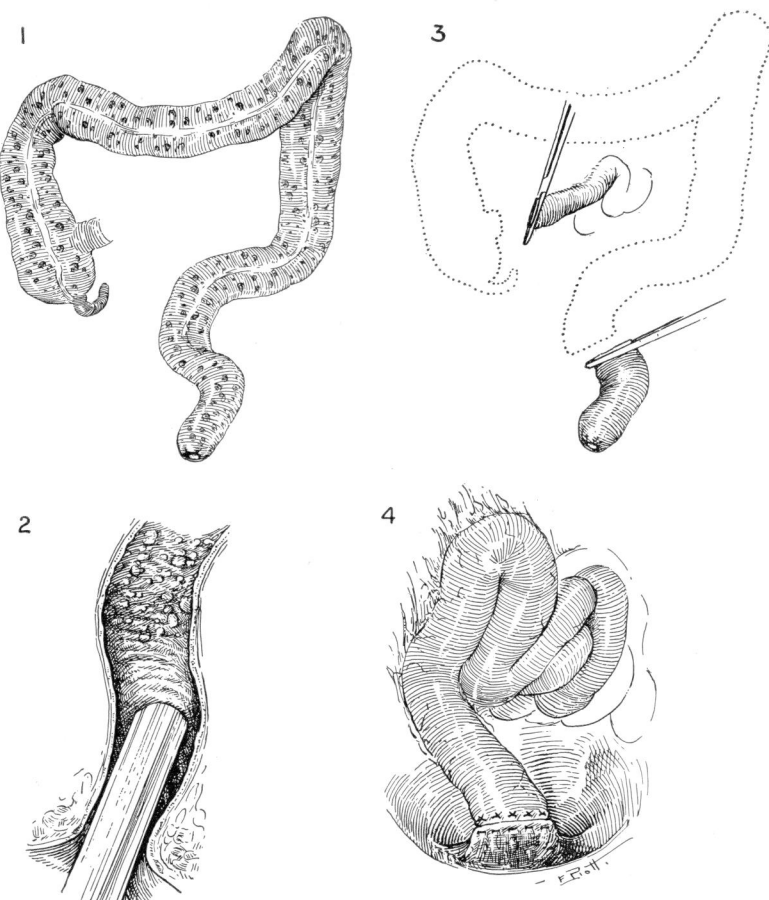

Fig. 174. General method recommended for treatment of extensive polyposis of colon. 1. Distribution of polyps, scattered from cecum to anus. 2. *First stage,* Removal of polyps from rectum (in one or more sittings). 3. *Second stage,* Removal of entire intra-abdominal portion of colon. 4. Establishment of ileo-proctostomy.

In those subjects with extensive polyposis, it has been necessary to resort to extensive resection of portions of colon or rectum to treat the lesions adequately; in two of these a permanent ileostomy (complete resection of rectum and colon) has been required. One child, twelve years of age, was treated for superimposed carcinoma of the rectum with lymph node metastases; she has been apparently cured for six years.

REFERENCES

1. Bartlett, R. W. and Peck, M. E.: The Management of Multiple Polyposis of the Colon. Surg., Gynec. & Obst., *90:*547, 1950.
2. Black, B. M. and Hansbro, G. L.: The Treatment of Familial Polyposis of the Colon. S. Clin. North America, *30:*1013, 1950.
3. Coffey, R. J. and Bargen, J. A.: Intestinal Polyps: Pathogenesis and Relation to Malignancy. Surg., Gynec. & Obst., *69:* 136, 1939.
4. Colvert, J. R. and Brown, C. H.: Rectal Polyps: Diagnosis, Five Year Follow-up, and Relation to Carcinoma of the Rectum. Am. J. M. Sc., *215:*24, 1948.
5. David, V. C.: Pathology and Treatment of Bleeding Polypoid Tumors of Large Bowel. Ann. Surg., *100:*933, 1934.

 6. Devine, J. and Webb, R.: Resection of the Rectal Mucosa, Colectomy, and Anal Ileostomy with Normal Continence. Surg., Gynec. & Obst., *92:*437, 1951.
 7. Erdmann, J. F. and Morris, J. H.: Polyposis of the Colon. A Survey of the Subject. Surg., Gynec. & Obst., *40:*460, 1925.
 8. Estes, W. L., Jr.: Familial Polyposis and Carcinoma of the Colon. Ann. Surg., *127:*1035, 1948.
 9. Hedin, R. F.: Polypoid Disease of Colon, Anatomical Measurements of Colon Including Description of Colonoscope. Surgery, *6:*909, 1939.
10. Helwig, E. B.: Adenomas of the Large Intestine in Children. Am. J. Dis. Child., *72:*289, 1946.
11. Jackman, R. J. and Mayo, C. W.: The Adenoma-carcinoma Sequence in Cancer of the Colon. Surg., Gynec. & Obst., *93:*327, 1951.
12. Jeghers, H., McKusick, V. A. and Katz, K. H.: Generalized Intestinal Polyposis and Melanin Spots of the Oral Mucosa, Lips and Digits. A Syndrome of Diagnostic Significance. New England J. Med., *241:*993, 1031, 1949.
13. Jones, T. E. and Turnbull, R. B., Jr.: Familial Polyposis of the Colon: Diagnosis and Treatment. S. Clin. North America, *28:* 1171, 1948.
14. Lamson, O. F.: Treatment of Solitary Polyp of Colon. Northwest Med., *38:*119, 1939.
15. McKenney, D. C.: Multiple Polyposis: Congenital Heredofamilial, Malignant. Am. J. Surg., *46:*204, 1939.
16. Mayo, C. W. and Butsch, W. L.: Surgical Consideration of Solitary Polyps of Colon. Ann. Surg., *107:*540, 1938.
17. Mayo, C. W. and Smith, C. H.: Transcolonic Removal of Polyps. Surgery, *5:*942, 1939.
18. Miller, R. H. and Sweet, R. H.: Multiple Polyposis of the Colon. A Familial Disease. Ann. Surg., *105:*511, 1937.
19. Pfeiffer, D. B. and Patterson, F. M. S.: Congenital or Hereditary Polyposis of the Colon. Ann. Surg., *122:*606, 1945.
20. Swinton, N. W.: Diagnosis and Treatment of Mucosal Polyps of the Rectum and Colon, with Early Malignant Change. Am. J. Surg., *75:*369, 1948.
21. Swinton, N. W. and Warren, S.: Polyps of Colon and Rectum and Their Relation to Malignancy. J.A.M.A., *113:*1927, 1939.
22. Welch, C. E.: The Treatment of Polyps of the Colon. Surg., Gynec. & Obst., *93:*368, 1951.

CHAPTER 22

Chronic Ulcerative Colitis

Chronic ulcerative colitis is a poorly understood disease for which little more than palliative treatment has yet been devised. While the condition is more common in early adult life, it is also found during childhood and may even appear in infancy. The onset is frequently acute but it may be rather insidious. The course is frequently severe; it leads to rapid emaciation, loss of strength, and possibly to a fatal termination. In most instances the disease is very debilitating, persists for a long period of years, and seriously handicaps the health of the individual. However, not all cases are so serious; prolonged attacks may be followed by temporary remission.

ETIOLOGY

Numerous theories have been advanced to explain the etiology of chronic ulcerative colitis; none seems to be entirely satisfactory. It is not impossible that the initial pathology or abnormal physiology is masked or overshadowed by secondary infection and inflammatory reaction.

Infection Theory

Some investigators believe the disease to have an infectious origin; numerous organisms have been considered to be the causative agents. Bargen and his associates[1, 8] have described a gram-positive diplococcus, which can also form chains of three or four, which is thought to be the responsible organism. While the Bargen diplococcus can be obtained from a very high percentage of the lesions, it can also be found in an appreciable number of normal individuals; it is difficult to accept it as the primary factor in the disturbance.

Detailed bacteriologic studies have been made on many of our patients, cultures were taken from stools at frequent intervals and generally they were made directly from ulcerations during proctoscopic examination. The results of these investigations have been very disappointing, because no single bacterium, or group of bacteria, of particular significance has been consistently isolated.

Neurogenic Theory

Lium[11, 12] has pointed out the possible neurogenic factor in chronic ulcerative colitis, and has put forth evidence to suggest that spasm of the colonic musculature compresses the perforating blood vessels so that local ischemia or hyperemia leads to necrosis and sloughing of the subjacent mucosa. It is very difficult to be sure whether such a mechanism is actually a factor in human cases of ulcerative colitis.

Psychogenic Factors

Study of children with ulcerative colitis indicates that a large proportion of them have a very complicated sociologic background or marked instability of personality.

Without doubt, behavior problems, familial maladjustments, highly emotional states, or other complex psychologic disturbances can manifest themselves by physiologic and later organic changes in some part of the alimentary tract, particularly in the colon. Whether or not mental aberrations can initiate chronic ulcerative colitis is a question, but they certainly can aggravate the condition when it has once begun.

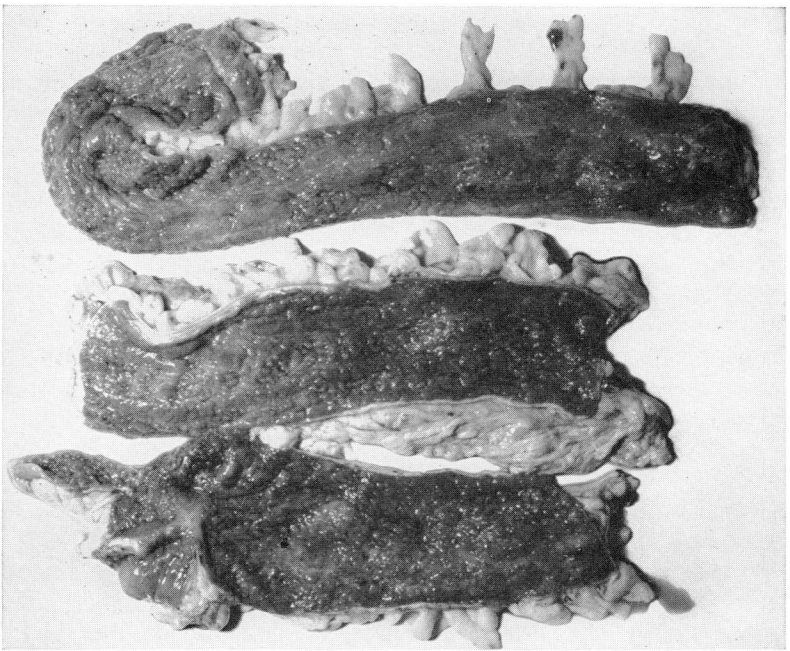

Fig. 175. Colon removed from a ten-year-old girl who had intractable diarrhea and malnutrition in spite of an ileostomy. Colon shows diffuse and marked changes of chronic ulcerative colitis and polypoid hyperplasia of the mucosa. Child restored to good health after subtotal colectomy.

PATHOLOGY

The ulcerative process is subject to great variation in severity and distribution of the lesions. It usually originates in and is more advanced in the rectosigmoid and descending colon, but a disease of some standing generally involves the entire colon. The early appearance is that of a hyperemic and granular mucosa with small punctate *hemorrhages* and a loss of the normal glistening, moist surface. The mucosa has a diminished number of folds and it bleeds after the slightest trauma; in many patients these are the only changes found by proctoscopy. *Ulcerations*, when they appear, are small and are placed quite close together, so that little unaffected mucous membrane remains between them. As the disease progresses, ulcerations become deeper and extend into the muscularis, which is destroyed or extensively scarred. All layers of the bowel can be penetrated. *Perforation* with abscess formation or generalized peritonitis is the cause of death in many subjects. A large part of the colonic lining may slough away, leaving only islands of shaggy, swollen mucosa, so that initial inspection of the specimen suggests a polyposis of the colon. However, closer examination, verified by histologic study, shows that these nubbins are the only remaining remnants of mucosa.

The terminal ileum may be involved in the ulcerative process, and perforation of the ileum is a not uncommon cause of fatality.

When the ulcerative process has been of long standing, malignant degeneration and carcinoma can appear. While such sequelae are more prone to appear in adult life, cancer has been found even in late childhood.

CLINICAL FINDINGS

Symptoms

In occasional patients the disease has a rather abrupt onset with what is thought to be an acute enteritis or entero-colitis. More commonly there is an insidious beginning and the first change is a gradual increase in *frequency of bowel movements*, which subsequently become more and more loose. They are accompanied by intermixtures of *mucus* and *pus* and, later, of *blood. Tenesmus* can be severe and exhausting. In advanced stages, discharges consist mostly of watery, hemorrhagico-purulent mucus, with very little fecal material in them. The defecations may be as often as fifteen or twenty times per day. *Abdominal cramps* and discomfort are common. A persistent low-grade *fever* is often observed, and higher temperatures appear if there is abscess formation or free perforation. *Pallor, weakness,* and *poor weight gain* are almost universal. In advanced cases there is extreme *weight loss,* emaciation, and retardation of physical development. The symptoms continue for many months or years. The disease can be a most debilitating one; constant loss of fluids and electrolytes can lead to virtual collapse and even to death. Remissions and exacerbations are often observed, but the symptoms seldom completely disappear during the periods of improvement.

Physical Findings

On physical examination the patient appears tired, fretful, and chronically ill. Pallor, weakness, and subnormal weight are evident. *Cachexia* and *wasting* are typical of advanced cases. There are few diseases which can produce the degree of emaciation which is characteristic of severe and longstanding ulcerative colitis. The abdomen is apt to be *tender,* particularly along the course of the colon. The firm tube-like bowel can sometimes be felt through the thin abdominal wall. Moderate or severe anemia is the rule. Tenesmus is great; actual incontinence is sometimes seen. There are frequent dejections of fluid material from the rectum. They contain blood, mucus, and pus in variable amounts.

Proctoscopic Examination

Such examination is preferably done under general anesthesia, for only in this way can one be certain that the end of the instrument will not damage the diseased and friable wall of the colon and perforate it. Furthermore, tenesmus and discomfort make it impossible to insert a sigmoidoscope for an adequate distance while a child is awake. Grayish, mucopurulent, or hemorrhagic material may be found on the rectal or sigmoidal wall. When this is gently removed, the underlying membrane is congested and rough; punctate hemorrhagic areas are scattered over it. Ulcers are seen in advanced cases. The mucus membrane bleeds easily on the slightest trauma. These changes are diffuse and no normal mucosa is found between the lesions—a point of some importance in ruling out certain other ulcerative processes.

ROENTGENOLOGIC EXAMINATION

Chronic ulcerative colitis gives rather typical appearances by barium enema examination (Fig. 176). The haustrations are partly lost, and there is often complete disappearance of segmentation. Because of spasticity or scarring of the wall, the lumen of the colon is greatly diminished. It is rather uniform in caliber; the colon is tube-like in

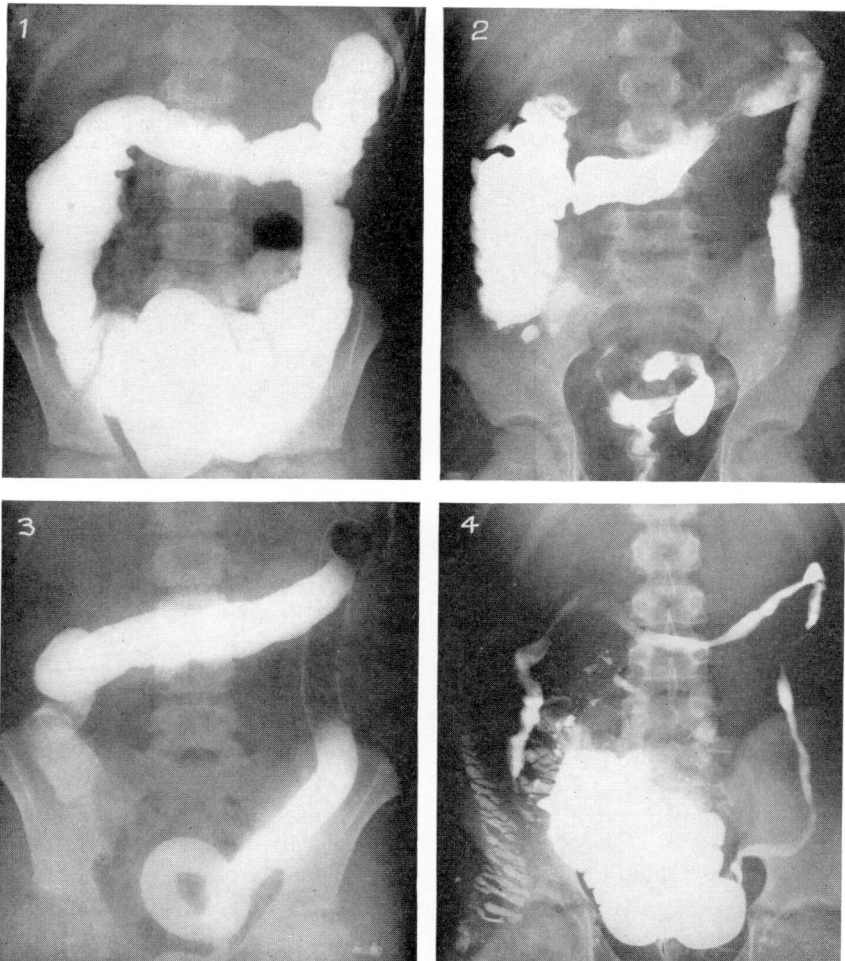

Fig. 176. Barium enema examinations from four children with different stages of chronic ulcerative colitis. 1. Nine-year-old girl. Slight loss of haustrations. Serrations of mucosal surfaces, particularly in and below splenic flexure. In spite of these seemingly mild changes, this child's disease progressed, required an ileostomy a year later, and colectomy five years after that. 2. Eight-year-old girl, three years after establishment of ileostomy. In the distal two-thirds of the colon there are moderately advanced changes of ulcerative colitis. In spite of ileostomy, the disease continued to advance and required a subtotal colectomy a year after this film was taken. 3. Eleven-year-old girl. Complete loss of haustrations, and a narrow-tube-like contour of the colon. In spite of this advanced picture, this child did exceedingly well with an ileostomy alone. 4. Twelve-year-old boy, seven years after an ileostomy. In spite of the extreme changes in the colon by x-ray visualization, this child was in very satisfactory health.

contour and becomes shortened. The wide distribution of these changes throughout the colon is quite characteristic of the condition. If there is any difference in the intensity of the findings, they are apt to be more marked in the left half of the colon. This serves to differentiate the condition from amebic colitis, which is more advanced in the right half of the colon, and is generally limited to the cecum and ascending colon.

DIFFERENTIAL DIAGNOSIS

Chronic ulcerative colitis can be suspected in any child with a history of recurrent

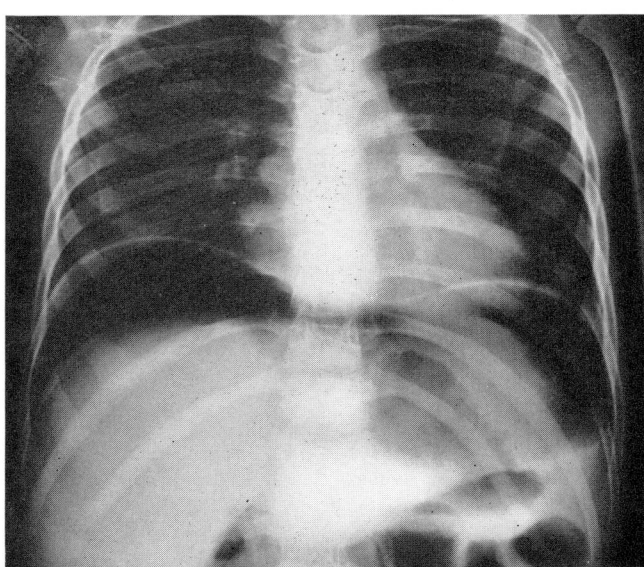

Fig. 177. Film from a seven-year-old boy with severe ulcerative colitis (of only a few months' duration), who developed multiple perforations of the terminal ileum and generalized peritonitis. Note extensive collections of free air under both diaphragms. Successful treatment by laparotomy, resection of terminal ileum, and establishment of ileostomy.

discharge of bloody mucoid material for a protracted time. Several conditions must be considered in the differential diagnosis.

Acute diarrhea, such as is caused by the dysentery bacilli and some members of the paratyphoid group, is usually typified by a sudden onset, short duration, and minimal general systemic reaction. The occurrence of diarrhea in other members of the family further suggests a self-limited, acute, and infectious type of colitis or enteritis.

Deficiency diseases, such as pellagra, beriberi, and sprue, must be considered when there is a history of marked dietary insufficiency. These conditions can be ruled out by adequate x-ray and proctoscopic studies.

Amebic dysentery can generally be excluded by careful examination of several stool specimens by someone who is familiar with the cysts and the vegetative forms of Endamoeba histolytica. Such examinations must be made upon a warm stage and upon freshly collected material. If there is any question about the possibility of amebic dysentery, a therapeutic trial with an emetine preparation is in order. By x-ray examination, the lesions are limited to the right half of the colon, or certainly are more severe there.

Tuberculous enteritis or *cecitis* can give rise to a chronic diarrhea with discharge of blood and pus in the stool. The *tuberculin test* is of great value in ruling out tuberculous enteritis in children. If the cutaneous test is negative with injection of 1 mg. of the substance, it is reasonably certain that tuberculous enteritis does not exist. If this reaction is positive, the patient must be carefully studied to determine whether lesions of other systems are responsible for the positive reaction. Tuberculous enteritis or cecitis is most apt to involve the Peyer's patches of the ileum and the lymphoid follicles of the cecum and ascending colon, and hence can usually be differentiated from idiopathic ulcerative colitis by suitable x-ray examination. If tuberculous enteritis can be reasonably suspected, properly prepared stool should be injected into guinea pigs for recovery and identification of the tubercle bacillus.

The diagnosis of idiopathic chronic ulcerative colitis is established only when the above-listed conditions have been excluded. Patients should have *serum agglutination tests* for Bacterium dysenteriae Shiga, B. dysenteriae Flexner, B. dysenteriae Hiss-Russell, B. dysenteriae Sonné, B. paratyphosum A and B, B. enteritidis, and B. abortus. Finally, barium enema examination and proctoscopic study (under anesthesia) should always be done and the latter two procedures should be repeated if the findings are equivocal.

TREATMENT

There is a wide divergence of teaching concerning the most acceptable method of treatment for idiopathic ulcerative colitis. From the outset it must be recognized that the disease may have varying degrees of severity. In its mildest form, a well regulated *medical regimen* can effect a complete and apparently permanent cure. More aggravated states can also be cared for medically; the symptoms and general health of the patient can be improved, even though some evidence of colonic disease persists. In severe cases *surgical relief*, by means of an ileostomy and possibly by resection of a part or all of the colon, can lead to great and possibly permanent improvement. Finally, in the most advanced forms, neither medical nor surgical management has much to offer and the mortality rate is extremely high.

Just where the line will be drawn between medical and surgical treatment is a matter of individual opinion. It is probably true that internists in general have leaned too far toward the conservative side, and have held patients under their care who might be improved by an ileostomy. Conversely, some surgeons have been too radical and have maintained that an ileostomy should be performed for the majority of these patients. In the Children's Hospital series, approximately half of the patients have been under medical guidance, while the remaining ones have had medical care following an ileostomy.

Medical Treatment

Adequate medical treatment requires *rest* and good general hygienic supervision, which in most instances can be obtained only by prolonged *hospitalization*.

Diet. A low-residue diet will diminish mechanical irritation of the colon. Bland and simple foods are desirable; elimination of condiments is essential. Small feedings are sometimes better tolerated than large ones. Foods which are known to aggravate the symptoms should be scrupulously avoided. Attention must be paid to the adequate administration of *vitamins*, particularly the B complex. *Crude liver extract*, 0.5 to 1 cc., and *vitamin B_{12}*, 15 to 30 micrograms, should be injected intramuscularly two or three times per week. We have seen these apparently have dramatic effects in some patients.

Drugs. Anemia is combated by iron or in severe cases by transfusion. Paregoric or other opiates have no beneficial effect or else give only temporary relief. Soothing substances, such as bismuth subcarbonate, have very little to recommend them. Substances with a broad spectrum of activity, such as sulfasuxidine or terramycin, should always be tried for their antibacterial effects; in some cases they seem to be helpful, generally they do not. It is important to try a course of *ACTH* or preferably *cortisone*. In a few patients this has marked beneficial effects, but in the majority it does not. If no benefits have been derived in a matter of weeks, there is probably little point in continuing the administration longer. Autogenous vaccines made from cultures of the Bargen diplococcus isolated directly from the patients have had no therapeutic value in our hands.

Colonic irrigations are worthless and painful; the possibility of perforating the bowel must be borne in mind.

Psychiatric Care. Since many of these children have important psychologic disturbances, every effort should be made to ferret out their troubles and to put them in rapport with their environment. Not infrequently this involves considerable readjustment on the part of the parent as well as the child. There can be no doubt that these patients are deplorable and have many deep-rooted and severe psychologic problems. Theoretically, attempts to untangle these should be of benefit, but on the whole we have been disappointed with what has been accomplished by such efforts. Whether the emotional disturbances are the cause or are the sequel of the colitis is generally impossible to determine; the mental and physical miseries become hopelessly intermingled. In spite of this dismal picture, it is often impressive to see how cheerful, happy, and well adjusted these children can become when they get rid of their exhausting diarrhea by establishment of an ileostomy or by a colectomy.

Surgical Treatment

Indications for Ileostomy. Surgery may be necessary for the treatment of perforation, abscess, peritonitis, stricture, or superimposed malignancy. Aside from these complications, which must be handled according to the requirements of the individual case, one must consider the possible benefits of procedures which are designed to alleviate the colitis itself. It is now agreed that *cecostomy* and lavage of the colon by this route has little or nothing to offer, and it has been generally abandoned. On theoretical grounds, supported by practical experience, placing the colon at complete rest by diversion of the fecal stream is of great value. An *ileostomy* will ameliorate the symptoms in most cases, and indeed it may be a lifesaving procedure for the patient who is rapidly declining because of uncontrollable diarrhea. The establishment of an ileostomy unquestionably introduces several disagreeable features and some dangers, yet in properly selected cases the advantages far outweigh the disadvantages.

Ileostomy should never be performed without an adequate trial on a well supervised medical regimen, during hospitalization, for at least two or three months and possibly longer. If permanent changes are beginning to appear in the colon, as roentgenologically indicated by shortening, loss of haustrations, and poor distensibility of the colon, surgical treatment should be advised. Arrest of the disease before important structural changes have taken place gives the only hope of sparing the colon and allowing it to heal so that it can be ultimately reconnected with the intestinal tract. Unfortunately, permanent damage to the colon cannot always be avoided, even by early ileostomy.

There are some surgeons who have proposed the use of an ileostomy *early* in all cases of ulcerative colitis. We do not agree with this view since it means the subjection to surgery of a considerable proportion of patients who would get along reasonably well under medical care. On the other hand, ileostomy should not be employed solely for terminal, desperate cases as an eleventh-hour effort to save life; when used in this way, it carries very high fatality rates. A middle ground seems to be most desirable in the selection of cases for operation. When it is certain that good medical supervision is not gaining much headway in control of the disease, establishment of an ileostomy while the patient still has some reserve is accompanied by mortality rates which are negligible. An elective ileostomy is a serious undertaking, but it is vastly safer than an emergency one.

Naturally, there is much revulsion from the idea of an ileostomy and all its disagreeable features. It is wise to have the patient (and family) live with the disease long enough so that he understands its ravages and disagreeable course; he is then in a better frame of mind to tolerate an ileostomy, for only then does he realize that it is a reasonable price to pay for rehabilitation.

It is important to emphasize that the surgeon who makes an ileostomy assumes a long-term and tedious responsibility in follow-up and care.

Technique of Performing Ileostomy. At the time of establishing an ileostomy, temptations to explore the abdomen and examine the colon must be assiduously resisted, because one never knows when the gut will rupture from even the simplest manipulations. The manner and care with which an ileostomy is established has much to do with the ease with which it can be cared for later by the patient. A right rectus incision should be employed. A loop of terminal ileum is picked up, and a point selected which is above any disease process. To give the best possible stoma, the upper bowel should not be brought out of the rectus incision, for the abdominal-wall scar will give some irregularity of skin surface which is difficult to keep clean and to which it is impossible to fit or cement an ileostomy bag snugly. These points have been clearly emphasized by Lahey.[10]

The site for the ileostomy should be carefully chosen; it should be kept away from the umbilicus, the anterior superior spine, and the groin. The proximal end of the ileum should therefore be brought out through a stab wound (Fig. 178) well to the right of the rectus muscle and at, or just below, the level of the umbilicus, placing the opening far enough above the anterior superior spine so that an ileostomy bag will not strike against this prominence and thereby be lifted off the abdominal-wall skin. A button of skin, the diameter of the ileum, should be cut out. After this stab wound has been made, a Kocher clamp can be passed in through it, the ileum grasped and severed; the proximal end of ileum is drawn out through the stab wound and appropriately anchored. The ileum should be made to project 2 or 3 cm. beyond the skin. This will shrivel down subsequently and give a nice length to fit into a bag. It is not necessary to place a Thiersch skin graft around the exterior of the presenting limb; the mucosa invariably folds back and grows over this to provide an adequate covering. The distal end of ileum is brought out through the upper end of the rectus incision. The ileum should never be transected and the distal loop closed and dropped back into the abdomen. It is well to have the distal loop opening on some portion of the abdominal wall, because one does not know when future developments in chemotherapy might bring forth a drug which can be conveniently run into the colon by this route.

Postoperative Care of Ileostomy Patient. When an ileostomy has been established, water and electrolyte loss through the orifice may be excessive and at first difficult to control, but with adequate administration of *parenteral fluids* a satisfactory balance can be reestablished quickly in most cases. During this time, it is highly important to have frequent checks on the blood chemistries so that the parenteral therapy can be guided in a manner which allows rapid reconstitution of the serum sodium, chloride, potassium, and acid-base balances. Withholding of solid food and fruit juices, and the limitation of the diet to clear fluids, such as water, soups, beef broth, salt and sugar solutions, for the first four or five days will greatly diminish the tendency of an ileostomy to discharge excessive amounts of intestinal contents. *Paregoric* at three- or four-hour intervals during the early postoperative period is of some value in slowing down the intestinal peristalsis. While the ileostomy discharges are at first quite thin, green, and watery, there is a tendency for the ileum to take over some of the drying functions of the colon so that the material later assumes a semisolid form. In some cases where the discharge continued to be fluid in nature, we have found that the material could be thickened by feeding small amounts of Kaopectate every four or six hours.

Protection of Abdominal Wall. One of the most troublesome features of an ileostomy

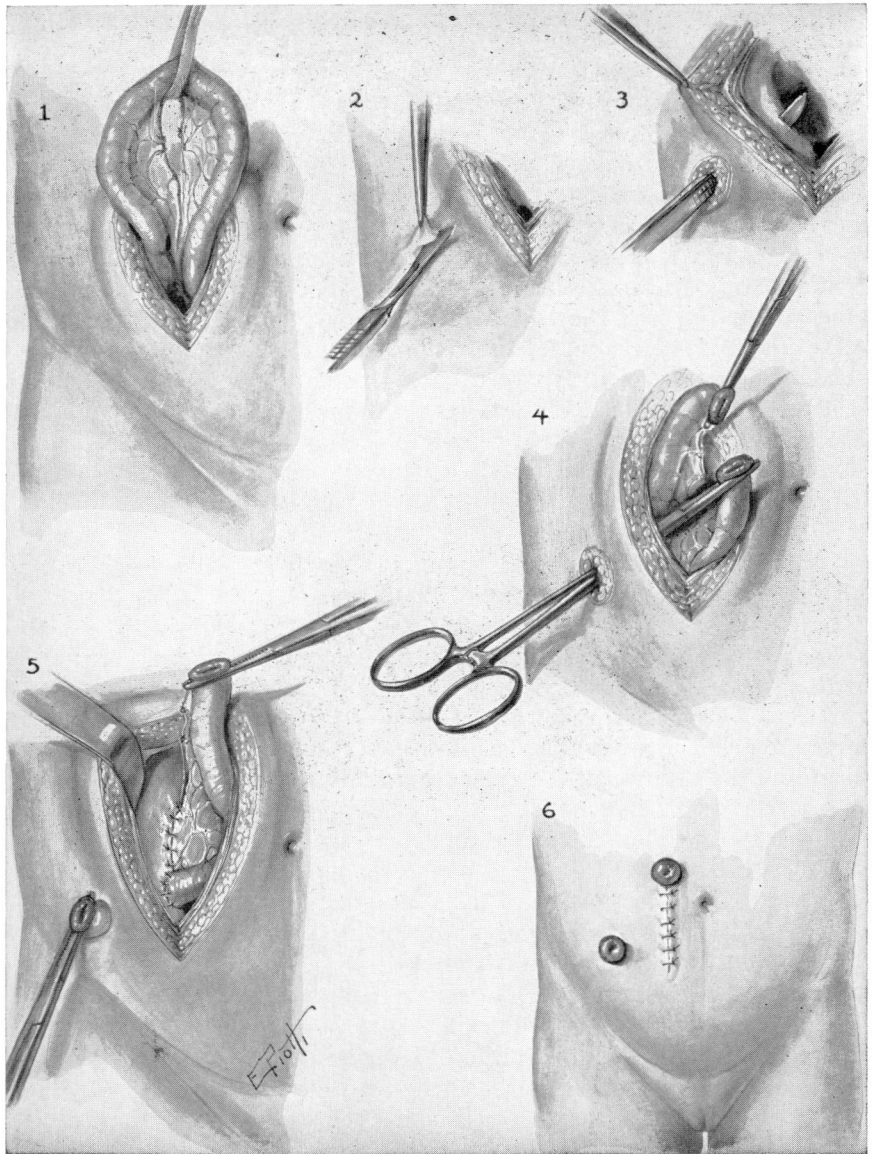

Fig. 178. Method of establishment of stab wound ileostomy (after Lahey). 1. Severance of mesentery at an appropriate distance from the ileocecal valve. The proximal ileum will be brought through a stab wound and the end of its divided mesentery will be sutured to the parietal peritoneum (as shown in 5) to prevent prolapse of the ileum. 2. Making of stab wound. Skin tented up and cut off to produce a circular defect. Remainder of abdominal wall pierced by a knife. 3. Stab incision carried through the entire thickness of abdominal wall. 4. Ochsner clamps applied and ileum divided by cautery. Proximal end should be cleansed as carefully as possible before dragging it through the abdominal wall. 5. Proximal end of ileum brought out through the stab wound, anchored to the surrounding peritoneum, and the mesentery likewise sutured to the parietal peritoneum. The non-functioning distal end of ileum is brought out the upper end of the rectus wound, where it is most easily dealt with if a colectomy is to be performed subsequently. 6. Operation completed. The permanent ileostomy is situated in a smooth area of skin where it is easiest to cement an ileostomy bag to the skin. In small children it is sometimes necessary to make the ileostomy at a slightly higher level than shown, to get away from the navel and the prominence of the anterior-superior spine.

is concerned with the irritation or erosion of the abdominal wall by intestinal juices. The skin should be protected by some sticky, soothing ointment, for which a combination of zinc oxide ointment, castor oil, and Aristol, made up into a thick paste, serves admirably. It is well to point out that cutaneous lesions are best treated by avoiding them; if the skin is adequately protected from the first, erosion seldom occurs. Thorough cleansing and painting of the skin every few days with tincture of benzoin and then cementing on the ring of the ileostomy bag will keep the cutaneous surface in good condition in most instances. If ulceration ever develops, it is most quickly cured by placing the individual in a face-down position on a Bradford frame so that the ileostomy discharges can fall directly into a receptable placed beneath the frame. The skin is thus kept completely dry and can be coated with medications to best advantage.

Fitting of an Ileostomy Bag. Much improvement has taken place in recent years in the manufacture of ileostomy bags; these enormously reduce the difficulties in caring for the intestinal discharges and they are infinitely superior to the older appliances. The Rutzen bag, or one of the modifications of it, is made so that a rubber or plastic ring is cemented to the skin around the ileostomy, thereby providing a leak-proof attachment. To this can be fitted inexpensive plastic sacs, which when filled are discarded. This arrangement gives a minimum of mess, odor, and inconvenience. It is generally possible to get a bag fitted into place within a week or two after establishment of an ileostomy.

Subsequent Closure of Ileostomies. The establishment of an ileostomy for chronic ulcerative colitis in the adult has been conceded generally to be an irrevocable step. A slightly more optimistic view can be taken when one is dealing with patients in childhood, for in an occasional case the ileostomy can be closed after a number of years, and the fecal current returned through the colon without lighting up the local disease. It is impossible to predict which patients will be candidates for subsequent closure of an ileostomy. A short duration of symptoms before the establishment of an ileostomy does not necessarily imply that there will be a greater likelihood of subsequent closure of the opening. Indeed, some children with the longest standing lesions can have the ileostomy closed, whereas some who are surgically treated very early must have the ileostomy permanently. No prediction can be made regarding the length of time an ileostomy must be left open before it can be closed. In some cases there is sufficient improvement within a year to justify reestablishing the continuity of the alimentary tract; in others four or five years or more will be required before the stoma can be closed with any hope of success. In the majority of subjects the colon, while greatly improved, will never stand having the fecal stream turned back into it.

Criteria for Determining Time of Closure. The criteria for determining when an ileostomy can be closed are somewhat vague and as yet are poorly defined. Study and reevaluation of the condition of the colon should be made at six-monthly or yearly intervals. Roentgenologic examination by barium enema may be of little importance in this regard, because fibrosis within the colonic wall will permanently keep its lumen small and tube-like. The clinical course of the individual is quite important. Adequate weight gain and establishment of a good general physical condition are essential but not sufficient. Rectal discharges of blood or pus indicate that the colon is still in a precarious state. Proctoscopic examination gives the best information concerning the repair in the colonic mucous membrane. Closure of the ileostomy should not be contemplated unless the rectal and sigmoidal mucosa appear reasonably normal by direct observation.

As suggested by Stone,[17] the gentle introduction of a catheter into the anus and instillation of about a pint (depending upon the size of the individual) of physiologic saline which is then retrieved will give considerable information. If the returned fluid is bloody by gross or microscopic study, active lesions can be assumed to exist in the lower colon. Only when the various factors indicate that the colon is quiescent should one entertain any thought of closing an ileostomy.

Colectomy. For adults, there has been rather widespread recommendation of removal of the colon (and in some cases, the rectum) in all cases after an ileostomy has been established for chronic ulcerative colitis. For children, we take a more conservative view toward colectomy. When there is persistence of fever, infection, toxicity, or debilitating rectal discharges after an ileostomy has been established, it is clear that the child will be better off by removal of the colon (or the colon and rectum). However, such cases are distinctly in the minority. It is much more common experience, after diversion of the fecal stream, to have the colon quiet down reasonably well and to have the child blossom dramatically in health and in weight gain; under such circumstances we see little need for routine removal of the colon. Furthermore, there is an occasional patient for whom the ileostomy can subsequently be closed and the colon again made to function. Therefore we believe that, whenever possible, the colon should be spared so that the child can have this opportunity of having the continuity of alimentary tract reconstituted—even though this hope is only a faint one.

In treating ulcerative colitis in childhood, there is frequently a dilemma regarding surgical excision of the colon. On one side are those who feel that the colon should be saved whenever feasible because it is possible in a few cases to restore the continuity of the intestinal-colonic tract; on the other hand are those who feel that, once an ileostomy has been established, the colon should always be removed to avoid the risk of subsequent development of cancer. It seems to us that a reasonable policy for children would be: (1) Establish an ileostomy whenever there are clear indications to do so. (2) Subsequently remove the colon (or colon and rectum) if toxicity has not been brought under control by ileostomy alone. (3) If the patient's improvement in health is satisfactory after establishment of the ileostomy, spare the colon for at least five or six years to see if it can be used again to receive the fecal stream. (4) Beyond pubertal years remove any colon or rectum which still gives evidence of any important degree of inflammatory disease.

RESULTS OF TREATMENT

It is impossible to compare the results from series of medically and surgically treated patients, because the type of cases are never quite analogous to one another. Within the medical group will be a certain number of individuals with exceptionally mild forms of the disorder; the surgical list will include advanced stages of the disease

Table 39

Summary of Data from 22 Children with Chronic Ulcerative Colitis Treated by Ileostomy (up to 1939)

Case	Sex	Duration of Symptoms	Age at Ileostomy	Result
				Fatal Cases
1	F	1 yr.	4 yrs.	For 2 years greatly improved. At 6 years ileostomy closed. Died 2 weeks later of peritonitis.
2	M	8 mos.	8 yrs.	Greatly improved. Three years later closure of ileostomy followed by colonic flare-up. Death 3 months later, respiratory infection.

Table 39 (continued)

Case	Sex	Duration of Symptoms	Age at Ileostomy	Result
3	M	4 mos.	8 yrs.	Some improvement. Nine months later colectomy, death from peritonitis.
4	M	2 yrs.	9 yrs.	Died 1 month later, perforation of ulcers in ileum.
5	F	7 mos.	9 yrs.	Died 7 days later, perforation of colon.
6	M	7 yrs.	10 yrs.	Excellent improvement for 2 years. Death from jejunal volvulus. Colonic mucosa almost normal at autopsy.
7	F	4 yrs.	11 yrs.	Some improvement, then death 3 years later from adhesions and intestinal obstruction.
8	M	7 yrs.	13 yrs.	Died, carcinoma of colon at 13 years.
9	M	8 mos.	14 yrs.	Died 5 days later.

Surviving Cases

Case	Sex	Duration of Symptoms	Age at Ileostomy	Result
10	F	2 mos.	4 mos.	Gradual improvement. Still had ileostomy and some symptoms at 6 years.
11	M	4 mos.	11 mos.	Very satisfactory. At 3½ years ileostomy closed. Well 16 years later.
12	F	5 yrs.	6 yrs.	Greatly improved, 15 months later ileostomy closed.* Entirely well in subsequent 5 years followed.
13	M	4 mos.	7 yrs.	Improved. No colon symptoms. Still had ileostomy at 12 years.
14	F	2 yrs.	8 yrs.	Excellent result. At 10 years ileostomy closed. No recurrences in subsequent 23 years followed.
15	F	3 mos.	8 yrs.	Some improvement. Still had colon symptoms 1 year later.
16	M	7 mos.	9 yrs.	Great improvement.
17	M	10 mos.	10 yrs.	Improving in 8 months followed.
18	F	3 yrs.	10 yrs.	Rapid improvement. At 18 years ileostomy closed.† Excellent health in subsequent 8 years followed.
19	F	5 yrs.	11 yrs.	Very satisfactory. At 13 years ileostomy closed. Well for 8 years followed.
20	F	9 mos.	11 yrs.	Greatly improved. Asymptomatic 3 years later.
21	F	11 mos.	11 yrs.	Great improvement.
22	M	4 yrs.	14 yrs.	Satisfactory improvement.

* Ileostomy and closure at another hospital.
† Closed at another hospital.

which have been refractile to all medical measures and which have been subjected to surgery in despair and even as a lifesaving measure. Therefore, the number of fatalities will probably always be higher in those treated surgically. A prolongation of medical treatment in any given case does not necessarily insure against a fatality, because colonic perforation, marasmus, and superimposed infection take an appreciable toll of patients treated solely by conservative measures.

Therapeutic Possibilities of Ileostomy

While there are certain advantages in the surgical treatment of this disease, the disagreeable nature of an ileostomy might make the treatment seem worse than the original complaints in the mind of patient or physician. Neglect of an ileostomy, development of cutaneous erosions around an intestinal opening, the change of habits required by a discharge of fecal material through an orifice other than the anus, can all be

Table 40

Data from 10 Cases with Chronic Ulcerative Colitis Treated by Ileostomy (1939 through 1950)

Case	Sex	Duration of Symptoms	Age at Ileostomy	Result
1	M	5 yrs.	8 yrs.	Only fair general condition in 7 years followed. Probably should have colectomy.
2	M	3 mos.	10 yrs.	Excellent result for 26 months, following which ileostomy was closed. In 8 months exacerbation of disease requiring right hemi-colectomy and reestablishment of ileostomy. Excellent health for subsequent 9 years followed.
3	F	1 yr.	11 yrs.	Excellent course for 2 years followed.
4	F	2 yrs.	10 yrs.	Fair course for 2 years, then severe exacerbation. Subtotal colectomy (elsewhere) 5 years after ileostomy; good course for 3 years after this.
5	F	3 mos.	5 yrs.	Up and down course for 5 years, with slow progression of disease. Subtotal colectomy 5 years after ileostomy. Excellent health 9 years after establishment of ileostomy.
6	F	2 yrs.	12 yrs.	Continued active disease without improvement for 16 months followed. Should have colectomy.
7	M	4 mos.	5 yrs.	Slow gradual improvement during 7 years followed.
8	M	2 yrs.	10 yrs.	Intermittent bouts of colitis; general condition poor. Because of revulsive attitude toward ileostomy, it was closed (elsewhere) at 6 years. Excellent for the year followed since then.
9	M	1 mo.	3 yrs.	Ileostomy established as an emergency procedure. Excellent course following this. Ileostomy closed 10 months later.
10	M	3 mos.	9 yrs.	Continued bloody diarrhea and failure to gain weight after ileostomy. 7 months later subtotal colectomy performed wh considerable improvement.

upsetting. However, with the proper fitting of a modern ileostomy bag (which can be cemented to the skin and which carries disposable plastic sacs) and with adequate supervision of its use, the disturbing features of an ileostomy can be minimized. It is most gratifying to see many of these deathly ill youngsters gain 40 to 50 pounds within a short space of time. In most instances the discharges of mucus, pus, and blood from the rectum will gradually diminish in number, and while they may not completely disappear they are reduced to a tolerable level.

Up to 1939, 22 children were subjected to ileostomy at the Children's Hospital; data from these patients are listed in Table 39. The ileostomy has been closed in 7 of these (from fifteen months to eight years later). One died of peritonitis incident to the closure and another died of pneumonia. The remaining 5 were in good health during the three years, five years, five years, eight years, and eight years respectively since closure of the openings.

From 1939 through 1950, 10 children were subjected to ileostomy (Table 40). As a whole, this group probably had better supportive care in the way of general supervision, vitamin administration, chemotherapy, etc. There have been no deaths. For one patient, a right hemi-colectomy was necessary. For two patients subtotal colectomies were done, with considerable additional improvement in their clinical pictures. One patient required complete removal of the colon and rectum. Two children have had closures of their ileostomies, six years and ten months respectively, after their establishment; they appear to be tolerating the closure very well.

REFERENCES

1. Bargen, J. A.: Chronic Ulcerative Colitis; Review of Investigations on Etiology. Arch. Int. Med., 45:559, 1930.
2. Beranbaum, S. L. and Waldron, R. J.: Chronic Ulcerative Colitis. Case Report in a Newborn Infant. Pediatrics, 9:773, 1952.
3. Cattell, R. B.: New Type of Ileostomy for Chronic Ulcerative Colitis. S. Clin. North America, 19:629, 1939.
4. Cave, H. W.: Chronic Intractable Ulcerative Colitis—A Surgical Problem. J.A.M.A., 113:549, 1939.
5. Elliott, J. M., Kiefer, E. D. and Hurxthal, L. M.: The Treatment of Chronic Ulcerative Colitis with ACTH. New England J. Med., 245:288, 1951.
6. Grace, W. J., Wolf, S. and Wolff, H. G.: Life Situations, Emotions, and Chronic Ulcerative Colitis. J.A.M.A., 142:1044, 1950.
7. Hart, J. A.: Ulcerative Colitis with Perforation in Newborn. Texas State J. Med., 42:286, 1946.
8. Jackman, R. J., Bargen, J. A. and Helmholz, H. F.: Life Histories of 95 Children with Chronic Ulcerative Colitis; Statistical Study Based on Comparison with Whole Group of 871 Patients. Am. J. Dis. Child., 59:459, 1940.
9. Ladd, W. E. and Fothergill, L. D.: Idiopathic Ulcerative Colitis in Children. M. Clin. North America, 19:1673, 1936.
10. Lahey, F. H.: Advantages of a Stab Wound Ileostomy. Surg., Gynec. & Obst., 95:29, 1952.
11. Lium, R.: Etiology of Ulcerative Colitis: II. Effect of Induced Muscular Spasm on Colonic Explants in Dogs, with Comment on Relation of Muscular Spasm to Ulcerative Colitis. Arch. Int. Med., 63:210, 1939.
12. Lium, R.: Observations on Etiology of Ulcerative Colitis. Am. J. M. Sc., 197:841, 1939.
13. McKittrick, L. S. and Miller, R. H.: Idiopathic Ulcerative Colitis. Ann. Surg., 102:656, 1935.
14. Patterson, H. A.: Surgery in Ulcerative Colitis. New York State J. Med., 51:2135, 1951.
15. Ravitch, M. M.: Total Colectomy for Benign Conditions, with Consideration of Anal Ileostomy with Sphincter Preservation. Virginia M. Monthly, 77:55, 1950.
16. Shands, W. C., Dockerty, M. B. and Bargen, J. A.: Adenocarcinoma of the Large Intestine Associated with Chronic Ulcerative Colitis. Clinical and Pathological Features of 73 Cases. Surg., Gynec. & Obst., 94:302, 1952.
17. Stone, H. B.: Surgical Problems in the Treatment of Chronic Ulcerative Colitis. Arch. Surg., 41:525, 1940.

CHAPTER 23

Congenital Megacolon (Hirschsprung's Disease)

While there were reports of megacolon in the literature antedating the publication of Hirschsprung in 1888, his description of and focus on the abnormality have led to widespread use of the term "Hirschsprung's disease" for congenital dilatation of the colon. This disease is certainly not uncommon. From the earliest weeks or months of life there is great difficulty in moving the bowels, and the colon becomes enormously distended and filled with gas and fecal material, leading to marked abdominal distention, poor nutrition, and even respiratory distress. Through the past few decades there have been numerous conflicting theories regarding the etiology of the condition, but there now seems to be rather universal recognition of the underlying etiologic factor. Within recent years clarification has come into the therapy of congenital megacolon; surgery now has much to offer those infants and children who are afflicted with advanced degrees of the abnormality.

PATHOLOGY AND ETIOLOGY

The entire colon, or portions thereof, may be many times normal caliber, and it is not uncommon to find loops 6 or 7 inches in diameter in older children. The greatly dilated gut contains tremendous accumulations of gas and inspissated fecal material. The colonic wall is greatly hypertrophied, has a leathery consistency, and may be thickened to as much as an eighth or a quarter of an inch. The haustrations are largely or completely lost. From pressure-erosion by the fecal masses, mucosal ulcerations are sometimes seen.

A view of the rectum and colon as a whole shows findings in their various portions which are of great importance in the understanding of the fundamental deficiency in this disease. The rectum and the rectosigmoid appear to have a normal caliber and thickness of wall, whereas the sigmoid above this is greatly distended and hypertrophied, and is filled with fecal material; the distention and thickening gradually become less marked as one progresses upward in the bowel. In some cases the enlargement is confined to the sigmoid loop itself, but it is more characteristic to have the changes extend up as high as the splenic flexure or the transverse colon; in advanced cases the entire colon, from the rectosigmoid upward, is enormously distended, the changes being most marked in the lower portion of the colon. In some instances the accumulations within the colon produce a backing-up and a distention of the terminal or even the mid-ileum.

At no point in the rectum or rectosigmoid is there a stenosis or scarring of the wall, but the entire picture in the colon above this consists of the changes which are characteristically found proximal to any point in the alimentary tract where there is

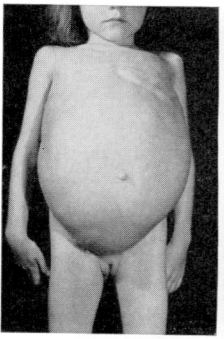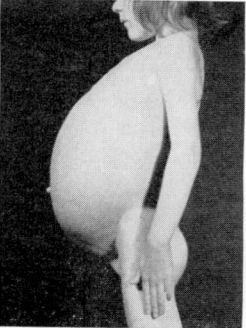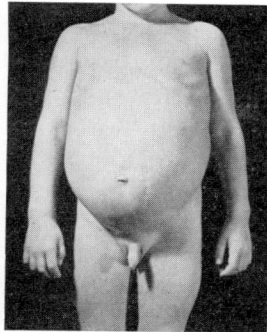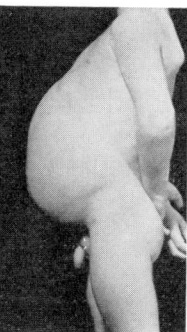

Fig. 179. Two children with marked Hirschsprung's disease. *Left,* Nine-year-old girl, with great abdominal distention and poor nutrition. *Right,* Four-year-old boy who had previously been treated with a colostomy, with prompt relief of the distention. Closure of the colostomy was quickly followed again by the colonic enlargement.

mechanical obstruction of long standing. It has become apparent that obstruction in patients with congenital megacolon is caused by a neuromuscular defect in the rectum, the rectosigmoid, or the lower part of the sigmoid itself; because of a local neuro-muscular deficiency, peristaltic waves are unable to pass properly through the recto-sigmoid area. This is an important change in the concept of the etiology of the disease; it used to be thought widely that the enlarged and thickened colon was the abnormal structure, whereas now there seems to be little doubt that these are merely effects which are secondary to the neuromuscular deficiency which exists in the bowel in the vicinity of the rectosigmoid junction.

The concept that there is a dyskinesia in the rectosigmoid area is supported by histologic examinations showing neural deficiencies. For many years studies of single cases, and more recently of series of specimens, have shown that there is a profound nerve cell defect in the rectum or rectosigmoid. As early as 1901, Tittel noted scantiness and also degenerative changes in ganglion cells of the myenteric plexus of the large

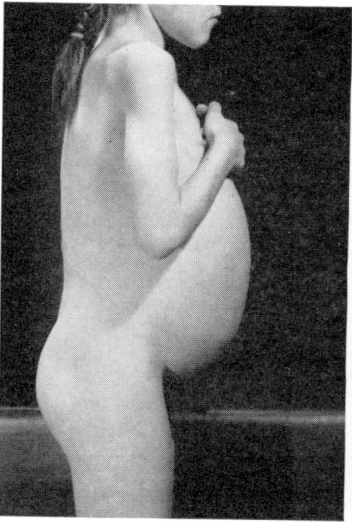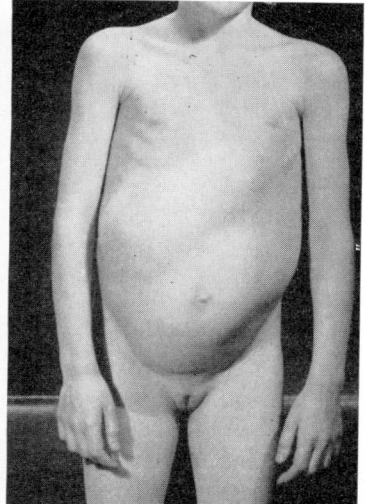

Fig. 180. Nine-year-old girl with advanced Hirschsprung's disease. In the right photograph the huge loops of colon are plainly visible.

intestine and concluded that the normal progression of peristalsis might have been influenced unfavorably by the neurologic abnormality. From this time until 1940, nine separate studies were published, all of which pointed out that the disturbances were of a neurologic nature in the colon wall. These papers were admirably summarized in 1948 by Whitehouse and Kernohan,[20] who also made an excellent pathologic study of 11 cases of congenital megacolon and found the myenteric plexus to be absent in the most

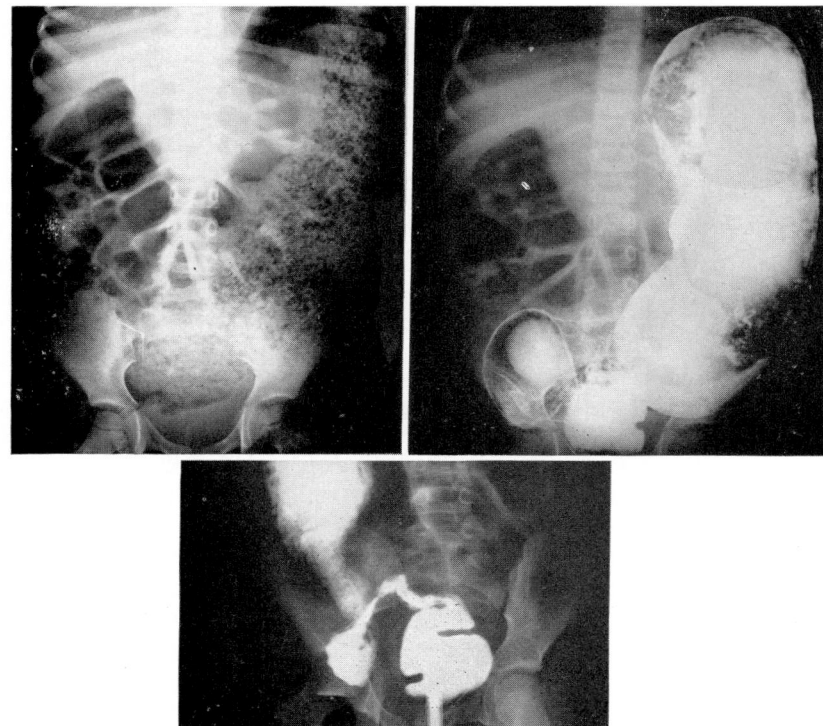

Fig. 181. Roentgenogram from an eight-year-old girl with well advanced congenital megacolon. The left upper film shows great accumulation of fecal material in the descending colon and sigmoid. The right upper film shows the enormous distention of the colon as visualized with a barium enema. *Below,* With a small amount of barium, attention is focused on the rectosigmoid junction, turning the patient in an oblique position to give best visualization of this region. The rectum has a normal caliber. The upper sigmoid is markedly dilated. The bowel at the rectosigmoid junction is narrow, and is the site of a dyskinesia. Peristaltic waves from the sigmoid would not pass through the abnormal rectosigmoid area. The narrowness is not due to stricture, but to neuromuscular incoordination.

distal part of the colon in all cases. In 1949 Swenson et al. confirmed such observations of neurologic deficit in the rectum or lower sigmoid, and on the basis of such observations made an important advance in the treatment of the disease, emphasizing that the therapy should be directed towards the removal of this segment which was neurologically deficient, rather than focusing attention on the dilated and hypertrophied portion of bowel above it.

Microscopic examination of blocks removed from various levels of the colon (Fig. 182) shows that in all cases of congenital megacolon there is a segment of bowel (usually in the rectum, rectosigmoid or lower sigmoid, but occasionally at a higher level) in which ganglions of the myenteric plexus are absent, are greatly reduced in number, or have within them only a small number of nerve cells (Fig. 183). This atrophy—or absence—of nerve cells is not accompanied by scarring, stricture, or other important change in the segment. Between the two muscular coats one can frequently find nerve fibrils, which indeed seem to be distinctly more prominent than those which are generally found in normal colons. There can be little doubt that the anatomic deficiency in nerve structures of the myenteric plexus is the factor which brings about disturbance of peristaltic motility in the area.

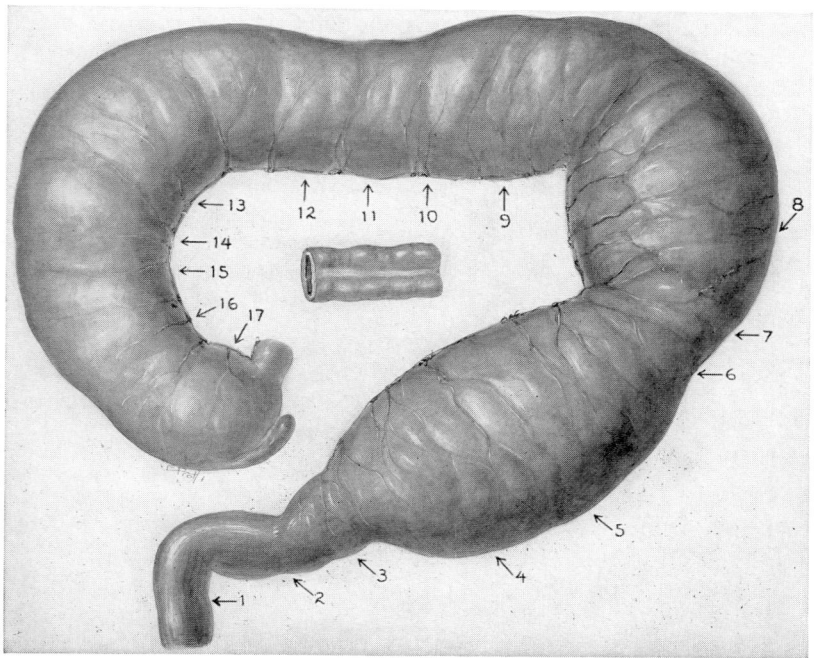

Fig. 182. Histopathologic observation from a case of congenital megacolon. (From Whitehouse and Kernohan.[20]) Note the normal size of the rectum and the great distention and hypertrophy of the colon proximal to this. (The segment of bowel in the center is normal colon for comparison in size.) The numbers indicate locations from which blocks of tissue were taken for microscopic study of the bowel wall. Areas 1 through 4 contained no ganglia, 5 through 7 contained a few, and 8 through 17 contained a normal number.

Nothing is known regarding the cause for the nerve cell changes in these cases. Whether the deficit reflects a congenital lack of development, or whether it is due to degeneration from hypoxia shortly before, or after, delivery of the baby has not been ascertained.

Occasionally, a megalo-ureter accompanies the condition of Hirschsprung's disease, and this suggests that there has been likewise a faulty neuromuscular balance in the ureter, in the bladder, or at the bladder outlet.

CLINICAL FINDINGS

History

Hirschsprung's disease is a congenital lesion and the initial symptoms appear shortly after birth or in early infancy. (In those children in whom colonic dilatation and obstipation first make their appearance after the second year of life, one should strongly suspect that the megacolon is not of the congenital variety.) From infancy, and progressing through the years, there is obstinate constipation and marked enlargement of the abdomen. There may be no bowel movements for many days, and some of the patients go as long as several weeks between defecations. While constipation is the rule, at times diarrhea may appear if fluid intestinal material is passed around inert solid fecal masses which lie in the colon. Distention, fetid odor of the breath, anorexia, lassitude, and malnourishment are the rule. The diaphragm may be displaced upward and cause compression-atelectasis of the lung bases; the distention may be so severe that respiratory and circulatory embarrassment culminate in death. Vomiting is seldom an outstanding feature. These individuals may have long periods with only mild or moderate complaints, superimposed upon which there are episodes simulating acute intestinal obstruction. Hospitalization or medical advice may be first sought during one of these attacks.

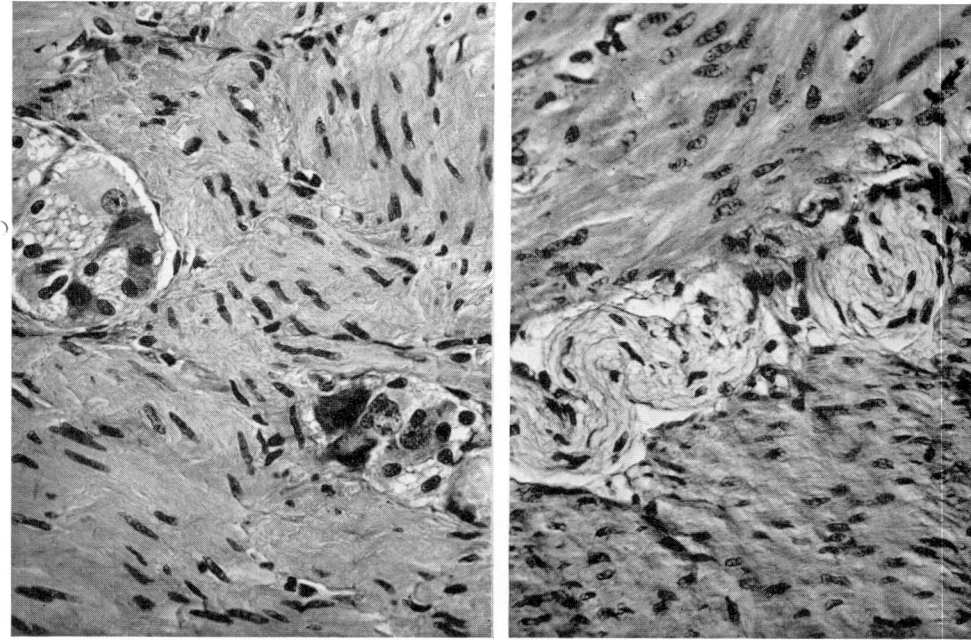

Fig. 183. Photomicrographs of the rectosigmoid at the interface of circular and longitudinal muscular coats. *Left,* From a normal colon, showing the nerve cells of the myenteric plexus. *Right,* From a patient with Hirschsprung's disease, showing absence of ganglion cells.

Physical Findings

Ninety per cent of the patients are males. On examination the abdomen is found protruding, and its skin is thin, tense, and shiny. Dilated veins may course over the wall. The umbilicus is often everted and pouting. Palpation shows massive accumulations of gas and fecal material in various parts of the abdomen. Not infrequently the colon, distended to several times its normal diameter, can be mapped out by palpation; in many cases the outlines of the bulging organ can be seen through the abdominal wall. It is sometimes possible to feel—even through the abdominal wall—that the colon is tremendously thickened and hypertrophied. Often the greatly distended abdomen appears to be an inert reservoir, but it is not uncommon to see or feel great waves passing along a dilated and hypertrophied colon which indicate that it is working against some sort of an obstruction in its distal portion. Auscultation often reveals increased and high-pitched peristaltic activity. During these peristaltic rushes the child may experience severe abdominal cramps, but generally the youngster has little sensation at these times. Rectal examination reveals no obstruction of a stenotic nature, either at the anus or within reach of the finger. In small subjects it is sometimes possible to introduce the index finger far enough to feel an area of spasm at the recto-sigmoid junction. The rectum may contain a good deal of fecal material, but rather commonly it is found to be empty. Such an observation, in the presence of huge palpable fecal masses in the colon above, is indicative of some sort of obstruction in the intervening rectosigmoid area. Edema of the legs may be seen in severe cases.

Varying degrees of the clinical picture are encountered. In less severe cases, constipation and slight abdominal distention are all that are noted. The child gets along reasonably well without a physician's care. The parents have generally learned that the child requires enemas, the frequent use of cathartics, large amounts of fruit juice and other measures to keep the bowel reasonably cleared out. In more severe cases the condition almost always calls for some form of medical or surgical supervision. In advanced states the patient's malnutrition, toxemia, and respiratory embarrassment combine to make a dire situation which demands urgent and effective therapy if a fatality is to be avoided.

Study of Urinary Tract

Before operation is undertaken on anyone with Hirschsprung's disease, it is quite important to investigate the urinary tract for neurologic deficits which are known to occur in a small percentage of patients. All of these subjects should have a measurement of the residual urine, should have visualization of the urinary tract by intravenous pyelography, and whenever any deficiency of bladder function is suspected there should be cystometrographic study.

ROENTGENOLOGIC FINDINGS

The correct diagnosis is often suggested by plain films of the abdomen which show a markedly distended colon, containing large volumes of gas or massive amounts of mottled, fecal material.

Examination with the use of a barium enema discloses no mechanical obstruction. The sigmoid, and to a lesser extent the entire colon above it, are tremendously enlarged, extremely capacious, and are thrown into great redundant loops. These overlie one another and seem to fill almost the entire abdomen. Haustrations are flattened out or are completely lost. Megacolon may be so marked that the bowel can receive literally quarts or gallons of fluid, making the abdomen quite opaque.

Examination with a barium enema must be done with some caution because the atonic gut may collect large amounts of the barium mixture which the patient is then unable to expel. Some children have great distress after such a study and, indeed, in one of our subjects it was necessary to resort immediately to a colostomy for prevention of what appeared to be impending death.

It is not necessary to fill the colon to the limit of its capacity to gain an accurate picture of the pathology; indeed, it is unwise to do so. Ballooning of the colon with a barium mixture not only may produce great distress in the patient, but it is also apt to obscure and make impossible an adequate examination of the rectosigmoid area, which Neuhauser has shown to be the zone of greatest importance during roentgenologic study. After it has been determined that the colon is enlarged and that there is no stricture as the cause of such enlargement, attention should be focused (either at this time or at a subsequent examination when the colon has been cleared of barium) on the rectum and rectosigmoid, injecting only a very small amount of barium into the rectum. The patient is examined in antero-posterior, lateral, and particularly in oblique views, to throw into relief and thereby visualize the terminal 6 to 10 inches. The caliber of the rectum and rectosigmoid is normal, or is possibly somewhat reduced in size. That this is not due to intrinsic stenosis or fibrosis is evident by the fact that from time to time these structures can dilate. The important finding is a dissociation of neuromuscular activity. The rectosigmoid area will frequently become spastic. Any peristaltic waves coming down the sigmoid will terminate abruptly at the rectosigmoid, there being a failure of normal progression of the wave across this zone. This dyskinesia in the rectosigmoid, or in the lower sigmoid, is found in all cases in which appropriate studies are made for its detection (Fig. 181).

TREATMENT

CONSERVATIVE TREATMENT

There can be no doubt that Hirschsprung's disease occurs in varying degrees of severity; by no means is it necessary to operate upon all individuals who have this condition. In those with a milder variety, the situation can be brought under control and the child can be carried along in a very satisfactory manner by appropriate medical management. Much can be accomplished if the diet is supervised, if mineral oil is constantly used, and if colonic lavage is systemically employed. This regimen can be conducted at home if the parent is intelligent and cooperative, but occasional periods of hospitalization may be necessary if fecal impaction becomes troublesome or if stricter management is required temporarily for deflation of the bowel.

The use of parasympathetic stimulants such as physostigmine has been rather disappointing. Doryl and Mecholyl bromide (acetyl-beta-methylcholine bromide) are potent activators of the parasympathetic system and have given promising results in a few cases. Acetylcholine derivatives have an enhanced activity when combined with neostigmine. While these drugs can have dramatic effects on the colon, they do not always produce an evacuation. We have observed some children with Hirschsprung's disease immediately after the administration of Mecholyl and have found a greatly augmented activity of the colon; within a few minutes the bowel begins to have violent contractions which are audible and are visible through the abdominal wall. Unfortunately, these contractions appear to be largely segmental ones and there is little or no advance of a peristaltic wave along the colon to produce a bowel movement. It is our impression that parasympathetic stimulants have a very limited use in treatment of Hirschsprung's disease, but in the milder forms of the condition, Mecholyl bromide has been shown[11] to have beneficial effects which are sufficient to give the child reasonably good elimination.

How long conservative measures should be employed must be decided from case to case, and depends upon the circumstances which exist. In the milder forms of the condition, such management is all that is required and can lead to fairly normal life and hea'th. In more advanced states, it may be obvious from the start that surgical therapy will eventually be necessary, but it is generally advisable to attempt handling the child first by conservative measures so that the parents and all concerned with the case can become convinced that more radical steps are required.

SURGICAL PROCEDURES

While many patients with this disease are relieved by supportive treatment, including dietary control, colonic lavage, and administration of drugs, there are a large number who must be treated by operative measures. Surgical procedures to be considered are: (1) Cecostomy or colostomy. (2) Sympathectomy. (3) Resection of a dilated loop, or a complete colectomy (preserving the rectum). (4) An abdominoperineal operation, removing the rectosigmoid which is the seat of a neurologic deficit and dyskinesia.

Sympathectomy

Observations on patients with Hirschsprung's disease have shown that elimination of the sympathetic control will increase the tone of the colon and will often produce evacuations. Such observations do not in any way vitiate the idea that the fundamental disturbance in megacolon is related to a dyskinesia in the rectosigmoid junction or lower sigmoid, which is brought about by local absence or diminution of nerve cells. Blockage of the sympathetic innervation merely augments the tone and peristaltic activity of the colon above the rectosigmoid area so that some fecal material is forced through the inert zone. To determine what effect removal of the sympathetic control might have, it is possible to give the patient a spinal anesthesia, which to be fully effective should reach as high as the nipples. During the subsequent hour observations are made to see if the colon has increased peristalsis, if flatus or feces are passed per anum, and if the colon becomes deflated. It is sometimes possible to gain dramatic results during such a test.

If a sympathectomy has produced a marked deflation of the colon, one is tempted to believe that a surgical removal (or the interruption) of the sympathetic apparatus might permanently give such a desirable change. The abdominal sympathetic chains have an outflow through the first, second, third, fourth, and fifth ganglia which lie on either side of the great abdominal vessels. Anatomic studies have shown considerable variation in the number, size, position, and connections of these ganglia. The chains coalesce and form a plexus over the promontory of the sacrum; the lower parts of this network, or the hypogastric nerves, course downward along the posterior walls of the pelvis, toward the rectum and genitalia. In males, it has been agreed generally that removal of the right and the left first lumbar ganglia produces sterility. Likewise, excision of the pre-sacral plexus will interfere with the ejaculatory apparatus. Therefore, if sympathectomy is to be performed in a male, it should be limited to the removal of the second, third, fourth, and possibly fifth lumbar ganglia on either side. In females, more extensive dissection is permissible without deleterious effects on the reproductive apparatus.

Sympathectomy for the treatment of Hirschsprung's disease is rapidly falling into disfavor. It is rare to attain the dramatic deflation of a colon which can be gained by a high spinal anesthesia; apparently the removal of that portion which is surgically available gives a much less extensive sympathetic blockage than can be accomplished temporarily by high spinal anesthesia. Whenever it has been performed in a series of cases, sympathectomy has generally led to much disappointment, though in an occasional case it will change the nerve balance in such a way that it gives fairly good relief of symptoms. On the whole, the operation has given such poor results that it is now seldom used.

Cecostomy or Colostomy

In those patients with acute retention or severe distress, cecostomy or transverse colostomy can bring immediate relief, and indeed may be a lifesaving procedure. Opening the gut in this manner permits a rapid deflation of the proximal portion of the colon and of the small intestine. It provides another route for the introduction of mineral oil, soapy solutions, and other fluids aimed at disintegration and removal of fecal masses which are impacted in the left half of the colon.

While we formerly believed that cecostomy might be used in some cases as a temporary decompression (over a period of one or two years), and that the colon would collapse or regain normal tone and activity making it possible for it to function reasonably well after closure of the colostomy, we now are sure that this is a forlorn hope. It is perfectly true that a cecostomy (or a transverse colostomy) can allow lavage and decompression of the distal colon, can permit deflation of the intestine, and can improve the child's nutritional status, comfort, and well being, but these improvements are merely temporary and they persist only as long as the vent is left open. When subsequently this opening is closed, we have found that the colon again becomes distended and that all of the disturbances of Hirschsprung's disease promptly return. Therefore, cecostomy (or colostomy) should be used only as a preliminary procedure to: (1) Permit deferral of operation on the rectosigmoid of small babies under six or eight months of age (when the rectal operation is technically difficult). (2) Serve as an emergency procedure for a child of any age who cannot be appropriately cleansed by enemas. (3) Act as an initial step in a few of the older children in whom it is desirable to improve the nutritional status or to gain better deflation of the colon prior to surgical removal of the rectosigmoid region (by abdomino-perineal operation).

Cecostomy (or transverse colostomy) may be performed under local or general anesthesia. For cecostomy, a McBurney incision is quite satisfactory. For right transverse colostomy, a short vertical incision with a rectus-splitting opening is adequate. The cecum or colon should, if possible, be withdrawn from the abdomen and sutured to the abdominal wall before it is opened. If the bowel can be handled in this way, soiling of the peritoneal cavity is completely avoided.

It is important to emphasize that the decision for or against subsequent resection of the rectosigmoid must always be made before any cecostomy or transverse colostomy is established. If it is not determined previously that there is a malfunctioning segment in the rectosigmoid area, it is almost impossible to demonstrate this (by x-ray) after a cecostomy or a colostomy has been made. Such vents allow the entire colon to collapse so that any subsequent examination (while the colostomy is still open) shows a colon of rather normal caliber throughout and no change which can be identified certainly as abnormal in the rectosigmoid area.

Transabdominal Resection

Local Resection. Removal of the dilated sigmoid loop (or more extensive portions of the colon) is an operation of considerable merit. Selected individuals have been given great relief for many years, through such procedures but there is always the possibility that the process might recur and that subsequently the remaining colon will become dilated and hypertrophied.

In the 1930's we had 9 patients who were treated by resection of the transverse colon or an enlarged sigmoid loop. One of these patients died of peritonitis. In one there was no change and in one there was slight improvement. One was in a very satisfactory state for fourteen years, after which there was recurrence and involvement of other parts of the colon. Five were greatly improved and in excellent condition when last seen one, four, seven, eleven and twelve years, respectively, after operation.

More recently State[14] has again revived this form of therapy and has treated patients with the method, excising the dilated portion of the colon, emphasizing removal of the narrowed rectosigmoid, carrying the dissection down to the peritoneal floor, where the bowel could be cut across. An anastomosis is then made between the remaining portion of colon and rectum, making this union below the peritoneal floor, at a level 6 to 10 cm. from the anal skin margin. The operation was performed on 15 subjects, with no deaths. Fourteen were greatly benefited, but the remaining patient had to resort to enemas on some occasions after operation. The follow-up periods ranged from six months to three years. It was State's feeling that the saving of the rectum is important, because it eliminates the danger of damage to the nervi erigentes, and hence there can be no question about interference with the ejaculatory apparatus in the male. It is our own opinion that a one-stage transabdominal operative procedure with resection of the narrowed terminal segment of sigmoid and the dilated colon above it, followed by an anastomosis of the remaining ends (beneath the peritoneal floor), will probably give a satisfactory result in a large proportion of cases, and that the pelvic nerves can be protected in all subjects, but that when followed for long periods of time there probably will be higher recurrence rates of megacolon than will be the finding in patients treated by an abdomino-perineal removal of the rectum and rectosigmoid. Therefore, at the moment, we strongly favor the abdomino-perineal operation, believing that it will result in a higher percentage of permanent cures. During the next decade or two it will be necessary to have more extensive observations following both types of operation to give a final evaluation of each and to determine which is the superior method.

Complete Colectomy. Late in the thirties we treated 3 children with megacolon by complete removal of the colon, anastomosing the terminal ileum to a stump of rectosigmoid, just above the peritoneal floor. Two of these children died shortly after operation, from disruption of the suture lines. The third patient was extremely well for one year, after which time he developed ulcerations just above the anastomotic area; these perforated and produced a fatal peritonitis. While we were initially encouraged by the last boy, the subsequent death of all three patients has now led us to abandon colectomy for treatment of this disease.

Abdomino-perineal Removal of the Rectosigmoid

The outstanding work of Swenson and his co-workers emphasized that the fundamental defect in Hirschsprung's disease was confined to a short segment of bowel, generally the rectosigmoid, wherein there was a neurologic deficiency which interfered with the propagation of peristaltic waves. This concept led to surgical removal of the neurologically deficient zone. It was felt that the dilated and enlarged colon above this need not necessarily be excised, since this would spontaneously deflate when the obstruction was removed. It is practically impossible to accomplish a low removal of the rectosigmoid and a major portion of the rectum, working solely through the abdomen. Hence a technique was perfected which allowed a low resection by a combined abdominal and perineal approach. The essential features of this operation are shown in Figure 185. While the various steps in the abdomino-perineal "pull-through" operation are depicted in the drawings, some comments here might be of some value.

After opening the peritoneal floor within the abdomen, the dissection is made around the rectum as far down as can be reached, carrying this as close to the rectal wall as possible, to minimize the danger of injury to surrounding nerves. While it might seem that the dissection has been extended far into the pelvis, approaching the anus, all too frequently it is found that the operator has not carried the liberation far enough. It is therefore always advisable to reglove and insert a finger into the anus (or have an assistant do this) so that while working from above it can be determined accurately just how far the mobilization has been done. *If the freeing is not carried well down toward the anus, there is little point in performing an abdomino-perineal "pull-through" type of operation,* because little more will have been gained than could have been accomplished by a transabdominal approach alone, and placing the anastomosis below the peritoneal floor.

After the rectum has been liberated, and an appropriate portion of mesosigmoid has been divided, it is sometimes possible to invert the sigmoid and pull it out through the anus as has been described by Hiatt.[8] However, we have found that in most patients the sigmoid loop is so bulky and thick that it is very difficult to pull it out through the anus, particularly in a baby or a small child. To facilitate matters, we therefore usually excise and discard the great sigmoid loop, a step which can be quickly performed by

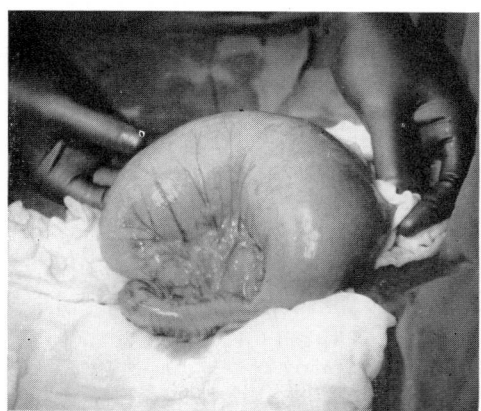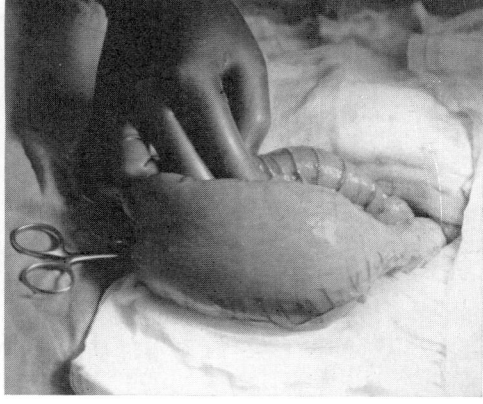

Fig. 184. Photographs taken at the operating table, showing great dilatation and thickening of the sigmoid. *Left,* From a seventeen-months-old boy. *Right,* From a four-year-old boy.

using von Petz clips at either end of the segment which is to be cut away. While this step has for its main purpose the removal of the unwieldy portion of bowel from the field, it also has the distinct advantage of allowing immediate, frozen section examination of the upper end of the specimen, to determine if the nerve cells are present. If such microscopic examination shows that nerve cells are absent, or greatly diminished in number, at this upper level, *it is essential to remove more of the sigmoid or the descending colon, cutting back to a point where nerve cells are found to be normal in number and size.* If such a precaution is not taken, a segment of colon is sometimes left in place which will not function properly and which might require more extensive excision at a subsequent time.

When the rectum has been freed, everted upon itself, and pulled out through the anus, its presenting membrane can be cleansed reasonably well with some solution such as aqueous Zephiran. The rectum is then opened close to the anus and the proximal portion of colon is drawn down through this rectal opening for establishment of an anastomosis. (Histologic examination of the rectal wall at the level where the anastomosis is performed almost always shows no ganglion cells because the neurologic defect generally extends down to the anus itself.) When the anastomosis is completed and the bowel is inverted into its normal alignment, digital examination should disclose a suture line which is no more than a centimeter or two above the anus. Every effort should be made to have the anastomosis as low in the rectum as possible, hoping in this way to

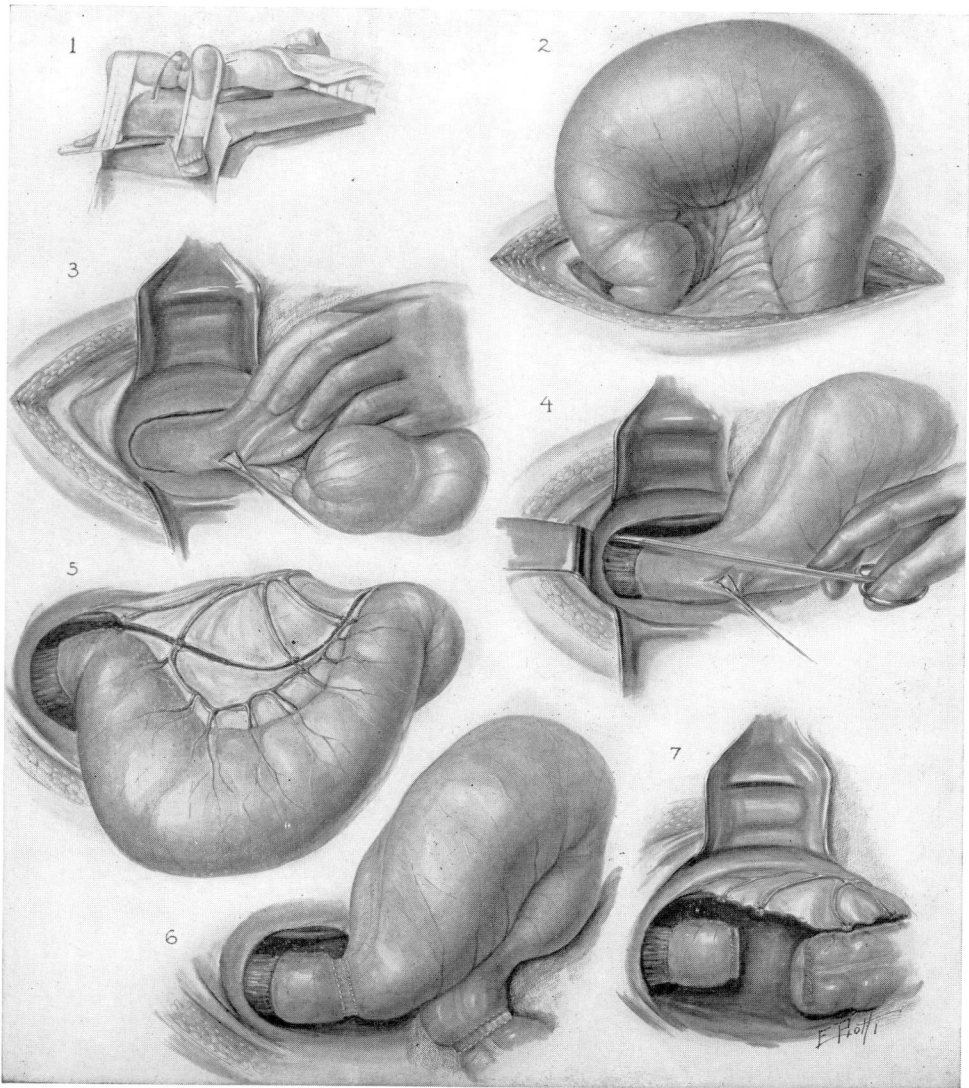

Fig. 185. Technique of abdomino-perineal resection of the rectosigmoid junction and removal of the distended sigmoid for treatment of Hirschsprung's disease. 1. Position of patient on the table, so that operation can be simultaneously carried out through the abdomen and the perineum. Urethral catheter in place. 2. Abdomen opened, showing the markedly thickened and dilated sigmoid loop which merges into the normal descending colon above and into bowel of normal caliber, without stenosis, in the rectosigmoid area. 3. Sigmoid held upward and peritoneal floor incised around the rectosigmoid. 4. Peritoneal floor opened. Ureters carefully avoided. With upward traction on the bowel, dissection is carried around the rectum well down toward the anus. 5. Mobilization of rectum completed. Meso-sigmoid divided. 6. Dilated sigmoid clamped below and above with von Petz clips. 7. Enlarged sigmoid loop removed. Remaining ends of the descending colon and rectum still closed with von Petz clips.

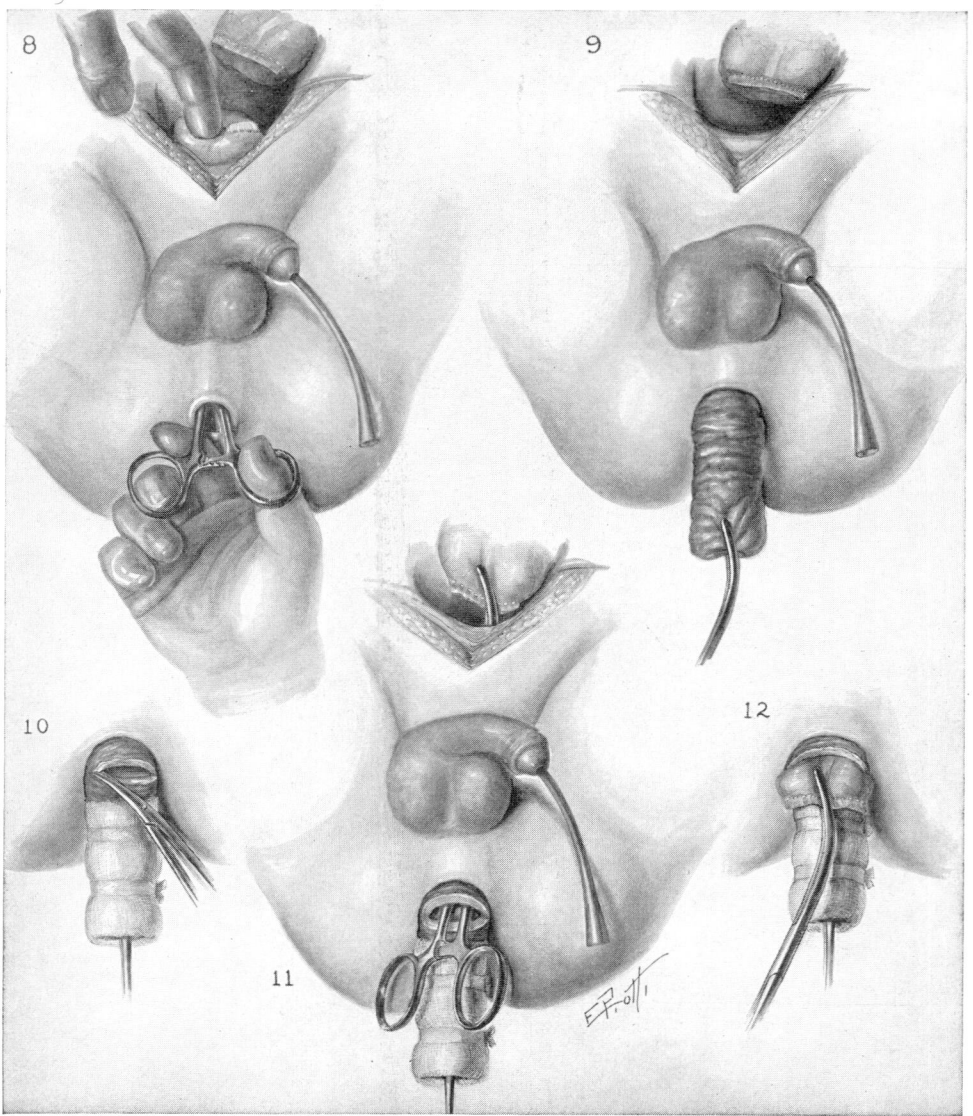

Fig. 185 (*continued*). 8. Full-length clamp introduced through the anus so the top of the rectum can be grasped. 9. Rectum completely prolapsed and everted. The presenting mucosa is then cleansed with antiseptic solution, such as aqueous Zephiran. 10. The lower portion of the everted rectum is covered with a gauze pad, the rectum being slit transversely, just outside of the anus. 11. Full-length clamp introduced through the rectal opening, to grasp the descending colon. 12. Descending colon pulled downward and out through the rectal opening.

leave a segment of minimal length which has neuro-muscular deficiency. If the anastomotic line is fairly close to the anus, a fecal bolus can be delivered to the anus and passed spontaneously.

It is generally possible to perform the abdomino-perineal "pull-through" operation without a preliminary cecostomy or transverse colostomy, provided the bowel is adequately lavaged, cleansed, and deflated prior to the time of operation. Such preparation might require a week or ten days. There are, however, two situations in which a prelimin-

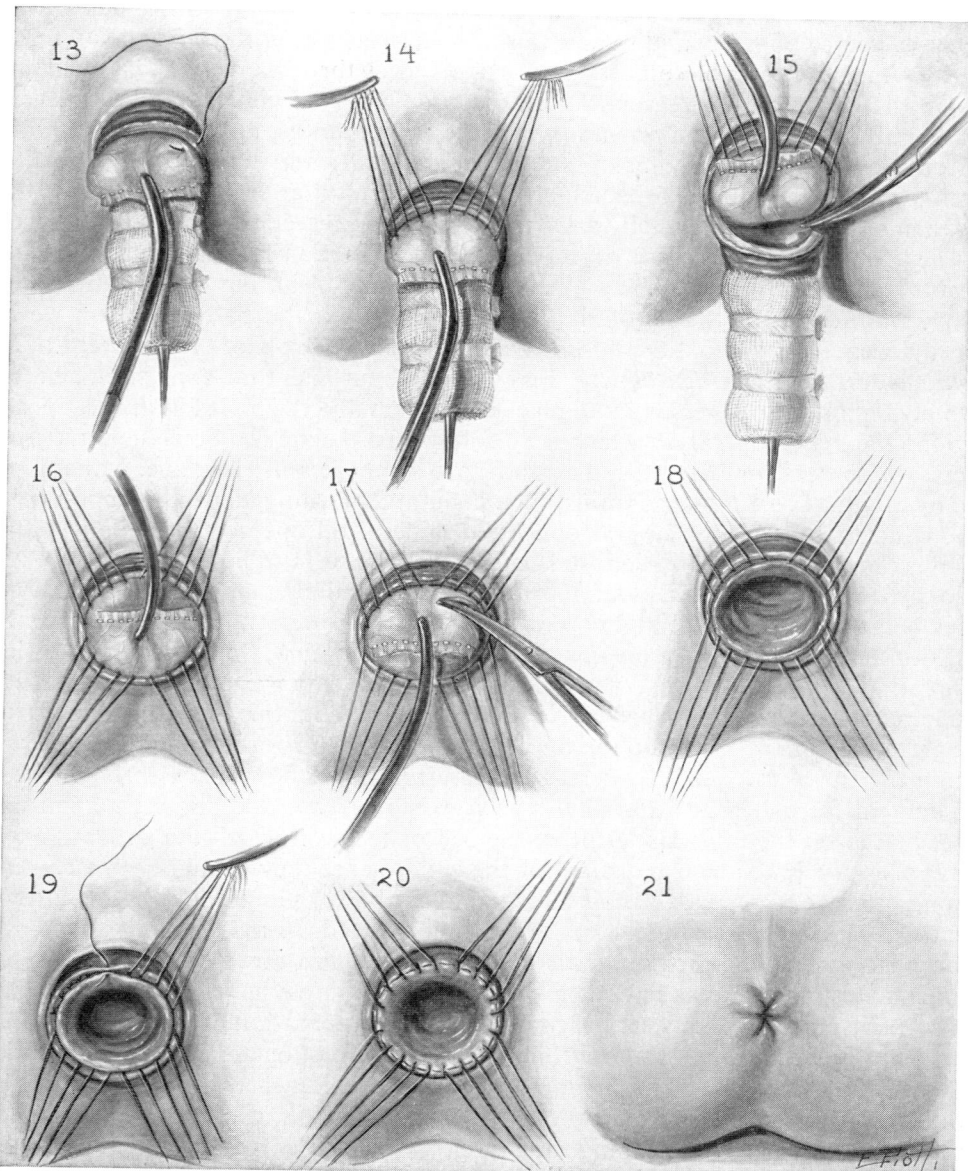

Fig. 185 (*continued*). 13. Anchoring rectum to descending colon. The sutures pass through the submucosa and muscularis of each segment. Sutures are 0000 Deknatel silk. 14. Anchoring completed in the two anterior quadrants, the silks of each quadrant are held in a hemostat. 15. The descending colon pulled forward to expose the back wall of the rectum, the posterior half of the rectum being cut off. 16. Row of sutures completed around posterior quadrants. 17. Descending colon being opened. The excess portion of it is cut away and discarded. 18. Excess descending colon has been completely cut off. 19. A quadrant of deep sutures has been trimmed off. Beginning of mucosal union. 20. Mucosal sutures completed around the entire circumference of bowel. 21. The mucosal sutures have been cut at their knots, and the bowel has been inverted up into the anus.

ary cecostomy or a transverse colostomy is desirable: (1) It is quite difficult to perform the abdomino-perineal operation in babies under six or eight months of age with any reasonable degree of safety and satisfaction. The narrowness of the rectal canal through the pelvis makes it troublesome to pull extra bowel through it and make a reliable anastomosis. If surgical intervention has been definitely decided upon, we generally avoid the abdomino-perineal operation in these early months, and prefer to establish a cecostomy or a transverse colostomy (if the individual cannot be carried on suitably with mineral oil and enemas) deferring the resection until after six or eight months of age, when it is technically much easier to perform the resection. (2) In an older child who is extremely malnourished, or in whom fecal impaction is great, it is occasionally desirable to establish a temporary opening to facilitate cleansing of the bowel and to improve the nutritional status of the individual. (Within the past few years we have generally been able to avoid a colostomy in patients who are more than a year of age.)

Preoperative preparation can be very troublesome and time-consuming, but it is extremely important. It is essential to place the patient and the bowel in the best possible states for the major operation which is to follow. To deflate the bowel is a messy and disagreeable ordeal for patient, nurse, and doctor, but it must be done. Mineral oil is given by mouth, 1 to 3 tablespoonfuls, each night and morning, depending upon the size of the child. Instillation of several ounces of mineral oil once or twice daily into the rectum is of some help. Warm soapsuds enemas at first seem to be ineffectual when only the soapy water returns, but after repeating them a number of times, the hard fecal masses begin to disintegrate and come away with the water. When the fluid has been instilled into the colon, gentle massage through the abdominal wall will help to dislodge and break up the fecal lumps. Colonic flushing with a Kemp irrigator is the best method of cleaning out a bowel which has been badly impacted. With this instrument, introduced through the rectum and up into the lower sigmoid, warm, irrigating fluid can be run in through the tip of the nozzle, whereas the returning fluid flows back through the side arms and can be collected externally in a large rubber tube and allowed to run into a bucket placed on the floor alongside of the bed or table on which the patient lies. Irrigations are very apt to be exhausting for the child, hence they should not be continued too long at any one time. Attempts at cleaning the bowel should be carried out two or three times in each twenty-four hours, repeating these for as many days as is necessary to completely deflate the colon. This will always require three or four days, and in stubborn cases may take as long as a week or ten days. We have seen no difference in postoperative results in cases with chemotherapeutic preparation of the bowel compared to those in which it was not given. When such reduction of bacterial flora is desired, the best combination seems to be neomycin and Sulfasuxidine. We prefer Sulfasuxidine (to Sulfathalidine) not only because of its high potency but also because it produces a diarrhea and thus helps in cleaning the bowel.

Following operation a few points are of importance. For a child to receive an adequate amount of nourishment, it is necessary to give support in the form of blood transfusions and intravenous or subcutaneous infusions of glucose and saline. Generally, this supportive treatment lasts from two to four days. The upper intestinal tract should be kept deflated with an inlying Levin tube, and the patient placed on constant stomach suction, until the gastric fluid becomes free of brownish or greenish colored material. Antibiotic therapy of intensive degree and with a wide spectrum of antibacterial activity should be used for four or five days. We have generally used parenteral administration of penicillin, streptomycin, and sulfadiazine; if good veins are available, aureomycin or terramycin is excellent. When fluids can be tolerated by mouth, it is generally best to give for five or six days only such liquids as have a low residue and will thereby give a minimum disturbance at the anastomotic line in the rectum. After the first week, soft solids, and later solids, can be added to the diet as desired.

RESULTS OF TREATMENT

There is no doubt that mild cases of Hirschsprung's disease can be treated under medical supervision and operation can be avoided. It has been pleasing to find that some children who had considerable accumulations within the bowel have been helped by the ingestion of mineral oil, by adequate colonic lavage, by some short periods of hospitalization, and possibly by the use of Mecholyl bromide; the family has learned to care for the child in an adequate manner (or an older youngster has been able to carry out the measures himself). The colon has regained reasonable activity and has not been allowed to reaccumulate inspissated material within it; the child has gone along in satisfactory health.

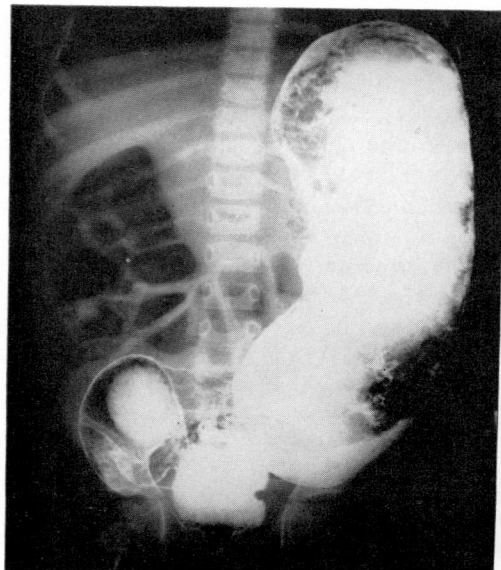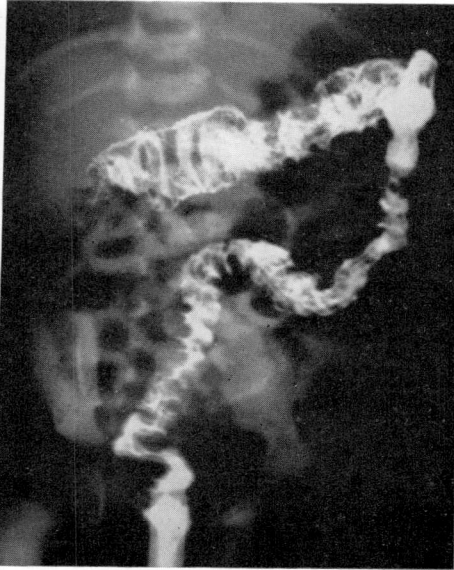

Fig. 186. Roentgenograms from an eight-year-old girl who was treated by abdomino-perineal resection of the rectosigmoid for Hirschsprung's disease. *Left,* Barium enema before operation, showing marked distention of the colon and loss of haustral markings. *Right,* Barium enema after operation, showing normal caliber, contour, and convolutions of the colon.

Sympathectomies have been abandoned by us, since we now feel that if the situation is serious enough to warrant operation, it is much better to perform some sort of resection, rather than to attempt to correct the situation by a rearrangement of the neurologic balance in the colon.

While we readily admit that transabdominal resection of most of the neurologically deficient rectosigmoid and some of the dilated colon above this has met with fair success in our hands and has considerable favor more recently in other clinics, it is our feeling that a longer follow-up on such cases will probably show a higher percentage of recurrence of megacolon than will be the finding when the abdomino-perineal "pull-through" procedure has been performed. The great advantage to the transabdominal approach is the preservation of the nerves supplying the ejaculatory apparatus in the male.

Whether or not these actually have been damaged by the abdomino-perineal operation has not yet been determined in any series of cases, and therefore it is impossible to state whether this factor is sufficient to warrant the routine use of transabdominal resections, which we believe are somewhat less effective for the treatment of megacolon than is the abdomino-perineal "pull-through" technique.

In the Children's Hospital material, up to December 31, 1951, 70 patients have been treated by the abdomino-perineal operation, with removal of the rectosigmoid and most of the rectum. This series was largely built up by Swenson and his associates. The excellent results which have been attained are largely due to his diligent supervision and management of these cases. Most of this material has been summarized previously in the various reports by Swenson et al. [16, 17, 18] There have been two deaths. One occurred in a six-weeks-old baby, in whom there was a fecal fistula from the suture line, leading to spreading peritonitis. The second was in a five-months-old child in whom there was postoperative perforation of the ileum and peritonitis. The surviving 68 patients have been followed for periods of time varying from eight months up to five years. Because of an insufficient resection, one child required a secondary removal of more bowel. There have been 4 who developed some degree of stricture at the anastomotic line; in 3 of these, the stricture could be readily dilated by digital probing, but in one it was necessary to cut a web of tissue and then dilate the tissues. The remaining patients have all had an adequate lumen at the anastomotic site. In one patient, there was development of a pelvic abscess, which was drained into the rectal lumen. Two patients have required rather frequent enemas to keep the bowel deflated, and in 6 others there have been a few occasions when it has been necessary to give one or several enemas to relieve temporary retention of fecal material in the colon. All of the remaining children have had amazing recovery; they have had spontaneous evacuation of the bowel and no reappearance of abdominal distention. They all have had excellent sphincteric control. These patients are taking a normal diet and require no laxatives or drugs. In 2 children there has been a hypotonia of the bladder. Whether this existed prior to operation (as a part of the neurologic deficit) or whether it was brought about by the operative procedure itself is uncertain.

The over-all picture with abdomino-perineal "pull-through" removal of the rectum and rectosigmoid represents a tremendous advance in the treatment of Hirschsprung's disease. We are extremely pleased with the results which have been obtained; while they are not completely perfect, the therapeutic gains have certainly been far superior to those which have been attained by any method of therapy which has thus far been undertaken. It has been shown that it is possible to carry out this operation with an extremely low fatality rate, with very little in the way of postoperative complications, and with a promise of curing the patient's complaints in well over 90 per cent of the cases.

REFERENCES

1. Aird, I.: A Companion in Surgical Studies. E. S. Livingstone, Ltd., Edinburgh, 1949, p. 72.
2. Bodian, M., Stephens, F. D. and Ward, B. C. H.: Hirschsprung's Disease. Lancet, *1:19*, 1950.
3. Cannon, W. B. and Burket, I. R.: The Endurance of Anemia by Nerve Cells in the Myenteric Plexus. Am. J. Physiol., *32:*347, 1913.
4. Caffey, J.: Pediatric X-ray Diagnosis. Year Book Publishers, Chicago, 1945, p. 467, Fig. 425.
5. dalla Valle, A.: Ricerche istologiche su un caso di megacolon congenito. Pediatria, *28:*740, 1920.
6. Ehrenpreis, T.: Megacolon in the Newborn. Acta chir. Scandinav., *94:*112, 1946.
7. Hiatt, R. B.: The Pathologic Physiology of Congenital Megacolon. Ann. Surg., *133:* 313, 1951.
8. Hiatt, R. B.: The Surgical Treatment of Con-

genital Megacolon. Ann. Surg., *133:*321, 1951.

9. Hirschsprung, H.: Stuhlträgheit Neugeborener in Folge von Dilatation und Hypertrophie des Colons. Jahrb. f. Kinderh., *27:* 1, 1888.

10. Hirschsprung, H.: Fortsatte Erfaringer Our den Medfodte Dilatation Og Hypertrofi of Tyktarmen. Hospitalstid., *43:*165, 1900.

11. Law, J. L.: The Treatment of Megacolon with Parasympathetic Drugs. J.A.M.A., *114:*2537, 1940.

12. Penick, R. M., Jr.: Problems in Surgical Treatment of Congenital Megacolon. J.A.M.A., *128:*423, 1945.

13. Scott, W. J. M. and Morton, J. J.: Sympathetic Inhibition of the Large Intestine in Hirschsprung's Disease. J. Clin. Investigation, *9:*247, 1930.

14. State, D.: Physiological Operation for Idiopathic Congenital Megacolon (Hirschsprung's Disease). J.A.M.A., *149:*350, 1952.

15. Swenson, O. and Bill, A. H., Jr.: Resection of Rectum and Recto-sigmoid with Pres-

ervation of Sphincter for Benign Spastic Lesions Producing Megacolon: An Experimental Study. Surgery, *24:*212, 1948.

16. Swenson, O., Neuhauser, E. B. D. and Pickett, L. K.: New Concepts of Etiology, Diagnosis and Treatment of Hirschsprung's Disease. Pediatrics, *4:*201, 1949.

17. Swenson, O., Rheinlander, H. F. and Diamond, I.: Hirschsprung's Disease: A New Concept of Etiology. New England J. Med., *241:*551, 1949.

18. Swenson, O.: A New Treatment for Hirschsprung's Disease. Surgery, *28:*371, 1950.

19. Tiffin, M. E., Chandler, L. R. and Faber, H. K.: Localized Absence of the Myenteric Plexus in Congenital Megacolon. Am. J. Dis. Child., *59:*1071, 1940.

20. Whitehouse, F. R. and Kernohan, J. W.: The Myenteric Plexus in Congenital Megacolon. Arch. Int. Med., *82:*75, 1948.

21. Zuelzer, W. W. and Wilson, J. L.: Functional Intestinal Obstruction on a Congenital Neurogenic Basis in Infancy. Am. J. Dis. Child., *75:*40, 1948.

CHAPTER 24

Malformations of the Anus and Rectum

Congenital anomalies of the anus and rectum are said to occur about once in every 5000 newly born babies. Some authors believe that such conditions appear as often as once in every 1500 infants, but this incidence is higher than is generally conceded. The malformations are frequent enough, and the problems concerned therewith are serious enough, to make this field one of the most important in the surgery of infancy and childhood. The Children's Hospital material includes 507 cases treated surgically up through 1951.

EMBRYOLOGY AND PATHOGENESIS

Embryology

In the 7.5 mm. embryo the tubular *allantoic duct* expands to form the bladder, which after receiving the *Wolffian ducts* continues caudally as the *urogenital sinus*. Posteriorly, this sinus has an extensive communication with the hindgut. Thus, there is a terminal cavity common to both the urogenital and intestinal tracts, which is called the *cloaca*. The cloaca is a narrow, laterally-compressed cavity which is closed off from the exterior of the body by the *cloacal membrane*. The intestinal tube extends beyond the cloaca into the tail, as the caudal intestine or *tail gut*. In either side of the cloaca, there is a longitudinal external groove with a corresponding internal ridge. Along this line of narrowing, the genito-urinary system will later become separated from the intestine.

In the 9.4 mm. stage there is further cleavage of the urogenital sinus from the intestine. This is accomplished by the downgrowth of a saddle of mesoderm between the urogenital sinus and the intestine, thereby reducing the opening between these two systems to a small passage called the *cloacal duct*. Normally, the process of separation continues so that this communication is closed off by the 16 mm. stage (seventh week).

In the 22 mm. stage (late in the seventh week) a primary perineum is present. The perineum develops by the division of the cloacal membrane into the *urogenital membrane* anteriorly and the *anal membrane* posteriorly, and by a downgrowth and ingrowth of the mesenchymal elements between these two membranes. Late in the seventh week, the urogenital sinus has acquired an external opening, but the anal membrane does not rupture till later. A small dimpling of the anal pit forms the *proctodeum*, which inpocketing continues until the proctodeum and rectum join their lumina by rupture of the anal membrane. There is apparently a slight variation in the normal time of this rupture, but usually it takes place in embryos of about 30 mm. (eighth week).

In young embryos the rectal tube has a spindle-shaped contour which persists up to birth, although its form changes greatly. This upper bulbous enlargement, termed the *bulbus analis*, has a position in the embryo which corresponds closely to that occupied by the rectal ampulla in the adult. Below the spindle-shaped portion just described, a second swelling develops which is much shorter and less well marked. It persists for only a brief period of embryonic life, and in specimens of 30 mm. it has largely disappeared. This lower enlargement, termed the *bulbus terminalis*, develops into the lower portion of the pars analis recti of the adult, namely the *zona intermedia*.

Pathogenesis

Many of the rectal and anal malformations can be interpreted as arrests or abnormalities of development in the seventh or eighth week of embryonic life. It is evident that an anomalous connection between the rectum and genito-urinary apparatus would be established if the cloacal duct failed to close. A rectoperineal fistula, however, would be formed if the anterior portion of the cloacal duct were obliterated, and if the remaining posterior portion were carried downward in the local growth of the region.

In the female, the rectal connections with the genital tract are doubtless formed in the following manner: The downward extension of the Müllerian ducts is at the expense of the posterior wall of the urogenital sinus, so that these ducts take over any fistula which already communicated with the rectum. The derivatives of the lower part of the Müllerian system, namely the vagina, can thereby attain a fistula to the rectum.

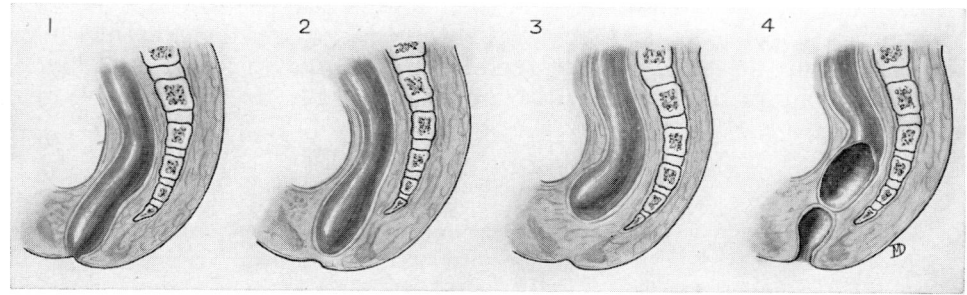

Fig. 187. Types of anal and rectal abnormalities. *Type 1*. Stenosis at the anus. *Type 2*. Imperforate anus. Obstruction only by a persistent membrane. *Type 3*. Imperforate anus. Rectal pouch ending blindly some distance above anus. *Type 4*. Anus and anal pouch normal. Rectal pouch ends blindly in hollow of sacrum.

Congenital anal stenosis (*Type 1*, Fig. 187) may occur at the anus or at a level 1 to 4 cm. above the anus. Such partial obstruction occurring at the anal level is the result of incomplete rupture of the anal membrane. A stenosis appearing within the terminal few centimeters of the rectum most likely arises because of incomplete development at the upper end of the bulbus analis or bulbus terminalis.

Membranous imperforate anus (*Type 2*, Fig. 187) results from a persistence of the anal membrane, an arrest at about the eight week.

In those abnormalities in which the rectum ends blindly at a considerable distance above the imperforate anus (*Type 3*, Fig. 187), the embryologic origin is still obscure. Possibly the sequence is similar to that which Boyden has carefully studied in the reduction of the hindgut of the ostrich. He has shown that as the tail gut disappears, excessive degeneration also involves the narrow, posterior, inferior part of the cloaca, which in man would correspond to the terminal portion of the rectum. Hence, if this resorptive process should extend to and involve the rectum, the upper portion of the rectum would end as a blind sac which is separated from the anus.

In those malformations in which the anus and anal pouch are normal, but the rectum ends blindly (*Type 4*, Fig. 187), an obliteration most likely occurs at the upper end of the bulbus analis, for this is the corresponding embryologic level. The occurrence of such anomalies 3 to 4 cm. above the anus suggests a relationship to this embryonic constriction, which by its form leads one to believe that concrescence could easily take place at this point.

It should be emphasized that the *external* anal sphincter muscle develops from the regional mesenchyma, and is not dependent upon the presence of the terminal bowel. Hence, this sphincteric muscle is generally present, regardless of the type of malformation under discussion.

TYPES OF ANAL AND RECTAL ABNORMALITIES

Rectal Abnormality

We have employed a classification of these cases which is valuable in determining the necessary form of treatment, and which is also useful for estimating the prognosis. All of our cases have been placed, irrespective of any associated fistulas, into four groups, as follows, and as illustrated in Figure 187: Classified as *Type 1* anomaly is the malformation having a patent anus and rectum, but with a stenosis either at the anus or in the rectum. As *Type 2* anomaly are grouped all conditions in which there is an imperforate anus, the obstruction being membranous in character. In *Type 3* malformation, the anus is imperforate, and the rectal pouch ends blindly some distance above it. In the *Type 4* group, the anus, sphincter, and lower portion of the rectum are all normal, but the upper point of the rectum ends blindly and is separated by a variable distance from the lower pouch.

Table 41

Distribution of Anal and Rectal Abnormalities in Males and Females

Type	Males	Females	Total
Type 1...............................	16	13	29
Type 2...............................	12	2	14
Type 3...............................	229	214	443
Type 4...............................	13	8	21
Totals...........................	270	237	507

Associated Fistulas

Three hundred and sixty-two of the patients (71 per cent of the series) had fistulas connecting the rectum with either the genito-urinary system or with the perineum; 67 per cent of the males and 81 per cent of the females had such fistulas. Four of these connections occurred in Type 1 cases, two in Type 2 malformations, and the remaining ones all had a Type 3 ano-rectal anomaly. Thus, of all the Type 3 cases, 80 per cent had an accompanying fistula of some sort. In no case was there a fistula with a Type 4 malformation, but embryologically such a combination might be expected.

In males, three kinds of fistulas are encountered (Fig. 188). The recto-vesical connections usually open into the trigone. The urethral fistulas open into either the prostatic or membranous portions. The perineal openings usually appear just behind the perineo-scrotal angle, but in one case there was a more anterior location with a bifid

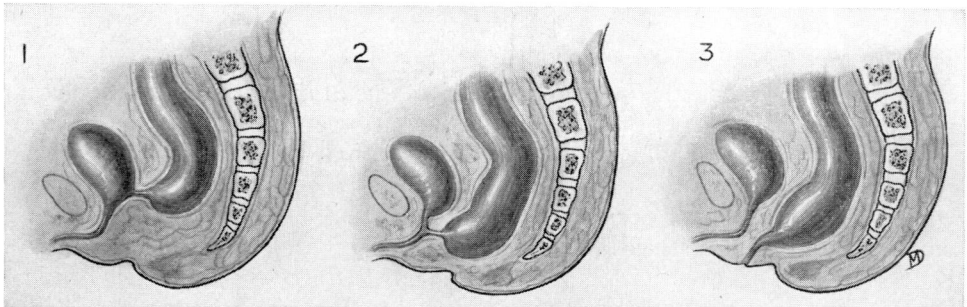

Fig. 188. Types of fistulas encountered in male patients. 1. Rectovesical fistula. 2. Recto-urethra communication. 3. Recto-perineal fistula (the opening being in front of the area where the anus should normally open).

scrotum. We have had no case similar to those in the literature in which the rectal fistula opened on the under surface of the penis.

In females (Fig. 189), a recto-vesical fistula is an extremely rare finding; our only example of this occurred in conjunction with a recto-vaginal one. The recto-vaginal connections open anywhere along the posterior vaginal wall from the posterior fornix down to the labia, though they are particularly apt to appear in the lower third of the vagina. In one child with a septate vagina, there were two separate fistulas, one to each side of the vagina. Many fistulas open into the fossa navicularis, just outside of the hymen. The perineal fistulas are seen from the fourchette back to the anal dimple.

Table 42
Distribution of Fistulas in Males and Females

Types of Fistula	Males	Females	Total
Recto-urethral.	59	0	59
Recto-vesical.	56	1	57
Recto-perineal.	54	49	103
Recto-vaginal.	0	143	143
Totals.	169	193	362

There may be considerable variation in the *size* of these tracts. The fistulas are often too small to permit evacuation of the rectum; only a small probe can be passed through them. In other instances (approximately half the patients with fistulas), the opening is large enough to permit defecation if the stools are kept soft or liquid.

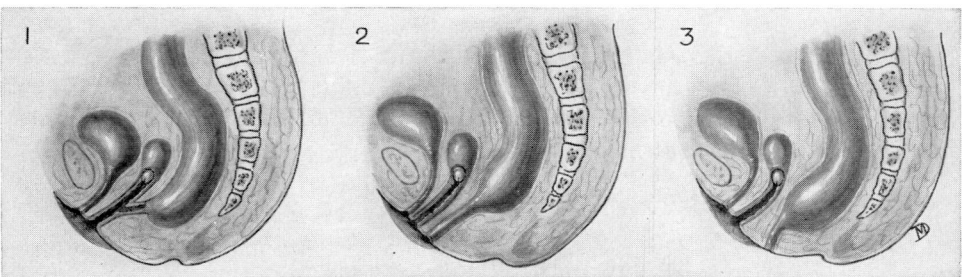

Fig. 189. Types of fistulas encountered in female patients. 1. Recto-vaginal fistula. 2. Recto-fossa navicularis fistula. 3. Recto-perineal fistula.

Complete Obstruction at Birth

Since about three-fourths of patients with anorectal malformations have complete (or nearly complete) obstruction from birth, they are seen in the first few days of life. It is usually apparent immediately that there is no anal opening, that stools have not been passed, or that meconium has come through an abnormal exit such as the penile urethra, vaginal outlet, or a perineal fistula. The anal abnormality is sometimes over-looked until the second or third day, when unsuccessful attempts are made to give the infant an enema or to take its temperature. When there is an associated fistula large enough to deflate the rectum, the regional malformation is sometimes overlooked for months or even years.

Type 1

These patients with stenosis of the anus or rectum come for medical care later than those with complete obstruction. The *age* when they are first seen varies from a few days to two or three years, with an average of nine months. The chief complaint is usually related to difficulty in defecation. *Obstipation* is severe when enemas or cathartics are not given. Not infrequently the stools are *"ribbon-like;"* forcing of a soft stool through a constricted anus makes it emerge like paste squeezed from a tube. The parent often points out that the enema nozzle can be inserted into the rectum only with difficulty or at times cannot be inserted at all. *Abdominal distention* is commonly found in these cases, but vomiting is not a prominent feature.

Type 2

These patients with an imperforate membrane are all seen within the first few days of life. The difficulty in each instance is apparent, for the physician or parent discovers a complete anal block. There is no meconium staining on the diaper. For the first twenty-four to thirty-six hours of life the absence of bowel movements is frequently the only symptom but after that time *abdominal distention, vomiting,* and other evidence of obstruction rapidly appear.

Type 3

In 264 of our 443 cases of this group, there was no associated fistula or else this tract was so small that it was ineffectual in emptying the rectum. Hence, these 264 babies had acute obstruction, and their symptoms were essentially the same as those of Type 2.

The remaining 179 patients had fistulous openings large enough to support life for considerable lengths of time and were not seen as early in life as those described in the last paragraph. The *age* when these first entered the clinic varied up to ten or eleven years, but the average age was about one year. Because of the relatively large size of the fistulas in these cases, there is rarely any complaint of nausea, vomiting, or distention. The patients are found to have *pain on defecation*, difficulty in moving the bowels, or else someone has discovered the abnormal position of the rectal outlet. The fistulous opening may be so large that incontinence develops.

Type 4

The normal-appearing anus tends to make the parent and the attending physician believe that there is no malformation of the rectum. Even with the giving of an enema the presence of a blind anal pouch is not always detected. Indeed, in only 2 of our 19 cases was the information elicited that an obstruction had been noted inside of the anus. Generally, there is considerable delay in recognizing that a mechanical blockage exists. Thus, while Type 2 and Type 3 patients are often seen within eight or twelve hours after birth, these Type 4 cases are more apt to be brought in on the third, or fourth, or even fifth day of life. Therefore, the usual history includes marked *abdominal distention, refusal of food, vomiting, dehydration*, and *"toxicity"* of prominent degree. As a result, these infants are much poorer surgical risks than those of Type 1, 2, or 3.

PHYSICAL FINDINGS

Complete Obstruction

A patient more than thirty-six or forty-eight hours old who possesses a complete occlusion has findings indicative of lower bowel obstruction. These include the classical signs of *abdominal distention, intestinal patterning, borborygmus, tympanites, vomiting, dehydration*, and even *respiratory* or *circulatory* collapse in the later stages. If the infant is seen within the first twenty-four hours of life, the signs of intestinal obstruction are seldom found. In each instance the local examination of the anal region gives practically all the information necessary for classification into one of the four main types.

More specific findings in the four types of rectal abnormalities are as follows:

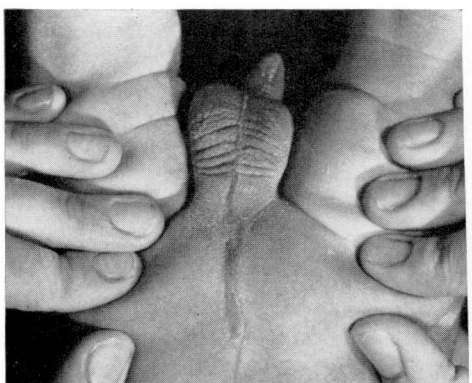 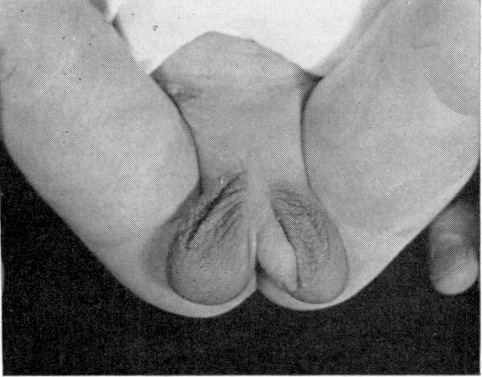

Fig. 190. *Left*, Male with imperforate anus. There is no crease between the buttocks. This laxity suggests a neuromuscular weakness of the levator ani muscles. *Right*, Child with an imperforate anus who also had a bifid scrotum and a retro-displacement of the penis.

Type 1

When there is an incomplete rupture of the anal membrane, the opening is often no more than 2 to 3 mm. in diameter. In those cases with an obstruction higher in the anal canal, the anus appears normal but the stricture is felt a few centimeters above the anal orifice. When the stenosis is marked, the *perineum* is often seen to bulge downward as the child strains, and at the same time a *ribbon-like stool* is produced. The entire colon occasionally exhibits marked enlargement because of this anal or rectal obstruction.

Type 2

The imperforate anal membrane is obvious. Because the obstruction is only membranous, a *dark discoloration* is imparted to the diaphragm by the meconium which lies against its inner side. The impaction of meconium against the membrane makes it bulge when the baby cries or strains.

Type 3

These patients present a considerable variety of findings. The *perineum* occasionally has a small ridge in the region where the anus should be, but a *dimple* at this site is a more common finding. This depression is of variable size and at times is large enough to admit a finger tip. *Puckering* of the surrounding skin can be seen whenever there is an external anal sphincter muscle which is contracting. Pinching of the buttocks or peri-anal skin will sometimes make the anal region contract, thereby giving evidence that a sphincter or levator ani muscle is present and can be made to function. If the blind rectal pouch is low in the pelvis, a finger placed on the anal region will detect an *impulse* when the baby strains or cries. A fistulous opening to the vagina, or the perineum, can give additional information concerning the position of the rectal pouch, because a probe may be passed along this tract and then directed downward toward a palpating finger held on the anal skin; local probing, inspection, and palpation in this way give more valuable information than does injection of the tract with barium and study by roentgenograms.

A fistula connecting the rectum with the bladder or urethra is usually discovered immediately because of the passage of meconium or flatus through the urethra, but it may evade detection even with careful observation. This failure of early recognition is presumably due to plugging of the small passageway by inspissated meconium or to temporary closure of the tract by a flap of mucous membrane. Microscopic examination of the urine may show fecal debris or evidence of urinary infection in some cases in which a fistula has not been suspected previously. It has been our practice to repeat the urine examinations from time to time, because one negative urine sediment examination does not necessarily rule out a communication between the rectum and urinary system.

Type 4

These cases elude detection at first because the clinical picture of low intestinal obstruction with a normal-appearing anus arouses suspicion of an atresia in the colon rather than in the rectum. However, digital rectal examination always reveals a complete block within reach of the little finger. The anal sphincter is always present and possesses contractile power.

ROENTGENOLOGIC EXAMINATION

Wangensteen-Rice Method

In 1930 Wangensteen and Rice published their ingenious method of determining the position of a blind rectal pouch in cases of imperforate anus by holding the infant with its head down and then making a reontgenogram of the abdomen and pelvis. Any gas in the colon will rise and outline the distal portion of the rectal pouch (Fig. 191), giving an indication of its position with relation to the anal membrane. Lateral films are better than anteroposterior ones for estimating the position of the rectal pouch. Information gathered in this way is extremely valuable when deciding which approach (abdominal or perineal) is to be employed. In some instances, colonic gas will pass through a fistula into the bladder and can be seen on lateral views.

Errors of Interpretation. A word of caution must be said regarding this method of investigation. When first making such examinations we made two errors in diagnosis, because gas had reached only to the terminal ileum in one instance, and to the mid-transverse colon in the other. We were therefore led to believe that atresias of the ileum

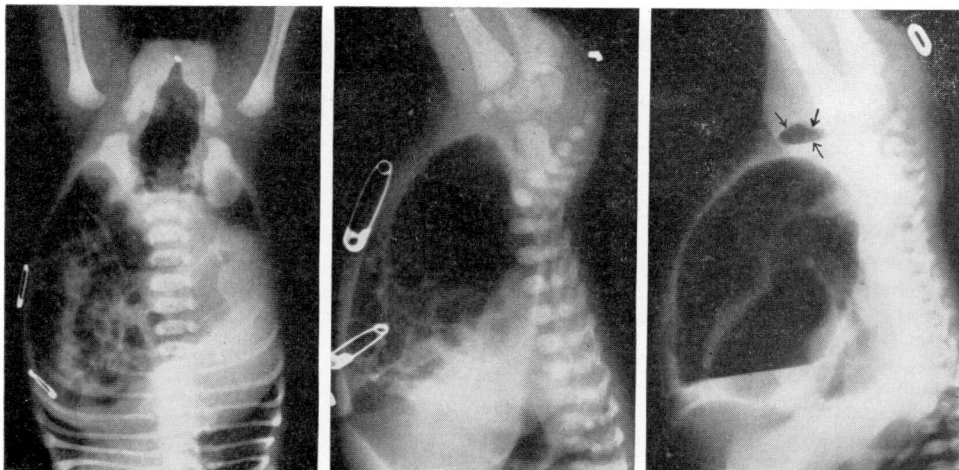

Fig. 191. Roentgenograms from three babies who had imperforate anus. In each subject, a lead marker is placed on the skin where an anus should be. Babies held in head-down position during film exposure, to allow gas to rise in the rectal pouch and outline its distal end. *Left,* The gas rises to the lead marker, indicating that the imperforate anus has only a membranous obstruction. *Middle,* The rectal pouch is a long distance from the anal marker. *Right,* The rectal pouch is far from the anus. The small bit of air (arrows) just distal to the rectum is air within the bladder, indicating the presence of a recto-vesical fistula. (For studies of the rectal position, lateral films are generally superior to those taken in an antero-posterior direction.)

and colon existed at these sites. Abdominal exploration of both these babies revealed the fallacy of these interpretations. The mistakes were made because gas had not yet been pushed along through all of the sticky meconium at the age of four and eight hours respectively. Thus, before fifteen to twenty hours of age, the absence of gas in the rectum should not be taken as evidence of intestinal or colonic obstruction. However, by the end of the first day of life, an x-ray picture of the abdomen is an accurate method of determining the position of the blind rectal pouch.

Barium in Colostomy Technique

Roentgenographic study can be useful in another way, when a sigmoidostomy has been established before repairing the rectum. Barium injected through the colostomy can give information regarding the distal extent of the same.

ASSOCIATED CONGENITAL ANOMALIES

One hundred ninety eight patients (39 per cent of the series) had other congenital anomalies (Table 43); some of these children had as many as seven or eight malformations. In 42 cases, this *other* abnormality was directly responsible for death; in the list of fatal conditions, congenital heart disease, atresia of the intestine, and atresia of the esophagus were particularly numerous.

TREATMENT OF STENOSIS OR ATRESIA OF ANUS AND RECTUM
Type 1

Repeated dilations of the stricture usually suffice to overcome the obstruction and permit normal anal function. Such dilations are performed with gum-elastic or metal dilators, the sizes of which are increased until the little finger can be employed. These dilations are continued daily until the stools pass readily and until there is assurance

Table 43

Associated Congenital Anomalies, with Frequency of Their Occurrence

Abnormality	Frequency of Occurrence	Abnormality	Frequency of Occurrence
Congenital heart disease	39	Bifid scrotum	7
Coarctation of aorta	2	Undescended testicle	5
Aplasia of lungs	2	Dermoid cyst of ovary	1
Hare lip and cleft palate	13	Bicornate uterus	5
Esophageal atresia	18	Atresia of vagina	2
Stenosis of esophagus	1	Vaginal stenosis	3
Hypertrophic pyloric stenosis	1	Septate vagina	6
Malrotation of intestines	4	Hydrometrocolpos	4
Annular pancreas	1	Malformation of vertebrae	24
Meckel's diverticulum	9	Spina bifida	7
Intestinal atresia or stenosis	8	Absence of radius	5
Duplication of ileum	1	Dislocated hip	5
Two appendices	1	Club feet	13
Atresia of colon	2	Sacral deformity	1
Duplication of sigmoid	1	Fusion of ribs	2
Absence of gallbladder	2	Supernumerary ribs	1
Situs inversus	1	Extensive deformity of leg	1
Horseshoe kidney	3	Supernumerary finger or toe	5
Both kidneys on left side	1	Syndactylism	1
Bilateral hydronephrosis	1	Absence of thumb	4
Absence of kidney and ureter	9	Bifid thumb	3
Polycystic kidney	4	Deformity of wrist	1
Ureteral valves	1	Absent metacarpal bones	1
Ureterocele	1	Absent metatarsal bones	1
Patent urachus	1	Pilonidal sinus	1
Urachal cyst	1	Myelomeningocele or meningocele	4
Megalobladder (neurogenic)	1	Deformed ears	4
Exstrophy of bladder	5	Congenital constriction of larynx	1
Absent bladder	1	Omphalocele	3
Blind fistula, base of bladder	1	Inguinal hernia	4
Double penis	1	Imbilical hernia	2
Ectopic penis	5	Mongolism	8
Hypospadias	10		

that the trouble will not recur. This generally requires several weeks, but at the end of this period the parent is instructed to continue the procedure two or three times a week for four to six months. When the opening in an anal membrane is markedly narrowed, the obstruction is readily relieved by incision of the remaining membrane and supplementing this with a few dilations. In rare cases, a plastic procedure is required to enlarge the constricted area which is either at the anus or at a point several centimeters above it.

Type 2

This form of imperforate anus is easily treated by cruciate *incision* of the membrane followed by occasional *dilations* with bougies or a finger. It is sometimes necessary to cut away all constricting tissue and then accurately bring mucous membrane to skin edges with interrupted stitches. The results following this are almost always better than mere incision of the membrane, hoping to make an opening large enough by dilations.

Type 3

The method of treatment depends upon the position of the rectal pouch. If the blind rectum is within a centimeter and a half of the perineal skin, almost always it can be repaired suitably by a perineal operation alone.

If the rectum is at a higher level, it is generally impossible (in a newborn baby) to reach it satisfactorily from below; one of two choices is open. Either a sigmoidostomy can be established and the rectum repaired when the child is one or two years of age, or else the malformation can be attacked immediately by abdomino-perineal approach. The former should be chosen if the child weighs less than 6 pounds, if there is a serious complication (such as congenital heart disease), or if the surgeon who is called upon to relieve the baby of obstruction has had little experience in this field. We much prefer the abdomino-perineal operation in all cases (with a high rectum), provided the child weighs more than 6 pounds and has no other serious abnormality. It is very unwise always to attempt perineal exploration and (if nothing can be accomplished) then to resort to an abdominal procedure of some sort. In the past we have had too many fatalities by such ill planned undertakings. Furthermore, even if a baby survives such a perineal exploration, the region usually becomes so damaged and scarred that it is very difficult at a subsequent date to get a satisfactory repair. For the successful correction of an imperforate anus, it is imperative to have an accurate evaluation of the malformation which is being treated and to plan a therapeutic approach which will correct the deformities and which is also within the operator's experience and capabilities; "exploratory" operations in the perineum have little to recommend them and they are apt to be quite destructive.

Technique of Perineal Operation. For a perineal operation, the baby is placed in the lithotomy position (Fig. 192). An antero-posterior incision is made in the midline of the perineal floor, extending from the scrotum or vagina backward to the tip of the coccyx. This incision divides the external anal sphincter into two lateral halves. This splitting of the anal sphincter is necessary to gain an adequate exposure. Dissection is now made through the levator ani muscle and is carried up into the space normally occupied by the rectum. Here the fat must be separated carefully; the dissection is carried close to the hollow of the sacrum to avoid injury to the genito-urinary tract. A catheter placed in the male urethra or a sound in the vagina will aid in identifying these structures, so that dissection may be kept away from them. In some cases, a narrow and ill defined fibrous cord leads upward and is attached to the blind rectum. When the pouch is identified, it is freed around its periphery so that later it can be pulled down to the perineum. Care is necessary at this stage to avoid opening the bowel, for if meconium leaks out, the operative field is obscured.

Three or four traction sutures are placed through the tip of the pouch, each passing through all layers except the mucosa. Pulling on these strings brings the rectum down to the proper position between the lateral halves of the sphincter. The edges of the anal sphincter muscle and the perineal skin are sewed together in front of and also behind the rectum which is being held down. The rectal wall is then sewed with fine silk stitches to the subcutaneous tissues. The rectal pouch is opened and any excess tissue is trimmed away. The mucosal edges are accurately sewed to the surrounding skin edges, either with 00000 silk or 0000 chromic catgut. We have found the latter very satisfactory. Thus, the rectum has an opening *through* the external anal sphincter, and there is continuity of the epithelial surfaces of the mucous membrane and the skin. *It cannot be emphasized too strongly that the rectum must be adequately freed so that all tension is avoided when it is sewed to the perianal structures.* If tension is present, the sutures will

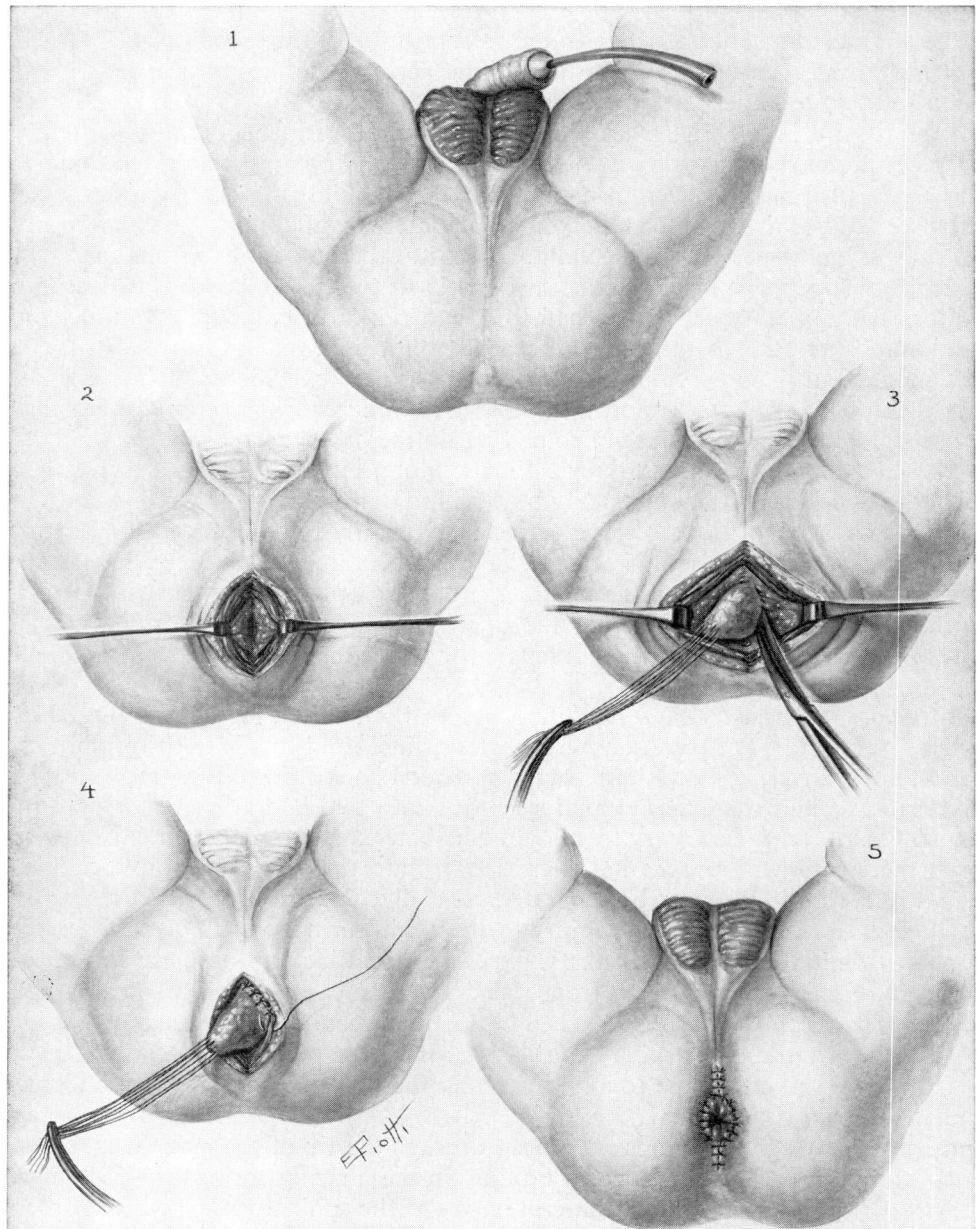

Fig. 192. Perineal operation for imperforate anus with a Type 3 abnormality, the rectum being low enough to reach from below. 1. Perineum viewed with legs drawn upward. Catheter in urethra so that later the urethra can be palpated deep in wound. 2. Midline incision exposing deep perineal fat. Sphincter muscle separated into lateral halves. 3. Blind rectal pouch identified and pulled downward with traction sutures. Dissection continued so that rectum may be better mobilized. 4. Rectal pouch drawn downward and being anchored with fine silk stitches to subcutaneous tissues. Rectum thus brought between the lateral halves of the sphincter muscle. 5. Rectal pouch opened, evacuated, and mucous membrane sewed to surrounding skin with 0000 chromic catgut sutures.

almost certainly pull out and in a few days' time the rectum will retract upward, leaving a strictured zone which is exceedingly difficult to cure by any subsequent operative procedure.

If a low fistula (to perineum, fossa navicularis, lower vagina, and possibly the male urethra) is present, it can be treated at the same time an imperforate anus is corrected. The dissection in the perineum must be carefully performed so that all anatomic structures are identified with certainty. The fistula can be divided, its anterior end suitably closed, and the rectal end displaced downward and backward to permit building up of a suitable perineal body. The fistulous end of the rectum is then pulled out beyond the level of the skin and the rectum anchored to surrounding tissues. Any excess of rectum (including the fistulous stump) is cut off and the rectal mucous membrane accurately apposed to the surrounding skin.

If an anal opening is made to appear relatively normal in dimensions, subsequent reaction and scarring will probably make it too small in a few months. Under these conditions, dilations—troublesome and disturbing—will be required for many months to establish an orifice of appropriate size. We have found it to be quite important to make the anus 40 to 50 per cent larger than normal at operation; with such intentional "overcorrection" it is found that the end results are infinitely superior and that rarely are postoperative dilations necessary.

Anal Dilations. In the vast majority of cases these are not required if the anoplasty has been made correctly, the anus has been made of sufficiently large size, and the operation has been carried out in a way that avoids subsequent scarring. Whenever anal dilations do become necessary, they can be started two or three weeks after operation. Once begun, anal dilations are continued until a functioning anus is obtained. The anal ring often becomes quite firm from postoperative reaction, and it seems that the anus will never be competent. But with persistence in dilations, it is surprising to find that after a few months the anal ring becomes pliable and possesses good muscle tone. The dilations are conducted daily by the hospital staff for two or three weeks to make certain that no undue tension is put on the line of suture, but after that time the parent can be instructed to perform the task several times a week. It is well to emphasize again that *if operation has been satisfactorily and properly performed*, dilations are completely unnecessary.

Dilation of Associated Fistulas. In rare cases, there are associated fistulas to the lower vagina or perineum which, because of their large size, can be used or can be dilated to permit defecation. Such patients can then be held over for operation on the anus and fistula until an older age. Not infrequently, dilation of a fistula has the great disadvantage of enlarging the opening and it is thus made more difficult to close it at a later date. Dilation of these fistulas should be done only if the child is in a precarious condition and cannot stand early operative attack on the rectum.

Technique of Abdomino-perineal Operation. In 1944 Rhoads[24] performed a combined abdominal and perineal operation in a newly born baby for treatment of an imperforate anus with a high rectum; he published a report of this in 1948. In 1944 we made an abdomino-perineal repair of an atresia of the rectum, as a secondary procedure; in 1948 we employed the procedure for the first time in our series as a primary operation in the newly born baby. In our group, 77 such operations have now been carried out.

Combined abdomino-perineal operation for treatment of these deformities has several disadvantages and also certain distinct advantages. It is certainly a major undertaking. It might be productive of shock, but we have found that is is possible to avoid this. It is apt to be followed in a few cases by loss of urinary or rectal control, because

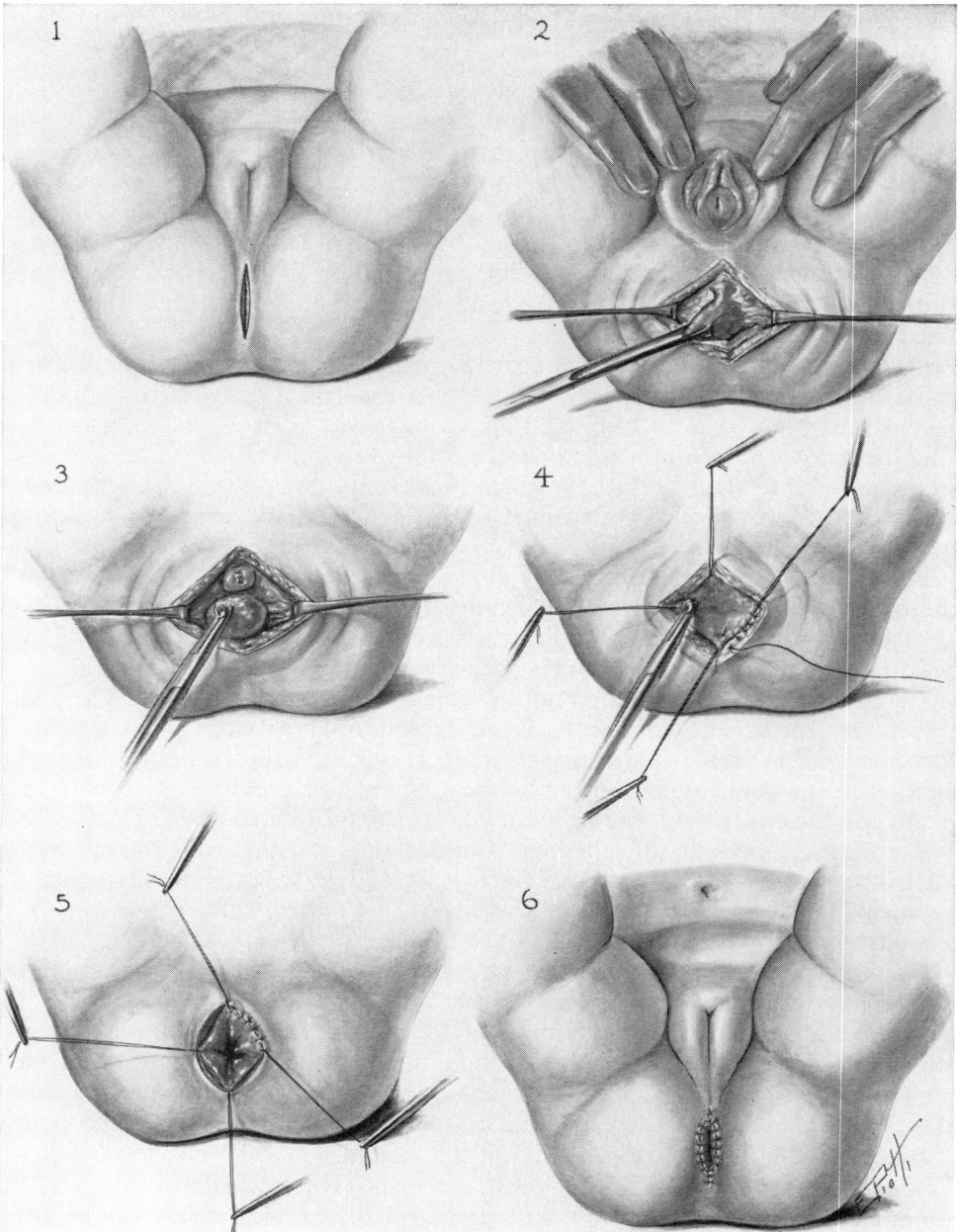

Fig. 193. Perineal repair of imperforate anus, when there is an associated low fistula. 1. Midline incision. 2. Wound opened and rectum freed sufficiently to identify the recto-vaginal fistula. 3. The fistula has been divided. A clamp is on the rectal end of the fistula. The rectum and vagina have been extensively separated. 4. Bowel is drawn downward and is being anchored to the subcutaneous tissues with fine silk sutures. Stitches are first placed in the four quadrants; two of these are held apart on tension, additional stitches are placed between them. 5. Bowel opened and excess trimmed away. Mucosa being sutured to skin with 0000 chromic catgut, beginning first at 3, 6, 9, and 12 o'clock. These can then be attenuated to fill in each quadrant. 6. Repair completed.

of injury to nerves during the extensive pelvic dissection; just how frequent are these complications must be determined by further study. On the favorable side is the fact that this operation makes it possible to mobilize any blind rectum or sigmoid—regardless of its high level—so that it can be brought down and opened at the anus. Furthermore the operation has just about solved completely the problem of treating any existing fistulas; in the past these were very troublesome and often required several operative attempts before some of them were closed permanently; now virtually all of them can be cured in one surgical step. In short, while the procedure has some drawbacks, particularly because of neuromuscular weaknesses which sometimes accompany it, it offers the tremendous advance of being able to remedy the most extensive rectal malformation and any coexisting fistula in one sitting, even for a newborn baby. While the operation has great merit, it should not be performed if it is possible to treat a particular anomaly by perineal operation alone.

Before starting an operation of this magnitude it is essential to have a metal cannula or a plastic tubing in an arm vein so that fluids and blood can be given during and after the operation. Rhoads recommended that the entire legs be prepared so that they could be included in the operative field; we prefer to keep the legs under the drapes, including only the perineum, genitalia, and abdomen in the operative field. During operation a catheter must always be placed (in the male) in the urethra, so that this can be identified in the depths of the wound and left uninjured. There is little point in attempting to insert a catheter into the urethra as an initial step; it is all too apt to pass through a fistula into the rectum. We have found it far better to incise the abdominal wall (down to the peritoneum) and then open the bladder so that a catheter can be passed from inside outward. At the same time a large suprapubic tube (for postoperative drainage) can be left in the bladder. Handling the matter in this way takes the least time.

Following opening of the abdomen, the various operative steps are as depicted in Figure 194. After the sigmoid (or rectosigmoid) is freed down to its fistulous attachment, the latter is divided. While the bladder (or urethral) end of this can be sewn over, there is danger that the sutures might turn in too much and give a stricture of the bladder outlet (or urethra). We have found it safer and completely satisfactory to leave the stump of the fistula open (where it has been cut off of the bladder or urethra). There need be no fear of recurrence of a fistula; subsequently a segment of normal bowel will be brought down opposite this fistulous end and there can be no chance of reestablishment of the channel. After a fistula has been severed and the lower end of the rectosigmoid has been freed, the subsequent dissection down into the pelvis should be largely by *blunt dissection*, hoping thereby to reduce the chances of cutting any important nerves which might run through the region. Likewise, after the initial midline incision has been made from below in the perineum, the upward dissection through pelvic structures is made by blunt dissection and *spreading* of tissues, rather than cutting them with scalpel or scissors. To permit threading the freed rectosigmoid down through the pelvic tunnel to the anus it is often necessary to divide the superior hemorrhoidal artery, and indeed it is sometimes necessary to cut the inferior mesenteric artery. If such a division is required, it is best to do it neither at the origin nor near the terminal branches of these vessels; section in their mid-portions will permit considerable flow through the arcuate channels. In no instance have we seen sloughing of the rectum or rectosigmoid in spite of the fact that these often have been extensively mobilized and their blood supply has been diminished. After the rectosigmoid is pulled down properly into its new position, the peritoneal floor must be repaired very carefully and the abdomen closed. Now attention can be turned again to the perineum and—under a lighter anesthesia—the bowel can be appro-

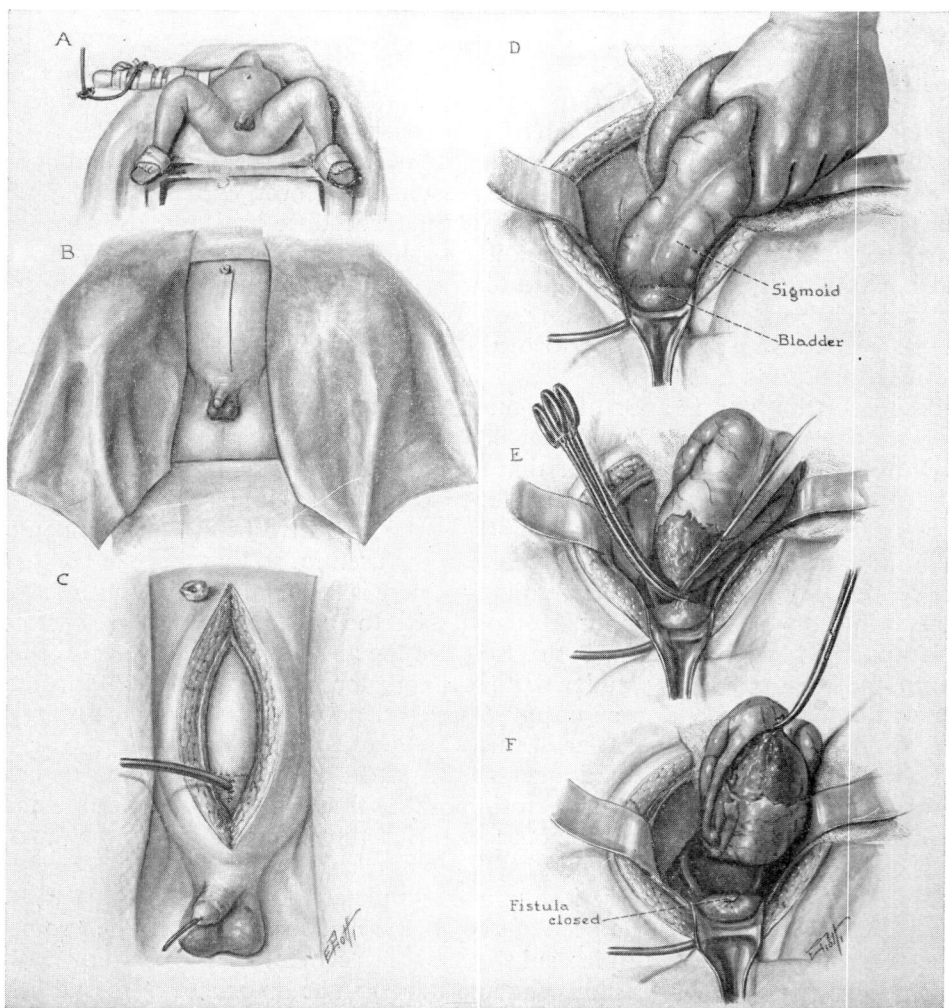

Fig. 194. Combined abdomino-perineal operation for imperforate anus having a high rectal pouch. A, Position of baby on table. Cannula (or plastic tubing) in an arm vein. Feet strapped to metal strips which are run in beneath the mattress. B, Abdomen, genitalia and perineum prepared; drapes in place. C, Abdominal incision down to peritoneum. Bladder has been opened, a small catheter passed out the urethra, and a large mushroom catheter (for post-operative drainage) left in place suprapubically. D, Abdomen opened. Intestines packed away. Sigmoid drawn upward. E, Peritoneal floor opened, lower sigmoid freed from surrounding structures, clamps placed across the fistula (which 80 to 90 per cent of these cases have), and fistula being severed. F, Liberated sigmoid drawn upward. If desired, the urinary end of the fistulous tract can be ligated or sutured; usually we do not close it.

priately anchored to the peri-anal tissues. While the urethral catheter can be withdrawn at this juncture, *the large suprapubic tube must be left open constantly for about eight or ten days* to permit sealing off of the vesical (or urethral) end of the old fistulous tract.

Type 4

These cases are most difficult to treat because the obstruction in the rectal pouch is frequently so high up in the pelvis that it cannot be reached by a perineal approach.

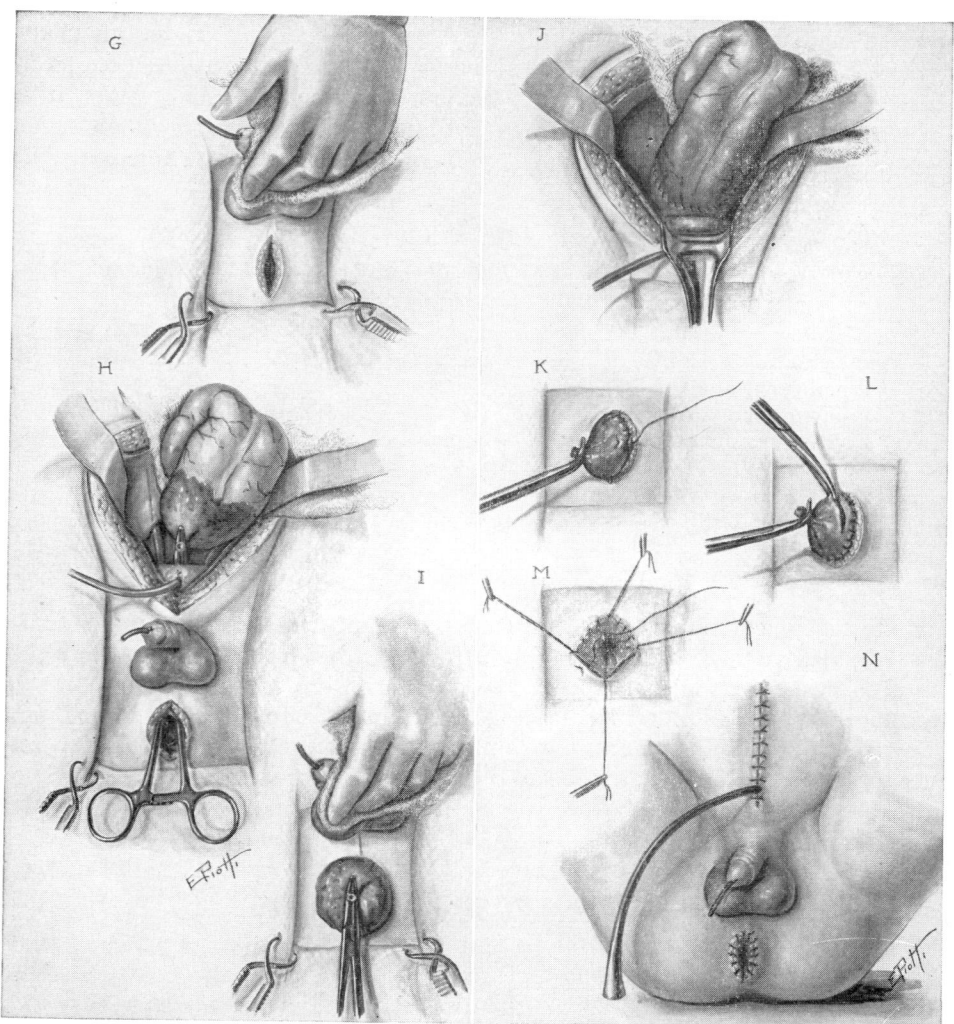

Fig. 194 (*continued*). G, Perineal part of operation begun. Midline incision. H, After the pelvic tissues have been bluntly dissected and a tunnel created, a clamp is passed up through it to grasp the rectosigmoid. I, Bowel pulled out through anal area. J, Peritoneal floor carefully closed to sigmoid. The abdominal wound is then closed. K, Continuation of anal repair. Bowel being sewed to subcutaneous tissues with interrupted silk stitches. L, Excess bowel being trimmed off. M, Mucous membrane being sewed to surrounding skin edges with interrupted 0000 chromic catgut stitches. N, Operation completed. The urethral catheter can now be withdrawn. The suprapubic one must be left open for eight or ten days before withdrawal.

In the past, we have blundered through some of these cases, attempting to join the two pouches within the pelvis (below the peritoneal floor) by a perineal or by a transabdominal approach; the mortality rates were exceedingly high and the over-all results were poor because of the tendency to scar formation at the operative site We now believe that (for most cases) it is far better to mobilize the entire rectum by an abdominoperineal approach, discard the affected portion, and cleanly join the upper rectum (or lower sigmoid) to the anal structures.

Choice of Operative Procedures

The treatment of rectal abnormalities has been undergoing considerable change in recent years. Therefore it would be misleading to summarize the experiences from our entire series of 507 cases which have been treated over a span of many years. It would give a better picture of present-day therapy to indicate the procedures which have been employed in a recent period; for this purpose, Table 44 indicates the choices which were

Table 44

Choice of Treatment in 104 Cases of Malformation of the Rectum, 1949 through 1951

Treatment	Cases	Deaths
Proctoplasty alone	49	2
Primary abdomino-perineal repair	18	1
Colostomy; later abdomino-perineal repair	23	0
Perineal, then abdomino-perineal repair	4	0
Colostomy; later perineal repair	2	0
Colostomy only	5	4
No operation	3	2

made in the three-year interval, 1949 through 1951. In this group were 104 patients. It will be noted that there were 4 deaths in the colostomy group, this operation being performed in desperately ill children. Likewise, there were 2 deaths in the "no operation" group, these being children brought in in extremis and for whom it seemed nothing could be accomplished. In the entire group of 104 cases the over-all mortality was 8.6 per cent; the mortality directly related to other serious anomalies was 5.7 per cent, and the mortality which should be charged to operative treatment of the rectal abnormalities was 2.9 per cent.

TREATMENT OF RECTAL FISTULAS

The high incidence of recto-urethral and recto-vesical fistulas in males implies that the problems of curing fistulas are far greater in males than in females, where the communications to the lower vagina and to the fossa navicularis are relatively easy to close.

If fistulas are low (to the perineum, the vagina, and possibly to the male urethra), it is possible to attack them solely through a perineal approach with a high chance of success, provided the rectal pouch is within a centimeter (and not over 1.5 cm.) of the anal skin. Under these circumstances, the exposure is adequate, and it is possible to work on the various structures in a wound which is relatively shallow. However, when the lower end of the rectal pouch is more than 1.5 cm. above the anal skin, operation thereon solely by the perineal approach will almost certainly be doomed to failure because of inability to close the fistula or (having treated it improperly) of recurrence. It is therefore our firm conviction that all *high rectal pouches* (80–90 per cent of which have fistulas) should be operated upon by the combined abdomino-perineal approach. To tackle these difficult problems in any other way is meddlesome; to use the combined abdomino-perineal approach gives almost complete assurance that a fistula can be closed off permanently. Justification for this statement comes from our experience in the treatment of 362 fistulas from the rectum. Prior to 1945 our results were bad, recurrences of fistulas were common and three or four operations were sometimes required to close them; since 1946 when the abdomino-perineal operation has been used extensively, the fistula problem has just about disappeared and it is virtually possible to guarantee a cure of a fistula by one operation. The abdomino-perineal repair of a blind rectum and an associated fistula—while having certain drawbacks—has the enormous advantage of allowing a normal segment of bowel to be pulled down over the previous site of a fistula; this makes it almost impossible for a fistula to recur.

RESULTS OF TREATMENT

In summarizing the results of treatment in these complicated cases, emphasis must be placed not only upon the number of deaths and survivals, but also upon the anatomic and functional results which have been obtained in the correction of the various anomalies.

Considerable stress must be placed upon the establishment of continuity between rectal membrane and adjacent skin, because this is quite essential in the prevention of scar formation and subsequent constriction. Failure to appreciate this simple fundamental rule has led many an operator, inexperienced in the field, to obtain a poor result. We feel that a soft and pliable anus can be attained in nearly all cases if care, gentleness, and proper approximation of tissues without tension are employed.

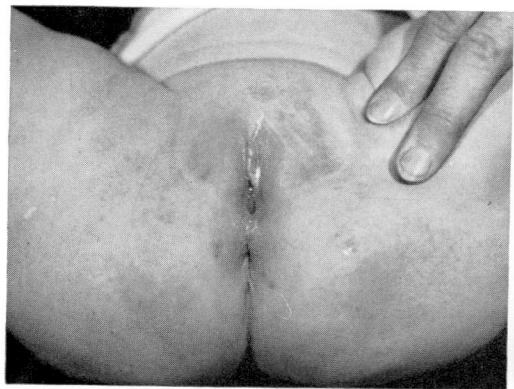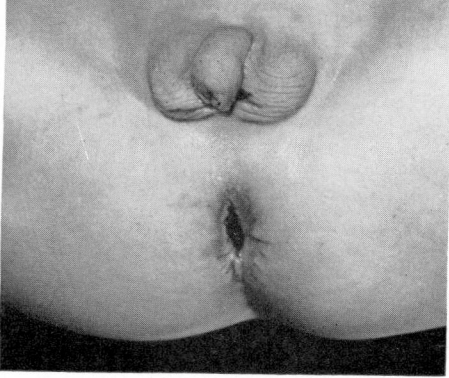

Fig. 195. Postoperative photographs of imperforate anuses. *Left,* Following repair by a perineal operation. *Right,* Following repair by an abdomino-perineal procedure.

The simpler types of abnormality (Types 1 and 2) should cause no apprehension regarding the postoperative result, for the outcomes can be made uniformly good.

For the common anomalies (Type 3) the situation becomes more complicated and disappointments occasionally appear. Yet the fact remains that well over 80 per cent of these subjects can be given an anus which functions in a very satisfactory manner.

The abdomino-perineal operation for repair of the more extensive abnormalities (Type 3 and 4) is still on trial regarding its final evaluation; yet we feel sure that it is an operation which now has a permanent place in the surgeon's armamentarium. Probably there will be some slight change in the selection of cases for which it is used. The magnitude of the operation does not seem to be forbidding, for it has been possible to keep mortality rates quite low. There does seem to be an associated chance of injury to nerves supplying the perineal musculature. It is sometimes difficult to say whether relaxation of the perineum and anal sphincter which follows some of these procedures has been due to a congenital lack which was present before operation or whether it was brought about by the operation itself. Because of the risk of producing neurologic deficits, abdomino-perineal operation should not be employed if there is a reasonable prospect of producing a satisfactory result by a perineal procedure alone. On the other hand, an operation limited to the perineal area which has been technically difficult to carry out can lead to subsequent anal scarring and other miseries which could certainly be avoided by a carefully done abdomino-perineal procedure.

Table 45

Survival Statistics for Combined Abdomino-perineal Repair of the Rectum

	Total	Dead
Primary abdomino-perineal operation................	20	1
Secondary abdomino-perineal operation..............	57	3
Totals..	77	4

In our series of 77 abdomino-perineal operations, the results are listed in Table 45. An analysis of the 4 deaths shows that the cause was undetermined in one, and that the other 3 resulted from other serious malformations.

In the 73 subjects who survived an abdomino-perineal procedure, the functional results have been summarized as follows:

Table 46

Functional Status of 73 Patients Who Survived an Abdomino-perineal Repair

BOWEL STATUS

Normal bowel habits..	23
Very satisfactory...	17
Only fair..	14
Anal stenosis..	1
Untrained yet (babies).......................................	11
Unknown...	7

URINARY STATUS

Entirely normal...	62
Urinary dribbling, with partial control........................	8
No apparent control...	2
Recurrence of fistula to skin.................................	1

To gain a view of over-all results in a series of cases treated in recent years for rectal malformations, our material has been analyzed for the years 1949 through 1951. There were 104 patients, 90 of whom had some sort of an associated fistula. The types of operation performed have been previously listed in Table 44. The over-all mortality was 8.6 per cent; the mortality directly stemming from serious anomalies in other parts of the body was 5.7 per cent, while the mortality attributable to surgical procedures was 2.9 per cent. Concerning the functional capacity after anal and rectal repair, the result was extremely satisfactory in 92 per cent of the survivors, while in the remainder it was unsatisfactory because of anal tightness or perineal laxity. Regarding the status of rectal fistulas, they have been cured in 87 and have recurred in 3.

In summary, a general survey of surgery for correction of malformations of the anus and rectum shows that: (1) There is a mortality rate (from all causes) somewhat over 8 per cent, but that the surgery itself carries a death rate slightly less than 3 per cent. (2) In surviving patients, well over 90 per cent can be given an anus which functions well. (3) It is possible to cure associated fistulas in one operation in about 97 per cent of the cases. (4) Only in rare cases is it necessary to perform secondary operations for relief of any residual anal deformity or persisting fistula.

REFERENCES

1. Ault, G. W., Castro, A. F. and Smith, R. S.: Clinical Study of Ligation of the Inferior Mesenteric Artery in Left Colonic Resections. Surg., Gynec. & Obst., 94:223, 1952.
2. Berman, J. K.: Congenital Anomalies of the Rectum and Anus. Surg., Gynec. & Obst., 66:11, 1938.
3. Bevan, A. D.: Imperforate Anus. Surg. Clinics Chicago, 4:21, 1920.
4. Bodenhamer, W. H.: Congenital Malformations of the Rectum and Anus. Wood, New York, 1860.
5. Boyden, E. A.: The Early Development of the Cloaca in Ostrich Embryos with Special Reference to the Reduction of the Caudal Intestine. Anat. Record, 24:211, 1922.
6. David, V. C.: The Treatment of Congenital Openings of the Rectum into the Vagina—Atresia Ani Vaginalis. Surgery, 1:163, 1937.
7. David, V. C. and Gilchrist, R. K.: Embryology and Malformations of the Rectum and Anus. Nelson New Loose-leaf Surgery. Thomas Nelson and Sons, New York, 1949, vol. 5, p. 141.
8. Dunphy, J. E.: Surgical Anatomy of the Anal Canal. Arch. Surg., 57:791, 1948.
9. Felix, W.: The Development of the Urinogenital Organs. In, Keibel and Mall: Manual of Human Embryology. J. B. Lippincott Co., Philadelphia, 1912, vol. 2, p. 752.
10. Hunter, R. H.: Observation on the Development of the Human Female Genital Tract. Carnegie Inst. of Washington, Publ., 414:91, 1930.
11. Johnson, F. P.: The Development of the Rectum in the Human Embryo. Am. J. Anat., 16:1, 1914.
12. Keibel, F.: Zur Entwicklungsgeschichte des menschlichen Urogenitalapparatus. Arch. f. Anat. u. Entwcklngsgesch., 1896, p. 55.
13. Keibel and Mall: Manual of Human Embryology. J. B. Lippincott Co., Philadelphia, 1912.
14. Keith, Sir A.: Malformations of the Hind End of the Body. Brit. M. J., 2:1736, 1908.
15. Keith, Sir A.: Malformations of the Human Body from a New Point of View. Brit. M. J., 1:489, 1932.
16. Ladd, W. E. and Gross, R. E.: Congenital Malformations of Anus and Rectum. Am. J. Surg., 23:167, 1934.
17. Lewis, F. T.: The Development of the Digestive Tract. In, Keibel and Mall: Manual of Human Embryology. J. B. Lippincott Co., Philadelphia, 1912, vol. 2, p. 306.
18. Mayo, C. W. and Rice, R. G.: Anorectal Anomalies. A Statistical Study of One Hundred Sixty Five Cases with Special Reference to "Distal-loop Trouble." Surgery, 27:485, 1950.
19. Norris, W. J., Brophy, T. W., III, and Brayton, D.: Imperforate Anus: A Case Series and Preliminary Report on the One Stage Abdominoperineal Operation. Surg., Gynec. & Obst., 88:623, 1949.
20. Parin, B.: Atresia Ani Urethralis. Arch. f. klin. Chir., 166:386, 1931.
21. Pohlman, A. G.: The Development of the Cloaca in Human Embryos. Am. J. Anat., 12:1, 1911.
22. Politzer, G.: Ueber die Entwicklung des Dammes beim Menschen. Ztschr. f. Anat. u. Entwcklngsgesch., 97:622, 1932.
23. Retterer, M. E.: Mode de cloisonnement du cloaque chez le cobaye. Bibliog. Anat., 1:184, 1893.
24. Rhoads, J. E., Pipes, R. L. and Randall, J. P.: Simultaneous Abdominal and Perineal Approach in Operations for Imperforate Anus with Atresia of Rectum and Rectosigmoid. Ann. Surg., 127:552, 1948.
25. Rosenblatt, M. S. and May, A.: Malformation of Anus and Rectum. Surg., Gynec. & Obst., 83:499, 1946.
26. Stieda, A.: Ueber Atresia ani congenita und die damit verbundenen Missbildungen. Arch. f. klin. Chir., 70:555, 1903.
27. Thunig, L. A.: Atresia Ani Urethralis. Arch. Surg., 38:501, 1939.
28. Wallace, F. T. and Colvin, E. M.: Complications of Imperforate Anus Repair. Surgery 24:832, 1948.

29. Wangensteen, O. H. and Rice, C. O.: Imperforate Anus—A Method of Determining the Surgical Approach. Ann. Surg., *92:*77, 1930.

30. Wilson, A. K.: Roentgen Examination in Congenital Intestinal Obstructive Defects in Infants. Its Aid in Planning Suitable Surgical Approach and Procedures for their Correction. Am. J. Roentgenol., *54:* 498, 1945.

31. Young, H. H.: Imperforate Anus: Bowel Opening into Urethra; Hypospadias. A Presentation of New Plastic Methods. J.A.M.A., *107:*1448, 1936.

CHAPTER 25

Rectal Bleeding in Infants and Children

In pediatric practice it is not uncommon to hear of complaints of rectal bleeding. In the vast majority of cases it is small in amount, has little significance, and does not require extensive investigation or operative therapy; in a minority of cases it is the initial or the outstanding symptom of an important pathologic process which requires surgical treatment. In those babies and children who pass considerable amounts of blood per rectum, one can sometimes find and treat the lesion which is causing it; in an astounding proportion of patients the cause for the bleeding is never found, even after extensive investigation and laparotomy.

Mild Bleeding

In office or out-patient department practice, most of the children who have rectal bleeding pass but small amounts of blood which is generally accountable on the basis of anal fissure or the passage of firm constipated stools. In either of these situations the damaged anal or rectal mucosa is given the best chance to heal if the child is given adequate amounts of milk of magnesia, or preferably mineral oil, once a day for two or three weeks; seldom is other therapy required. In only an occasional case is it necessary to dilate the anus (under anesthesia); this will paralyze the anal sphincter for a week or ten days, make the anus quite lax during such a period, and will give any crack of the mucosa time to heal.

Extensive Bleeding

For the infant or child who has rectal bleeding of sufficient degree to cause concern, one's ingenuity is often taxed in handling the problem. Investigation (such as proctoscopy and barium enema) might show a lesion (such as rectal polyp) which can be treated quickly and effectively. All too often, proctoscopy, barium enema, hematologic studies show no abnormalities and there is a quandary regarding the advisability of laparotomy. Certainly *some* of these children should be operated upon because this may be the only means of detecting a condition such as Meckel's diverticulum, small duplication of the intestine, intestinal polyp, et cetera. However, not all of these children need surgery because so frequently abdominal exploration reveals nothing; the parents and surgeon are disappointed in having undertaken a major operation from which little or no benefit is derived. In dealing with children with rectal bleeding of obscure origin it is sometimes exceedingly difficult for even the most experienced physician or surgeon to decide—in an objective and honest manner—whether to operate or not.

In children, bleeding by rectum can be so variable in amount, frequency, and importance that no dogmatic rules can be made regarding the therapeutic handling of it.

Page 369

It is necessary to view each case individually, and to make the decision for or against surgery upon the evidence which is presented. To give some idea of the extent of the problem, the types of pathology which are apt to be found, and the number of cases in which no satisfactory diagnosis is ever made, it seems desirable to give a cross-section of material by listing and discussing all patients who entered our hospital in a one-year span primarily because of rectal bleeding.

CLINICAL MATERIAL

During the year 1950, 65 children were admitted to the Boston Children's Hospital with a presenting symptom of bleeding per rectum. In each instance the bleeding was thought to be serious enough by the parent or the referring doctor to warrant hospital study. This material does *not* include patients who were seen only in the out-patient department with minor bleeding. Furthermore, it does *not* include patients who might have had rectal bleeding as a part of a picture which could be readily recognized, such as intestinal bleeding when there was known leukemia, or bleeding from an obvious intussusception. It includes only the 65 children who entered the hospital with rectal bleeding which was a diagnostic problem. After appropriate studies, consultations, and (for some) exploratory operation, a final diagnosis could be conclusively established in many; in others it could not. Data regarding the 65 patients are given in Tables 47 and 48. This material for the year 1950 gives a fairly representative picture of most of the causes of rectal bleeding of moderate or marked degree in infants and children; this particular year did not happen to include any examples of rare conditions such as multiple polyposis of the colon, hemangioma of the intestine, or benign intestinal polyp.

The children varied in age from a few days to thirteen years. Forty per cent of them were a year, or less, in age; another 20 per cent were between one and four years. Males outnumbered females two to one. Some had had repeated episodes of bleeding, others only a single bout. The extent of bleeding varied greatly; 6 patients were in shock and were described as "bled out." The various diagnoses which were finally made are listed in Table 47; discussions of the various conditions appear in the following sections.

Benign Polyp of Rectum or Colon

Eleven of the children were discovered to have benign polyps of the large bowel. In two instances more than one polyp was present, but no cases of true multiple polyposis were encountered during this one-year interval. Bright red streaking, particularly on the outside of the stools, had been noticed in all patients for a period varying from one to eighteen months. All but two patients had been otherwise entirely asymptomatic; the two exceptions each had associated complaints of occasional crampy abdominal pain. Despite the long duration of bleeding in several of these children, all had normal blood counts. All 11 patients were proctoscoped and, in 7 cases, polyps were visualized in the rectum or lower sigmoid, and could be removed through the proctoscope. All patients had barium enemas and in 4 instances polyps of the colon, above the rectosigmoid level, were demonstrated. In these latter 4 patients, the polyps were fairly high in the colon, so that a transabdominal approach was required for their removal.

Malignant Intestinal Polyp

One child, a boy aged two years, had had rectal bleeding of three weeks' duration. He then passed per rectum a small globular mass which was retrieved by the parents, and was sent for pathologic examination by the family physician. A histologic diagnosis of *adenocarcinoma* was made by competent pathologists. While the bleeding had ceased

Table 47

Data from 65 Patients Who Were Admitted to Hospital because of Rectal Bleeding During the Year 1950

Final Diagnosis	Number of Cases	Ages	Sex		Number "Bled Out"
			M	F	
Benign polyp of rectum (7 cases)* or of colon (4 cases)*	11	2, 3, 3, 5, 5, 6, 7, 7, 8, 8, 8 yrs.	7	4	
Malignant intestinal polyp	1	2 yrs.	1		
Proctitis, papillitis, anal fissure, etc.	6	7, 11 days; 1, 2, 2, 10 yrs.	5	1	
Gastritis or enteritis	5	1 mo.; 1, 1, 2, 3 yrs.	2	3	
Ulcerative colitis	4	4, 9, 12, 13 yrs.	3	1	
Intussusception*	1	11 yrs.	1		
Meckel's diverticulum*	3	2, 8, 20 mos.	3		1
Duodenal ulcer*	1	2 days (premature)	1		
Intestinal duplication*	1	13 yrs.		1	1
Systemic hemorrhagic disease	4	26 days; 3, 4, 8 yrs.	2	2	3
Hemorrhagic disease of newborn	10	1, 1, 1, 1, 2, 2, 2, 3, 7, 14 days	5	5	1
Gastro-intestinal bleeding of unknown etiology†	18	1, 1, 3, 7, 9, 11 mos.; 1, 2, 2, 3, 3, 3, 4, 4, 4, 7, 7, 7 yrs.	14	4	
Totals	65		44	21	6

* All of these patients were operated upon for definitive treatment.

† Fourteen of these patients were not operated upon. Four were operated upon and no pathology found. Further data concerning all 18 of these cases are listed in Table 48.

following the passing of this tumor, the child was admitted to hospital for investigation. The stools were repeatedly negative for occult or gross blood. Proctoscopy and barium enema failed to reveal any lesion whatsoever. The patient has now been followed for one and one-half years. No further bleeding has occurred, and barium enemas and proctoscopies performed every three months have been repeatedly negative. (We assume he had a malignant polyp which fortunately was sloughed off.)

Fissures or Mild Inflammatory Disease of the Anus and Rectum

Proctitis, papillitis, stercoral ulceration, et cetera were found in 6 patients. The rectal bleeding in these cases was small in amount, and generally had been present inter-

Table 48

Follow-up Data on the 18 Children from Table 47 Who Had Been Discharged from Hospital with Diagnosis of "Rectal Bleeding of Unknown Etiology"

Case No.	Age	Sex	Length of Follow-up	Results
1	1 mo.	F	1½ yrs.	Later had a small rectal prolapse. Now well, with no further bleeding.
2	1 mo.	M	1½ yrs.	No further bleeding. Died March 1952 of septicemia. Autopsy revealed no lesion of the G. I. tract.
3	3 mos.	M	1½ yrs.	No further bleeding.
4*	7 mos.	M	1 yr.	No further bleeding.
5	9 mos.	M	1½ yrs.	No further bleeding.
6*	11 mos.	M	1 yr.	Continues to have occasional bleeding. Repeat investigation negative. Sister also has rectal bleeding.
7	13 mos.	M	1 yr.	No further bleeding.
8	2 yrs.	F	1½ yrs.	No further bleeding.
9	2 yrs.	F	1½ yrs.	No further bleeding.
10	2 yrs.	M	1 yr.	No further bleeding.
11*	3 yrs.	M	1½ yrs.	No further bleeding.
12	3 yrs.	M	1½ yrs.	No further bleeding.
13	3 yrs.	M	1½ yrs.	No further bleeding.
14	3 yrs.	M	1½ yrs.	No further bleeding.
15	4 yrs.	M	1½ yrs.	No further bleeding.
16*	7 yrs.	M	1½ yrs.	No further bleeding.
17	7 yrs.	M	1½ yrs.	No further bleeding.
18	7 yrs.	F	1½ yrs.	Continues to have occasional bleeding. Brother also has rectal bleeding. Investigations negative.

* These four patients were the ones who had been explored during the previous hospitalization, and in whom no pathology had been found.

mittently for considerable periods of time. Two patients gave a history of chronic constipation, while two others had had recent episodes of diarrhea. The diagnosis was made on proctoscopy in each case. Barium enemas were performed on these 6 patients and all results were negative. These children were placed on soft, low-residue diets and were given daily small doses of mineral oil. Four patients have had no further bleeding, while in two there has been an occasional recurrence. These two children have been reinvestigated, but no other lesions have been discovered.

Gastritis or Enteritis

This was found in 5 infants and young children. In general, the bleeding was of short duration, the longest having been one month. All had mild gastro-intestinal symptoms consisting of occasional abdominal cramps, diarrhea, or vomiting. All diagnoses were made on a clinical basis except for one infant, in whom a diagnosis of antral gastritis was made roentgenologically by barium meal, and was later confirmed at laparotomy. The other 4 children have subsequently done well on medical management, and none has had a recurrence of bleeding.

Ulcerative Colitis

This was discovered in 4 children. In each case the bleeding had been noted for several months, the shortest history being of two months' duration. Two of the children had associated mild diarrhea, one had excess mucus in the stools, and one was otherwise asymptomatic. The diagnoses were made either by barium enema, proctoscopy, or both. All cases were mild and have been treated medically; two received cortisone with marked improvement.

Intussusception

This condition was found in one boy. He had previously been seen in the out-patient department because of episodes (during two months) of rectal bleeding associated with crampy abdominal pain and occasional vomiting. Physical examination as well as hematologic and roentgenologic investigations was negative. During a subsequent more severe attack, he was admitted to the hospital and this time an ileal intussusception was demonstrated both by barium enema and by gastro-intestinal series. At operation the intussusception was easily reduced; a small Meckel's diverticulum had been the leading point. Apparently there has been recurrent intussusception from time to time.

Meckel's Diverticulum

A diverticulum (without intussusception) was found in 3 male infants who had recurrent rectal bleeding (without other symptoms) for one week to two months. One of these patients was markedly anemic, but the others were not. Investigations of these 3 children, including barium enemas, barium meals, and proctoscopy were entirely negative. All had laparotomy, at which time the Meckel's diverticula were found and excised. All diverticula contained either aberrant gastric or pancreatic tissue.

Duodenal Ulcer

One premature male infant, weighing 3 pounds, 14 ounces, was admitted to the hospital on the second day of life with severe rectal bleeding and abdominal distention. A roentgenogram of the abdomen revealed free air under both leaves of the diaphragm. At operation a perforated and bleeding duodenal ulcer was found and closed. Unfortunately, the baby did poorly after operation and died on the third postoperative day.

Intestinal Duplication

This was the cause of serious rectal bleeding in one case. This anemic girl of twelve years had been bleeding by rectum for five months. On admission, the hemoglobin was 5.0 gm. per cent and the red cell count was 1.28 million. Physical examination was negative except for great pallor and sweating. By barium meal a large diverticulum arising high in the small intestine was demonstrated. Following correction of the anemia by transfusion, abdominal exploration was performed and a large jejunal duplication containing gastric mucosa was found. Because of a blood supply common to the intestine it was necessary to resect a portion of the jejunum along with the diverticulum. There was an uneventful recovery.

Systemic Hemorrhagic Disease

This condition was discovered in 4 children. The youngest, a male infant one month of age, had a marked hypoprothrombinemia which responded immediately to the administration of vitamin K. There has been no recurrence of this patient's bleeding since that time. One boy, aged seven years, fainted after passing a large amount of blood per rectum five hours prior to admission. On physical examination petechial hemorrhages and subcutaneous ecchymotic areas were found. Following blood studies, a diagnosis of non-thrombocytopenic (Henoch's) purpura was made. The third child had rectal bleeding of five months' duration accompanied by intermittent fever. On admission to hospital his platelets numbered only 60,000 and a diagnosis of thrombocytopenic purpura was made. He was treated conservatively without splenectomy and now—one and one-half years later—is well, with no evidence of hemorrhagic disease. The fourth child, a girl of three years, had had bleeding per rectum since the age of six weeks. At that time investigation, including laparotomy, had been entirely negative. On admission to the hospital in 1950, she was severely anemic, with a red cell count of 1.94 million, and a hemoglobin level of 6.0 gm. per cent. Hematologic studies were performed and have been reported by Alexander, Goldstein, Landwehr, and Cook.[1] They revealed a deficiency of "serum prothrombin conversion accelerator," and she since has been carried along improved, although still intermittently bleeding, by means of occasional whole blood and serum transfusions.

Hemorrhagic Disease of the Newborn

This disease was found in 10 infants, all under two weeks of age. The diagnosis was made, although only two of the babies were definitely shown to have low prothrombin levels. In 8 infants the bleeding stopped soon after the institution of treatment with vitamin K. None of these has had any further bleeding. One infant suffered a serious intracranial hemorrhage from which he died. Another had a barium enema performed at an outside hospital, seeking the source of the bleeding. During examination the transverse colon was unfortunately perforated and he was admitted here for laparotomy. The disrupted transverse colon was exteriorized by a Mikulicz procedure. No lesion other than the perforation was demonstrated and on vitamin K therapy no further bleeding occurred. The colostomy was subsequently closed, and the child recovered.

Gastro-intestinal Bleeding of Unknown Etiology

In 18 older children no cause for rectal bleeding could be discovered. Symptoms had been present on an average of six weeks, varying from one day to five months. Only one child had any significant degree of anemia. All patients had complete blood studies; 17 patients had barium enemas; 4 had barium meals; 11 were studied by proctoscopy; none of these tests or examinations disclosed any lesion. Four of these 18 children were subjected to laparotomy; still no cause for bleeding was found thereby. These 18 patients with rectal bleeding of unknown etiology have all been followed for more than a year Their courses following hospitalization are listed in Table 48. Fifteen of the children in the group have remained in good health with no further rectal bleeding. Two children have continued intermittently to have small amounts of bright red blood in the stool; one of them has been reinvestigated, again with negative results. One other child continued to pass occasional small amounts of blood per rectum for several weeks; then one day while straining at stool a small prolapse of the rectal mucosa appeared. He was given small doses of mineral oil for several weeks to soften the stool and reduce straining, the mother was taught how to reduce a prolapse if it should reappear, and after institution of this regimen the prolapse and rectal bleeding have ceased.

EVALUATION AND MANAGEMENT OF RECTAL BLEEDING

The investigation and management of children admitted to hospital because of rectal bleeding varies somewhat from patient to patient but certain general statements can be made. From the history of the illness, from the amount, type, and duration of the bleeding, from the family history, from the physical examination, and from inspection of the stools, important leads may be obtained toward making the correct diagnosis.

General Statements

Fissure-in-ano is the commonest cause of rectal bleeding in children. In these patients there is almost always a history of constipation and generally of pain during defecation. The bleeding is usually small in amount, is bright red, is streaked on the outside of the stool, and occurs during or just after a bowel movement. *Polyps* give bleeding which is usually painless, and generally is fairly copious. On digital rectal examination a polyp can frequently be felt within reach of the finger, and the diagnosis thus quickly established. In other instances, it cannot be identified in the rectum until proctoscopy is performed or cannot be seen in the colon until barium enema visualization is done. *Intussusception* commonly gives rectal bleeding, but the presence of intermittent abdominal pain, and possibly a palpable abdominal mass in a child who is obviously quite ill, are usually sufficient to recognize the condition; a barium enema may be required in some cases to be certain of the diagnosis. A *Meckel's diverticulum* tends to cause bleeding which starts suddenly and silently, persists for a day or two, and then terminates abruptly. It is usually quite large in amount, is typically dark in color or actually tarry, and is mixed throughout the substance of the stool. *Intestinal duplication* is an occasional source of massive bleeding, particularly if much of the blood is dark in color. Hemorrhage of this type is usually painless but may be accompanied by a vague dull ache or mild tenderness in the region of the umbilicus. *Lesions high in the intestinal tract*, i.e., peptic ulcer, esophageal varices, diaphragmatic hernia, esophagitis, almost always give symptoms referable to the upper abdomen, a stool which is black (or strongly positive on guaiac test), and are usually associated with hematemesis; in those cases in which there is bleeding from portal hypertension, the spleen and possibly the liver are enlarged. *Blood dyscrasias*, including leukemia, frequently cause rectal bleeding but they are usually accompanied by hemorrhagic tendencies in other parts of the body; complete hematologic studies will establish the correct diagnosis. *Hemorrhagic disease of the newborn* appears only in the first two or three weeks of life. Rectal bleeding can be a part of the picture; there is prompt response to the administration of vitamin K.

Preparation for Transfusion

All infants and children who are admitted to the hospital with rectal bleeding should immediately have blood grouping and matching, so that blood for transfusion is readily available at all times. On several occasions we have seen children, who previously had had only insignificant bleeding, suddenly develop massive hemorrhage to such a degree that exsanguination occurred within twenty to thirty minutes. Under such circumstances, it is very helpful to have blood available immediately for supporting them.

Study

In the more common, milder cases of rectal bleeding, investigation may be carried out in a systematic manner. For all patients it is routine to have counts of red cells, white cells, and platelets and also determination of prothrombin, bleeding, and clotting times. A barium meal or small bowel study is not performed unless (from history or physical examination) an upper gastro-intestinal lesion is suspected. The demonstration of a Meckel's diverticulum by means of a barium meal is so rare that we do not attempt to make this diagnosis roentgenologically. Barium enema and proctoscopy should be performed almost routinely; generally we prefer to make the barium enema examination first. The radiologist cannot properly visualize the rectum and lower sigmoid; barium enema without proctoscopy constitutes an incomplete examination of the colon. Proctoscopy is seldom useful in a child if done without general anesthesia. It is safer, more informative, and much more satisfactory to give a light general anesthesia for this examination; if a polyp is found in the rectum or lower sigmoid it can be removed, or if nothing is found, laparotomy can be carried out immediately (if the symptoms had been sufficient to warrant this step).

Laparotomy

As a general rule, laparotomy should not be performed merely because of the history that a parent has seen blood. To a layman, a little blood is apt to look like an alarming hemorrhage. Furthermore, color in the stool from beets, chocolate, or the like is sometimes mistaken for blood. It is best not to perform a major operation unless some doctor has seen the blood in the stool and can estimate that the amount was considerable. (Whenever a parent actually did see large amounts of blood passed by rectum, there will still be more of it for the doctor to see when he arrives and makes a rectal examination.)

In those cases in which bleeding has obviously been of serious degree, and all methods of study have not established the cause for bleeding, laparotomy should be advised and performed. In some of these cases a congenital malformation or other lesion will be found in the abdomen; in others nothing will be discovered.

In those cases in which the bleeding has been of only slight degree, and no cause for it can be demonstrated, we are inclined to discharge the patient from the hospital and follow him carefully at home. Frequently the bleeding stops and does not recur. If, however, bleeding does recur in serious amount, then the child can be brought back for laparotomy. This general policy is adopted in the effort to avoid unnecessary operations.

REFERENCE

1. Alexander, B., Goldstein, R., Landwehr, G. and Cook, C. D.: Congenital SPCA Deficiency: A Hitherto Unrecognized Coagulation Defect with Hemorrhage Rectified by Serum and Serum Fractions. J. Clin. Investigation, *30*:596, 1951.

CHAPTER 26

Omental Cysts and Mesenteric Cysts

OMENTAL CYSTS

Cysts of the omentum presumably originate in the same manner as do those of the mesentery, namely, by obstruction of an existing lymphatic channel or by growth of congenitally misplaced lymphatic tissue which fails to communicate with the vascular system. These cysts are thin-walled, rounded, or lobulated, and contain serous fluid. Microscopically, they are lined by a flattened layer of endothelial cells. The cysts may be small and embedded within the substance of the omentum, or they may be huge and largely replace this structure. One specimen we have excised measured 13 x 8 x 6 cm.; a second was larger, and contained more than 1000 cc. of fluid; a third was of such size that it extended from the greater curvature of the stomach down into the pelvis and out into either flank so that it entirely covered the intestines. Of the 6 examples we have encountered, 2 were multilocular and the other 4 were unilocular.

Symptoms and Signs

The symptoms are usually those of a slowly enlarging abdominal mass which gives little or no discomfort. Our patients varied from three months to eight years of age. Physical examination discloses little more than a prominent or protuberant abdomen within which an elastic, non-tender, forward-lying mass can be palpated. The rounded or slightly lobulated cyst can often be dislodged from side to side, and if it is large, a fluid wave can be elicited.

Diagnosis

The diagnosis of an omental cyst is usually suggested by the physical findings and by the silent nature of the swelling. It may be difficult to differentiate between mesenteric and omental cyst, but the latter diagnosis is suggested if the mass is found by roentgenologic studies to lie in front of the intestines.

Treatment

This can be easily carried out by simple excision. Large cysts may require amputation of almost the entire omentum. Smaller ones can be dissected out from the surrounding omental fat, which should be saved because of its usefulness in combating any infection which might arise in the peritoneal cavity at a subsequent time. Some data from our cases are presented in Table 49.

ISOLATED MESENTERIC CYSTS

Cysts may arise in any portion of the mesentery or the mesocolon. They may reach enormous proportions and because of their slow growth they may give symptoms over long periods of time.

Page 377

Etiology

Mesenteric cysts could conceivably arise by obstruction of a pre-existing lymphatic trunk, but the absence of demonstrable inflammation or other fibrosing lesion in the mesentery generally makes this theory improbable. It is more than likely that mesenteric cysts develop from misplaced bits of lymphatic tissue which proliferate and then accumulate fluid because they do not possess communications which allow them to drain properly into the remainder of the lymphatic system.

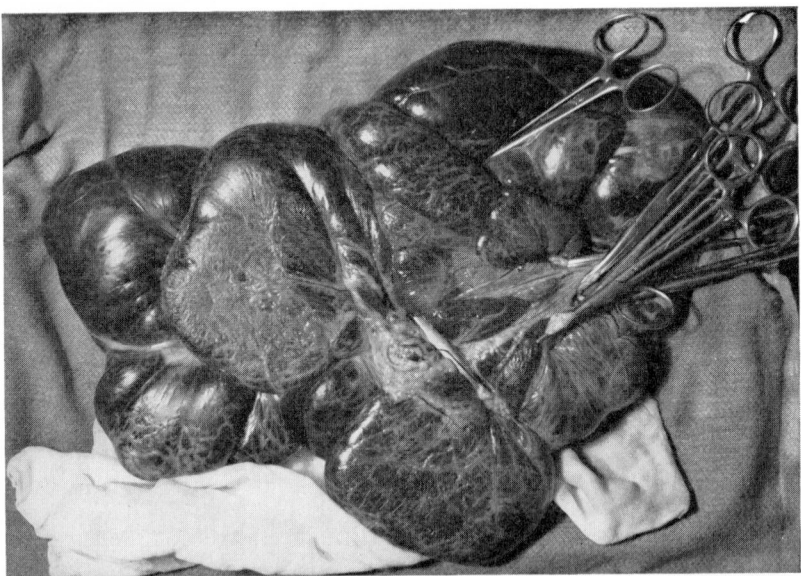

Fig. 196. Huge multilocular omental cyst from a child of three years (Case 4). It contained 1300 cc. of fluid.

Pathology

Mesenteric cysts are most commonly found in the mesentery of the jejunum or ileum, but in two of our cases they appeared in the transverse mesocolon and in the mesosigmoid, respectively. The cysts obviously must pass through a stage when they are quite small, but by the time that they have produced symptoms requiring operation usually they have reached a very large size. Not infrequently they are as large as an orange or a grapefruit, and indeed they may fill a major portion of the abdominal cavity. One specimen contained 1200 cc. of fluid. They are usually not tensely filled, and indeed tend to have a flabby consistency. It is common for them to have a dumb-bell shape (Fig. 198) and to project out from either surface of the mesentery, sometimes partly surrounding the adjacent intestine in the form of a saddle. A structure of such conformation can strangle the adjacent loop of intestine and obstruct it. In the majority of cases only one cyst is present, but in two of our patients the main cyst was accompanied by several smaller ones in the base of the mesentery.

The cysts lie between the peritoneal leaves of the mesentery (or mesocolon) and may be situated anywhere from its base out to the enteric border. Their walls are quite thin, rarely more than a millimeter or two in thickness. The inner surfaces are smooth. By microscopic examination the walls are found to consist of connective tissue. There is no muscular coat or mucosal lining. In well preserved specimens a layer of flattened endothelial cells can be identified on the inner surface.

Fluid within the cysts may be of two sorts. In most instances it is serous and color-less, but in others it is chylous and has the appearance and consistency of whitish or yellowish white milk. In our 12 examples of isolated mesenteric cysts, 7 had a *serous* and 5 a *chylous* fluid. All of the chylous cysts arose from the mesentery of the jejunum or upper ileum, where material draining from the intestinal tract presumably contained a high percentage of fat. Fluid from a serous cyst of the mesocolon was found by chem-ical examination to contain the following: sodium, 133 mEq. per liter; chloride, 101 mEq. per liter; non-protein nitrogen, 31 mg. per cent; total protein, 4.9 gm. per cent; cholesterol, 68 mg. per cent. The concentration of these substances was approximately the same as that of plasma. Chemical examination of the chylous fluid from the cyst illustrated in Figure 198 showed: chlorides, 108 mEq. per liter; non-protein nitrogen, 29 mg. per cent; total protein, 2.1 gm. per cent; fat, 1 per cent.

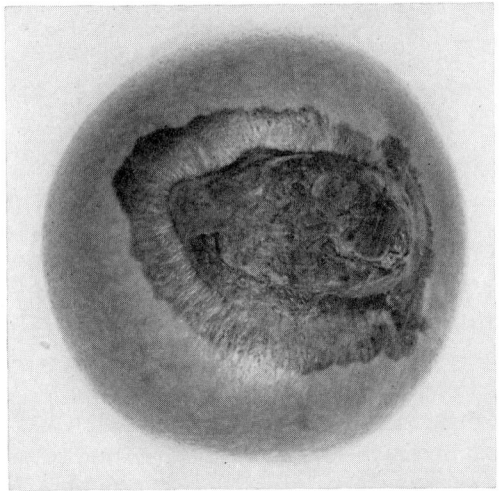

Fig. 197. Omental cyst 6 cm. in diameter, which had become twisted and infarcted. Child one year of age (Case 2).

Differential Diagnosis

There are many descriptions in the literature which confuse true mesenteric (lym-phatic) cysts with *enteric* cysts (duplications) (see Chapter 17). These two lesions can have somewhat similar positions in the mesentery, but it is desirable to distinguish between them because they are pathologically different and because they require quite different forms of therapy. A *duplication* is a thick-walled structure which has a serous coat, layers of smooth muscle, and a mucous membrane lining. It usually lies imme-diately adjacent to the bowel between the folds of the mesentery, and the musculature of the duplication is so intimately associated with that of the intestine that the two can-not be separated easily from one another. Furthermore, the blood supply of a duplica-tion is the same as that of the intestine to which it is adjacent, so that the duplication cannot be removed without impairing the blood supply of the intestinal segment. In contrast, a *mesenteric cyst* is thin-walled and has no muscular coat or mucosal lining. While it may lie against the mesenteric surface of the intestine, there is a line of cleavage so that it can usually be excised without injuring the bowel or its bloods upply. It is generally impossible to distinguish between mesenteric cyst and duplication prior to operation, but once an abdomen is opened the two lesions can be distinguished easily by their gross characteristics.

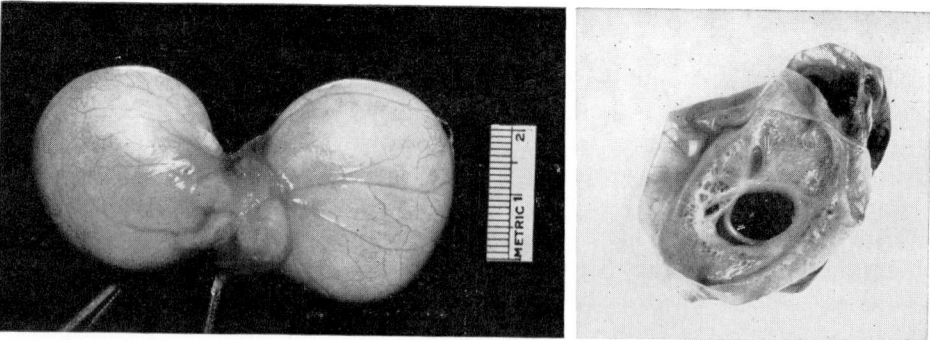

Fig. 198. *Left*, Chylous cyst removed from the jejunal mesentery of a seven-week-old baby (Case 2). The cyst had a dumb-bell shape and bulged out on both sides of the mesentery. *Right*, Multilocular lymphatic cyst removed from mesentery of an infant.

Clinical Findings

Mesenteric cysts can be found in infancy, but they are more apt to appear in childhood. The ages of our thirteen patients varied from three days to ten years. The symptoms may be of three sorts: (1) In the typical case a painless, slowly *enlarging abdomen* is the only complaint. The progressive enlargement is sometimes noted for a year or two before surgical advice is sought. (2) There may be recurring attacks of mild to moderate *abdominal pain*, at times associated with vomiting. These usually last for a day or two and appear only at infrequent intervals. There may be reduced appetite and poor weight gain. (3) In occasional patients (e.g., No. 9 of Table 49), the symptoms are those of acute *intestinal obstruction* if the cyst lies at the free border of the mesentery where it can press upon or angulate the gut.

Whether or not a mesenteric cyst can be felt through the abdominal wall depends somewhat upon its size and tenseness. If the child is examined within the first few months of illness, abdominal *palpation* may reveal no abnormality. Indeed, even the largest cysts sometimes may elude detection because they are so flabby that their borders can-

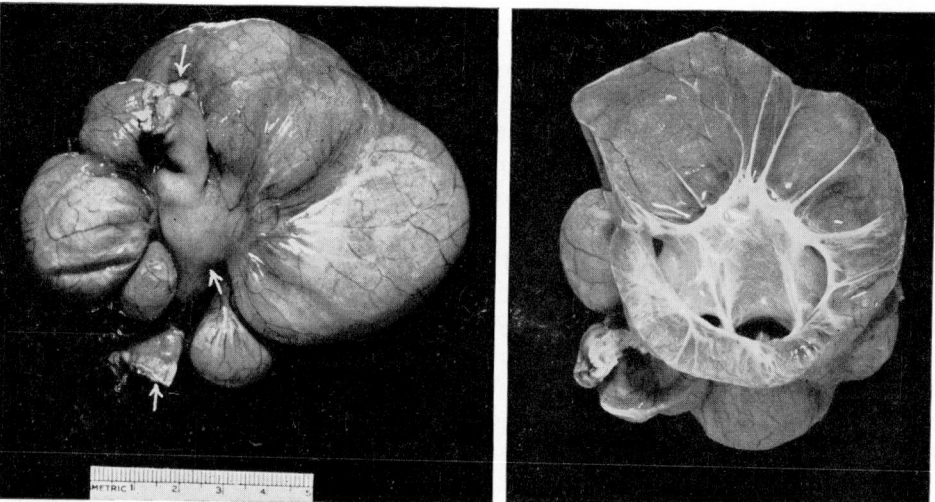

Fig. 199. *Left*, Large mesenteric cyst from a four-year-old child (Case 9). A segment of ileum (arrows) had to be removed along with the cyst. *Right*, The specimen transected, to show its multilocular structure.

not be mapped out. However, in most cases a fairly well-defined, fluctuant, soft mass can be palpated. This can be shifted within the abdomen and it is more freely movable in a lateral than in a vertical direction. If the cyst is large, a fluid wave or even shifting dullness may be detected.

Roentgenologic Findings

Films of the abdomen, with or without a barium meal, often give a valuable lead, for a gasless shadow will be found which displaces intestines into other parts of the abdomen. Fluoroscopic study shows that the mass can be pushed into different parts of the abdomen. Since these lesions seldom produce obstruction, dilated intestine is rarely found.

Treatment

Surgical treatment can be effected in one of three ways: (1) If the cyst is unduly adherent to intestine, it may be excised along with the portion of intestine, performing a primary anastomosis of the remaining ends. (2) The cyst may be *marsupiaiized*, but there is little to recommend this form of therapy; it should be abandoned. (3) The cyst may be *dissected* out from the mesentery. This is the preferred method of treatment.

Excision of a cyst is carried out by peeling away the peritoneal leaves of the mesentery from the underlying mass and by displacing all important blood vessels to one side. It is usually not difficult to dissect the sac from the intestine or colon. The surrounding cleavage planes are easier to find if the cyst is not opened or ruptured. When the mass has been removed, a considerable rent may be left in the mesentery, which is now repaired with interrupted sutures of fine silk or catgut. If dissection is carefully done, the blood supply of the adjacent gut will not be interfered with. If the major portion of a cyst has been dissected away, but it appears too dangerous to remove a small bit which remains against an important blood vessel or against the intestine, this can be left and can be cauterized with carbolic acid (followed by alcohol) according to the suggestion of Peterson.

Twelve patients with isolated mesenteric cysts have been operated upon at the Children's Hospital. Some data from these are summarized in Table 49. Two patients died, both of whom had had a volvulus which gave rise to extensive infarctation of intestine.

MULTIPLE CYSTIC DISEASE OF THE MESENTERY

The foregoing section dealt with *isolated* mesenteric cysts which usually carry an excellent prognosis. In sharp contrast are the cases (fortunately rare) in which the entire mesentery, or a large portion thereof, is filled with myriads of cysts, either lymphatic or chylous in nature. The mesentery is irregularly swollen to as much as one or several centimeters in thickness by literally hundreds of cystic lesions which vary greatly in size from those which are barely discernible to others which are many centimeters in diameter. In addition to these cysts between the mesenteric leaves there is usually considerable edema and possibly some fibrosis of the mesentery, both of which contribute to its thickening.

It is utterly impossible to remove surgically all of the cysts and clean out the mesentery; some of the larger ones can be cut away, but there remains so much of the abnormal tissue in the edematous and scarred mesentery that the operator wonders just how much good has been accomplished. It is sometimes possible to remedy the situation to sufficient degree so that the individual's health is reasonably good over a

Table 49. Data from Cases of Omental and Mesenteric Cysts

Case	Age and Sex		Symptom Duration	Position of Cyst. Type of Fluid in Cyst	Size of Cyst	Operation	Result
Omental Cysts							
1	3 mos.	M	None	Omentum. Serous	11 x 4 mm.	Excision	Cured
2	1 yr.	F	48 hrs.	Omentum. Serous	6 cm. in diam.	Excision	Cured
3	3 yrs.	M	?	Omentum. Serous	Filled entire anterior abdomen	Excision	Cured
4	3 yrs.	M	6 mos.	Omentum. Serous	1300 cc.	Excision	Cured
5	8 yrs.	F	3 mos.	Omentum. Serous	1000 cc.	Excision	Cured
6	8 yrs.	F	5 days	Omentum. Serous	13 x 8 x 6 cm.	Excision	Cured
*Mesenteric Cysts**							
1	3 days	F	24 hrs.	Ileum. Chylous	6 x 4 x 3 cm.	Excision	Cured
2	7 wks.	M	12 hrs.	Jejunum. Chylous	Size of 2 golf balls	Excision. Reduction of volvulus	Died
3	2 mos.	M	1 day	Jejunum. Serous	5 x 4 x 4 cm.	Excision	Cured
4	3 mos.	M	2 days	Jejunum. Serous	7 x 4 cm.	Reduction of volvulus	Died
5†	7 mos.	F	7 days	Ileum. Cystic lymphangioendothelioma	17 x 10 x 6 cm.	Excision and resection of ileum	Died
6	2½ yrs.	M	1 yr.	Transverse colon. Serous	Size of grapefruit	Excision	Cured
7	3 yrs.	M	2 yrs.	Jejunum. Chylous	Orange size	Excision. Intestinal resection	Cured
8	3 yrs.	M	2 yrs.	Jejunum. Serous	Size of 3 fists (dumbbell shape)	Excision	Cured
9	4 yrs.	M	5 days	Terminal ileum. Serous	Lobulated (dumbbell shape)	Excision. Resection of ileum	Cured
10	6 yrs.	F	5 mos.	Sigmoid. Serous	10 x 8 x 8 cm. 875 gm.	Excision. Resection of sigmoid	Cured
11	6 yrs.	F	6 mos.	Jejunum. Chylous	30 x 30 x 15 cm.	Excision	Cured
12	7 yrs.	M	2 yrs.	Ileum. Serous	Size of 2 fists (dumbbell shape)	Excision	Cured
13	10 yrs.	F	3 yrs.	Ileum. Chylous	12 cm.	Excision	Cured

* This does not include duplications, which are listed in Chapter 17.
† This child had multiple cystic disease of the mesentery.

period of years, even though there is apprehension about the possibility of progression of the underlying condition, which can subsequently give rise either to hopeless intestinal obstruction or to irremediable accumulation of fluid in the wall of the intestine or in the peritoneal cavity. Multiple cystic disease of the mesentery is an extremely distressing condition which, on the whole, carries a rather poor prognosis in most cases.

REFERENCES

OMENTAL CYSTS

1. Beahrs, O. H. and Dockerty, M. B.: Primary Omental Cysts of Clinical Importance. S. Clin. North America, *30*:1073, 1950.
2. Berger, L. and Rothenberg, R. E.: Cysts of Omentum, Mesentery and Retroperitoneum; Clinical Study of 18 Cases. Surgery, *5*:522, 1939.
3. Birnkrant, M.: Traumatic Serous Cyst of the Lesser Omentum. Radiology, *42*:74, 1944.
4. Dowd, C. N.: Cyst of the Omentum. Ann. Surg., *54*:617, 1911.
5. Guernsey, C. M.: Primary Tumors and Cysts of Omentum. Proc. Staff Meet. Mayo Clin., *14*:694, 1939.
6. Hall, D. P.: Lymphangiomata of the Great Omentum. Ann. Surg., *111*:605, 1940.
7. Horgan, J.: Cysts of Omentum; Review and Report of Case. Am. J. Surg., *29*:343, 1935.

MESENTERIC CYSTS

8. Block, F. B.: Chylous Mesenteric Cyst. Ann. Surg., *128*:158, 1948.
9. Carter, R. M.: Cysts of the Mesentery. Surg., Gynec. & Obst., *33*:544, 1921.
10. Dowd, C. N.: Mesenteric Cysts. Ann. Surg., *128*:158, 1948.

11. Flynn, C. W.: Mesenteric Cysts, With Report of a Case of Cystic Lymphangioma. Ann. Surg., *91*:505, 1930.
12. Gale, J. W. and Keeley, J. L.: Mesenteric Cysts Causing Intestinal Obstruction. Am. J. Surg., *40*:647, 1938.
13. Messer, F. C.: Analysis of Fluid from Chylous Mesenteric Cyst. J. Lab. & Clin. Med., *23*:596, 1938.
14. Oberhelman, H. A. and Condon, J. B.: Hemorrhagic Cyst of the Mesentery of the Ileum. Arch. Surg., *57*:301, 1948.
15. Peterson, E. W.: Mesenteric and Omental Cysts. Ann. Surg., *96*:340, 1932.
16. Peterson, E. W.: Cysts of the Mesentery. Ann. Surg., *112*:80, 1940.
17. Swartley, W. B.: Mesenteric Cysts. Ann. Surg., *85*:886, 1927.
18. Vaughn, A. M., Lees, W. M. and Henry, J. W.: Mesenteric Cysts. A Review of the Literature and Report of a Calcified Cyst of the Mesentery. Surgery, *23*:306, 1948.
19. Warfield, J. O.: A Study of Mesenteric Cysts with a Report of Two Recent Cases. Ann. Surg., *96*:329, 1932.

CHAPTER 27

Primary Peritonitis

"Secondary peritonitis" is a term which can be used to indicate those peritoneal inflammations which originate from some abdominal organ, such as an inflamed appendix, a perforated Meckel's diverticulum, an ulcerated colon, or a ruptured viscus. Quite distinct from these is the condition, generally known as "primary" or "idiopathic" peritonitis, which has no focus of infection within the peritoneal cavity and which, in the vast majority of cases, probably arises from a bacteremia. A considerable proportion of these infections are in patients who are known to have nephrosis.

Primary peritonitis has been described in all age groups and has been observed even in elderly individuals, but it is largely a disease of infancy and early childhood. The responsible organism in most cases is a pneumococcus or a hemolytic streptococcus, the latter being somewhat more common than the former.

Primary peritonitis is a type of infection which was rather common prior to 1938–1940, but since that time has had a diminishing incidence so that we now see on an average only three or four cases per year. This falling off in frequency of the disease is almost certainly related to the widespread use of antibiotics and chemotherapy which in many instances probably prevents bacterial invasion by way of the blood stream, or, if a primary peritonitis has begun, aborts it in early stages. In spite of this favorable turn of events, full-blown primary peritonitis still presents a difficult problem of diagnosis and treatment; it still carries a rather high mortality rate and hence, in spite of its rarity, demands considerable attention and thought.

PATHOLOGY AND ETIOLOGY

Exudate

The inflammatory process diffusely affects the parietal and visceral peritoneum; small accumulations of fluid appear between the intestinal loops. The mesenteric lymph glands are pale, swollen, and usually very prominent. The peritoneal exudate is thin, slightly cloudy, and contains flecks of fibrin if a streptococcus is present. When a pneumococcus is the causative organism, the fluid tends to be a little thicker; later on the material becomes fibrinopurulent or even plastic, so that the visceral and parietal peritoneum is coated with a layer of yellow, shaggy exudate.

Sequestration of exudate into isolated pockets occurs much less frequently in cases of primary peritonitis (especially when a streptococcus is the offending organism) than it does in those of a secondary type. Walled-off abscesses are occasionally formed but it is more characteristic for the peritoneal infection to kill the individual quickly, or to disappear completely and leave no traces.

Not infrequently, a surgeon opens the right lower quadrant of one of these abdomens and, finding the appendix red and injected, will suppose that the peritonitis originated there. The appendix in such cases is no more involved than are other viscera, and appendectomy is a useless, and indeed often a harmful procedure.

Causative Organisms

In a series of 158 patients at the Children's Hospital, the responsible bacteria were as follows:

Hemolytic streptococcus............................ 99
Pneumococcus................................... 50
Colon bacillus..................................... 5
Unknown... 4

In 31 of our pneumococcus patients for whom typing was performed, there were 8 of Type VI, 7 of Type I, 2 each of Types IV, V, VII, XI, XIV, and one each of Types VIII, X, XVIII, XIX, XX, and XXII. No conclusions could be drawn relating the type of pneumococcus to the severity of peritonitis, or the prognosis thereof. In those patients who developed a primary peritonitis during the course of nephrosis, the pneumococcus was by far the most common infecting organism.

An analysis of our 38 cases of primary peritonitis from 1940 through 1950 shows the following statistics:

Infecting Organism	Patients without Nephrosis	Patients with Nephrosis
Streptococcus	11	1
Pneumococcus	8	9
Colon bacillus	3	2
Undetermined	2	2

Paths of Invasion

The avenues by which organisms enter the celomic cavity cannot be accurately determined. Some authors have conjectured that bacteria can invade the female *genital tract* and ascend by way of the uterus and its tubes into the pelvic peritoneum. This theory, of course, utterly fails to explain the mode of infection in males. It is our belief that invasion by way of the uterus occurs but rarely, because autopsy examination in our fatal female cases has never shown evidence of ascending genital tract infection. The *gastrointestinal tract* may serve as a source of infection in rare cases, for sometimes pathologic examination has shown a severe inflammation of all of the enteric coats. The *transdiaphragmatic lymphatics* have also been incriminated; they certainly cannot be a common portal of infection because a preceding pneumonia or empyema is rarely a part of the picture. The *blood stream* is probably the path by which bacteria reach the peritoneum in most cases. This belief is supported by the frequent occurrence of an upper respiratory infection during or just preceding the peritonitis and by the number of bacteremias which can be demonstrated by cultural means. Such evidence is particularly convincing because, if an organism is recovered from the blood stream, the same one is nearly always found in the peritoneal exudate. In about half of our cases a definite blood stream infection could be demonstrated by culture; earlier or repeated studies would probably have uncovered more instances of transient bacteremia.

SYMPTOMS AND SIGNS

Primary peritonitis appears in about equal numbers in males and females. The somewhat higher incidence of primary peritonitis among charity patients than among private ones suggests that lowered standards of living and a diminished resistance may play a role in susceptibility to this type of infection.

Symptoms

Infants or young children are most frequently affected; 75 per cent of our patients have been less than five years of age. The illness commonly, but not always, begins with a head cold or other *respiratory tract infection.* The onset of abdominal symptoms is sometimes masked by the respiratory infection. When the abdominal involvement has become established, the symptoms are severe and rapidly progressive. Older children may complain of diffuse *abdominal pain;* babies show this by crying, restlessness, or irritability. *Vomiting* is frequent and may produce marked *dehydration.* A *fever,* higher than that found in secondary peritonitis, and excessive perspiration are common. *Diarrhea* is observed in about half of the cases, particularly during the first day of intestinal irritation, but it is apt to be followed by constipation.

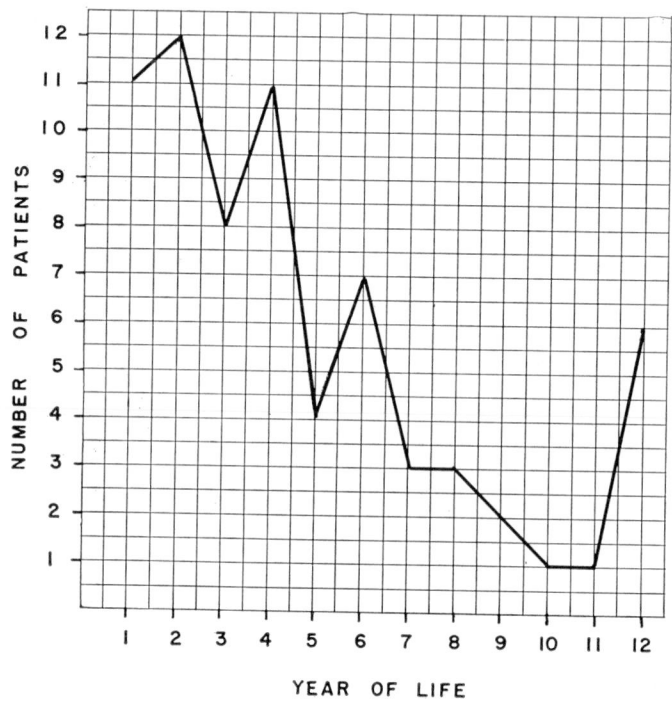

Fig. 200. Graph showing age incidence of primary peritonitis in a series of patients. The disease is most common in infancy and early childhood. About three-fourths of the patients are less than five years of age.

Physical Findings

The individual appears extremely ill. The *facies* are drawn and worn, and the eyes are sunken and listless. An upper respiratory infection may be present. The *temperature* is generally elevated to 104° or 105° F. and the pulse is correspondingly rapid. The abdomen is diffusely *tender.* Should an inguinal hernia be present, there may be thickening and tenderness along the sac which extends downward into the canal or scrotum. In older individuals the abdomen may have a boardlike rigidity, but in babies it is more apt to be soft and *"doughy."* Some degree of *distention* is the rule, and a protuberant and slightly tender abdomen may be the only local finding if the patient is an infant. Shifting dullness of abdominal fluid can be made out but rarely. Peristaltic activity may be found to be increased by auscultation during early stages of the infection, but it is greatly diminished in later periods. Sticky mucous membranes, sunken eyes, inelastic skin, and dry, coated tongue are evidences of dehydration. Rectal examination reveals diffuse tenderness, but usually there is no pelvic mass.

Laboratory Data

The *white blood count* is almost invariably elevated, and generally ranges between 20,000 and 50,000; the polymorphonuclear leukocytes are 80 to 90 per cent or more. The *red blood count* may be slightly or moderately depressed, particularly in the streptococcal infections of several days' standing. Urinalysis commonly shows an acetonuria, but is otherwise not remarkable.

DIFFERENTIAL DIAGNOSIS

Primary peritonitis is most likely to be confused with *generalized peritonitis* which is secondary to a ruptured appendix. In the latter condition the symptoms and signs are maximal on the right side of the abdomen at the beginning of the illness, whereas in primary peritonitis the pain and tenderness are generalized from the outset. An age of less than three years, initiation of the illness by a chill, and a very stormy course from the start, are all suggestive of a primary type of infection. Fever and leukocytosis are usually higher with the primary form. It is uncommon for patients having peritonitis of appendiceal origin to have a temperature over 103° F., while those having a primary peritonitis commonly have temperatures of 104° or even 105° F. and rarely one below 103° F. In dealing with peritonitis patients, we have found that it is possible preoperatively to recognize and diagnose correctly the primary form in about two-thirds of the cases.

The other lesion which is particularly difficult to differentiate from primary peritonitis is *pneumonia* in its early stages. This is especially so in small infants and, in fact, it is not too uncommon for the two conditions to coexist. In early pneumonia all the symptoms found in peritonitis are likely to be present—vomiting, chill, high temperature, and high leukocyte count. The chest signs in pneumonia may be slight and hard to demonstrate, and the abdomen is often distended and resistant. An unduly elevated respiratory rate and a lack of abdominal tenderness are the two most important factors lending support to a diagnosis of pneumonia. An x-ray examination will usually help to clarify this confusing diagnostic puzzle.

TREATMENT

Forms of treatment advocated for primary peritonitis vary from abdominal exploration and appendectomy on the one hand to more recent suggestions of chemotherapy (and no operation) on the other. We do not agree with either of these extremes and believe that a middle course is usually productive of the best results. Certainly, there can be no question about the harm inflicted by extensive packing, retraction, and manipulation within the abdominal cavity in the attempt to find a source of peritoneal infection. Appendectomy is to be condemned. Such operative measures are apt to be followed by forbidding mortality rates.

Operation versus Chemotherapy

The present tendency to advise against operation and to rely entirely on chemotherapy and antibiotics (along with other appropriate supportive measures) can give many favorable results, but we feel strongly that operative therapy should not be abandoned. We still advise surgery—of a very limited sort—for most patients who are suspected of having a primary peritonitis. It seems much the safest policy to adopt. Our only deviations from it have been in: (1) Patients who are known nephrotics, whose peritonitis would almost certainly be of the primary type, and who seem to be progressing satisfactorily on chemotherapy and other supportive measures. (2) Patients who are overwhelmingly ill (such as one with acute leukemia, pneumonia, empyema, or meningitis) when it is obvious that the child is dying from generalized sepsis, of which the peritonitis is only one part.

Under most circumstances we have found it very desirable, quite safe, and of great help to perform a laparotomy through a tiny wound to: (1) Verify the diagnosis of primary peritonitis. (2) Obtain some of the exudate for immediate smear and culture. (3) Drain the abdominal cavity, which in many instances reduces the patient's toxicity. (4) Proceed with a more extended opening and exposure if exudate is found which is odoriterous or which by smear is shown to contain gram-negative organisms, either one of which intimates that there is a ruptured appendix which should be removed.

Abdominal Exploration and Drainage

A small incision—no more than $\frac{3}{4}$ inch or an inch in length—can be made under local procaine infiltration of the abdominal wall, or preferably under general anesthesia if the child is not too ill. A rectus-splitting opening is made in the right lower quadrant (Fig. 201). With two narrow finger retractors to separate the wound edges, the peritoneum can be exposed and slit open for about $\frac{1}{2}$ inch. Without disturbing intestinal loops, the operator is now able to obtain a sample of peritoneal fluid on a swab, or to suck it up in a syringe. If this has no odor a primary form of peritonitis should be suspected at once, and *nothing further done until an assistant can smear, stain, and microscopically examine some of the pus.* If pneumococci or streptococci are thus identified, a single Penrose (cigarette) drain is gently inserted down into the pelvis and a sterile dressing is applied. If this minor procedure is properly done it is not shocking. If the incision has been kept short as recommended, the abdominal opening will be just large enough to accommodate a drain without placing a single suture in any layer of the wound. The information gained from this simple exploration permits immediate institution of intelligent specific therapy for primary peritonitis.

It is hardly necessary to state that any such exploration and drainage should not be done until there has been adequate preoperative support in the form of gastric intubation and decompression, parenteral administration of saline and glucose, and initiation of chemotherapy.

After-care

The after-care of these patients is of utmost importance. A high Fowler's position should be constantly maintained. *Morphine* every four hours by the clock for a day or two will give much-needed rest. *Constant gastric siphonage* should be continued as long as there is any intestinal or bile-stained fluid returning through the tube. Water may be sipped as desired, for it helps to moisten the mouth and, by flushing back through the gastric tube, keeps the apparatus cleared and working. A flaxseed poultice or *hot-water bottle* on the abdomen every two or three hours is helpful. A tent with high concentration of *oxygen* (90 to 95 per cent) is a valuable adjunct in the treatment of abdominal distention. *Blood transfusions* are liberally employed for anemia, and plasma or human albumin will help correct any hypoproteinemia.

Constant gastric suction may be necessary for four or five days or more. After it is discontinued, nourishing fluids and then semi-solid food should be started *with caution.* Physicians sometimes interpret a falling temperature and a flat abdomen as sure signs of recovery, and hence prescribe the return to a normal diet. All too often this decision is followed by reappearance of distention and fever which might have been avoided by

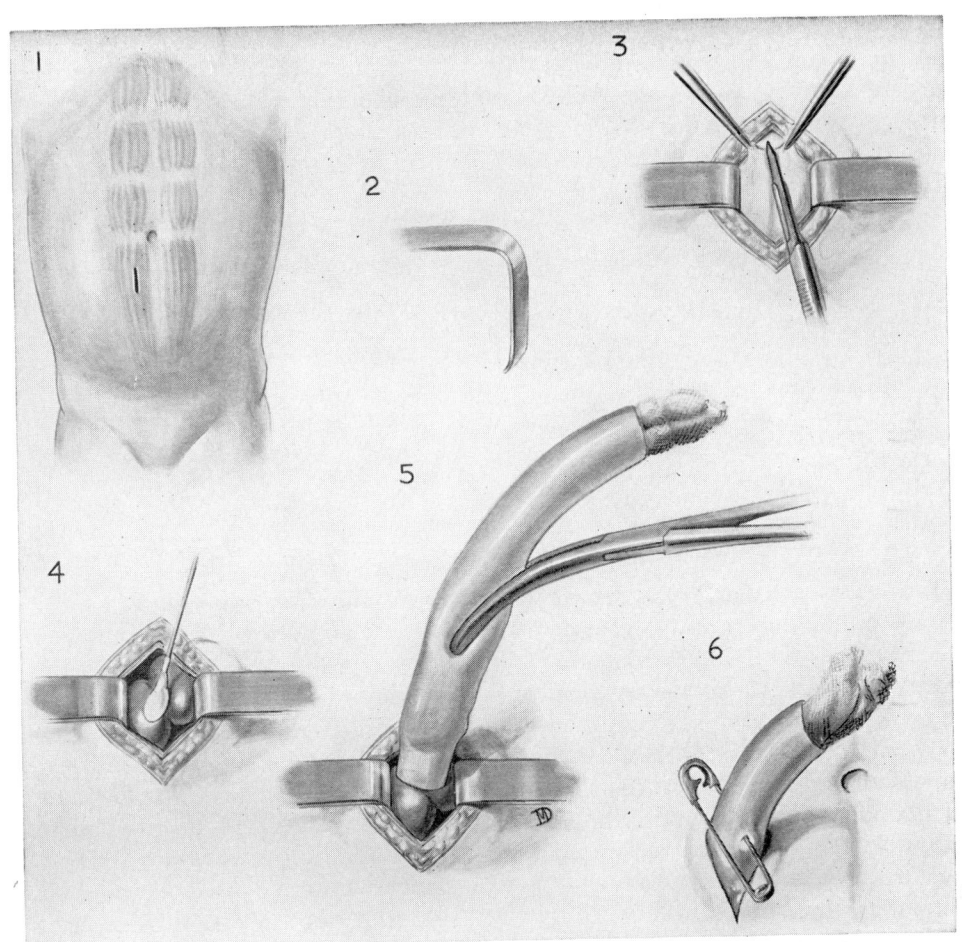

Fig. 201. Surgical treatment of primary peritonitis. 1. A right rectus muscle-splitting incision not over 2 or 3 cm. long. If this is made below the inferior tendinous inscription (which is opposite the umbilicus), very little bleeding is encountered. 2. Right-angle retractor, 1 cm. wide. 3. Muscles retracted. Peritoneum being opened. 4. Intestines presenting; these are not disturbed. Exudate taken for culture and immediate smear. 5. If pure pneumococcus or streptococcus is seen on smear, nothing more is done except to insert a drain down into the pelvis. 6. Soft cigarette drain just fills the wound. No sutures are necessary.

restricting the intake of food for several additional days. The *wound* should be dressed frequently enough to keep it reasonably clean. The *abdominal drain* should be loosened from its bed on the fourth or fifth day and pulled out a little each succeeding day so that it is completely removed by the seventh or eighth day.

Antibiotics or *chemotherapy* must be given from the very beginning of the therapeutic regimen. This must be intensive and sustained. It should be continued until all evidence of infection has disappeared, and should probably be carried on in reduced dosage for four or five days thereafter. Parenteral penicillin is by far the drug of choice.

RESULTS OF TREATMENT

For students today, it is difficult or impossible to realize the tribulations which plagued the treatment of primary peritonitis in the not-too-distant past. Disappointments were numerous, complications were frequent, mortality rates were high. The following table lists a few of the results from publications in the last twenty-five years; they give an idea of the changing picture during this period. With fairness, the results of therapy of one author cannot be contrasted with those of another, because methods of surgical handling were undergoing evolution. The figures do reflect the seriousness of primary peritonitis before the days of modern therapeusis, and they indicate that enormous strides have been made in the treatment of this condition.

Table 50

Mortality Rates in Pneumococcal and Streptococcal Peritonitis

Author	Year Reported	Pneumococcal Peritonitis %	Streptococcal Peritonitis %
Lipshutz and Lowenburg[11]	1926	100	100
Ladd[6]	1930	66	65
Donovan[5]	1934	75	78
Cole[3]	1937	54	..
Leopold and Kaufman[10]	1937	..	91
Ladd and Gross[8]	1940	12	22

In our own material, there have been 158 instances of primary peritonitis. The first 120 of these, up to 1940, were analyzed by Ladd and Gross. (In the latter part of that series, 1937 to 1940, the mortality in primary peritonitis had been reduced to 17.1 per cent—a figure which was remarkable for that day.) From 1940 through 1950 there have been 38 cases of the condition; 14 of these had nephrosis and 24 did not.

The 38 patients in the last decade have been treated by surgical measures in 22 instances and by non-surgical approach in 16; antibiotics and chemotherapy have been used liberally in both groups. In general, all cases entering the hospital because of peritonitis have been given the surgical therapy; in addition there was operation on 4 known nephrotics who were quite ill or in whom there was some question about the possibility of appendiceal peritonitis. In the non-surgical group there were 10 nephrotics in whom there seemed little question about the peritonitis being a primary one; there were 2 patients without nephrosis; and there were 4 patients, seriously ill with leukemia, meningitis, empyema, or other overwhelming sepsis, in whom the peritoneal infection was a terminal event in a complicated and deteriorating picture. The two series—surgical versus non-surgical—are therefore composed of different materials and the results of therapy should not be compared with one another. In the surgical group, the mortality rate was 18.1 per cent; in the medical group the mortality rate was 37.5 per cent. From these figures it becomes quite clear that the treatment of primary peritonitis is not simply a matter of administering miracle drugs. There can be no doubt that the use of cautious operative measures, outlined above, add to the number of favorable results. Even with all therapeutic weapons that can be used, there is still a mortality rate which is quite high. It is noteworthy that our fatality figures are no lower than those which we obtained in the years before penicillin became available!

In considering the group of 14 nephrotics with peritonitis, 4 of whom were treated "surgically" and 10 "medically," there were 10 recoveries and 4 deaths (surgical: 3

alive, 1 dead; medical: 7 alive, 3 dead). While the figures are not sufficient to warrant any sweeping conclusions, the fact that generally the milder peritonitis cases were kept on medical therapy and that in spite of this the surgical mortality rates were lower, would seem to indicate that a surgical approach to the problem of primary peritonitis in nephrotics is the one which should be preferred.

REFERENCES

1. Barnett, H. L., Hartmann, A. F., Perley, A. M. and Ruhoff, M. B.: The Treatment of Pneumococcic Infections in Infants and Children with Sulfapyridine. J.A.M.A., *112*:518, 1939.
2. Carey, B. W., Jr.: The Use of Para-Amino-benzenesulfonamide and Its Derivatives in the Treatment of Infection Due to the Beta Streptococcus Hemolyticus, the Meningo-coccus, and the Gonococcus. J. Pediat., *11*:202, 1937.
3. Cole, W. H.: Pneumococcus Peritonitis. Surgery, *1*:386, 1937.
4. Donovan, E. J.: Surgical Aspects of Primary Pneumococcus Peritonitis. Am. J. Dis. Child., *48*:1170, 1934.
5. Glazier, M. M., Goldberg, B. I. and Weinstein, A. A.: Primary Pneumococcic Peritonitis: Recovery of the Acute Serous Type Following Type I Serum Treatment Without Surgical Intervention. Ann. Int. Med., *10*:1042, 1937.
6. Ladd, W. E.: The Acute Surgical Abdomen in Children. Pennsylvania M. J., *34*:153, 1930.
7. Ladd, W. E., Botsford, T. W. and Curnen, E. C.: Primary Peritonitis in Infants and Children. A More Effective Treatment. J.A.M.A., *113*:1455, 1939.
8. Ladd, W. E. and Gross, R. E.: Abdominal Surgery of Infancy and Childhood. W. B. Saunders Company, Philadelphia, 1940, P. 188.
9. Leonardo, R. A.: Primary Pneumococcus Peritonitis. Ann. Surg., *83*:411, 1926.
10. Leopold, J. S. and Kaufman, R. E.: Acute "Primary" Streptococcus Peritonitis. J. Pediat., *10*:45, 1937.
11. Lipshutz, B. and Lowenburg, H.: Pneumococcic and Streptococcic Peritonitis. Report of Twenty-three Cases in Infancy and Children. J.A.M.A., *86*:99, 1926.
12. McCartney, J. E. and Fraser, J.: Pneumococcal Peritonitis. Brit. J. Surg., *9*:479, 1922.
13. Mazal, V.: Le Traitment de la péritonite à pneumocoques par la penicilline. Ann. paediat., *170*:253, 1948.
14. Pahmer, M.: Pneumococcus Peritonitis in Nephrotic and Non-nephrotic Children. J. Pediat., *17*:90, 1940.
15. Shands, H. R.: Pneumococcus Peritonitis. Mississippi Doctor, *24*:223, 1947.
16. Török, G.: Le diagnostic et le traitment actuel de la péritonite pneumococcique. Ann. paediat., *170*:263, 1948.

CHAPTER 28

Iliac Adenitis

CLINICAL FINDINGS

Symptoms

Staphylococcal or streptococcal infection of the perineum, anus, or leg may give rise to inflammation in lymph glands of the iliac fossa. Iliac adenitis manifests itself as an acute process with symptoms primarily of *abdominal pain* or of *restriction in leg movements*. There are fever, restlessness, and constant abdominal discomfort which is more severe in one of the lower quadrants. Nausea and vomiting are minimal and indeed usually absent—a point of some importance in differentiating a right-sided adenitis from acute appendicitis. The iliopsoas muscle is thrown into spasm by the inflamed nodes which lie upon it, so that a *limp* or a *flexion deformity* of the thigh is produced. Not infrequently these patients come to the attention of the orthopedist because of an altered gait, which suggests a hip infection, an osteomyelitis at the upper end of the femur, or a psoas abscess originating in the spine.

Physical Examination

These patients show deep, lower-abdominal *tenderness* which is most marked just above the inguinal region. If the infection has been of short duration no swelling can be detected, but in later stages it is possible to feel a palpable mass medial to and below the anterior-superior spine. As an abscess mass increases in size, it extends forward toward Poupart's ligament, and closely approaches the inguinal canal. In longer-standing cases there is *edema* and *induration* of the subcutaneous tissues of the area. By *rectal examination* nothing abnormal can be detected, or a swelling may be felt high on one side of the pelvis, depending upon the size of the lesion. A *portal of entry* of the infection may be found on the leg or possibly around the anus, but the initial lesion is often healed and not discernible by the time the patient seeks advice for abdominal complaints or limp. In most cases the infection has skipped the femoral and inguinal glands and lodges solely in the iliac group. The temperature ranges from 101° to 104° F. The white blood count is elevated to 15,000 or 25,000, but it may be as high as 30,000 or 40,000.

Differential Diagnosis

Iliac adenitis differs from *appendiceal abscess* in that it usually has no intestinal symptoms, and that its area of maximum tenderness is closer to Poupart's ligament. It is contrasted to the *psoas abscess* of spinal origin in that it develops more rapidly, has less flexion deformity of the thigh, and has no demonstrable spinal lesion. It is to be differentiated from *infection of the hip joint* because rotation of the hip is less disturbed, the tenderness or mass is above Poupart's ligament, and roentgenograms do not show any increased width of the hip joint.

Clinical Course

Iliac adenitis will spontaneously disappear in about half of the cases. This subsidence can be aided by bed rest, sedation, chemotherapy, and application of heat to the lower abdomen. In the remaining patients *suppuration* occurs, and as much as several hundred cubic centimeters of exudate may become pocketed in the iliac fossa behind the peritoneum. It is a great rarity for this to break into the general abdominal cavity, but in one case we have seen it force its way around in front of the peritoneum and finally rupture into the urinary bladder. The exudate in most cases tends to dissect along outside of the peritoneum and point at or near the internal inguinal ring. The resulting swelling may be mistaken for a tender, incarcerated, inguinal hernia, but the fever, leukocytosis, duration of the lesion, and absence of intestinal symptoms should exclude that diagnosis.

TREATMENT

Surgical Drainage

While it is possible for less severe infections to disappear spontaneously, or with the aid of appropriate chemotherapy, suppuration should be treated by surgical drain-

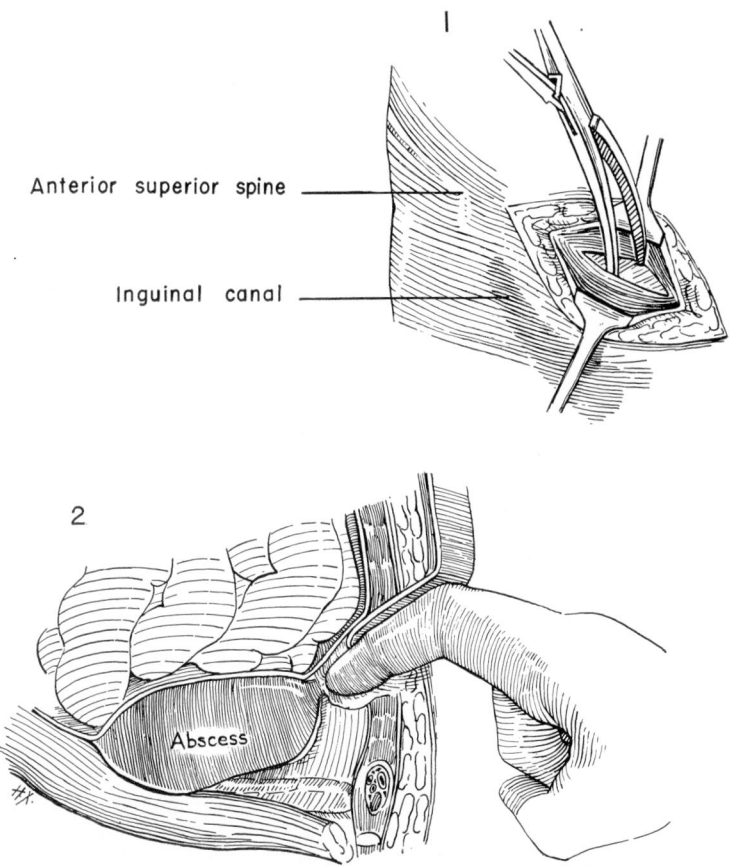

Fig. 202. Method of draining right, suppurative iliac adenitis. 1. The external oblique fascia has been split and retracted. Muscles are being bluntly separated with a half-length clamp. 2. Parasagittal section showing peritoneum pushed inward with a retractor and finger being passed outside of this to reach the abscess cavity.

age for this certainly provides the best method of assuring a rapid convalescence. If it becomes obvious that inflammation is advancing, the problem arises of choosing the correct time for incision and drainage. It is best to wait until adequate walling off from surrounding structures has taken place, and until the mass has assumed considerable size and has dissected the peritoneum away from and above the inguinal canal. While the dissecting pus can pierce the deeper tissues of the abdominal wall, it is stopped by the external oblique fascia. Hence, fluctuation is almost never found and operation should not be delayed in the hope that it will develop.

Surgical drainage is readily effected through a short *incision* below and medial to the anterior-superior spine (Fig. 202); care should be taken to keep the wound above the inguinal canal so that its structures will not be exposed to infection. The external oblique fascia is split in the direction of its fibers and the underlying muscles are bluntly separated. When the pyogenic membrane comes into view, it is pierced by the tip of a hemostat, the jaws of which are then separated. Purulent material usually gushes out at this stage, and the tip of an exploring finger can be passed extraperitoneally into the abscess cavity in the iliac fossa. When an adequate opening has been made, a soft rubber wick or a cigarette drain is inserted into it and the wound left open. These patients do extremely well after proper drainage has been instituted. The suppuration rapidly subsides and hospitalization is seldom necessary for more than a week or two.

Results of Therapy

In the Children's Hospital series, 20 patients, ranging in age from one to eleven years, have been operated upon and all of them recovered. Nineteen other children were believed to have iliac adenitis without suppuration which subsided under conservative treatment.

REFERENCES

1. Coutts, W. E.: Acute Inflammation of Deep Iliac Lymph-Nodes. Ann. Surg., *86*:782, 1927.
2. Frank, L.: Suppurative Adenitis of Iliac Lymph Nodes of Hemolytic Streptococcal Origin. Ann. Surg., *105*:975, 1937.
3. Hyman, A.: Suppurative Retroperitoneal Pelvic Lymphadenitis. Ann. Surg., *91*:718, 1930.
4. Irwin, F. G.: Acute Iliac Adenitis; Report of 18 Cases. Arch. Surg., *36*:561 1938.

Omphalitis

In recent years there has been tremendous improvement in the care of newly born babies; among the many ways in which this has been reflected in better health for the baby is the great reduction in the incidence of omphalitis. In spite of this important advance, infections of the umbilicus, and their sequelae, are still frequent enough to merit the attention of obstetricians, pediatricians, and surgeons. Inflammation around the navel in the first two months of life is exceedingly dangerous because bacteria can readily progress inward through the abdominal wall and give rise to regional or distant infections which are a serious menace to life.

Contamination of the umbilical cord may occur even before delivery of a child, if there has been premature rupture of the membranes. Organisms may also gain access to the cord during descent of the baby in the birth canal, particularly if vaginal examinations have been made by the attending physician. Most umbilical infections begin when the cord is severed and tied, or when insufficient care is used during the subsequent dressings.

In most cases of omphalitis, the organism concerned is a *Staphylococcus aureus*. Next in importance is the *hemolytic streptococcus*, while the *colon bacillus* or mixed bacteria are the responsible agents in a minority of cases. Particularly troublesome are the *anaerobic* or *micro-aerophilic* organisms which may give rise to extensive undermining and sloughing of skin.

ANATOMIC CONSIDERATIONS

The umbilicus has certain anatomic features which have an important bearing on the routes along which infections may spread from this area. The *umbilical vein* pierces the abdominal wall and continues inward at the inferior edge of the falciform ligament. It then branches and communicates with the portal veins, and also with the inferior vena cava (via the *ductus venosus*). After birth, the ductus venosus becomes obliterated and forms the ligamentum venosum; the anterior portion of the umbilical vein becomes obliterated and forms the ligamentum teres. Portions of these channels may retain a lumen for some weeks after delivery of the child, and it is obvious that bacteria which enter them can have easy access to the portal system and the inferior vena cava.

The two *umbilical arteries* pierce the abdominal wall and then course downward, as the paired *hypogastric vessels*, between the transversalis fascia and the peritoneum to join the internal iliac arteries in the pelvis. They pass along the inner surface of the anterior abdominal wall on either side of the bladder. While they normally become obliterated soon after birth, a lumen has been known to persist for several weeks. Like the venous channels, these degenerating arteries are able to serve as pathways through which, or along which, bacteria from the umbilicus can reach the blood stream or give rise to suppuration on the inner aspect of the lower abdominal wall.

Since the hypogastric arteries and the umbilical vein are separated from the abdominal cavity only by a layer of peritoneum and thin areolar tissue, it is at once evident that any infection along these vessels can easily spread to the peritoneal cavity and can set up a generalized peritonitis.

The *lymphatic drainage* of the umbilical region is of some importance. The cutaneous channels run downward and outward toward the inguinal nodes, but the deeper ones drain upward and fan out over the pectoral regions. Infections which affect the internal structures of the navel have a tendency to spread along these deep lymphatics and along the various fascial planes and thus give a widespread cellulitis of the upper abdominal and the lower thoracic wall.

PATHOLOGY

Granulation tissue frequently persists in the navel several weeks or months after the cord stump has fallen away. Droplets of serous or even purulent fluid may appear on the surface of such granulations from time to time. These lesions rarely give rise to any important sequelae, and they can be quickly treated by application of silver nitrate to the exuberant granulations. The resulting raw area will then be rapidly closed over by the surrounding proliferating skin.

In distinct contrast to the benign, weeping, or granulating umbilicus is the *peri-umbilical cellulitis* or *abscess*, which must be regarded as a serious problem. Infections of this sort are usually limited to the first few weeks of life. Redness and induration may appear in the surrounding skin or pus may exude from the folds of the umbilical depression.

Severe omphalitis may take four different courses: (1) The infection may remain locally. An *abscess* may form in the abdominal wall, along the falciform ligament, or particularly along the hypogastric arteries. (2) Inflammation may extend along the fascial planes or lymphatics of the outer layers of the abdominal wall, so that a *necrotizing lesion* gives sloughing over the epigastrium or lower chest wall. It is not uncommon for the infection to burrow beneath the immediate peri-umbilical skin and leave this intact while destroying the skin of the upper abdomen. (3) There may be *blood stream invasion*. When this occurs, the bacteremia becomes manifest by overwhelming illness and by development of multiple foci of suppuration in divers parts of the body. (4) Infection may pass inward through the umbilicus and directly produce a spreading *peritonitis*.

CLINICAL FINDINGS

The clinical findings in a case of omphalitis will depend upon which of the above four conditions exist.

1. If there is only *regional* infection, then local edema, reddening, tenderness, and serous discharge are the rule. Gentle pressure above or below the umbilicus may express a droplet or two of purulent exudate, and thus indicate that there is an abscess alongside one of the major extraperitoneal blood vessels.

2. When a *cellulitis* extends along the lymphatics or fascial planes, then edema, tenderness, redness, or duskiness appears in the upper abdominal skin. Subsequent examinations show a deeper red or purplish color indicative of an impaired blood supply and within a few days actual necrosis may begin. When sloughing has once started, it has a tendency to extend with great rapidity. The cutaneous edges become widely undermined and melt away. The musculature and fasciae of the abdominal and thoracic walls become exposed, and subsequently become covered by granulation tissue.

3. When *bacteremia* exists, dactylitis, deep-tissue abscesses, high fever, jaundice, or severe toxicity may overshadow what appears to be a rather minor umbilical infection.

4. In those individuals with peritonitis, the complaints include vomiting, marked abdominal distention, high fever, and either diarrhea or constipation. The white blood count may range from 20,000 to 40,000. The child's general appearance is that of prostrating infection.

TREATMENT

Because of the extreme hazard to life which omphalitis carries, all patients with such infection should be given intensive chemotherapy. To gain immediate and adequate effects, penicillin should be started promptly and should be given in high dosage by intramuscular injection. While this will probably be all that is required for most patients, because of the fact that some of the patients have mixed infections in which gram-negative organisms play a part, all of the babies should have antibiotics which have a wide range of antibacterial activity. Sulfadiazine or terramycin should also be employed routinely; these can generally be given by mouth. In addition to these general measures, treatment of the omphalitis and its complications depends somewhat upon the conditions which are present.

1. Application of hot, moist compresses will help to clean up the local infection. They will aid in softening and removal of any crusts, beneath which exudate is dammed up. If gentle pressure on the abdominal wall expresses purulent material from the navel, a deep-lying *abscess* should be suspected. To investigate this possibility, a probe can be *gently* passed inward through the tiny umbilical opening. If a sinus leads downward along the course of either hypogastric artery, then a grooved director can be inserted into this tract and the full thickness of the abdominal wall (anterior to the director) is laid open with scissors or scalpel. Extreme delicacy must be exercised to avoid perforation of the thin areolar tissue and the peritoneal layer which alone protect the abdominal cavity.

2. Extensive *ulcerations* of the abdominal wall are best treated with large, warm, wet, boric acid compresses. Changing of the pack every hour or two will carry away loose debris and will rapidly clean the wound. If there is undermining of the cutaneous edges, the wound can be cleaned with hydrogen peroxide solution. It is helpful to apply a zinc peroxide paste, then covering this with a sufficiently airtight dressing which will allow slow liberation of nascent oxygen which retards the growth of anaerobic and microaerophilic organisms. Dressings of this type can be changed at daily intervals. It is essential to employ a zinc peroxide powder which has been dried in an oven at 140° C. for four hours, and to prepare the paste freshly just before it is applied to the wound.

3. Infants with a *bacteremia* will require local applications of heat in the various sites of metastatic infection and possibly incision and drainage of some of these if suppuration occurs.

4. The treatment of the *peritonitis* cases is a disappointing procedure from the first, because of the extremely grave prognosis. However, proper drainage of the umbilicus should be instituted if there is any suspicion that an abscess is pointing inward rather than out through the skin. If there is an appreciable collection of peritoneal exudate, simple incision and insertion of a drain may reduce the individual's toxicity. Supportive measures in the form of a gastric suction, abdominal heat, Fowler's position, parenteral fluids, and transfusion should all be undertaken.

RESULTS OF THERAPY

At the Children's Hospital there have been a large number of minor umbilical infections which were treated in the out-patient department or which were incidental findings during hospitalization for some other illness. The outlook for all of these has been excellent. In addition, there have been patients with infections of the umbilicus which have been serious enough to demand hospitalization and treatment. Over the years the picture has changed greatly; whereas formerly the condition was rather common, was very difficult to treat, and carried high mortality rates, it is now a disappearing disease and it is accompanied by fewer complications and by lower risks of fatality. These dramatic changes have been brought about by better *prophylaxis* in protecting the cord stump of newborn babies, and also by better *therapy* with chemotherapeutic agents or antibiotics in those subjects who have developed any navel infection. Therefore it is well to divide and analyze our material into two periods which reflect these changes in prevention and treatment.

Material through 1939

In 60 cases an omphalitis or its complications was the primary illness for which hospitalization was advised. Of these 60 babies, 12 could be classified as having a local infection; all of them recovered. Five had extensive ulceration of the abdominal wall; 4 survived and 1 died. Thirty-seven developed a bacteremia; 6 of them survived and 31 died. Six had omphalitis and peritonitis; all of them succumbed. Most of these 60 babies were treated prior to the time when chemotherapeutic agents were available. The deaths of 38 gave a fatality rate of 63 per cent.

Material from 1939 through 1951

During this period, 31 patients entered the hospital primarily for treatment of umbilical infection. There were 10 males and 21 females. The ages varied from one to forty days, with an average of thirteen days. Most of them had a localized abscess or cellulitis. There was a notably lower incidence of the more severe types of complication (bacteremia, peritonitis) than had been the experience in the earlier series of cases up through 1939. All of the patients received sulfadiazine, penicillin, streptomycin, or aureomycin, either singly or in combinations; in addition they had such local treatment as was required. There were 5 deaths, 3 of which were without doubt attributable to general extension from the acute omphalitis. The two other babies had additional serious diseases (erythroblastosis, severe nutritional disturbance, and electrolyte imbalance) which were regarded as the major cause of death. Aside from these 5 in whom there was fatality, all remaining patients recovered uneventfully.

REFERENCES

1. Adair, F. L.: Care of the Umbilical Stump. A Bacteriologic Study. J.A.M.A., *61*:537, 1913.
2. Chamberlain, J. W.: Omphalitis in the Newborn. J. Pediat., *9*:215, 1936.
3. Creadick, A. N.: The Frequency and Significance of Omphalitis. Surg., Gynec. & Obst., *30*:278, 1920.
4. Hunt, A. B.: Diseases of Umbilicus of Newborn Infant. S. Clin. North America, *17*:1187, 1937.
5. Siddall, R. S.: The Significance of Inflammation of the Umbilical Stump. Am. J. Obst. & Gynec., *14*:192, 1927.
6. Weitzman, C. C.: Omphalitis of the Newborn. Am. J. Obst. & Gynec., *26*:117, 1933.

CHAPTER 30

Rare Conditions of the Umbilicus and Abdominal Wall

The most common lesions of the navel of surgical significance are omphalocele, omphalitis, and umbilical hernia; each of these is discussed in a separate chapter. Six other conditions of the abdominal wall which are rarely seen, but which deserve brief mention, are cyst of the umbilical cord, cyst of the navel, weeping umbilicus, patent urachus and urachal cyst, persistent vitelline duct, and neoplasms of the abdominal wall.

CYST OF THE UMBILICAL CORD

Within any portion of the cord, and particularly toward its attachment at the abdominal wall, there may be a large collection of *Wharton's jelly* which locally distends the structure and gives rise to a cyst. This may be large enough to interfere with descent of the baby through the birth canal. If it appears at the very base of the cord, there is no space between the cyst and the abdominal wall for proper placement of the ties by the obstetrician. When this occurs, the ligatures must be applied distal to the cyst and the latter must then be surgically removed subsequently from the abdominal wall—a dissection which can be done with little difficulty. Inasmuch as the cyst wall has a poor blood supply, there is a tendency to rapid necrosis and sloughing; hence surgical removal should be done within the first twenty-four hours of life.

CYST OF THE NAVEL

During the development of the navel area, epidermal tissues can become included in the subcutaneous tissues so that a cyst develops in the region. These are lined by squamous epithelium and accumulate material just as with any sebaceous or dermoid cyst. Usually they become no larger than a few millimeters or, at most, a centimeter in size. They can be easily excised.

WEEPING UMBILICUS

A mass of granulation tissue, usually no more than a few millimeters in diameter, occasionally is found in the depths of a navel. Its surface is apt to be moist and the skin which lines the navel may become macerated. Such findings are most common in the early weeks of life, just after the cord has dropped off. They usually disappear promptly with appropriate local attention of cleaning with an antiseptic (as alcohol or Zephiran), drying with a dusting powder (as Aristol), and covering it with a dry dressing. However, some granulation tissue may persist for a long time and require the repeated application of silver nitrate to burn down the excess tissue. In a rare case, the local granulation mass remains so long and is so annoying that excision of it is necessary to effect a rapid and permanent cure.

PATENT URACHUS AND URACHAL CYST

A patent urachus may give rise to considerable annoyance because of recurring umbilical discharge of urine, and a urachal cyst can be a source of real danger if it should become infected. Fortunately, these abnormalities can be treated by recourse to surgery.

Pathogenesis

The urachus is derived from the superior part of the allantois. In embryos of 10 to 24 mm. the bladder normally extends up to the umbilical region, but subsequently it descends along the anterior abdominal wall. During this downward migration its upper portion becomes more and more attenuated to form the narrow, tube-like *urachus* which subsequently becomes obliterated. If this entire tract persists, the urinary bladder retains an opening at the navel in postnatal life. If only a segment of the tract remains, a cyst (lined by transitional epithelium similar to that of the bladder) develops anterior to the peritoneum, somewhere between the umbilicus and the superior surface of the bladder.

Symptoms and Diagnosis

Patent Urachus. Patent urachus manifests itself by an *intermittent escape of variable amounts of urine* at the umbilicus. If the cutaneous opening is tiny, there is little more than a recurring moisture of the navel, but if the orifice is large a great deal of urine is emitted by this route. The visible part of the opening is lined by skin or by a pouting and reddened mucous membrane (Fig. 203).

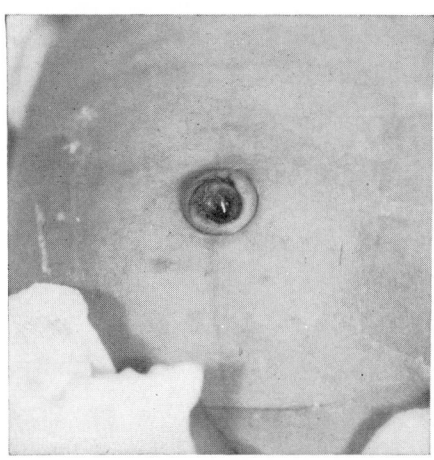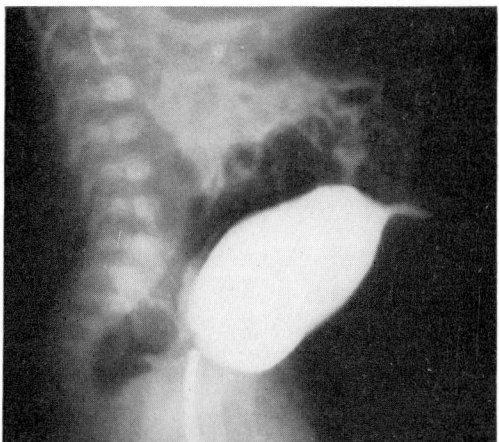

Fig. 203. Patent urachus. Navel of one-month-old child from which urine intermittently discharged. Cystogram shows the narrow tract running upward through the umbilicus. (From Mahoney and Ennis; New England Journal of Medicine.)

A patent urachus must be differentiated from a *granulating umbilicus* (which generally yields to local applications of silver nitrate) and from a *persistent vitelline duct*. The latter usually communicates with the intestinal tract and the character of the umbilical discharge should suggest the proper diagnosis. Furthermore, gentle injection of Lipiodol into the presenting tract before taking lateral roentgenograms will quickly tell whether the connection is with the intestine or the bladder. A cystogram, made by injecting iodide solution through the urethra, will visualize any urachal tract running forward and upward to the navel. In 3 patients (all in the newborn period) the persistence of a bladder opening at the umbilicus was accompanied by some form of obstruction of the urethra; in a large group of patients the discharge of urine at the navel was not secondary to obstruction in the bladder neck or urethra.

Urachal Cyst. Urachal cyst manifests itself as a deep, midline *swelling* below the navel which has a definite and broad attachment to the internal part of the abdominal wall. This may appear in infants or children, but it occasionally escapes notice until adult life. The 9 in our series were 2 to 5 cm. in greatest dimensions, but larger ones have been described. Not infrequently the mass arises very quickly—a fact which depends upon the sudden closing off of a tiny opening which previously existed between the urachal tract and the bladder proper.

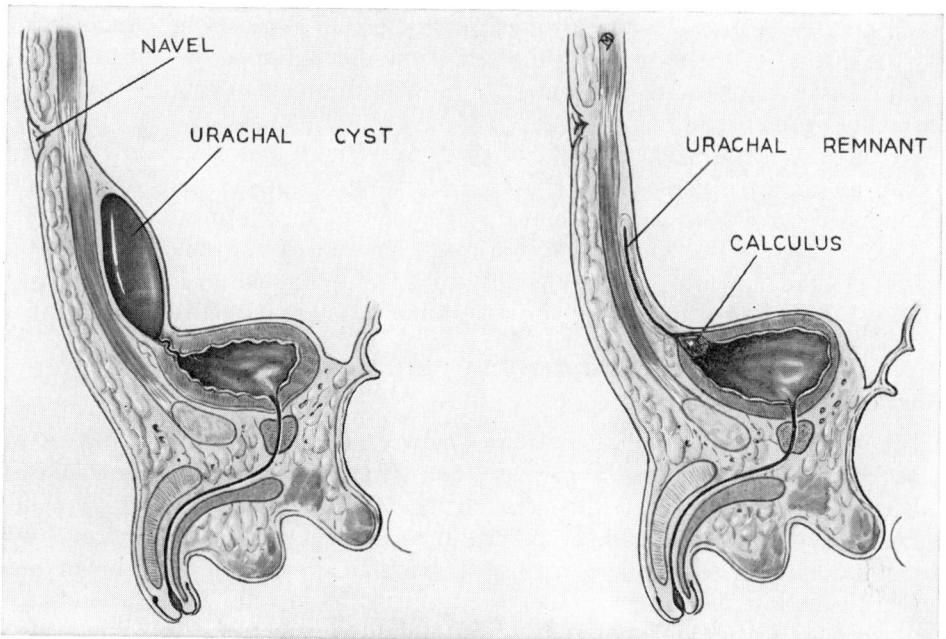

Fig. 204. *Left,* Sagittal view of a urachal cyst which connected with the bladder by a pin-hole opening. *Right,* Sketch from seven-year-old boy with calculus in lower end of a urachal tract. Eneuresis cured by excision of the tract and stone.

Urachal cysts are apt to become infected, and when they do so the clinical features are those of a deep, midline *abscess* of the lower abdominal wall; the urine may or may not contain pus cells. In one of our cases, a *calculus* formed in this pouch above the bladder.

Lateral *roentgenograms* can aid in making the diagnosis of urachal cyst. No intestines will be found interposed between the mass and the anterior abdominal wall. Furthermore, a cystogram will show the mass to abut directly against the upper surface of the bladder.

Treatment

Removal of urachal cyst or a patent urachus is not difficult if operation is performed *before infection occurs.* The possibility of superimposed infection is so great that surgical excision should always be done as soon as the diagnosis is made. These operations should be done in such a way that the peritoneum is not opened, for if this pre-caution is heeded the dangers of peritonitis are largely avoided.

Operative Technique. A midline incision below the umbilicus, separating the rectus muscle bellies, gives an excellent exposure, and with gentleness the lesion can be freed up and then peeled away from the peritoneum which is its sole posterior covering. The dissection is continued superiorly so that connections with the umbilicus can be severed, and it is then carried inferiorly to allow separation from the bladder. If an opening is made in the bladder, this is closed with inverting sutures, and an inlying suprapubic or urethral catheter is left in place for about a week to allow the bladder to heal.

Results of Treatment

In the Children's Hospital there have been 10 patent urachuses. Eight of these were excised; one (early in the series) died of peritonitis. In a ninth the child died (from polycystic disease of the kidney). In the tenth, the urachal sinus has been closed, but the child has required long-continued suprapubic drainage because of a coexisting abnormality of the urethra.

We have seen 9 urachal cysts (3 of these were small and discovered at autopsy; they had no clinical significance). Of the 6 which gave clinical signs and symptoms, one contained a calculus and the entire structure was successfully dissected out; the others were infected. For these 5 infected cysts, incision and drainage were employed for each; in 4 the sepsis fortunately destroyed the linings so that no further removal was necessary, but in the last case there was recurrence which required excision of the mass.

PERSISTENT VITELLINE DUCT

Pathogenesis

The vitelline duct, extending as it does between the ileum and the yolk sac in the base of the umbilical cord, may remain as a *sinus* after the cord has been separated from the abdominal wall. In this way the intestine may attain an opening at the navel by way of a small mucosa-lined channel several centimeters in length. If a segment of this vitelline duct becomes closed off, a *cyst* forms which has an attachment to the lower intestine and also to the internal aspect of the anterior abdominal wall. The persistent duct is occasionally the seat of inflammation, but it is more apt to be bothersome because of a disagreeable and malodorous discharge at the navel.

Diagnosis

The proper diagnosis can be readily suspected by local examination and by judicious probing. It can be established beyond doubt if injection of Lipiodol into the tract shows a communication with the intestine by fluoroscopic or film studies.

Treatment

The entire tract (including the umbilicus) can be *excised*; it must be detached from the ileum, and a suitable closure then made of the intestinal wall. If care is taken in cleansing the abdominal skin and in walling off the peritoneal cavity, little soiling results and the dangers of peritonitis are minimal. From 1940 through 1950, 11 of such anomalies have been encountered; all patients survived operative correction.

NEOPLASMS OF THE ABDOMINAL WALL

Tumors may appear on any portion of the anterior abdominal wall and are found in infants as well as older children. The *prognosis* in any given case varies with the type

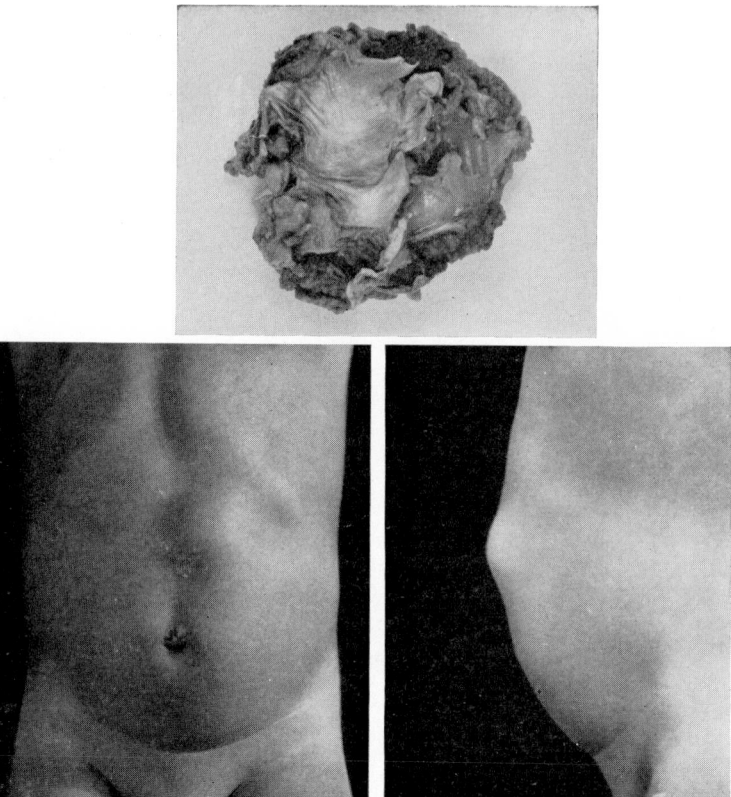

Fig. 205. Mass in left upper quadrant of abdominal wall; a seventeen-month-old child. Lesion was a desmoid (peri-neural fibrosarcoma of rectus sheath). Treated by excision; child well ten years later.

of neoplasm, the rate of cell growth, and the size of the neoplasm when treatment is undertaken. Benign growths are more numerous than malignant ones, yet a localized swelling in the abdominal parietes should not be regarded lightly. Any mass, particularly if it has been noticeably increasing in size, should be immediately and widely removed. Only in this way can the malignant neoplasms be picked up and treated while in an operable stage.

Hemangioma

Hemangioma is the most common tumor of the abdominal wall. The rounded, flat discoid varieties are relatively numerous; they often appear in conjunction with similar cutaneous lesions in other parts of the body. They can be readily treated with applications of carbon dioxide snow or by x-ray therapy. Less common and more important to the surgeon are those hemangiomas which are bulky and which extend through most of the abdominal wall. These usually have some hemangiomatous tissue showing on the skin surface which makes the diagnosis obvious, but they may reside in the deeper structures of the abdominal wall without involving the skin. The vast majority of blood vessel tumors are capillary and cavernous hemangiomas, and are entirely benign; an occasional one shows the more rapid growth of a hemangioendothelioma. In either case total excision of the mass and suitable fascial repair of the abdominal defect is the treatment of choice.

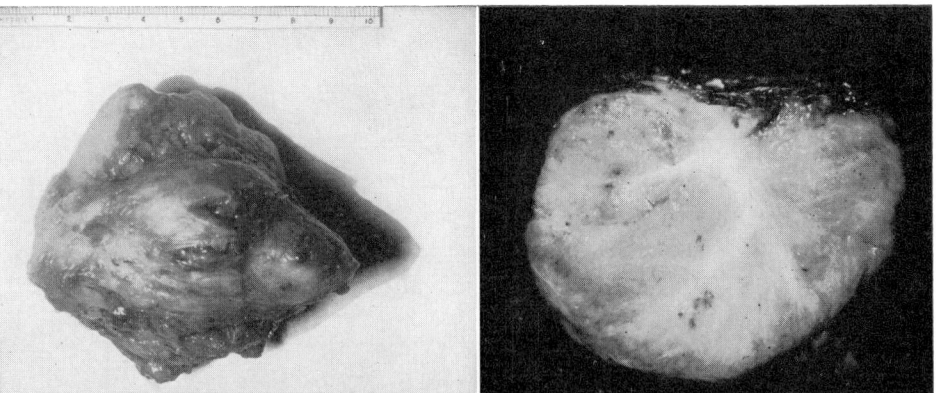

Fig. 206. External and cross-section views of a perineural fibroblastoma (desmoid) removed from lower abdominal wall of a three-year-old girl. This was a recurrent tumor; cure after this secondary incision.

Lipoma

Lipomas of the anterior and lateral abdominal wall are not uncommon. They may reach quite large proportions; they may be accompanied by some similar fatty tumors in other parts of the body. They can be readily treated by simple excision.

Desmoid Tumors

Desmoids have been observed in childhood (Figs. 205 and 206). They tend to occur along the rectus muscles, and are more frequently encountered below the umbilicus than above it. They are hard, painless, non-tender, flattened growths with poorly defined borders and with an obvious wide attachment to the rectus fascia or muscle. Some pathologists believe that desmoid tumors are perineural fibroblastomas, since the histology frequently suggests such an origin, in spite of the fact that the mass generally seems to arise from the anterior rectus fascia. These neoplasms tend to recur locally, and hence every effort should be made to remove a rim of normal tissue around the entire tumor, to insure a complete removal. Failure to do this in one patient resulted in a recurrence which necessitated a subsequent and more difficult dissection.

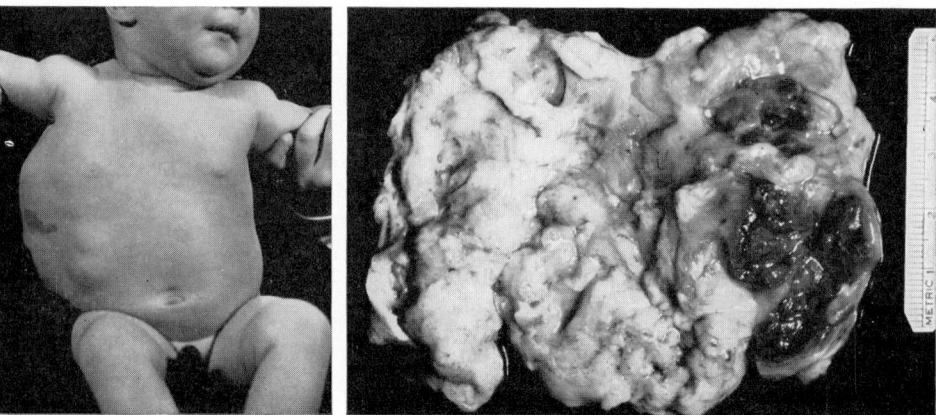

Fig. 207. Huge cavernous lymphangioma of abdominal wall; thirteen-month-old child.

Teratoma

Teratomas of the abdominal wall are rare. They may carry a poor prognosis if some of their elements are rapidly growing. We have removed a large one from an eight-day-old baby, but this child unfortunately died at a subsequent time from congenital heart disease. In another year-old boy a growth of the upper abdominal wall, which was largely a myxofibroma, was excised on two occasions only to recur and extend locally into the abdomen so that death ensued from intestinal obstruction.

REFERENCES

CYSTS OF UMBILICAL CORD

1. Haas, H.: Beitrag zur Lehre von den Cysten der Nabelschnur. Beitr. z. Geburtsh. u. Gynaek., *10*:483, 1906.

PATENT URACHUS AND URACHAL CYST

2. Begg, R. C.: The Urachus and Umbilical Fistulae. Surg., Gynec. & Obst., *45*:165, 1927.
3. Dudgeon, H., Jr.: Treatment of Patent Urachus. Surg., Gynec. & Obst., *71*:302, 1940.
4. Garvin, E. J.: Patent Urachus. J. Urol., *42*: 463, 1939.
5. Kantor, H. I.: Cysts of Urachus; Report of 2 Cases. Ann. Surg., *109*:277, 1939.
6. Mahoney, P. J. and Ennis, D.: Congenital Patent Urachus. New England J. Med., *215*:193, 1936.
7. Wyatt, G. M. and Lanman, T. H.: Calculus in a Urachus. Report of a Case with Enuresis. Am. J. Roentgenol., *43*:673, 1940.

PERSISTENT VITELLINE DUCT

8. Hudson, H. W., Jr.: Meckel's Diverticulum in Children. New England J. Med., *208*: 525, 1933.
9. Ratnayeke, M.: Umbilical Fistula Caused by Patent Meckel's Diverticulum. Brit. J. Surg., *24*:402, 1936.

NEOPLASMS OF THE ABDOMINAL WALL

10. Booher, R. J. and Pack, G. T.: Desmomas of the Abdominal Wall in Children. Cancer, *4*: No. 5, 1052, 1951.
11. Klot, B.: Bauchdeckentumoren. Beitr. z. klin. Chir., *123*:28, 1921.
12. Meade, W. H. and Brewster, W. R.: Tumefactions of the Abdominal Wall. Am. J. Surg., *45*:419, 1939.
13. Pfeiffer, C.: Die Desmoide der Bauchdecken und ihre Prognose. Beitr. z. klin. Chir., *44*: 334, 1904.

CHAPTER 31

Omphalocele
(Umbilical Eventration)

Umbilical hernia is a weakness of the abdominal wall which is frequently encountered in childhood. The rectus fascia is deficient and permits a small, forward protrusion of peritoneum between the bellies of the rectus muscles, so that the peritoneum is covered solely by skin. Akin to this is the rather rare malformation, *omphalocele*, which has a very large peritoneal sac which is *not* covered by skin. An omphalocele is a herniation of abdominal viscera into the base of the umbilical cord; the pouch is a thin, translucent structure consisting only of peritoneum and amniotic membrane. These two layers become fused and make a delicate avascular wall, which is less than a millimeter in thickness. It is evident that this type of abnormality must be considered separately from the common umbilical hernia because the surgical problems of the two conditions are entirely different.

This malformation has been designated by many names, such as "tunicular hernia of the umbilicus," "hernia into the umbilical cord," "umbilical eventration," "amniotic hernia," "exomphalos," or omphalocele. We have long chosen to employ the last term.

EMBRYOLOGY

From the sixth to the tenth weeks of fetal life the *celomic cavity* has a forward expansion into the base of the umbilical cord, this pocket containing loops of intestines and other abdominal viscera (Fig. 208). Such an anatomic arrangement presumably takes place because the abdominal organs have grown at a greater rate than has the peritoneal cavity itself. After the tenth week the abdomen enlarges at an accelerated pace and the organs are withdrawn into it.

If, for any reason, there should be a permanent disparity in size between the viscera and the abdomen, the intestines or a portion of the liver may continue to remain out in the base of the umbilical cord. Such a disproportion could arise if the liver or intestinal tract is abnormally large, or if the abdominal parietes have a retarded development. A study of our patients gives the impression that the latter explanation is the correct one in most instances.

CLINICAL FINDINGS

Physical Characteristics

An omphalocele sac has a translucent or transparent membranous wall which has very much the same appearance and physical characteristics as the fetal membranes which normally surround a baby. Through this thin structure the intestines, liver, and possibly other abdominal organs are directly exposed to view, as if they were exhibited in a showcase.

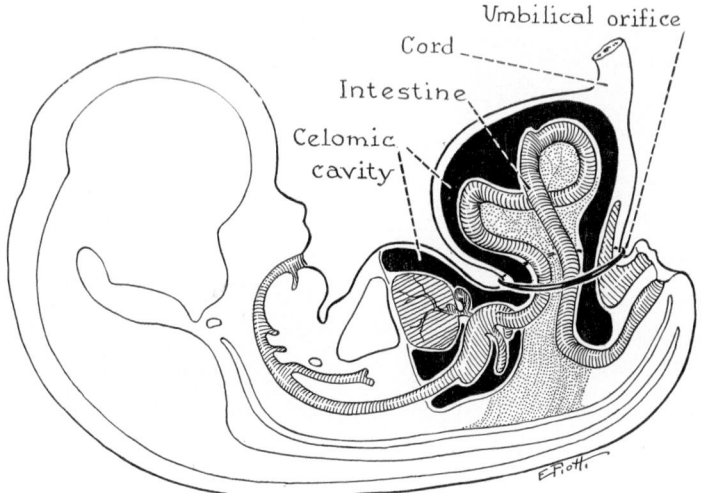

Fig. 208. Sketch of a normal 17 mm. human embryo (after Mall and Prentiss). The celomic cavity normally extends out into the expanded base of the umbilical cord in this early period. A persistence of this state gives rise to an omphalocele.

An omphalocele may be several centimeters in diameter or may be as large as a grapefruit. Average ones are 6 to 8 cm. in cross dimensions; some are much smaller, while some have a cubic capacity which is actually larger than that of the baby's abdominal cavity. The stump of the cord is attached to the apex of the sac, over which the three umbilical blood vessels course to enter the abdominal wall. Aside from these three large channels, the sac wall is notable for its avascularity. The defect in the abdominal wall has no direct relationship to the size of the presenting mass. The fascial opening is usually 4 or 5 cm. in diameter; it may be smaller or it may be much larger than this. The abdominal skin usually stops just at the base of the omphalocele, but in some cases it extends up a centimeter or so beyond this. Loops of small intestine are almost always extruded into the sac, while portions of the stomach, spleen, pancreas, and the urinary bladder may also be displaced here. The transverse colon is dislocated in about

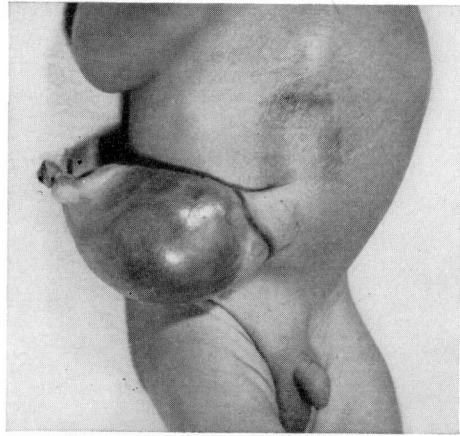 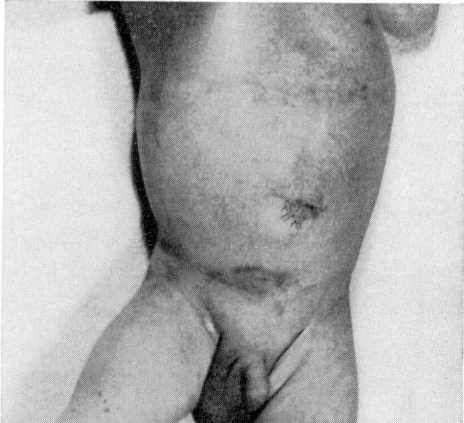

Fig. 209. *Left,* Three-hour-old baby with omphalocele containing only small intestines. *Right,* Same patient eleven days after operation; satisfactory repair of abdominal wall. (From Gross and Blodgett: Surgery, Gynecology and Obstetrics, vol. 71.)

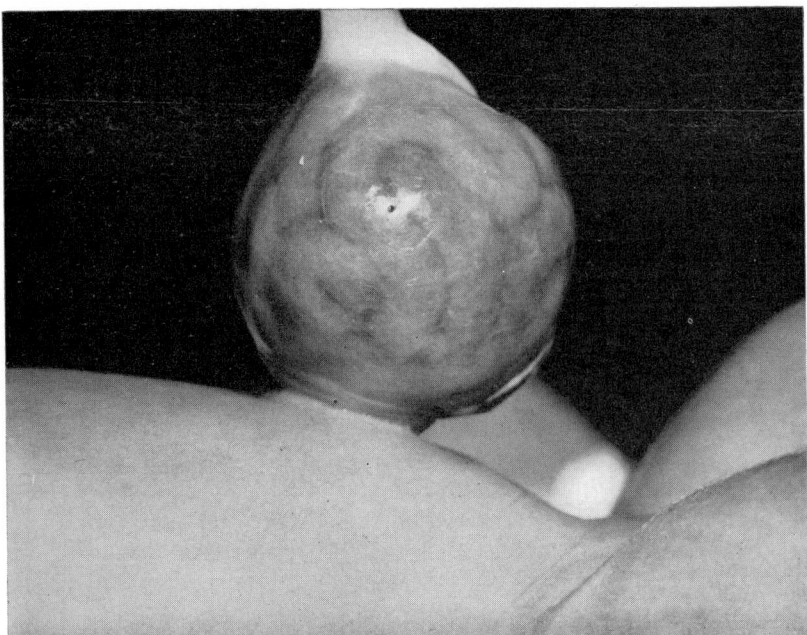

Fig. 210. Newly born baby with an omphalocele which has a very thin, transparent sac. The orifice in the abdominal wall is only 3 cm. in diameter; the prognosis for surgical repair is excellent.

a third of the cases, and some part of the liver passes out through the abdominal opening in almost half of them.

In the first twenty-four hours of life the sac wall is moist and pliable. After this it tends to become shriveled, opaque, dried, and somewhat friable. During the first day it will stand a certain amount of gentle handling, but subsequently it is apt to rupture and allow evisceration (Fig. 214). Indeed, in some cases the sac has ruptured before birth. The membrane, even if unbroken, has a very low resistance to bacterial invasion. These tendencies of the sac to undergo necrosis or to become infected are presumably related to its extremely poor blood supply. These various factors make it imperative to perform a surgical correction of the anomaly as soon as it is possible. Photographs of typical cases are shown in the accompanying illustrations.

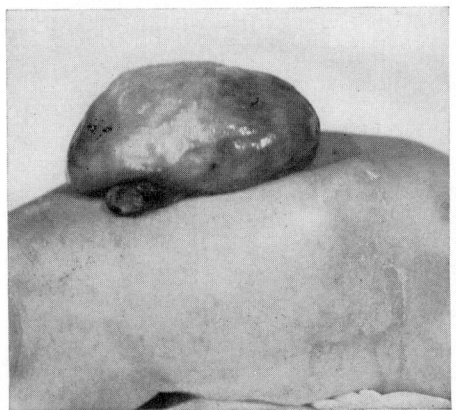 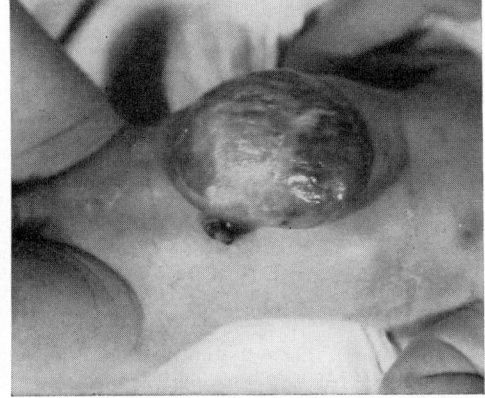

Fig. 211. Omphalocele in a two-day-old boy. The sac is thicker than is usually the case. (From Gross and Blodgett: Surgery, Gynecology and Obstetrics, vol. 71.)

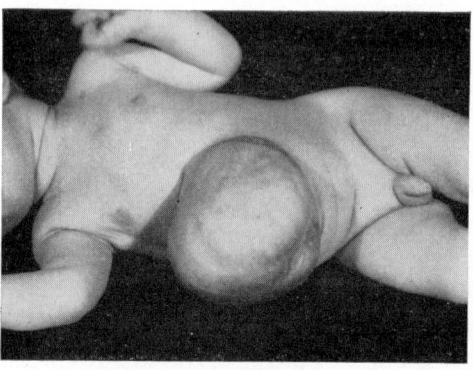 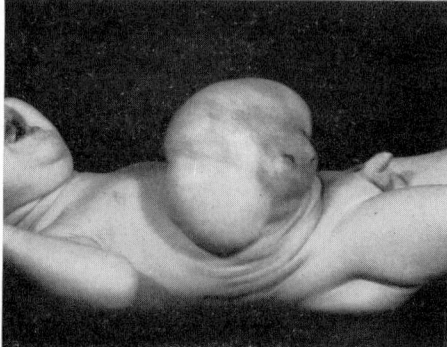

Fig. 212. Large omphalocele which contained almost half of the abdominal viscera. (From Gross and Blodgett: Surgery, Gynecology and Obstetrics, vol. 71.)

Symptoms

During the first twelve or eighteen hours these babies rarely show any evidence of pain or altered physiology from the displacement of viscera and the exposure of them to a lower temperature. It is rare to find respiratory difficulties or signs of intestinal obstruction. In no instance has jaundice been observed, in spite of dislocation of the liver and distortion of the extra-biliary passages in some subjects. Indeed, the omphalocele appears to act as a compensatory decompression which permits the baby to be quite comfortable.

Associated Anomalies

Congenital anomalies in other parts of the body occur with more than coincidental frequency. Fifty-nine per cent of our babies had some other anomaly; occasionally these were serious, such as congenital heart disease, imperforate anus, or the like, but in the majority of cases they were of a minor sort and did not threaten the life of the individual. Of particular importance was the fact that 28 per cent of the babies had malrotation of the intestine and colon which gave intestinal obstruction and had to be treated at the time of omphalocele repair or subsequent thereto. Defects in mesenteric attachments and failure of the abdominal wall closure occur at about the same embryologic time, hence it is not surprising to find a high incidence of association of these two conditions. The clinical importance of the relationship lies in the fact that vomiting

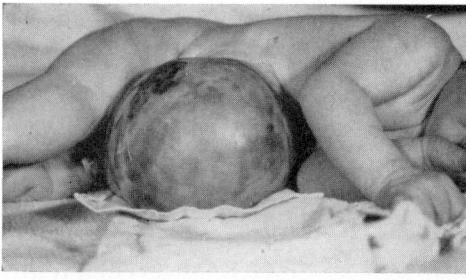 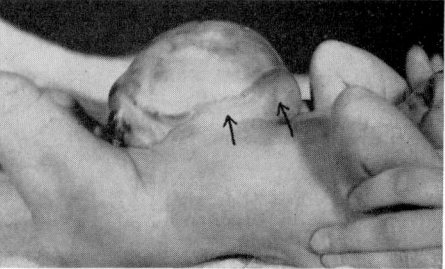

Fig. 213. Very large omphalocele in a two-day-old baby. The mass is composed of intestines, a large portion of the colon, and a part of the liver. Arrows indicate narrow rim of skin at base of omphalocele. In a deformity of this extent, repair by a single stage would almost certainly be fatal because of abdominal crowding. A two-stage repair should be done (Figs. 217 and 218). (From Gross and Blodgett: Surgery, Gynecology and Obstetrics, vol. 71.)

during the postoperative period of an omphalocele repair is sometimes a clear sign of obstruction for which another urgent operation is required for correction of a malrotation. Six of our omphalocele patients had to be operated upon again some time after the omphalocele repair so that a malrotation could be corrected.

TREATMENT

Indication for Radical and Immediate Operation

Treatment by any means other than immediate operation exposes the child to risk of a fatal rupture of the thin sac or a spreading infection of the abdominal wall. Without operation the mortality is extremely high, and most infants succumb within a few days. In one of our cases the skin of the adjacent abdominal wall had started to grow up over the margins of a (small) sac, and we were encouraged to believe that this would continue until the whole structure was covered. Operation was therefore deferred, but infection supervened in the second month and the baby died. There is now quite general agreement that radical and immediate operation offers practically the only hope for

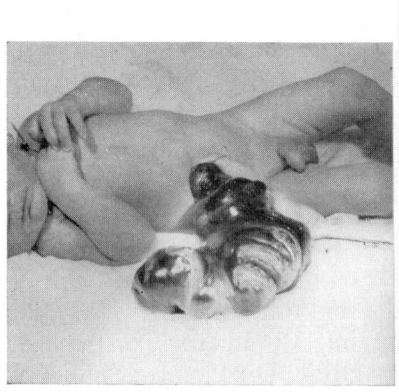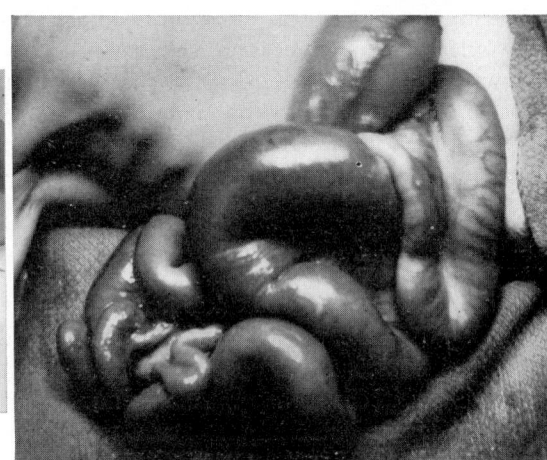

Fig. 214. Two babies with rupture of an omphalocele. *Left*, Rupture had taken place *in utero*. The intestines are thickened, edematous, and matted together. *Right*, Rupture took place after delivery. The loops of intestine are smooth, moist, and are not adherent to one another. (A situation of this sort has a more favorable outlook than does that in which rupture has occurred before birth.)

sustained life. The surgical repair should be performed on the first day, and preferably within the first few hours after birth. Indeed, it has been aptly said that the baby should pass from the obstetrician's hands onto the operating table. Early operation is advantageous because the stomach and intestines are not yet distended by food and gas, and hence the abdominal wall repair can be made with the least difficulty.

Technique of One-Stage Operation

The plan of operation for a one-stage repair need not be a set one. The procedure consists essentially of replacement of the various viscera, excision of the sac, and suitable closure of the abdominal wall (Fig. 215). In cutting away the sac it is best to freshen the edges of the presenting ring to obtain the strongest postoperative healing of the wound. Particular attention must be paid to the two umbilical arteries and the umbilical vein, each of which must be ligated carefully. It is not always possible to free up muscle and fascial layers around the ring, but if this is done a better repair can be made. The

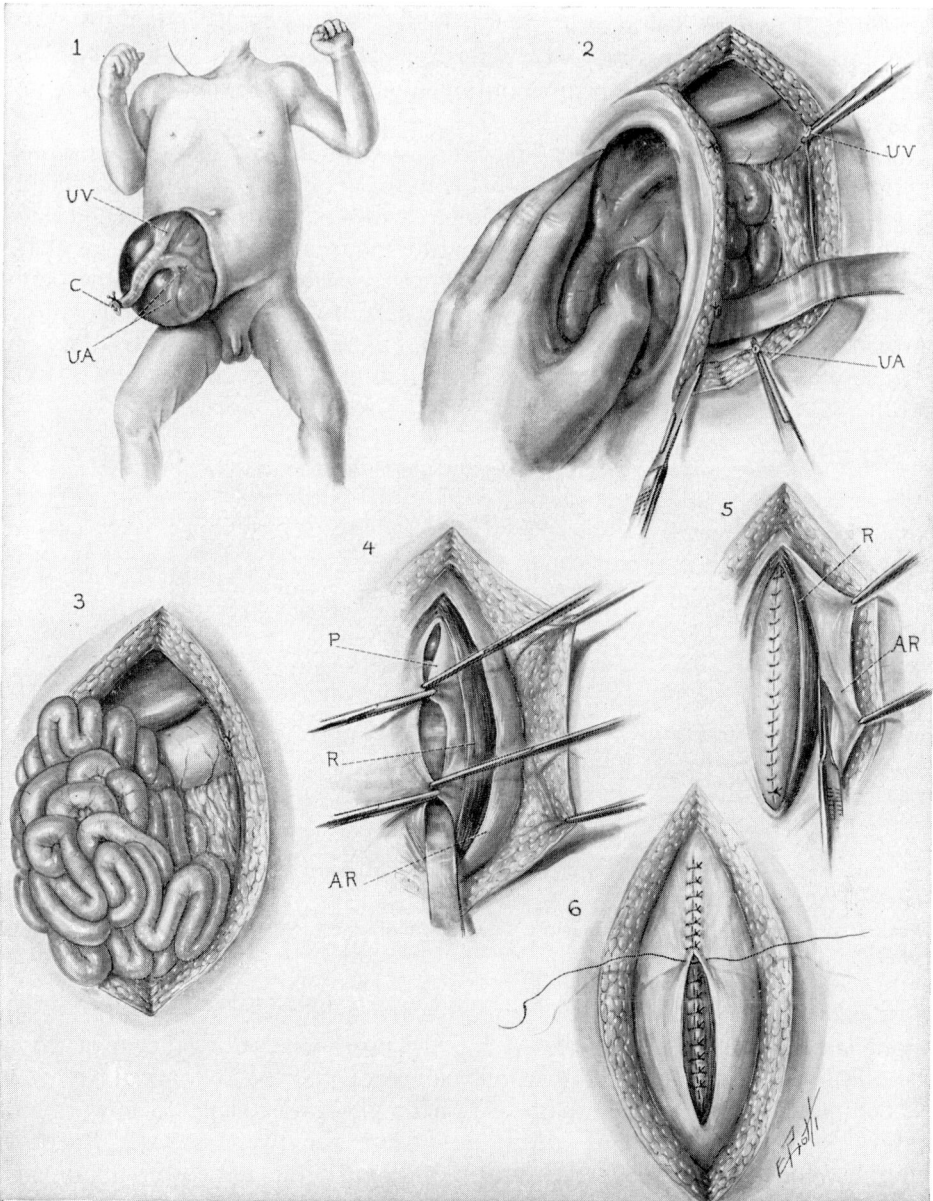

Fig. 215. Method of one-stage correction of an omphalocele. 1. Preoperative appearance. 2. Cutting away the sac; removing a narrow rim of the adjacent skin and abdominal wall to freshen their edges. The umbilical vein and arteries are clamped to avoid bleeding. 3. Sac removed. Umbilical vein and arteries ligated. 4. Intestines replaced in abdomen. Peritoneum freed up. 5. Peritoneum closed. Rectus muscles and anterior rectus fascia are cleared. 6. Rectus muscles have been approximated. The anterior rectus fasciae are being brought together with interrupted silk sutures.

AR, Anterior rectus fascia   R,   Rectus muscle
C,   Cord   UA, Umbilical artery
P,   Peritoneum   UV, Umbilical vein

peritoneum and posterior rectus sheath should be closed simultaneously, by a continuous suture. The rectus muscles should be mobilized so that they can be approximated in the midline. Likewise, the anterior rectus fasciae should be dissected out and then joined or overlapped (if possible) with interrupted stitches. It is preferable to repair these last two layers with silk to insure continued tensile strength until adequate fibrous union takes place.

The *closure of the abdominal wall* is the most difficult part of the operation. The viscera, having forfeited their right of domicile in the abdominal cavity, are difficult and at times impossible to replace. If a satisfactory closure of the wall is obtained, the tension within the abdomen may be so great that respiratory and circulatory embarrassments occur. Considerable judgment must be exercised in determining how perfect a closure should be attempted. If necessary, some part of the abdominal wall can be left unapproximated for the moment, leaving this gap to be repaired at a secondary operation. On several occasions this choice has permitted us to treat successfully a situation which otherwise looked hopeless.

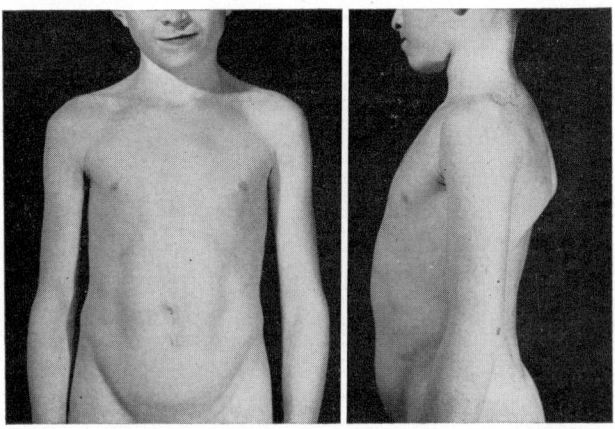

Fig. 216. Photograph of patient nine years after single-stage removal of an omphalocele. There is no weakness of the abdominal wall. (From Gross and Blodgett: Surgery, Gynecology and Obstetrics, vol. 71.)

Postoperative Complications. The operative shock imposed by one-stage repair of an omphalocele is usually not excessive, but the postoperative condition of the baby may be precarious. If viscera are unwittingly squeezed into the abdominal cavity, three serious complications are apt to arise. (1) the diaphragm is displaced upward so that respiratory disturbance, severe cyanosis, and death rapidly appear. (2) Pressure on the inferior vena cava impedes the return of blood from the lower abdomen and legs, so that death follows from circulatory collapse. (3) Pressure on the stomach and intestines may bring about partial or temporary obstruction. These various complications are of such a nature that death, when it occurs, follows within twelve to thirty-six hours. The crisis is within the first day or two. Indeed, it may be stated that if a child lives for forty-eight hours after one of these procedures the chances of a successful outcome are excellent.

Need for Two-Stage Operation

If omphaloceles are small, there is no real surgical problem in repairing them by the procedure above described. In distinct contrast, large omphaloceles present formidable surgical problems and are attended by high fatality rates. When herniation is great, the surgeon will find that the abdominal cavity is relatively small and will not receive the various displaced viscera and simultaneously permit a satisfactory closure of the abdominal wall. A review of a series of 88 babies treated for omphalocele at the Boston Children's Hospital showed that the size of the omphalocele sac had some prognostic value. In those patients with a sac less than 7 cm. in diameter, there was about a 75 per cent chance of survival following surgery. When the sac was 7 to 9 cm. in diameter, survivals were cut to about 30 per cent. When the sacs were larger than 9 cm., the survivals were reduced to about 15 per cent. Whenever a large portion of the liver was found in an omphalocele, a grave outlook could be expected.

If there is to be any reduction in the fatality rates in the treatment of the larger omphaloceles, it is essential to devise some method whereby intra-abdominal crowding is avoided at the first operation. With this thought in mind, a two-stage repair has been designed for managing the extensive lesions. The essential feature of this therapy is to leave intact the omphalocele membrane (taking care to cleanse it thoroughly), cut free and widely undermine the surrounding skin, and then bring together huge cutaneous flaps to cover over the bulging omphalocele sac. By this maneuver the intestines retain their smooth membranous covering which resembles a normal peritoneum, the intestines have not been exposed to the air nor have they been touched by any instrument or gauze, the intestinal viscera have been given the added protection of a cutaneous coat, and the pressure within the abdominal cavity has not been increased appreciably. While the child may be left with an enormous, bulging, and weird-looking mass on the anterior abdominal wall, this is compatible with life and will permit a secondary repair some months later when the abdominal cavity has grown sufficiently to receive the intestines easily and permit a secondary closure of the muscles and fasciae. The soundness of these principles is demonstrated by several cases in which both stages have been completed. I am reasonably sure that in all these infants a fatal outcome would have followed any attempt at a one-stage repair of the large omphaloceles in the newborn period.

Technique of Two-Stage Operation

The various steps in the first stage of the repair are shown in Figure 217. Following this, it is usually possible to discharge the baby from the hospital in about two weeks. The mother is apt to be somewhat apprehensive about the possibility of rupture of the bulging mass; it distends considerably during acts of straining or crying. It is necessary to reassure her that such an accident has not happened in other babies. The child may be bathed. The trunk can be kept wrapped in an elastic binder, for which a 4 or 6-inch-wide Ace bandage serves admirably.

Just how much delay is necessary between the two operations will vary from case to case. We have performed the second stage as early as three months and as late as eighteen months; in some instances the interval may have to be even longer. *The important point is to wait until the abdominal cavity has grown large enough so that it can receive the intestines without crowding*. The child should be examined at intervals of one to two months; whenever manual pressure shows that the viscera can be easily pushed back into the abdominal cavity, and when the sac wall can be readily picked up between the examining fingers, then the appropriate time has arrived for the secondary operation. The various steps of the second procedure are shown in Figure 218.

Possible Complications from Two-Stage Repair. A two-stage repair would appear to have certain theoretical hazards, none of which, however, has materialized in our patients. (1) The omphalocele sac is obviously not sterile and to bury it (minus the stum of the cord) beneath the skin carries certain risks of infection. Yet a careful cleansing of the sac, followed by application of half-strength tincture of iodine (tincture of iodine diluted with an equal volume of 70 per cent alcohol) has been sufficient to sterilize it in all our subjects. (2) It is possible that wide undermining and mobilization of skin might lead to sloughing, particularly when the cutaneous flaps are applied to an underlying membrane which has no important vascularity. However, this has not proved to be troublesome. (3) There is some possibility that the amniotic membrane might not grow

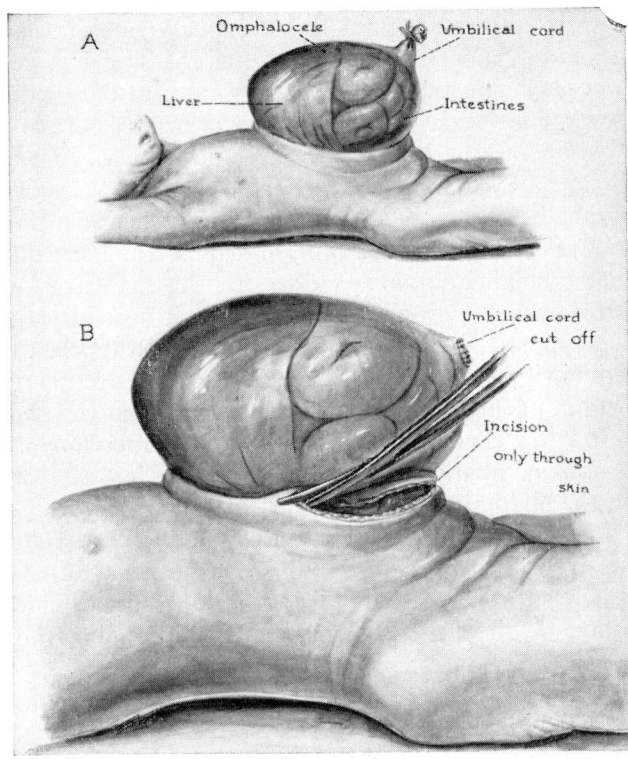

Fig. 217. Initial operation in a two-stage repair of large omphaloceles. A, Drawing of omphalocele showing large size of the presenting mass, which is covered by a thin, transparent sac. The sac contained many loops of small intestine, part of the colon, and a large part of the liver. B, Stump of umbilical cord has been cut away. Skin edge is being cut away from base of the omphalocele sac, taking great care to avoid opening the sac.

to the skin which is applied to it, but instead might allow accumulation of fluid between these two layers and form cysts which would be difficult to treat. No cystic accumulation occurred in any of our cases; possibly the tincture of iodine solution caused sufficient reaction to destroy the smooth external surface of the amniotic sac, a process which might not have occurred if a milder type of antiseptic had been employed. (4) It is possible at the first operation, when the skin is cut away from the base of the sac for raising of the cutaneous flaps, that small islands of epidermis may be left on the base of the sac and covered up, which presumably could give rise to subsequent inclusion cysts. This objection has minimal importance, since it is possible to remove such inclusion cysts during the secondary operation. (5) It might be possible for a strong antiseptic to penetrate the thin amniotic membrane and set up adhesions between its inner surface and the subjacent intestines. However, at the secondary operations which have

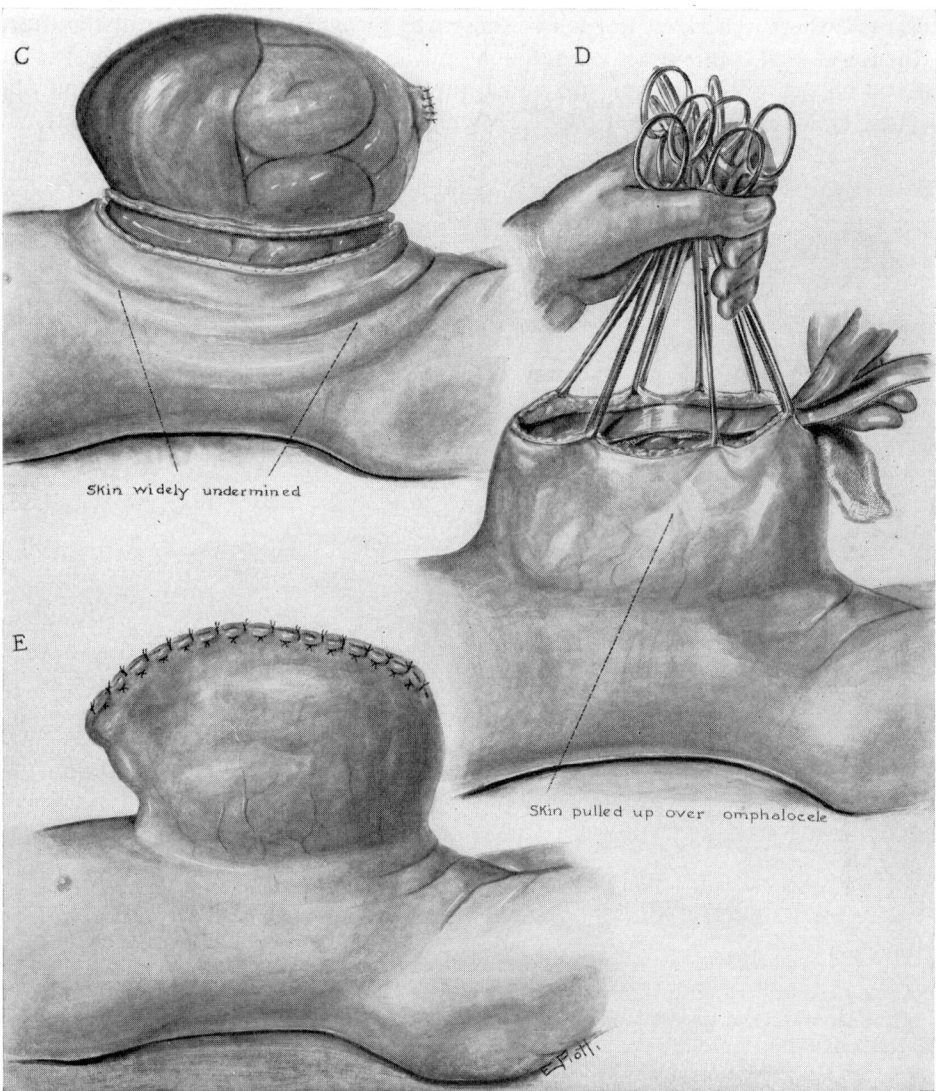

Fig. 217 (*continued*). C, Skin has been freed from entire circumference of base of omphalocele sac. The skin has then been widely undermined as far down as the pubes, well around to both flanks, but *no farther up on chest than is necessary*. D, Skin edges grasped by Allis clamps and pulled up over the intact omphalocele sac. E, Closure of skin, using buried interrupted silks to subcutaneous tissues, and then mattress stitched to the skin. These give apposition of broad subcutaneous surfaces for optimum healing. They can be interspersed with other stitches to bring the skin edges together accurately. *There is no crowding of viscera back into the small abdominal cavity.*

now been done it has been most gratifying to find the peritoneal cavity completely free of adhesions.

We have seen several patients (one to two years of age) who had had the first stage of repair elsewhere. The liver in each of these was displaced up in *front* of the thoracic cage, the lower part of the cage being thereby pushed back against the vertebral column. There was no sub-phrenic fossa into which the liver could be fitted at a second operation. These children now present problems which almost seem to be insoluble. It would

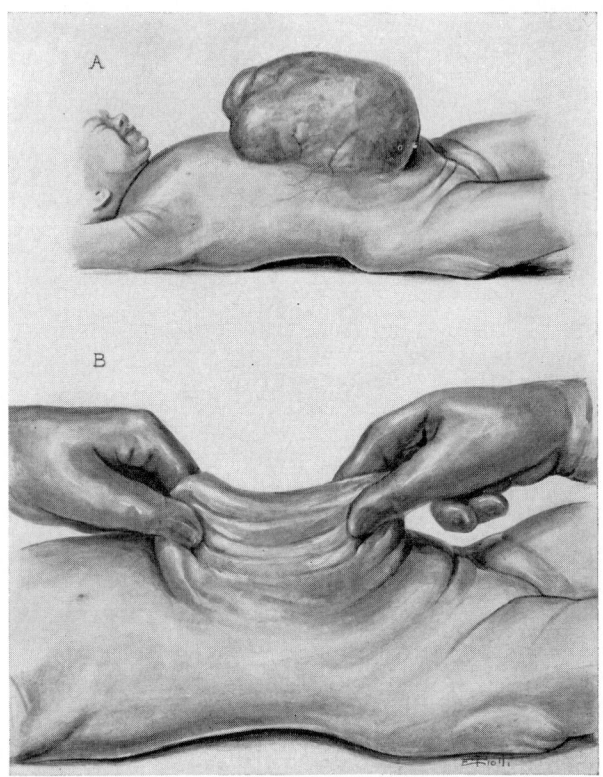

Fig. 218. Second operation in a two-stage repair of a large omphalocele. A, Appearance of the skin-covered mass at beginning of second operation (many months after the first one). B, Showing the laxity of the sac wall. The viscera have been squeezed back into the abdomen, following which the sac can be grasped and its looseness demonstrated.

appear that (at the first operation) skin was dissected too far upward off the chest, thus making a pre-thoracic pocket up into which the liver had slipped and had forfeited its right of intra-abdominal residence completely. It would therefore seem to be a very important principle and precaution at the first operation *never to free skin up over the chest any farther than is necessary* to gain coverage of the omphalocele membrane.

Rupture of an Omphalocele Sac

Prior to 1940, rupture of an omphalocele sac (Fig. 214) was a uniformly fatal accident. It was often possible to gather up the intestines, return them to the abdomen, and close the abdominal wall, but such an emergency operation was always followed by fatal peritonitis. Since the advent of chemotherapy and antibiotics, this outlook has now completely changed; whenever evisceration has taken place, every effort should be made to cleanse the exposed viscera and perform some form of suitable repair of the wall. A reasonable percentage of subjects so treated will survive if given postoperative decompression of the alimentary tract, appropriate chemotherapy, and supportive measures. From 1940 through 1950 we have had 17 such patients, of whom 6 recovered. If the rupture and evisceration had taken place after birth, the outlook was far brighter than in those cases where the rupture had occurred during intra-uterine life and the intestines had become edematous, swollen, and matted together.

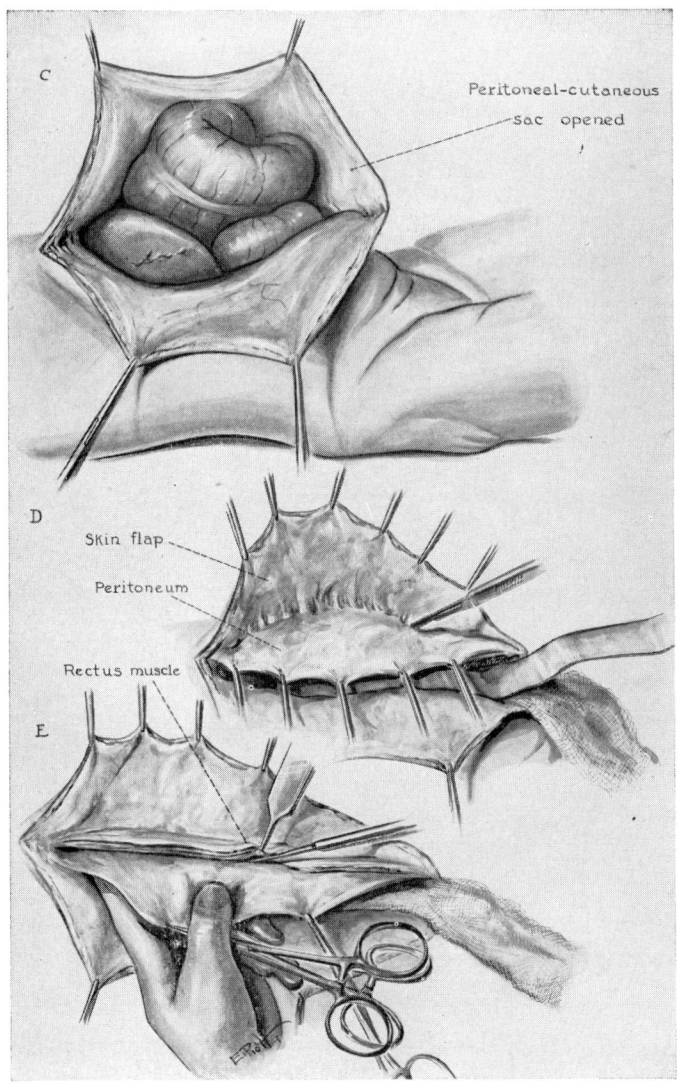

Fig. 218 (*continued*). C, Thin sac opened, showing lack of adhesions between viscera and interior of the sac. D, Left side of abdominal wall flap held so that peritoneum can be separated from skin. E. Separation of flap components continued until left rectus muscle is identified and isolated.

RESULTS OF TREATMENT

In a series of 88 cases at the Boston Children's Hospital, 10 patients were not operated upon because they were in extremis or the deformities (at times combined

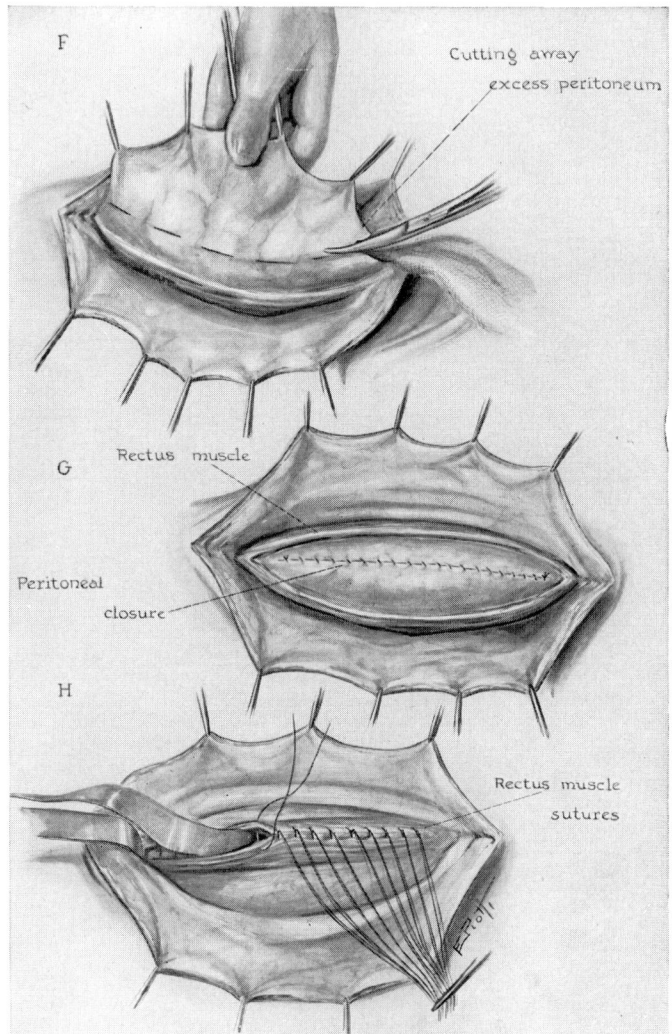

Fig. 218 (*continued*). F, Right side of sac has been split into its component layers. Excess peritoneum will be cut off at the dotted line. G, Peritoneum easily closed, with running fine catgut suture. H,
Rectus muscle bellies being approximated with interrupted silk sutures.

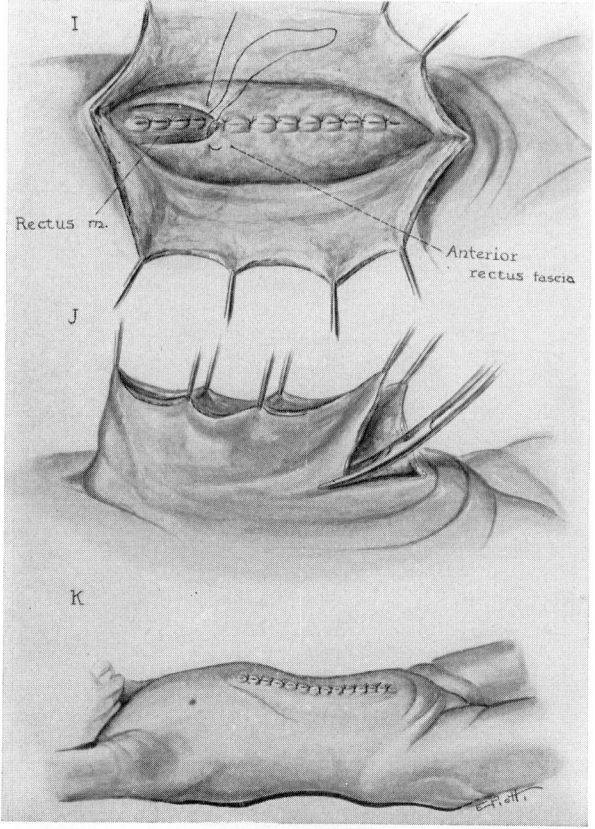

Fig. 218 (*continued*). I, Anterior rectus fascia dissected away from underlying muscle, and then repaired with interrupted fine silk sutures. J, Excess skin being cut away. K, Closure of skin.

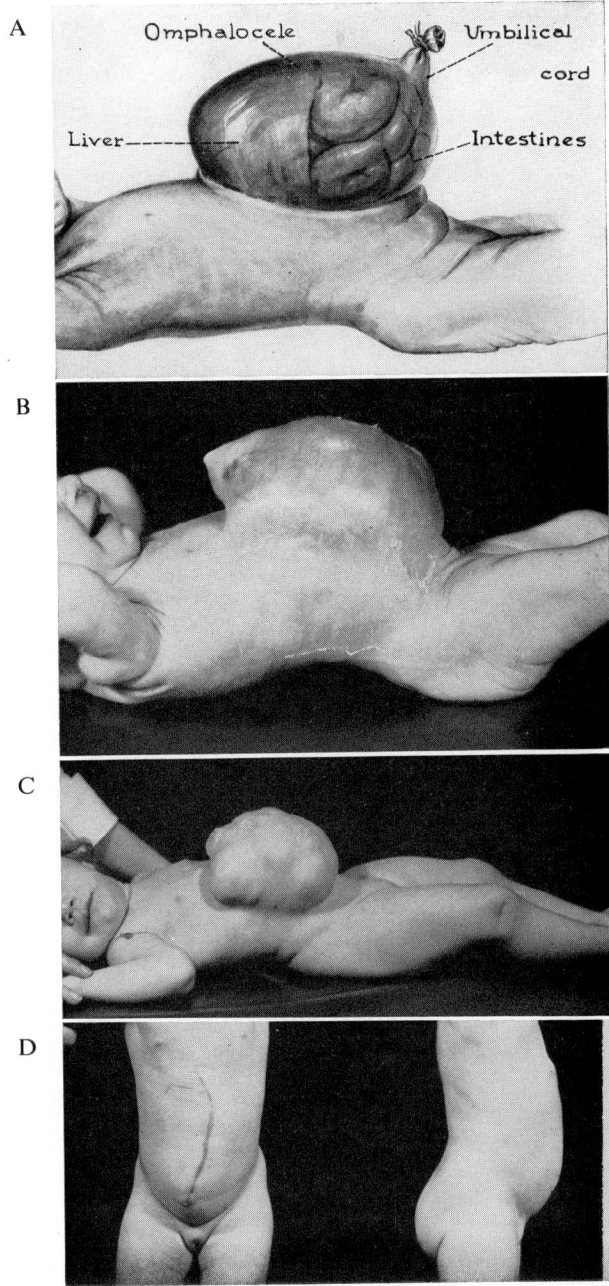

Fig. 219. Progress in omphalocele repair when a two-stage reconstruction has been performed. A, Drawing of original lesion before operation. The presenting mass is about the same size as, or possibly a little larger than, the general abdominal cavity. B, Photograph two weeks after first-stage operation. C, Photograph nine months after first operation, and immediately before second-stage operation. D, Photograph two months after completion of the second-stage operation.

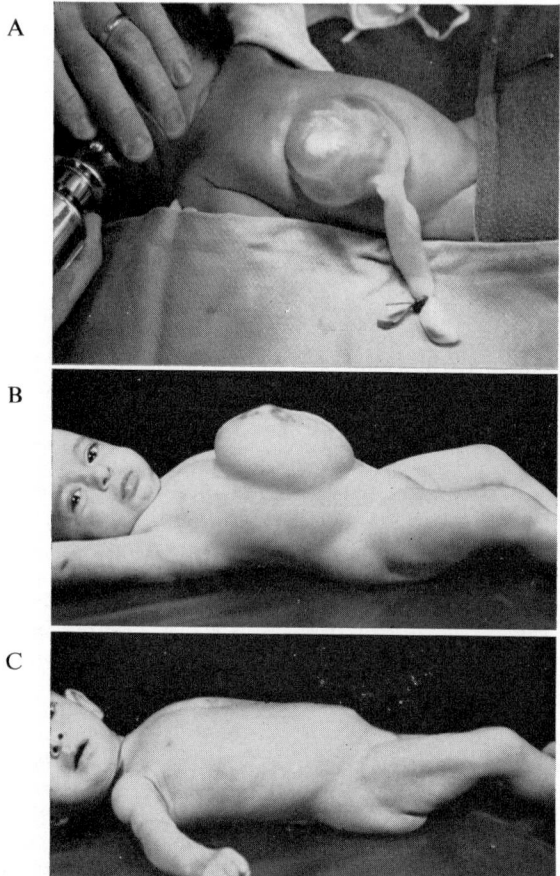

Fig. 220. Omphalocele repair for a child wherein a two-stage repair was employed. A, Preoperative photograph of omphalocele in premature infant weighing 3 pounds, 5 ounces. B, Photograph six months after primary operation, and immediately before the secondary repair. C, Photograph after the secondary repair of the abdominal wall.

with other serious anomalies) presented a hopeless situation; all 10 of them died. In the 78 surgically treated babies there were 30 deaths and 48 survivors, giving a mortality of 38 per cent in those who were accepted for surgery. For the more recent portion of the series, patients treated from 1940 through 1950, the mortality rate was 34 per cent for those accepted for surgery. Analysis of the deaths in this eleven-year period shows them to be due to the following:

Congenital heart disease	4
Respiratory embarrassment	2
Perforation of bowel	2
Pneumonia	2
Peritonitis	1
Intestinal obstruction from adhesions	1
Subdural hemorrhage	2
Shock	1
Atelectasis	1
Volvulus	1
Infected meningocele	1
Diarrhea	1
Nephritis	1

Those children who survived have abdominal walls which are very satisfactory (Figs. 216, 219, and 220). In 6 of them a subsequent operation was necessary for treatment of intestinal obstruction resulting from malrotation of the intestines and colon.

REFERENCES

1. Arey L. B.: Developmental Anatomy: a Textbook and Laboratory Manual of Embryology. Ed. 5. W. B. Saunders Co., Philadelphia, 1946.
2. Bardeen, C. R.: Critical Period in the Development of the Intestines. Am. J. Anat., 16: 427, 1914.
3. Cullen, T. S.: Embryology, Anatomy and Diseases of the Umbilicus. W. B. Saunders Co., Philadelphia, 1916.
4. Cutler, G. D.: Prolapsus of the Bowel through a Patent Omphalomesenteric Duct Opening on the Side of the Umbilical Cord: Report of a Case with Operation. Boston M. & S. J., 190:782, 1924.
5. Dott, N. M.: Clinical Record of a Case of Exomphalos, Illustrating Embryonic Type and Its Surgical Treatment. Tr. Edinburgh Obst. Soc., 39:105, 1932.
6. Gross, R. E.: A New Method for Surgical Treatment of Large Omphaloceles. Surgery, 24:277, 1948.
7. Gross, R. E. and Blodgett, J. B.: Omphalocele (Umbilical Eventration) in the Newly Born. Surg., Gynec. & Obst., 71:520, 1940.
8. Herbert, A. F.: Hernia Funiculi Umbilicalis; With Report of Three Cases. Am. J. Obst. & Gynec., 15:86, 1928.
9. Iason, A. H.: Congenital Eventration at Umbilicus. Surgery, 16:950, 1944.
10. Jarcho, J.: Congenital Umbilical Hernia. Surg., Gynec. & Obst., 65:593, 1937.
11. Kahle, H. R.: Omphalocele. Analysis of 21 Cases from Charity Hospital of Louisiana at New Orleans. Am. Surgeon, 17:947, 1951.
12. Keibel, F. and Mall, F. P.: Manual of Human Embryology. Vol. II. J. B. Lippincott Co., Philadelphia, 1912.
13. Klopp, E. J.: Amniotic Hernia. Ann. Surg., 73:642, 1921.
14. Ladd, W. E. and Gross, R. E.: Congenital Diaphragmatic Hernia. New England J. Med., 223:917, 1940.
15. Michelson, E. and Raffel, W.: Repair of Large Umbilical Hernia. Surgery, 10:999, 1941.
16. Niebuhr, W. D., Dresch, C. A. and Logan, F. W.: Hernia into the Umbilical Cord Containing the Entire Liver and Gall Bladder (Successfully Treated Surgically). J.A.M.A., 103:16, 1934.
17. Stein, J. L. and Gerber, A.: Congenital Omphalocele. J. Pediat., 14:89, 1939.
18. Watson, L. F.: Hernia. Ed. 2. C. V. Mosby Co., St. Louis, 1938, Chap. XXIV.
19. Williams, C.: Congenital Defects of the Anterior Abdominal Wall. S. Clin. North America, 10:805, 1930.

CHAPTER 32

Umbilical Hernia

Pathology

Umbilical hernia is extremely common in infants and young children. It results from muscular and fascial defects of the abdominal wall at the point where it has been pierced by the blood vessels of the umbilical cord. The forward-projecting peritoneum is covered only by subcutaneous fat and skin. The hernial ring has an edge of firm connective tissue which represents the fused posterior rectus, anterior rectus, and transversalis fascia. While the separation of the muscle bellies is usually confined to the periumbilical region, it not infrequently extends upward, even as far as the ensiform process, as a diastasis recti. Umbilical hernias are about twice as common in girls as they are in boys—a fact possibly related to the less well developed musculature of the female. Most of these weaknesses can be detected in the early months of life, but they may escape attention until the child assumes an erect posture and the bulging becomes more marked.

Physical Findings

The *size* of an umbilical hernia depends upon the extent of the fascial defect and upon the length of time that the sac and overlying skin have been stretched. In infants under one year, the bulge is rarely more than 1 or 2 cm. in diameter. In older children, hernias 3 to 4 cm. in cross dimensions are often encountered, and larger ones are sometimes seen. The pocket rarely contains more than omentum or a single knuckle of small intestine. Adhesions seldom form between these viscera and the sac wall.

Symptoms

In most cases the patient's or the parents' complaints are concerned with the *swelling* which becomes larger and more tense during crying, standing, straining, or other exercise which raises the intra-abdominal pressure. There may be a mild, local discomfort of a vague sort. *Cramps* may appear if a loop of small intestine enters the hernia and becomes partially obstructed. Omentum is sometimes caught in the hernial ring, but intestine is rarely incarcerated. These findings are in distinct contrast to the frequency of incarceration with inguinal hernias in childhood.

TREATMENT

Adhesive Strapping

Before initiating any measures for treatment of an umbilical hernia, it is well to remember that the majority of them will be *spontaneously cured* as the individual grows older and the rectus muscles constrict and finally obliterate the hernial orifice. Thus, small hernias often disappear as the child is observed over a period of several years. This natural tendency for small hernias to vanish can be augmented by proper adhesive strapping during the early months of life. This should be done in such a way that the lateral tension of the abdominal wall is diminished and the hernial ring is allowed to shrink. Furthermore, the sac must be kept empty so that nothing interferes with its collapse and obliteration. These requirements are not fulfilled by strapping a metal coin over the protruding navel. Neither are they met by spring trusses or rubber belts fitted with a small projection which is intended to press into the hernial opening.

The most satisfactory support for a small umbilical hernia is by adhesive strapping. Two pieces of 2-inch adhesive tape are cut, one with a hole and the other with a tongue, so that they can be interlaced. The abdomen is painted with tincture of benzoin to enhance the sticking qualities of the tape and to protect the skin from ulceration. The straps are placed on either side of the abdomen and the narrow tongue is threaded through the hole of the opposite piece. The free ends are then grasped and pulled in a forward and outward direction until the skin becomes lax and wrinkled in the umbilical area. If necessary, an assistant can simultaneously push the hernia inward with the tip of a finger. While the pull is still maintained, the free ends of the adhesive straps are stuck down. If this has been done properly, the umbilical skin will still have longitudinal wrinkles.

While the above-described method of strapping seems to be about the best which has been devised, it is reasonably satisfactory to use a simpler method which consists merely of applying a single strip of 2-inch adhesive tape across the abdomen, making sure as this is applied that the umbilical mass is folded inward and the skin of the navel area is thrown up into small folds as the tape is drawn into place so that all lateral tension is taken off of the region.

The strapping is renewed every week or two. Continued support must be maintained for a period of several months. If no appreciable improvement is noticed by the end of six months, it is useless to continue this form of treatment. A great deal can be accomplished with strapping during the first six months of life, but after this time it has a diminishing value. It has practically no merit for a baby more than a year old.

Umbilical Herniorrhaphy

Many umbilical hernias cause little nuisance except for the slight disfigurement and the worry to the parent. After the first year of life a swelling which is 1 cm. or less in size should cause little concern, particularly if the palpable fascial ring is less than 7 or 8 mm. in diameter. Such a small sac will generally become obliterated as the child grows. Hernias 1.5 to 4 cm. or more in cross dimensions should be repaired, particularly if there has been recurrent discomfort or a tendency for the hernia to increase in size. Umbilical herniorrhaphy in a child is a rather minor procedure. For small hernias, operation is seldom an urgent matter and it can usually be deferred until the age of one or two years to see if the defect will diminish without a surgeon's aid. If, however, there is a sizable hernia, with a ring more than 8 to 10 mm. in diameter in a small baby, the chances of spontaneous cure are quite small; hence it is advisable to repair the defect at an early age.

There is more reason for repairing an umbilical hernia in a female than in a male. It is well known that in adults, umbilical hernias carry a particular hazard for the female, where there may be incarceration, strangulation, and appreciable risks of fatality. This picture in later life, when the abdomen of the female may be filled and tense with a pregnant uterus, makes it somewhat more important to treat umbilical hernias in the female child than in the male.

Techniques. Operative repair should always restore the normal navel depression.

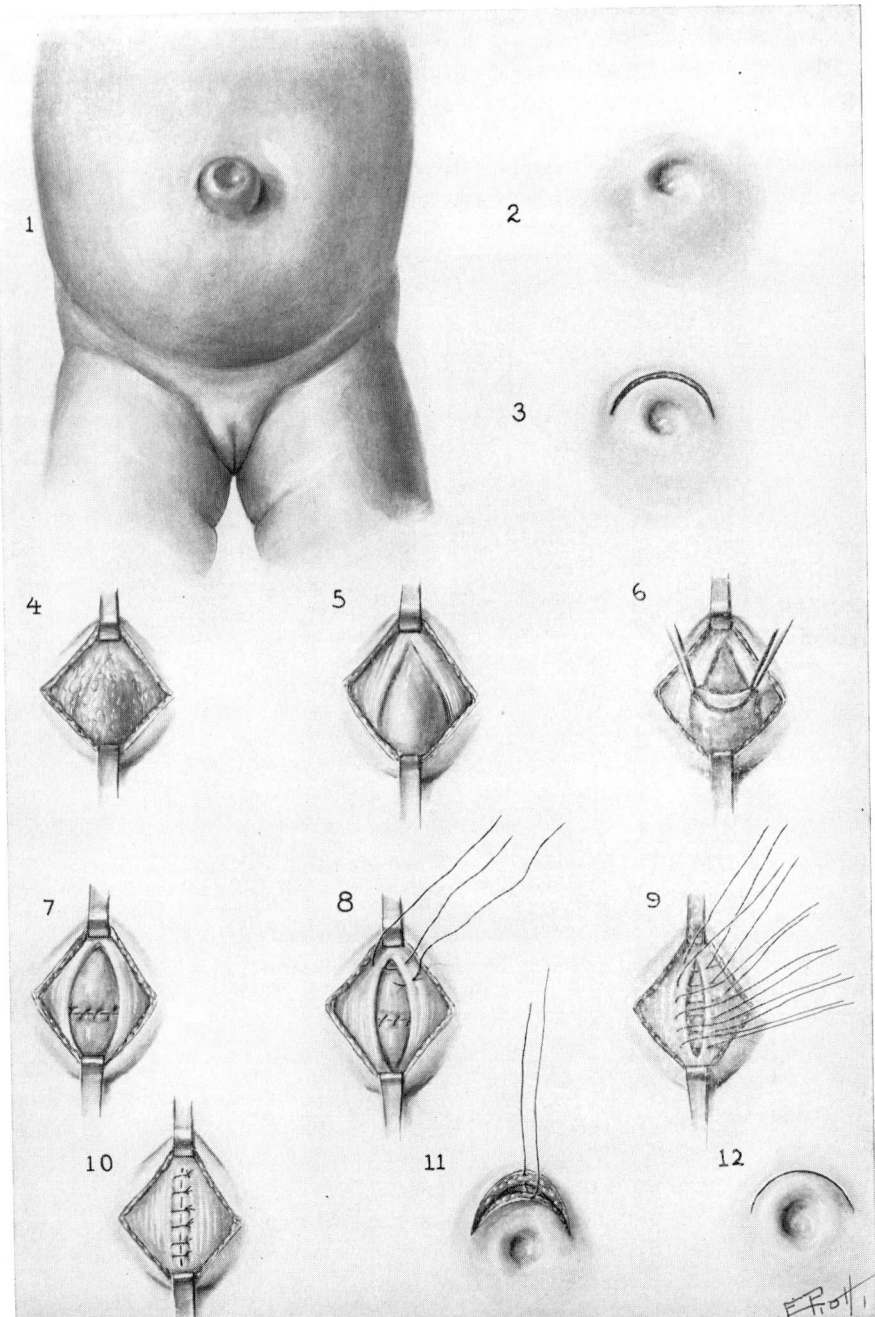

Fig. 221. Recommended technique for umbilical herniorrhaphy in a baby or child. 1. Showing the navel swelling. 2. When relaxed under anesthesia, the navel becomes depressed. 3. Position of the curved incision in skin just above navel. 4. Skin flaps freed from underlying tissues and retracted. 5. Rectus sheaths cleared of overlying fat. Hernial sac cleared. 6. Hernial sac cut away from under surface of navel skin. 7. Peritoneum (hernial sac) closed. 8. Stitches (of silk) being taken in the edges of the rectus sheaths. 9. Rectus sheath stitches in place. 10. Rectus fasciae brought together in midline. 11. Subcuticular stitches (of 000000 Deknatel silk) just beneath the corium. Skin edges brought together, by the subcuticular stitches. 12. No cutaneous sutures are necessary.

To do so does not appreciably complicate the technical procedure and it gives an appearance to the abdominal wall which is more natural and pleasing.

For the repair of an umbilical hernia of any size in childhood, we have employed the method of repair shown in Figure 221. Under general anesthesia, a small curved incision is made in the upper part of the umbilical swelling. The sac is dissected free from the under surface of the navel, and is turned inward. The small cutaneous orifice can be stretched to give an opening of adequate size. The rectus fascial sheaths must be

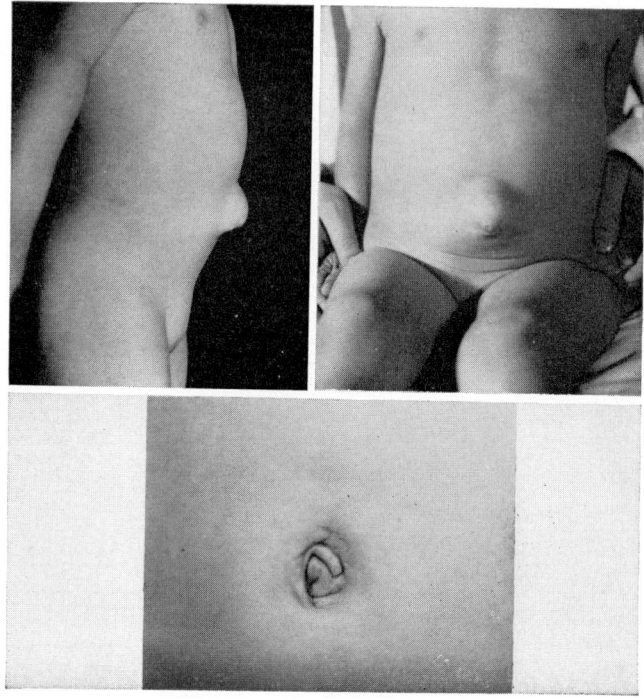

Fig. 222. *Above*, Photographs of umbilical hernia in a three-year-old boy. *Below*, Photograph after herniorrhaphy with incision which lies in the umbilical folds. The cosmetic effect is excellent.

cleared of any overlying fat. The sheaths are brought together in the midline by a vertical row of interrupted silk sutures. The skin is brought together by three or five interrupted silk sutures (000000 Deknatel) placed on the under side of the corium. A sterile dressing is applied and an adhesive strapping is used which removes all lateral tension and which wrinkles up the skin in the navel area.

The child can be discharged from the hospital within a few hours, as soon as there has been recovery from the anesthesia. A baby can be allowed to cry; an older child can be permitted normal activities. The dressing can be taken off in eight or ten days. There are no skin stitches to remove (Fig. 222).

Results of Treatment

At the Children's Hospital more than 1500 umbilical hernias were observed during the twenty-five-year period from 1915 through 1939. Most of these were the primary reason for admission to the out-patient department or the house service; others were insignificant and were discovered during routine examination for some other condition. Many of the smaller hernias in babies were cured by strapping. Out of the entire number, 360 were operated upon, and 3 recurrences have been noted. There was one death, which occurred on the fourth postoperative day from pneumonia.

From 1940 through 1951, a total of 439 umbilical hernias were operated upon, almost all of them by the technique shown in Figure 221. There were no deaths. There was one recurrence, which was satisfactorily treated by a secondary procedure.

REFERENCES

1. Barrington-Ward, L. E.: The Abdominal Surgery of Children. Oxford University Press, London, 1937, p. 25.
2. Blodgett, J. B.: Transumbilical Repair of Congenital Umbilical Hernia. Surg., Gynec. & Obst., *72*:632, 1941.
3. Gorelow, M. A.: Zur Anatomie des Nabelkanals. Arch. f. klin. Chir., *181*:395, 1934.
4. Herzfeld, G.: Hernia in Infancy. Am. J. Surg., *39*:422, 1938.
5. Power, R. W.: Preservation of Umbilicus in Radical Cure of Umbilical Hernias in Children. Brit. M. J., *2*:353, 1934.

CHAPTER 33

Congenital Hernia of the Diaphragm

Diaphragmatic hernia is a not uncommon defect in children and in the newly born. It can be easily detected by physical examination and roentgenologic study. It can be satisfactorily and permanently cured by appropriate surgical procedures.

An extensive literature has accumulated on the general subject of diaphragmatic hernia but relatively little attention has been paid to the condition as it occurs in the first few weeks or months of life. During these periods the therapeutic problems pertaining to such defects are quite different from those encountered in older children or adults. It is preferable to use therapeutic techniques which are somewhat different from the surgical measures which have proved to be so effective in repair of acquired (traumatic) diaphragmatic hernias of adults.

Various authors have stressed the fact that congenital hernia of the diaphragm is a serious lesion which menaces the life of the individual. In 1925 Hedblom reviewed the literature and found that most physicians and surgeons preferred to avoid surgical attacks on small subjects, hoping to have the child grow and be in better condition to withstand a major surgical procedure; with this "conservative" approach, 75 per cent of patients died before the end of the first month. In contrast, practically everyone agrees today that generally the best method of treating diaphragmatic hernia is to repair it immediately, regardless of how small the child might be and regardless of how much respiratory distress might exist. With this complete reversal in therapeutic policy, babies and children with diaphragmatic hernias can now be cured of their malformation in 90 to 95 per cent of the cases. The following sections have been written on the basis of material drawn from the literature and from experience at the Children's Hospital in operating upon 91 of these subjects, 76 of whom are alive and cured.

EMBRYOLOGY

In the young embryo the thoracic and abdominal portions of the body cavity communicate freely with each other. The ventral part of the diaphragm is formed from the *septum transversum*, which separates the heart from the abdominal viscera. This septum is joined posteriorly by a proliferation of mesodermal cells at the upper end of the dorsal mesentery to make a bridge across the celomic cavity from front to back, but openings are left in both postero-lateral parts of the diaphragm which are known as the *pleuroperitoneal canals*. These canals are later closed by a double-layered membrane, consisting of peritoneum on one side and pleura on the other. Striated muscles then develop between these two serous coats to complete and strengthen the partition between the peritoneal and pleural cavities.

The formation of the diaphragm is sufficiently complicated so that there is little wonder that congenital defects are apt to appear. If arrest in development occurs early in embryonic life, a child is born (as is typical of most cases) with a free communication between a pleural cavity and the abdomen. If arrest of development occurs after the pleural and peritoneal membranes have closed the defect, but before the muscle has appeared, the child is born with a thin hernial sac which covers the upward-protruding intestines.

PATHOLOGIC ANATOMY

Congenital hernia may appear in one of several areas of the diaphragm: (1) In either *postero-lateral portion*, along the old pleuroperitoneal canal (the foramen of Bochdalek). This is by far the most common site. They are about five times more common on the left than on the right. In very rare cases the opening may be so large that the diaphragm is virtually absent; only a small rim is found around the periphery. (2) At the *esophageal hiatus*. (3) In the *retrosternal area* (the foramen of Morgagni). The frequency of occurrence of these various types in our material is summarized as follows:

Left postero-lateral.......................... 69 cases
Right postero-lateral......................... 13 cases
Esophageal hiatus............................. 5 cases
Retrosternal area............................. 4 cases

It is almost unknown to find adhesions between the abdominal viscera and the parietal pleural surfaces—a situation quite different from that found in acquired (traumatic) hernia.

Postero-lateral Hernias

In about nine-tenths of the postero-lateral herniations, *no hernial sac* exists; the affected pleural cavity is filled to its very apex with intestines, a portion of the colon, and (depending upon the side involved) a part of the liver or else the stomach and spleen. The lung on the affected side is completely collapsed, the heart is apt to be pushed to the opposite side of the chest, and the contralateral lung is generally partially compressed. Great *displacement of abaominal viscera* is facilitated by a rudimentary attachment of the mesentery to the posterior abdominal wall. Indeed, malrotation (incomplete rotation) of the intestine occurs in a rather high proportion of cases. The kidney may lie in a position somewhat higher than normal; a portion or indeed all of it can reside above the level of the posterior diaphragmatic attachment.

The prenatal displacement of abdominal viscera into the chest implies that they have "forfeited their right of domicile" and hence (in the larger herniations) the peritoneal cavity is smaller than normal. In a minority of postero-lateral herniations there is a *hernial sac*; the various displacements or derangements are less extensive; the apex of the sac may reach a quarter, a half, or two-thirds of the way up the chest. It is very rare for a sac to extend all the way to the apex of a pleural cavity.

Hiatus Hernias

Hernias which appear at the esophageal hiatus always have a *sac* which greatly limits the upward progression of abdominal viscera. While a loop or two of intestine might project into this, the sac seldom contains more than the stomach. The gastric fundus may be above the general level of the diaphragm; in larger hernias, a considerable part of the stomach is above the level of the diaphragm and may be folded upon itself and obstructed. Because of therapeutic considerations, a sharp differentiation must be made between the hiatus hernia with an esophagus of normal length (and the stomach or intestine prolapsed up alongside of it) and that type of hiatus hernia in

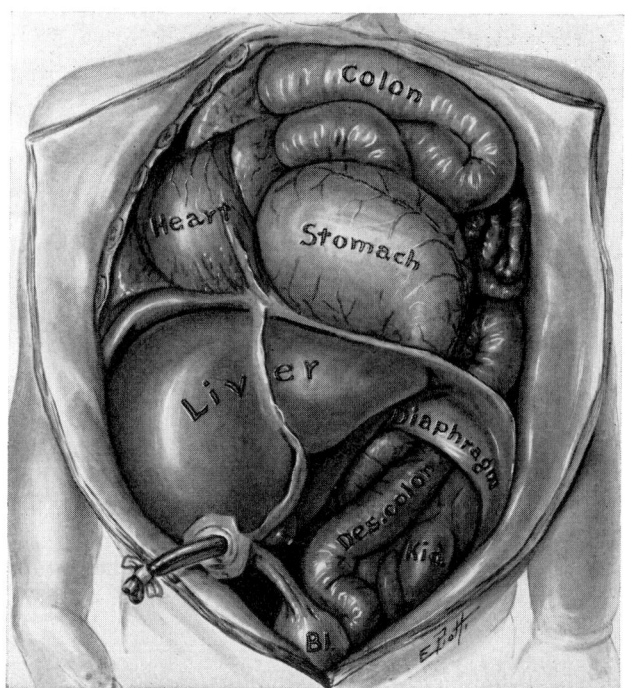

Fig. 223. Drawing made at postmortem examination of a baby with a left diaphragmatic hernia. Four hours following delivery the child died, after severe cyanosis and respiratory distress. As in most congenital diaphragmatic hernias, there is no sac surrounding the extruded abdominal viscera.

which a portion of the stomach is drawn upward by an esophagus which is shorter than normal (the so-called *congenitally short esophagus*).

Retrosternal Hernias

Hernias which occur behind the sternum (through the foramen of Morgagni) have a sac in about half of the cases. Even if there is no sac, there is never a very extensive displacement of abdominal viscera up into the chest. The available space behind the sternum is limited on either side by the pleural envelopes and above by the adherence of pericardium to the upper part of the sternum. Seldom is there upward protrusion of more than a tip of the liver, part to the stomach, some of the transverse colon, or a loop or two of intestine. While these herniations are almost upward in front of the pericardium, one of our patients had a defect in the diaphragmatic portion of the pericardium so that there was herniation into the pericardial sac itself.

CLINICAL FINDINGS

Common Symptoms

Diaphragmatic hernias may give findings referable to the respiratory, circulatory, or digestive systems; some are tolerated with amazingly little disturbance. The severity of symptoms depends upon the number of abdominal viscera which are displaced into the thorax, whether there is kinking or constriction of hollow viscera, and whether the lungs are seriously collapsed. A newly born infant who exhibits *cyanosis, dyspnea*, or *vomiting* should be studied with diaphragmatic hernia in mind.

Cyanosis may be evident immediately after delivery. It may be transient and may appear only during nursing or crying, but in some cases it is so severe that constant use of an oxygen tent is necessary to sustain life. Occasionally it can be relieved by turning the baby so that the side of the hernia is downward; in this position the mediastinum falls toward the affected side, giving better expansion of the other lung.

Vomiting may be only occasional, or it may follow most of the feedings. In patients who survive for a month or two, it is common to find poor weight gain and even weight loss.

The *postero-lateral hernias* are very apt to have extensive displacements of viscera into the thorax and hence give important symptoms early in life. Occasionally one of them is tolerated very well and goes undiscovered for many months or years.

The *hiatus hernias* seldom give trouble in infancy, except for those which have free reflux of gastric contents into the esophagus and vomiting or regurgitation therefrom. Generally this type of defect is apt to show up in older children, or even adults, because reflux of gastric juice into the esophagus produces esophagitis, from which can come esophageal spasm, dysphagia, hematemesis, or melena. If the diaphragmatic ring constricts the stomach, there may be signs of high obstruction or of bleeding from the upper part of the alimentary tract.

The *retrosternal hernias* give symptoms which are of a vague sort, are seldom very intense and which are generally related to partial compression of some hollow viscus.

Physical Examination

With the *more extensive postero-lateral herniations*, physical examination shows respiratory and pulse rates to be increased. By *inspection* the affected side of the chest is seen to move less than the normal side. *Percussion* of the chest on the side of the hernia may give a dull or tympanitic note, depending upon which viscera are residing in the pleural cavity and whether the trapped intestines contain fluid or air. The heart is displaced away from the affected side. By *auscultation* the breath sounds are distant or absent. If intestinal gurgles are heard instead of breath sounds, the correct diagnosis should be suspected at once. When a major part of the alimentary tract is in the thorax, tympany is lacking on abdominal percussion, and the abdomen is scaphoid.

In the *hiatus* type of hernia nothing abnormal is found on physical examination. In the *retrosternal* type of hernia the physical findings are not striking.

ROENTGENOLOGIC EXAMINATION

Roentgenologic studies quickly establish the diagnosis and give a rough method of estimating what abdominal viscera are herniated into the thorax. Film or fluoroscopic examination without the use of contrast media will usually give all the information that is required.

The *chest findings* may at first be very bizarre. In the common type of herniation into one of the pleural cavities, the unaffected side generally has a poorly expanded lung because the mediastinum and heart are shifted in this direction. The affected pleural cavity contains intestines and viscera whose shadows are continuous with those in the abdomen. Thus, a liver or stomach shadow may extend above and below the level where the diaphragm should be, or else the intestines and colon can be traced from the abdomen into the chest. If a hernial sac is present, some lung tissue can be seen in the upper part of the chest and the intestines will not extend the entire way up to the apex. If, however, there is no hernial sac, abdominal viscera can be seen to the very top of the pleural cavity.

In the *pleural herniations in babies*, it is important to emphasize that examination of the *gastro-intestinal tract* with barium should be omitted if possible. This is rarely necessary to establish the diagnosis, and while it is interesting to determine accurately what viscera are in the chest and what is the position and size of the diaphragmatic defect, such information has little practical value. It does not alter the operative approach or procedure; the obtaining of such data may be dangerous for the baby.

In *esophageal hiatus hernias* it is very important to study by barium swallows the esophagus and the stomach so that an accurate appraisal can be made of the length of

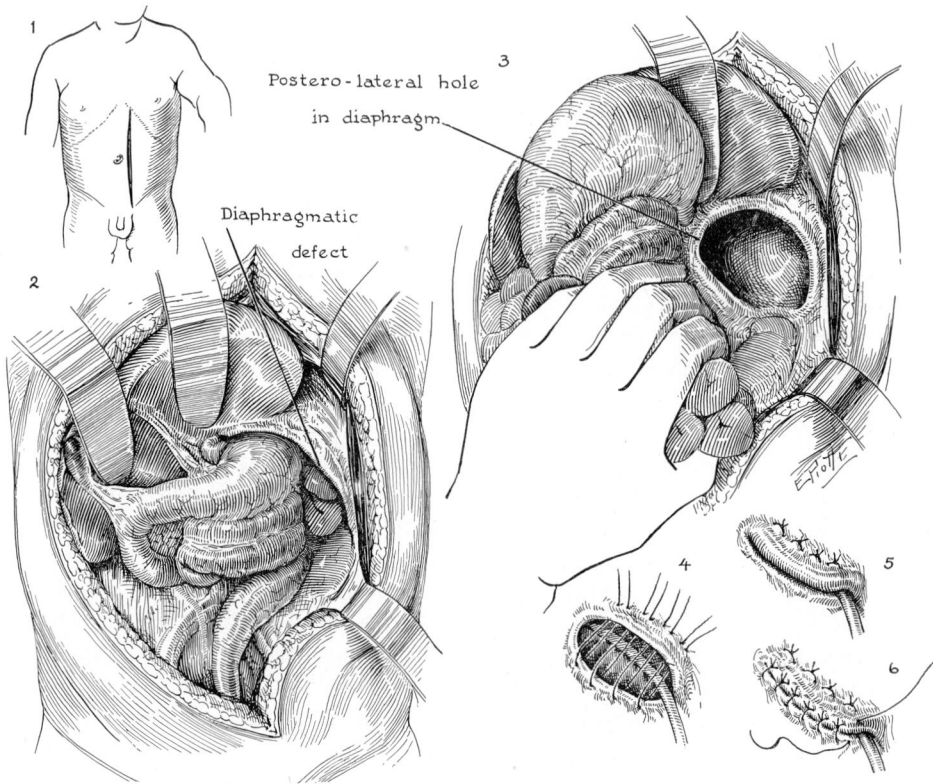

Fig. 224. Repair of left diaphragmatic hernia by a transabdominal approach. 1. Long left rectus incision, retracting the muscle belly laterally. 2. View inside the abdomen. The spleen, a portion of the stomach, much of the colon, and most of the small intestine are prolapsed through the diaphragmatic orifice up into the chest. 3. All of abdominal viscera have been withdrawn from the chest, giving a good view of the postero-lateral diaphragmatic opening. 4. Mattress sutures of silk are placed. A catheter has been run up into the pleural cavity. 5. Mattress stitches tied down. 6. The flap of diaphragm is anchored down with interrupted silk sutures. Just before tightening the last stitch, all air will be withdrawn from the chest with the catheter, which is then withdrawn.

the esophagus, the position of the esophago-gastric junction, the alignment of the stomach, and the degree of gastric constriction.

The *retrosternal hernias* are almost always found in older children. Because of the overlying heart shadow which alters the picture, a clear understanding of the derangement is seldom possible without the use of a barium enema and gastro-intestinal barium series.

TREATMENT

Importance of Immediate Operation

There can be no question that surgery is the treatment of choice in all these patients, except the occasional ones with a small esophageal hernia. There is sufficient evidence, from our own failures and from the literature, to show the futility of "expectant" or medical measures. The general condition of the patient may be improved temporarily by supportive therapy but no enduring benefit can be expected therefrom. The risks are great if operation is unduly deferred. The policy of waiting until a child is older and stronger is responsible for the loss of a great many lives which might have been saved by early operation. We are convinced that operation should be undertaken as soon as the diagnosis is made (except for minimal hiatus defects).

On a theoretical basis, an operation performed *in the first forty-eight hours* of life is very advantageous, and we have had the opportunity of proving this in many cases. It is our experience that infants stand major surgical procedures extremely well in the first day or two of life—in fact, far better than they do at the end of a week or ten days. Within the initial twenty-four or forty-eight hours the operator has the added advantage of dealing with an intestine which is not yet distended. This can easily make the difference between the possibility or impossibility of replacing intestines into the abdominal cavity.

Preoperative Measures

Preoperative treatment should be directed toward attainment of proper hydration and toward deflation of the alimentary tract. This latter can be accomplished by enemas, by constant gastric suction, and by placing the infant in a tent with 90 to 95 per cent oxygen.

Anesthesia

If available, the anesthetic of choice is cyclopropane. It is justifiable to assume the slight risk of explosive hazard which its use entails, because it gives a gaseous mixture with a very high content of oxygen. This is highly important for a baby whose respiratory apparatus is seriously handicapped and it also facilitates the operation by decreasing the respiratory excursions of the chest and diaphragm. If cyclopropane is not available, ether (with a high oxygen mixture) in a closed system is fairly satisfactory.

There must always be provision for giving *positive pressure anesthesia* if the need should arise. It is desirable to use an intratracheal tube because positive pressure can be more readily given if such a tube is in place. The small respiratory exchange of a baby will not produce a flow of gas through the large and long rubber tubes which connect a face mask to the flap-valve chamber of the average gas machine. It is therefore helpful to have an attachment whereby the soda-lime chamber is brought close to the infant's mask. With this closed apparatus, the single tube has only a one-way flow as it brings oxygen or gaseous mixture from the gas machine.

Technique of Operative Repair

Abdominal Approach. A thoracic approach is without doubt the best one for exposure and treatment of diaphragmatic hernias in adults or older children, but the abdominal approach is far superior in babies. In infants, adhesions are seldom found between intestines and pleural structures. In the absence of adhesions, it is much easier to *pull* the abdominal viscera out of the chest from below than it is to *push* them down from above. In fact, in most infant cases it is impossible (or very difficult) to reduce the hernia through a thoracic wound, because the abdominal cavity is too small to receive all of its viscera without crowding.

While Johnson et al. have recently advocated a transpleural approach for repair of diaphragmatic hernia in babies, we still feel that—while a better view of the dia-

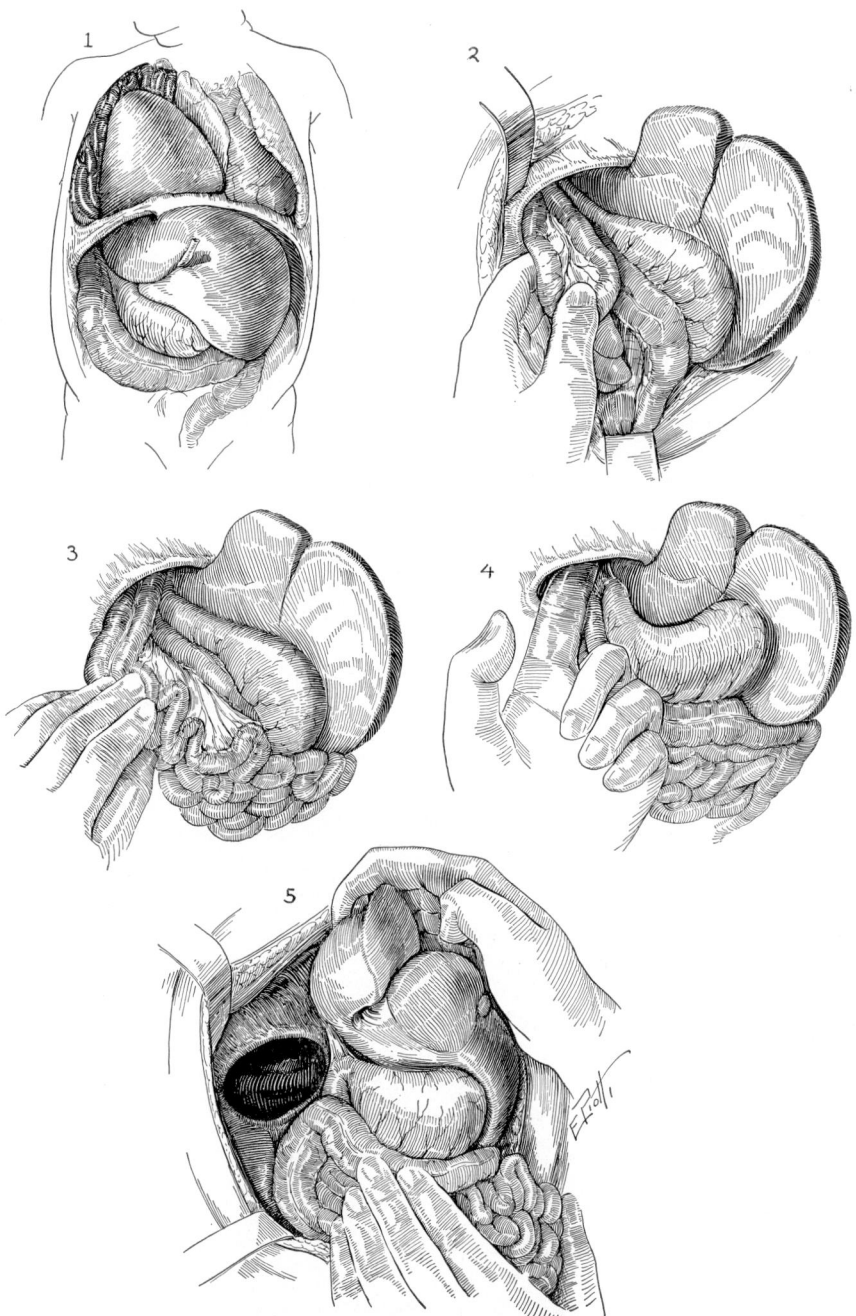

Fig. 225. Operative reduction of a right diaphragmatic hernia by a transabdominal approach. 1. Orientation sketch showing position of the viscera in the abdominal and right pleural cavities. A large part of the liver is above the diaphragm. Its substance has a deep fissure imposed by the diaphragmatic shelf. 2. Starting reduction by withdrawing loops of small intestines. 3. Small intestines delivered, colon being pulled out. 4. Finger passed up into the pleural cavity to engage and withdraw the thoracic portion of the liver. 5. Liver entirely withdrawn and hernial ring completely exposed. Withdrawal of the liver should be left until the *last* part of the reduction. (Diaphragmatic defect is now repaired as illustrated in Fig. 224.)

phragm is obtained from above—it is often difficult to compress intestines into the small abdomen and keep them out of the way while the diaphragm is being repaired. Further, and of great importance, is the fact that in about one case out of six there is an associated malrotation of the intestinal mass (with intestinal obstruction) which is utterly impossible to correct through a thoracic approach. Conversely, working through the abdomen *all* of the abdominal viscera can be pulled out through the diaphragmatic hole, and can be temporarily held outside of the abdominal wall while the diaphragmatic defect is being repaired with ease. Furthermore, if any malrotation of intestines exist (as it has in 12 of our last 72 cases) it can be corrected immediately and adequately. For these various reasons we feel strongly that a transpleural approach should be used only for (1) primary repairs in children above one year of age; (2) treatment of recurrent hernias at any age; or (3) treatment of hiatus hernias.

For an abdominal approach, the incision may be subcostal or preferably paramedian with a lateral rectus retraction on the affected side. We have much preferred the *rectus incision,* as it destroys less of the nerve supply to the abdominal wall.

Withdrawal of Abdominal Viscera from Thorax. After the peritoneum is opened, one may see at once what viscera are in the peritoneal cavity and deduce what is in the thorax. Often it is helpful to introduce a blunt instrument or a finger through the hernial ring so that air can enter the chest. If this is not done, the intestines tend to be sucked back into the chest as fast as the operator pulls them out. After the abdominal viscera are withdrawn, they are placed outside of the abdominal wall where they are wrapped in a warm, moist gauze or are protected within a wet rubber bag.

If a hernial ring is small, it will be found easier to withdraw the abdominal viscera if a definite procedure is followed. For example, in a *left-sided* hernia, the stomach is first brought down, then the small intestine, then the cecum, ascending and transverse colon, and finally the splenic flexure and spleen. In dealing with a *right-sided* hernia when the liver is partly or wholly in the pleural cavity, attempts should *not* be made to withdraw this most anterior and presenting organ first, for it will be found that there is insufficient room to pull the liver down without damaging it. It is essential to withdraw the intestines first, then the colon, and finally the liver.

Closure of the Hernial Opening. In repair of a diaphragmatic defect, it is not necessary to denude the edges of the ring to insure good union of them. It is highly important to use some permanent suture material, such as silk; this is *no* place for catgut. It is very desirable to imbricate (overlay) the edges of flaps in a repair, thus providing broader surfaces for sealing and fibrosis. To accomplish this, mattress stitches are first inserted in a row, which leave a free flap 4 or 5 mm. in width. After the mattress stitches have been drawn up snugly, the remaining free flap is sutured down with a number of interrupted fine stitches along its edge.

Expansion of the Ipsilateral Lung. Before placement of the final stitches in the diaphragmatic repair, a small catheter is led up into the chest. Just as the last suture is tightened, suction is applied to the catheter, all air is evacuated from the pleural cavity, and the catheter is then withdrawn. This *immediate expansion of the lung* puts the child in the best possible condition.

Replacement of Abdominal Viscera and Closure of Abdominal Wound. The abdominal viscera—which had been kept out on the abdominal wall during the herniorrhaphy—are now replaced into the peritoneal cavity and the abdominal wound is closed carefully *in layers.* Oftentimes the abdomen is poorly developed because it has never contained all of its viscera; hence the operator may have great difficulty in finding room for the intestines and other organs. This might seem to be an insuperable problem, but it can generally be accomplished if patience and care are exercised. If the closure is a tight one, it may be difficult to use a running peritoneal stitch; it is better to use interrupted sutures of fine silk, gradually inserting and compressing intestines as the closure progresses.

In a few of our earlier cases it was impossible to replace all the intestines into the abdomen and then approximate all layers of the abdominal wall. Under these desperate

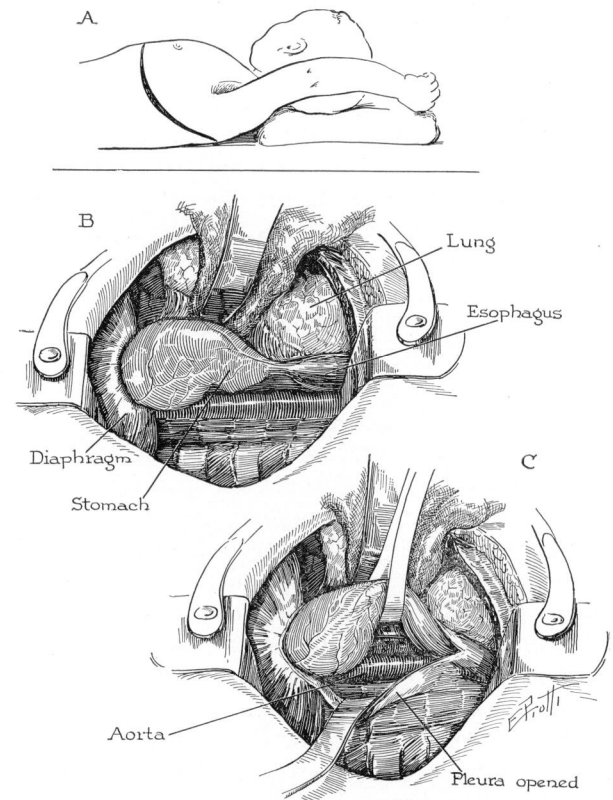

Fig. 226. Repair of hiatus hernia in which there is a congenitally short esophagus. A, Position of incision. B, View in the chest. A considerable portion of the stomach is above the diaphragm. The esophago-gastric junction is in the mid-thorax. C, Parietal pleura opened to expose the stomach and esophagus, which are being liberated from their bed.

circumstances only the skin could be brought together over the bulging intestinal mass. As the abdominal cavity stretched, it was possible to reopen the wound five or six days later, completely place the viscera within the abdomen, and then close all layers of the abdominal wall. This two-stage closure seemed to have great merit; babies survived it who almost certainly could not have been treated by any other method. Fortunately, we have not had to use this two-stage closure since 1945, probably because: (1) we are receiving cases earlier (before the alimentary tract is extensively distended); and (2) when marked intestinal distention exists, it is combated by deflation before operation is undertaken.

Treatment of Patients with True Hernial Sacs

Patients with a true hernial sac can also be treated satisfactorily by a *transabdominal approach*. After the sac has been emptied of its contents, a small incision is made in it to allow air to enter the pleural cavity. After this has been done, the sac can be delivered into the abdomen and its margins trimmed away appropriately. A denuded edge will then show all the way around the circumference of the hernial ring. The defect is now closed with two rows of silk sutures, as already described for cases having no sac. It is very important to place the sutures into substantial (muscle) tissue; at least the first layer (mattress stitches) should grasp such firm substance. Failure to do this is very apt

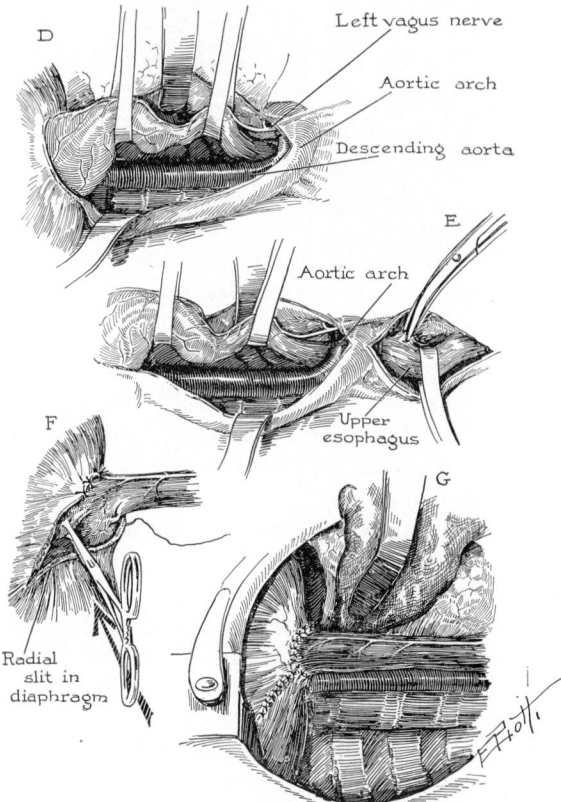

Fig. 226 (*continued*). D, Presenting portion of stomach freed. The esophagus has been liberated all the way up to the aortic arch, being careful to preserve the vagi. E, Mediastinal pleura opened above the aortic arch to free the esophagus up to the apex of the chest. F, Diaphragm opened and stomach being pushed down into abdomen. The edges of the diaphragmatic orifice being anchored with silk sutures to esophagus. G, Diaphragm completely closed. Stomach and esophagus are now in normal positions.

to be followed by recurrence of the hernia, because the employment of thin flaps (pleura and peritoneum) gives the repair very little holding-power.

Treatment of Esophageal Hiatus Hernias

Individuals with esophageal hiatus hernias should be operated upon only if there are important symptoms such as recurrent lower thoracic or epigastric pain, gastric obstruction at the hernial ring, or sufficient constriction of the stomach by the hernial ring to cause mucosal ulceration and bleeding.

If the symptoms are serious enough to warrant operation, much can be gained by operative repair. The approach should *always* be a left transpleural one. Whenever the

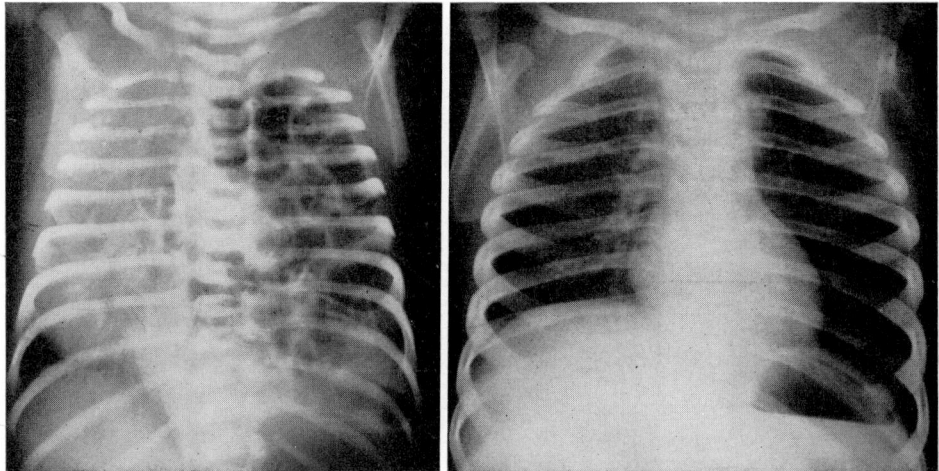

Fig. 227. Roentgenograms of a baby with left diaphragmatic hernia, operated upon during first day of life. *Left*, Preoperative film. *Right*, Film one year after operation.

esophagus is of normal length (the esophago-gastric junction lies at or below the level of the diaphragm), it is not difficult to open the hernial sac, free up the fundus or body of the stomach, displace them down into the abdomen and then repair the muscular edges of the diaphragm in constructing a new hiatal ring of proper size. Whenever there is a short esophagus, the repair is a much more difficult task, but still can be accomplished (Fig. 226). It is possible to free the cardia completely from surrounding structures and to mobilize the esophagus from its bed well up to the aortic arch (or even above this if necessary). Great care must be taken to avoid unnecessary injury to branches of the vagi. In one case we freed the esophagus to the very apex of the chest, isolating and keeping intact the vagus nerves and their recurrent laryngeal branches. After such extensive mobilization, the stomach can be replaced below the level of the diaphragm and the muscular ring of the diaphragm can be closed. It is very important to grasp the lower esophageal wall with a row of silk sutures, anchoring it around the entire periphery of the new diaphragmatic opening to prevent subsequent withdrawal of the esophago-gastric junction up into the chest. If the esophageal freeing has been adequate in extent, we believe it possible to replace the stomach into the abdomen in virtually all cases of "short" esophagus.

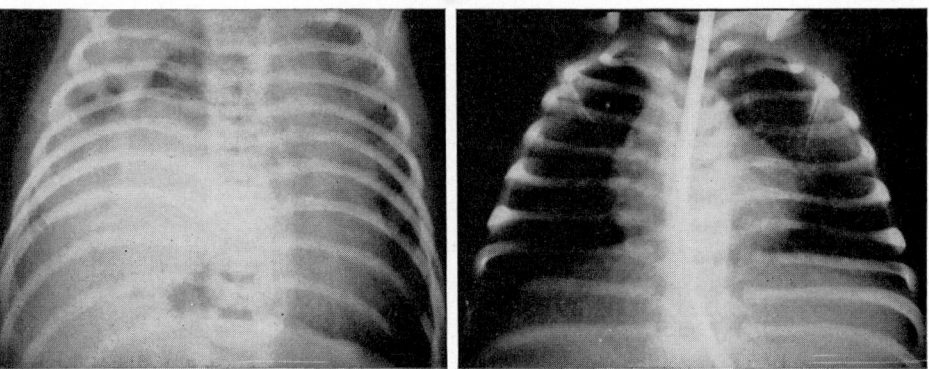

Fig. 228. Extensive right-sided hernia in a newborn baby who was dyspneic and cyanotic. Operation on first day of life. *Left*, Preoperative film. *Right*, Film after the diaphragmatic repair.

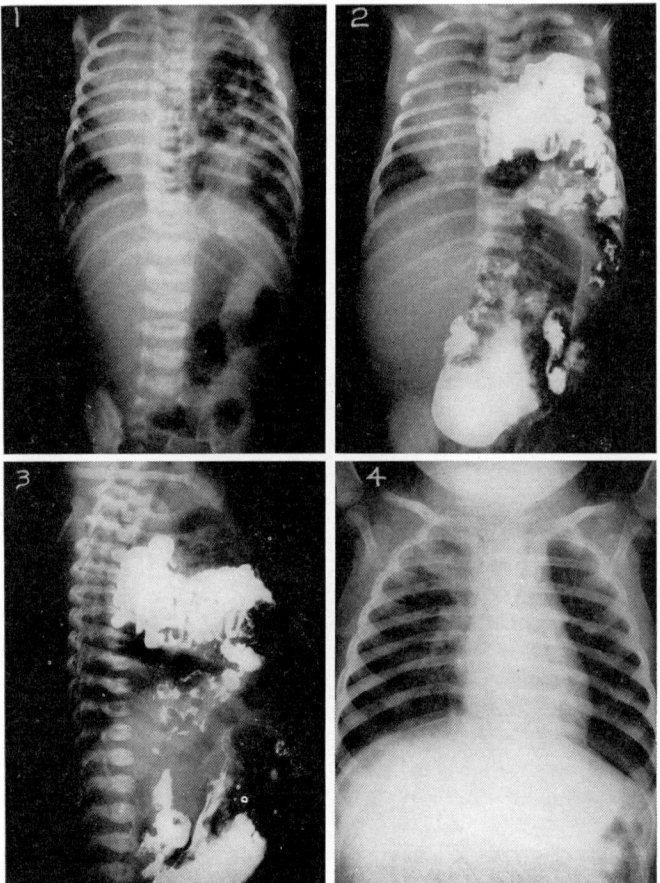

Fig. 229. Barium studies in a newly born child with left diaphragmatic hernia and extensive displacement of viscera. 1. Right lung greatly compressed, heart pushed to patient's right, left side of chest filled with intestines. The liver is displaced downward and toward the midline. 2. Barium series, showing the stomach within the abdomen and many loops of intestine in the thorax. 3. Lateral view taken during the barium series. 4. Roentgenogram one year after the surgical repair.

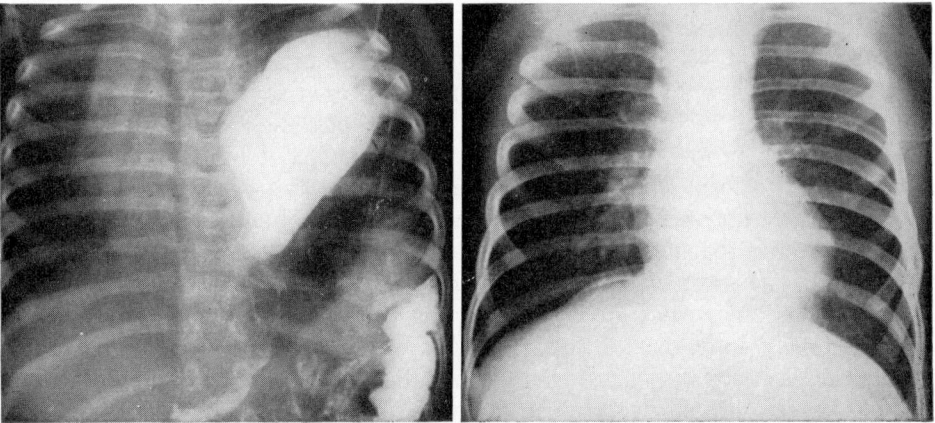

Fig. 230. Hernia on left side of diaphragm; two-year-old girl. *Left*, Preoperative film, after a barium meal, showing barium-filled stomach and gas-filled intestines in the left pleural space. *Right*, Postoperative film, twenty-one months after surgical repair of the hernia.

In two patients we have had the disagreeable experience of pushing the stomach down into the abdomen, to find during the postoperative period that its function was impaired because the stomach was twisted or angulated upon itself. Therefore, it would seem desirable in all hiatal hernial repairs to extend the lateral thoracic incision across the costal margin into the abdomen, so that the abdomen can be entered, the viscera can be viewed and can be made to lie in normal positions.

Crushing of the Phrenic Nerve

While there are some theoretical advantages in temporary interruption of the nerve supply so that a diaphragm can be put at rest during the healing stage, we have abandoned this long ago. If a good repair has been made, it will always heal! Crushing the

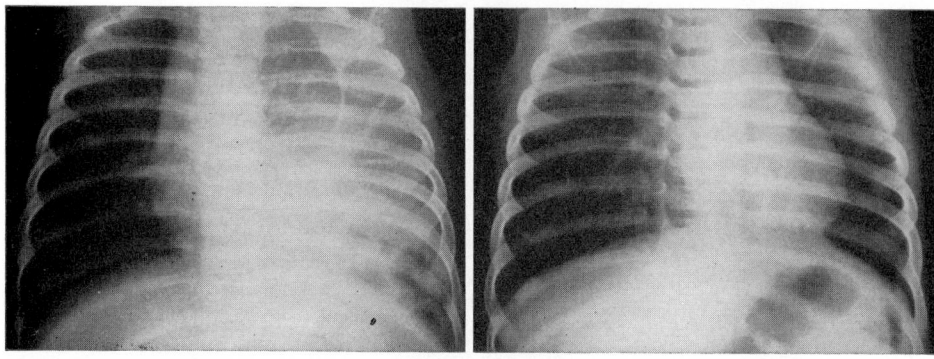

Fig. 231. Films to demonstrate that a collapsed lung can be quickly and fully expanded at the operating table. *Left,* Preoperative film (seven-month-old girl) showing multiple loops of intestine in the left pleural cavity, with a slight shift of the heart to patient's right. *Right,* Film taken fifteen minutes after termination of operation, showing satisfactory repair of the diaphragm and full expansion of the lung.

nerve helps but little—if any—in the healing of the suture line; it certainly increases the child's respiratory embarrassment (unnecessarily) after operation by reducing the pulmonary ventilation.

Postoperative Care

The postoperative care of these patients is important, but can be made relatively simple. A *blood transfusion* should be given at the end of operation. This should be large enough to replace any blood which has been lost, and to control any bleeding tendency which might exist. It should be small enough to avoid any risk of embarrassing the right side of the heart, which is a very real danger in some of these individuals. *Feedings* are regulated so that a proper water balance is maintained, but little attempt should be made to fulfill the caloric requirements for the first few days. If sufficient fluids cannot be given by mouth, they are supplemented by parenteral routes.

We now believe that it is seldom necessary to place these patients in oxygen tents after operation. The great *emphasis should be on immediate and complete expansion of the lung at the operating table by aspirating all air from the pleural cavity* (Fig. 231). If this is meticulously done, the respiratory apparatus is put in its best possible state and oxygen therapy is completely unnecessary. Our abandonment of oxygen tents for these patients has greatly simplified the postoperative care and has reduced the expense. It is seldom necessary to hospitalize these patients for more than eight or nine days after operation.

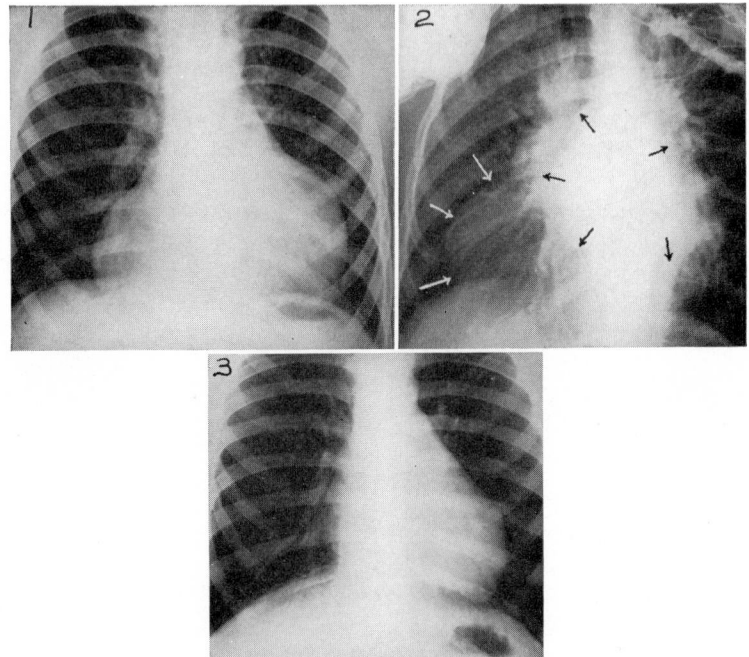

Fig. 232. Diaphragmatic hernia into the pericardial sac. 1. Preoperative roentgenogram showing the bulge of the cardiac shadow projecting into the lower part of the right pulmonary field. 2. Angio-cardiogram, after injection of a 70 per cent aqueous solution of Diodrast into a vein of the left arm. The black arrows indicate the opaque medium in the cardiac chambers. The white arrows indicate the mass (not containing Diodrast). At operation this mass alongside the heart was found to be a lobe of the liver which had protruded up through a hole in the diaphragm and the pericardium. 3. Post-operative roentgenogram, after replacement of the liver in the abdomen and repair of the diaphrag-matic defect.

RESULTS OF THERAPY

In 1925 Hedblom[11] reviewed the literature and found that it was the general consensus of opinion that babies with diaphragmatic hernia should not be operated upon; with this "conservative" therapy 75 per cent of patients had died before the end of the first month. In a review of the literature up to 1940 we[14] were able to find only 31 cases treated by operation in the first year of life, and in but 17 of these did the patient survive; to this list could be added our own series at that time of 19 operative attempts with 12 cures.

Since 1940 better pediatric care and more careful handling of the surgical problems have led to the cure of a large number of babies and young children in the hands of many surgeons and clinics. Our own material from 1940 to January 1, 1951, includes 72 patients treated by surgical means. The type of the congenital hernias and the results obtained are tabulated in Table 51. In the 72 cases there were eight deaths (11 per cent) and 64 cures (89 per cent).

Table 51
Diaphragmatic Hernia, Data from Children's Hospital Material, 1940 to 1951

Position or Type of Hernia	Total Cases	Deaths	Cures
Left postero-lateral	53	7	46
Right postero-lateral	10	1	9
Esophageal hiatus	5	—	5
Foramen of Morgagni	4	—	4
Totals	72	8	64

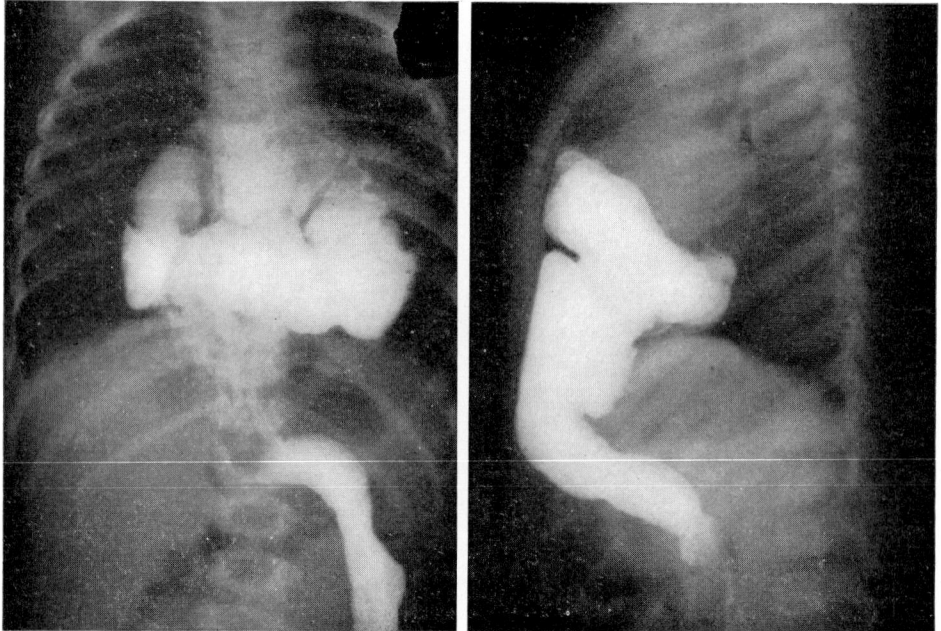

Fig. 233. Antero-posterior and lateral views of a retrosternal hernia.

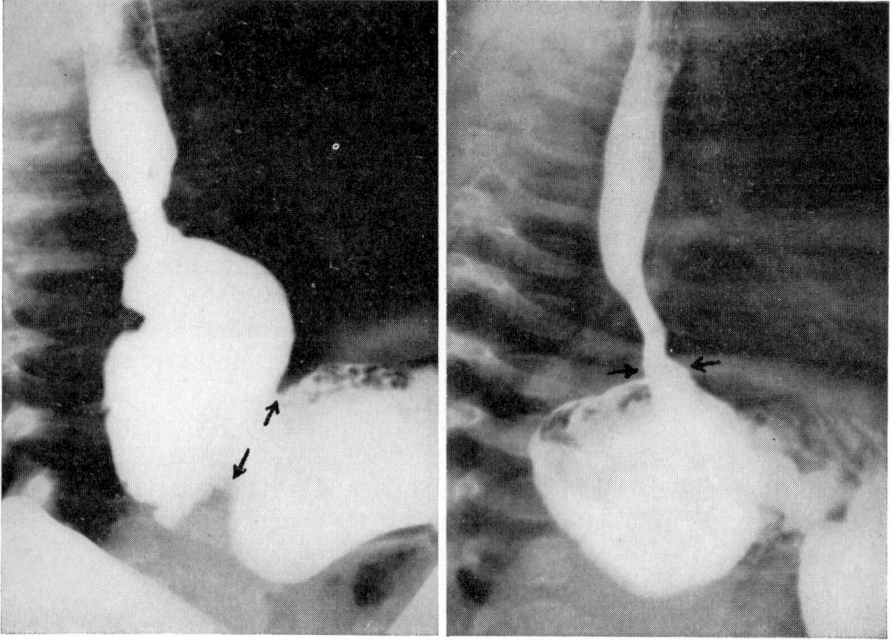

Fig. 234. Films from a child with hiatus hernia and a congenitally short esophagus, repaired by the technique shown in Figure 226. *Left*, Preoperative film, showing a large part of the stomach above the diaphragm. The esophago-gastric junction is nearly half way up the chest. Arrows indicate position of diaphragm. *Right*, Study after operation. The stomach is now entirely below the diaphragm.

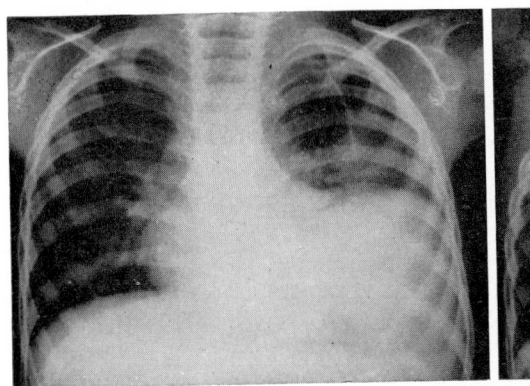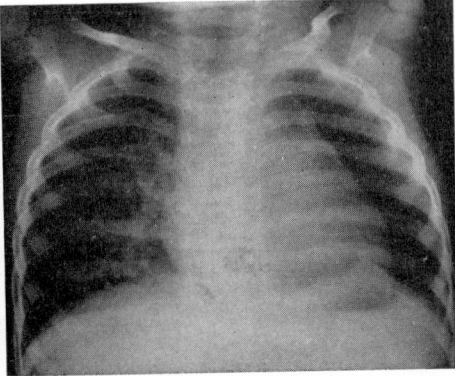

Fig. 235. Films before and after repair of eventration of diaphragm. *Left*, Eventration of left side of diaphragm, before operation. *Right*, Five days after plication of the eventration.

In all of the postero-lateral hernias except two, the approach employed was through the abdomen. In 3 of the retrosternal hernias the approach was through the abdomen, while in 1 it was through the right pleural cavity and pericardium (there had been a herniation into the pericardial sac). In the esophageal hiatus hernias the exposure was always through the left pleural cavity.

In 2 patients there was a small recurrence of a diaphragmatic hernia (or better termed an incomplete removal of the hernial sac at the initial operation). One of these was in a left postero-lateral and the other in a right postero-lateral hernia. In each instance, a secondary operation was undertaken within three weeks, by a transpleural approach, and the hernia cured.

An analysis of the 8 fatal cases shows that 3 of the deaths were related primarily to other congenital defects; 5 of them were directly attributable to the diaphragmatic hernia and its complications.

In the 5 patients treated for esophageal hiatus hernia and short esophagus, there were 2 subjects who developed neuromuscular incoordination of the esophagus (with either atony of the esophagus or spasm of the cardia) and 1 in whom there was pyloro-spasm. All of these complications presumably arose from disturbance of the vagi during the esophageal liberation. These were severe enough to make us strongly consider the need for operative relief; with conservative therapy all of these neuromuscular inco-ordinations disappeared in five or six weeks.

In the 72 patients there were 12 in whom a malrotation of the intestines was detected and treated at the time the abdomen was open for treatment of a diaphragmatic hernia.

Two patients developed ileo-ileal intussusception and required abdominal opera-tion on the fifth and twelfth days respectively; both recovered.

In summary, it is to be emphasized that the surgical therapy of congenital diaphrag-matic hernia is highly satisfactory, regardless of the extent of the herniation and the apparent critical condition of the child. Except for small hiatus defects which are asymp-tomatic at the time, it is our belief that all congenital diaphragmatic hernias should be operated upon as soon as the condition is recognized. Certainly those babies or children who are having symptoms should be given operative relief. In addition, those who have herniation through some part of the diaphragm (other than the hiatus) are best operated upon even if asymptomatic, because this is the best way to avoid subsequent complica-tions in the way of intestinal obstruction or incarceration. With this general policy, we have found over an eleven-year period that in 72 cases there were 3 deaths from other serious congenital defects and 5 deaths from the hernia or one of its complications; 64 of the patients (89 per cent) survived and have been cured of the diaphragmatic anomaly.

REFERENCES

1. Barrett, N. R. and Wheaton, C. E. W.: Pathology, Diagnosis and Treatment of Congenital Diaphragmatic Hernia in Infants. Brit. J. Surg., *21:*420, 1934.
2. Chisholm, T. C.: Transthoracic Repair of Large Diaphragmatic Hernias; Experimental Study. J. Thoracic Surg., *16:*200, 1947.
3. Donovan, E. J.: Congenital Diaphragmatic Hernia. Ann. Surg., *108:*374, 1938.
4. Donovan, E. J.: Congenital Diaphragmatic Hernia. Ann. Surg., *122:*569, 1945.
5. Dunhill, T.: Diaphragmatic Hernia. Brit. J. Surg., *22:*475, 1935.
6. Effler, D. B. and Collins, E. N.: Complications and Surgical Treatment of Hiatus Hernia and Short Esophagus with Thoracic Stomach. J.A.M.A., *147:*305, 1951.
7. Evans, C. J. and Simpson, J. A.: Fifty-seven Cases of Diaphragmatic Hernia and Eventration. Thorax, *5:*343.
8. Gross, R. E.: Congenital Hernia of the Diaphragm. Am. J. Dis. Child., *71:*579 1946.
9. Harrington, S. W.: Diaphragmatic Hernia of Children. Ann. Surg., *115:*705, 1942.
10. Harrington, S. W.: Various Types of Diaphragmatic Hernia Treated Surgically. Report of 430 Cases. Surg., Gynec. & Obst., *86:*735, 1948.
11. Hedblom, C. A.: Diaphragmatic Hernia. J.A.M.A., *85:*947, 1925.
12. Johnson, H. and Bower, A. G.: Strangulated Diaphragmatic Hernia in an Infant. California & West. Med., *36:*48, 1932.
13. Ladd, W. E.: Congenital Absence of the Pericardium. New England J. Med., *214:*183, 1936.

14. Ladd, W. E. and Gross R. E.: Congenital Diaphragmatic Hernia. New England J. Med., *223:*917, 1940.
15. Lauenstein, H.: Zur Symptomatologie und Diagnostik der Zwerchfellhernien im Sauglings—und Kindesalter. Ztschr. f. Kinderh., *54:*117, 1932.
16. Morton, J. J.: Herniation through the Diaphragm. Surg., Gynec. & Obst., *68:*257, 1939.
17. Ochsner, A., deBakey, M. and Murray, S.: Absence of the Anterior Mediastinum with Report of Case Associated with Congenital Diaphragmatic Hernia. Surgery, *6:*915, 1939.
18. Orr, T. G. and Neff, F. C.: Diaphragmatic Hernia in Infants under One Year of Age Treated by Operation. J. Thoracic Surg., *5:*434, 1935–36.
19. Schonbauer, L. and Warkany, J.: Zur Frage der Behandlung angeborener Diaphragmalhernien. Ztschr. f. Kinderh., *50:*125, 1930.
20. Sweet, R. H.: The Repair of Hiatus Hernia of the Diaphragm by the Supra-diaphragmatic Approach. Technic and Results. New England J. Med., *238:*649, 1948.
21. Truesdale, P. E.: Diaphragmatic Hernia in Children with a Report of Thirteen Operative Cases. New England J. Med., *213:*1159, 1935.
22. Weinberg, J.: Diaphragmatic Hernia in Infants; Surgical Treatment with Use of Renal Fascia. Surgery, *3:*78, 1938.

CHAPTER 34

Intra-Abdominal Hernia

Sites

Concealed, or intra-abdominal, hernia is one of the rarer causes of acute intestinal obstruction. The sites at which these are likely to occur are indicated in Figure 236. Herniation through the *foramen of Winslow* or through preformed openings in the *broad ligament* and *omentum* deserves only passing mention. Congenital rents may appear in any part of the *mesentery*, particularly in that of the *terminal ileum*, and through such holes loops of small intestine can pass and become incarcerated. This is the most common intra-abdominal hernia in the childhood period. A similar but much rarer opening is found in the *ascending mesocolon*, which leads in behind the cecum or ascending colon. Finally, there are *paraduodenal hernias*, the orifices of which are situated just below the ligament of Treitz.

Paraduodenal (Mesentericoparietal) Hernia

Pathology. A considerable literature has accumulated regarding paraduodenal or "mesentericoparietal" hernia—an escape of intestines through a small posterior-wall opening, to gain access to the space behind the mesentery or behind the descending mesocolon. As the midgut rotates in fetal life, the mesentery becomes fused to the posterior abdominal structures from the ligament of Treitz downward and outward toward the right iliac fossa. This process of attachment may be complete except for a small zone just below the junction of duodenum and jejunum where the former emerges from its retroperitoneal position. The pocket thus formed may extend to the right behind the mesentery, behind the ascending colon, or up behind the transverse mesocolon. Conversely, the pocket may extend to the left behind the descending mesocolon and descending colon. When intestines enter these two spaces the resulting lesions are called, respectively, right and left mesentericoparietal (paraduodenal) hernia. Generally, only a loop or two may be caught in these hernias, but in some cases the major part of the small intestine may be confined within them. When the latter is true, the mass of intestines appears to be covered by an enveloping membrane, which in reality is a leaf of either mesocolon.

Etiology. It was formerly thought that these lesions were *acquired*, and that the sacs were produced by intestines forcing their way into some small recess or indentation below the ligament of Treitz. Such a theory is scarcely plausible because there is insufficient differential pressure within the confines of the abdominal walls to allow such a dissection to take place. More recent studies rather conclusively support the view that these pouches are always *congenital* in origin and that they result from an incomplete posterior fixation of the mesentery and mesocolon. This "congenital" theory is not vitiated by the fact that when intestines once enter such a sac they can accumulate increasing amounts of fluid and gas and can thereby distend a small preexisting sac into one of considerable proportions.

Anatomic Considerations. Mesentericoparietal hernia on the left is about three times as common as that on the right. The left-sided hernia has a mass lying largely to the left of the vertebral column and an orifice facing toward the right. Coursing in the

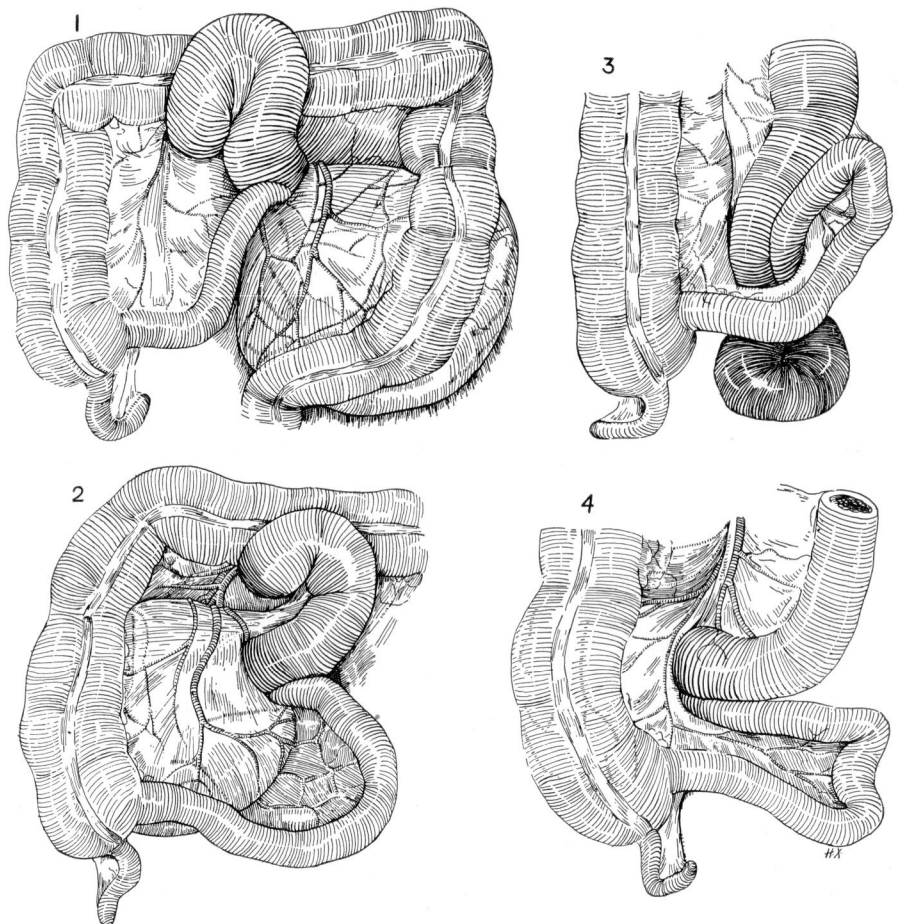

Fig. 236. Forms of the more common intra-abdominal hernias. 1. Left mesentericoparietal hernia. The inferior mesenteric artery and the inferior mesenteric vein course along the neck of the sac; hence, the neck must not be cut when the hernia is being reduced. 2. Right mesentericoparietal hernia. The superior mesenteric artery and vein course near the orifice of the sack, so the neck cannot be slit to reduce the hernia. 3. Mesenteric hernia with intestine prolapsing through the defect. 4. Hernia into ascending mesocolon with intestines prolapsed in behind colon.

inferior and anterior edge of this opening are the *inferior mesenteric artery and vein,* an anatomic fact which precludes slitting of the constricting ring in the surgical reduction of the hernia. The locations of these arteries and veins are important for two reasons: First, stretching of the hernial ring by entrapped viscera may compress the blood vessels and bring about extensive infarction of intestine or colon. Second, although it is permissible for the surgeon to open the presenting, less vascular dome of a hernial sac to release tension before pulling intestines out of the hernial orifice, in no case should he continue the incision close enough to the orifice to endanger these vessels.

Symptoms of Intra-abdominal Hernia

The symptoms of all forms of intra-abdominal hernia are primarily those of intestinal obstruction. *Nausea* and *vomiting* combined with diminishing passage of flatus and stools are the rule; severe *abdominal pain* is observed in most cases. Pain may be intermittent and referred to the umbilicus, or it may be more continuous and maximal in other regions. If the intestine or colon has been infarcted below the obstructed segment, variable amounts of *blood* appear in the stool. In one of our patients this was the outstanding symptom. The history may include previous minor episodes of vomiting or pain, presumably related to temporary bouts of incarceration which were spontaneously relieved.

Physical Findings

The physical findings are those of an acutely and seriously ill patient. *Vomiting, dehydration,* and abdominal *tenderness* are usually observed. A *localized mass* can often be felt, corresponding to the entrapped group of intestines, though dilatation of intestine above the point of obstruction may be sufficient to make abdominal palpation unsatisfactory. Increased peristalsis and borborygmi may be heard. The pulse is elevated. The white blood count is apt to be raised, particularly if infarction is present.

Roentgenologic Examination of the abdomen in some cases gives valuable aid in suggesting the diagnosis. Dilated intestine appears above the obstructed point, or (in the mesentericoparietal type of hernia) a group of intestines may appear to be crowded into and encapsulated in one section of the abdomen, while the remainder of the abdomen is more or less empty.

Treatment

It is almost impossible to establish the correct diagnosis in these patients before operation. Indeed, it is not necessary to do more than make a diagnosis of acute intestinal obstruction and to explore the abdomen on this basis. It is important, however, to be familiar with the types of hernia which have been discussed, because this knowledge will enable the operator to recognize more quickly the lesion at hand and to institute the proper therapeutic measures without delay. Reduction can be effected in most cases with little difficulty, but resection will be necessary when the delivered intestine is not viable.

Results of Treatment. Our familiarity with these lesions in children is limited to 7 cases which were of the following types: mesenteric defect hernia, 3 (with one death); ascending mesocolic hernia, 1; right mesentericoparietal hernia, 2; left mesentericoparietal hernia, 1 (died). Both of the fatalities were in children with extensive intestinal gangrene who died in shock.

REFERENCES

1. Alexander, F. K.: Roentgen Diagnosis of Intraabdominal Hernia. Am. J. Roentgenol., *38:*92, 1937.
2. Baty, J. A.: Internal Strangulation through Aperture in Mesentery. Brit. M. J., *1:*671, 1938.
3. Callander, C. L., Rusk, G. Y. and Nemir, A.: Mechanism, Symptoms, and Treatment of Hernia into the Descending Mesocolon (Left Duodenal Hernia). Surg., Gynec. & Obst., *60:*1052, 1935.
4. Chamberlain, J. W.: Acute Intestinal Obstruction Following Hernia into Ascending Mesocolon; Case Report. New England J. Med., *216:*299, 1937.
5. Cutler, G. D.: Mesenteric Defects as a Cause of Intestinal Obstruction. Boston M. & S. J., *192:*305, 1925.

6. Dowdle, E.: Right Paraduodenal Hernia. Surg., Gynec. & Obst., *54*:246, 1932.

7. Halpert, B.: Right Retromesocolic Hernia. Surgery, *3*:579, 1938.

8. Halpert, B.: Left Retromesocolic Hernia. Surgery, *5*:379, 1939.

9. Hansmann, G. H. and Morton, S. A.: Intra-abdominal Hernia; Report of Case and Review of Literature. Arch. Surg., *39*:973, 1939.

10. Longacre, J. J.: Mesentericoparietal Hernia. Surg., Gynec. & Obst., *59*:165, 1934.

11. Martzloff, K. H.: Prolapse of the Intestine through a Preformed Opening in the Great Omentum. Surg., Gynec. & Obst., *50*:899, 1930.

12. Masson, J. C. and Atkinson, W.: Hernias into Broad Ligament and Remarks on Other Intraabdominal Hernias. Am. J. Obst. & Gynec., *28*:731, 1934.

13. Mitchell, G. F.: Acute Intestinal Obstruction in Baby 15 Months Old; Hernia through Foramen of Winslow. Brit. J. Surg., *26*:648, 1939.

14. Moynihan, B. G. A.: On Retroperitoneal Hernia. William Wood & Co., New York, 1906.

15. Paul, M. and Hill, W. C. O.: Right "Duodenal" Hernia. Brit. J. Surg., *25*:496, 1938.

16. Short, A. R.: On Retroperitoneal Hernia; With a Report of the Literature. Brit. J. Surg., *12*:456, 1925.

17. Snyder, J. W.: Paraduodenal Hernia. Surgery, *5*:389, 1939.

18. Watson, J. R.: Acute Intestinal Obstruction Due to Mesenteric Defect. Ann. Surg., *106*:1097, 1937.

CHAPTER 35

Inguinal Hernia

Inguinal hernia in a child is almost invariably of the indirect type and represents a persistence of the fetal condition in which the peritoneum has a funicular outpocketing along the inguinal canal. In embryonic life the testis develops high on the posterior wall of the abdomen, whence it gradually descends to its final resting place in the scrotum. This migration is apparently initiated and facilitated in some poorly understood way by the *gubernaculum*, a mass of tissue containing smooth muscle which is attached to the lower pole of the testicle. Before the testis enters the inguinal canal, the peritoneal outpocketing (*processus vaginalis*) projects down through the various muscle and fascial planes but still retains a communication with the general peritoneal cavity. The fully developed testicle rests alongside of this sac, the lowermost bit of which is eventually pinched off to form the ensheathing *tunica vaginalis*. The upper part of the processus vaginalis normally atrophies and closes, but if it does not do so the sac remains as a congenital indirect inguinal hernia. If the entire processus vaginalis remains patent, the resulting hernia extends downward as far as the lower tip of the testicle, forming a scrotal hernia.

The right testicle descends at a somewhat later date than does the left, and accordingly the right processus vaginalis is closed off at a later time than is the one on the left. This delayed series of events probably accounts for the greater frequency of congenital indirect inguinal hernia on the right side.

In the female, the processus vaginalis develops in a similar manner and can persist into postnatal life. Along the inguinal canal, the hernial sac is contiguous with the round ligament of the uterus.

The following remarks are based on experience gained from the surgical treatment of more than 8000 inguinal hernias in infants and children at the Children's Hospital of Boston.

CLINICAL FINDINGS

A hernia is frequently discovered at or shortly after birth, and some of the largest scrotal varieties are found during the neonatal period. The majority, however, are first noted during the early months of life when the child becomes stronger; straining or crying forces intestine down into the preexisting sac. Not infrequently, a hernial mass does not appear until a child is some years of age. About 60 per cent of inguinal hernias are right-sided, 15 per cent are bilateral, and 25 per cent are left-sided. Ninety per cent of all hernias appear in males.

Size and Contents

A hernial bulge may be small and appear only at the internal ring, or it may be elongated and extend through the entire canal. Less often, the mass fills the scrotum

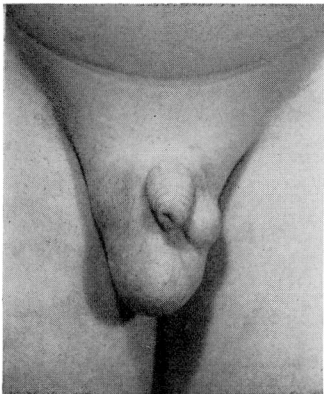
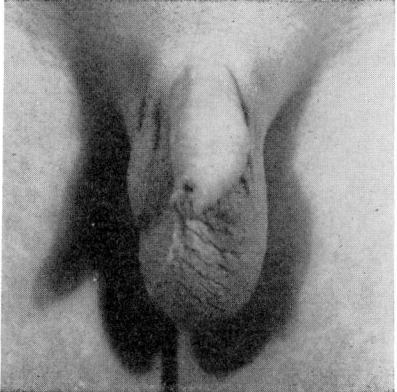

Fig. 237. Photographs of two children with right and left inguinal hernias.

on the involved side. The size of the swelling depends upon the dimensions of the sac and the degree to which it is distended. In a neglected case, the hernia has a tendency to become progressively larger and permit more and more loops of intestine to enter it. Most hernias in infancy and childhood contain only small bowel. In babies the omentum is usually quite short and cannot reach this far, but in older children it occasionally projects out through the internal ring. On the right side the appendix sometimes extends down into a hernia. A fallopian tube or ovary can prolapse into the sac on either side in a female.

Subjective Symptoms

Varying degrees of *discomfort* are observed, according to the tenseness with which structures are crowded into the narrow space. Some children show little concern and have surprisingly little disturbance; others are quite fretful, have a loss of appetite, and gain weight poorly. In the majority of cases the existence of a swelling is the only com-

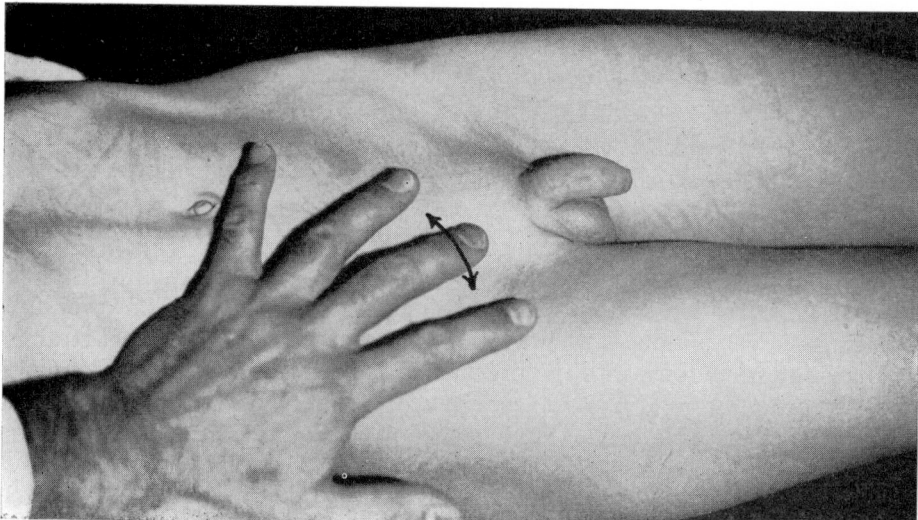

Fig. 238. Method of examining a child with a suspected inguinal hernia. The middle finger rests lightly over the canal and is rubbed gently from side to side in the direction of and within the limits of the arrows. If the canal contains a hernial sac, an increased thickness can be felt, and there is a sensation of silken surfaces sliding over each other.

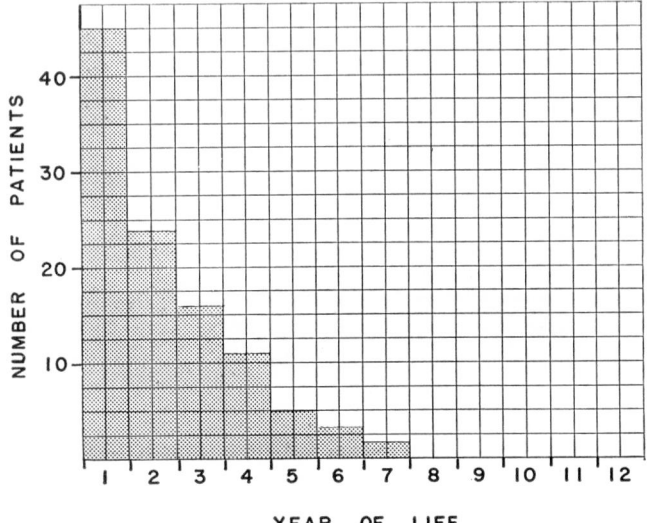

Fig. 239. Age incidence of 106 children who had incarcerated inguinal hernias.

plaint. The hernial sac is usually large enough to permit easy ingress and egress of intestinal loops; the mass therefore appears frequently and is easily reduced by local pressure or by assuming a recumbent position. A history of recurring swelling in the groin or scrotum is the most important factor in making a diagnosis of inguinal hernia.

Incarcerated Hernia

Incarceration occurs with considerable frequency. It is most often seen in the first six months of life (Fig. 239); it becomes less common after the second year and is relatively rare after the fifth or sixth year. About 80 per cent of incarcerated hernias are on the right, and 95 per cent are in males. Thorndike and Ferguson[10] studied a series of these cases at the Children's Hospital. In one decade, 106 patients with incarcerated or strangulated hernias were treated, and during the same period 1740 individuals were operated upon for inguinal hernia, giving an incidence of 6 per cent for this complication. During a subsequent period, 1940 through 1951, there were 63 incarcerations and there were 3874 patients treated for inguinal hernia, giving an incidence of 1.6 per cent. In about one-third of these children an inguinal hernia had not been recognized prior to the time of incarceration. When incarceration occurs, the local swelling is quite *painful*, and the youngster shows evidence of intense discomfort or agony. *Vomiting* is common, and, indeed, all the major symptoms of obstruction may appear if intestine is caught for several hours.

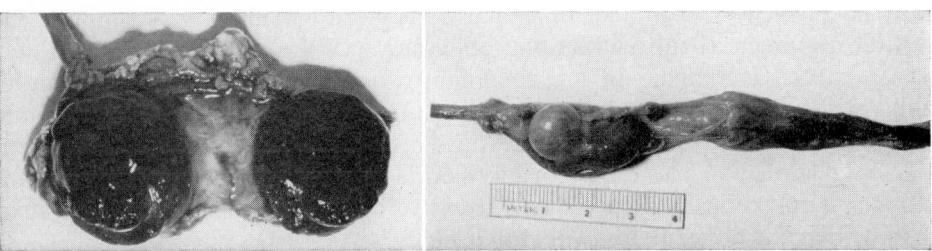

Fig. 240. *Left*, Hemorrhagic testis (cut open) from a one-month-old baby. It has been damaged by hernia. *Right*, Infarcted testicle removed from a four-month-old boy who had an incarcerated hernia.

Physical Findings

The examination for an inguinal hernia must be quite different from that which is generally employed for adults. It is useless to invert the scrotum and to poke a finger up through the external ring, in the hope of feeling a hernial sac. Such manipulations are very disturbing to a child and important information is seldom gained in this way.

Inspection. Everything possible should be learned from inspection before the patient is touched. The appearance and regression of an inguinal swelling during coughing or straining may be all that is required to make the diagnosis. A baby should be allowed to cry, or an older child should be allowed to stand up if he so desires, because these efforts may produce sufficient intra-abdominal pressure to bring out the inguinal bulge. When a hernial mass is found, gentle pressure should be exerted on it from below upward to see if it can be reduced. When the lump is reducible the diagnosis of hernia is definite, and other local lesions such as inguinal adenitis, suppurative iliac adenitis, or hydrocele of the cord are at once ruled out.

Palpation over the Cord. In many instances the parent gives a convincing story that a recurrent swelling has been seen in the scrotum or inguinal area, but it is impossible to make such a mass appear when the physician inspects the child. Under such circumstances a great deal can be learned by laying a single finger (preferably the middle one) parallel to and over the inguinal structures (Fig. 238) and then lightly rubbing from side to side across the cord. This will not disturb the child and yet a good estimate can be gained of the thickness of tissues within the canal. When compared to the normal, a side with a hernia is found to be distinctly thicker, even though the hernial sac is empty at the moment. In addition, there is often imparted to the finger a sensation similar to that obtained by rustling together two surfaces of silk. With a little experience, this simple examination is found to be most valuable and informative.

Findings with Incarcerated Hernia. When a hernia is incarcerated, an elongated mass can be felt along the inguinal canal which usually does not extend beyond the external ring, though in some cases it may fill the scrotum on the same side. This is quite tender; the subcutaneous tissues may be edematous; the child is very fretful. If incarceration has been of some standing, then vomiting, abdominal distention, borborygmi, and intestinal patterning may give evidence of intestinal obstruction. With gentle pressure the examiner may be able to reduce the inguinal mass; generally this is not possible.

Hydrocele (most frequently of the tunica vaginalis) was found in 586 out of 3874 of our patients operated on for hernia from 1940 through 1951, an incidence of 15 per cent.

TREATMENT

Possibility of Spontaneous Cure

Parents often inquire about the possibility of spontaneous cure of an inguinal hernia if no therapy is instituted, or if a truss is worn for temporary support. There can be little argument about the fact that obliteration of the processus vaginalis (which should have been completed in late fetal life) can continue into the first months of postnatal existence, but such a spontaneous closure of a hernia is distinctly uncommon. While some of the smaller hernias in babies have been known to disappear, it is extremely rare for large hernias in babies, or for any hernia in youngsters beyond a year of age, to seal over spontaneously. Hence, there seems to be little merit in putting off surgery in the hope that the abnormality will cure itself.

Use of Trusses

It was formerly our policy to avoid surgery whenever possible in subjects under a year and a half or two years of age, feeling that for various reasons surgery was too difficult or hazardous in such young subjects. It was therefore accepted treatment to operate immediately upon all older children, but to defer surgery in babies by utilizing a yarn truss until the child was more than a year or two of age. Since 1940 we have

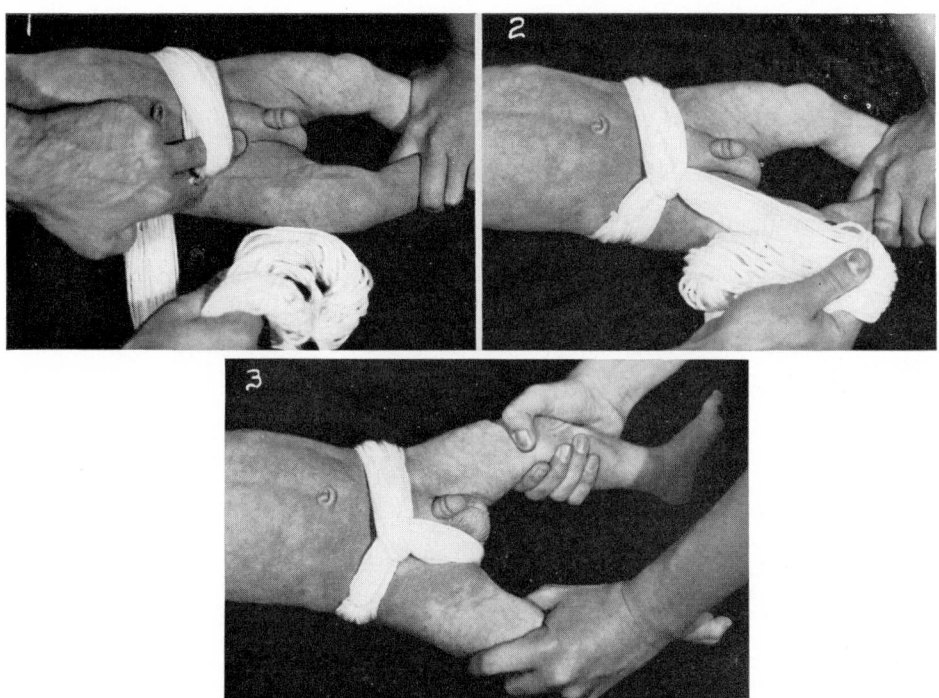

Fig. 241. Method of applying a yarn truss to a baby for inguinal hernia. 1. The hernia has been reduced and is held back with the finger as shown. 2. The wool truss has been threaded through the first loop. This makes a lump which is brought to rest over the internal ring. 3. The yarn presses down over the inguinal canal and is passed up over the buttocks to be tied posteriorly. It must be tied near the midline posteriorly to prevent slipping of the truss when the thigh is flexed.

completely changed this policy, and now feel that even the smallest babies can be operated upon with safety and satisfaction if competent anesthetists are available and if the surgeon has experience in this field and is willing to make a delicate dissection and a careful handling of the parts. We now operate upon all babies, regardless of age, and have had exceedingly satisfactory results therefrom; operation is deferred in only the occasional child who is premature or who has some serious malady which contraindicates operation. Except for these latter two situations, we have virtually abandoned the use of trusses.

If a truss is ever to be used, it should not be a rubber, spring, or leather appliance which is so apt to be irksome to the child and which may do harm by placing too much pressure on the spermatic cord. A reasonably satisfactory support can be quickly and cheaply fashioned from ordinary soft white knitting yarn. A loop is prepared so that it is about 24 inches long and contains about 15 strands of yarn. For older babies and young children the loop may be longer and thicker; its dimensions depend, of course, on the size of the patient. To apply this truss the child is placed in a recumbent position and the hernia is reduced. A finger is passed through one end of the yarn loop and the tip of the finger is then placed over the internal inguinal ring (Fig. 241). The free loop of yarn is then passed medially and completely around the trunk so that it can be threaded

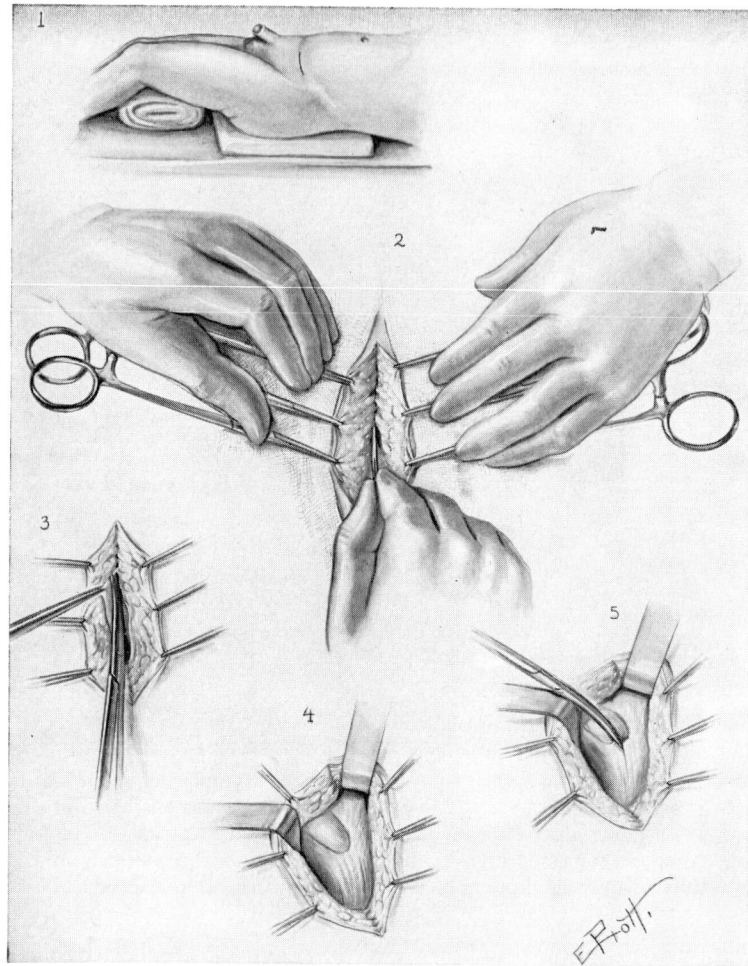

Fig. 242. Operative repair of a left inguinal hernia. 1. Position of child on table with a roll under knees. Incision will be made in the crease of the skin as shown. 2. Three hemostats on subcutaneous tissues of upper and lower sides of wound. Traction on these helps to separate and open up the wound. 3. Superficial fascia being opened. 4. External oblique fascia cleaned off, to expose the external ring. One retractor pulls tissues toward midline; the other retractor pulls tissues inferiorly. 5. External oblique fascia being split upward and outward in the direction of its fibers.

through the end where the finger is. This will make a knot or lump directly over the internal ring. The free end of yarn is now turned downward along the inguinal canal, then between the legs, so it can be tied up posteriorly to that portion which runs across the back. Such a truss can be easily and quickly applied. It gives firm but yielding pressure over the canal, and if snugly applied it prevents intestines from entering the hernial sac. If the skin is powdered, there is practically no chafing. This form of truss is cheap; it can be washed; and when badly soiled it can be replaced by a fresh one.

Surgical Therapy

The *Mitchell-Banks operation* has long had widespread favor in England and Scotland for hernial repairs in infants and young children; it has gained only slight favor in this country. By this simple technique a short incision, no more than 1 to 2 cm. in

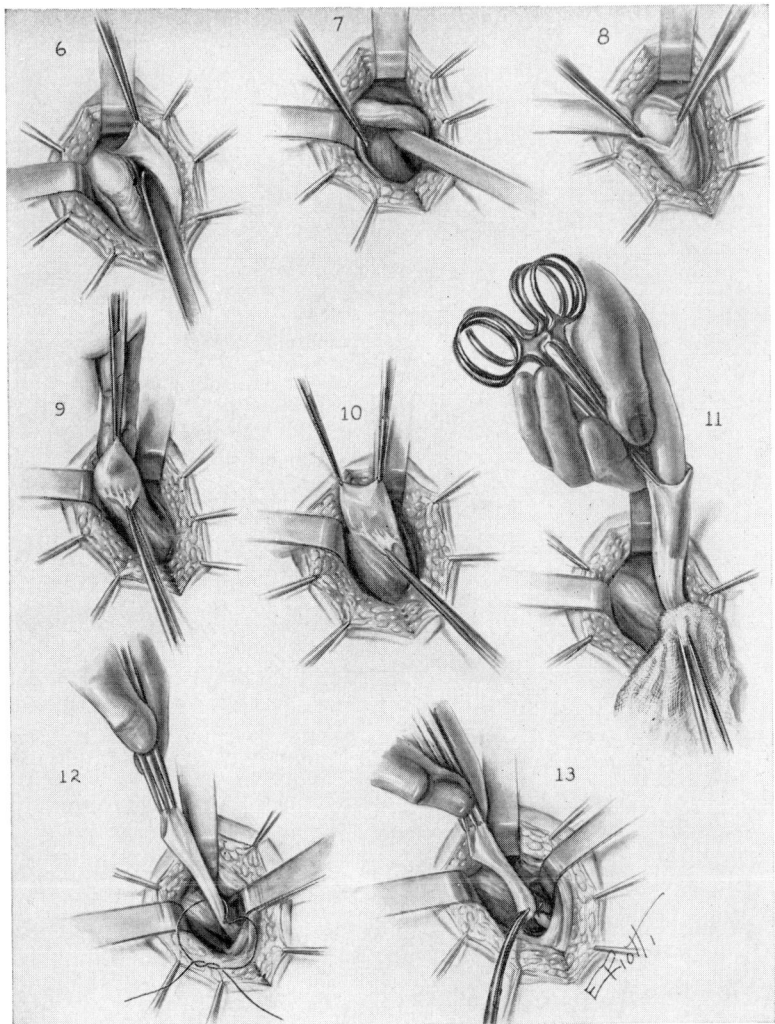

Fig. 242 (*continued*). 6. External oblique fascia being freed superiorly. 7. Lower flap of external oblique fascia being freed downward to expose Poupart's ligament. 8. Structures of cord being teased apart with blunt forceps to expose the hernial sac. 9. Sac grasped with hemostat; tissues of cord being stripped away from sac. 10. Two hemostats on tip of sac. 11. Sac opened at its apex and edges held with three hemostats. Finger inserted in sac, while blunt dissection with gauze is made toward neck of sac. 12. Neck of sac transfixed and being ligated with silk suture. 13. Excess sac being cut away.

length, is made in the skin over the inguinal canal, the hernial sac is teased out through the external ring, is then tied off, and the excess sac cut away. No effort is made to repair the inguinal canal. The success of this simple procedure is based on the widely accepted principle that removal of a hernial sac, or closure of its neck, is the most important single step in curing an indirect inguinal hernia. While the method gives satisfactory results in a very high percentage of cases, it would sometimes seem to be inadequate, particularly in those infants in whom the walls of the canal have been greatly thinned and stretched out by a large hernial mass. We have not used this operation, having always preferred to employ a more thorough opening of the canal and repair of the same.

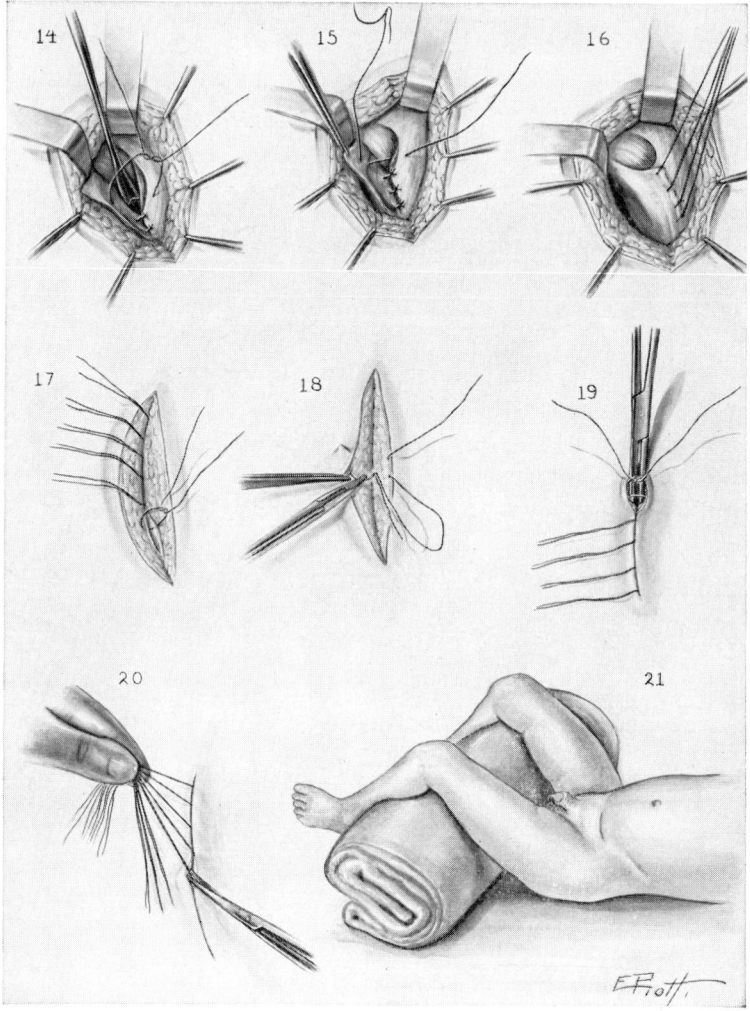

Fig. 242 (*continued*). 14. Beginning reconstruction of canal by simultaneously bringing external oblique fascia and internal oblique muscle down to Poupart's ligament with interrupted silk stitches. This repair is started from above and runs downward towards the external ring. 15. The last suture in this deep repair is not taken down to Poupart's ligament (for fear of making the ring too tight) but Instead grasps the undersurface of the external oblique fascia a short distance away from Poupart's iigament. 16. The lower flap of external oblique fascia has been imbricated upwards with interrupted silk sutures. 17. Interrupted silk sutures to the superficial fascia. 18. Approximation of the skin by the use of 000000 Deknatel silk which grasps the undersurface of the corium, 7 or 8 mm. back from its edges. 19. Method of keeping fat from protruding between skin edges. A hemostat holds down sub-cutaneous tissues as each suture is being tied. 20. These subcuticular silk stitches must be cut just on the knot so that no silk protrudes. 21. After the drapes are removed, the knees are held up in acute flexion by placing a large roll under them. This takes tension off of the skin edges. (Legs held in this position for some minutes while collodion dressing is drying.)

Ferguson Herniorrhaphy. The principles of a Ferguson repair—or modification thereof—include opening of the canal throughout its entire length, closure of the sac neck at a high level, removal of the hernial sac, replacing the cord in its normal anatomical position, and reconstruction of the canal to appropriate size. This operation is adequate and is extremely satisfactory for babies and children; the various steps are depicted in Figure 242. Several general remarks regarding the operation are in order.

Such operations are much more difficult in babies than in older children, because of the delicacy of the hernial sac and the cord structures. The peritoneum is very apt to

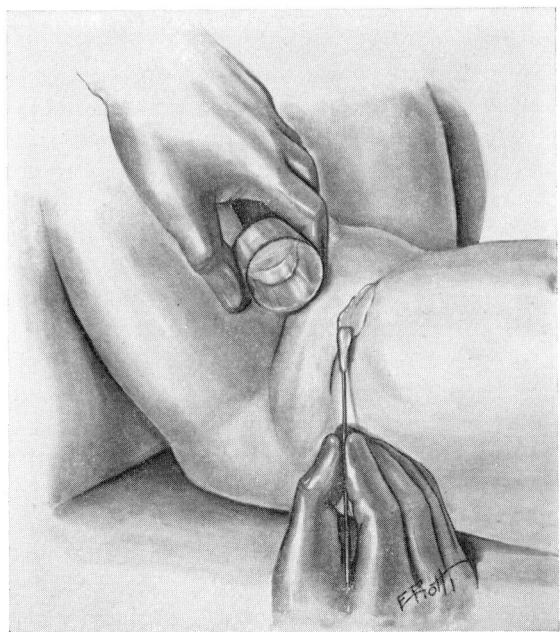

Fig. 242 (*continued*). Collodion being applied to the wound with a cotton applicator. (The collodion is of thick consistency and barely runs when the glass container is tilted.)

tear and the closure at the internal ring may be troublesome because the tissue splits if handled roughly. However, these obstacles can be overcome if the operator is deliberate, light-handed, and treats the structures with extreme care. We do not now have the slightest hesitation in operating upon any baby who is otherwise in good general condition, and who weighs more than 6 pounds. On some occasions the procedure has been done on prematures.

Cutaneous incisions made in an oblique manner, parallel to and over the inguinal canal, provide the best possible exposure, but do not give the best scar. Transverse incisions of the skin, preferably in a crease of the skin, give a less wide, but adequate, exposure; they heal much better and give a better looking wound. Because of the pleasing appearance of the fine hair-line scar, which generally is almost invisible, we routinely use the transverse wound for all babies and children.

After opening the canal, the hernial sac can be identified and its mobilization begun. If this extends only part way down the cord, its tip can be raised first and dissection started from here up to the internal ring where the neck is ligated and the excess sac cut off. In those long sacs which communicate with the tunica vaginalis, it is sometimes easier to pick up the sac, divide it in its mid-portion, carry the dissection upward until the neck is ligated, then returning to the lower portion of the sac and proceeding with its liberation and excision.

When there is an associated *hydrocele* of the tunica vaginalis, the hydrocele mass should be drawn up into the wound and then its superficial vestments peeled back until the hydrocele sac proper is seen (identified by its thin and avascular structure). This peeling-back need not be carried around the *entire* hydrocele sac; nor does the testicle need to be separated from its posterior attachments to the dartos. This limitation of the dissection is expressly for the purpose of avoiding undue bleeding which is all too apt to accompany the more extensive liberations which have been employed in the past. When a hydrocele sac has been properly cleared over 50 to 75 per cent of its anterior surface, this portion of the sac is trimmed off and discarded; it is practically avascular and can be cut off without any important bleeding. More extensive removal of the sac is completely unnecessary and is all too apt to give troublesome bleeding, either during operation or in the postoperative period. (It is quite unnecessary to sew the remnants of tunica vaginalis around behind the testis; it not only does no good, but may even be harmful. We have completely omitted this step for the last fifteen years in the treatment of hydrocele of the tunica.) The testicle, devoid of a half or three-quarters of its tunica, is now pushed back down into its normal position in the scrotum.

In reconstruction of the *canal*, a modified Ferguson technique is employed, whereby the cord is replaced in its normal anatomic position and the canal is reduced to proper size. (It is very rarely necessary to employ a stronger repair, such as a Bassini reconstruction.) Rather than bringing them down as separate layers to Poupart's ligament, the external oblique fascia and the internal oblique muscle can be included in the same stitches and anchored to the inguinal ligament. Three or four stitches are usually sufficient. For this repair 0000 Deknatel silk is excellent. *It is highly important to make sure that the closure is not too tight at the lower end of the canal.* The inexperienced operator, in the effort to make a snug closure and avoid recurrence, is prone to make this opening too tight and thereby constrict the spermatic veins, producing a swollen testicle postoperatively, and ending up with an atrophied organ later on. Such testicular injury and atrophy can be completely avoided if the canal, particularly its lower third, is left sufficiently large. It is our invariable custom after repairing the canal to insert up through the external ring a blunt periosteal elevator (about 6 mm. wide and 3 mm. thick). If this can be pushed up into the canal, the orifice is large enough; if it will not go into the canal, one or two of the lower stitches must be removed to relieve the constriction.

If hernias are present on both sides, we have no hesitation in repairing both of them at one operation.

To get these babies and children home early (which we routinely do the following day), it is essential to close the wound with subcuticular stitches so that the wound can be kept clean, no gauze dressing is required, and no skin sutures need be removed at a later date. Time used in subcutaneous closure of the skin is well spent. The deeper or under part of the corium is approximated with fine silk sutures. These grasp the tissues 7 or 8 mm. back from the edges of the incision; the pull from these positions drags together the edges of the corium and also the overlying epidermis. For these subcuticular stitches the suture material should always be 000000 Deknatel silk. If this fine material is used, and the stitches are placed sufficiently deep, the stitches do *not* show and they do *not* extrude subsequently. Such a wound heals beautifully and gives a scar which is minimal and sometimes invisible.

For coverage of the wound, a little collodion is spread on it and allowed to dry. Clothes can be put on over this the following morning when the child goes home. The collodion usually peels off in a few days; if any remains, it can be easily pulled off when the child returns for a follow-up visit one week later.

Treatment of Incarcerated Hernia

Conservative Measures. While it is possible to operate upon all incarcerated inguinal hernias immediately, the dissection and repair are most difficult because edema and engorgement of structures makes accurate recognition of the various tissues somewhat troublesome. Therefore, it is generally best to reduce, if possible, the hernia by conservative measures and then allow the local reactions to subside for twenty-four or forty-eight hours before proceeding with the operative repair. Of course, if conservative measures will not reduce an incarcerated hernia within a short time, operation must be undertaken forthwith in spite of the fact that the repair is not being done under optimum conditions.

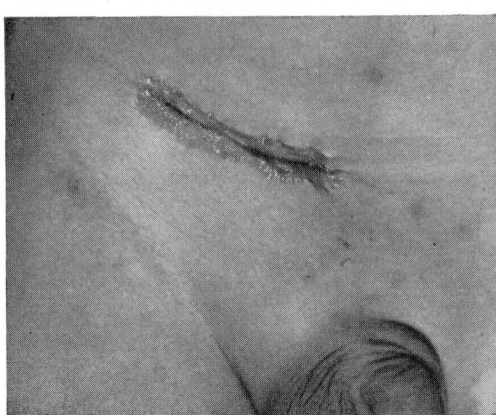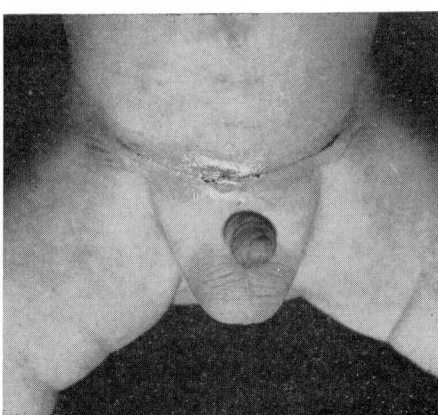

Fig. 243. *Left*, Postoperative appearance of collodion on a right inguinal herniorrhaphy wound. *Right*, Postoperative appearance of collodion on bilateral inguinal herniorrhaphy wounds.

If light local pressure will not reduce an incarcerated hernia, no forceful effort should be made to accomplish this. The child should be given an adequate dose of morphine to abolish pain, to induce sleep, and to relax the abdominal wall. The patient should then be placed on his back in a bed, the foot of which is elevated so that the mattress is inclined at an angle of about 20 degrees with the horizontal. An ice bag placed over the scrotum and inguinal region will help to reduce local edema. When this position has been maintained for an hour or two, the intestines may spontaneously return to the abdomen, or they will do so when the fingers gently press upon the mass With this management, 80 per cent of incarcerated inguinal hernias can be reduced, and operation can be put off for a day or two. If conservative management will not reduce the hernia within three or four hours, operation should be undertaken promptly, because of the danger of strangulation of trapped intestine.

Operation. If operation is necessary for an irreducible, incarcerated hernia, general anesthesia should always be employed and an adequate exposure provided for. The external oblique fascia and internal oblique muscle should be slit upward and outward from the external ring. The intestine must not be allowed to slip back into the abdominal cavity until it can be thoroughly examined, because a necrotic loop may thus disappear and evade all efforts to locate it again through the small peritoneal opening. In occasional cases of incarceration the pressure against the adjacent spermatic vessels is sufficient to bring about infarction of the testicle, and orchidectomy may be required. In general, it is our policy to leave a damaged testicle, in spite of the fact that it will almost certainly atrophy, hoping that it might be able to maintain a trace of spermatogenic or hormonal activity in later years.

Strangulation of intestine is relatively rare. In the 106 cases of incarcerated hernia studied by Thorndike and Ferguson, there was strangulation with gangrene in only 4 instances. When it is necessary to resect a portion of dying or perforated intestine, an adequate peritoneal opening is essential. This can be obtained by enlarging the internal ring outward and upward.

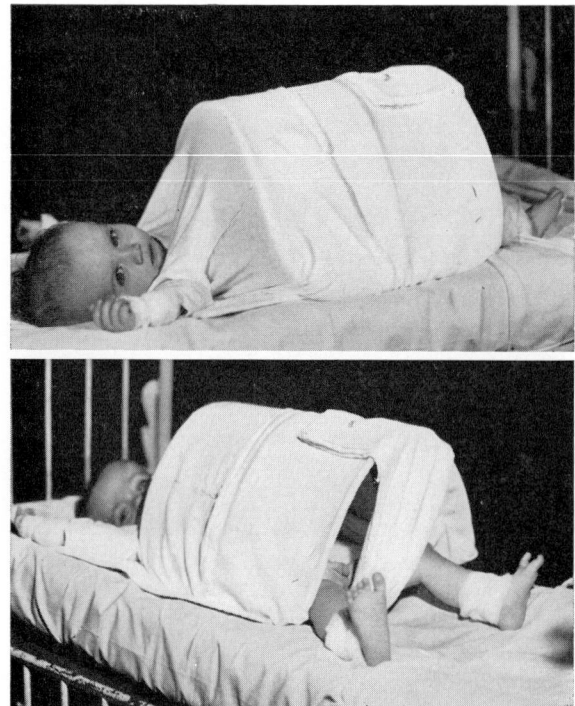

Fig. 244. Stiles' dressing for postoperative herniorrhaphy in an infant or child. The cradle keeps bed clothing off of the body. A diaper is suspended from the lower end of the cradle to catch any urine which is passed. The wound is thereby kept dry. The arms and legs are restrained.

POSTOPERATIVE CARE

A most important consideration in the postoperative care of these cases is keeping the wound dry and clean for twenty-four hours after operation while it is being sealed off. This is easily accomplished with a *Stiles dressing*, consisting of a cradle from which a diaper is hung down between the patient's thighs (Fig. 244). When the child voids, the urine will be directed against this diaper, which absorbs it. The child should be restrained and kept on his back for the twenty-four hours after operation. During this time adequate amounts of morphine should be given as required.

Since 1940 we have been discharging these patients from the hospital twenty-four hours after operation. There have been *no* wound infections, a situation we ascribe to the use of a meticulous asepsis in the operating room. At home, the babies can be immediately treated as normal, can be picked up, can be allowed to be in any position they desire, can cry or kick at will, and need not be restrained or restricted in any way. The wound area should be kept as dry as possible by omitting tub baths. After one week, when any residual collodion is removed from the wound, water baths can be resumed. For older children, it is our custom to have them remain in bed at home on the first postoperative day, except for trips to the toilet. In bed, they can lie on the back, abdomen, or side; they can sit up, yell, or kick if they so desire. The parent should always be told that there is no danger of straining or damaging the wound, *regardless* of the activity of the child. On the following day the child can be allowed out of bed an hour in the morning and in the afternoon; during this time he can stand, walk, go up and down steps, and partake of any activity desired while in the house. Each day thereafter, the time is increased by one hour, so that by the end of four or five days the youngster is up the entire day. At the end of one week he can go outside, return to the doctor for a check-up visit, and thereafter is allowed *any* outside activity he desires. This regimen is remarkably simple, acceptable, devoid of danger, and agreeably cheap.

RESULTS OF TREATMENT

During the twenty-five year period 1915 through 1939, 4133 patients with inguinal hernia were operated upon on the public and private services of the Children's Hospital. From January 1, 1940, through December 31, 1951, 3874 additional patients were treated surgically by various members of the visiting and house staffs of the hospital; a few statistics regarding this latter group are shown in Table 52. These figures do not include

Table 52

Data from 3874 Patients Operated upon for Inguinal Hernia, 1940 through 1951

	Males			Females			Totals	
Right	Left	Bilat.	Right	Left	Bilat.	Right	Left	Bilat.
2034	946	529	193	108	64	2227	1054	593

Total males—3509	Total females—365
Associated hydroceles, 586	Incidence, 15 per cent
Incarcerated hernias, 63	Incidence, 1.6 per cent

herniorrhaphies which were done during operations for undescended testes (which would add nearly 900 other herniorrhaphies). In these 8007 patients there was one death (a strangulated hernia in 1946).

There have not been long-time follow-up observations on all of these subjects for an evaluation of the final results of operation. However, nearly all of them have been seen for at least a year, and a large number of them have returned to the hospital at later times for other medical or surgical ailments. It is therefore possible to give a fairly accurate idea of their condition after the hernial repairs. Since 1940, there have been only 6 instances of *recurrence*. In one of these, the baby had an exstrophy of the bladder and extreme thinness of regional tissues. In the other 5, the repair was apparently done in an improper manner; the external oblique fascia and internal oblique muscle were sewed to the lower flap of external oblique fascia, rather than to Poupart's ligament. In all 6 subjects, there was a satisfactory course after secondary repair.

Since 1940 we have seen no atrophy of a testicle after operation, a fact which we

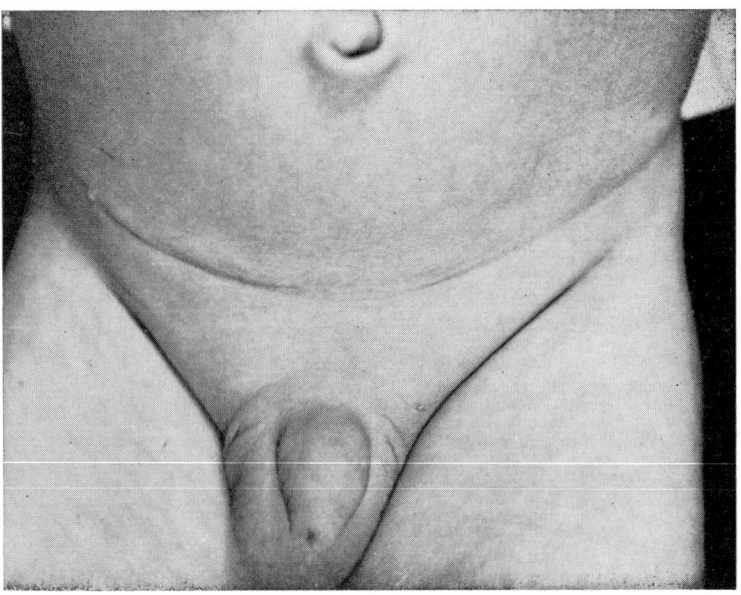

Fig. 245. Photograph taken two months after bilateral inguinal herniorrhaphies, showing the satisfactory appearance of the wounds. The skin incisions had been made in the skin creases.

attribute to the constant stressing of the importance of carefully preserving the testicular blood supply and also of reconstructing an inguinal canal which is large enough to accommodate the spermatic cord without undue constriction.

In an occasional patient, the repair of a hernia (particularly if it has been done on the left side) is followed by the subsequent appearance of a hernia on the opposite side, requiring a second operation. Experiences of this sort led us for a time to explore *both* sides in all subjects. In some of these patients a hernia was found on the second side, more frequently it was not. Therefore, at present we open the second side only when there is something in the history or physical examination which suggests that a hernia might be present on the second side.

REFERENCES

1 Anson, B. J. and McVay, C. B.: Inguinal Hernia; Anatomy of Region. Surg., Gynec. & Obst., 66:186, 1938.

2. Caulfield, P. A.: Congenital Hernias in Infancy and Childhood. Postgrad. Med., 10: 327, 1951.

3. Goldberg, S. L.: Strangulated Inguinal Hernias in Premature Infants. Am. J. Surg., 32:478, 1936.

4. Herzfeld, G.: Hernia in Infancy. Am. J. Surg., 39:422, 1938.

5. Iason, A. H.: Inguinal Hernia in Infants. Gen. Practitioner, 5:67, 1952.

6. MacLennan, A.: The Radical Cure of Inguinal Hernia in Children. Brit. J. Surg. 9:445, 1922.

7. Potts, W. J.: Truss for Inguinal Hernia in Infants. J.A.M.A., 117:1440, 1941.

8. Potts, W. J., Riker, W. L. and Lewis, J. E.: The Treatment of Inguinal Hernia in Infants and Children. Ann. Surg., 132:566, 1950.

9. Rea, C. E.: Sterility Following Injection Treatment of Hernia; Determination of Its Incidence. Ann. Surg., 105:351, 1937.

10. Thorndike, A. Jr. and Ferguson, C. F.: Incarcerated Inguinal Hernia in Infancy and Childhood. Am. J. Surg., 39:429, 1938.

CHAPTER 36

Hydrocele

In fetal life the peritoneum has a downward, finger-like projection—the *processus vaginalis*—which reaches into the scrotum. The inferior tip of this sac precedes the descending testicle and then becomes pinched off and surrounds the testis to form the *tunica vaginalis*. Accumulation of fluid within this forms a *hydrocele of the tunica*. The upper part of the processus vaginalis lies alongside of the spermatic cord (or the round ligament in the female) and normally atrophies. If it persists, and still maintains a communication with the peritoneal cavity, the individual has an indirect inguinal hernia. If it persists and is closed off from the peritoneum, the child has a *hydrocele of the spermatic cord* (or *hydrocele of the canal of Nuck* in the female).

SYMPTOMS AND DIAGNOSIS

Hydroceles are frequently encountered in infants and young children. They are rounded or oblong, cystic, and rather soft. In order of decreasing frequency they are found around the testicle, along the spermatic cord, and in the canal of Nuck. Hydroceles usually give rise to few symptoms other than those of mild local *discomfort*. Even this may be very slight in proportion to the large dimensions which some of them attain. A hydrocele of the spermatic cord (or of the canal of Nuck), constricted as each is by the inguinal canal, is seldom more than 1 cm. in diameter and possibly 2 cm. in length. In contrast, hydroceles of the tunica vaginalis may be very large, and can greatly distend the scrotum on the affected side (Fig. 246).

A hydrocele of the tunica vaginalis seldom causes any difficulty in diagnosis. The mass is soft, non-tender, and envelops the testicle. The structure can be transilluminated quite readily, and in some instances the shadow of the encased testicle can be faintly outlined by passing light (from a flashlight) through the mass. A hydrocele of the tunica vaginalis is accompanied very frequently by an indirect hernia; hence inspection and palpation should always be extended to include the inguinal canal. A "hydrocele" of the tunica which has been observed by the parent to change in size from time to time is almost certainly accompanied by a hernia; there must be a small pin-hole through which fluid escapes back into the peritoneal cavity on various occasions.

A hydrocele of the spermatic cord (or of the canal of Nuck) may be confused with an *incarcerated inguinal hernia*. In the central part of the inguinal canal is a mass which cannot be reduced and cannot be moved upward or downward. The known persistence of the mass over a long period of time, and the absence of local pain, tenderness, and vomiting are more suggestive of a hydrocele. These lesions of the cord do not transmit light readily, since they are small and are covered by the external oblique fascia.

TREATMENT

Spontaneous Cure

A hydrocele of the *tunica vaginalis* seldom requires operation within the first year of life. Small accumulations of fluid will often disappear without treatment, and infants need not be operated upon unless the mass is large enough or tense enough to cause discomfort. Hydroceles of the tunica which persist after the first year of life, or which appear after this age, usually have little tendency to regress spontaneously, and hence they should be treated.

It is seldom necessary to treat a hydrocele of the *canal of Nuck* or of the *spermatic cord* in the first year of life. These lesions result from a pinching off of the upper end of a small, unsuspected hernia, and if left alone they usually obliterate spontaneously in several months' time. In contrast hydroceles of the canal of Nuck or of the spermatic cord appearing after the first year usually persist, and will require operative removal.

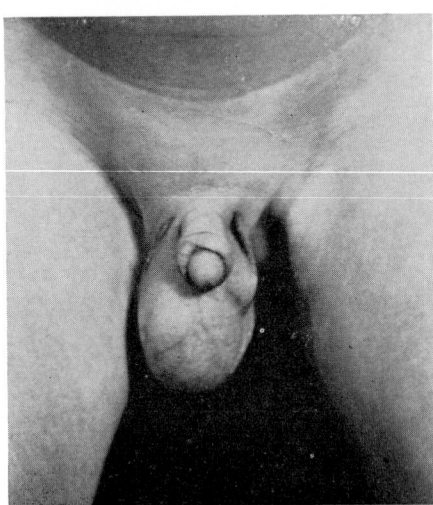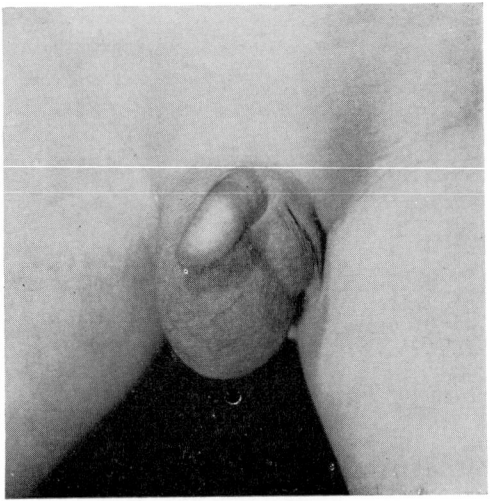

Fig. 246. Hydrocele of the right tunica vaginalis; two boys who were two and five years of age respectively.

Aspiration

Aspiration of a hydrocele should never be done in a baby or child. Recurrence almost invariably takes place and the dangers of sepsis are slight but real. The injection of sclerosing fluids is valueless and even harmful. The local accumulation of fluid may be increased and the testis or spermatic cord is apt to be permanently injured. The reaction which follows such injections is certainly more troublesome and painful than that which follows surgical excision. While aspiration of a hydrocele under local anesthesia is frequently a satisfactory procedure in adults, we have seen many serious complications when it has been attempted in small subjects.

Operative Treatment

In the operative removal of a hydrocele from the *canal of Nuck* or from the *spermatic cord*, a transverse incision is made in the fold of the skin over the inguinal region. The superficial layers of the inguinal canal are teased apart, the hydrocele is freed, and the sac is removed from its attachments.

A hydrocele of the *tunica vaginalis* should likewise be exposed through a transverse incision over the inguinal canal (Fig. 247). Rather than make the wound in the wrinkled skin of the scrotum, which is difficult to sterilize and to approximate accurately, it is better to make the cutaneous opening high as recommended and then draw the hydrocele up into the operative field. Any hydrocele can be grasped and drawn up through the high cutaneous opening—a process which sometimes can be aided by inversion of the scrotum by a finger pressing upward through the draping sheet. It is

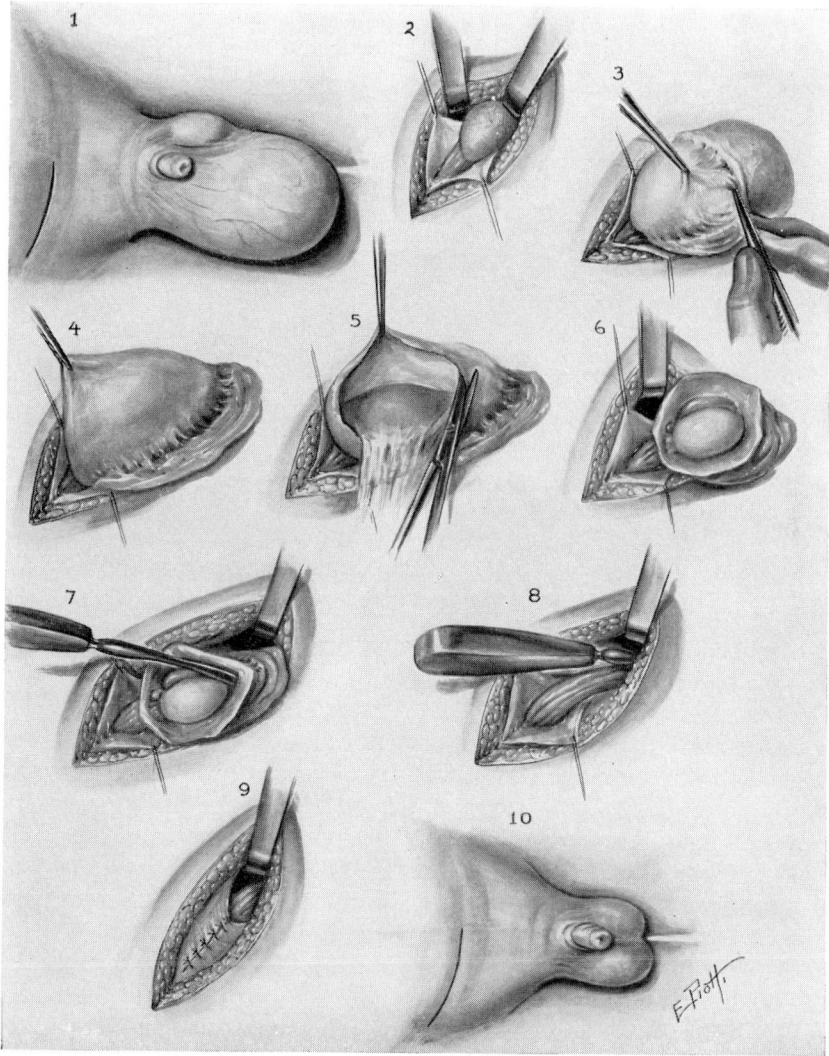

Fig. 247. Operative treatment of a hydrocele of the right tunica vaginalis. 1. Transverse incision in a fold of the skin. 2. Inguinal canal opened. The cord should be inspected for an indirect hernia, and repair undertaken if one is found. Upper portion of hydrocele bulges into lower portion of wound. 3. Hydrocele mass has been drawn up out of the scrotum, so that it presents outside of wound. Dartos and areolar tissue being peeled back off of the serous sac. This inner layer has few if any blood vessels. 4. Serous sac largely cleaned of the surrounding structures. It is *not* necessary to peel this back entirely off of the testis. 5. Sac being opened, and excess wall being cut away. 6. Sac cut off. It is not necessary to remove all of the sac completely back to the testis. 7. Lower end of wound held up with retractor, opening up the pathway into the scrotum. With a blunt instrument the testis will be pushed down into the scrotum. 8. Testis is pushed all the way into scrotum, straightening out the cord. 9. Inguinal canal repaired by method shown in Figure 242. 10. Wound closed with subcuticular stitches. No skin sutures are necessary.

never necessary to dissect the hydrocele entirely away from the inverted scrotum. The cremasteric fibers and fasciae are pushed posteriorly by sharp and blunt dissection, to lay bare the thin, innermost serous layer of the sac. This delicate membrane is now opened and the major portion of it is trimmed away.

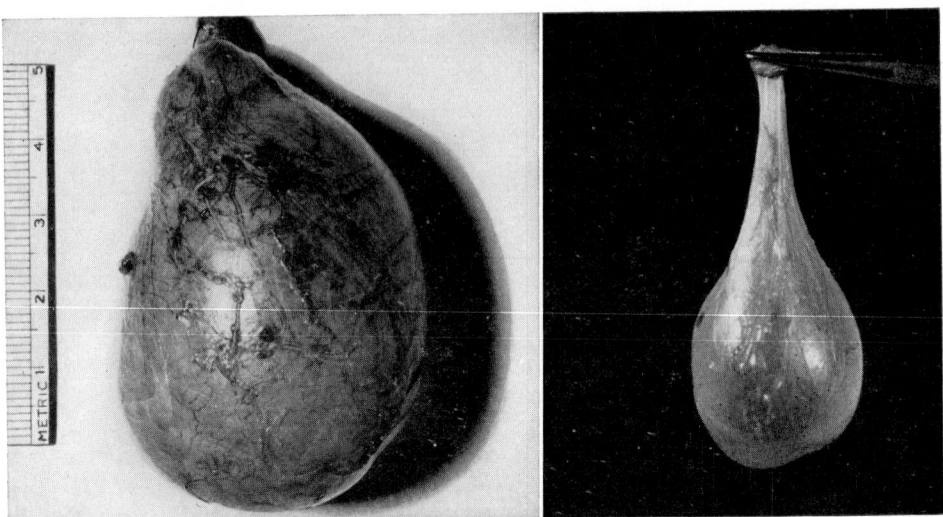

Fig. 248. Hydrocele of the cord, from two boys.

Some operators prefer to leave two narrow edges and sew these back behind the epididymis—the so-called *bottle operation*. We believe that this is completely unnecessary. It is simpler and also is quite satisfactory to trim away the membrane close to the testicle. If this incision is not carried too near the testicle, there are usually no vessels to tie. The field should be made completely dry. There is no excuse for postoperative oozing into the scrotum.

Whenever a hydrocele is being operated upon, the spermatic cord should be inspected for an inguinal hernial sac, which if found should be excised. An accompanying hernia is found in the majority of cases.

The testicle is returned to the scrotum, the inguinal canal repaired, and the superficial parts of the wound then closed. After suturing the subcutaneous fascia, the skin edges are approximated with 000000 Deknatel silk sutures placed in the under side of the corium. There are no sutures showing externally; the wound can be painted with a little collodion. We discharge all these babies and children on the day after operation.

Results of Operation

From 1915 through 1939, 507 patients with hydrocele were operated upon at the Children's Hospital. From 1939 through 1951, 586 babies or children were operated upon primarily for a hydrocele; a considerable number of these children were found at operation to have an inguinal hernia which was repaired at the same time. In the earlier and in the latter series there has been no mortality from operation and in no case has there been recurrence of a hydrocele.

REFERENCES

1. Greene, L. B.: Hydrocele and Varicocele: Operative and Injection Treatment. Am. J. Surg., *36*:204. 1937.
2. Langer, M.: Über die Hernie und Hydrokele des Kindesalter. Arch. f. klin. Chir., *18*:418, 1934.
3. Rolnick, H. C.: Hydrocele, Spermatocele, Varicocele. S. Clin. North America, *15*:757, 1935.
4. Young, H. H.: Radical Cure of Hydrocele by Excision of Serous Layer of Sac. Surg. Gynec. & Obst., *70*:807, 1940.

CHAPTER 37

Undescended Testicle
(Cryptorchidism)

The testicle develops in a rather high position in the posterior part of the abdomen, from which it normally descends along the retroperitoneal tissue-planes to pass along the inguinal canal into its resting place within the scrotum. This migration may be interrupted at any point so that the testicle remains within the abdomen or, more commonly, stops somewhere in the inguinal canal. Regardless of the presence or absence of the testis in the canal, the finger-like *processus vaginalis* extends as an outpocketing from the peritoneum through the inguinal canal. Therefore, an undescended testicle is almost always associated with an *indirect inguinal hernia*.

Complications

When a testicle does not normally complete its descent, several complications may arise. First, and not the least important, is the *cosmetic* deformity. For some individuals this may, in later life, be a source of considerable anxiety because of the feeling of physical or sexual inferiority. Second, a testicle which lies within the canal has an increased *danger of trauma*, because the rather rigid posterior wall of the canal does not afford the cushioning which is provided by the soft and elastic scrotum. Third, an undescended testis may become twisted. In childhood we have seen more *torsions of the testicle* in undescended testes than in normally placed ones. Fourth, a testicle which resides within the canal, and particularly one within the abdomen, has a *diminished spermatogenic* activity which may advance to complete deterioration of the germinal epithelium. These retrogressive changes are presumably related to the higher temperature of the testis when it is not inside the cooling scrotum. Finally, an undescended testicle is said to be subject to *malignant degeneration* in a slightly higher percentage of cases than is a normally placed one.

Material

The following remarks, while embodying many facts and principles which are widely known about the condition, are drawn largely from experiences gained from observations on 933 patients (1164 undescended testes), of whom 722 boys have been operated upon (for 827 undescended testes, for 36 absent testes, and 16 perineal testes).

DIFFERENTIAL DIAGNOSIS

True cryptorchidism must be clearly distinguished from ectopic testis and from retracted testis.

The term *ectopic testis* is used to describe a gonad which has progressed normally through the inguinal canal, but after emerging from the external ring has been directed away from the scrotum and has assumed a position up in front of the external oblique fascia (about 10 per cent of our cases) or else has traveled downward and ended its migration in the upper thigh or within the perineum (Fig. 249). Those testes which, after passing through the external inguinal ring, have turned up and lodged in the superficial tissues of the abdominal wall, can sometimes be recognized by physical examination. Conversely, examination may show only that the testis is high and it is often impossible (particularly in an obese boy) to distinguish it from one which is within

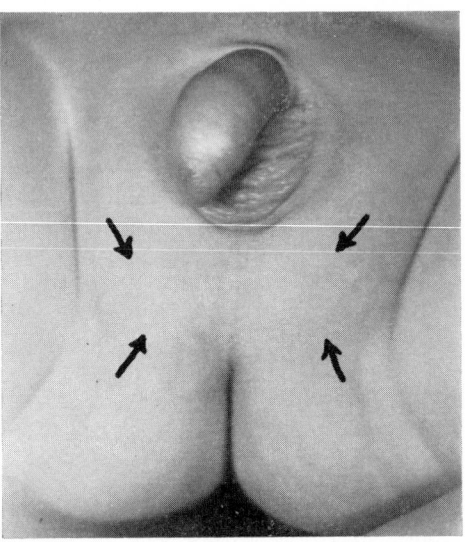

Fig. 249. Five-month-old baby with bilateral ectopic testes which reside in the perineum. They could be palpated in the area indicated by the arrows. Perineal testes should be operated upon in infancy—so that the child will not injure them when he sits up.

the canal. Ectopic testes, whether outside of the external oblique fascia, within the thigh, or within the perineum, can always easily be placed surgically into the scrotal sac since they all have spermatic cords of sufficient length to permit this.

By the term *retracted testis* attention is directed to the strong cremasteric reflex, so frequently observed in infants and young children, which can withdraw the testicle momentarily or for protracted periods of time into the upper part of the scrotum or even into the canal. By this muscular action, which must be regarded as completely normal, the testis is spontaneously held high, particularly during periods when the thigh or abdomen is touched or when the child is exposed to cold. As the boy grows older, the testicle enlarges, the cremasteric muscle becomes less active, and the testicle drops permanently into the scrotum.

CLINICAL FINDINGS

In about 50 per cent of the patients, undescended testes are right-sided, in 20 per cent they are bilateral, and in 30 per cent they are left-sided.

Patients with undescended testes are usually brought to the physician because a small scrotum has been noticed and the parent is concerned about the future development of the sexual apparatus. An undescended testicle is rarely the cause of discomfort, but a concomitant inguinal hernia can give recurrent swelling or pain.

Inspection shows that the entire scrotum, or one side of it, is smaller than normal and has an incompletely developed appearance. Before palpation, careful inspection in a proper light may show a slight bulge along some part of the canal, indicating the position of a testicular mass.

Palpation

If it cannot be felt anywhere, a testis is presumably atrophied or else resides within the abdomen. Most commonly, a gonad can be felt at the external ring or along the canal. The finger tips should be placed at the upper lateral edge of the mass and attempts made to push it obliquely downward toward and into the scrotum. With this maneuver some idea may be gained about the mobility of the organ. If it is fixed by adhesions, it can be displaced but little. If it is merely held in a high position by an overactive cremasteric reflex, generally it can be pushed downward along the canal toward the scrotum or even into it. (With the latter findings it is at once clear that the testis will eventually lodge in the scrotum spontaneously and will not require any medical or surgical therapy.)

If, in a given case, a testis cannot be felt anywhere, dogmatic statements regarding "absence" should not be made from a single examination. In many subjects, a high testis can momentarily slip up the canal into the abdomen and elude detection; at subsequent visits it probably will come out through the internal ring and can be felt. If, on multiple occasions, no testis is felt, the physician has reason to feel gloomy because it is highly probable that no gonad is present, or else it is so high in the abdomen that it may be surgically impossible to bring it into the scrotum.

Associated Hernia

Well over 90 per cent of patients with an undescended testis have an associated indirect inguinal hernia, the *processus vaginalis* of the peritoneum directly communicating with the *tunica vaginalis*, and even extending beyond this as an empty sac into the upper scrotum. In some instances the hernia is so troublesome that it must be repaired in the first year or two of life, in spite of the fact that the delicacy and shortness of the cord generally make this age unfavorable for performing an orchidopexy satisfactorily. If at all possible, correction of a hernia should be deferred until there is a favorable size for correcting the incomplete descent of the testicle, which circumstances are generally found between the ages of ten and twelve years. Just how long operation can be put off for a given child depends entirely upon the exigencies of the situation. If the repair can be delayed until the boy is sizable, the surgeon has the best chance of attaining an excellent result. If a troublesome hernia dictates that operation be done at an age which is less than optimum as far as operation on the testis is concerned, one compromises somewhat on the result which might be gained in repositioning the testicle. In spite of this, it is often possible to repair a hernia and to get a satisfactory correction of the testicular position in the first years of life.

If a child with an undescended testis and an associated hernia is being carried along for several years in the effort to reach a more satisfactory age for performing the surgery, under no circumstances should a truss be employed during this time, for fear of damaging the testis. If a situation is so critical that something certainly must be done about an existing hernia, it is best to repair it, even though this might entail only partial correction of the testicular malposition.

TREATMENT

Spontaneous Descent

A testis which is undescended in infancy or early childhood does not necessarily always stay in this position. In most individuals the normal processes of descent are completed before birth, but they can be delayed and can continue during childhood years. In all cases sufficient time should be allowed to make sure that the testicle will not ultimately assume its proper position without the clinician's aid. Oftentimes an undescended testicle does not enter the scrotum until or just before puberty. This fact is the main basis for adoption of the policy of "watchful waiting" during infancy and early childhood. There is little or no advantage in getting a testis into the scrotum before the years just preceding puberty. In general, a testis which has not yet reached the scrotum by the age of ten or eleven years should be given appropriate therapy to attain this goal.

Hormone Treatment

The treatment of undescended testicles raises the question of therapy by injection of various hormones. The mechanism of descent, which is sometimes accelerated by gonadotropic hormones, is poorly understood. It is difficult to believe that the testicle plummets downward solely because it is larger and heavier. It is possible that the hormones have some effect on contracting smooth musculature within the gubernaculum, thus aiding in pulling the testicle downward. It is likely that the increased size and length of vessels of the spermatic cord which certain hormones are known to produce can let the gonad drop more easily.

The literature contains myriads of reports of so-called triumphs for the treatment of undescended testicles by injection of gonadotropic substances, but a careful evaluation of the results makes one develop considerable skepticism. First of all, it is well known that many testicles will descend spontaneously in the prepubertal years. Without doubt, this descent can at times be brought on at an earlier age with injections. One cannot deny that in a certain number of cases the testicle will enter the scrotum under hormone therapy, but this is undoubtedly the type of testicle which would descend anyway when the boy reaches pubertal years and produces his own hormones in sufficient quantity. Second, the surgeon who has had any breadth of experience with these patients knows that fibrous adhesions often hold a testicle to various parts of the inguinal canal and to the posterior abdominal wall; it is unbelievable that injected hormones could produce any downward movement of the testicle under these circumstances.

The hormone treatment of undescended testicles has several *disadvantages:* (1) The injections must be repeated several times a week over a period of some months; they are disturbing to a child and the cumulative discomfort is far worse than that experienced in the few days after a properly performed surgical orchidopexy. (2) While the cost of these drugs has diminished, it is still considerable. This usually approximates that of surgical therapy, and in many instances exceeds it. The problem of expense is doubly important to those individuals who, after a long course of injections without results, must submit to a surgical procedure. (3) Hormone treatment accomplishes little or nothing of permanent value. It precipitates the descent of only those testicles which would spontaneously descend if left alone for a few more years. (4) Excessive stimulation of the testicle by gonadotropic hormones is not without danger, because an atrophy has at times followed the cessation of injections.

If gonadotropins are to be tried, some predetermined limit should be set beyond which they will not be used; there is no point in continuing them indefinitely. If a desired result is not attained in five or six weeks of adequate therapy, no favorable outcome will come from larger doses or longer courses. Accepted doses have been 500 to 1000 units of Antituitrin S, three times per week.

Several staff members of the Children's Hospital have accumulated considerable unpublished data from cases treated by various preparations of hormones. An objective study of the results has led us to abandon the use of hormone treatment for undescended testicles. The only exception to this rule would be the boy who is overly fat and has generalized underdevelopment of the genitalia. Administration of gonadotropic substances (40,000 to 50,000 units over a period of six months to a year) for this *Fröhlich type* of individual has some slight value when subsequently followed by orchidopexy.

Orchidopexy

In general, orchidopexy is a double operative procedure, combining treatment of an indirect inguinal hernia and repositioning of a testis. The former can be done satisfactorily at any age; the latter can be accomplished only when the spermatic vessels and the vas are long enough to permit the placement of the testis in a lower position.

The operative correction of undescended testis can be performed by the two-stage Thorek procedure—in which the testis is brought down and anchored to the thigh fascia and then some months later liberated and allowed to reside in the scrotum—or the entire undertaking can be completed in one sitting. We much prefer the latter, and do not employ the Thorek operation under any circumstances. If the dissection of the cord is adequate and if the spermatic vessels and vas are widely liberated from behind the peritoneum, the testis can almost always be brought down into the scrotum. *Laying great stress on this extensive dissection is the factor which makes a one-stage operation both possible and satisfactory.*

Optimal Age for Operation. It has been shown that the intra-abdominal testicle will continue to produce small numbers of spermatozoa for some years, but that, if both testicles are thus retarded, sterility will occur in 90 per cent of individuals. One of the prime reasons for placing a testicle in the scrotum where the temperature is lower is to maintain spermatogenic function of the organ. Therefore, it is not necessary to treat these cases in early childhood, but certainly the testicle should be given its optimum conditions for function before the onset of puberty. If an associated hernia is troublesome and demands earlier treatment, herniorrhaphy might be required in the first few years of life, but the operator should be prepared to perform orchidopexy at the same time. If dissection is exacting and delicate, this combination has fair promise of success, but the results of the orchidopexy are not as favorable as those following operation at an older age. It has been found that the best age for operative placement of the testicle in the scrotum is *between the ninth and twelfth years.*

Skin Preparation and Draping. The skin preparation, for which we prefer half-strength tincture of iodine, must extend well beyond the inguinal area. To reach an intra-abdominal testis, the incision might have to be extended well up above the anterior superior spine. In all cases the scrotum will have to be handled, and hence must be completely prepared.

Exposure and Separation of Testicle and Cord from Surrounding Structures. The operative steps are shown in Figure 250. A long cutaneous incision is made over the inguinal canal. The external oblique fascia is opened, and under the edge of the internal oblique muscle the testis will usually be found lying alongside of a patent processus vaginalis. This entire mass is lifted up and the gubernaculum is completely severed from its lower and surrounding attachments. While the testis is being held downward under tension, the hernial sac is completely transected just above the upper pole of the testis, and is then dissected upward and away from the cord, often a very delicate job. After the hernial sac has been freed, its peritoneal orifice is closed.

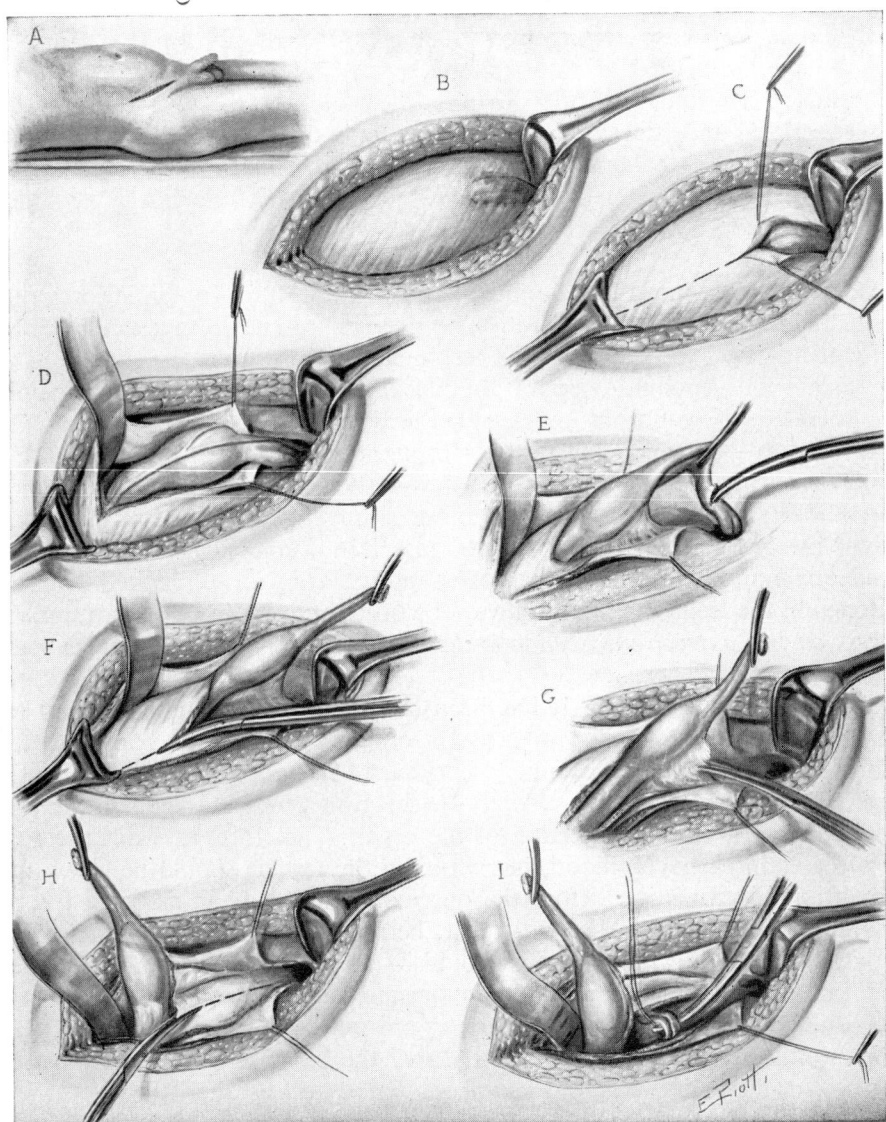

Fig. 250. Surgical procedure for simultaneous herniorrhaphy and orchidopexy. Operation for right undescended testis. A, Position of incision. B, External oblique fascia cleaned. C, Opening external oblique fascia. D, Testicle found in lower end of canal. E, Gubernaculum grasped with clamp, and being divided below this. F, Internal oblique muscle being slit upward and outward. G, Testicle being raised from its bed by severing surrounding adhesions. H, Testis held so that back wall of canal (transversalis fascia) can be taken down. I, Division of inferior epigastric vessels.

Adequate Exposure and Liberations. It is possible to carry out the subsequent retroperitoneal dissections through a normal internal ring, but these can be facilitated tremendously by widening the exposure, which we accomplish in all cases by slitting open the back wall of the canal (the transversalis fascia) and by dividing the inferior epigastric vessels.

Severance of Adhesions from the Cord. Attention is now turned to the area around the internal inguinal ring. The peritoneum is held upward and medially by a malleable retractor. By blunt dissection the peritoneum is pushed forward, away from the pos-

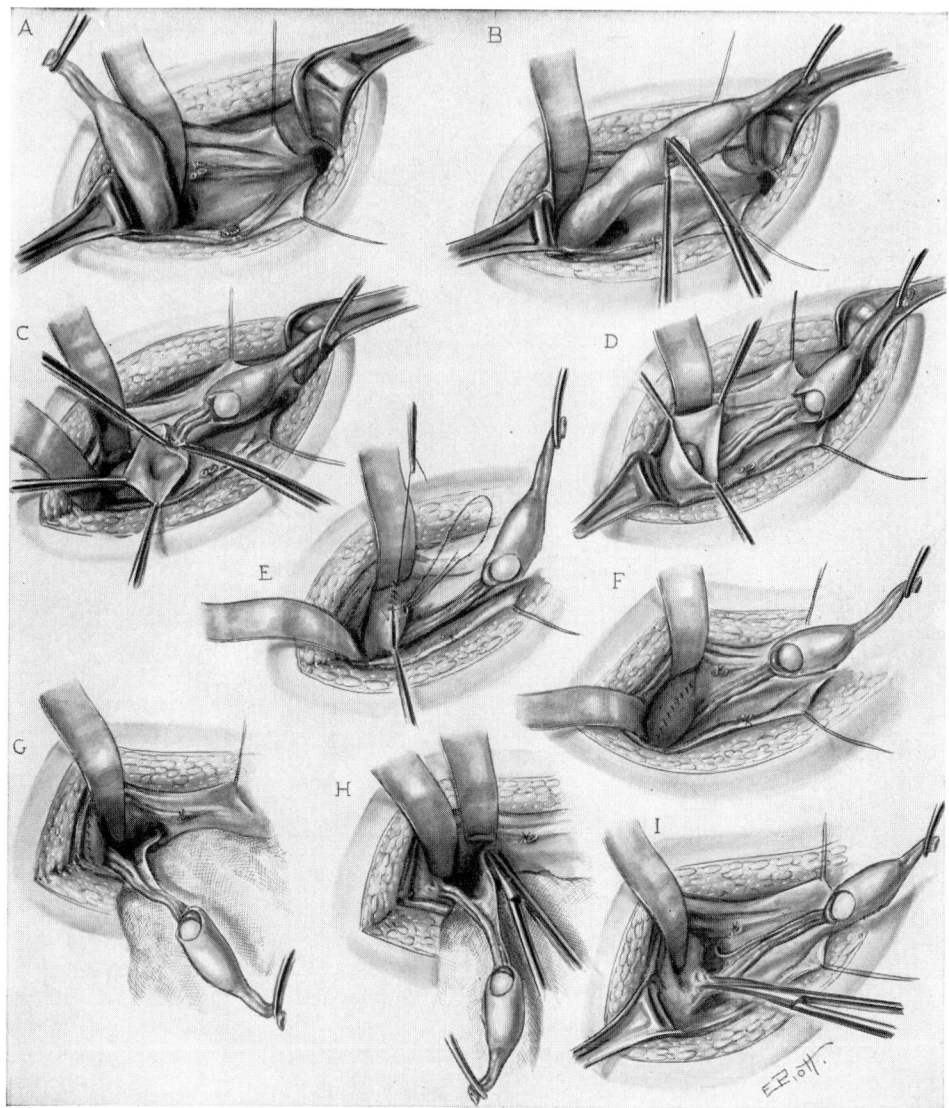

Fig. 250 (*continued*). A, Back of canal widely opened. B, Hernial sac being divided, leaving enough for a tunica vaginalis. C, Hernial sac freed upward from the cord. D, Upward dissection of hernial sac completed. E, Closure of peritoneal orifice of hernial sac. F, Peritoneal closure completed. G, Peritoneum held forward and medially by retractor so that retroperitoneal dissection can be started. The vas and the spermatic vessels disappear into the depths of the wound. H, The vas being freed from behind the bladder. I, Dissecting spermatic vessels away from posterior peritoneum.

terior pelvic wall. When this is accomplished, the spermatic artery and vein can be seen coursing upward and disappearing in the depths of the wound. Likewise the vas deferens will be found running inferiorly and disappearing behind the bladder.

Because it is most accessible, the vas is freed first, liberating it well down behind the bladder, tracing it nearly to the seminal vesicle.

By gentle downward traction on the testis, the spermatic vessels can be made to stand out clearly. By sharp and blunt dissection they are freed from behind the posterior peritoneum and off the ilio-psoas muscle, so that they stretch like a bow-string

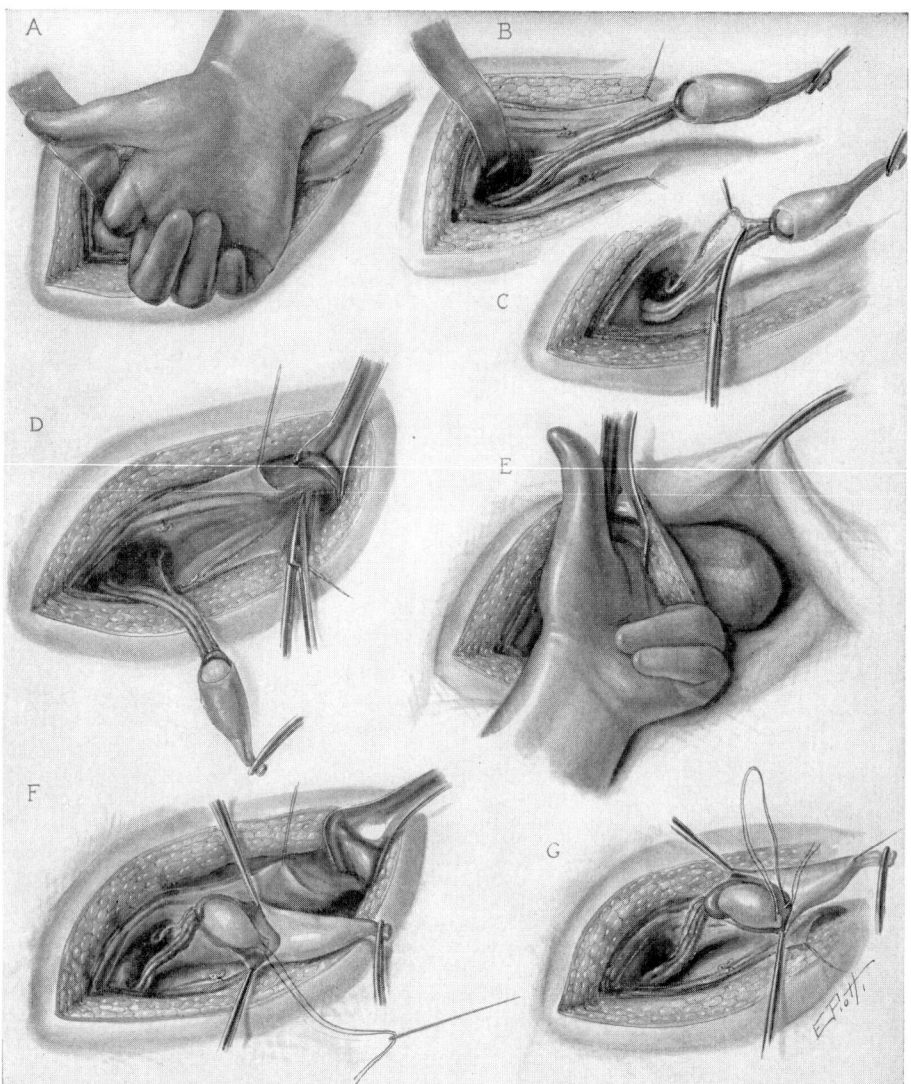

Fig. 250 (*continued*). A, With a finger deep in the wound, the vessels can be further freed. B, Retroperitoneal dissection completed, having obtained maximum liberation of the vas and the vessels C, Individual portions of cord being freed of any kinks or bands, so that maximum length can be obtained. D, Beginning of scrotal dissection. E, Scrotum forcibly stretched with finger. F, Testicle being threaded with a traction suture. G, Stitch being passed through apex of the tunica.

across this very deep cavity. As dissection is carried up behind the peritoneum, the testicle will be found to have attained a longer and longer pedicle. This dissection above the internal ring generally has to be carried 5 or 6 inches or more into the depths of the wound. *It is this extensive freeing which gives sufficient length to the cord and allows the testicle to move into a scrotal position without undue tension.* The vas deferens is generally of adequate length. Any difficulties which are encountered are more apt to be related to shortness of the spermatic blood vessels.

Preparation of Scrotum. Traction Suture to Testis. After sufficient mobility and lengthening of the cord have been obtained, the scrotum must be prepared for receiving the testicle. Inasmuch as this sac has been underdeveloped, it must be *forcibly stretched;*

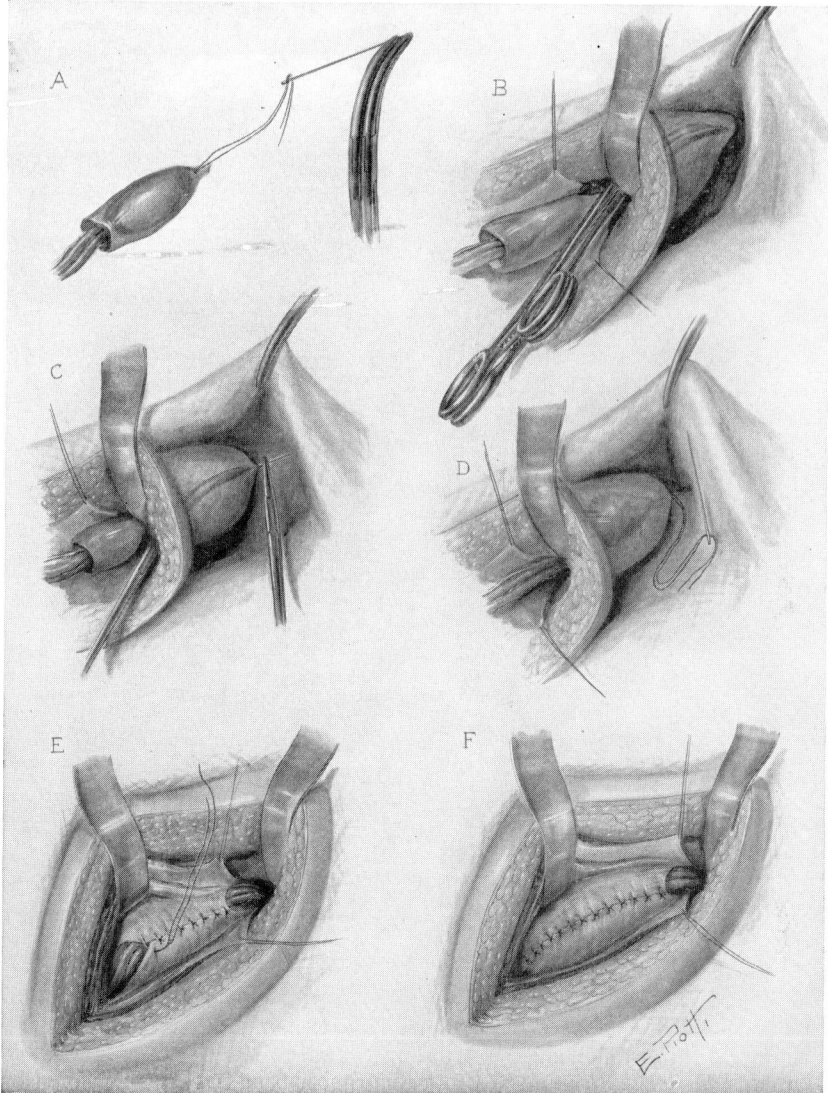

Fig. 250 (*continued*). A, Needle of the traction-suture is held by a full-length clamp just covering its point, a second clamp placed just above this. B, Clamps inserted along malleable retractor down into depths of scrotum. C, Protecting distal clamp is removed and needle pushed through scrotum by the remaining clamp. D, Testes drawn into scrotal sac. E, Posterior wall of canal repaired by closure of transversalis fascia over the cord, making the internal ring just above and lateral to the pubic spine. This dislocation of the internal ring to a more inferior and medial position allows the spermatic cord to lie in a more direct line, and therefore allows the testis to reside lower in the scrotum. F, Completion of repair of transversalis fascia.

this is best done by passing two fingers down through the operative wound, and then very extensively distending the dartos and scrotal skin.

A stitch of silk is now placed through the lower pole of the testis; this is to be used subsequently as a *traction suture*. If the stitch is passed through the gubernaculum, this might subsequently stretch and allow the testis to ride up rather high in the scrotum; it is therefore better to take the suture through the lower 2 or 3 mm. of the testicle itself. This traction stitch can be passed through the tunica vaginalis, which had been saved

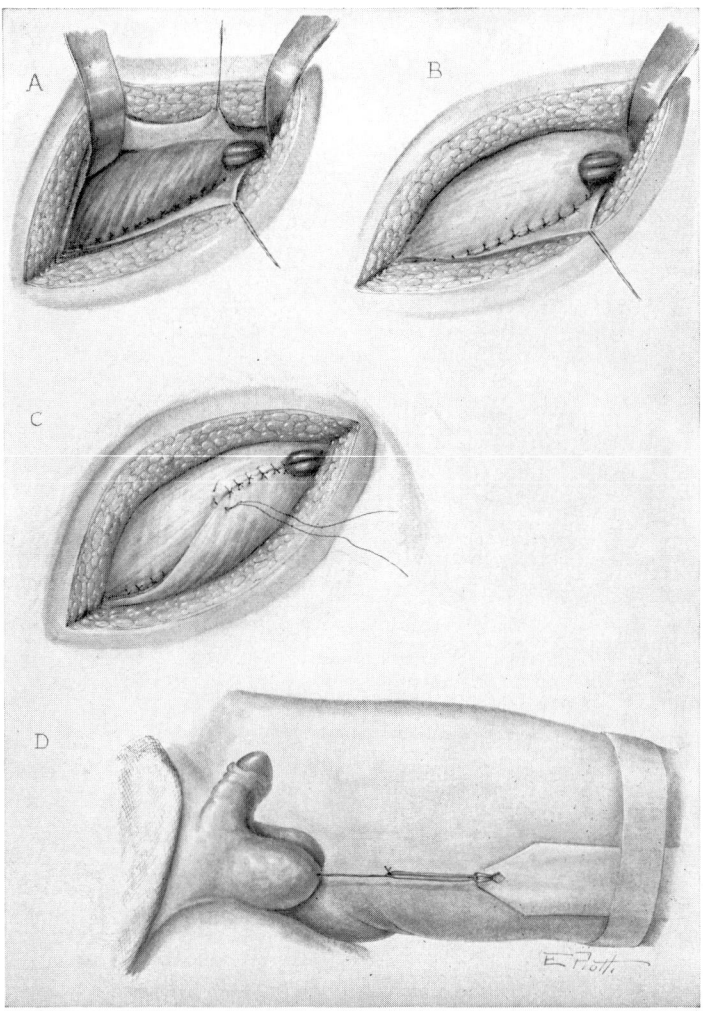

Fig. 250 (*continued*). A, Internal oblique muscle brought down to Poupart's ligament with inter-rupted silk sutures. B, External oblique fascia brought down to Poupart's. C, Lower flap of fascia imbricated upwards. D, Traction suture tied to a thin rubber band, which is anchored by adhesive tape to the opposite thigh.

to make a covering for the testicle. Both threads are put through the eye of the needle and this is passed downward (its point covered by a full-length clamp). When the bottom of the scrotum is reached, the shielding clamp is removed and the needle then thrust (by the second full-length clamp) out through the very bottom of the scrotal skin. A gentle pull on the suture will pull the testicle down into the scrotum. As the testicle is pulled into its bed, the cord must be kept from twisting.

Repair of Canal. The inguinal canal is closed by first carefully repairing the trans-versalis fascia. The cord is permitted to drop inferiorly and medially so that, by closing the transversalis superiorly and laterally, a new internal ring is made just above and lateral to the spine of the pubis. This makes it come to lie almost exactly behind the area where the external ring will be reconstructed. Presumably, this arrangement would be conducive to the production of a direct hernia through this zone, but we have not yet observed any such complication.

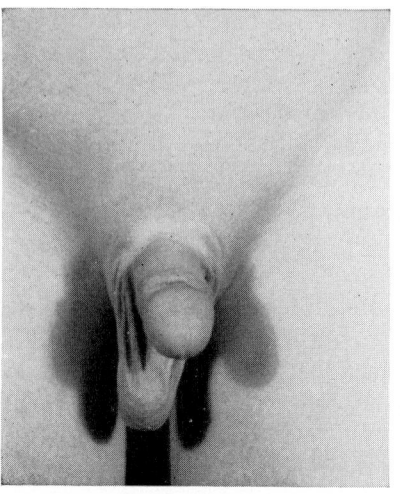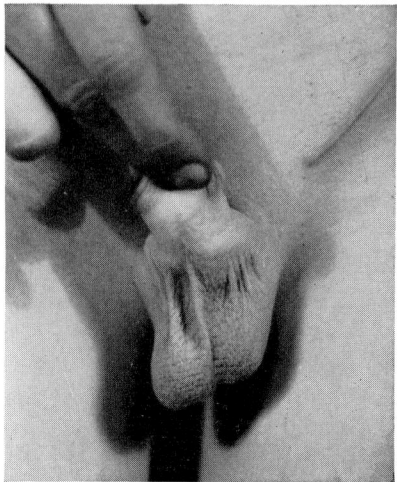

Fig. 251. Left undescended testicle in an eight-year-old boy before operation and six months after orchidopexy. The testicle resides in a satisfactory position in the scrotum.

Next, the internal oblique muscle is brought down to Poupart's ligament with interrupted silk sutures. Over this, the edges of the external oblique fascia are joined by interrupted silk suture. (All of the repair is made with 0000 Deknatel silk.)

Anchoring of Testicle. After the cutaneous wound has been closed and dressed, the tension suture (piercing the scrotum) is attached to a thin rubber band, the lower end of which is anchored to the lower part of the opposite thigh by adhesive tape. This tension apparatus is left in place for about six days, and is then removed. This appliance is not used with the idea of stretching the cord. The success of an orchidopexy depends on adequate surgical freeing of various structures so that the testicle can lie in the scrotum without much tension on its cord. If, after operation, a testis were not anchored in its sac it might retract a little and become fixed at a high level. Hence, a traction suture should always be used to hold the testicle until it becomes adherent in its scrotal position.

Two-Stage Mobilization

In a very small percentage of patients, the spermatic vessels and the vas are so short that it is impossible to bring a testis anywhere near the scrotum, even by the most extensive dissection and traction. Possibly it can be brought down only to the

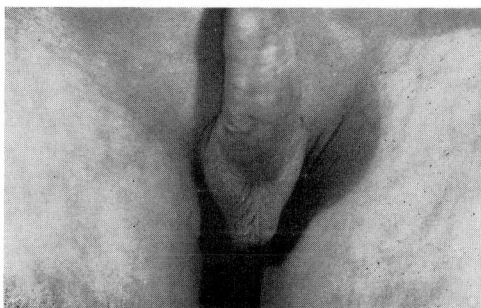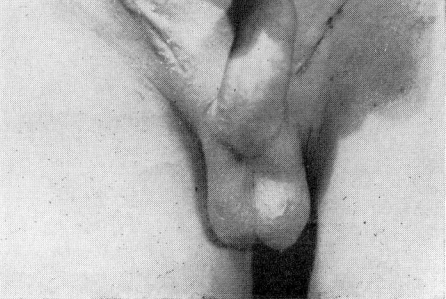

Fig. 252. *Left*, Bilateral undescended testes in a ten-year-old boy. The scrotum is underdeveloped. *Right*, Postoperative picture. The testes lie within the scrotum.

lowermost part of the canal or just outside the external ring. There is still the possibility of achieving a satisfactory result by allowing it to stay in this position for a year or two, and then attempting a secondary liberation, at which time the entire cord is again mobilized from the canal and from the retroperitoneal areas. During this time interval of a year or two, the blood vessels and the vas can elongate sufficiently so that now the testis can be brought into the scrotum without tension. We have used this two-stage mobilization in a few cases with highly satisfactory results (Fig. 254).

Bilateral Operations

When both testes must be operated upon, it is very inadvisable to attempt both procedures at one sitting; this causes the surgeon to feel hurried, and therefore to make inadequate dissection. It is always better judgment to treat bilateral cases with two separate operations, which, however, may be completed during one hospitalization. We have sometimes done the second operation four or five days after the first one. More commonly, we undertake it a year later.

RESULTS OF TREATMENT

Surgical Statistics

During the thirty-year period up to January 1, 1951, a total of 933 boys with abnormalities of the testes have been examined at the Children's Hospital. Of this number, 211 are yet too young for operation, and are being followed until such time that this can be done most advantageously. Of the entire group, 722 patients have been operated upon (for 827 undescended testes, for 36 absent testes, and for 16 perineal testes). The distribution of the various anomalies were as shown in Table 53.

Table 53

Conditions Found in 722 Boys Who Were Operated upon Because of Testicular Abnormalities

Undescended testis		
Bilateral	147	
Left	218	
Right	315	
Total		680
Absence of testis		
Bilateral	6	
Left	18	
Right	6	
Total		30
Perineal testis		
Bilateral	4	
Left	3	
Right	5	
Total		12
Total number of patients		722

In the entire group of 722 patients, there have been no deaths. Hospitalization has seldom been for more than six or seven days.

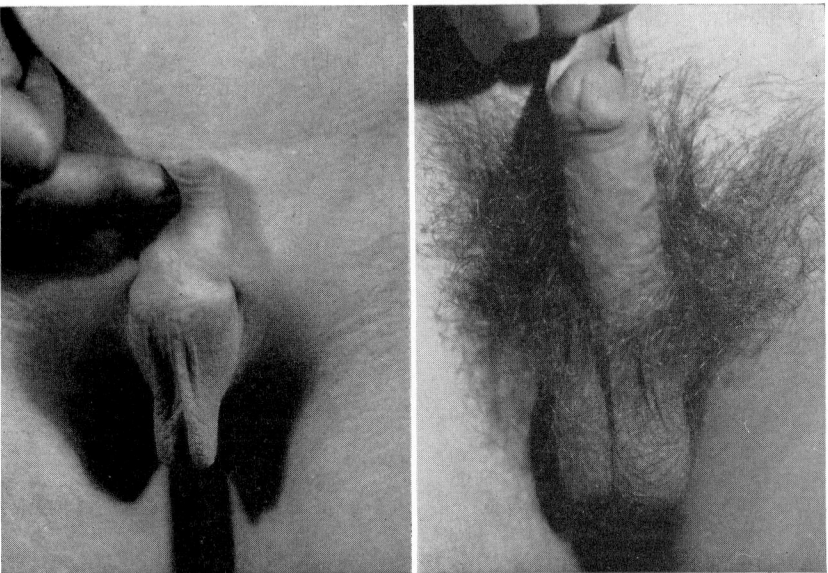

Fig. 253. *Left,* Boy with bilateral undescended testes. *Right,* Photograph four years after operation, showing normal-sized testes in the scrotal sac.

Absence of Testis. Perineal Testis

In the entire series of exploration of the groin and retroperitoneal areas, there were 30 subjects in whom no testis could be found. (This is slightly more than 4 per cent of the entire series.) Also, included in our material were 12 babies or older boys with perineal testes who were operated upon for placement of these gonads into the scrotum.

Poor Results

In any large series of patients who are treated for undescended testicles, a certain number of disappointments are bound to occur. (1) Sometimes a testicle is found which

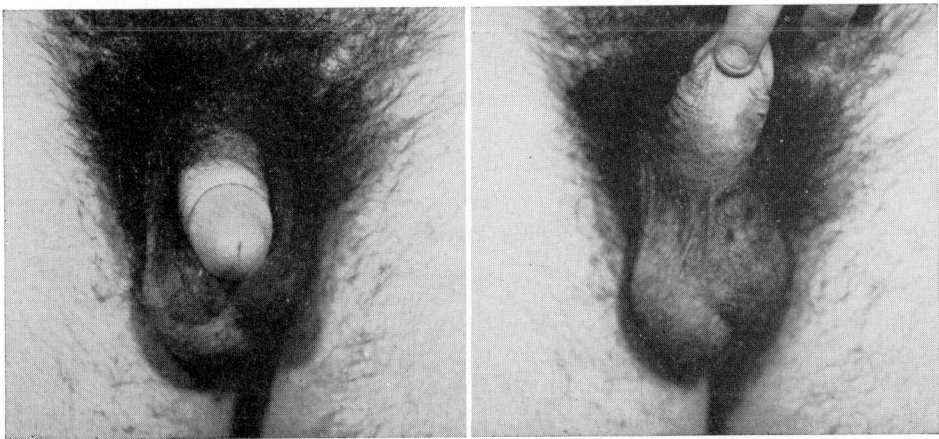

Fig. 254. Boy treated by two-stage mobilization of a very high left testis which was just at the nternal ring. During operation at twelve years the testis could be brought only to the external ring. Dnring operation at thirteen years, it could easily be brought into the scrotum. Both photographs at fifteen years.

is small and underdeveloped at the time of operation, and it always remains so thereafter. (2) In a few patients, a testicle which appears normal at the time it is brought down into the scrotum subsequently becomes *atrophied* because of interference with its blood supply. (3) Occasionally there is postoperative hematoma in the scrotum which gives pressure atrophy of the testis. (4) In a few cases the structures of the cord are so short that the testicle cannot be brought into the scrotum by any means. (5) In occasional patients the testicle does not become firmly anchored in the scrotum and will retract up to the external ring or even higher. These various disappointing results have totaled about 6 per cent of our series.

Favorable Results

For those patients who have been proved to have a testis, and do not have damage to it at operation or in the postoperative convalescence, the final results of operation have been judged by postoperative observations on the *size* of the testicle, the *consistency* and *contour* of the testis, and the ultimate *position* of the organ. In about 90 per cent of all cases operated upon, the scrotum has been made to hold a testis (or testicles) of apparently normal size and consistency.

Functional Capacity of Testicle after Operation

Engberg[7] has made studies which indicate that men with cryptorchidism have a reduced androgen excretion. Likewise, they have a higher excretion of gonadotropin (because the pituitary gland is not suppressed by testicular hormones). There was very little change in these figures in a second group of men who had been subjected to orchidopexies. From a clinical point of view, the secondary characteristics (development of pubic hair, enlargement of penis, growth of beard, deepening of voice) all appear whether bilateral undescended testes are operated upon or not. Therefore, the testes (even if intra-abdominal) presumably produce satisfactory amounts of male hormone, and this function is not changed appreciably by operation.

It is difficult and almost impossible to estimate what power the unilateral surgically treated testicle possesses for producing spermatozoa and testicular hormones, because the contralateral normal organ simultaneously carries on these functions. However, in cases of bilateral cryptorchidism the postoperative functional results are susceptible to analysis. It has been stated that there is only 10 per cent fertility in persons with bilateral cryptorchidism who have not been treated. MacCollum[15] studied 22 adults who had previously been treated by bilateral orchidopexy; he found definite fertility in 15 and potential fertility in 3 others (who had reduced counts but yet had more than 25,000,000 actively motile spermatozoa per cubic centimeter of ejaculate). The percentage of probable fertility could then be computed as 82 per cent. These studies showed conclusively that not only can good cosmetic results be obtained by operation, but that formation of spermatozoa is likewise made satisfactory.

Malignancy in Testis after Surgical Placement in Scrotum

In no patient of our series have we yet seen malignancy in a testis which has been placed surgically in the scrotum; such a complication must therefore be quite rare. Gilbert[8,9] has collected from the literature 58 cases of malignancy in testes after orchidopexy, the tumor becoming evident, on an average, about ten years later. Therefore, the surgical placement of a testis into the scrotum apparently has little effect in changing the likelihood of subsequent malignant degeneration. However, it is important to emphasize that a testis which resides in the abdomen (of an adult) and becomes malignant has little chance of being discovered until tumor extension or metastases have occurred, whereas a testis which has been brought down into the scrotum has the possibility of early detection and treatment of any tumor which might arise in it.

REFERENCES

1. Bigler, J. A., Hardy, L. M. and Scott, H. V.: Cryptorchidism Treated with Gonadotropic Preparations; Surgical Repair of Cryptorchidism with and without Gonadotropic Therapy. Am. J. Dis. Child., *56:* 989, 1938.

2. Campbell, H. E.: Incidence of Malignant Growth of the Undescended Testicle. A Critical and Statistical Study. Arch. Surg., *44:*353, 1942.

3. Carroll, W. A.: Malignancy in Cryptorchidism. J. Urol., *61:*396, 1949.

4. Christofferson, W. G. and Owen, S. E.: Neoplasms in Cryptorchids. Am. J. Cancer, *26:*259, 1936.

5. Eisenstaedt, J. S.: Imperfect Descent of the Testis and Its Management. S. Clin. North America, *30:*141, 1950.

6. Eisenstaedt, J. S., Appel, M. and Fraenkel, M.: The Effect of Hormones on the Undescended Testis: An Experimental and Clinical Study. J.A.M.A., *115:*200, 1940.

7. Engberg, H.: Investigations on the Endocrine Function of the Testicle in Cryptorchidism. Proc. Roy. Soc. Med., *42:*652, 1949.

8. Gilbert, J. B.: Studies in Malignant Testis Tumors. V. Tumors Developing After Orchidopexy. J. Urol., *46:*740, 1941.

9. Gilbert, J. B. and Hamilton, J. B.: Studies in Malignant Testis Tumors. III. Incidence and Nature of Tumors in Ectopic Testes. Surg., Gynec. & Obst., *71:*731, 1940.

10. Hansen, T. S.: Fertility in Operatively Treated and Untreated Cryptorchidism. Proc. Roy. Soc. Med., *42:*645, 1949.

11. Hinman, F. and Benteen, F. H.: Relationship of Cryptorchidism to Tumor of Testis. J. Urol., *35:*378, 1936.

12. Jones, A. E. and Lieberthal, F.: Perineal Testicle. J. Urol., *40:*658, 1938.

13. Lopin, J. H., Klein, W. and Goldman, A.: Cryptorchidism. J. Pediat., *22:*175, 1943.

4. Lowsley, O. S. and Curtis, H. C.: Surgical Treatment of Ectopic Testes. Surg., Gynec. & Obst., *71:*811, 1940.

15. MacCollum, D. W.: Clinical Study of the Spermatogenesis of Undescended Testicles. Arch. Surg., *31:*290, 1935.

16. Mason, W. R., Jr., and Lehman, E. P.: Undescended Perineal Testis; Report of Case. Surgery, *5:*932, 1939.

17. Pace, J. M.: The Histologic and Pathologic Anatomy of the Retained Testis. Proc. Staff Meet. Mayo Clin., *10:*726, 1935.

18. Rea, C. E.: Treatment of Undescended Testis; with Special Reference to Therapy with Hormones. Surgery, *4:*552, 1938.

19. Rea, C. E.: Functional Capacity of Undescended Testis. Arch. Surg., *38:*1054, 1939.

20. Rea, C. E.: Histologic Character of the Undescended Testis After Puberty. Its Significance with Reference to the Performance of Orchidopexy. Arch. Surg., *44:*27, 1942.

21. Rea, C. E.: Is Hormonal Therapy of Value in the Treatment of Undescended Testes? Tr. West. Surg. Assoc., *56:*195, 1949.

22. Smith, R. E.: Observations on Descent of Testicle with Special Reference to Spontaneous Descent at Puberty. Arch. Dis. Childhood, *14:*1, 1939.

23. Thompson, W. O. and Heckel, N. J.: Undescended Testes; Present Status of Glandular Treatment. J.A.M.A., *112:*397, 1939.

24. Wangensteen, O. H.: The Undescended Testis. An Experimental and Clinical Study. Arch. Surg., *14:*663, 1927.

25. Wangensteen, O. H.: The Surgery of the Undescended Testis. Surg., Gynec. & Obst., *54:*219, 1932.

26. Wangensteen, O. H.: The Undescended Testis. Its Fate After Satisfactory Scrotal Anchorage. Ann. Surg., *102:*875, 1935.

27. Zelson, C. and Steinitz, E.: Treatment of Cryptorchidism with Male Sex Hormone. J. Pediat., *15:*522, 1939.

CHAPTER 38

Torsion of the Testis and the Appendix Testis

TORSION OF THE TESTIS

Etiology. Torsion of the testis is less frequent in childhood than in adult life. It may be produced by a sharp blow to the scrotum or by the individual's being jounced in a roughly riding vehicle. Torsion may occur spontaneously without history of trauma.

Symptoms. There is sudden onset of excruciating local *pain* and *tenderness. Nausea* and *vomiting* are rare. The testicle rapidly becomes swollen and *edema* may extend up along the cord. As infarction of the testicle proceeds, the local symptoms become more severe and low-grade *fever* can appear.

Differential Diagnosis. Diagnosis of the condition rarely offers any difficulty. The absence of urethral discharge and seminal vesicle tenderness, as well as the rarity of gonorrheal infection in young boys, should rule out *epididymitis* in most cases.

The finding of a testicular mass might in some cases suggest a *neoplasm,* but the history of pain and sudden onset of symptoms would suggest torsion as a more likely diagnosis.

Treatment

The treatment of testicular torsion consists of *immediate exploration* of the organ as soon as the diagnosis is made. The longer that operation is delayed, the greater are the chances of irreparable infarction. Exploration should be done through a low, oblique incision just above the scrotum, and the inguinal canal should be laid open if necessary. Inspection of the spermatic cord will quickly indicate in which direction a twist has taken place. The surrounding structures are edematous and the tissues distal to the twist are hemorrhagic or dusky in color. *Reduction* of the torsion may permit a return of circulation if the injury has been of short standing. Slitting open the tunica vaginalis and directly viewing the testicle allows a better estimate of its viability. When the state of the circulation is in doubt, five or ten minutes' observation, to find out how much the color will improve, is preferable to performance of an *orchidectomy* too hastily. If the testicle is extensively damaged and its viability is lost, it should be removed. On several occasions we have left a testis of questionable viability, feeling that it had probably been destroyed but there was a bare possibility that it might retain some slight endocrine function.

A few surgeons feel that if there has been torsion of one testis, there is enough possibility of developing eunuchism from subsequent twist of the other testis to justify operation on the remaining one, tacking it down so that it cannot twist. In our limited experience with torsion of the testis, we have not seen a patient with involvement of a second side, hence we have not performed such anchoring operations, but admit there is a certain attractiveness to the proposal.

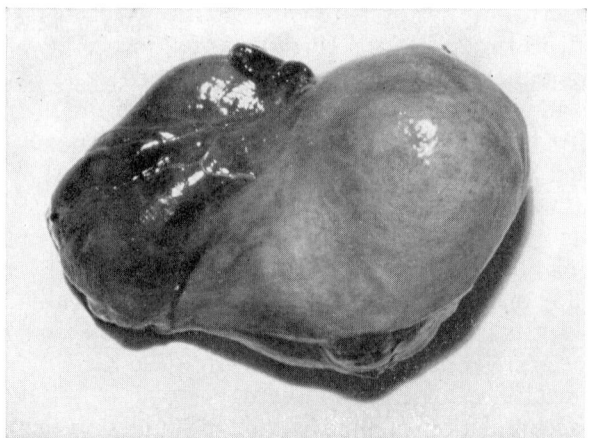

Fig. 255. Infarction of testis from torsion of the cord; fourteen-year-old boy.

Twenty cases of torsion of the testis have been treated at the Children's Hospital. About half of these appeared before the age of two months; the youngest patient was two days of age and the oldest was fourteen years. Three of these torsions occurred in undescended testes. In 7 of the cases, the torsion was reduced and the testes not removed; in 11 an orchidectomy was performed; in 1 the testis was found to be quite atrophic (apparently there had been earlier attacks of torsion); in 1 no operative treatment was carried out.

TORSION OF THE APPENDIX TESTIS

The appendix testis, or hydatid of Morgagni, is a small, pedunculated structure several millimeters in diameter arising from the superior portion of the testis and lying within the tunica vaginalis. It represents a remnant of the degenerated Müllerian system.

Symptoms. The appendix testis occasionally becomes twisted upon its pedicle (Fig. 256) and the resulting infarction produces symptoms somewhat the same but

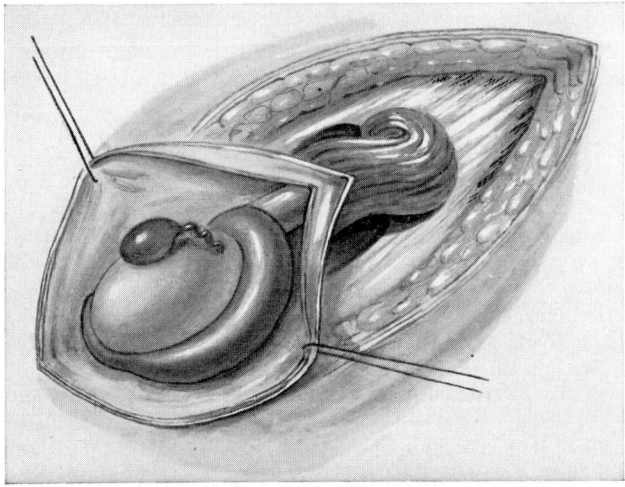

Fig. 256. Torsion and infarction of an appendix testis. The darkly discolored appendix testis is seen in the upper pole of the normal testis.

possibly not as severe as those of torsion of the testicle. While torsion of the appendix testis has been reported in infancy, it is chiefly a condition of boys and young adults. Eighty per cent of the patients are between five and fifteen years of age; our youngest was fourteen months and the oldest was fifteen years. The disorder is marked by sudden onset of sharp *pain*. At first this is of moderate severity, but later it tends to subside— a fact possibly related to the gradual killing of the nerves which pass through the twisted pedicle. *Local swelling* and *tenderness* follow within a few hours and are sharply confined to the affected side of the scrotum. *Redness* of the overlying skin may appear in thirty-six to forty-eight hours. If the condition is not relieved by surgical means, the swelling may persist for many days. It has been said that nausea and vomiting are less frequent than in cases of twisted testis, but a review of our material shows the opposite to be true. The temperature is normal, or only slightly elevated. In some instances the swollen and tender hydatid can be felt at the upper pole of the testicle, but in most cases there is early accumulation of fluid within the tunica vaginalis which prohibits accurate palpation of the structures within it.

Differential Diagnosis. Torsion of the appendix testis may be confused with *torsion of the testicle* itself. The mildness or the absence of general reaction and the less striking local changes suggest that the process is limited to the appendix. In some instances the past history will indicate that there have been similar episodes of minor pain or swelling which probably represented slight twists of the appendix testis which were spontaneously reduced. In many cases this recurrence of symptoms is a noteworthy feature.

Treatment

The treatment in all cases should be *operative removal* of the appendix testis. It is important to know that this condition can exist, for all too often orchidectomy has been performed in the belief that the patient actually had a torsion of the testicle. In the exploration of one of these cases, edema and vascular engorgement along the cord without a frank twist of the cord should always arouse one's suspicions regarding torsion of the appendix testis. *When there is any question about the pathology concerned, it is best to open the tunica vaginalis and inspect the hydatid.* If this is twisted and infarcted, it can be rapidly excised and the testicle can be spared. In the first patient we encountered with this lesion (a sixteen-month-old boy), regional vascular engorgement was believed to indicate infarction of the testicle. Hence, this organ was removed. However, postoperative examination of the surgical specimen showed that the important pathology was confined to the twisted appendix. Accordingly, in 12 subsequent cases precaution was always taken to open the tunica at operation so that the gangrenous appendix testis could be removed and the testis saved.

REFERENCES

1. Allen, P. D. and Andrews, T. W.: Torsion of the Spermatic Cord in Infancy. Am. J. Dis. Child., *59:*136, 1940.
2. Ewert, E. E. and Hoffman, H. A.: Torsion of Spermatic Cord. J. Urol., *51:*551, 1944.
3. Foshee, C. H.: Torsion of the Appendix Testis; Report of Two Cases. J.A.M.A., *99:*289, 1932.
4. Heslin, J. E. and Allyn, R. E.: Torsion of the Appendix Testis. Urol. & Cutan. Rev., *47:* 210, 1943.
5. Howser, J. W. and River, L. P.: Torsion and Gangrene of Hydatid of Morgagni. Review of Literature and Case Report. Am. J. Surg., *59:*571, 1943.
6. McFadden, G. D. F.: Torsion of Appendix of Testis. Lancet, *1:*320, 1939.
7. Randall, A. J.: Torsion of Appendix Testis (Hydatid of Morgagni). J. Urol., *41:*715, 1939.
8. Rolnick, H. C.: Torsion of Hydatid of Morgagni. J. Urol., *42:*458, 1939.
9. Turley, H. K.: Torsion of the Testicle and Its Appendages. South. M. J., *35:*828, 1942.

10. Vermeulen, C. W. and Hagerty, C. S.: Torsion of the Appendix Testis (Hydatid of Morgagni): Report of Two Cases with a Study of the Microscopic Anatomy. J. Urol., *54*:459, 1945.

11. Whittington, C. T.: Undescended Intra-abdominal Testicle with Torsion of the Cord and Embryonic Cell Carcinoma. Case Report. Am. J. Surg., *60*:304, 1943.

CHAPTER 39

Tumors of the Testicle

Tumors of the testicle in infants and immature boys are rare, but they deserve consideration because many of them are of a high degree of malignancy but still in many instances can be permanently cured if surgical therapy is instituted promptly. The following remarks are based largely on experiences gained from observation and treatment of 12 subjects (Table 55) with various types of testicular tumors in infancy and childhood.

PATHOLOGIC TYPES

Four or five rather distinct types of tumors should be considered, listing these in order of increasing malignancy: (1) Interstitial cell (Leydig) tumor; (2) teratoma; (3) seminoma; (4) adenocarcinoma; (5) embryonal carcinoma. In some specimens there is a tendency for combinations of these to occur, the prognosis depending on the more malignant components which are present. Multiple sections of each testicular lesion are necessary to give a true picture of the pathology in any given case.

All of the tumors of the testis tend to be well encapsulated and to expand the tunica albuginea in a rather spherical or slightly lobulated manner. The tumors are firm to hard and generally have a dark reddish or purplish red discoloration, when viewed through the intact scrotum. Most of the masses are several centimeters in greatest dimension; it is rather rare for them to be larger than a golf ball or a small lemon. It is impossible by external, local examination to distinguish the malignant from the benign neoplasms of the testicle. A malignant testicular tumor may give extensions which can be palpated along the inguinal canal, but in many cases metastases skip this region and show up initially within the abdominal cavity, particularly along the iliac vessels or posterior abdominal wall. In some of the malignant lesions, metastases can appear in the skeleton or in the lungs in the terminal stages, but early extensions or metastases are very apt to be limited to the abdomen.

CLINICAL PICTURE

History

While in some patients the regional swelling of the testicle has from the very first aroused the suspicions of the family or the doctor regarding neoplasm, a review of our records indicates that in the vast majority of instances the local swelling was thought to be related to a hernia (which indeed in some cases was also present) or to a hydrocele of the tunica. When the latter was the opinion of the physician, much valuable time was often lost because the lump was thought to be a hydrocele which did not demand any immediate therapy. Indeed, it was amazing to find that several of these masses had been tapped, being thought to contain fluid, and only after unsuccessful needling was the true nature of the mass suspected. It is difficult to believe that these lumps did not from the very first have a certain hardness, a darkish discoloration, and a failure to transilluminate light, all of which should have ruled out the possibility of hydrocele to even the most casual observer.

Fortunately, a testicle is so situated that any neoplasm within it should be readily apparent because of the exposed position of the organ. Thus there should always be an excellent chance for detection and removal of the mass in the early stages of the disease. In spite of these favorable circumstances, it is distressing to find that a rather high percentage of the babies and children have had a mass which had been present for many months before surgical therapy was instituted.

Generally, testicular tumors cause little or no pain or discomfort; a rather solid mass is the only complaint. This situation has often been known to exist for many weeks or months before metastases have appeared. In only one of our cases was the initial complaint related to abdominal neoplastic disease, with no history of a mass having previously been noticed in the testicle; the latter was initially discovered at the time of physical examination.

Since tumors of the testis tend to remain localized for an appreciable period of time before metastases occur, it is reasonable to stress an optimistic note in the treatment of these neoplasms, for early surgery should lead to higher percentages of cure in the future than has been the record in the past.

While the endocrinologically active tumors of interstitial cell origin are quite rare, they form a particularly interesting group. They have been described in children from two to six years of age. Some data regarding them are summarized in Table 54. These

Table 54

Cases of Testicular Interstitial Cell Tumor Reported in Children[2]

Author	Age at Onset	Age at Operation	Pseudo-precocious Puberty	Postoperative Course
Sacchi............	5 6/12	9 6/12	Present	Voice reverted; considerable regression
Rowlands et al.....	6	9	Present	No regression
Stewart et al.......	4	5	Present	Pubic hair disappeared
Somerford........	5	11	Present	No regression
Huffman..........	4	6	Present	No regression
Urban	5	5 1/12	Present	Pubic hair disappeared
Werner et al.......	5 6/12	6 9/12	Present	Moderate regression
Sandblom........	2 3/12	3 6/12	Present	Regression
Cook, Gross, et al..	4 7/12	5 3/12	Present	Slight regression

boys present a picture of marked precocious development of the entire body and especially of the genitalia. This picture of macrogenitosomia praecox may be so striking that the family has regarded the small mass in one testicle as incidental.

Physical Findings

A mass is found in one testicle, occurring with about equal frequency in each of the two organs. The child seems to be quite comfortable and to have no particular pain or discomfort from a lump which may be several times the size of the opposite normal testicle. In some instances the tumor may be 4 to 5 cm. in greatest dimensions but rarely is it larger than this. The mass is generally smoothly rounded or slightly lobulated. It is firm to hard and almost always has a darkish discoloration. It is impossible by external examination to differentiate benign from malignant lesions. Generally

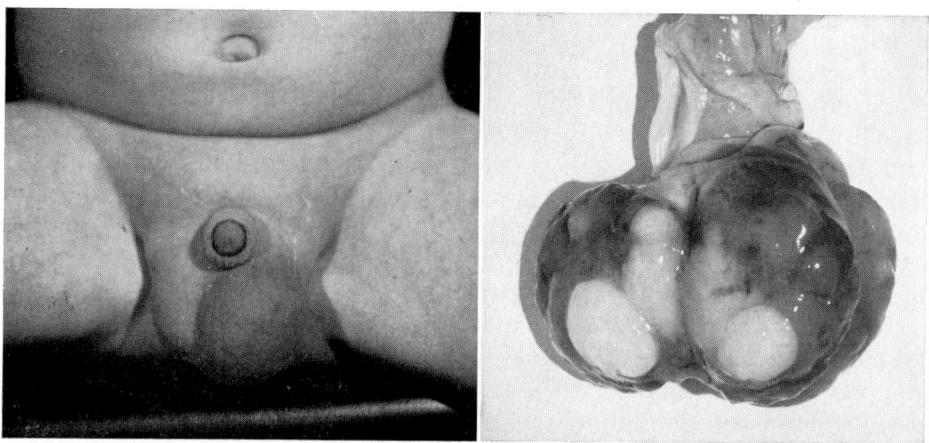

Fig. 257. Embryonal carcinoma of the testis in a fourteen-month-old boy. Case 3, Table 55. Alive, well, and without evidence of metastasis one year after surgical removal.

no extensions can be felt up along the spermatic cord. The abdomen should be care-fully palpated for any masses along the posterior wall of the pelvis or the paravertebral gutter because it is in these regions that metastases of the malignant lesions are so apt to appear.

In those rare cases with some endocrine activity of an interstitial cell tumor of the testis, the changes of precocious growth and masculinization are obvious. The overall size of the body is far beyond the expected normal and the skeletal musculature is

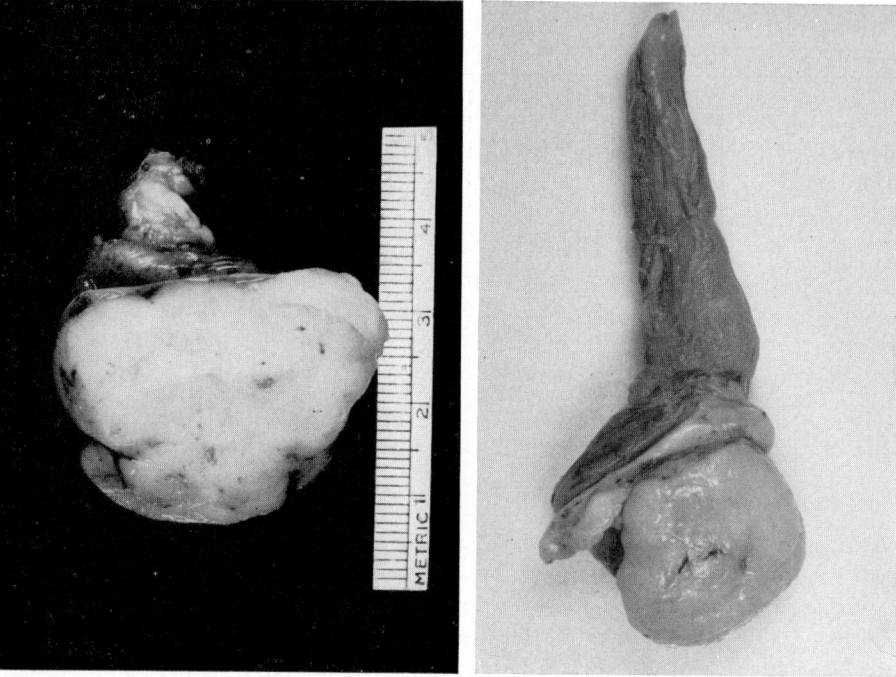

Fig. 258. *Left,* Embryonal carcinoma of testis from a year-old child. Case 1, Table 55. Patient entirely well three and one-half years later. *Right,* Embryonal carcinoma of testis from fifteen-month-old child. Case 4, Table 55. Patient entirely well ten years later.

exceedingly well developed; the boy has a very solid and massive muscular development, at times accompanied by ceaseless physical activity. Acne of the skin, particularly about the shoulders and face, is very common. The voice is deepened. There may be an excessive growth of hair on the face. The penis, scrotum, and prostate are greatly enlarged. There is increased skeletal growth and maturation. In our single case (Table 56), mild hypertension, elevation of the serum sodium to 154 mEq. per liter and an elevation of the serum chloride to 112 mEq. per liter, as well as an eosinopenia to 0–27, were probably related to androgenic activity. The excretion of urinary 17-ketosteroids was elevated in our patient to 16.8 mg. (normal upper limit being 1 mg.).

Diagnosis

There should be little difficulty in recognizing immediately a neoplasm of the testis. The hardness of the mass, the darkish discoloration, and the inability to transmit light should at once rule out hydrocele. In the smaller tumors the darkish, rather firm lump might be confused with an infarction of the testicle; an infarcted testis is seldom much larger than the other normal testis and is generally accompanied by the history of an episode suggesting torsion. Certainly a discolored mass which is increasing in size over a period of time cannot be regarded as infarction. In those rare cases in which the changes are minimal, there might be difficulty in differentiating between testicular hemorrhage (or infarction) and neoplasm. Under these circumstances the only safe course of management is to biopsy the mass (by incision) and to be prepared for immediate orchidectomy if neoplasm is found.

TREATMENT

Excision

In the absence of demonstrable metastases in the abdomen (by palpation) and in the lungs (by x-ray film), there can be no doubt that immediate orchidectomy is the therapy of choice. The field should be widely prepared so that the scrotum, inguinal regions, and indeed the entire anterior abdominal wall are suitably sterilized and draped in anticipation of an extensive procedure if this seems to be wise. A very generous incision over and parallel to the inguinal canal should be made, extending this well up above the level of the anterior-superior spine. The canal should be laid open by cutting the external oblique fascia upward and outward from the external ring, carrying this incision well above the region of the internal ring. The internal oblique and transversalis muscles should be split upward and outward for several centimeters to give adequate exposure of the field beyond the internal ring. The peritoneum can be opened and a finger passed into it to palpate the regions along the iliac vessels. If nodes are found in this area, the incision should be enlarged so that the abdomen can be extensively entered and tumor tissue along the great vessels or brim of the pelvis thereby removed. If the original, small exploratory incision through the internal ring area reveals no palpable masses in the pelvis, the peritoneum can be closed and orchidectomy proceeded with, ligating and dividing all the structures of the cord just at the internal ring, turning of the cord downward, carrying along with it all adventitial structures and thus giving as liberal and extensive removal of the cord tissues as possible.

When the entire cord has thus been resected from its bed, gentle traction from above, along with finger pressure on the tip of the scrotum, will bring the testicular mass up into the wound, with the scrotum inverted. The dartos can then be cut away from the mass so that the entire tunica vaginalis is removed along with the testicular lump. After this excision of the neoplasm and the structures of the cord, the abdominal

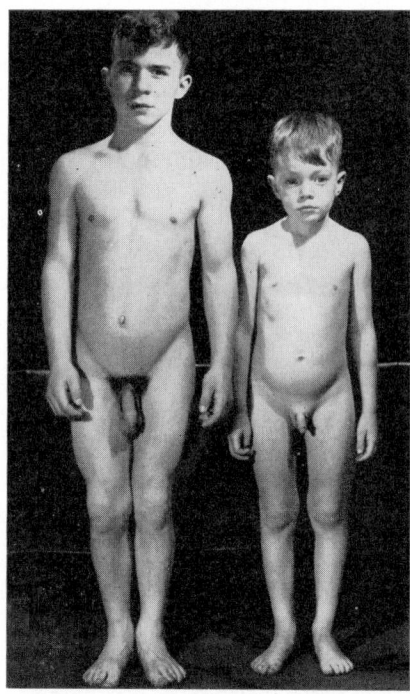

Fig. 259. On *left* a boy of five years with an interstitial cell tumor of his right testicle. Note growth of genitalia, pubic hair, massive development of skeleton, and body musculature. Case 11, Table 55. On *right*, a normal boy of the same chronologic age for comparison.

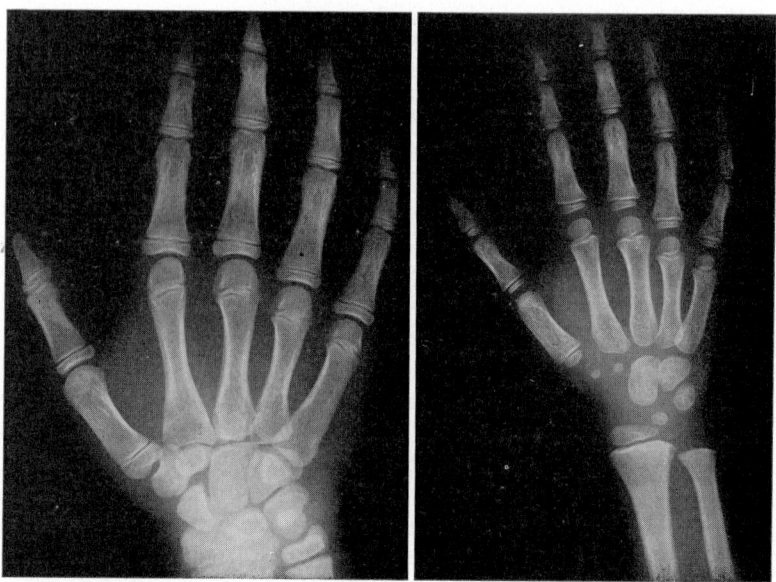

Fig. 260. *Left*, Roentgenogram of hand and wrist of a five-year-old boy with an interstitial cell tumor of the testis. Case 11, Table 55. The bony development and maturation is that of a thirteen-year-old male. *Right*, Hand and wrist of a normal five-year-old boy for comparison.

wall can now be repaired by bringing the transversalis fascia down to Poupart's ligament with interrupted silk stitches. Over this the internal oblique muscle is likewise brought down to Poupart's ligament. The external oblique fascia is then closed. Suture of these various layers gives a most satisfactory repair of the wall.

No definite statements can be made for or against the value of x-ray irradiation in neoplasms of the testis in infancy and childhood. Our own material is certainly too limited to give any conclusive evidence regarding the value of such an adjunct. Two infants (with apparently clean excisions of the tumors) were given 2600 and 3000 r

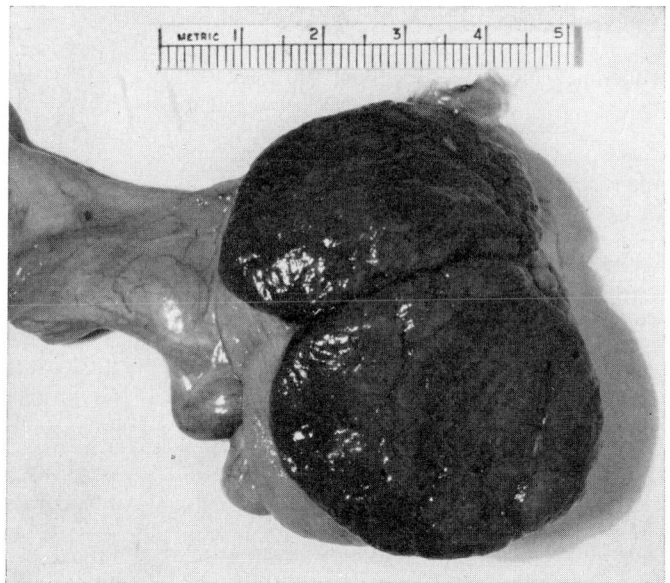

Fig. 261. Leydig cell tumor of the testis which had caused psuedo-precocious puberty in a five-year-old boy; the tumor had a brownish color. Case 11, Table 55.

respectively over the scrotum or over the pelvis and abdomen; both of these children have apparently been cured. However, other neoplasms of the same histologic type and in the same age groups have been excised and no x-ray therapy given; cures have also resulted therefrom. We are rather skeptical about the value of x-ray irradiation over the pelvis and abdomen of children with carcinomas of the testis; there might be some plausibility in giving it to those who have had a seminoma, which is a more radiosensitive tumor.

One child has been given 2300 r over known abdominal extensions of an embryonal carcinoma of the testis, possibly with some temporary benefits, but followed by widespread and enlarging recurrences, leading to death some months later. We have a rather skeptical opinion of what can be accomplished by x-ray irradiation over known abdominal metastases of these neoplasms.

RESULTS OF THERAPY

Some pertinent data regarding our 12 patients with neoplasms of the testicle are recorded in Table 55.

Teratoma. One child, a year of age, with teratoma of the testicle treated by excision, followed by irradiation of 800 r to the scrotum, is entirely well and apparently free of disease four years later.

Table 55

Testicular Tumors in Children's Hospital Series

Case	Age in Years	Type of Tumor	Therapy	Results. Remarks.
1	1	Embryonal carcinoma	Excision. 2600 r to scrotum	Entirely well 3½ yrs. later
2	1	Teratoma	Excision. 800 r to scrotum	Entirely well 4 yrs. later
3	1 2/12	Embryonal carcinoma	Excision	Entirely well 1 yr. later
4	1 3/12	Embryonal carcinoma	Excision. 300 r over chest. 3000 r over pelvis and abdomen	Entirely well 10 yrs. later
5	1 5/12	Adenocarcinoma	Excision (elsewhere)	Well for the 6 mos. he has been followed
6	1 7/12	Embryonal carcinoma	Excision	Entirely well 6 yrs. later
7	2 5/12	Seminoma	Excision	Entirely well 3 yrs. later
8	2 5/12	Carcinoma	Excision (elsewhere)	In 6 mos. widespread metastases to abdomen, lungs, skeleton. Dead
9	2 9/12	Embryonal carcinoma	Biopsy only	Widespread metastases to abdomen when first seen. Dead
10	4 2/12	Embryonal carcinoma	Excision (elsewhere)	In 4 mos. widespread metastases in abdomen and chest. Impending death
11	5	Leydig cell tumor	Excision	Tumor had marked endocrine function. Patient well 2 yrs. after excision
12	9	Embryonal carcinoma	Excision (elsewhere). 2300 r over abdominal extensions	In 6 mos. widespread abdominal recurrence. Dead in 1 yr.

Seminoma. One child, two and five-twelfths years of age, was treated by excision of the testicular mass, and is known to be entirely well three years later.

Interstitial Cell Tumor. One child, five years of age, with marked endocrine changes from one of these functioning tumors of the testicle, was treated by excision. The patient has been followed two years since then and has shown marked regression in acne and the improvements in laboratory data noted in Table 56.

Carcinomas. Of the 9 lesions, either adenocarcinoma or embryonal carcinoma, that we have seen, one had extensive metastases in the abdomen when first examined (proved by biopsy of the testicular tumor) and there was death within a few months. The remaining 8 patients were all treated by excision of the testicular mass (one of these being known to have intra-abdominal extension at the time of operation). Of these 8 patients, 2 were given x-ray therapy as a precautionary measure over the

Table 56

Pertinent Laboratory Data from Case 11 (Table 55)
(Interstitial Cell Tumor of Testis)

	Before Surgery	After Surgery	1 Month Later	13 Months Later
Blood pressure, mm. of mercury	138/90	120/78	128/88	108/84
Serum sodium, mEq. per liter	154	151	146	
Serum chloride, mEq. per liter	112	98	107	
Nonprotein nitrogen, mg. per 100 cc.	35.4			
Blood sugar, mg. per 100 cc.	102			
Eosinophils per cubic millimeter	0–27	88	99	
Urinary 17-ketosteroids, mg. excreted in 24 hr.	16.8	1.13	0.273	0.99

scrotum and abdomen, and 1 was given x-ray therapy over the abdomen for the known abdominal extensions. Of the 8 patients, 3 are known subsequently to have had wide-spread metastases or death, and 5 are presumably cured of their neoplasms.

REFERENCES

1. Campbell, M.: Clinical Pediatric Urology. W. B. Saunders Co., Philadelphia, 1951.
2. Cook, C. D., Gross, R. E., Landing, B. H. and Zygmuntowicz, A. S.: Interstitial Cell Tumor of the Testis. Study of a Five Year Old Boy with Pseudo-Precocious Puberty. J. Clin. Endocrinol., *12:*725, 1952.
3. Gray, C. P., McDonald, J. R. and Thompson, G. J.: Chorio-epitheliomatous Elements Occurring in Teratoma of the Testis. Am. J. Surg., *79:*653, 1950.
4. Hoffman, M. M.: The Urinary 17-Ketosteroids of a Patient with an Interstitial Cell Tumor of the Testes (Abstract). Endocrinology, *35:*215, 1944.
5. Haines, J. S. and Grabstald, H.: Tumor Formation in Atrophic Testes. Arch. Surg., *60:* 857, 1950.
6. Kimbrough, J. C. and Denslow, J. C.: Malignant Disease of the Testicle. J. Urol., *65:* 611, 1951.
7. Kretschmer, H. L.: Embryoma of the Testicle in a Five-Year Old Child. Am. J. Surg., *76:* 99, 1948.
8. Melicow, M. M., Robinson, J. N., Ivers, W. and Rainsford, L. K.: Interstitial Cell Tumors of Testis. J. Urol., *62:*672, 1949.
9. Merren, D. D., Vest, S. A., and Lupton, C. H., Jr.: Treatment of Malignant Tumors of the Testis. J. Urol., *65:*128, 1951.
10. Moore, R. A.: Teratoid Tumors of Testis. J. Urol., *65:*693, 1951.
11. Rowlands, R. P. and Nicholson, G. W.: Growth of the Left Testicle with Precocious Sexual and Bodily Development (Macrogenito-somia). Guy's Hosp. Rep., *79:*401, 1929.
12. Sauer, H. R. and Burke, E. M.: Prognosis of Testicular Tumors. J. Urol., *62:*69, 1949.
13. Sobel, E. H., Sniffen, R. C. and Talbot, N. B.: The Testis. V. Use of Testicular Biopsies in the Differential Diagnosis of Precocious Puberty. Pediatrics, *8:*701, 1951.
14. Twombly, G. H. and Pack, G. T.: The Relationship of Hormones to Testicular Tumors. In, Endocrinology of Neoplastic Diseases. Oxford University Press, New York, 1947, p. 228.

CHAPTER 40

Diseases of the
Female Genital Tract

HYDROMETROCOLPOS

Etiology

Enormous distention of part of the genital tract sometimes appears in female babies during the first month of life. This occurs when there is: (1) a complete obstruction of the vagina (at an *imperforate hymen* or at an *atresia* just above it); and also (2) an excess secretion of fluid from the uterine glands, the latter being stimulated by estrogenic hormones which have been absorbed from the baby's mother. (Obstruction *alone* does not give symptoms in girls until puberty, when bloody material accumulates and produces a hematocolpos.) By way of the placental circulation from the mother, estrogens can accumulate in a baby in sufficient concentration to stimulate the baby's cervical and endocervical glands into abnormal secretory activity before birth and for a few weeks thereafter, much in the same manner that breasts can develop in the newborn (male and female) and give witch's milk. Excess secretion of the uterine or cervical glands goes unnoticed unless there is an obstruction in the lower vagina, in which event the uterus and upper vagina accumulate enormous amounts of fluids.

Pathology

In hydrometrocolpos the vagina (which is normally but 1 or 2 cm. in length and 5 or 6 mm. in width at this age) reaches the proportion of a golf ball or a tennis ball, or may even be larger (Fig. 262). The accumulated fluid may stretch the uterine body and the cervical canal to such extent that their contours are greatly distorted. The ballooned genital tract may assume a dumbbell shape and rise from the pelvic floor into the abdominal cavity, with the constricted portion representing the junction of the uterus and the vagina. At operation, it may be impossible to recognize the true nature of the lesion until the more or less normal uterine tubes and ovaries are identified at the upper pole of the mass. When such a lesion is opened, the vagina is found to be obstructed by a thin diaphragm across its lower third, or by an imperforate hymen. The uterine and vaginal cavities are filled with clear or brownish mucoid fluid. The cervix is widely patulous. The stagnation of entrapped fluid gives a favorable medium for bacterial invasion and growth; the fluid may become muco-purulent. Microscopic examination shows an overproduction of mucus by the cervical glands, which have been stimulated by estrogens. Keratinization of the vaginal epithelium likewise gives evidence of an increased hormone activity.

Clinical Findings

This condition appears as a pelvic or lower abdominal swelling (Fig. 263) which may produce: (1) Anterior pressure and *urethral* obstruction; (2) posterior pressure and *rectal* obstruction; or (3) upward displacement of intestines and *respiratory* embarrassment. The *enlarged uterus* may be palpable, and can reach up to or beyond the navel. It is apt to be tensely filled and give the impression of a smoothly rounded, solid tumor. Not infrequently it is mistaken for a distended bladder, until drainage of the bladder with a urethral catheter fails to diminish the size of the abdominal mass.

The enlarged vagina and uterus may so impinge upon the ureters and obstruct them that marked ureterectasia and hydronephrosis appear.

By *rectal examination* the pelvis is found filled by a mass projecting backward against the hollow of the sacrum. Gentle separation of the labia and inspection of the vaginal orifice or canal shows a bulging membrane either at the hymen or at a slightly higher level.

Treatment

It is important to recognize this condition, because the unwary operator may open the abdomen, excise the presenting lesion, and not realize until it collapses that he has removed the uterus and a large part of the vagina. In most instances treatment is possible by simply *nicking the membrane* which presents at or near the vaginal orifice. A small needle should be inserted through the membrane and some of the fluid aspirated to make certain of the diagnosis before plunging a knife into the structure. If mucoid fluid (which may be slightly hemorrhagic or even purulent) is obtained, the occluding diaphragm can be slit and the opening dilated with a hemostat. There will be an immediate discharge of the entrapped fluid; the pelvic or abdominal mass will collapse like a pricked balloon.

In some cases there is so little room between the urethra in front and the rectum behind that it is quite dangerous (for fear of injuring the urethra or rectum) to operate solely from below to relieve the obstruction. Under these circumstances it is safer to open the abdomen and—working well down behind the bladder—open the bulging anterior wall of the vagina. In this way probing instruments can be passed down the vagina from above, while investigation is made from below upward. The combination of abdominal and perineal approaches permits exact delineation of the obstructing membrane which can then be opened with relative safety. The anterior wall of the vagina (which was incised through the abdomen) can now be repaired appropriately. Incisions in the obstructing vaginal membrane are quite apt to seal over and give recurrence of the blockage; it is therefore important to keep a small piece of rubber catheter through this orifice for some weeks or months to prevent such contracture and closure; the short piece of catheter can be left lying in the vagina, its lower end strapped and anchored to the vulva with adhesive tape.

HEMATOCOLPOS

In girls with an *imperforate hymen* the uterine discharge of blood from the uterus at puberty leads to a collection of hemorrhagic material within the vagina.

Clinical Findings. These patients, eleven to thirteen years of age, have *abdominal* or *pelvic pain* which may be constant or crampy. Constitutional symptoms are absent or minimal; nausea and vomiting are rarely observed. *Tenderness* is found by rectal examination or by suprapubic midline pressure. Rectal examination discloses the ballooning of the vaginal tract.

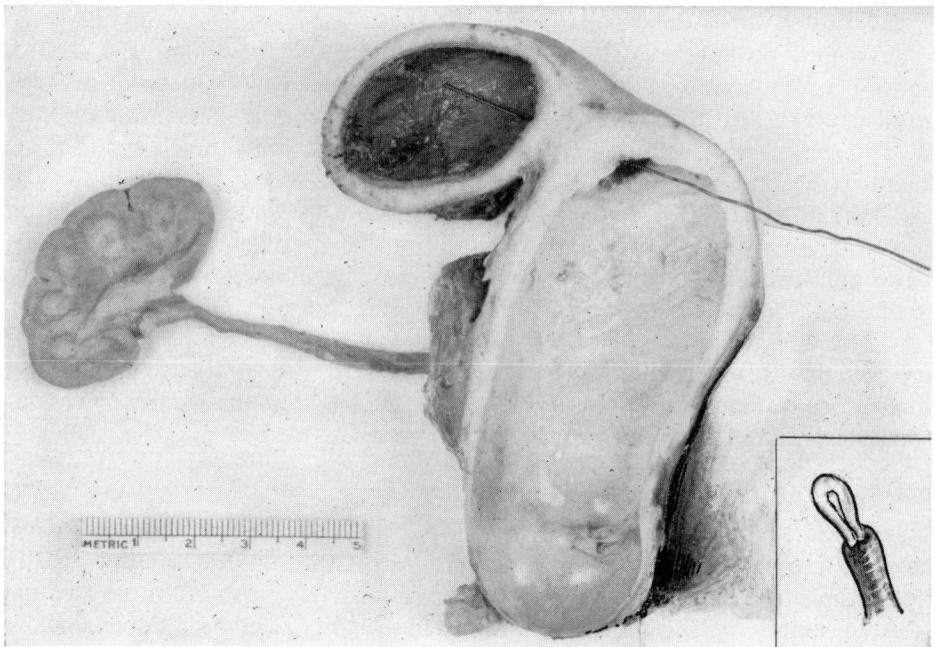

Fig. 262. Photograph of hydrometrocolpos removed at autopsy in a week-old baby. The specimen had contained mucoid fluid. The vagina and uterus are greatly distended. (For comparison, the outline at the right indicates the relative size of a uterus and vagina from a normal baby of this age.)

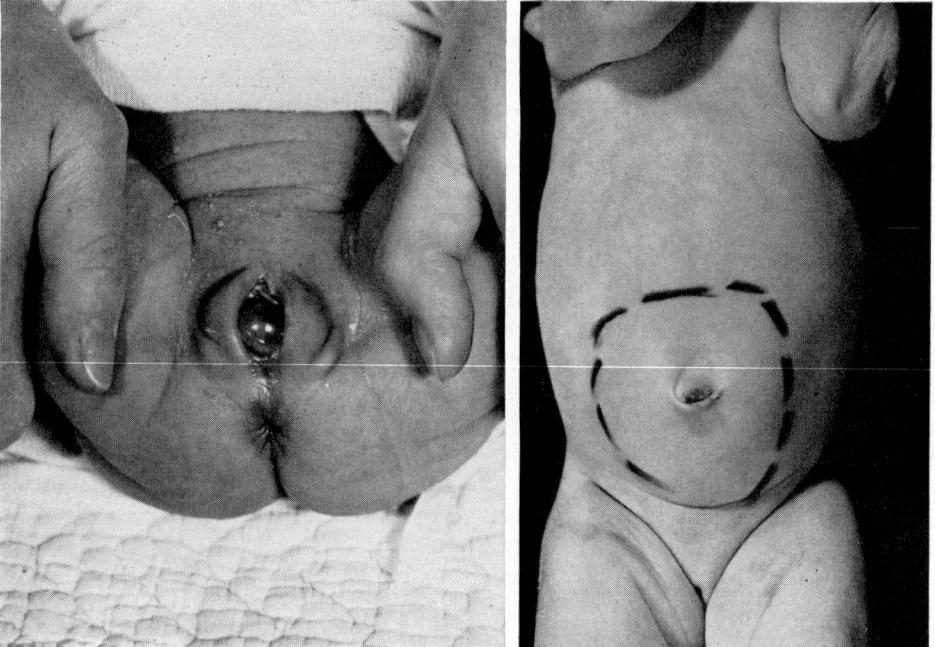

Fig. 263. *Left*, Photograph of an eighteen-day-old baby with hydrometrocolpos, showing very clearly the bulging vaginal membrane. *Right*, Photograph of a two-week-old baby with hydrometro-colpos. The pencil outlines show the extent of the palpable and enormously distended uterus.

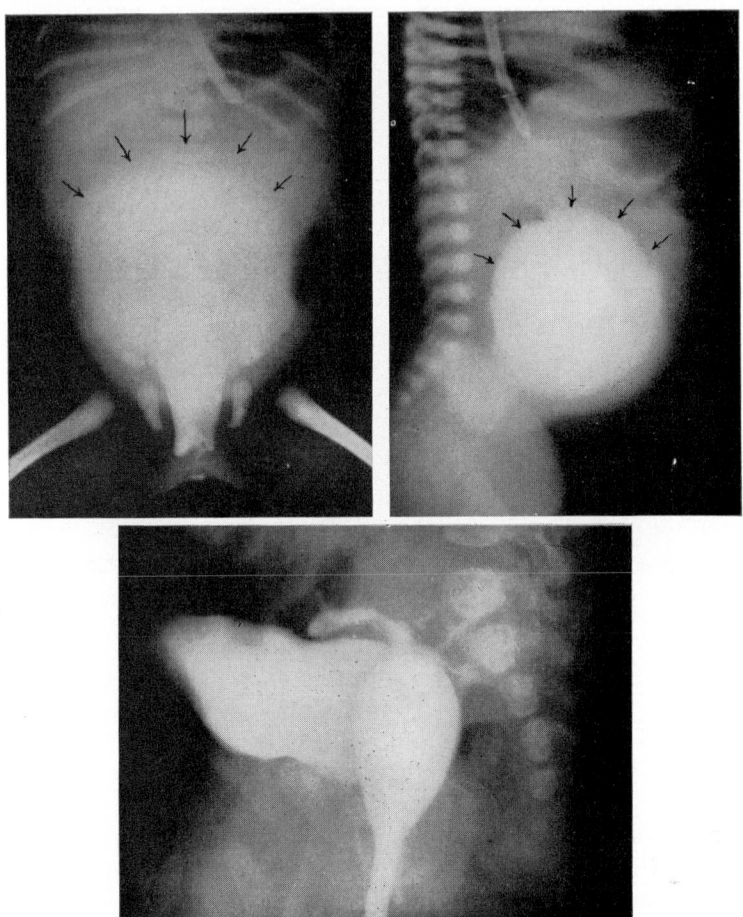

Fig. 264. *Above*, Roentgenograms of a hydrometrocolpos in a two-day-old baby made by injection of iodide into it through the vaginal membrane. (From Mahoney and Chamberlain: New England Journal of Medicine.) *Below*, Four-day-old baby with instillation of iodide into a hydrometrocolpos, showing the huge vagina and uterus.

Diagnosis. Intraperitoneal pathology, such as appendicitis, may be suspected, and it is well to remember that lower abdominal pain in a female of this age can be caused by a distended vagina. This possibility is to be especially considered if the individual has not yet menstruated but has other signs of beginning sexual maturation, such as appearance of pubic hair and enlargement of the breasts. Examination of the vaginal outlet immediately establishes the correct diagnosis (Fig. 265). The occluding vaginal membrane will be bulging and will have a dark color because of the blood which is dammed up behind it.

Treatment. A simple incision of the imperforate hymen permits escape of the entrapped fluid and brings immediate relief to the girl.

OVARIAN CYSTS

Cysts of the ovary are not uncommon prior to the age of puberty. They have been found at birth, shortly afterward, or at any period of childhood. They attract attention by intermittent *lower abdominal discomfort*, by progressive *enlargement of the abdomen*,

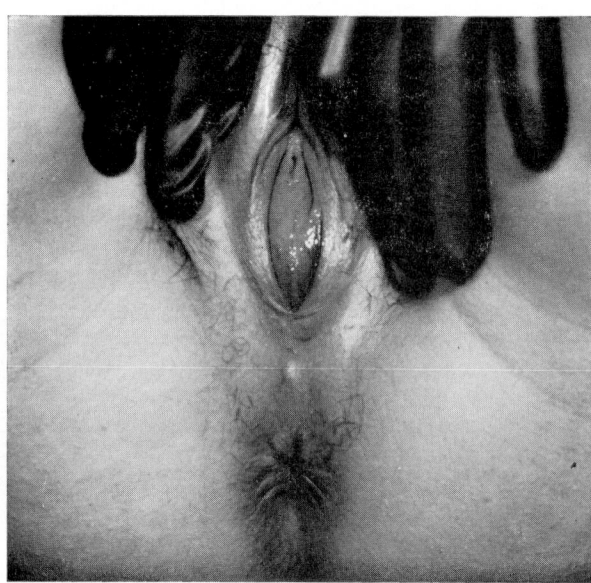

Fig. 265. Photograph of a twelve-year-old girl with hematocolpos, showing the bulging hymen.

or by acute episodes of severe *abdominal pain* resulting from torsion of the pedicle. Abdominal or rectal examination reveals a mass, which is usually not tender but which may be very much so if the cyst is twisted and infarcted. In some cases a cyst rides up out of the pelvis and is thought to originate from some other structure, such as the mesentery or omentum. Some data from 12 cases of ovarian cyst in childhood surgically treated at the Children's Hospital are summarized in Table 57.

Dermoids are more common than *simple cysts*. Dermoids contain hair, sebaceous material, teeth, or other tissues which can arise from ectoderm. When a dermoid cyst contains teeth, they can be detected by roentgenologic studies. Some pathologists feel

Table 57

Ovarian Cysts in Children

Case	Age	Type of Cyst	Size
1	6 mos.	Simple (with torsion)	16 x 13 x 11 cm. 1100 cc. of fluid
2	3 yrs.	Dermoid	1470 gm. 19 x 14 x 9 cm.
3	4 yrs.	Dermoid (with torsion)	74 gm. 6.5 cm. diameter
4	6 yrs.	Dermoid	7 x 3 x 3 cm.
5	6 yrs.	Multilocular (with torsion)	6.5 x 4 x 3 cm.
6	8 yrs.	Dermoid	6.5 x 7 x 4 cm.
7	9 yrs.	Dermoid	5.5 x 4 x 4 cm.
8	10 yrs.	Dermoid	12 x 10 x 9 cm.
9	11 yrs.	Dermoid (with torsion)	10 x 7.5 x 6.5 cm.
10	11 yrs.	Multilocular pseudo-mucinous	3750 gm. 30 x 18 x 18 cm.
11	12 yrs.	Dermoid (with torsion)	12 x 8 x 8 cm.
12	13 yrs.	Simple	4 cm.

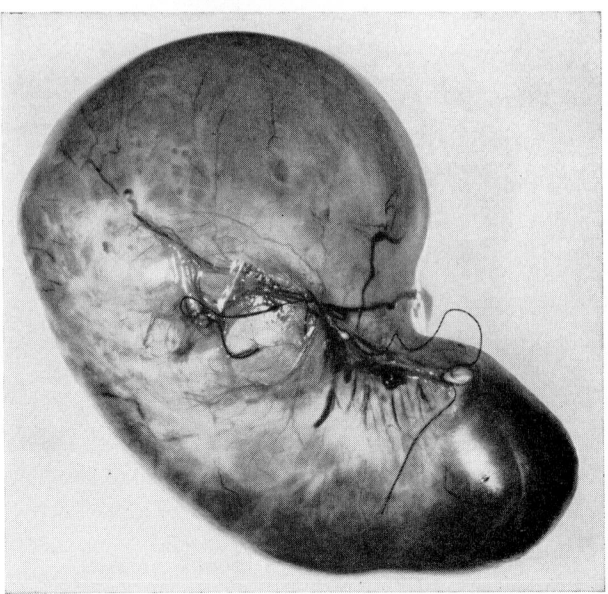

Fig. 266. Pseudomucinous cyst of the ovary, weighing 3750 gm., from an eleven-year-old girl.

that if a sufficient number of microscopic sections are taken for study from dermoid cysts, elements of all three germ layers can be found and hence they are all essentially teratomas.

Simple cysts are filled with serous fluid; only rarely are they mucinous. Cysts are generally monolocular, seldom are they multilocular.

NEOPLASMS OF THE OVARY

Many examples of ovarian neoplasms in girls have been recorded in the literature. Of all the tumors and cysts of ovarian origin which have been described, roughly 35 per cent are malignant neoplasms, about 50 per cent are dermoids or benign teratomas, and about 15 per cent are simple cysts. Data from 13 cases of ovarian neoplasm from the Children's Hospital material are listed in Table 58.

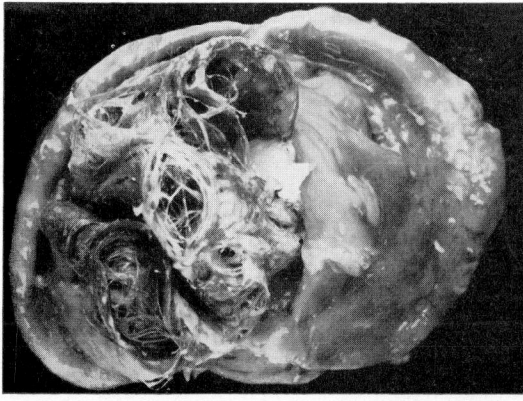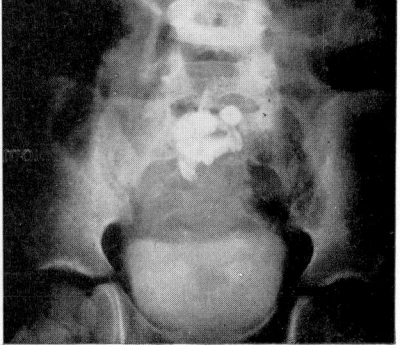

Fig. 267. *Left,* Dermoid cyst of the ovary removed from an eight-year-old girl. *Right,* Roentgenogram from a four-year-old girl showing teeth in a dermoid cyst of the ovary.

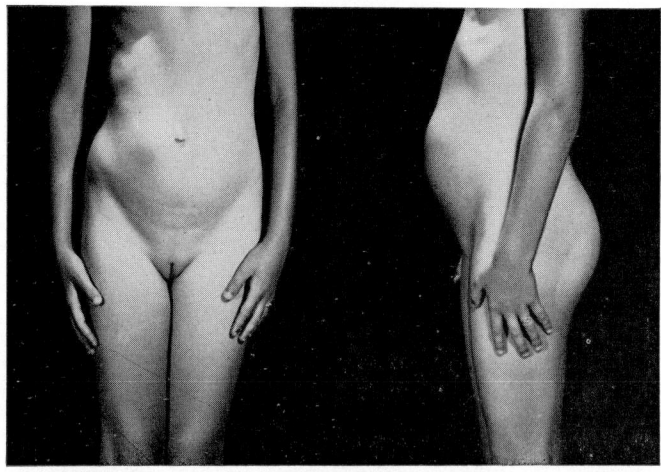

Fig. 268. Abdominal swelling in a nine-year-old girl who was found to have bilateral teratomas of the ovaries. (See Fig. 269.)

Sarcoma

Sarcoma of the ovary is one of the rarest of malignant tumors in this age group. It proliferates rapidly and tends to metastasize early. In fortunate cases the incidental discovery of the mass during an abdominal examination, or the torsion and infarction of the growth, has led to early detection, excision, and permanent cure.

Teratomas

Teratomas are not uncommon. They are well encapsulated. They may be largely composed of sebaceous material, but microscopic study of the solid portions shows other forms of tissue which indicate a derivation from ectoderm, mesoderm, and ento-

Table 58

Ovarian Neoplasms in Children, Occurring in the Children's Hospital

Case	Age	Type of Growth	Size	Postoperative Result
1	13 mos.	Granulosa cell carcinoma	15 x 11.5 x 12 cm.	No recurrence 4 yrs. later
2	19 mos.	Thecoma	7 x 5 x 5 cm.	No recurrence 21 yrs. later
3	5 yrs.	Fibrosarcoma (torsion)	11 x 6 x 4 cm.	No recurrence 10 yrs. later
4	5 yrs.	Adenocarcinoma	12 x 9 x 6 cm.	No recurrence 3 yrs. later
5	5 yrs.	Granulosa cell carcinoma	418 gm. 16 x 9.5 x 7 cm.	No recurrence 3 yrs. later
6	6 yrs.	Teratoma	5 x 4 x 4 cm.	No recurrence 14 yrs. later
7	9 yrs.	Bilateral cystic teratomas	Rt: 8 x 12 x 16 cm. Lt: 11 x 8 x 7 cm.	No recurrence in 3 mos.
8	10 yrs.	Malignant teratoma	1500+ gm.	Metastases in 3 mos.
9	10 yrs.	Carcinoma	Inoperable	Died 1 mo. later
10	11 yrs.	Teratoma	2055 gm.	No recurrence in 7 yrs.
11	11 yrs.	Adenocarcinoma	700 gm.	Metastases. Death in 6 mos·
12	11 yrs.	Teratoma	?	Metastases. Died in 5 mos.
13	11 yrs.	Dysgerminoma	2060 gm. 22 x 14 x 10.5 cm.	No recurrence 2 yrs. later

derm. Abortive teeth or bones can be frequently identified by roentgenologic examination of the abdomen. These lesions vary considerably in size; they may become extremely large and still retain rather benign features. In some, excision is followed by a permanent cure, in others surgery is followed by recurrence and metastasis.

Carcinoma

Carcinoma is the most common solid tumor of the ovary in childhood. It has most of the characteristics found in such neoplasms in women. The lesion is usually unilateral. It is apt to be solid, though portions may be cystic or necrotic. While growth is rapid, encapsulation may exist for a considerable period of time, a fact which enhances

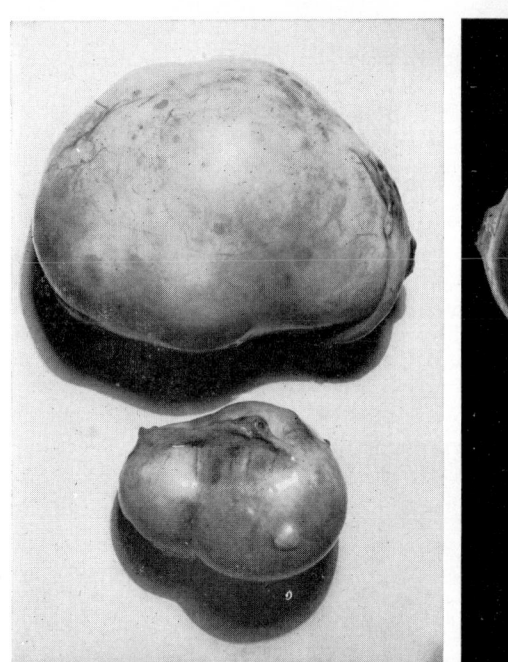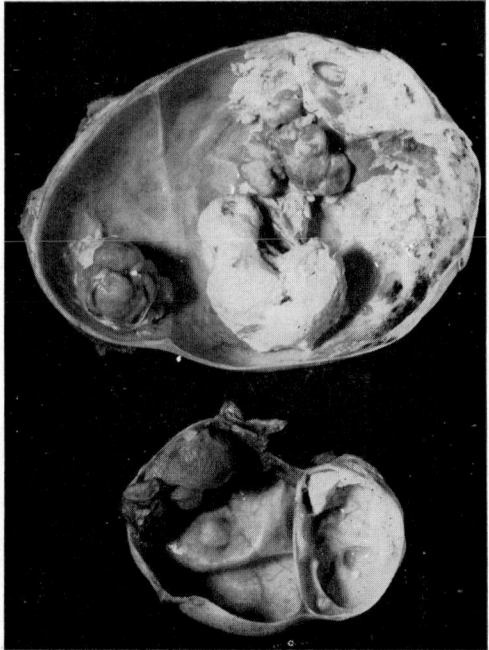

Fig. 269. Bilateral teratomas of the ovaries removed from a nine-year-old girl.

the possibility of cure if early removal can be performed. These tumors may be an *embryonal* type of epithelioma, a more slowly growing *adenocarcinoma*, or even the more highly differentiated *granulosa cell* neoplasm. With the latter type so much estrogenic substance may be produced that menstrual periods appear, breasts develop, and the bone growth is ahead of normal.

Clinical Findings in Ovarian Tumor

Clinical features of ovarian tumors are those of an enlarging lower abdominal or pelvic mass which may or may not be fixed. *Pain* is rare unless torsion has occurred or peritoneal implantations have taken place. *Sexual precocity* (Figs. 270 and 271) and *uterine bleeding* appear if the neoplasm produces sufficient amounts of estrogenic substance. In patients 1 and 5 (Table 58) there had been slight development of the breasts and some menstrual flow. While a few functioning tumors in the adult may be so small that they cannot be felt in the abdomen, or with bimanual palpation, as a general rule sexual precocity in a female child should not be regarded as arising from

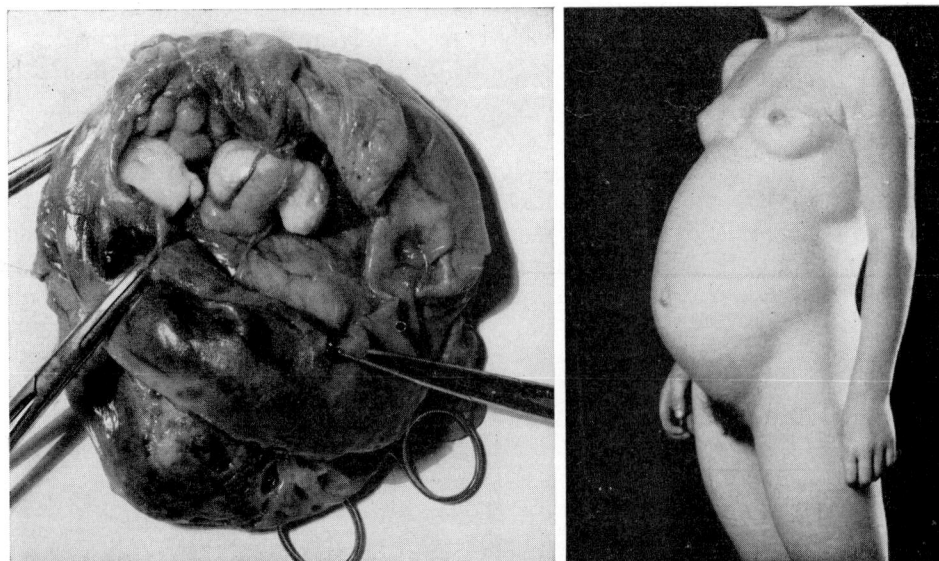

Fig. 270. *Left*, A granulosa cell carcinoma of the ovary from a thirteen-month-old child, showing cystic portions and the internal pedunculated solid tissue. This baby entered the hospital because of uterine bleeding. (Urinary excretion of 17,500 international units per 24 hours before operation.) *Right*, Photograph of a seven-year-old girl with granulosa cell carcinoma of the ovary, showing pubic hair, enlargement of the breasts, and advanced physical development. (From Bland and Goldstein: Surgery, Gynecology and Obstetrics, vol. 61.)

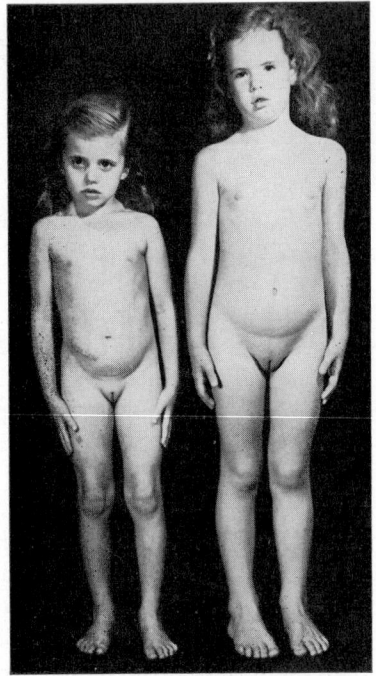

Fig. 271. Photograph of five-year-old girl (*right*) who had a granulosa cell tumor of the ovary; some enlargement of the breasts and areola for six months, and menstruation for two weeks. Her bone age was advanced (four years beyond her chronological age). She is considerably larger than the five-year-old girl (*left*) placed here for comparison.

an ovarian neoplasm unless a pelvic mass can be felt by combined (rectal and abdominal) palpation. In short, if an ovarian tumor in a child is large enough to give endocrine disturbance, it can always be felt.

Treatment

If physical examination and roentgenologic study do not demonstrate metastases, *exploration* should always be performed, because the neoplasm may be a comparatively benign teratoma or else a malignant growth with an unbroken capsule. In either situation the chances of complete cure are better than has been generally supposed.

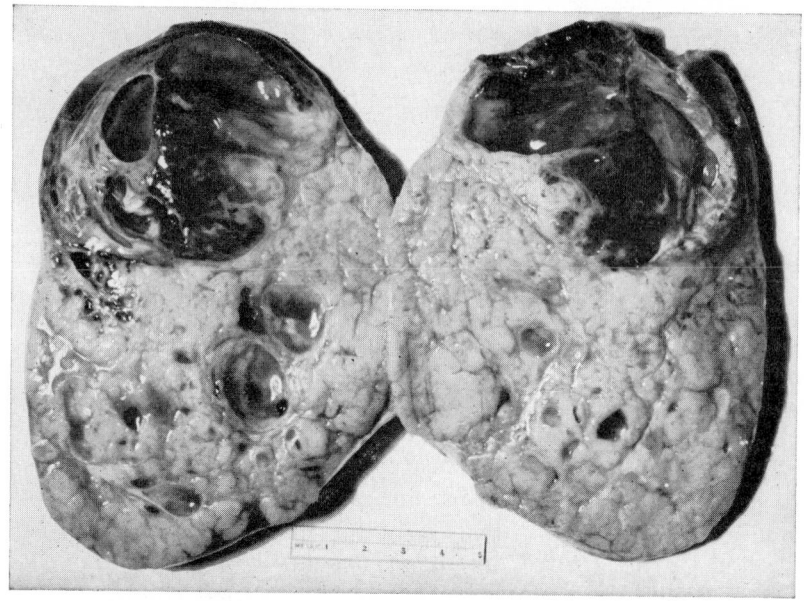

Fig. 272. Granulosa cell carcinoma of the ovary, removed from a five-year-old girl (Fig. 271). Patient alive and well three years later.

When a malignant ovarian neoplasm has been found at operation and has been apparently completely removed, the question arises whether *x-ray irradiation* should be given postoperatively over the abdomen and pelvis as a precautionary measure. We customarily withold postoperative irradiation because it will permanently sterilize and will prevent the full maturation of the individual. If malignant cells have been left in the operative field, x-rays will probably not destroy all of them; if neoplasm has not been left, x-ray treatment is superfluous and will bring on the detrimental effects of destruction of the remaining ovary.

NEOPLASMS OF THE UTERUS OR VAGINA

Sarcoma Botryoides

Fortunately rare, but yet representing a definite and easily recognizable entity, are those highly malignant tumors of the uterus and vagina which occur in children and especially in babies. Rhabdomyosarcomas are of extreme malignancy. They present themselves as a bunch of colorless, grape-like, cystic masses extruding from the vaginal outlet which at first appearance may seem to be innocuous. These multi-cystic lumps can be curretted out of the vagina on many occasions, usually without much bleeding,

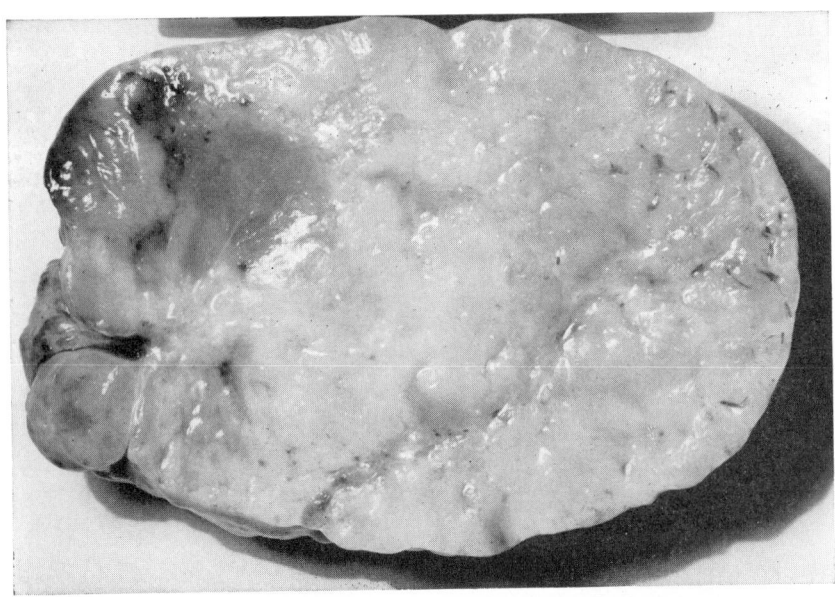

Fig. 273. Dysgerminoma removed from an eleven-year-old girl.

only to be followed in a few weeks or months by prompt recurrence. Within a short time thereafter, the neoplasm grows wildly, invades pelvic organs and intra-abdominal structures, killing by extensions which can be widely disseminated but which are generally found mostly within the abdomen. Roentgen therapy has practically no effect in limiting the growth of these neoplasms. Surgery, early and extensive, holds the only hope of cure.

Ulfelder and Quan[19] treated this highly malignant tumor by hysterocolpectomy; the child was alive and free of neoplasm five years later.[18] Schackman[17] treated a three-

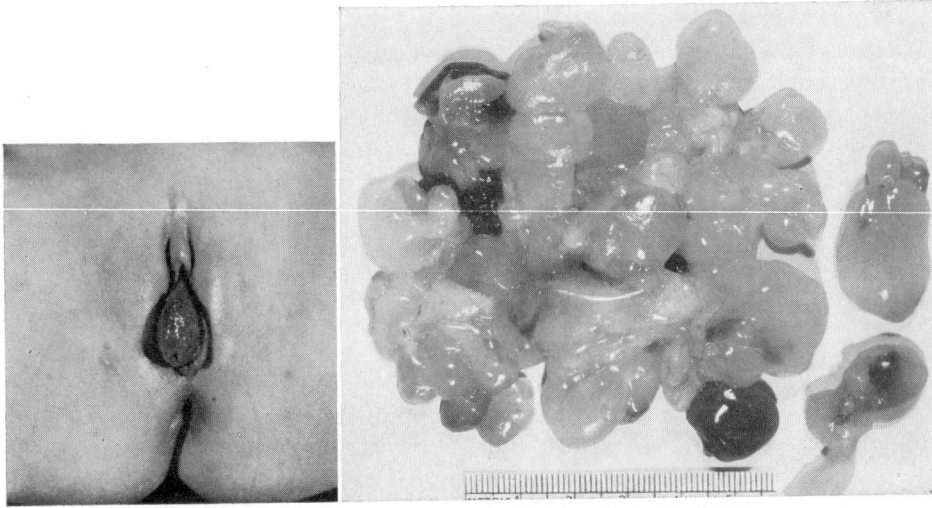

Fig. 274. *Left*, Photograph of cystic mass protruding from vagina of a two-year-old girl; highly malignant rhabdomyosarcoma. *Right*, Grape-like tumor (sarcoma botryoides) which extruded from vagina of a two-year-old girl with highly malignant rhabdomyosarcoma of uterus.

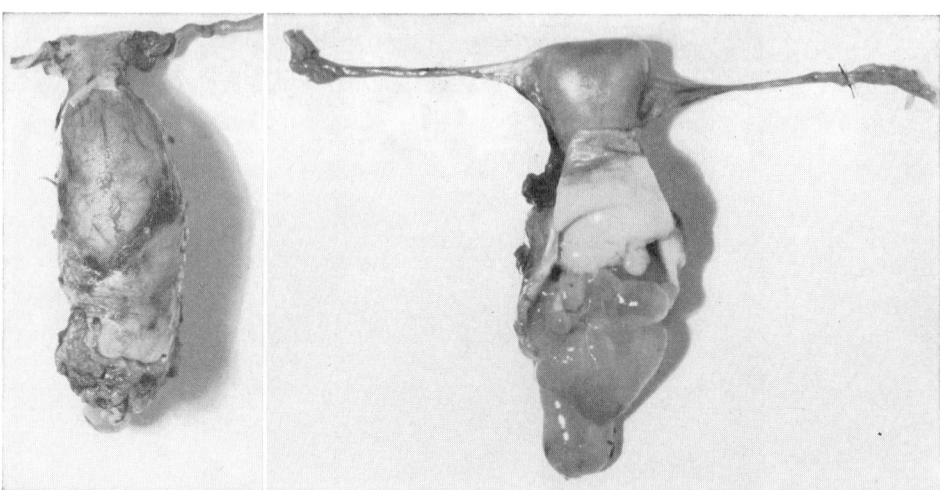

Fig. 275. Malignant rhabdomyosarcoma removed from a sixteen-month-old girl, by combined abdomino-perineal excision (in one mass) of tubes, uterus, and vagina. *Left*, Specimen unopened. *Right*, Vagina cut open to show the grape-like tumor which filled the cavity. (See Fig. 276.)

year-old girl by transplanting the ureters into the sigmoid, and at the same operation excising in one lump (through a long incision extending from the navel down into the perineum) the vulva, vagina, uterus, urethra, and bladder together with the right pubic ramus. The child was in excellent condition and without evidence of recurrence two

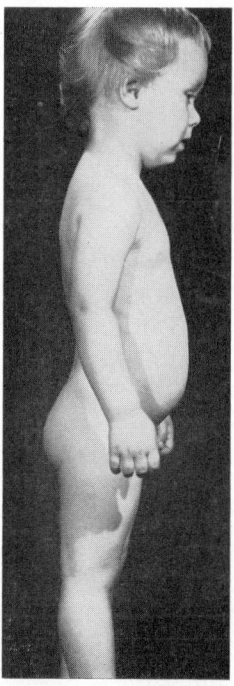

Fig. 276. Photograph of four-year-old girl, two and one-half years after removal of uterus and entire vagina for rhabdomyosarcoma of the uterus (Fig. 275). She is apparently cured of the neoplasm.

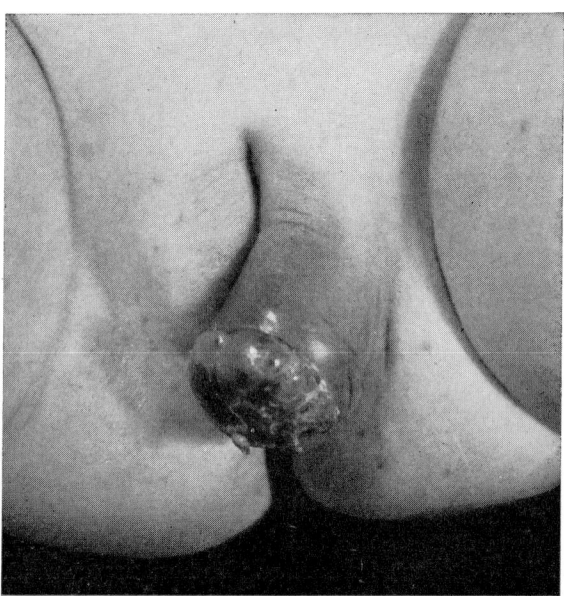

Fig. 277   Thirteen-month-old child with rhabdomyosarcoma of the vulva. (Removal was followed by pulmonary metastases.)

and one-half years later. We have treated 6 of these children, ranging from one to three years of age, by inadequate excision; all have had subsequent recurrence and extension, and death. More recently we have treated a sixteen-month-old girl by one-stage removal of the uterus and entire vagina (leaving the ovaries). The vaginal orifice was dissected free from the labia majora, leaving the urethral meatus undisturbed. The cuff of vaginal orifice, thus freed, was sewed closed and the uterus and vagina were removed in toto (Fig. 275), without opening into either of these, employing a combined abdominal and perineal approach. The child is in excellent health, without evidence of recurrence three years later (Fig. 276).

VAGINITIS

Vaginitis is occasionally found in young girls and has been described in epidemic form in foundling homes where there are inferior toilet facilities and poor hygienic care. Gonococcal vaginitis and purulent discharge is uncommon but yet is a well recognized entity.

Foreign bodies of various sorts may be introduced by a child into her vagina; their presence is often unsuspected until persistent discharge leads to an adequate vaginal examination. Such foreign objects can usually be felt by rectal examination.

Most cases of vaginitis in children will permanently subside with proper attention to local *cleanliness*, occasional vaginal *irrigations*, and possibly instillation of mild *antiseptics* such as aqueous Zephiran (which can be given by inserting a small catheter into the vagina and flushing the solution through this). If local irritation has been produced by a *foreign body*, the removal of this object is the principal therapeutic measure which is necessary. If gonococcal infection is recognized by examination of a smear, systemic treatment by intensive penicillin therapy is specific. In all inflammatory lesions of the vulva or vagina, hot sitz baths, once or twice a day, are beneficial.

REFERENCES

HYDROMETROCOLPOS

1. Cranwell, D. J.: Congenital Hydrocolpos. Rev. de gynéc. et de chir. abd., 9:635, 1905
2. Mahoney, P. J. and Chamberlain, J. W.: Hydrometrocolpos in Infancy. Congenital Atresia of the Vagina with Abnormally Abundant Cervical Secretions. J Pediat., 17:772, 1940.
3. Spencer, H. F.: Imperforate Hymen in a Baby. Lancet, 1:823, 1916.

HEMATOCOLPOS

4. Calvin, J. K. and Nichamin, S. J.: Hematocolpos Due to Imperforate Hymen. Am. J. Dis. Child., 51:832, 1936.
5. Tompkins, P.: Treatment of Imperforate Hymen with Hematocolpos; Review of 113 Cases in Literature with Report of Five Additional Cases. J.A.M.A., 113:913, 1939.

OVARIAN CYSTS AND NEOPLASMS

6. Bland, P. B. and Goldstein, L.: Granulosa Cell and Brenner Tumors of the Ovary. Surg., Gynec. & Obst., 61:250, 1935.
7. Costin, M. E., Jr., and Kennedy, R. L. J.: Ovarian Tumors in Infants and Children. Am. J. Dis. Child., 76:127, 1948.
8. Dargeon, H. W.: Ovarian Tumors in Childhood. Pediatrics, 3:773, 1949.
9. Gordon, V. H. and Marvin, H. N.: Theca-cell Tumor of Ovary in Child One Year of Age with Review of the Literature. J. Pediat., 39:133, 1951.
10. Gross, R. E.: Neoplasms Producing Endocrine Disturbances in Childhood. Am. J. Dis. Child., 59:579, 1940.
11. Mayo, C. W. and Butsch, W. L.: Ovarian Tumors Among Young Girls. Minnesota Med., 21:256, 1938.
12. Mazzola, V. P. and Ryan L. M.: Dermoid Cyst of Ovary in Child 5 Years Old with Comments on Value of X-ray in Diagnosis. Am. J. Obst. & Gynec., 35:696, 1938.
13. Pray, L. G.: Sexual Precocity in Females. Report of Two Cases, with Arrest of Precocity in the McCune-Albright Syndrome After Removal of a Cystic Ovary. Pediatrics, 8:684, 1951.
14. Schaeffer, M. H. and Cancelmo, J. J.: Cavernous Hemangioma of Ovary in Girl 12 Years of Age. Am. J. Obst. & Gynec., 38:722, 1939.
15. Trout, H. F. and Marchetti, A. A.: A Consideration of So-called "Granulosa" and "Theca" Cell Tumors of the Ovary. Surg., Gynec. & Obst., 70:632, 1940.
16. Wilkins, L.: The Diagnosis and Treatment of Endocrine Disorders in Childhood and Adolescence. Charles C Thomas, Springfield, Illinois, 1950, Chapters IX and X.

NEOPLASMS OF UTERUS AND VAGINA

17. Shackman, R.: Sarcoma Botryoides of the Genital Tract in Female Children. Brit. J. Surg., 38:26, 1950.
18. Ulfelder, H.: Personal Communication.
19. Ulfelder, H. and Quan, S. H.: Sarcoma Botryoides Vaginae. Complete Excision of the Tumor in an Infant by the Combined Abdominal and Perineal Approach. S. Clin. North America, 27:1240, 1947.

VAGINITIS

20. Burpee, C. M., Robinow, M. and Leslie, J. T.: Gonorrhoeal Vaginitis in Girls Treated with Estrone (Theelin), Fever, and Sulfanilamide. Am. J. Dis. Child., 57:1, 1939.
21. Hoffman, S. J., Schneider M., Blatt, M. L. and Herrold, R. D.: Sulfanilamide in Treatment of Gonorrheal Vulvovaginitis. J.A.M.A., 110:1541, 1938.
22. Jacoby, A., Madonia, D. E., Till, S. M. and Wood, T. H.: Treatment of Gonococcal Vaginitis by Estrogenic Hormone. Am. J. Obst. & Gynec., 38:140, 1939.
23. Schauffler, G. C., Kanzler, R. and Schauffler, C.: Management of 256 Cases of Infection of Immature Vagina; Practical Deductions with Study of Use of Sulfanilamide in Treatment. J.A.M.A., 112:411, 1939.

CHAPTER 41

Obstructive Jaundice in Infancy

Obstructive jaundice in the early months of life can arise from four different conditions. (1) There may be erythroblastosis fetalis, excessive destruction of red cells, and a temporary blockage of the biliary ducts by pigment debris. (2) There may be blockage of the ductal system from inspissated mucus or bile, in the absence of erythroblastosis. (3) Rarely, there may be pressure on the extra-biliary ducts by enlarged lymph nodes or by neoplasm. (4) By far the most common of all, there may be atresia of the intra-hepatic or extra-hepatic bile ducts. In the first two categories the biliary obstruction may be complete or partial, it may be constant or intermittent, it may relieve itself spontaneously, or it may require the employment of cholagogues or even surgical flushing of the biliary passages. In the third and fourth categories, in which there is a complete block (atresia) of some part (or all) of the biliary passages, medical therapy has nothing to offer in the relief of jaundice; the only hope for cure lies in surgical exploration, looking for the small percentage of cases in which it is possible to find some situation which can be relieved by operative means.

Congenital obstruction of the bile ducts will always be associated with the name of John Thomson for his careful analysis of 50 cases in 1892.[13] However, it was the detailed study of more than 100 examples of biliary anomalies by Holmes in 1916[5] that called attention to the fact that many of these babies presented conditions which might be correctable by surgical means. Following the publication of Holmes' work, we began to explore routinely all infants with such pathology. In 1927 operation was first performed successfully by Ladd for the relief of congenital atresia of the bile ducts.

It was the contention of earlier writers that relief of biliary obstruction—when it was possible—would be a futile procedure because the extensive *biliary cirrhosis* which is generally present would militate against full recovery of the patient. We have now learned that this is not true, for babies with such cirrhosis have been given operative relief of biliary obstruction for periods as long as twenty-four years and have not developed hepatic insufficiency. Considerable evidence has now accumulated to show that the liver has extraordinary powers of regeneration; if biliary obstruction can be relieved, the liver can heal in an astounding manner and can perform all of its physiologic functions in a completely satisfactory way.

In many reports the emphasis on treatment of obstructive jaundice in infancy has been placed on the absorption of fats, the digestion of food, and the various other chemical and digestive problems that occur as a result of the absence of bile from the intestinal tract. Although such considerations are important, they are greatly overshadowed by the therapeutic possibilities of relieving the biliary obstruction by surgery in about one-quarter of the cases. The following remarks are based almost entirely on the Children's Hospital material, in which 198 babies with obstructive jaundice have been treated by medical or surgical means.

DIFFERENTIAL DIAGNOSIS

When the clinician is faced with a jaundiced baby, the first problem is concerned with determining whether there is jaundice on the basis of: (1) The several conditions which can occur in the first month of life which are not primarily diseases of the liver; (2) hepatitis, which in recent years seems to be of increasing incidence and importance; or (3) one of the obstructive types of jaundice which are listed in the first paragraph of this chapter.

Icterus Neonatorum can usually be ruled out without difficulty. The jaundice usually diminishes by the end of the second week of life and has certainly disappeared by the end of the first month. Such an infant does not have hepatic enlargement, acholic stools, or heavily pigmented urine, all of which are found in cases of biliary obstruction.

Erythroblastosis Fetalis, sometimes classified under the name of *icterus gravis* or *erythroblastic anemia*, may present a clinical picture partially simulating that of biliary obstruction. The jaundice may be of like intensity, the liver may be of equal or greater size, and it is common to have an associated splenomegaly. A golden-colored vernix caseosa and a hypertrophied placenta should make the obstetrician suspect the presence of erythroblastosis. The findings of an anemia of marked degree and a large number of immature red cells, including nucleated forms, are important factors in recognizing the disease. The condition is produced by anti-Rh factors built up by an Rh-negative mother to a Rh-positive baby; these antibodies cross the placenta and reside in the child in sufficient concentration to destroy the baby's circulating red cells. Erythroblastosis can be readily recognized by accurate hematologic study of the mother and child, by a positive Coombs' test on the baby, by the baby's blood picture, and by finding from time to time that some small amounts of bile get through into the stools. The condition may be mild and self-limited since the antibodies become washed out of the baby's system in a month or two. In some cases the condition is so severe that it rapidly leads to fatality if the hematologic disorder is not recognized and treated promptly. Most of these babies can now be satisfactorily treated by "exchange transfusions," the purpose of which is to reduce quickly the baby's circulating antibodies, and thereby abate the hemolytic process. Erythroblastosis fetalis can be accompanied by serious liver damage. It can also be followed by plugging of the biliary drainage system to such a degree that some relief, either by cholagogues or by surgical flushing, becomes necessary.

Jaundice of Sepsis can appear from an overwhelming bacteremia, the causative organism most commonly being a *hemolytic streptococcus* or the *colon bacillus*. While jaundice may be intense there are also signs which point to the presence of infection, such as fever, leukocytosis, progressive anemia, and positive blood cultures. It is important to point out that an overwhelming infection in a small infant may show no febrile reaction, yet such babies have a profound toxicity which is not found in individuals with biliary obstruction. Patients with hemolytic sepsis do not have acholic stools or bile-stained urine.

Congenital Syphilis should be mentioned in the differential diagnosis, but it is rarely a source of confusion. A careful maternal history, a Wassermann test on the mother and child, and roentgenologic studies of the long bones usually give sufficient data to rule out syphilis as a cause of hepatic enlargement and jaundice.

Hepatitis, the origin of which is sometimes completely obscure, is not uncommon in small babies. It is much less common than the biliary obstructions in the same age group. It can generally be recognized by abnormalities in one or several tests, as the cephalin flocculation test, the bromsulphalein retention test, a reduced prothrombin level of the serum, or a lowered serum protein. In addition, the child appears to be more ill than is generally the case with biliary obstruction, and the stools are seldom acholic. While it is important to recognize the baby with hepatitis and to avoid surgery therein because of the disastrous consequence sometimes incurred by anesthesia and exploration, the fact remains that in an occasional case the clinical and laboratory pictures are very bizarre and it is virtually impossible to make an accurate differential diagnosis without surgical exploration of the ducts and biopsy of the liver.

As a general working rule, it may be stated that if one delays in making a positive diagnosis of congenital biliary obstruction until the infant is four to six weeks of age, the chance of error is not great. Generally, it is better not to operate upon patients with biliary obstruction before the end of the first month. Nothing is lost by this delay, and the assurance of a more accurate diagnosis is gained.

BILIARY OBSTRUCTION FROM ERYTHROBLASTOSIS

Erythroblastosis fetalis, particularly in its more severe forms, is often accompanied by jaundice. This may result from: (1) An extremely rapid breakdown of red cells, the pigment of which cannot be cleared from the blood stream promptly by even a normal liver; (2) a derangement of the liver itself, with pathologic changes therein, the exact nature of which is poorly understood; or (3) a plugging of the bile ducts by pigment debris which has accumulated from the enormous destruction of red cells. This latter condition apparently occurs with considerable frequency; it generally requires no specific therapy since the ducts tend to become flushed out spontaneously. In an occasional patient the obstruction is of such degree or duration that active measures must be taken—by medical or surgical means—to dislodge the material.

To recognize the underlying erythroblastosis usually does not present any serious problem. To determine whether any accompanying jaundice is due to hepatic damage or to accumulations within the ducts may be exceedingly difficult even with a battery of liver function tests and with repeated examinations of the stools, looking for the presence or absence of bile. When jaundice is largely on the basis of ductal obstruction, one is dealing with a child in the period after the blood picture has largely corrected itself (or has been corrected by transfusions). The jaundice is of mild or only moderate degree. The stools may at times be quite white, but on other days they do have considerable yellowish color and also positive tests for bile. *Intermittency* is generally an outstanding feature of the degree of jaundice and the intensity of color in the stools. There is no sharp borderline between the milder cases which in time will correct themselves and the more severe cases which should call for active measures in relief of the partial biliary obstruction. In general, there is little need for hurry, and it is permissible to let several weeks or more pass before instituting specific measures for increasing the biliary flow. Little or no damage is incurred by this policy; it will avoid operation for some patients who can in time clear the ducts themselves.

Medical and surgical therapy are discussed in a following section.

OBSTRUCTIVE JAUNDICE FROM INSPISSATED BILE OR MUCUS IN THE BILIARY PASSAGES

Infants with obstruction of the biliary passages from inspissated mucus or bile have jaundice which appears in the first few weeks of life and which may be present at birth. The jaundice may reach a high intensity. Nutrition is usually well maintained, but there may be some slight intolerance to fat. The *stools* are clay-colored or white, and have a puttylike consistency. The *urine* is deeply colored with pigments. Some *bleeding tendency* may be in evidence, though this is not the rule.

Generally, the histories of these babies closely simulate those of babies who have congenital obliteration of the bile ducts. In a few cases, however, one finds that the jaundice has *changed* in intensity from time to time, and that on some occasions there has been a faint green or yellow color to the stools. Therefore, a history of *jaundice of varying degree*, particularly when associated with *intermittent* appearance of bile pigments in the stool, should make one suspect partial obstruction of the ducts by inspissated mucus or bile plugs. However, it must be emphasized that a history of intermittent symptoms is not always obtained in these cases, and in many instances it is impossible to differentiate the condition from atresia of the bile ducts until the baby is explored.

The age of these infants when entering the clinic has varied from one week to three months, with an average slightly under two months. In all of them the outstanding feature has been a marked jaundice. The lowest recorded *icteric index* was 85, and the highest was 120, with an average around 100. Thus, the intensity of the jaundice cannot be used as a factor to differentiate the lesion from congenital obliteration of the bile ducts. In each case there was an *enlarged liver*, usually associated with accumulation of some intra-abdominal fluid, and in some cases the *spleen* has been palpable. In all of these babies the *stool* was acholic at the time of hospitalization (though in some instances the parent or family physician had noted some color in the stool on previous occasions).

Plugs in the biliary passages can produce important obstruction, and, indeed, can completely impede the flow of bile into the intestinal tract. With this degree of blockage, one finds in the liver most of the changes which are associated with congenital obliteration of the bile ducts. The organ is *enlarged*, quite *cirrhotic*, and is deeply *stained* with retained biliary pigments. This hepatomegaly may induce partial portal obstruction which manifests itself clinically by the accumulation of abdominal ascitic fluid and by enlargement of the spleen.

Without doubt, some of these patients have symptoms of only mild degree and spontaneously clear their ducts. Our material includes only those in whom the symptoms were of such intensity or duration that they led to hospitalization for study and treatment.

The presence of plugs in the ducts does not infer that some other serious malady exists. In a few of these patients, observations at the operating table made us feel that possibly the extra-hepatic ducts were smaller than normal; but even these, after a flushing out, have functioned quite well. While an occasional patient in this group subsequently exhibits evidence of profound disturbance of hepatic or pancreatic function which leads to serious illness or even death, about three-quarters of the babies have developed as normal children after the ducts have been washed out. Therefore, it is important to recognize and treat jaundice from inspissated material because the over-all outlook is excellent.

Methods for medical or surgical clearance of the ducts are discussed in a following section.

CONGENITAL ATRESIA OF THE BILE DUCTS

The term *atresia* is used to mean complete closure of a duct. This may be in the form of a *block* within the liver itself, in the main hepatic duct, or in the common duct. It can also be used to describe those cases in which there is obliteration of all the ducts

of the intra-hepatic or the extra-hepatic system. The position and extent of such obliteration, of course, determines the operability in each case. If the atresia is in the lower
part of the hepatic duct or anywhere in the common duct, there remains above this
point a small bulbous enlargement of the ductal system which can be anastomosed to
the alimentary tract. The positions and extents of obliteration as found in 146 babies

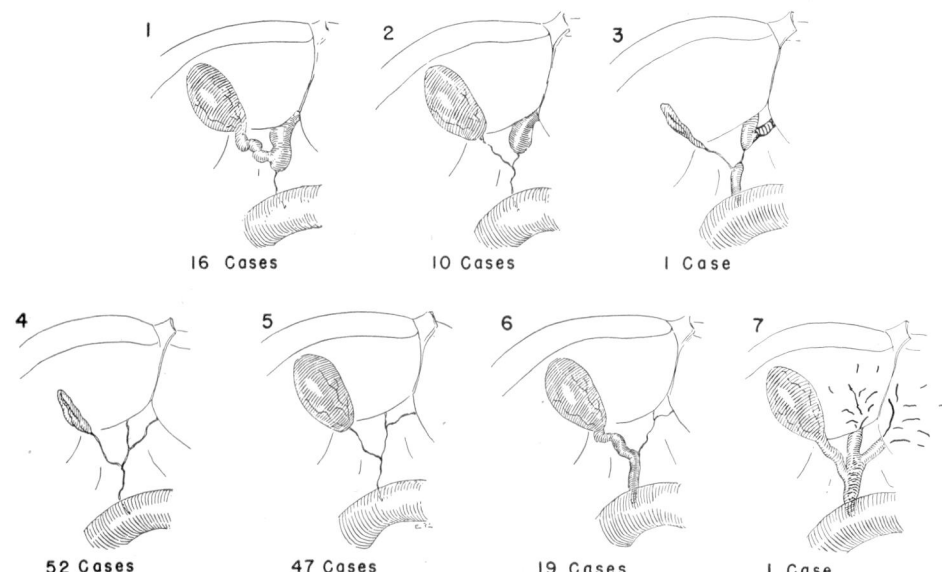

Fig. 278. Sketches of types of atresia of the bile ducts, with frequency thereof, as found in surgical
exploration of cases. 1. Hepatic duct, cystic duct, and gallbladder patent. Common duct obliterated.
2. Hepatic duct patent, other extra-hepatic ducts obliterated, gallbladder normal. 3. Hepatic duct
patent in its upper portion, but atretic below. Common duct patent. Gallbladder atretic. 4. Gallbladder and all ducts atretic. 5. Gallbladder containing mucoid material, all ducts atretic. 6. Hepatic
duct atretic. Gallbladder connects with duodenum. 7. All extra-hepatic structures normal. There is
atresia of the intra-hepatic ducts. The conditions in the upper row are operable, those in the lower
row are inoperable.

we have operated upon are summed up in Figure 278. Of these 146 patients, 27 had a
condition which presumably could be remedied by some anastomotic procedure; thus
18 per cent could be termed "operable."

Gallbladder

The gallbladder may be found in one of several states: (1) It may be completely
atretic and may be represented by only a cord of fibrous tissue 3 or 4 mm. thick and
2 or 3 cm. in length. (2) It can contain a *lumen*, yet be so small that it is not more than
7 or 8 mm. in diameter and 2 or 3 cm. in length. Such a gallbladder usually contains a
little clear mucoid material. (3) (Very rare.) It may be quite large and tensely filled with
accumulated *secretory products* of its own mucosal glands. Such contents may be
described as "white bile." (4) It may be relatively normal in appearance and may contain *bile*, indicating that the obstruction is in the common duct.

Liver

The liver always shows a well advanced portal *cirrhosis* of the obstructive type.
The organ is two or three times its normal size. It is very firm, and is stained a *dark-*

green color by the accumulation of bile pigments. The surface is diffusely nodular (Figs. 279 and 280). In the depressions between these nodules there is a firm, grayish, fibrous substance representing an increased amount of interlobular connective tissue. The cut surface shows further evidence of extensive cirrhosis. There is diffuse destruction of liver substance, accompanied by regeneration. The intense green color is strikingly contrasted to the light gray connective tissue which abounds in the peri-portal regions. Macroscopic enlargement of the ducts within the liver is rarely seen, in spite of the complete obstruction which has existed for many months.

Microscopic examination shows widespread degeneration of hepatic lobules and distortion of lobular architecture, accompanied by active liver-cell regeneration. In the peri-portal zones, there are usually large numbers of small bile ducts with considerable ductal regeneration and proliferation. This network of ducts is embedded in a dense fibrous tissue. There may be mild inflammatory cell reaction in these peri-portal zones, but this is not a striking feature. Biliary stasis is shown by the marked accumulation of pigments within the ductal lumina and within liver-cell cytoplasms.

Spleen

The spleen may be slightly or moderately enlarged, a change presumably dependent upon portal obstruction which is set up by the biliary cirrhosis. Further evidence of portal obstruction is exhibited by the collection of fluid within the abdominal cavity.

Etiology

Numerous theories have been proposed to explain the origin of congenital atresia of the bile ducts. It was once thought that *fetal peritonitis* produced local inflammatory reactions which were responsible for the obliterative process. The absence of adhesions or of inflammatory lesions in other parts of the abdomen in most cases tends to discredit this view.

Congenital *syphilis* has often been listed as the etiologic factor. The absence of histologic evidence of syphilis and the finding of a negative Wassermann reaction in both child and mother in most cases make it clear that congenital obliteration of the bile ducts is not the result of luetic infection.

Ylppö has pointed out that the extra-hepatic bile ducts are always patent in early fetal life, but they normally subsequently lose their lumina by epithelial concrescence, and that they become patent again at a later time. It is highly probable that an *arrest of development* during the solid stage is the proper explanation for congenital atresia of the bile ducts. Certainly this view explains the pathologic findings far better than any other theory does.

Symptoms and Signs

The outstanding symptom in congenital atresia is jaundice of a high degree. It is usually present at birth or shortly thereafter. Not uncommonly, two or three weeks elapse before there is sufficient staining of the skin or scleras to make the jaundice conspicuous. After jaundice once appears, it is persistent and progressive unless operative relief is possible. Furthermore, the intensity of the color never subsides, a point which is helpful in ruling out several other diseases.

The presence of obstruction in the extra-biliary tree implies that bile pigments are absent from the intestinal tract. Therefore, *the stools are always clay-colored or white from birth*, even though jaundice may not have been noticed until the second or third

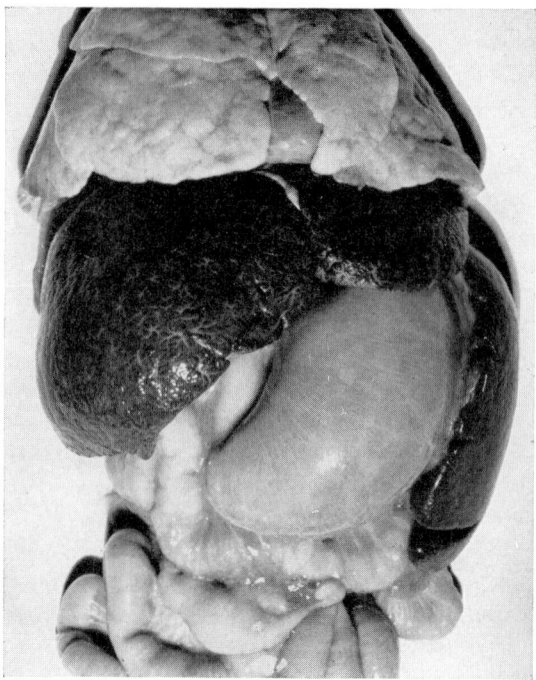

Fig. 279. Photograph taken at autopsy table to show enlargement of liver and spleen in a baby who died with inoperable atresia of the extra-hepatic ducts at five months. The liver showed marked bile stasis (green) but had only slight cirrhosis.

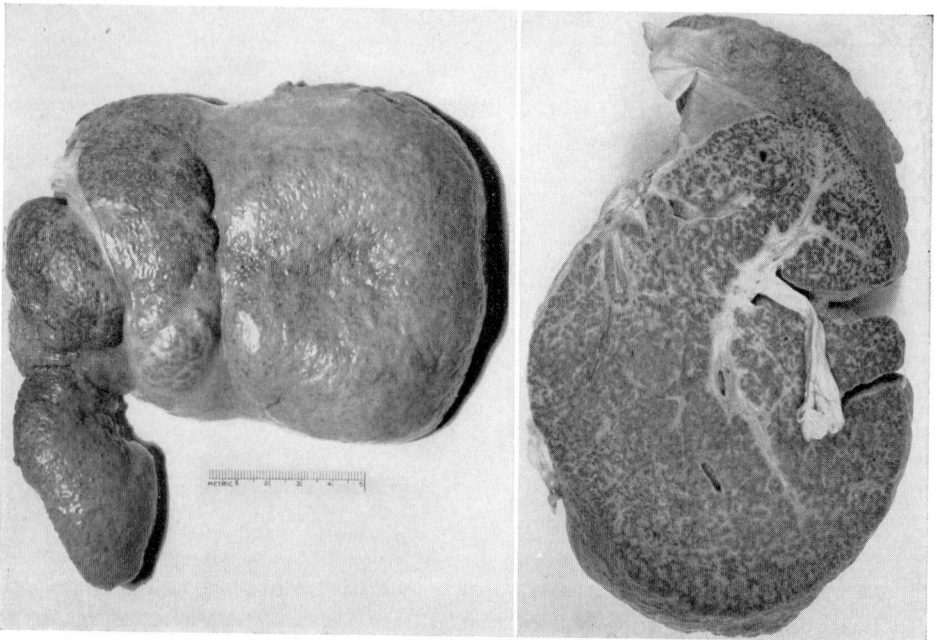

Fig. 280. Photographs of livers with typical cirrhosis from patients who died with atresia of the extra-hepatic bile ducts. The livers were dark green in color because of biliary stasis. *Left*, Child died at seventeen months. External view to show pebbly surface. *Right*, Child died at eleven months. Cut surface showing increased fibrous tissue in periportal zones. (There is no duct large enough to permit junction to the intestine by the Longmire technique.)

week of life. As the condition progresses and the child reaches an older age, there is an increasing saturation of the blood plasma and various organs of the body with excess pigment. Some of this material is excreted in small amounts by glands of the intestine and colon, so that a faint yellowish tint may be imparted to the stools. Pigments which are excreted in the stool by this route have a low concentration; the stool is putty-like in consistency and is still predominantly white in color. The presence of light-colored stools from birth onward contrasts the condition from other forms of biliary obstruction which have an intermittent character.

The *nourishment* of these babies is usually better than might be expected. The absence of bile from the intestinal tract might cause some difficulty with absorption of fats. Hence, there is usually a history that the formula has been changed on several occasions and often a fat-free or low-fat mixture has been suggested and has been better tolerated. These babies tend to be somewhat lethargic and slow in their physical movements and mental reactions. Taken as a whole, the babies are somewhat below par in their physical development, but yet nutrition may be fairly good if the child is not more than three or four months of age.

A *bleeding tendency* (because of reduced serum prothrombin) may be observed. Our cases show a striking rarity of this symptom in the babies who were less than six months old, but serious deficiencies in this regard can appear in older subjects.

The salient finding is *jaundice*, the degree of which may be appreciated by an average icteric index of 125 in our cases. The lowest icteric index we encountered was 50 and the highest was 325. When the jaundice is deep, even the tears and saliva may be yellow.

Examination of the *stool* is important, for it is strikingly whitish in color, and has a pasty or putty-like consistency. The *urine* is highly colored and gives a positive test for biliary pigments.

Fullness of the *abdomen* is produced by enlargement of the liver and by accumulation of ascitic fluid. The presenting liver edge may extend well down toward the umbilicus. The spleen may be slightly enlarged. In two cases there was *situs transversus* of all the thoracic and abdominal viscera.

The *blood* findings are usually not remarkable. There may be a slight anemia, with a red cell count rarely below 3,500,000 or 4,000,000. The clotting time may be increased to six or seven minutes, but rarely longer.

MEDICAL TREATMENT FOR BILIARY OBSTRUCTION

The introduction of concentrated magnesium sulfate into the duodenum (via a tube) can produce an increased flow of bile in those cases in which the ducts are patent but are plugged by pigment concretions or inspissated material. In one of our babies this therapy was quite effective, but in general the depressant effects on the central nervous system, or the purging action on the alimentary tract, is so marked that this material has been abandoned as a cholagogue.

Within recent years Dr. Paul Patterson in our clinic has shown great interest in the study and medical treatment of babies with biliary obstruction. In his hands, the use of certain choleretics has been very helpful, and without doubt a flow of bile has been obtained in some babies who in previous years would have been subjected to surgical exploration. While his failures have been many, the number of cases with successful medical treatment now makes us feel that it is probably advisable to attempt the use of cholagogues in all babies having biliary obstruction before resorting to surgical therapy. The methods employed are as follows:

A duodenal tube is put in place and duodenal fluid collected for determination of bile content. If none, or reduced amount, is present, 5 cc. of Decholin* (20 per cent solution of sodium dehydrocholic acid) is given intravenously (2 cc. for patients weighing less than 8 pounds). Fluid collected by the tube is observed for at least one and one-half hours afterward for the appearance of bile, and the tube then removed. The Decholin injections are repeated three times per week. For infants under two months of age, a one-week trial is sufficient. For older infants (seven to nine months) three weeks may be required. Orally, 250 mg. of Ketochol† (desiccated bile salts) is given with each feeding (125 mg. for infants under 8 pounds). The dosage of Ketochol is maintained (even though bile has been subsequently demonstrated in the duodenal fluid and Decholin has been stopped) unless vomiting or diarrhea has occurred or the patient's jaundice has practically disappeared. If these materials do not produce a good flow of bile within one to three weeks (depending upon the age of the child), little hope should be entertained that they will be effective with more prolonged administration.

SURGICAL TREATMENT FOR BILIARY OBSTRUCTION

Preoperative Measures

If any anemia exists before operation, *transfusions* should be given to put the baby in the best possible condition for the operative procedure. *Vitamin K* should always be given by injection to combat any bleeding tendency which might exist. For many years these children were fed *ox-bile salts* with the purpose of improving the digestion, but there is probably little to recommend this procedure.

Anesthesia

Operation in all of our cases has been performed under *ether* narcosis given by the drop and open mask method. There has been only one death during or immediately following operation; the extent of the operative manipulations was probably sufficient to explain the death on the basis of shock without blaming the anesthesia as a contributing factor. Great relaxation of the abdomen is necessary for a generous exposure, and this cannot be obtained with local anesthesia of the abdominal wall.

Exploration of Biliary System

A long incision is made from the costal margin well down below the umbilicus, laterally retracting the belly of the rectus muscle. More recently we have been employing a transverse incision which gives a somewhat better exposure. Great care must be taken to *ligate all bleeding points*, but it is surprising to find how rarely oozing of blood is a troublesome factor. The enlarged liver is retracted upward, and the extra-biliary system examined. The gallbladder is usually small and deeply embedded in liver substance which has mounded up around it. The peritoneal covering of the gastrohepatic ligament is opened, to expose the region of the common and hepatic ducts. Great care must be exercised in the subsequent dissection to avoid injury to small vessels in the gastrohepatic ligament, hemorrhage from which will obscure the field. The position and size of the ducts are now carefully estimated. Should the hepatic and common ducts appear to be atretic, one must turn attention to the gallbladder itself.

If the gallbladder possesses a lumen, its tip is now opened. The presence of bile in the bladder implies that the hepatic and cystic ducts are patent, even though they

* Ames Company, Inc.
† G. D. Searle & Co.

might not appear so by external examination. Into the gallbladder a small catheter is tightly sewed so that it can be distended with salt solution. By this irrigation a lumen may be found in the hepatic and common ducts which might otherwise elude detection. The injection of a methylene blue solution through the catheter and into the ductal system helps to outline those ducts which possess a lumen.

After this examination, which perforce will require considerable time and delicacy, the operator must decide whether he is dealing with obliterated cords of ducts, for which nothing can be accomplished, or whether there is some small remnant of a duct which can be joined with the alimentary system. If some patent duct is available (which joins with the liver), it is much better, as a general rule, to anastomose the hepatic or common duct, rather than the gallbladder, to the duodenum, in spite of the fact that the latter is technically easier to accomplish.

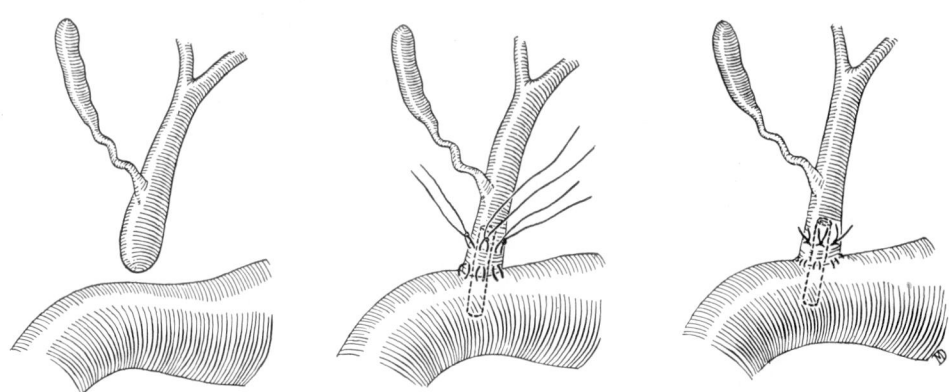

Fig. 281. Sketch of method of anastomosis of common (or hepatic) duct to the duodenum. The union is made over a short piece of ureteral or urethral catheter which is threaded into the duct and also into the duodenum. Anastomosis is made with interrupted silk sutures.

Hepatico-duodenostomy

In 11 cases we have found an obliteration of most of the extra-biliary system, with only a small nubbin of hepatic duct with a lumen presenting at the porta of the liver. In each instance this duct was but 3 to 5 mm. in diameter, yet it could be joined to the duodenum (Fig. 281). This is best accomplished by placing several silk ligatures to anchor the mobilized duodenum to the presenting nubbin of duct before opening the hepatic duct or duodenum. A small piece of No. 8 or 10 catheter about 1.5 cm. long is then threaded up into the hepatic duct and also down into the duodenum. With this tube in place, an anterior row of sutures is placed so as to anchor the anterior wall of the duct to the duodenum and complete the union. With so small a duct and with such limited exposure one can rarely place more than a single row of interrupted stitches around the line of anastomosis. It is imperative to use silk to insure permanent fixation of the two structures until proper healing has taken place.

It is important to make the anastomosis over a *small piece of tubing*, to prevent constriction of the lumen during the operative procedure. If the tube is too long, it may not pass spontaneously into the intestine. In one case a tube 7 to 8 cm. in length was employed, which did not move during the following two months when observed by x-ray examination. This child subsequently died of peritonitis, presumably from pressure necrosis and perforation of the opposite wall of the intestine. Following this disastrous experience we have always employed a piece of tubing no more than 1.5 or

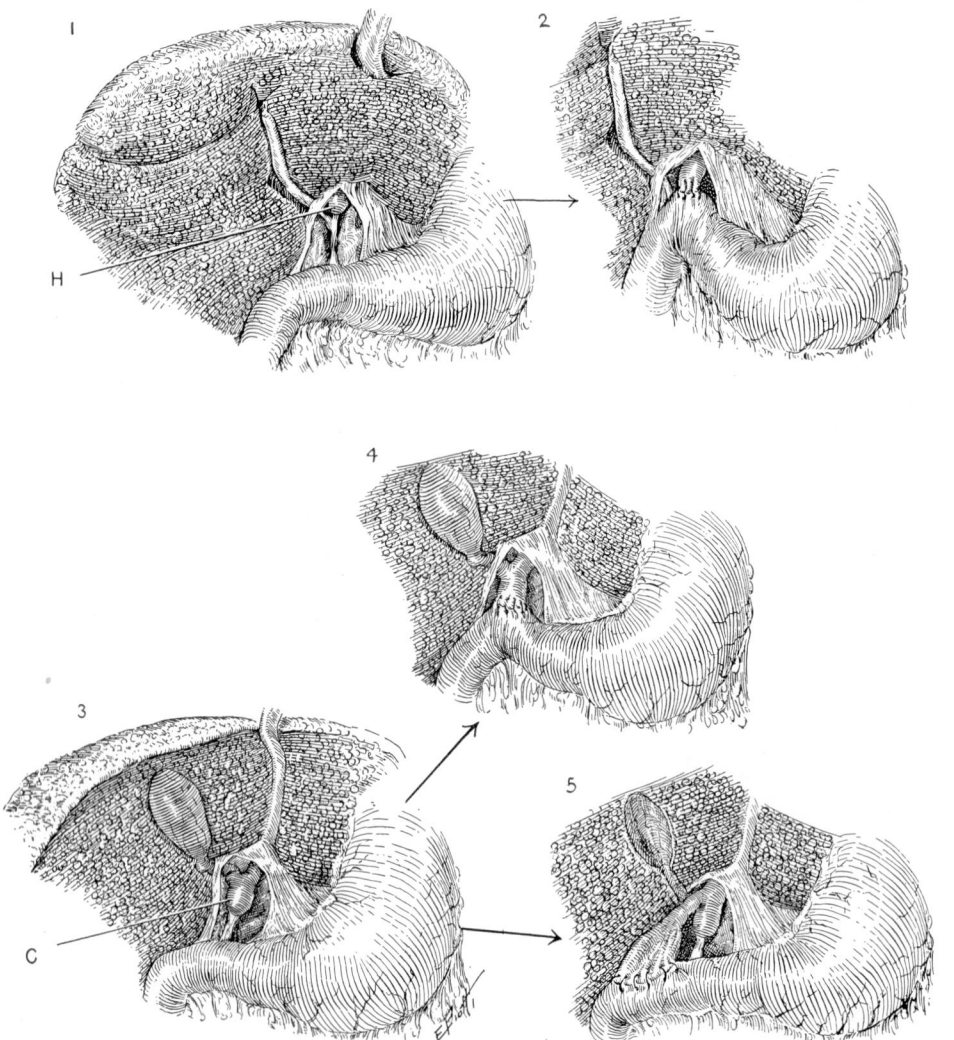

Fig. 282. Types of operative relief which have been effected for atresia of the extra-hepatic bile ducts. 1. Atresia of the hepatic duct. 2. Treatment of hepatic atresia by hepatico-duodenostomy. 3. Atresia of the common duct. 4. Treatment of common duct atresia by choledochoduodenostomy. 5. Treatment of common duct atresia by cholecystoduodenostomy. (Choledocho-duodenostomy is believed to be the better procedure). H, Blind end of hepatic duct. C, Blind end of common duct.

2 cm. in length, and have found that this always passes spontaneously within several days.

Cholecysto-duodenostomy

When a block exists in the *common duct* (16 of our cases), two procedures are available (Fig. 282). If the common duct is so small that there will be great technical difficulty in anastomosing it to the intestine, the gallbladder—if it connects with the biliary tree—may be freed from its bed, turned over, and joined to the duodenum.

Choledocho-duodenostomy

If the common duct can be mobilized, choledocho-duodenostomy is the operation of choice and has proved most successful in our hands. It is believed to be preferable to a cholecysto-duodenostomy. The technique employed depends upon the size of the presenting common duct. If it is large enough, a double layer of sutures may be placed, using an external row of interrupted silk and an internal continuous suture of very fine catgut to join the mucosal edges of duct and duodenum. However, the duct is usually only a few millimeters in diameter and one is rarely able to insert more than a single row of stitches.

All anastomoses should be made over a piece of *catheter* to insure that the lumen at the anastomotic site is not constricted during placement of the last sutures. In one case the cystic and common ducts were large enough to permit passage of a catheter down the gallbladder, through the cystic and common ducts, through the anastomosis,

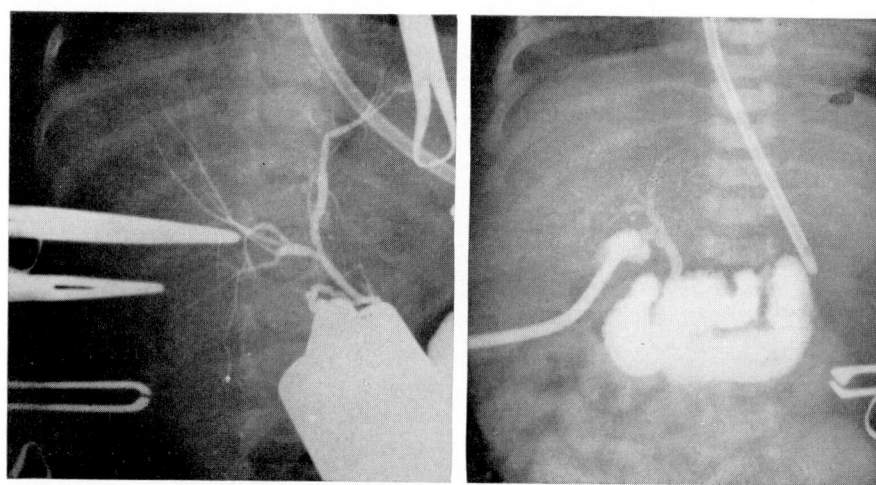

Fig. 283. From two babies, x-ray visualization of bile ducts at operating table by injection of Diodrast through the gallbladder. The infants had been deeply jaundiced; inspissated plugs were flushed out of the ducts, following which the visualizations were made, showing normal appearance and arrangements of ducts.

and into the duodenum. After the anastomosis had been completed, the catheter was withdrawn through the gallbladder. The small size and the tortuosity of the cystic duct does not often permit the employment of a catheter in this way.

Irrigation of Ducts

For those cases with patency of all the extra-biliary ducts but with biliary obstruction because of inspissated material within the ducts, much can be accomplished by opening the peritoneal covering, exposing the ducts freely to view, gently manipulating and massaging them, and frequently irrigating with saline (via a tube tied into the gallbladder). At first, it may be found that fluid will not run easily into the ductal system, but then as the common duct obstruction is relieved there is a free passage of liquid into the duodenum.

X-ray Visualization of Ducts

During operation this is sometimes helpful when it is found that all of the extrahepatic ducts are apparently present and have been cleared by washing detritus out of them. Injection of Diodrast, or other water-soluble iodide solution, through a tube which is sewed into the gallbladder will fill the ductal system (Fig. 283) and give a clear picture of the ductal ramifications.

RESULTS OF THERAPY

Medical Treatment

One baby with jaundice was given a trial with duodenal instillation of 25 per cent magnesium sulfate, which produced an excellent flow of bile into the duodenum. This happy outcome proved that the ductal system was patent and that it had probably been temporarily plugged with inspissated material; operation could be avoided. This therapy is apt to have drastic effects on the child; hence we have abandoned it in favor of using other cholagogues.

Thirty babies with biliary obstruction have been treated with the use of intravenous Decholin and oral Ketochol. In 14 of these a satisfactory flow of bile could be obtained and the jaundice cleared; one of these subsequently died of hepatic disease and insufficiency, all of the others appear to be in excellent health. In 16 babies no flow of bile could be obtained and all were then subjected to surgical exploration of the biliary system.

With the more frequent use of these medical techniques in the future, it is quite likely that successful medical therapy can be given to that group of patients (with blockage of ducts by inspissated material) for whom we have in the past used surgical exploration and ductal irrigation.

Surgical Treatment

Up to January 1, 1952, a total of 183 babies have been explored for biliary obstruction.

Of those who have been explored, 32 were found to have patent extra-biliary systems, but with blockage because of inspissated material in them. The ducts were manipulated and irrigated. Three babies who were thought at operation to have only cord-like threads representing the ducts were given a hopeless prognosis, but much to our surprise subsequently cleared their jaundice and have since been entirely well; they must have had patent but tiny ducts, with plugs therein. They have therefore been listed with the "inspissation" cases. Twenty-six of these 35 children were relieved of jaundice and have subsequently been in excellent health; some of these have been followed for more than a decade. Nine of the babies could be cleared of their jaundice, but died subsequently from a variety of causes; at least 4 of these were known to have some evidence of hepatic insufficiency.

Two babies were found to have jaundice because of external pressure on the extra-hepatic ducts. In one there was an extensive hemangio-endothelioma in the head of the pancreas and in the gastro-hepatic ligament, for which nothing could be done. In the other there were greatly enlarged nodes in the gastro-hepatic ligament, the removal of which relieved the biliary obstruction; pathologic examination of the nodes showed Niemann-Pick's disease, from which the child died some years later.

One hundred forty-six babies were found to have atresia of one or of all the extra-hepatic ducts, the details of which are summarized in Table 59. Out of these 146 cases, 27 were found to have available some part of a ductal structure which communicated with the liver and which could be joined surgically to the duodenum. Of the 27 patients with anastomoses, 12 have been completely relieved of jaundice, have livers which have diminished to normal size, and are in excellent health, the oldest now being twenty-four years of age. The remaining 15 patients have died; 9 of them succumbed while still in the hospital and 6 expired later from various causes amongst which a high proportion had evidence of serious hepatic disease. The remaining 119 babies had obliteration of the intra-hepatic ducts, the main hepatic duct, or all the extra-hepatic ducts—conditions about which nothing could be done by surgical means. In 5 of these cases, subsequent attempts were made to get relief by cutting off most of the left lobe of the liver and sewing its stump into a slit in the stomach wall, hoping there might be some small

Table 59

Findings and Methods of Treatment for Obstructive Jaundice in Early Months of Life
(To January 1, 1952)

Findings and Treatment	Total Number Cases	Cases without Relief of Biliary Obstruction	Cases with Relief of Biliary Obstruction	
			Died of Various Causes	Surviving and in Good Health
MEDICAL THERAPY (31 cases) by duodenal MgSO₄ or intravenous Decholin..........................	(16)(15)*	16	1	14
SURGICAL THERAPY				
1. Inspissated mucus or bile in ducts.	35	...	..	..
Manipulation or irrigation of ducts.....................	...	...	9	26†
2. External pressure on bile ducts..	2	...	..	..
Hemangio-endothelioma....	...	1	..	..
Niemann-Pick's lymph nodes.	...	...	1	..
3. Atresia lower end of hepatic duct	11	...	..	..
Hepatico-duodenostomy....	...	...	7	4
4. Atresia of common duct......	16	...	..	..
Choledocho-duodenostomy..	...	...	5	6
Cholecysto-duodenostomy...	...	...	2	2
Cholecystostomy..........	...	...	1	..
5. No ducts found leading from the liver...................	119	...	..	..
Biliary exploration........	...	114	..	..
Excision left lobe of liver, attempting to establish a fistula to stomach.........	...	5	..	..
Totals......................	198‡	120	26	52

* Of the 31 patients with attempts at medical therapy, 15 were treated successfully and 16 unsuccessfully. The failures were all submitted to surgery; they appear in the figures for surgical therapy.

† At operation, 3 of these babies were thought to have obliteration of the extrahepatic ducts, but subsequent to operation had passage of bile and clearance of jaundice. They must have had exceedingly tiny ducts which, subsequent to the regional manipulations, did open up.

‡ This total figure of 198 patients includes the 15 who were successfully treated medically and the 183 who were subjected to surgery.

intra-hepatic ducts which could deliver bile into the stomach; in none of these was a flow of bile produced. In no case have we ever seen an intra-hepatic duct more than pin-point in size; hence we cannot believe it will ever be possible to employ the Longmire technique (which has been developed for cases of biliary obstruction in the adult, by anastomosing a large intra-hepatic duct to the jejunum). In these inoperable cases, death usually came on an average of six to eight months later; 8 lived for a year, 2 lived for three years, and at the present writing there is one still alive at four and one-half years with intense jaundice, hepatic insufficiency, and a Banti's syndrome—a most deplorable sight. In most instances death followed a downhill course, characterized by progressive jaundice and inanition, sometimes with marked ascites, occasionally with hepatic rickets and fractures, usually terminated by superimposed infection and in a few cases by fatal hemorrhage.

Over-all Results

The list of fatal cases is long and most discouraging, yet the fact remains there has been an over-all salvage rate of 26 per cent of the 198 babies who were treated (medically and surgically) for obstructive jaundice in the early months of life. This ray of light makes it evident that surgical exploration should be undertaken for all babies with biliary obstruction, in the hope of picking out and saving those who have a remediable situation.

Table 60

Results of Treatment in 198 Cases of Obstructive Jaundice in First Year of Life
(To January 1, 1952)

	No Relief of Jaundice	Jaundice Relief. Death from Related or Unrelated Cause	Jaundice Cured. Good Health
MEDICAL by THERAPY duodenal MgSO$_4$ or intravenous Decholin.............................	16*	1	14
SURGICAL FINDINGS OR THERAPY			
External pressure on ducts (tumor or enlarged nodes)...................................	1	1	..
Inspissated plugs washed out of ducts.........	...	9	26
Obliteration of ducts (nothing could be done)...	119	..	..
Nubbin of hepatic or common duct available for anastomosis...............................	...	15	12
Totals (198 cases).........................	120	26	52
Percentage (of 198 cases) with permanent cure.................................			26%

* These 16 patients, unsuccessfully treated by medical means, were all operated upon and hence appear in the surgical figures below.

REFERENCES

1. Ahrens, E. H., Harris, R. C. and MacMahon, H. E.: Atresia of the Intrahepatic Bile Ducts. Pediatrics, 8:628, 1951.
2. Craig, J. M.: Sequences in the Development of Cirrhosis of the Liver in Cases of Erythroblastosis Fetalis. Arch. Path., 49:665, 1950.
3. Donovan, E. J.: Congenital Atresia of the Bile Ducts. Ann. Surg., 106:737, 1937.
4. Gray, H. K. DuShane, J. W. and Heneger, G. C.: Cholecystogastrostomy for Congenital Atresia of the Common Bile Duct. Report of a Case. Proc. Staff Meet., Mayo Clin., 23:473, 1948.

5. Holmes, J. B.: Congenital Obliteration of the Bile Ducts: Diagnosis and Suggestions for Treatment. Am. J. Dis. Child., 11:405, 1916.
6. Ladd, W. E.: Congenital Atresia and Stenosis of the Bile Ducts. J.A.M.A., 91:1082, 1928.
7. Ladd, W. E.: Congenital Obstruction of the Bile Ducts. Ann. Surg., 102:742, 1935.
8. Ladd, W. E. and Gross, R. E.: Surgical Anastomosis Between Biliary and Intestinal Tracts of Children. Follow-up Studies. Ann. Surg., 112:51, 1940.
9. Lightwood, R. and Bodian, M.: Biliary Obstruction Associated with Icterus Gravis

Neonatorum. Arch. Dis. Childhood, *21:* 209, 1946.

10. Patterson, P.: The Etiology and Treatment of Biliary Obstruction in Children. Pediatrics. In Press.

11. Rosemond, C. P., Burnett, W. E. and Beecher, R. M.: Congenital Atresia of the Common Bile Duct. Am. J. Surg., *78:*903, 1949.

12. Sweet, L. K.: Congenital Malformation of the Bile Ducts: A Report of Three Cases in One Family. J. Pediat., *1:*496, 1932.

13. Thomson, J.: On Congenital Obliteration of the Bile Ducts. Edinburgh M. J., *37:*523, 1892.

CHAPTER 42

Miscellaneous Conditions of the Liver and Biliary Passages

By far the most common disturbance of the liver and biliary passages requiring surgery in infancy and childhood is biliary obstruction and chronic jaundice in the early months of life. Because of the frequency and importance of these conditions, they have been separately considered in the preceding chapter. Other conditions of the liver, gallbladder, and biliary passages are described in the present chapter.

IDIOPATHIC DILATATION OF THE COMMON BILE DUCT

Cystic dilatation of the common bile duct is a congenital lesion in which there is tremendous enlargement of the lower part of the extra-biliary passages, the origin of such dilatation often being quite obscure. In some cases there is a demonstrable stenosis, angulation, or valve-like fold in the ampulla of Vater or in the lower part of the common duct, but in other well studied specimens the outlet of the common duct shows no apparent abnormality. The dilated duct may be as large as an orange or a grapefruit and in exceptional cases it has even been larger. Once the "cyst" has appeared, it tends to become ever bigger because its weight makes it hang to one side and thus angulate the inferior end in such a way that stasis and further obstruction follow. Excellent reviews of this subject have been made by Judd and Greene,[5] Zinninger and Cash,[12] and others. Nearly 200 examples have been reported in the literature. The present author[4] reviewed a series of 52 cases observed in childhood; the list has now grown much longer.

Pathology

Dilatation of the common duct is the characteristic finding and takes the form of a striking spherical enlargement of a part or of the whole of the ductus choledochus. This distention may involve only the common duct proper, or it may also include the junction of the cystic, hepatic, and common ducts. Thus, there may be only one duct entering the cyst (the upper part of the common duct), or the hepatic and cystic ducts may enter the cyst separately and their orifices may be 2 or 3 cm. apart (Fig. 284). In either instance, the cyst is connected to the duodenum by the lower segment of the common duct. In rare cases the enlargement may involve such a low portion of the common duct that the pancreatic duct opens directly into the choledochal cyst.

This *localized* dilatation of the biliary system is unique and is to be differentiated from enlargements which obtain in purely obstructive lesions of the lower common duct, such as those found with carcinoma at the head of the pancreas in the adult. Dilatations which result solely from obstruction tend to extend through the entire biliary tree, and the common duct is seldom larger than a loop of small intestine.

Also, in the purely obstructive lesions, the gallbladder is markedly dilated. Contrary to such conditions, a true choledochal cyst represents a localized dilatation, primarily of the common duct, while the gallbladder is seldom enlarged.

The *dimensions* of such a cyst may be very great, especially when one considers the size of the patient in whom the abnormality exists. Many of them have had a capacity of 1 or 2 liters; frequently they are described as being as large as a "fist," or the size of a "child's head." In an adult, Sheldon et al. mention ones which contained 5800 cc. of bile! There is no constant correlation between the size of the cyst and the duration of the symptoms or the age of the patient, although the larger ones tend to be found in older individuals.

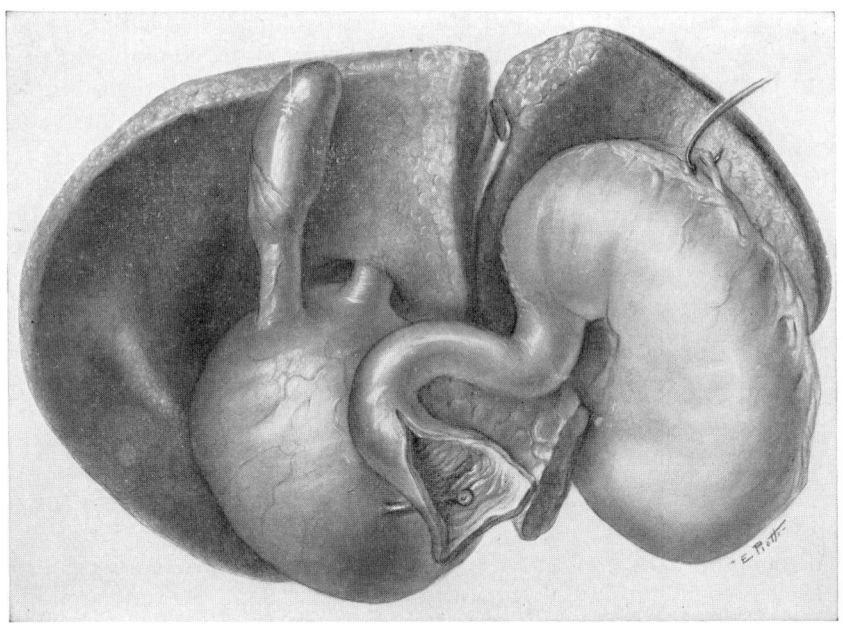

Fig. 284. Cystic dilatation of the common bile duct, as found in a three-year-old girl. Cystic and hepatic ducts are somewhat dilated and enter the "cyst" separately. Lower portion of the common duct is normal in caliber and normally enters the ampulla of Vater. The dilated portion of the common duct measured 7 cm. in diameter and 12 cm. in length. (From Gross: J. Pediatrics, vol. 3.)

The *cyst wall* is quite tough and varies from 2 to 4 mm. in thickness. It is composed of a dense connective tissue in which elastic substance and smooth muscle are often lacking. Epithelium has usually disappeared from the lining of the cyst, which is commonly represented by only a dense layer of connective tissue. The inner surface may be roughened and irregular, may be covered by heavy deposits of inspissated bile pigment, and occasionally there is a purulent exudate indicative of severe secondary infection. The cyst wall generally has evidence of some inflammatory reaction.

At the *outlets* of these cysts there are a great variety of findings. Valve-like folds have been described in a few. Stenosis of the lower part of the common duct has been observed, but is by no means a universal finding. In some specimens it was noted that the lower part of the common duct was angulated, and could not be probed. The common duct below the dilated portion may be normal in size and appearance, and in a few cases has actually been abnormally large—a fact which dispels the idea that obstruction is the sole factor in the causation of the choledochal cyst.

The *cystic duct, hepatic duct, and gallbladder* may have minor degrees of dilatation, but these changes are minimal when compared to the great size of the common duct.

The *liver* is frequently enlarged and cirrhotic. In a minority of cases the intra-hepatic ducts are grossly dilated. Microscopically, there is often a cirrhosis with increased peri-portal connective tissue, proliferation of the bile capillaries, and rarely some bile stasis. Infection is common, and leukocytic infiltration of the portal areas may be marked. Cholangitis may reach an advanced stage, and intraductal suppuration has been seen.

Etiology

While it is certain that obstruction in some form has been found in many of the cases, the great enlargement of the common duct, compared to the remainder of the biliary tree, suggests that there is some local deficiency in the common duct wall which allows it to balloon out. Many hypotheses have been advanced regarding the underlying cause for the production of this malady and the following include some of the leading views:

1. An anomalous direction of the common duct through the duodenal wall kinks the duct and produces obstruction to biliary flow.

2. A congenital stenosis of the lower part of the common duct causes back pressure sufficient to produce dilatation.

3. The dilatation may be due to an achalasia, namely, a failure of Oddi's sphincter to relax at the proper time, which would cause obstruction by a neuromuscular incoordination.

4. The cyst represents a developmental anomaly which is present before birth, and is due primarily to weakness of the common duct wall which allows dilatation under normal intraductal pressure. The condition has been compared to a congenital idiopathic hydronephrosis or ureterectasia, and, similar to these conditions, there may be no demonstrable obstruction.

5. The common duct wall lacks contractile elements and balloons out locally following obstruction in the lower portion of the duct. Some writers support this and claim that the obstruction is due to valve formation from redundant membrane of the duct secondary to cholangitis. Others postulate the congenital weakness of the duct wall, but believe the obstruction to be due to fibrosis of the lower part of the duct from a preceding cholangitis.

6. The cyst is of "congenital origin" and represents a malformation of the duct, while the valve formation is entirely secondary. Thus, a cyst can be displaced downward (because of its size and weight), and the resulting angulation will produce a valve. Such a valve, after it is once formed, may give obstruction and aggravate the symptoms, but it is not the primary cause of the ductal dilatation.

7. The cystic dilatation may spring from an abortive diverticulum of the common duct similar to the one which gives rise to the ventral pancreas.

With such a multiplicity of explanations it is entirely possible that we are dealing with a heterogeneous group of lesions which may be produced in several ways, for while many of the theories are plausible, no one explanation fulfills the conditions found in all cases.

In review, the most feasible theory is that which accepts a congenital weakness of the duct wall, a weakness not in itself producing dilatation unless there is a second factor of obstruction which raises the intraductal pressure. Such obstruction has been shown to come from a number of lesions in the lower part of the common duct.

Symptoms and Signs

The outstanding clinical feature of a choledochal cyst is the triad of abdominal pain, tumor, and jaundice.

Pain is observed in a large majority of cases. It is usually located in the epigastrium or in the right upper quadrant, but in some instances it is referred to the umbilicus. It may be of a colicky type, but more often it is of a "dragging" nature, or is described as pressure or a vague fullness. The pain is usually not very severe, and while it may cause considerable discomfort, it is rarely sufficient to make the patient "double up" or cry out. Pain is occasionally accompanied by nausea, but vomiting has occurred in only a few instances. There is no correlation between the size of the cyst and the severity of the pain.

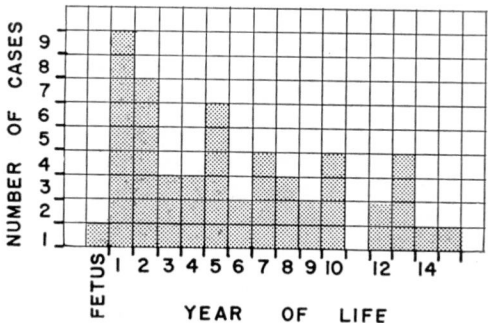

Fig. 285. Ages of 50 children (from literature) at onset of choledochal cyst symptoms. The number of patients in each group is indicated by the height of the columns. (One case occurring in a fetus is also indicated.)

Abdominal tumor is found in about 90 per cent of the cases. In about half of the cases a well defined and circumscribed mass has been palpated just below the liver edge, but there may be only a resistance to palpation in the right upper quadrant. When the cyst can be felt, it is often farther to the left than might be expected, because an enlarged liver can push the dilated common duct over beyond the midline of the body. In occasional cases the mass had been designated as "definitely cystic," "elastic," "tensely cystic," or some such term which indicates its physical nature, but not infrequently it has been so tense that it has been described as firm or solid. Hence, the clinician may have the impression that it represents a neoplasm or an enlarged lobe of the liver.

The *size* and *tenseness* of the cyst may vary from time to time, depending upon varying degrees of obstruction at the cyst outlet or upon quantitative changes in the production of bile. It is quite likely that this is a sign which has been present more often than recorded.

Jaundice is a prominent symptom and is seen in about 90 per cent of the cases. Acholic stools and highly colored urine have been noted from time to time in about one-third of the patients.

Fever is occasionally found, and is probably a reflection of cholangitis or hepatitis. The temperature range is usually to 101° or 102° F., but has been recorded as high as 104° F.

The *order of appearance* of pain, tumor, and jaundice varies in different cases. Any one of these may occur first, may exist alone, or may persist in combination with the others. One of these may exist for a long period of time before additional ones are evident. The *duration of symptoms* before the condition is recognized varies over a wide range, but the *chronicity* of complaints is noteworthy. The average duration of symptoms has been about three years before the underlying condition is found, but in some cases it has been much longer than this. The severity of symptoms bears no constant relationship to the duration of complaints.

The *intermittency of symptoms* should be emphasized. When it is stated that symptoms are "intermittent," it is meant that the general course of the illness has been one of exacerbations and remissions, even though one or more of the symptoms may have been rather constant.

The condition is about four times as common in females as it is in males. In a series of cases collected from the literature, the *ages* of the patients at time of hospitalization were as follows: 44 from birth to ten years, 31 from 11 to 20 years; 32 from 21 to 30 years; 11 from 31 to 40 years; and ten over 40 years.

Differential Diagnosis

Echinococcus cyst of the liver may give symptoms and physical findings similar to those of a choledochal cyst, but more often there is a palpable mass in the liver which causes little disturbance to the patient's health. The swelling is usually of long standing and is the only complaint; but if suppuration occurs, there are the additional indications of infection, and if the tumor is very large, there may be associated jaundice. An echinococcus cyst is stationary or progressive in size, whereas the choledochal cyst tends to vary in size, especially after the ingestion of food. A hydatid cyst of the liver moves with respiration and rarely produces pain. The presence of echinococcus cysts in other organs is of aid in detecting the parasitic infection. The geographic location of the patient in countries where the disease is rare, the absence of these parasites in dogs of the community, and the lack of intimate contact with dogs, all tend to exclude echinococcus cysts as a probable diagnosis. Where facilities are available, negative complement-fixation tests or precipitation reactions should rule out echinococcus infection.

Cholelithiasis is rare in children and its exclusion should be made with ease. X-ray studies may aid in indicating the presence of stones. Furthermore, gallstones in children usually result from some blood dyscrasia in which there is an abnormal hemolytic process. The absence of hematologic disorder makes a diagnosis of cholelithiasis unlikely.

Abdominal neoplasms in childhood, without treatment, generally run a rapidly progressive and fatal course. Thus, if a child has had symptoms of an abdominal mass for a year or more and still maintains fair nutrition and vitality, neoplasm as a causative agent is unlikely. Therefore, when this differential diagnosis is in question, a long duration of symptoms should tend to exclude malignancy. Neoplasms may certainly be excluded if the subhepatic mass has been found to vary in size.

Congenital atresia of the bile ducts should give no difficulty, chiefly because of the different age groups into which the two classes of patients fall. The average age of patients with congenital atresias of the extrahepatic ducts is from one to several months. In those cases not amenable to operative relief, the expectancy of life is generally less than a year. In contrast, only about 5 per cent of patients with a choledochal cyst have had symptoms before six months of age. Thus, the older age incidence of patients with choledochal cysts (Fig. 285) sharply differentiates the two conditions.

Treatment

The results of operation have depended in large measure upon the time when the nature of the cystic lesion was first recognized. In many cases exploration has been continued unduly long so that therapeutic procedures had to be curtailed because of onset of surgical shock. It is therefore pertinent to emphasize that *the surgeon must be familiar with the pathology of this condition* for only then can he quickly recognize the lesion and rapidly promote drainage of the biliary system into the intestine which has proved to be so efficacious in curing these individuals. Even if the diagnosis is not made preoperatively, the probabilities of a cure are high if the condition is recognized promptly at the operating table and proper treatment is *immediately* instituted.

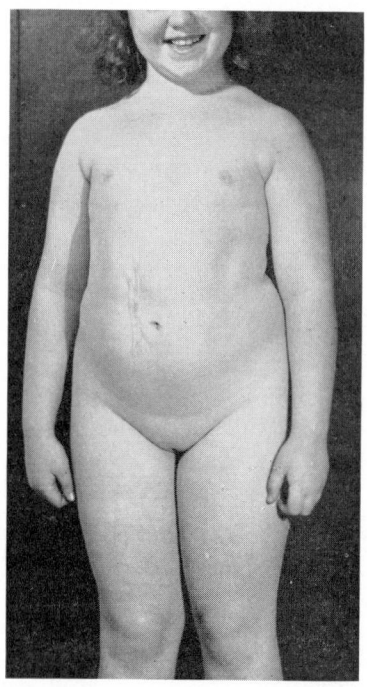

Fig. 286. Photograph of patient seven years after choledocho-duodenostomy for treatment of a large choledochal cyst. The child is in excellent health, and at no time has there been evidence of ascending cholangitis or hepatitis.

In a number of patients the dilated common duct has been *drained externally* in the hopes of joining the ductal system and intestine on a later occasion. Such external drainage of the choledochal cyst has been followed by exceedingly high mortality rates.

Excision of the cyst should never be attempted, for it is unnecessary and it is productive of dangerous surgical shock. Abdominal *tapping* is to be avoided, because of the danger of producing a leak from the cyst into the abdominal cavity, and because of the possible injury to other viscera.

Without question, the treatment of choice is to perform a *primary anastomosis* between the biliary system and the intestinal tract at one operation. *There has been ample opportunity to demonstrate the potentiality of the cyst to shrink to small dimensions when adequate drainage has been instituted.* The gallbladder may be united to the stomach or duodenum, but the best treatment of all is to anastomose the cyst directly to the duodenum. If desired, a cystostomy may be established in addition as a temporary outlet to relieve tension on the suture line of the choledocho-duodenostomy. While this extra step may be omitted, it doubtless has some merit as a safety factor. We do not eblieve it is necessary to connect the cyst to a side-arm of the jejunum, in a Roux-Y manner, though this has been suggested and has been used in the hopes of preventing cholangitis.

Results of Treatment

In a group of 52 childhood patients[4] the total mortality was 69 per cent, but in those treated by primary anastomosis of the biliary tract and intestine there was a mortality of only 9 per cent. These findings are summarized in Table 61.

Table 61

Results of Treatment in 52 Cases of Choledochal Cyst in Childhood (Collected from the Literature)

Treatment	Died	Recovered
1. No operation	9	0
2. Type of operation not stated	1	0
3. External drainage of the biliary system:		
(a) Drainage of choledochal cyst	15	1
(b) Drainage of gallbladder	1	0
(c) Drainage of hepatic duct and excision of cyst	3	0
(d) Drainage of gallbladder and excision of cyst	1	0
4. Drainage of cyst at first operation, and anastomosis to intestine at second operation	5	5
5. Anastomosis of biliary system and intestine at one operation:		
(a) Hepatico-enterostomy with cholecystectomy and excision of choledochal cyst	0	1
(b) Cholecystenterostomy	0	2
(c) Choledocho-enterostomy	1	7
Totals	36	16

We have treated 9 children with various types of operation (Table 62). Seven of these survived and were restudied 19, 16, 14, 11, 6, 4, and 3 years respectively after operation, to determine their general health and the condition of their biliary systems. One of them, 16 years later, is still having recurring cholangitis and jaundice. Since this anastomosis had been performed with a Murphy button (in 1925), we believe that the poor clinical result was dependent upon the establishment of too large a communication through which intestinal contents could regurgitate into the biliary tract. In each of the other 6 patients who had anastomoses by direct suture, the follow-up study has shown excellent physical development in each and biliary disease in none.

CHOLECYSTITIS

Cholecystitis in childhood, while still a curiosity, has been assuming increasing importance in recent years, for it is evident that it is not as rare as was once thought. Over 500 cases of gallbladder disease in children have been recorded in the literature, and the number which are discovered each year appears to be steadily growing. While cholecystitis is admittedly uncommon, the present-day success in treating this lesion by surgical means makes it important to recognize it.

Symptoms

The symptoms of acute cholecystitis in the child vary but little from those in the adult. They consist of severe, poorly localized, right upper quadrant *pain, nausea,*

Table 62

Results of Treatment in Idiopathic Dilatation of the Common Bile Duct
(Children's Hospital Series)

Treatment	Died	Recovered
Choledocho-duodenostomy...	0	4
Cholecysto-duodenostomy...	0	2*
Cholecysto-gastrostomy..	0	1
Dilated common duct excised; hepatic duct externally drained................	1	0
Exploration begun: cardiac arrest (coarctation of aorta)....................	1	0
Totals...	2	7

* One of these patients (in whom anastomosis was performed with a Murphy button) has recurring cholangitis.

vomiting, and *fever*. Localized, right upper quadrant tenderness or mass can be found. The general picture often leads to a diagnosis of intestinal obstruction. Hence, the presence of biliary disease may not be suspected until the abdomen is opened.

Treatment

In adults cholecystitis is commonly initiated by irritation from a stone or by blockage of the cystic duct with a calculus, whereas in children it is more apt to be a bacterial inflammation (particularly by the pneumococcus, the colon bacillus or the Salmonella group) unaccompanied by stones. Hence, in a child the process will often subside without resort to surgical means, and the treatment can be more conservative than that generally employed in adults. If the diagnosis appears to be fairly clear, the individual can be tided over the acute episode with chemotherapy, sedation, application of heat to the abdomen, a fat-free diet, and gentle saline purging.

If the fever and white blood count are rising and the local symptoms are advancing, exploration is advisable to arrest the spread of infection. If, under these circumstances, an acutely inflamed gallbladder is found, *cholecystectomy* is the procedure of choice. If edema around the neck of the gallbladder prevents easy isolation and ligation of the cystic duct and cystic artery, *cholecystostomy* is safer and preferable.

CHOLELITHIASIS

Symptoms

Cholelithiasis, though rare, is more common than acute cholecystitis in children The symptoms are largely those of recurrent upper abdominal *pain*, *nausea*, and *vomiting*. Calculi may enter the diminutive cystic and common ducts and produce intermittent biliary obstruction with resulting *jaundice* and severe vomiting. It is rare for a child to complain of the pain in the back or shoulder which is so frequently found in the adult.

The most common cause of cholelithiasis in children is related to the excessive excretion of pigments during a *hemolytic anemia*. In fact, the association is so frequent that cholelithiasis in childhood should always arouse one's suspicions concerning a *blood disorder*. The 6 patients (aged 3, 4, 7, 9, 10, and 14) we have operated upon for cholelithiasis were studied in this regard and 3 were found to have a hemolytic anemia. Cholelithiasis should never be treated without due regard for the blood picture, for not only must the stones be removed, but the reason for their formation must also be corrected.

Diagnosis

Gallstones in children are composed mostly of pigment, but sufficient calcium may be precipitated to cast positive shadows on x-ray films of the abdomen. When this is not true, *cholecystography* will show negative shadows in the dye-filled gallbladder.

Children with *congenital hemolytic anemia* have recurring bouts of jaundice due to temporary over-saturation of the blood stream with liberated pigments. If biliary obstruction is superimposed on this picture, it may be quite difficult to decide whether the jaundice depends solely upon a hemolytic crisis or upon a combination of hemolytic crisis and common duct obstruction. Acholic stools and a higher icteric index, particularly when associated with abdominal pain and vomiting, suggest that biliary obstruction is present.

Treatment

When the diagnosis of cholelithiasis has been confirmed by roentgenologic means or by unequivocal signs of biliary obstruction, exploration and removal of the stones is in order. If the calculi lie wholly within the gallbladder, *cholecystectomy* can be done, but if the bladder wall is not thickened, *cholecystostomy* and removal of the stones may be all that is necessary. This is particularly true if the patient has congenital hemolytic anemia which has been corrected (or is going to be corrected) by splenectomy. Under these circumstances the chance of future formation of stones is minimal and the gallbladder can be saved with impunity. If there has been obstructive jaundice, the common duct must be thoroughly explored for any calculi it might contain.

In the individual with both hemolytic anemia and cholelithiasis the question arises of whether it is preferable to correct the hemolytic process or to remove the biliary calculi first. This decision must necessarily depend upon the conditions in any given case. In general, *it is better to perform the splenectomy first, and then remove the calculi at a subsequent operation*. If, however, the patient has a high grade of common duct obstruction, the operator must explore the common duct first and leave the splenectomy for a subsequent time. *In no case should cholecystectomy (or common duct exploration) be combined with splenectomy, because this combination carries too high a risk of severe and even fatal shock.*

HEPATIC TUMORS

Pathologic Types

Neoplasms of the liver are rare, but several pathologic types have been found in infancy and childhood. Primary liver-cell *carcinoma* is the most common of the malignant forms and carries the worst prognosis. This grows at a rapid rate, replaces a large part of the normal hepatic tissue, and ultimately has widespread metastases. Small *hemangiomas* of the liver are not infrequently listed as incidental findings at autopsy. A few have been large enough to be of clinical significance. *Hamartomas* of the liver are rare, but it is important to recognize them because surgical removal can be followed by a fairly good prognosis. These are really not neoplastic growths; they should be regarded rather as developmental abnormalities of liver tissues which are attempting to form liver substance but yet not attaining the complete pattern of the normal organ (Fig. 287). Hence, the mass contains imperfectly formed hepatic lobules, biliary ducts, and possibly blood vessel networks in purposeless arrangements. Mitotic figures are rare; there is no tendency to invasion of surrounding tissues; metastases do not occur. The mass may be encapsulated or it may merge widely with adjacent liver substance.

Symptoms and Signs

The symptoms and signs of a liver tumor depend upon the size of the lesion, the site at which it appears in the liver, and the rapidity of growth. *Abdominal discomfort,*

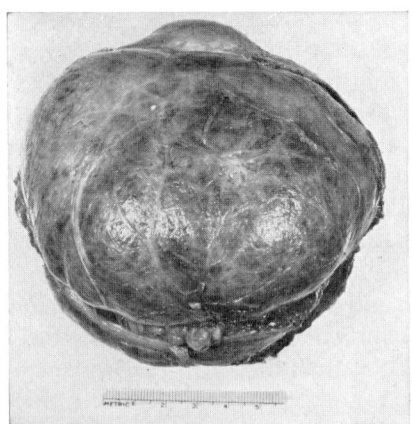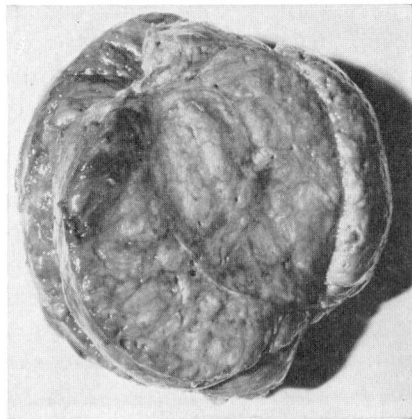

Fig. 287. Hamartoma of the liver from a three-year-old girl. Specimen weighed 400 gm.

nagging pain, and a palpable mass are the rule. If the liver tissue is largely replaced, or if intrahepatic bile ducts are compressed, varying degrees of *jaundice* are encountered. The nutritional state of the patient may be good or there may be advanced *cachexia.*

Prognosis

Steiner in 1938 reviewed 77 cases of malignant liver tumors occurring in children; the ages of the patients varied from one day to sixteen years, 41 being under two years of age. There were about twice as many males as females. The average duration of symptoms before diagnosis was about four months. Metastases were observed in about a third of the cases. All the patients died.

Singleton[29] in 1935 reported the case of a seventeen-day-old infant from whom a carcinoma of the liver had been excised. Packard and Stevenson[24] in their excellent review of hepatomas in infancy and childhood reported the case of a thirteen-month-old male infant who had a malignant hepatoma of the right lobe enucleated, and who did well for three years, but then developed recurrence.

Hamartomas are benign and may be successfully removed, as reported by Patton,[25] and by Benson and Penberthy,[18] but it has been suggested that it is possible for them to occur in malignant form (McRae[22]).

Hemangiomas are more common in the liver than in any other internal organ. They are usually small, give no symptoms, and are only incidentally discovered at operation or autopsy. Occasionally, however, they may be large enough to give symptoms, or they may rupture and cause intra-abdominal bleeding. Hendrick[20] reported such an occurrence in a newborn infant with death resulting. In some cases, hemangiomas are in a position where they may be excised. Others are diffusely scattered through liver substance and may require x-ray therapy.

Treatment

This is primarily surgical. Enucleation of a tumor or, better, partial hepatectomy of the tumor-bearing portion of the liver, cutting through normal tissue beyond the neoplasm, is the method of choice in treatment of these lesions. In some the tumor may be pedunculated, in which case resection and control of bleeding is easy, while in others the tumor may be inaccessibly buried within the substance of the liver and may replace so much of the viscus that excision is difficult or even impossible. In partial hepatectomies, the control of hemorrhage is the main obstacle that the surgeon is required to surmount. Tinker and Tinker,[31] Pickrell and Clay,[26] and Duckett and Montgomery[19] have all written extensively about this problem. In general, hemorrhage from the liver may be controlled by through-and-through hemostatic mattress sutures placed proximal to the line of incision, by cutting away the liver substance with the endothermy unit, by individual suture of major vessels, by temporary occlusion of the hepatoduodenal ligament, by the use of hemostatic agents such as Oxycel or Gelfoam, and by sewing closed the surface of the liver defect, possibly with omentum interposed between the edges of the liver capsule. With these adjuncts, it is amazing how much of the liver tissue can be lopped off without serious blood loss or shock.

Blood for transfusion must be available and should be administered throughout the operation by means of an intravenous cannula or polythene tube. Preoperative therapy by oral and parenteral means should be instituted to build up liver reserves as much as possible. The use of agents noxious to the liver must be avoided. A liver in which the blood supply is already compromised by tumor and operation is particularly susceptible to anoxia, and this must ever be kept in mind both by the surgeon and the anesthetist.

In cases of multiple hemangioma, x-radiation therapy is indicated.

Clinical Material and Results

In the Children's Hospital material there have been 18 patients with tumors of the liver. Eleven of them (5 were under one year of age, 1 was one year, 2 were three years, 2 were five years, and 1 was seven years of age) had primary malignant hepatomas. One (eight months of age) had a large adenoma of the liver. Two (aged one year and two years) had hamartomas, one of which had hemangiomatous elements. One (aged eight months) had multiple hemangiomas of the liver. One (three years old) had a malignant hemangio-endothelioma. One (age one year) had an extensive lymphangioma, and one (aged six months) had a widespread myxosarcoma of the liver. The youngest patient was two days old at the time of operation, and his tumor, a malignant hepatoma, had obviously developed during intra-uterine life.

In all cases a palpable mass was present, and in most instances it was of such a size that it had been noticed by the parents. Other symptoms and signs were loss of appetite, vomiting, irritability, and weight loss. In only one case was there jaundice, and this occurred in a patient with diffuse involvement of the liver by hemangio-endothelioma. In all cases the duration of symptoms was very short, averaging four weeks, and varying from two days to four months. All patients were explored and their tumors biopsied, and in 5 resection was performed. In only 2 instances has the patient survived. One was an eight-month-old girl who at operation was found to have multiple hemangiomas of the liver which were biopsied and treated with x-radiation (1600 r over an eight-day period). This child has been followed for seven years, is in excellent health, and shows no evidence of tumor or of liver damage. The other patient was a two-year-old boy in whom a small hamartoma was found and removed incidental to repair of a diaphragmatic hernia. This child has been followed for ten years. One other patient lived more than a year following excision of a hemangiomatous hamartoma and then succumbed to intestinal obstruction from adhesions. At autopsy a small remnant of the hamartoma was found, but was inactive, and was causing no trouble. All other patients died, either due to the effects of operation or due to the continued growth of their tumors.

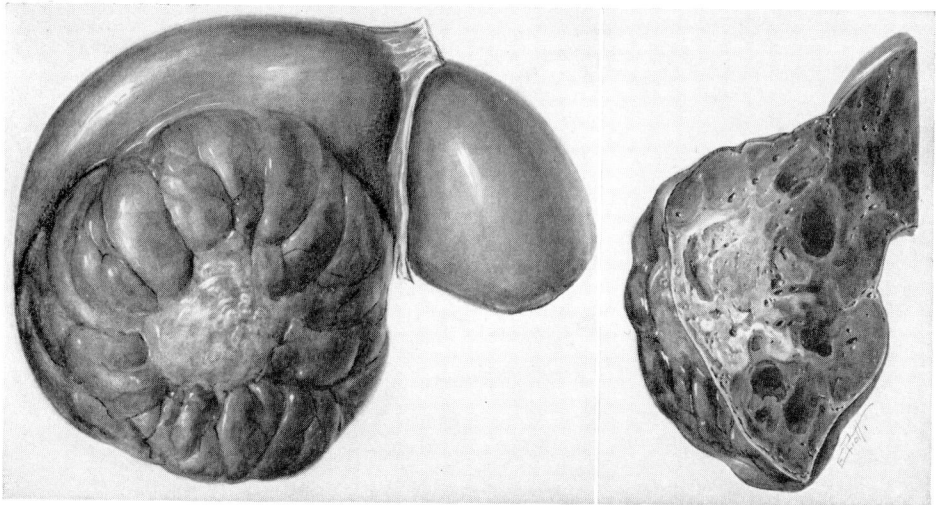

Fig. 288. Malignant hepatoma in a two-day-old male. *Left*, The isolated mass projecting from the right lobe of the liver. *Right*, A para-sagittal section of the tumor, merging into normal liver substance above.

CONGENITAL ANOMALIES OF THE GALLBLADDER

Anomalies of the gallbladder are rare, but the surgeon and roentgenologist should be familiar with them. In 1936 Gross reviewed 148 cases of such abnormalities which had been previously recorded in the literature. Histologic studies on these specimens were usually lacking and notes on the blood supply to the liver and gallbladder were very poor. The various conditions which might be briefly described are: *double gall-bladder, bilobed gallbladder, diverticulum of the gallbladder, floating gallbladder, anomalous position of the gallbladder*, and *absence of the gallbladder*.

Double Gallbladder

The term "double gallbladder" is used to describe 28 examples of duplication of the vesica fellea in each of which there were two separate bladder cavities and two separate cystic ducts (Fig. 289). The paired cystic ducts either join as a V-shaped structure or else open separately into the extra-hepatic bile ducts. The accessory gallbladder may be alongside the normal one or it may rest in some unusual location, for instance, under the left lobe of the liver or along the gastrohepatic ligament. In one case (Fig. 290) the accessory bladder was globular and was largely embedded within the right lobe of the liver. The accessory bladder usually is about the same size as the normal one, but it may be much larger or it may be diminutive.

Duplicate gallbladders have been discovered *roentgenologically* in a few cases, either by observing two rows of positive-shadow gallstones or by finding two distinct shadows of dye by cholecystography.

These patients do not have any characteristic *symptoms or signs* which might make the physician suspect the presence of a congenital anomaly before operation or autopsy. When the accessory organ is the seat of inflammatory change or stone formation, the symptoms and signs are indistinguishable from those occurring with cholecystitis or cholelithiasis in a normally formed organ.

Whether or not an accessory organ is more likely to be involved by *disease* is difficult to state, but the fact that most of these anomalies have been found at the operating

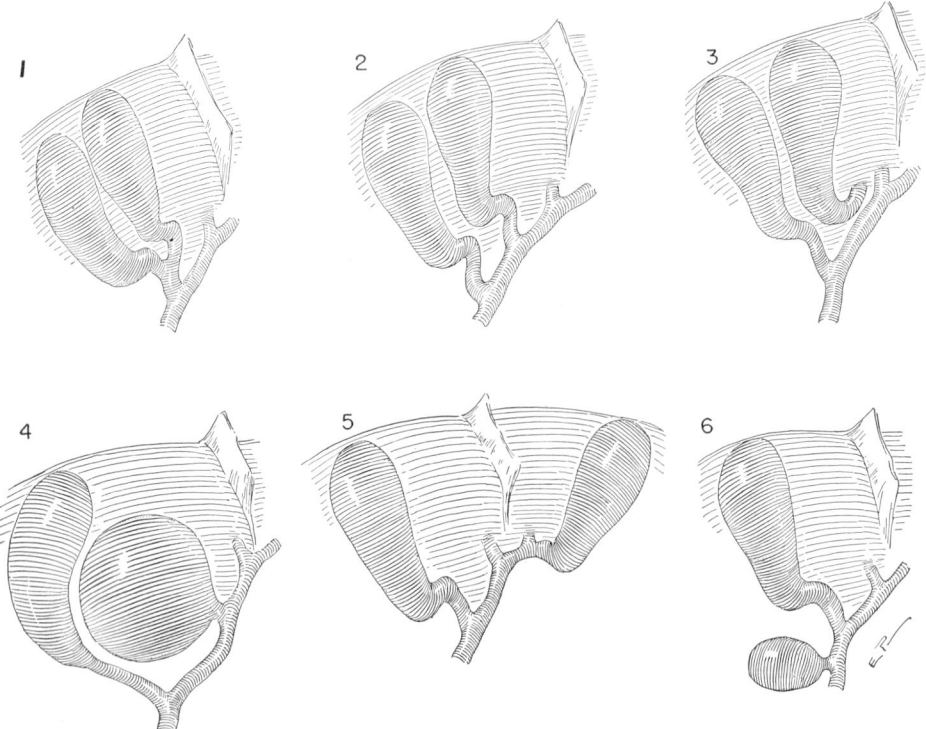

Fig. 289. Types of double gallbladder, showing positions of the accessory organ and the distribution of its cystic duct. 1. In the normal fossa with Y-shaped cystic duct. 2. In the normal fossa with a separate cystic duct. 3. In the normal fossa with cystic duct directly to the liver. 4. Partially embedded in the liver (see Fig. 290) with cystic duct entering main hepatic duct. 5. Under the left lobe of liver and communicating with left hepatic duct. 6. In the gastrohepatic ligament and emptying into the common duct. (From Gross: Arch. Surg., vol. 32.)

table and only a few at postmortem examination tends to show that the accessory structure is more prone to have pathologic changes than is a normally formed one.

Bilobed Gallbladder

A bifid or partially divided gallbladder, which is so common in many of the higher vertebrates, is seldom encountered in the human. About 6 examples have been described. Included in this category are those specimens which have two cavities, both of which are drained by a single cystic duct. Two types are found (Fig. 291). In one, the bladder has a normal external appearance, but contains an internal longitudinal septum which divides it into two chambers. In the other type there is a complete division of the fundic portions and a fusion of these at the bladder neck.

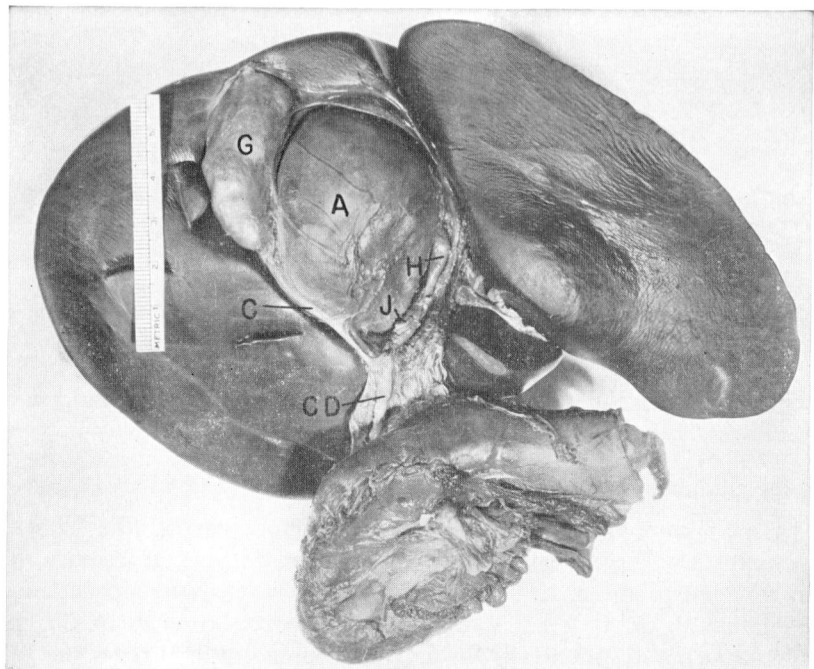

Fig. 290. Photograph of liver and accessory gallbladder from a three-year-old boy. (From Gross: Arch Surg., vol. 32.)

A, Accessory bladder   G, Normal gallbladder
C, Normal cystic duct   H, Hepatic duct
CD, Common duct   J, Junction of accessory gallbladder to the hepatic duct

Diverticulum of the Gallbladder

A diverticulum may be found anywhere along the free surface of the bladder from the fundus to the neck (Fig. 292). In the 10 cases studied, the diverticula varied from $\frac{1}{2}$ to $1\frac{1}{2}$ inches in diameter. Only a small number have been observed at operation, but they are occasionally recognized by cholecystography as incidental findings. A calculus may form in such a pouch.

Floating Gallbladder

The bladder may hang from the liver on a sort of "mesentery" (Fig. 293). The peritoneal fold may run the entire length of the gallbladder and cystic duct, or it may support only the cystic duct and allow the gallbladder to hang free and thus be movable. Gallbladders with this type of attachment are fairly common. It is not difficult to foresee the clinical significance of this anomaly, because an organ which is so mobile is apt to become twisted; infarction will supervene from impairment of its blood supply. Cases of this sort have been frequently listed in the literature (mostly occurring in adults). The *symptoms* are those of severe local pain, nausea and vomiting, collapse, and even fatal peritonitis if the gallbladder ruptures.

Anomalous Positions of the Gallbladder

These are rare, but at least three locations (Fig. 294) should be mentioned because of the interest they have had for surgeons and the technical difficulties they have some-

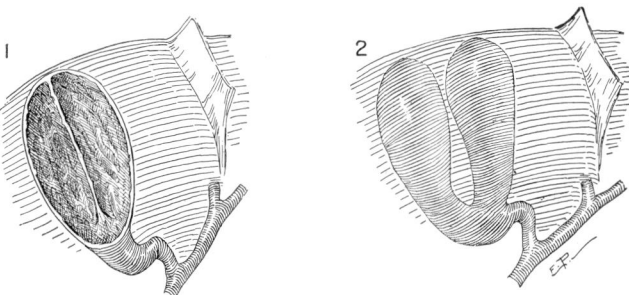

Fig. 291. Forms of bilobed gallbladders. 1. With an internal septum. 2. Paired at the fundic portion and joined at the bladder neck. (From Gross: Arch. Surg., vol. 32.)

times presented at operation. These are respectively: *intrahepatic, left-sided*, and *retro-displaced* positions.

Absence of the Gallbladder

More than 400 cases of atresia of the extrahepatic bile passages have been recorded in the literature, and about one-sixth of these had an associated absence of the gall-bladder. In addition to these, no less than 38 cases have been reported in which the hepatic and common ducts were normal and congenital absence of the gallbladder was the only abnormality noted. As far as could be determined from the reports, the absence of the bladder did not in any way impair the health or digestive functions of these persons. The absence of the gallbladder, *per se*, was rarely accompanied by any compensatory dilatation of the hepatic or common ducts.

TRAUMA TO THE GALLBLADDER AND BILE DUCTS

The gallbladder of a child is relatively small, is rather well protected beneath the inferior surface of the liver, and rarely sustains important trauma. The extra-hepatic bile ducts in the gastrohepatic ligament are less well protected and may be lacerated or even completely severed during severe abdominal injuries.

A *rupture of the gallblaader* is easily treated by cholecystectomy.

A *transection or extensive laceration of the common or hepatic ducts* should be repaired if possible by end-to-end suture or by suitable reconstruction over a piece of small catheter to insure the continuity and patency of the ductal lumen. If the common duct is extensively damaged the gallbladder can be anastomosed to the duodenum, but

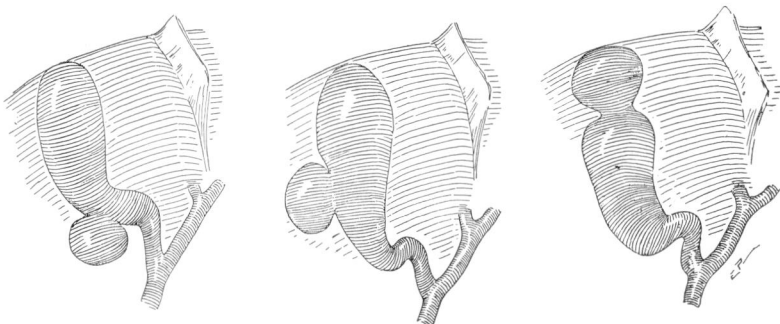

Fig. 292. Forms of congenital diverticula occurring in different parts of the gallbladder. (From Gross: Arch. Surg., vol. 32.)

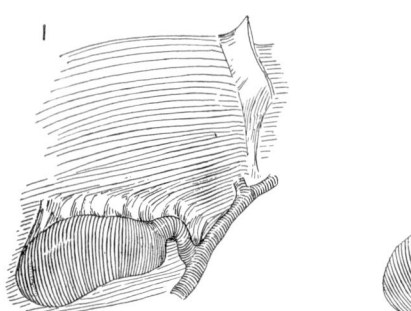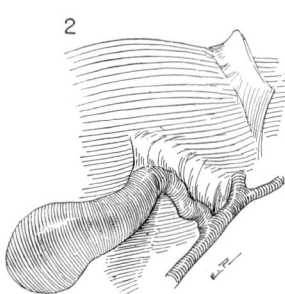

Fig. 293. Floating gallbladders, suspended by a "mesentery." 1. Mesentery supporting both bladder and cystic duct. 2. Mesentery supporting only the cystic duct, allowing the bladder to hang freely. (From Gross: Arch. Surg., vol. 32.)

it is always preferable to reestablish the continuity of the common duct if this is at all feasible.

The only two instances of injury to the extra-biliary passages that we have encountered were in girls four years of age. In one of these the child fell to the ground and was then struck in the abdomen by a falling board. The hepatic duct was torn but not severed. It was impossible to suture the torn edges accurately; an abdominal drain was merely inserted to this region. Copious amounts of bile escaped through the drain for some weeks, but the sinus then spontaneously closed and the continuity of the biliary passage was presumably reestablished, since the child became and remained symptomless.

In the second case the child's abdomen was crushed by the bumper of an automobile and the common duct was completely divided. A large amount of bile escaped into the abdomen, which was greatly distended. Hemorrhage, edema, and disruption of tissue in the gastrohepatic ligament made a repair of the lacerated common duct extremely difficult. Subsequent stenosis appeared at this point, and to relieve the biliary obstruction a cholecysto-duodenostomy was performed. This child developed recurring cholangitis, cirrhosis, and bleeding esophageal varices, from which she died eight years later.

As a commentary on these cases of *extravasation of bile into the abdomen*, it is to be noted that bile, as long as it is *sterile* and from the common duct, seems to be comparatively innocuous. This material in the abdomen causes little discomfort or pain and there is rarely more than a degree or two of fever. However, if bile has been con-

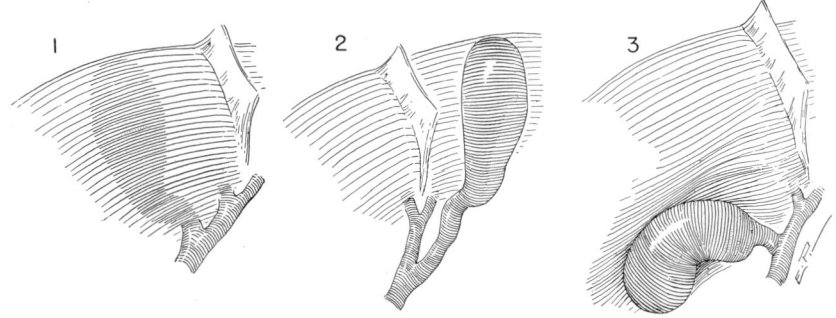

Fig. 294. Abnormal positions of the gallbladder. 1. Within the substance of the liver. 2. Under the left lobe of the liver. 3. On the posterior-inferior surface of the right hepatic lobe. (From Gross: Arch. Surg., vol. 32.)

centrated in the gallbladder before it escapes into the abdominal cavity, its relatively high osmotic pressure may draw forth a considerable amount of fluid from the various peritoneal and intestinal tissues, and in this way produce a greater accumulation of fluid than can be accounted for purely on the basis of extravasated bile.

The results of our meager experience with these cases tend to show the same conclusion as does a review of the literature; namely, that ductal injuries are usually best treated by merely *draining* the damaged area and possibly the biliary system. This form of therapy appears to be the preferable one unless a duct has been completely severed, in which case a plastic procedure or a short-circuiting operation must be resorted to.

REFERENCES

CHOLEDOCHAL CYST

1. Archambault, H., Archambault, R. and Lasker, G. W.: Choledochus Cyst. A Case Treated by Y-Roux Type Anastomosis of Jejunum to the Cyst. Ann. Surg., *132*:1144, 1950.
2. Blocker, T. G., Jr., Williams, H. and Williams, J. E.: Traumatic Rupture of a Congenital Cyst of the Choledochus. Arch. Surg., *34*:695, 1937.
3. Davis, C. E.: Choledochus Cyst. Ann. Surg., *128*:240, 1948.
4. Gross, R. E.: Idiopathic Dilatation of the Common Bile Duct in Children. J. Pediat., *3*:730, 1933.
5. Judd, E. S. and Greene, E. I.: Choledochus Cyst. Surg., Gynec. & Obst., *46*:317, 1928.
6. Keeley, J. L.: Congenital Cystic Dilatation of the Common Bile Duct. Arch. Surg., *56*:508, 1948.
7. McWhorter, G. L.: Congenital Cystic Dilatation of the Bile and Pancreatic Ducts. Necropsy Thirteen Years after Hepaticoduodenostomy. Arch. Surg., *38*:397, 1939.
8. Shallow, T. A., Eger, S. A. and Wagner, F. B., Jr.: Congenital Cystic Dilatation of the Common Bile Duct. Ann. Surg., *123*:119, 1946.
9. Smith, B. C.: Cyst of the Common Duct. Arch. Surg., *44*:963, 1942.
10. Swartley, W. B. and Weeder, S. D.: Choledochus Cyst with a Double Common Bile Duct. Ann. Surg., *101*:912, 1935.
11. Wright, A. D.: X-ray Appearances Produced by Congenital Cystic Dilatation of the Common Bile Duct. Brit. J. Radiol., *8*:227, 1935.
12. Zinninger, M. M. and Cash, J. R.: Congenital Cystic Dilatation of the Common Bile Duct. Arch. Surg., *24*:77, 1932.

CHOLECYSTITIS AND CHOLELITHIASIS

13. Hamilton, H. B., Rich, C. O. and Bisgard, J. D.: Cholecystitis and Cholelithiasis of Childhood. J.A.M.A., *103*:829, 1934.

14. Penberthy, G. C. and Benson, C. D.: Surgery of the Biliary Tract in Infants and Children. Am. J. Surg., *40*:232, 1938.
15. Potter, A. H.: Biliary Disease in Young Subjects. Surg., Gynec. & Obst., *66*:604, 1938.
16. Seidler, V. B. and Brakeley, E.: Gallstones in Children. Report of a Case Diagnosed by Roentgen Examination and Confirmed at Operation. J.A.M.A., *114*:2082, 1940.
17. Swing, A. T. and Bullowa, J. G. M.: Acute Cholecystitis Complicating Scarlet Fever. Am. J. Dis. Child., *55*:521, 1938.

LIVER TUMORS

18. Benson, C. D. and Penberthy, G. C.: Surgical Excision of Primary Tumor of Liver (Hamartoma) in Infant Seven Months Old with Recovery. Surgery, *12*:881, 1942.
19. Duckett, J. W. and Montgomery, H. G.: Resection of Primary Liver Tumors. Surgery, *21*:455, 1947.
20. Hendrick, J. G.: Hemangioma of the Liver Causing Death in a Newborn Infant. J. Pediat., *32*:309, 1948.
21. Keen, W. W.: Report of a Case of Resection of the Liver for the Removal of a Neoplasm, with a Table of Seventy-Six Cases of Resection of the Liver for Hepatic Tumors. Ann. Surg., *30*:267, 1899.
22. McRae, F. W.: Unusual Tumor (Malignant Adenoma) of Liver in Baby. Am. J. Surg., *28*:575, 1935.
23. Montgomery, A. H.: Solitary Nonparasitic Cysts of the Liver in Children. Arch. Surg., *41*:422, 1940.
24. Packard, G. B. and Stevenson, A. W.: Hepatoma in Infancy and Childhood. Discussion and Report of Patient Treated by Operation. Surgery *15*:292, 1944.
25. Patton, R. J.: Hamartoma of the Liver. Ann. Surg., *127*:180, 1948.
26. Pickrell, K. L. and Clay, R. C.: Lobectomy of the Liver. Report of Three Cases. Arch. Surg., *48*:267, 1944.

27. Schmelling, J. W.: Rare Case of Congenita Multiple Tumors of Liver (Hamartomas) in Infant Four Months Old. Nederl. tijdschr. v. geneesk., *78*:3566, 1934.

28. Shumacker, H. B., Jr.: Hemangioma of the Liver. Discussion of Symptomatology and Report of Patient Treated by Operation. Surgery *11*:209, 1942.

29. Singleton, A. O.: Discussion of: McRae, F. W.: Unusual Tumor (Malignant Adenoma) of Liver in Baby. Am. J. Surg., *28*:581, 1935.

30. Steiner, M. M.: Primary Carcinoma of the Liver in Childhood. Report of Two Cases with a Critical Review of the Literature. Am. J. Dis. Child., *55*:807, 1938.

31. Tinker, M. B. and Tinker, M. B., Jr.: Resection of the Liver. Conditions Favorable for Operation; Methods; Experimental Studies. J.A.M.A., *112.2*:2006, 1939.

32. Warvi, W. N.: Primary Tumors of the Liver. Surg., Gynec. & Obst., *80*:643, 1945.

33. Wilens, G.: Adenoma of Liver. Am. J. Dis-Child., *55*:792, 1938.

ANOMALIES OF THE GALLBLADDER

34. Boyden, E. A.: The Accessory Gall-Bladder: An Embryological and Comparative Study of Aberrant Biliary Vesicles Occurring in Man and the Domestic Animals. Am. J. Anat., *38*:177, 1926.

35. Eisendrath, D. N.: Anomalies of the Bile Ducts and Blood Vessels. J.A.M.A., *71*: 864, 1918.

136. Gross, R. E.: Congenital Anomalies of the Gallbladder. A Review of 148 Cases, with Report of a Double Gallbladder. Arch. Surg., *32*:131, 1936.

37. Murray, J. F.: Torsion of the Gall Bladder. Brit. J. Surg., *20*:687, 1933.

38. Schachner, A.: Anomalies of the Gall Bladder and Bile Passages. Ann. Surg., *64*:419 1916.

INJURY TO BILIARY PASSAGES

39. Harkins, H. N., Harmon, P. H. and Hudson, J.: Lethal Factors in Bile Peritonitis. I. "Surgical Shock." Arch. Surg., *33*:576, 1936.

40. Hicken, N. F. and Stevenson, V. L.: Traumatic Rupture of the Choledochus, Associated with an Acute Hemorrhagic Pancreatitis and a Bile Peritonitis. Ann. Surg., *128*:1178, 1948.

41. Ladd, W. E.: Toxicity of Bile, with Report of an Unusual Case. Boston M. & S. J., *168*: 166, 1913.

42. Rudberg, H.: Traumatic Rupture of Common Bile Duct. München. med. Wchnschr., *68*: 1650, 1921.

43. Walters, W.: Strictures and Injuries of Bile Ducts; Study of Results of Operations in 80 Cases. J.A.M.A., *113*:209, 1939.

44. Waugh, G. E.: Traumatic Rupture of the Common Bile-Duct in a Boy Six Years Old. Brit. J. Surg., *3*:685, 1916.

CHAPTER 43

Diseases of the Spleen

Much has been written about the physiology and the pathologic states of the spleen in relation to abnormalities of the blood and circulation; the field is one which has grown with extraordinary rapidity in recent years. The following sections discuss those disorders which can be cured or alleviated by surgical measures; they also include brief mention of some for which splenectomy has been found to be of little or no value. For the past twenty-five years Dr. Louis K. Diamond has made extensive studies on the Children's Hospital patients with various hematologic disorders or diseases of the spleen; most of the observations and opinions recorded in this chapter have been taken from

Table 63

Splenectomies (January 1, 1931, to September 1, 1952)

Diagnosis	Number of Cases
Congenital hemolytic anemia	59
Acquired hemolytic anemia	12
Idiopathic thrombocytopenic purpura	23
Secondary thrombocytopenic purpura	3
Portal hypertension (with or without hypersplenism)	24
Rupture of spleen	18
Lipoid storage diseases	17*
Incidental splenectomy (during pancreatectomy, gastrectomy, etc.)	10
Leukemia	12
Hypoplastic or aplastic anemia	7
Cooley's anemia	4
Sarcoid	3
Tuberculosis of spleen	1
Cyst or tumor of spleen	2
Splenic infarction (wandering spleen)	1
Splenic neutropenia	1
Sickle cell anemia	1
Agnogenic myeloid metaplasia	1
Total	199

* Gaucher's disease 9, Niemann-Pick's disease 4, Letterer-Siwe's disease 1, Hurler's syndrome (lipochondrodystrophy) 2, Unclassified 1.

his reviews. Table 63 lists the conditions for which 199 splenectomies have been performed in this hospital from January 1, 1931 to September 1, 1952.

CONGENITAL HEMOLYTIC ANEMIA

Symptoms and Physical Findings

This condition, also known as "familial hemolytic anemia," "chronic hemolytic jaundice," "acholuric jaundice," etc., is characterized by a chronic or recurring anemia, hemolytic crises, and by abnormalities in the blood picture which permit recognition of the disease with great certainty. It must be distinguished from acquired hemolytic anemia which is usually secondary to infection, to drug or chemical sensitivity, or to transfusion of mismatched blood.

The *anemia* may be discovered at any age. It can be of moderate or marked degree. The red count ranges between 2,000,000 and 4,000,000 but has been found as low as 1,000,000 cells per cubic millimeter. Following crises, the red blood count rises slowly; it may reach normal levels, but it is more characteristic for some degree of anemia to persist. It is typical for the disease to have periods of exacerbation and remission.

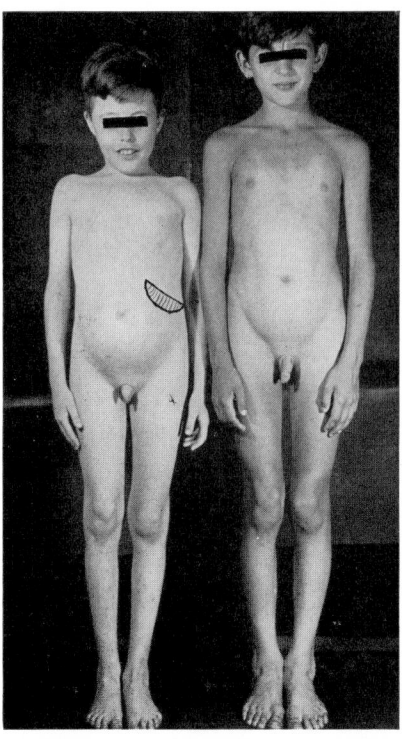

Fig. 295. Photograph of boy (*left*) with congenital hemolytic anemia, showing retardation in growth compared to a normal boy of the same age. Lower border of the enlarged spleen is outlined. (From Diamond: Am. J. Surg., vol. 39.)

Hemolytic crises with fever, abdominal pain, pallor, jaundice, and weakness occur at varying intervals. At such times there is excessive destruction of red blood cells, as is shown by a falling red count, a rising icteric index, and an increased excretion of urobilinogen in the stools and urine. A mild *jaundice* may be present most of the time, or it may appear only when there is excessive erythrocyte destruction. Crises may be of a minor sort, or they may be so severe that the patient dies with profound anemia and anoxemia, in spite of repeated transfusions. In general, the younger the individual, the more severe are the crises.

The *spleen* is generally enlarged mildly or moderately. *Retardation of growth* is often seen in these children; they may be somewhat underweight; it is common for them to be smaller in stature than the expected normal (Fig. 295).

Girls are apt to be slightly more numerous than males in any series of cases. An adequate search often shows that other members of the family have had the same disease, yet a familial incidence is not found in all. In about 70 per cent of our cases, other members of the family were known to have congenital hemolytic anemia, the inheritance being about equally divided between the maternal and the paternal sides of the family. In about one-third of the families of our patients, other members had had a splenectomy.

Laboratory Data

An anemia of varying degree is always found, this being most marked during or immediately after any crisis.

Microscopic examination of the blood shows a tendency for the erythrocytes to be globular (so-called *spherocytosis*)—a point of some diagnostic importance. The cells often appear to be microcytic, but detailed studies show the cell volume to be within a normal range. *Reticulocytes* appear in the peripheral blood with great prominence; counts of 20 to 30 per cent are common, but much higher values have been observed. The appearance of reticulocytes in such great numbers at once suggests that the anemia is not due to a failure of blood formation, but that it has resulted from excessive hemolysis of red cells; the marrow is actively trying to replace erythrocytes which have been destroyed. Nucleated erythrocytes may appear in the circulating blood during a crisis. The leukocytes and platelets are within normal limits except in a crisis, at which times they may be depressed.

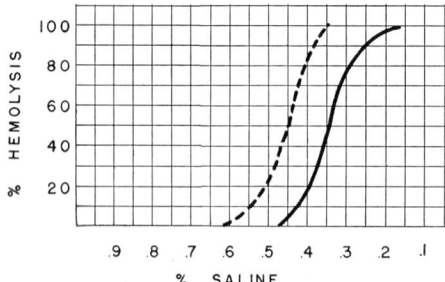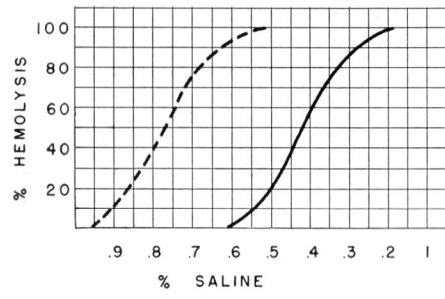

Fig. 296. Fragility test of red cells, from a case of congenital hemolytic anemia. The *solid* curved lines represent normal; the *broken* curved lines represent findings from the patient being studied. *Left,* Test which was conducted at room temperature. *Right,* Test which was conducted by setting up cell suspensions and then incubating them at 37° for twenty-four hours. The patient's cells show increased fragility at room temperature and markedly so after incubation.

Increased fragility of the red cells, when placed in salt solutions of different concentrations, is a diagnostic feature. Normal red cells begin to hemolyze in solutions of about 0.45 per cent sodium chloride and the hemolysis will be complete in concentrations of about 0.20 per cent. In contrast, cells from an individual with hemolytic anemia may begin to disintegrate in much higher concentration and the hemolysis is usually complete in concentrations of 0.40 per cent (Fig. 296). It might be necessary to incubate the blood (while suspended in the salt solutions) to bring out evidence of increased fragility (Fig. 297). Whenever tests for fragility are made, a simultaneous examination of normal blood should always be set up as a control observation.

The *icteric index* can rise to 40 or 50, but it does not increase to the high values observed in most cases of biliary obstruction. The total serum bilirubin is similarly elevated to 8.0 or 10.0 mg. per cent, giving a predominantly indirect van den Bergh reaction.

The *Coombs test,* by which an abnormal coating of the patient's erythrocytes by auto-antibodies can be demonstrated, is positive in erythroblastosis fetalis, is usually positive in acquired hemolytic anemia, but is generally negative in congenital hemolytic anemia.

Urobilinogen is excreted in the urine and stools in amounts which may be as much as thirty or forty times normal; this elimination goes hand in hand with the excessive destruction of red cells and liberation of their pigments. Increases in urobilinogen excretion are particularly evident during or immediately after hemolytic crises, at which times the urine may have a very dark yellow or orange color. Quantitative determinations of this substance can be made on the stool, but it is easier to study the urine by testing it with Ehrlich's reagent.

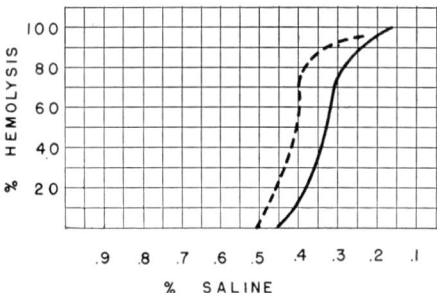 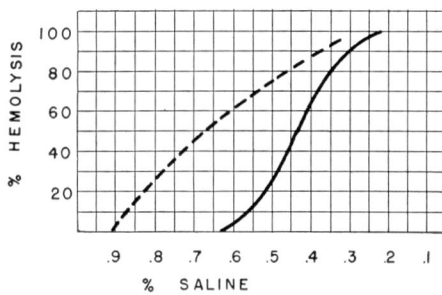

Fig. 297. Fragility test of red cells, from a case of congenital hemolytic anemia, showing particularly the value of the incubation method. The solid curved lines represent normal; the broken curved lines represent findings from the patient under study. *Left*, Test conducted at room temperature. *Right*, Test conducted with incubation of tubes at 37° for twenty-four hours. The test conducted at room temperature shows only slight evidence of increased fragility, but the one conducted with incubation clearly shows a marked increase of fragility.

Roentgenologic Examination

X-ray studies may show some relevant changes which, however, are not characteristic of the condition. The bones may have retardation of growth, a point which is best determined by examination of the wrist. When the bone marrow is overactive and hyperplastic, the medullary substance is expanded so that there is a concurrent thinning of the adjacent cortical bone. These readjustments are best observed in the long bones where there is thinning of the cortex or in the skull where there is a striate or fuzzy appearance of the tables. These changes are similar to, but not as common or as marked as, those which are found with Mediterranean anemia.

Course

The severity of the anemia, the frequency of the crises, and the ultimate prognosis are all somewhat related to the age at which the disease begins. Individuals whose symptoms *first appear in late childhood or early adult life* may have but slight disability and exhibit only mild anemia or jaundice. *When the disease starts in infancy* or the first few years of life, there is a more fulminating process, and death not infrequently occurs during a crisis, even during the initial one. In such individuals the destruction of blood may be so rapid that repeated transfusions will not tide them over the acute episode. In short, the earlier in life that the disease begins, the poorer is the outlook and the more urgently should splenectomy be advised.

Increased excretion of blood pigments by way of the biliary tract not infrequently leads to development of *gallstones*, even in pre-adolescent years. Such calculi are largely of the pigment variety but calcium and cholesterol can also be found in small amounts. The discovery of cholelithiasis in any child should always make one suspect the possibility of congenital hemolytic anemia.

Treatment

Splenectomy is specific therapy for congenital hemolytic anemia; it gives quick and permanent relief. If possible, operation should not be done during a crisis. Following splenectomy there is a gradual fall in the reticulocytes and an increase in the number of circulating red blood cells. Erythrocytes still retain their increased fragility but the abnormal destruction of red cells ceases. The changes in red count, white count,

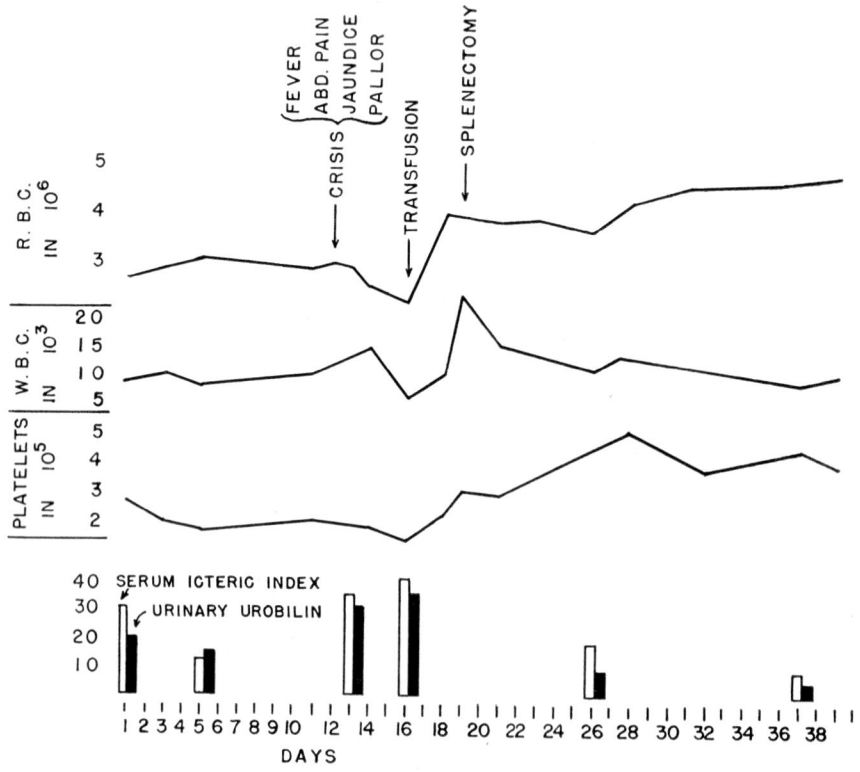

Fig. 298. Chart from a child with congenital hemolytic anemia who was treated by splenectomy.

platelet count, icteric index, and urobilinogen excretion before and after operation in an eleven-year-old girl are graphically set forth in Figure 298.

Coller et al.[1] and others have observed reactions following preoperative transfusion, and they recommend delaying transfusion until splenectomy is completed or at least until the splenic artery has been clamped. In our experience we have seen no serious untoward reaction from transfusion and in no case has hemolysis appeared to increase as the result of transfusion. Hence it is our policy to treat preoperatively any anemia below 10 gm. per cent by transfusion, preferably by the use of washed, packed, red blood cells.

In those occasional patients in whom one must treat anemia (by splenectomy) and cholelithiasis (by cholecystectomy and possibly common duct exploration), no attempt should be made to perform both of these procedures at one operation. In general, it is far better to remove the spleen first, and shortly thereafter the gallstones. If evidence of common duct obstruction is great, it is preferable to perform the biliary operation first, and then remove the spleen a week or two later.

Results of Treatment

At the Children's Hospital, from 1930 to September 1, 1952, 59 children and babies with congenital hemolytic anemia have been subjected to splenectomy. The average age of patients at operation has been five years, with a wide spread from thirty-seven days up to puberty; 11 of the subjects were under one year of age. At operation, accessory spleens were found in 7 instances. This is a relatively low figure compared to the data of Curtis and Movitz,[40] who found accessory spleens in 57 per cent of their patients with congenital hemolytic anemia who were operated upon in the first decade of life.

One child died during operation for cholecystectomy, common duct exploration, and splenectomy (1939). This combination of operations on opposite sides of the abdomen at one sitting should be avoided because the operative shock is too great. One patient developed intracranial venous thrombosis from which she eventually recovered.

In our experience splenectomy, even when performed in the first year of life, has few or no deleterious side effects on the future development and progress of the child. King and Shumacker[42] have expressed the opinion that removal of spleens in the first year of life alters the reaction of babies in such a way that they are more prone subsequently to develop serious infections; we have found little evidence to support this view.

The over-all results of operation have been most gratifying. There has been a striking improvement in growth and development, when these were previously retarded. Of the 58 children who survived operation and were discharged from the hospital, 2 are known to have died subsequently; one six-year-old boy from meningitis six months later and one infant from acute tracheo-bronchitis seven months later. In only one case was there a continuation of hemolytic crises, but even here the attacks were much less frequent and less severe. Of the remaining 55, 7 have been lost to follow-up, but were well at the time of their discharge from the hospital. All others are known to have had no recurrence of anemia; they have been followed for an average of two years, varying from a few months to as long as sixteen years.

ACQUIRED HEMOLYTIC ANEMIA

Acquired hemolytic anemia, as opposed to congenital hemolytic anemia, is a condition in which excessive hemolysis of red cell occurs as a result of abnormal antibodies found free in the blood or adsorbed to the surface of red cells. This antibody is ordinarily more active against the patient's own red cells (auto-antibody) than against those of other persons (iso-antibody). On the basis that antibody formation may be decreased by splenectomy, removal of the spleen has been extensively tried. However, poor results generally follow, there being some striking exceptions. Since the disease is subject to spontaneous remissions, it becomes exceedingly difficult to evaluate the results of splenectomy. Lahey and Norcross[43] reported splenectomy in 6 cases of acquired hemolytic anemia; and in only one was there improvement. Cole, Walter, and Limarzi[38] have had similar disappointments in 5 patients with acquired hemolytic anemia; 2 died, 2 continued their course unaltered, and 1 improved, but only after numerous transfusions. It appears that in the future, relief for these patients is more likely to be obtained by the use of ACTH or cortisone, with or without splenectomy, as reported by Dameshek, Rosenthal, and Schwartz[3] and by Gardner, McElfresh,

Harris and Diamond,[4] than by splenectomy alone. It appears that ACTH or cortisone is useful in preparing patients for splenectomy; they seem to have only transient value in controlling hemolytic activity, beneficial effects disappearing soon after the drugs are stopped.

At the Children's Hospital we have operated upon 12 children for acquired hemolytic anemia. Following operation, 5 showed marked improvement, 4 had further hemolytic episodes which eventually ceased, and 3 died within a year after surgery of continued hemolysis.

IDIOPATHIC THROMBOCYTOPENIC PURPURA

Thrombocytopenic purpura is a disease in which there is a bleeding tendency because of a diminished number of circulating platelets. Blood smears show a paucity of platelets which by counts may be depressed to 75,000 or less per cubic millimeter. The bleeding time tends to be prolonged, although it may be normal. The clotting time is not lengthened, but retraction of the clot is delayed and poor. Other than the diminished platelets, the blood usually shows no abnormalities except those which can be attributed to blood loss.

The vast majority of thrombocytopenic purpuras are of the *secondary* variety; the depression of circulating platelets is caused by infection, by drug poisoning, by aplasia involving all the elements of the hematopoietic system, by leukemia or other neoplastic infiltration which replaces bone marrow and thereby crowds out platelet-forming tissue. In a minority of cases, a thrombocytopenia is of *idiopathic* type, for which no etiologic factor can be demonstrated. Two clinical types of *idiopathic thrombocytopenia* can be distinguished: *acute*, self-limited thrombocytopenia and *chronic* thrombocytopenia. In the former, spontaneous recovery usually occurs within four months of the onset. In the latter, while clinical remissions are also the rule, thrombocytopenia persists and exacerbations are common. It is usually possible to distinguish between the two entities. The diagnosis of thrombocytopenia, particularly of the chronic idiopathic type, must be considered whenever a child has excessive bleeding, even in the absence of petechiae or purpura.

The means by which the spleen might be involved in bringing about a depression in the circulating blood platelets is not entirely clear. Apparently, it not only filters them out of the circulation but it also appears to have a depressing influence on the *megakaryocytes* of the bone marrow from which the platelets have their origin. As a result of the experimental work of Troland and Lee[11] (in which extracts of spleen obtained from patients suffering from thrombocytopenic purpura were injected into normal experimental animals, thereby causing thrombocytopenia), a "hormonal role" has been attributed to the spleen in the control of platelet formation.

Symptoms and Findings

Idiopathic purpura appears at any age; about 60 per cent of the patients have been between three and seven years. There may be spontaneous *oozing* from the mucous membranes from time to time, and such bleeding may be profuse. *Epistaxes* and subcutaneous *extravasations of blood* are particularly common. *Ecchymoses* may be induced by the slightest trauma, but they can also appear without injury. Excessive oozing may complicate minor surgical procedures. In females, the menstrual periods may be prolonged and the bleeding profuse. *Retinal hemorrhages* are frequently encountered. Mild fever may accompany the more extensive lesions. Placement of a tourniquet around a limb usually produces *petechial hemorrhages* in the extremity within a few minutes. The spleen may be somewhat enlarged, particularly in the chronic forms.

Diagnosis

The diagnosis is usually made without difficulty, and is based on a history of recurring purpuric manifestations, the finding of low platelet counts, and the absence of conditions which might depress the number of circulating thrombocytes. Examination of the bone marrow by sternal aspiration will help rule out many of the secondary thrombocytopenias. In idiopathic thrombocytopenic purpura, large atypical megakaryocytes are numerous.

In a series of more than 400 cases of thrombocytopenic purpura observed on the medical service of the Children's Hospital, only about 15 per cent were finally considered to fall into the "idiopathic" group.

Medical Treatment

When the diagnosis of idiopathic purpura has been established, the form of therapy must be decided upon. Symptomatic treatment includes *bed rest,* proper *sedation,* local *control of blood loss* by styptics or thromboplastic substances, and possibly *blood transfusions* (of fresh blood) to increase temporarily the available platelets and to replace blood which has been lost. Transfusion may tide the individual over for a few days, but it has no permanent influence on the course of the disease. Of greatest benefit are platelet-rich transfusions, using silicone-coated equipment for the infusions.

Dameshek, Rosenthal, and Schwartz[3] treated 11 patients (children and adults) with acute and chronic idiopathic thrombocytopenic purpura, by giving corticotropin (ACTH) or cortisone. The results were not dramatic, but were considered to be worthwhile. Although no permanent remission of the disease was obtained in any of the patients studied, these hormones: (1) reduced in most cases the spontaneous bleeding manifestations; (2) improved the capillary fragility; and (3) shortened the bleeding time and prolonged the phase of initial vasoconstriction that followed an incision of the skin. It appeared that corticotropin and cortisone might be useful in patients with idiopathic thrombocytopenic purpura: (1) to control severe bleeding, especially in those with the acute type of the disease when an expectant attitude may be rewarded by the occurrence of spontaneous remission; (2) prior to splenectomy, when this procedure is considered necessary, to reduce the loss of blood at operation; (3) when splenectomy has been unsuccessful and severe spontaneous bleeding manifestations continue.

Jacobson and Sohier[8] showed that the administration of ACTH or cortisone in 3 patients (adults) with idiopathic thrombopenic purpura was followed by prompt increases of platelets from purpuric levels to normal and even abnormally high levels. Bethell, Miller, and Myers[5] reported that 6 cases of idiopathic thrombocytopenic purpura treated with ACTH or cortisone responded with rises in platelet counts; in several instances the remissions persisted months after completion of treatment. We have found that cortisone can be of considerable value in the control of this disease (Fig. 299).

Splenectomy

In evaluating therapy it is necessary to differentiate clearly between acute thrombocytopenia and the chronic form. In acute thrombocytopenia the evaluation of any treatment, including splenectomy, is frequently impossible because of the self-limited

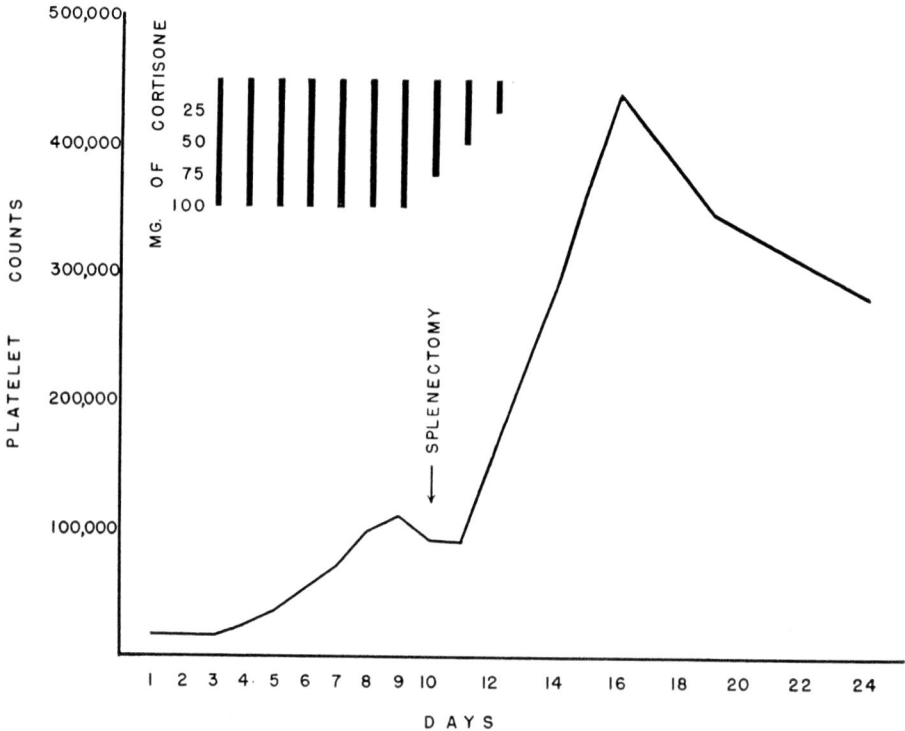

Fig. 299. Chart from a one-year-old child with idiopathic thrombocytopenic purpura, showing the beneficial effects of cortisone and also of splenectomy on the platelet counts. Feeding of cortisone was an excellent method of preparing the child for surgery. Removal of the spleen gave lasting improvement in the number of circulating platelets.

nature of the disease. In chronic idiopathic thrombocytopenia, because of the frequency of spontaneous clinical remissions that often are of many years' duration, and because of the spontaneous fluctuations in thrombocyte count, treatment can be considered successful only if the platelet counts are normal over a significant period (at least four to six months after operation). Although it is difficult to make a decision for or against splenectomy in an individual case during an attack of acute purpura, it is usually best to treat such episodes solely by supportive measures. It is generally conceded that splenectomy is valuable in the chronic form of idiopathic purpura hemorrhagica. If the symptoms have been severe and have recurred over a long period of time, removal of the spleen has beneficial effects in a high percentage (possibly two-thirds) of cases, but it is by no means always curative. It is well to bear in mind that many children have this disease in a mild form and that they tend to have diminishing symptoms with the passage of years. Therefore, splenectomy should be reserved for those whose hemor-rhagic tendencies are severe enough to justify the slight but definite dangers of lapar-otomy. It is always important to examine the bone marrow in these cases; the finding of a few or no megakaryocytes signifies a poor outlook as far as the results of a splenec-tomy are concerned. When splenectomy has been decided upon, it is only fair to warn the parents that relief from the disease does not invariably occur.

Results of Splenectomy

The results of splenectomy will vary tremendously, depending upon the cases which have been selected for surgical therapy. If patients with "acute" forms of the disease are operated upon, the postoperative results might look very good; most of such patients would have recovered spontaneously if left alone. If only those are selected for surgery who have "chronic" forms of the disease, the over-all successes of surgery are apt to be less favorable. The sharp distinction between acute and chronic forms is somewhat artificial, and in individual cases it is sometimes difficult to know into which group a patient should be classified. In general a case is termed "chronic" only after the disease has persisted for many months.

At the Children's Hospital, from 1931 to September 1, 1952, nearly 400 children have been treated for thrombocytopenic purpura. About one-sixth of these were thought to have the idiopathic form. Only 23 were subjected to splenectomy; generally, only those were selected who had had more than two or three episodes of bleeding, a course of more than six or eight months, and who were frequently being knocked about and hence in danger of trauma. Males and females were about equally represented. The average age of patients at the time of operation was nine years; it varied from two to fifteen years. The average duration of symptoms prior to operation was three years, varying from three weeks to eight years. Preoperative platelet counts were uniformly low, varying from 6000 to 54,000. At operation accessory spleens were found in 5 cases. There were no deaths in the group of 23 patients. Of the 23 children operated upon, 18 had an excellent result following splenectomy; 2 had an apparently satisfactory clinical result but had a poor hematologic response in that their platelets increased only slightly; 3 remained unimproved, continuing to show purpuric manifestations. (In one of these latter cases, a poor result had been anticipated preoperatively because of the absence of megakaryocytes in the bone marrow.)

SECONDARY THROMBOCYTOPENIC PURPURA

In 3 patients, we have performed splenectomy for secondary thrombocytopenic purpura. (In two of these, operation was undertaken with a diagnosis of idiopathic disease, but pathologic examination of the spleen revealed tuberculosis in one case and Boeck's sarcoid in the other.) The first patient obtained an excellent response following splenectomy, while the second continued to bleed, finally improving one year later. A third patient had splenectomy because of purpura associated with rheumatic fever and subacute bacterial endocarditis; her purpura improved following surgery, but she died one year postoperatively from endocarditis.

PORTAL HYPERTENSION

Hypertension in the portal system can be caused by thrombosis in the veins themselves or by obstruction in the liver which is secondary to a cirrhosis. Portal hypertension which first shows up in adult life has generally followed hepatic disease; that which comes in childhood can arise from either cause, with a predominance of cases appearing after old thrombosis of various branches of the portal system. While Banti did much to focus attention on these conditions, the term "Banti's disease" connotes such a multiplicity of lesions to different physicians that it is best to avoid confusion by completely abandoning the appellation.

Portal hypertension can prove to be fatal within a few years, or it may have a course extending over several decades. In discussing it three general pictures have to be considered: (1) Hemorrhage from some portion of the alimentary tract, especially the esophagus, because of rupture of dilated collateral venous channels (varices). (2) Hypersplenism, wherein overactivity of the spleen gives depression of any or all of the circulating blood elements. (3) Hepatic insufficiency or failure (in some of the cases in which portal hypertension is secondary to liver disease). Each of these three features can exist alone, or they can appear in any set of combinations; when all of them exist together in a given patient, there can be any order of appearance as they come into the picture.

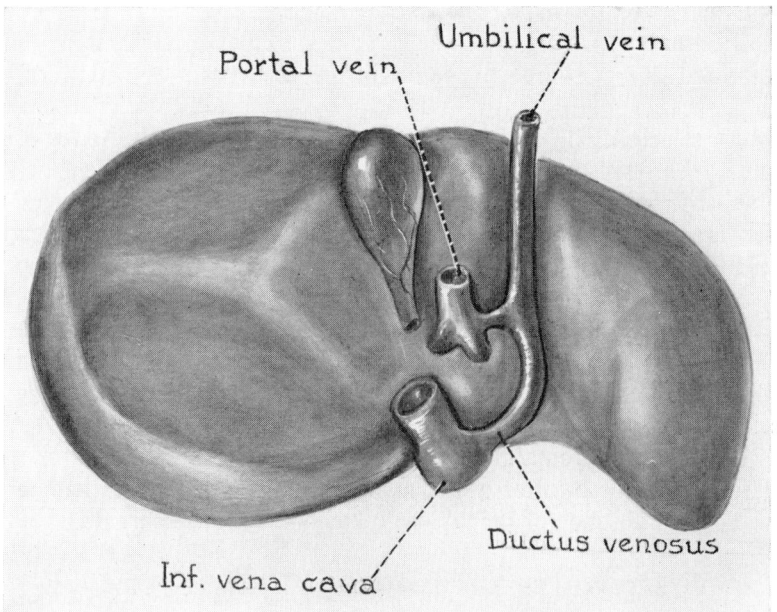

Fig. 300. Sketch of fetal circulation. The umbilical vein (returning oxygenated blood from the placenta) has communication with branches of the portal vein within the liver; most of the blood passes through the ductus venosus to the inferior vena cava. In the newborn period, before the umbilical vein is completely thrombosed, any severe infections of the navel can pass along the umbilical vein and involve the portal system.

Etiology. Pathologic Considerations

Portal obstruction may be intrahepatic or extrahepatic. Any process, either congenital or acquired, which causes liver cirrhosis is capable of producing intrahepatic block. Hepatitis may be of an infectious or poisonous origin; often the etiology is obscure. Liver damage may have been known to exist previously; not infrequently the symptoms of portal hypertension are the initial ones to indicate that there has been serious disease. Thrombophlebitis in the extra-hepatic veins may follow regional or distant infections. Omphalitis of the newborn is particularly liable to cause portal thrombosis, since organisms can proceed inward along the umbilical vein and invade the portal veins or the tissues immediately surrounding them (Fig. 300). In rare instances, abdominal injury can give rise to portal thrombosis and obstruction. Extra-hepatic block may be due to congenital venous "valves" or strictures, or to thrombosis of various radicles of the portal veins. Valves are found as normal structures in various portal channels during embryonic and early postnatal life; while they normally disappear, portions of them may persist and partly obstruct the vessels. "Cavernous transformation" of the portal vein might possibly be a congenital anomaly, but most observers believe it to represent recanalization of an old thrombus (Fig. 302).

As a sequel of portal hypertension, children develop a multitude of collateral

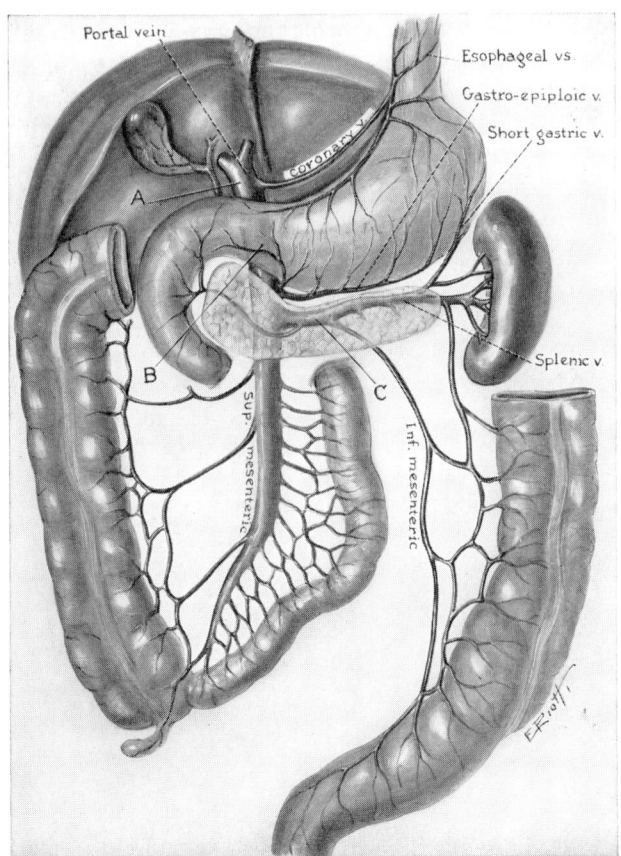

Fig. 301. Sketch of a typical portal system (some subjects show considerable variation in the way vessels empty into the splenic and portal veins). Obstruction occurring within the liver will produce engorgement of the entire system, enlargement of the collateral channels, and development of esophageal varices. Obstruction at A will produce the same changes. Obstruction at B will probably give the same changes. Obstruction at C will usually not lead to development of esophageal varices, but it can give splenomegaly and secondary hypersplenism.

venous channels in the effort to get blood back to the heart. Many of these pathways run over (or in) the wall of the stomach, course through the coronary and esophageal veins, then connecting with the superior vena cava by way of the azygos system. Many of the esophageal veins become dilated and tortuous; they can bulge into the esophageal lumen, covered only by mucosa. They are particularly vulnerable to trauma; rupture of them gives rise to exsanguinating hemorrhage. Baronofsky[13] has emphasized the role of the acid-pepsin factor in erosion of esophageal varices and causation of hemorrhage.

The back pressure and engorgement in the spleen can give rise to, destruction of any of the elements of the circulating blood, a form of secondary hypersplenism.

Symptoms. Physical Findings. Course

The clinical picture may include *hemorrhage from the esophagus and stomach*, *hypersplenism*, or *hepatic failure*. There may be any one of these alone, or there may be any combination of them. In some children a careful history indicates that there was— in the newborn period—an infection of the navel which might well have been the source of infection for a portal vein thrombosis. In others there is a definite history suggesting hepatitis in infancy or childhood. In either event, it is generally many years before symptoms subsequently appear which indicate the existence of portal hypertension. In a considerable number of cases no history of antecedent disease can be elicited.

Hemorrhage from the stomach and esophagus comes as an alarming emesis of blood, often in a child who was thought to be in reasonably good health up to this time. Bleeding is apt to be severe, persistent, and exhausting; pallor and collapse are the rule. Shock is common, and death is not infrequent during one of these harrowing episodes. The hemoglobin and red count can fall to extremely low levels. With this frightful

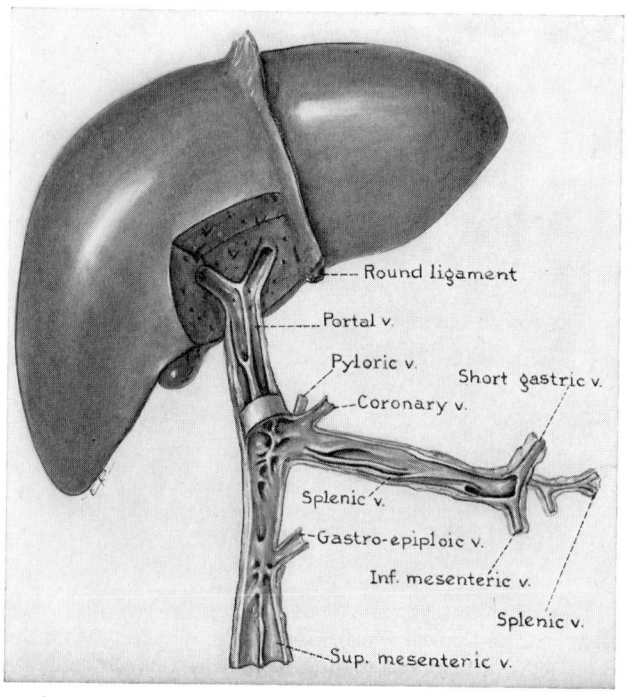

Fig. 302. Autopsy sketch of portal system from a ten-year-old girl who died of esophageal hemorrhage of Banti's disease (portal hypertension). There are old, extensive, and partially recanalized thrombi in the portal, superior mesenteric, and splenic veins, giving rise to extrahepatic venous obstruction. These presumably formed during the multiple severe infections which the child was known to have in the first year of life.

decompression of the portal system, the bleeding generally stops spontaneously; in other cases drastic measures are necessary to bring it under control. Bleeding from esophageal varices usually expresses itself in vomiting of large amounts of blood; it is usually also followed by passage of tarry stools. In some subjects, there is little or no hematemesis, but there is persistent or intermittent passage of blood in the bowel movement, which is evident by the abnormal color of the stools or by strongly positive guaiac tests on the material. The spleen is enlarged to great size (Figs. 304 and 305), but oftentimes it can be found to diminish greatly in size, like a pricked balloon, during or immediately after a bout of bleeding, only to assume its former large size some days later as the congestion in the portal system builds up again. Prominent veins can generally be found on the upper abdomen or lower thorax. The liver may or not be enlarged, depending upon whether the obstruction is within the organ itself or in the vessels outside of it. Patients with esophageal bleeding can run totally unpredictable courses. Bouts can be

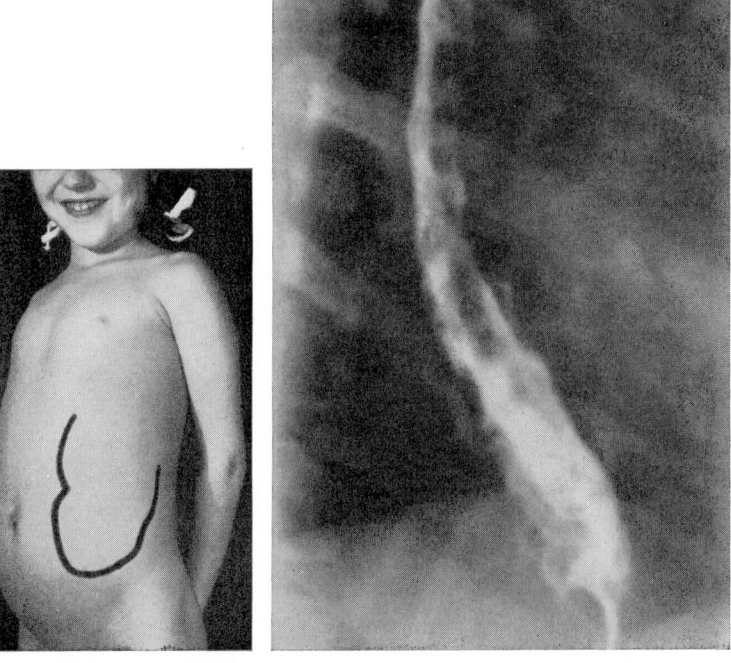

Fig. 303. *Left*, Photograph of nine-year-old girl with portal hypertension. The liver was normal; the block was in the portal vein. Outline of greatly enlarged spleen is shown. This was known to be big since one year of age. *Right*, Esophageal varices, from portal hypertension.

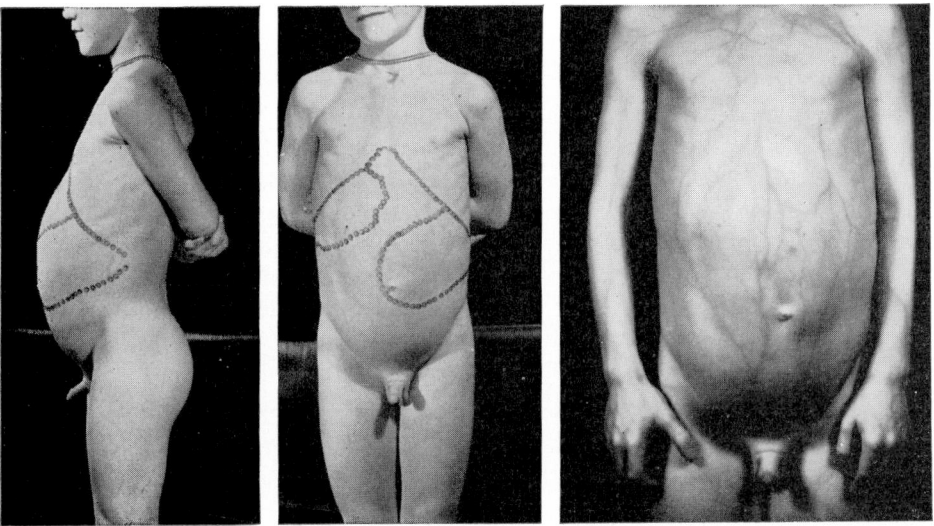

Fig. 304. Eleven-year-old boy with cirrhosis of liver, hepatomegaly, portal hypertension, spleno-megaly; symptoms of hematemesis and hypersplenism. *Left* and *middle* photographs show outlines of the greatly enlarged liver and spleen. *Right* photograph made by infra-red technique, showing the development of collateral vascular channels in the abdominal wall.

very common, recurring at short intervals, and massive in amounts; in other subjects an episode or two can be followed by many years or even decades of quiescence.

Esophageal varices can be suspected whenever there has been either hematemesis or strongly positive guaiac tests on the stools. Their presence can be proved with certainty by roentgenographic visualization (Fig. 303) of the esophagus and under some circumstances by esophagoscopy.

Hypersplenism becomes evident when there is depression to serious degree of the circulating red cells, white cells, or platelets. If the erythrocytes are most affected, there is weakness, pallor, and mild or moderate anemia. When the white cells are the most involved, there is a neutropenia and recurrent infections may be major complaints. When platelets are involved, there can be a variety of purpuric manifestations in any

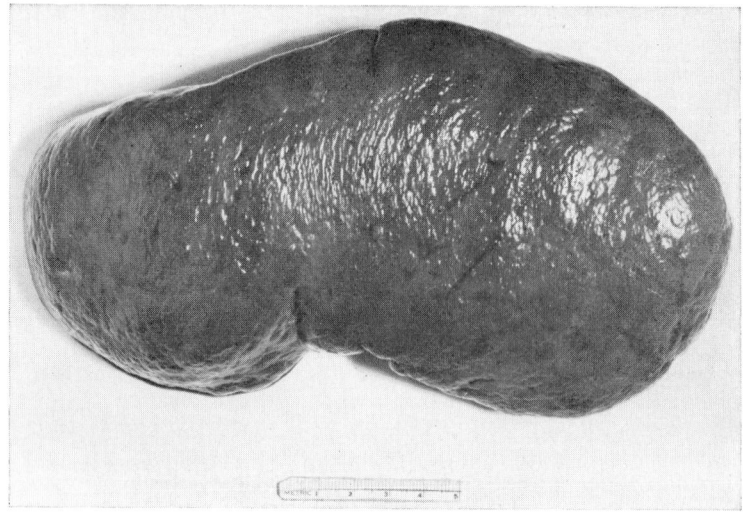

Fig. 305. A spleen weighing 449 gm. removed from boy with portal hypertension (Fig. 304).

part of the body. While the excess destruction can involve solely the erythrocytes, leukocytes, or platelets, generally there is some depression of all three elements. In any event, the spleen is palpably enlarged and examination of bone marrow shows active hematopoietic tissue; obviously the abnormal blood picture has been produced by excessive destruction and not by a failure of formation of the various blood elements.

Hepatic failure is manifestated by lassitude, weakness, malnutrition, anorexia, possibly jaundice or ascites, and inability to form certain substances normally manufactured in the liver, notably prothrombin and plasma albumin. Such a picture usually indicates an exceedingly poor outlook; it is the herald of impending death. Even at such a stage, it is still possible for the reparative powers of the liver to bring about some regeneration and to restore to a reasonable degree the greatly deranged liver functions, but generally such is not the case.

Determination of Source of Portal Hypertension

While it is sometimes impossible to do so, one can usually determine with reasonable accuracy whether a portal hypertension stems from an obstruction within the liver or outside of it. Factors favoring the latter are: (1) No history of liver disease. (2) A normal-sized liver. (3) Normal plasma prothrombin and albumin. (4) Normal liver-function tests. (5) When available by biopsy, a normal histologic liver architecture.

Conversely, the hypertension is almost certainly of hepatic origin if there are: (1) A history of important liver disease. (2) An enlarged (or a greatly shrunken) liver. (3) Strongly positive cephalin flocculation, thymol turbidity, or Bromsulphalein tests. (4) Diminished plasma prothrombin or albumin levels. (5) Abdominal ascites. (6) By biopsy, microscopic evidence of liver damage.

It is of great importance to determine whether or not liver disease is a part of the picture; it has considerable bearing on the prognosis. If the obstruction is from thrombosis of the portal vein (or its radicles), a splenectomy (or splenectomy and splenorenal shunt) can have great and permanent value. Conversely, if the obstruction is from a scarred and cirrhotic liver, treatment by some shunting operation such as a splenorenal or porto-caval anastomosis might have beneficial effects as far as relief of the portal hypertension is concerned, but these can be overshadowed by progressive and even fatal disease of the liver.

Treatment

Preoperative Measures. In those patients with any important degree of anemia, there should be transfusion, feeding of iron, and administration of vitamin K. If there is current, active bleeding from the esophagus, there should be bed rest, sedation, transfusions, and withholding of oral feedings. In some patients, administration of antacids may be of value, as acid-pepsin erosion is thought to be a factor in the initiation of hemorrhage.

Should the bleeding continue unchecked despite these measures, a triple-lumen tube carrying two separately inflatable balloons should be passed down the esophagus so that its distal end lies in the stomach. The distal small balloon is then inflated and by traction on the tube is snugged up against the cardia. The second balloon situated just proximal to it is then inflated and connected to a manometer so that constant pressure can be maintained against the walls of the lower esophagus and the varices which are located there. In this way, according to Sengstaken and Blakemore,[18] hemorrhage from esophageal varices may be effectively stopped. The third lumen of the tube is connected to a suction apparatus to empty the stomach. If this is not done, vomiting is likely to occur, with dislodgment of the tube. After the emergency has passed, but before the surgeon feels safe in removing the tube, feedings may be given cautiously through the third lumen of the tube. These tubes are large and bulky; they can be used with satisfaction for adults and older children; they are impractical for small children.

Emergency ligation of the splenic artery in the presence of acute severe hemorrhage has a little merit, but at times has been employed. Blain and Blain[35] have suggested, and gathered a small number of cases to support the contention, that splenic artery ligation (a relatively simple procedure and having the immediate effect of greatly reducing the amount of blood flowing into the portal circulation) is an operation of value in selected (poor risk) patients with splenomegaly due to portal hypertension. If spleno-renal anastomosis cannot be carried out because of the patient's poor condition or the surgeon's lack of experience with the operation, splenic artery ligation is far superior to splenectomy. There is less interference with the anastomotic venous pathways; subsequent spleno-renal anastomosis will be easier if the patient's improvement subsequently permits an attempt at this more extensive operation.

Before any surgery is undertaken, the current status of the liver must be evaluated and if this organ is damaged, intensive medical measures should be instituted to get it into the best possible condition. Whether or not the seriously ill patient will survive surgery is frequently determined by the degree of success of this preoperative care. Anemia and decreased blood volume must be corrected by transfusions. A high-protein, high-carbohydrate diet, supplemented by vitamins B_{12} and K and possibly by choline or methionine, is of great value in aiding liver recovery; continued bed rest as emphasized by Chalmers and Davidson[15] also appears to be worth-while.

The outlook for surgical treatment of portal hypertension is much better for those subjects whose block is outside of the liver and is poorer in the group in which the block is secondary to cirrhosis. In those with mild or arrested liver disease, surgery can be tolerated reasonably well; in those with advanced or with progressing hepatitis, the prognosis is grave. Especially bad prognostic signs are: (1) A plasma albumin less than 3 gm. per cent. (2) Ascites which fail to respond to medical treatment. (3) An elevated serum bilirubin. (4) A prothrombin time which remains more than 4 seconds above normal after adequate vitamin K therapy. (5) Cephalin flocculation tests of 3 plus or 4 plus. (6) A Bromsulphalein retention test showing more than 10 per cent dye retention after thirty minutes.

Splenectomy. Removal of the spleen has curative effects as far as hypersplenism is concerned. Therefore, the presence of neutropenia, thrombocytopenia or any important degree of anemia (other than on the basis of hemorrhage) is a clear indication for splenectomy. For the treatment of recurrent esophageal bleeding, splenectomy also has considerable value in that removal of the organ (or ligation of its artery) reduces by about 20 per cent the amount of blood which is flowing into the portal circuit. In rare patients, who have thrombosis of the splenic vein, splenectomy alone is followed by complete cessation of bleeding. More often, obstruction is in the portal vein or in the liver; splenectomy alone has little or no effect in reducing the severity or the frequency of the bleeding attacks. It is now generally stressed that limiting operation to splenectomy is poor judgment; closure and atrophy of the splenic vein prohibits the use of this vessel subsequently for establishment of any anastomosis. Certainly, *if any esophageal bleeding had been present before operation, if varices have been demonstrated by roentgenograms, or if any important degree of portal hypertension is found at operation (either by visible engorgement of the regional veins or by actual pressure readings with a manometer), splenectomy should always be combined with establishment of a splenorenal shunt.*

Measurement of venous pressures within the abdomen may be misleading; false values can be obtained because of tilting the operating table, fluctuations in the systemic blood pressure, artificial kinking of the veins by packs or instruments, etc. However, if the surgeon eliminates as many as possible of these factors and realizes the limitations of the method, the measurement of portal pressures is of value in determining the degree of the hypertension and possibly the position of the block. A plea for standardization in methods for obtaining portal pressures has been made by Taylor and Egbert[20]; serious discrepancies in pressure readings occur, depending upon the height the manometer is held above a vein. They suggest that the splenic vein, where it crosses the anterior surface of the vertebral column, be universally employed as the base-line for manometric readings. In a series of adults, they determined that portal pressures by this standard are normally below 225 mm. of water. Certainly, pressures above 250 mm. can be regarded as abnormally high.

Shunt Operation. Shunts can be made either of the porto-caval or the spleno-renal variety. In children there is rarely need for the former and indeed it is often impossible to perform them because the portal vein is the seat of disease and is unsuitable for a shunting operation. Spleno-renal anastomoses are adequate, are easier to perform, and can be made at the same time that a splenectomy is performed. About the only indication for anastomosis of the porto-caval type is for those children who previously had been subjected to a splenectomy (without a shunt), who still have esophageal bleeding, and who require further surgical attack on their problem.

For performance of spleno-renal anastomosis (Fig. 306), there is usually little difficulty in mobilizing the tail of the pancreas (with the splenic vein) and the kidney pedicle to allow them to come together without tension on the line of suture. Because of the small size of vessels, there is a limit, below which it is difficult to make a satisfactory union with reasonable hope that it will remain open; the dividing line is probably around three years, but this is not a fixed figure. Spleno-renal vein unions should never be made by the non-suture method, employing a vitallium cuff to bring vein ends together; it is far better to make an anastomosis by direct suture. It is never necessary to sacrifice the left kidney; the spleno-renal union can be made in an end-to-side manner, preserving the kidney.

Needless to say, the liver should always be biopsied to get a permanent and accurate record of its state.

It cannot be emphasized too strongly that a surgeon should not undertake splenectomy in a patient suspected of having congestive splenomegaly unless he is also prepared to measure vein pressures, and, if indicated, to proceed with a venous anastomosis. Should portal hypertension exist in a patient and splenectomy alone be performed, the golden opportunity has been lost; following splenectomy its vein usually thromboses or shrinks and thereafter cannot be employed for anastomosis.

Results of Therapy

The Children's Hospital material includes 24 patients who have been surgically treated for portal hypertension.

Eight patients, in whom hypersplenism appeared as the predominant symptom, were treated by splenectomy alone. While the follow-ups in several instances were of only short duration, 6 patients did well, one improved but still had mild symptoms, and one could not be traced.

In 16 cases, hemorrhage from the esophagus or stomach had been the predominating symptom, but in some there also had been a degree of hypersplenism. Nine patients (before the time spleno-renal anastomoses were developed) were treated by either splenectomy alone, or by splenectomy combined with omentopexy and vein ligations in the region of the cardia. Of these patients, one has done well, 4 are known to have had further hemorrhage and to have done poorly, while 4 are known to have died. Seven recent patients have had splenectomy combined with spleno-renal anastomosis (Table 64), all of them being operated upon within the last three years. They ranged from three to eleven years of age; 3 had normal livers, 1 had a mildly abnormal liver, 3 had markedly abnormal livers. One had mild recurrence of bleeding 6 months after operation; all the others appear to be doing very well and have not had further hematemesis. None of these 7 children has died.

HYPERSPLENISM

Hypersplenism is a term which has come into vogue in recent years,[24,25,26] to describe states in which an overactive spleen has produced significant depressions in the levels of circulating red cells, white cells, or platelets. These include a variety of pictures, which have been divided into *primary hypersplenism* and *secondary hypersplenism*.

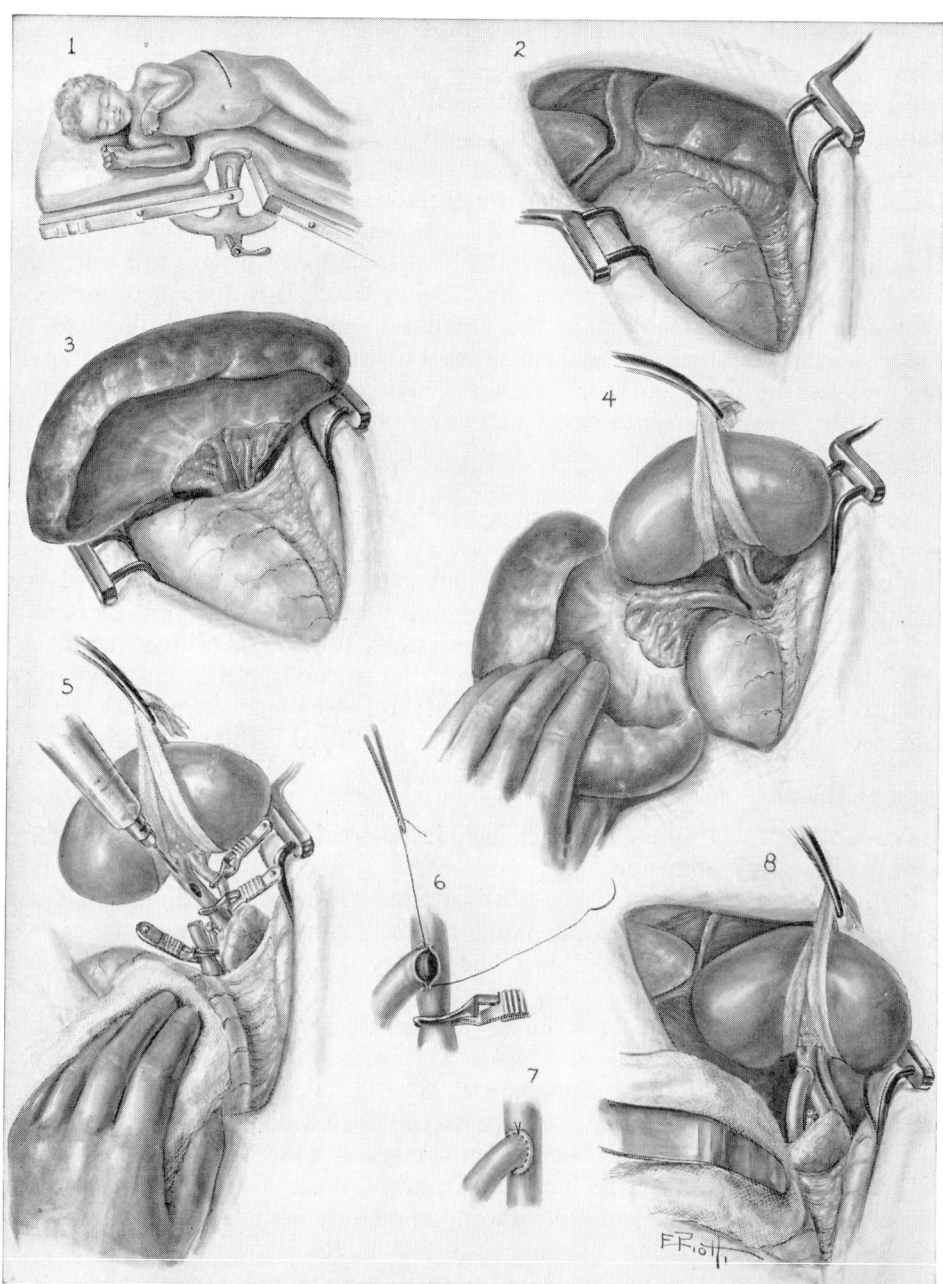

Fig. 306. Technique for establishment of spleno-renal shunt. 1. Position of patient on table, a roll under the right flank, the body leaned backward slightly. Incision in the ninth interspace, running obliquely downward through the abdominal wall. 2. Wound held open with self-retaining retractor. Excellent view of region obtained. 3. The spleen is mobilized and raised upward from its bed. To keep the splenic vein in best possible condition, the splenic pedicle will not be divided until after the kidney has been mobilized. (In some cases, the spleen is so large that it is necessary to remove it early to get exposure of the kidney.) 4. Kidney mobilized from its bed, attenuating its pedicle by pulling on the kidney tapes. 5. Spleen removed. Serrefine clamps on the splenic vein and the renal artery and vein. Ellipse of wall cut out of renal vein. Field kept moistened with heparin solution. 6. End-to-side union begun. Stitch (00000 Deknatel silk) goes through all layers, turning the edges outward. 7. Anastomosis completed. 8. Position of vessels after anastomosis is finished. Surrounding tissues will now be anchored to the renal pedicle, to make certain that there is no angulation or tension on the splenic vein or the anastomosis.

In *primary hypersplenism*, platelets, red blood cells, or neutrophils, or all three of these elements of the blood, may be destroyed by the spleen. Four resulting clinical diseases are recognized. Excessive destruction of platelets results in essential thrombocytopenic purpura. The destruction of red cells in primary hypersplenism produces congenital hemolytic anemia. The syndrome of primary splenic neutropenia is a consequence of increased destruction of the neutrophils. If all three of the blood elements

Table 64

Children Treated for Portal Hypertension by Splenectomy and Spleno-renal Shunt

Case	Sex. Age at Operation	Position of Portal Block	Date of Operation	Remarks and Follow-up
1	M 9 yrs.	In extra-hepatic veins. Secondary to trauma? Liver normal.	2/13/48	Last seen 9/17/52. Excellent condition. No more bleeding. 1 year after operation still had varices but smaller.
2	F 8 yrs.	In extra-hepatic veins. Had newborn umbilical infection. Liver normal.	11/15/49	Last seen 9/17/52. Was excellent at that time.
3	F 11 yrs.	Intra-hepatic. Liver mildly abnormal.	12/22/49	Excellent condition, Oct. 1952.
4	F 10 yrs.	Intra-hepatic. Liver markedly abnormal.	10/2/50	7/22/52. In excellent health. No more bleeding.
5	F 11 yrs.	Intra-hepatic. Liver markedly abnormal.	10/20/50	3/10/52. Excellent general condition. No bleeding.
6	M 3½ yrs.	In portal vein. Liver normal.	4/2/51	Bled 6 months later. Well 1 year after that.
7	F 11 yrs.	Intra-hepatic. Liver markedly abnormal.	2/26/52	7/10/52. Very satisfactory condition. No further bleeding.

are depressed as a result of hypersplenism, the clinical disease is known as primary pancytopenia. Splenectomy in any of these diseases will usually effect a cure of the hematologic disturbances.

Secondary hypersplenism produces a clinical picture identical with that of primary hypersplenism but occurs as a complication of a number of chronic disease processes, such as chronic leukemia, portal hypertension, Boeck's sarcoid, Hodgkin's disease, or certain infections. The astute hematologist has found that, during an unsatisfactory phase of one of the above-mentioned generalized systemic diseases, there may be a superimposed overactivity of the spleen, producing secondary thrombocytopenic pancytopenia. The spleen has been proved to be the offending organ in the production of these cytopenias. Splenectomy may prolong life in a patient with a secondary hypersplenism or it may establish a more favorable hematologic state; it will not alter appreciably the eventual outcome of the primary disease.

Results of Splenectomy

The common forms of *primary hypersplenism*, congenital hemolytic anemia and idiopathic thrombocytopenic purpura, are of sufficient interest to be described as separate entities. The results of treatment of them by splenectomy have been listed in preceding sections. Rarer forms, *primary splenic neutropenia* and *primary splenic pancytopenia*, can be identified only after elaborate blood and bone marrow studies, and verified after examination of the spleen shows no other disease. Splenectomy has been reported by Doan and his associates,[24,26] to give excellent results in improvement of the blood picture. Our one patient with primary splenic neutropenia did very well after splenectomy.

Secondary hypersplenism can sometimes be recognized before operation by the blood picture which shows depression of one or more elements, by the presence of an active marrow, and by the coexistence of some generalized or local disease such as tuberculosis, leukemia, Boeck's sarcoid, etc. In other instances, the underlying disease might not be found until the spleen is removed and examined histologically. In 12 patients we have removed the spleen, knowing that chronic leukemia existed; the children have felt better because of removal of a huge and weighty organ; their blood pictures have improved somewhat; the operative procedures can be regarded only as experimental in nature, the values of which are dubious. In 4 patients, who before operation were thought to have a primary form of hypersplenism, the surgically removed spleens were found to be the seat of localized tuberculosis or sarcoid; they must therefore be classified in the secondary group; considerable benefit in the hematologic picture appeared after removal of the spleens.

TRAUMATIC RUPTURE OF THE SPLEEN

Abdominal injuries, particularly those resulting from direct violence, such as a blow on the abdomen, a fall from a considerable height, or an impact from a moving vehicle, may rupture various viscera including the spleen.

Symptoms

When the spleen is torn, the important symptoms are primarily those of *hemorrhage*. The amount of blood lost into the peritoneal cavity depends upon the extent and position of the splenic laceration. Left shoulder *pain* may suggest some pathologic condition below the left diaphragm, but this symptom is not always present. Inasmuch as the violence usually produces some contusion of the abdominal wall, the physician often has difficulty in deciding whether the local *pain* and *tenderness* are due to trauma of the abdominal wall or to injury of organs within the peritoneal cavity. In such a quandary, a falling red blood count is of great importance in the differential diagnosis, if there is no other blood loss to explain a progressive anemia. Whenever there is known abdominal injury, rising pulse, declining blood pressure, pallor, thirst, air hunger, or a falling red count there are certainly indications for *exploratory laparotomy*. It is usually impossible to determine before operation the extent of the injury and what organs have been affected.

Roentgenological examination of the abdomen and chest is of little value in establishing a positive diagnosis of ruptured spleen, but serves to rule out other injuries such as diaphragmatic rupture or pneumothorax. However, Solis-Cohen and Levine[30] as well as O'Neill and Rousseau[28] have described roentgen findings which they consider practically pathognomonic of rupture of the spleen. These changes are due to extravasation of blood between the layers of the gastro-splenic ligament and include a

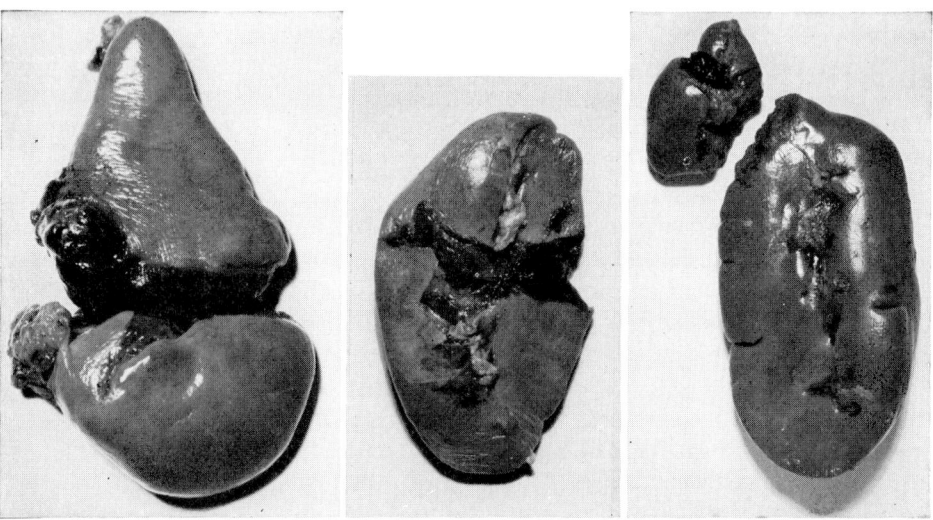

Fig. 307. Ruptured spleens removed from three children, thirteen, ten, and fifteen years of age.

dilated stomach with a serrated greater curvature and obliteration of the splenic shadow (Fig. 308). While we have seen these changes in some cases of splenic rupture, we have found them also in other conditions which can cause hemorrhage or edema of tissues adjacent to the stomach.

Treatment

When operations of this sort are undertaken, provisions for *transfusion* should always be made. It is a wise precaution to place a cannula in an arm or leg vein before opening the abdomen so that blood may be given promptly during the procedure, if this should be necessary. Not infrequently, more blood is found free in the peritoneal cavity than had been anticipated, and there may be additional loss before the site of

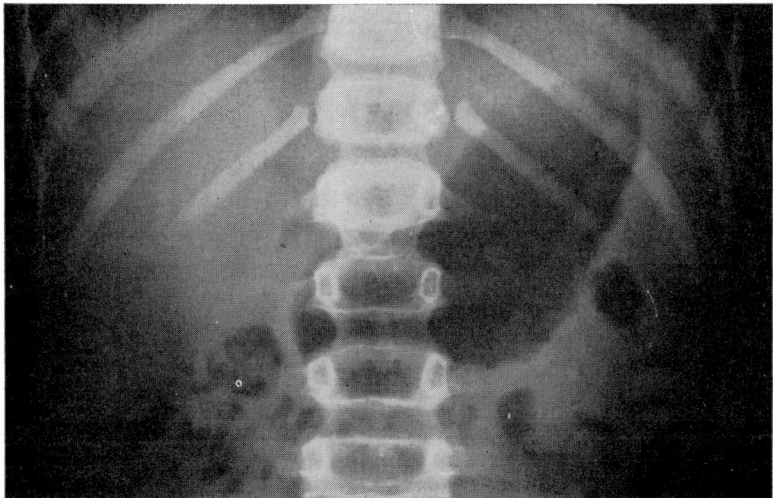

Fig. 308. Roentgenogram from a child with traumatic rupture of the spleen. There is atony and dilatation of the stomach. The serrations along the greater curvature are caused by extravasations of blood into the gastro-lienal ligament.

hemorrhage can be identified and the bleeding controlled. The operator's troubles are considerably lessened and the patient's chances for survival are greatly enhanced if transfusion can be given during this period.

For such operations, we always prefer a transverse incision, because of the ease of extending this to the right, if the liver is found injured, or back into the flank if a kidney must be treated.

The average spleen is so friable that once its capsule has been ruptured, fractures into its substance are apt to be deep and difficult to repair. *It is therefore easier and preferable to remove the entire organ.* The vessels of the splenic pedicle should be digitally compressed or else ligated as soon as possible to stop the loss of blood from the ruptured spleen. Whenever there is extravasation of blood into the gastro-lienal ligament, the division here must be made very carefully so the stomach will not be entered.

Results of Therapy

At the Children's Hospital, 18 patients have been treated for splenic injury. Nine ruptures of the spleen occurred as the result of falls, usually on the left side; 4 came from sledding accidents; 3 came from automobile accidents; 1 was sustained from a hard tackle in a football game, and 1 was from a bullet wound. In all but two cases, operation was performed within a few hours after injury. The others were operated upon at two days and five days following injury and in these the hemorrhage was relatively slight and came from small tears in the spleen. All the children made uneventful recoveries following splenectomy.

LIPID STORAGE DISEASE

There are three primary disorders of lipid metabolism which are closely allied to one another. According to the type of lipid involved, these may be grouped as: (1) *Gaucher's disease*, a cerebroside (kerasin) disturbance. (2) *Niemann-Pick's disease*, a phosphatide (sphingomyelin) disturbance. (3) *Schüller-Christian's* disease (generalized xanthomatosis), a cholesterol disturbance.

Gaucher's Disease

Gaucher's disease manifests itself by excessive accumulation of kerasin in cells, principally of the liver, spleen, lymph nodes, and bone marrow. In some instances a marked *splenic enlargement* dominates the picture and there is progressive abdominal distention, discomfort, anorexia, fatigue, and retardation of physical growth, and possibly some degree of secondary hypersplenism.

Whenever there is bony involvement there may be local pain, limitation of motion, and even pathologic fracture. The roentgenologic picture of localized destruction of bone is often mistaken for osteomyelitis. If such a bone lesion should be exposed at operation, removal of some of the yellowish brown material for *histologic examination* should establish the diagnosis. The large, lipid-laden cells have a wrinkled appearance and do not take the Smith-Dietrich stain as do the lipid-filled, foamy-appearing cells of Niemann-Pick's disease. Patients with Gaucher's disease may subsequently develop foci in other bones; it is important to recognize that these are lipoid accumulations, and that operation (for suspected osteomyelitis) is not necessary.

Treatment. The bone lesions, like those of Schüller-Christian's disease, can be effectively treated by exposure to x-rays. This induces fibrosis, healing, and symptomatic relief. Such changes may appear spontaneously in some cases, but they are speeded up and advanced by x-ray therapy.

If the spleen is large, its removal has been found to be of definite value. The indications for splenectomy are: (1) Discomfort from a progressively enlarging organ. (2) Development of anemia or thrombocytopenia with a tendency toward bleeding. (3) Retardation in growth and physical development of the individual.

Results of Treatment. Following splenectomy the abdominal discomfort is relieved, the anemia is improved, and physical growth becomes accelerated.

At the Children's Hospital 9 splenectomies have been performed on patients with Gaucher's disease with over-all results which are probably favorable but are difficult to evaluate. In one baby the course following splenectomy continued downhill without alteration; he died two months later with cerebral and pulmonary involvement. The other 8 patients were older and had a much better outlook. Particularly impressive has been the rapid increase in body growth, so that a retarded child reaches a normal average size for his age within a few years. When secondary hypersplenism has existed before operation, the blood picture has been improved by removal of the spleen. It might be argued that splenectomy would precipitate or accelerate the accumulation of the lipoid in the skeleton, but numerous roentgenologic observations on our cases lead us to believe that such is not the case. Although it may still be too early for final evaluation of splenectomy in this disease, it is our distinct impression that the operation has considerable merit.

Niemann-Pick's Disease

This condition is known to be most common in Jews. A familial tendency is frequently present. It is a disease of infancy. The children usually die before their third birthday, cerebral involvement and deterioration usually dominating the picture. In 4 infants for whom we performed a splenectomy, little or nothing was accomplished to stop or retard the ravages of the disease.

CYSTS AND TUMORS OF THE SPLEEN

Cysts

Small cysts of the spleen, 1 or 2 cc. in diameter, are occasionally observed at the autopsy table, particularly in conjunction with congenital cysts of the liver or kidneys. Cysts of the spleen which are large enough to be of clinical importance are very rare. Fowler[31] collected reports of 137 non-parasitic splenic cysts and of this group only 10 occurred in the first decade of life. Cysts may be of several sorts: (1) *Thin-walled serous cysts* which presumably arise from inclusion of a nest of peritoneal cells which have become pinched off in a cleft of the splenic surface. From this nidus there develops a small intrasplenic sac which accumulates and retains fluid. (2) *Lymphangiomas* of the spleen have often been described. These are usually multilocular and have a honeycombed appearance. They may be so large that they replace most of the splenic substance. (3) *Epidermoid cysts* are rare, usually do not attain a large size, and do not accumulate hair or sebaceous material. They are lined with squamous epithelium which does not keratinize. (4) *Parasitic cysts* are almost always of echinococcus origin. They may be found in conjunction with similar lesions of the liver, lung, or other viscera, but in some instances they develop solely in the spleen.

Tumors of the spleen are rare, but sarcomas and hemangiomas have been described.

Treatment

Removal of the spleen for treatment of a cyst is seldom necessary unless the lesion is large enough (Fig. 309) to cause local discomfort or to arouse suspicions regarding the presence of a neoplasm. Neoplasms are extremely rare, but if a mass is felt through the abdominal wall, or if it is discovered during laparotomy for some other condition, removal of the organ is indicated.

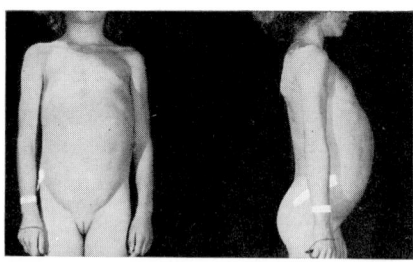

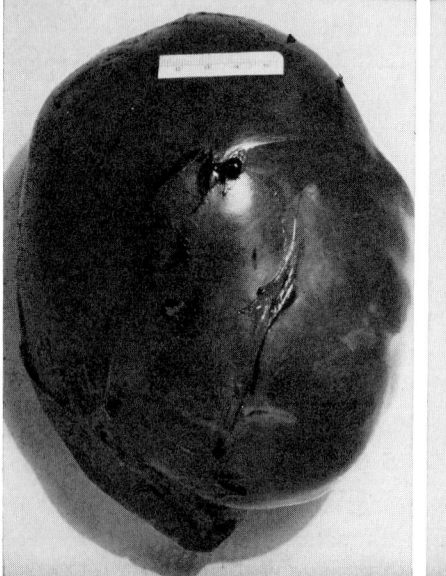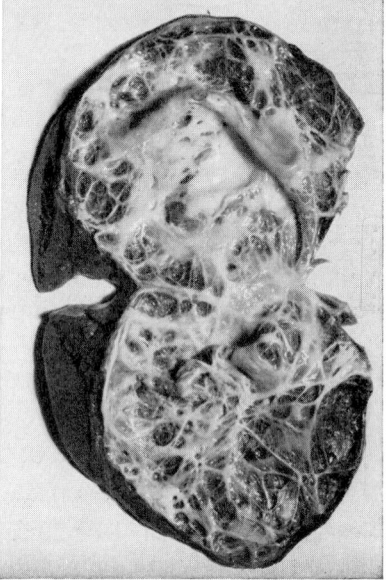

Fig. 309. Congenital cyst of spleen in an eight-year-old child. *Above,* Note marked prominence of the abdomen in the lateral view. *Below,* Photographs of the surgical specimen, which weighed 1400 gm. and measured 18 cm. in length and 10 cm. in diameter.

MISCELLANEOUS CONDITIONS

There are a variety of conditions which deserve only very brief mention.

For *hypoplastic or aplastic anemia,* splenectomy has no beneficial effects.

For *Mediterranean (Cooley's) anemia,* splenectomy is of no value, and may even aggravate the disease.

For *sickle cell anemia,* splenectomy is valueless.

For *agnogenic myeloid metaplasia,* splenectomy has not proved to be helpful.

TECHNIQUE OF SPLENECTOMY

The removal of a spleen can be made a simple procedure. *Mortality rates* for this operation have often been high, but with improved methods for controlling anemia by transfusions and with better operative exposures, fatalities have now been reduced to a negligible figure. In our series of 199 splenectomies there has been but one operative death; this occurred (in 1939) from shock in a child who was simultaneously treated

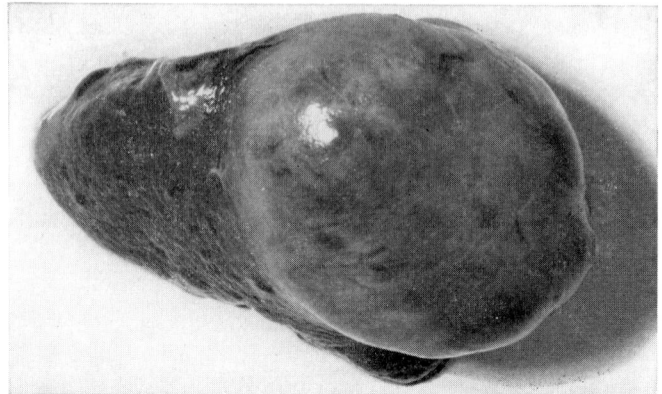

Fig. 310. Hemangioma of the spleen, removed from a three-month-old boy.

by splenectomy and removal of common duct stones. There have been no deaths from splenectomy in the thirteen years since then.

Preoperative treatment is important. When he patient has a bleeding tendency, it is desirable to *transfuse* him before operation and to be prepared to repeat this during or immediately thereafter. In those patients with anemias below 3,500,000 or 4,000,000 the red count should be brought up to adequate levels by medication and transfusion. Cleansing and *deflation of the stomach and colon* will make these organs less troublesome in the operative field and will enhance the exposure

Exposure of the Spleen

There is some variance of opinion concerning the type of incision which should be employed. There has been common use of a left paramedian or rectus incision for splenectomy; we believe this is a very poor approach. Using it, one finds the colon, the stomach, and many loops of intestines constantly in the field and requiring retraction and packing away. The splenic pedicle lies deep in the abdomen and is difficult to get at and work upon. The operation is needlessly tiresome and is often difficult. In contrast, a *transverse incision* below the costal border, extending forward from the posterior-axillary line is much to be preferred (Fig. 314). The incision should be made

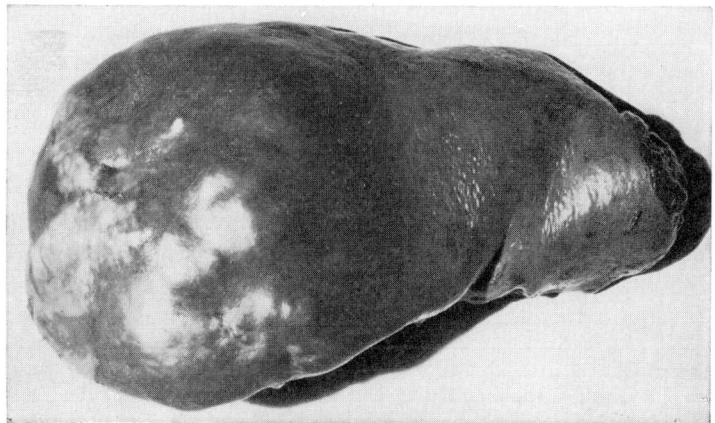

Fig. 311. Spleen with Hodgkin's disease, removed from a thirteen-year-old boy. Weight 430 gm.; normal for this age 93 gm.

so the tenth nerve is identified and can be protectively held in the posterior angle of the wound with a retractor. If the spleen is small, it is not necessary to divide the rectus muscle, but if it is large the rectus can be cut across with impunity. In the abdomen, rarely does one see or need to pack away intestines. While making gentle and constant downward traction on the spleen, *the various splenic ligaments can be cut, after which the spleen can be flopped up out of the wound and brought to rest outside the abdomen.* It is then exceedingly easy and safe to divide its pedicle. Transverse incisions heal extremely well. They give a narrow cutaneous scar and they are not followed by any weakness of the abdominal wall from division of nerves.

When treating portal hypertension, and contemplating splenectomy and establishment of a spleno-renal shunt, a thoraco-abdominal wound (Fig. 306) gives the optimum exposure.

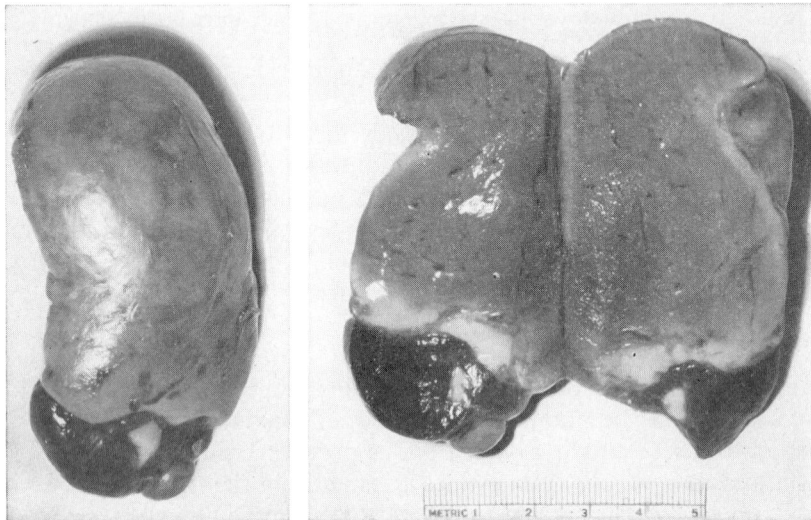

Fig. 312. Wandering spleen, removed from a seventeen-day-old baby. There had been torsion, with infarction of most of the splenic substance. Normal splenic substance remains at the bottom of the specimen; the remainder is infarcted.

POST-SPLENECTOMY THROMBOSIS

After splenectomy there is almost always some increase in the number of circulating blood platelets. These may reach 600,000 or 700,000 per cu. mm., and counts of 1,000,000 or more are occasionally found. Excessive rises are particularly apt to be found after removal of spleen for treatment of congenital hemolytic anemia and traumatic rupture of the spleen. Platelet rises begin within the first week after operation and have usually disappeared by the end of the second or third week (Fig. 315). The peak of rise generally comes within the second week. If the platelets become very numerous, *thrombi* can develop in various parts of the body, particularly in branches of the portal system. Unexplained abdominal pain and fever occurring in the first weeks after splenectomy should strongly suggest that thrombosis is occurring, particularly if the platelet count

---

need to be clamped or ligated. 7. Spleen completely freed of all its attachments, excepting the pedicle. When this is done, the organ flops *outside* the level of the abdominal wall. As the spleen is rotated backward by the assistant, an excellent view of the pedicle is obtained. The subsequent division on the pedicle can be done easily and safely because the pedicle is readily accessible. 8. Beginning division of splenic pedicle. 9. Spleen removed. Field inspected and left completely dry.

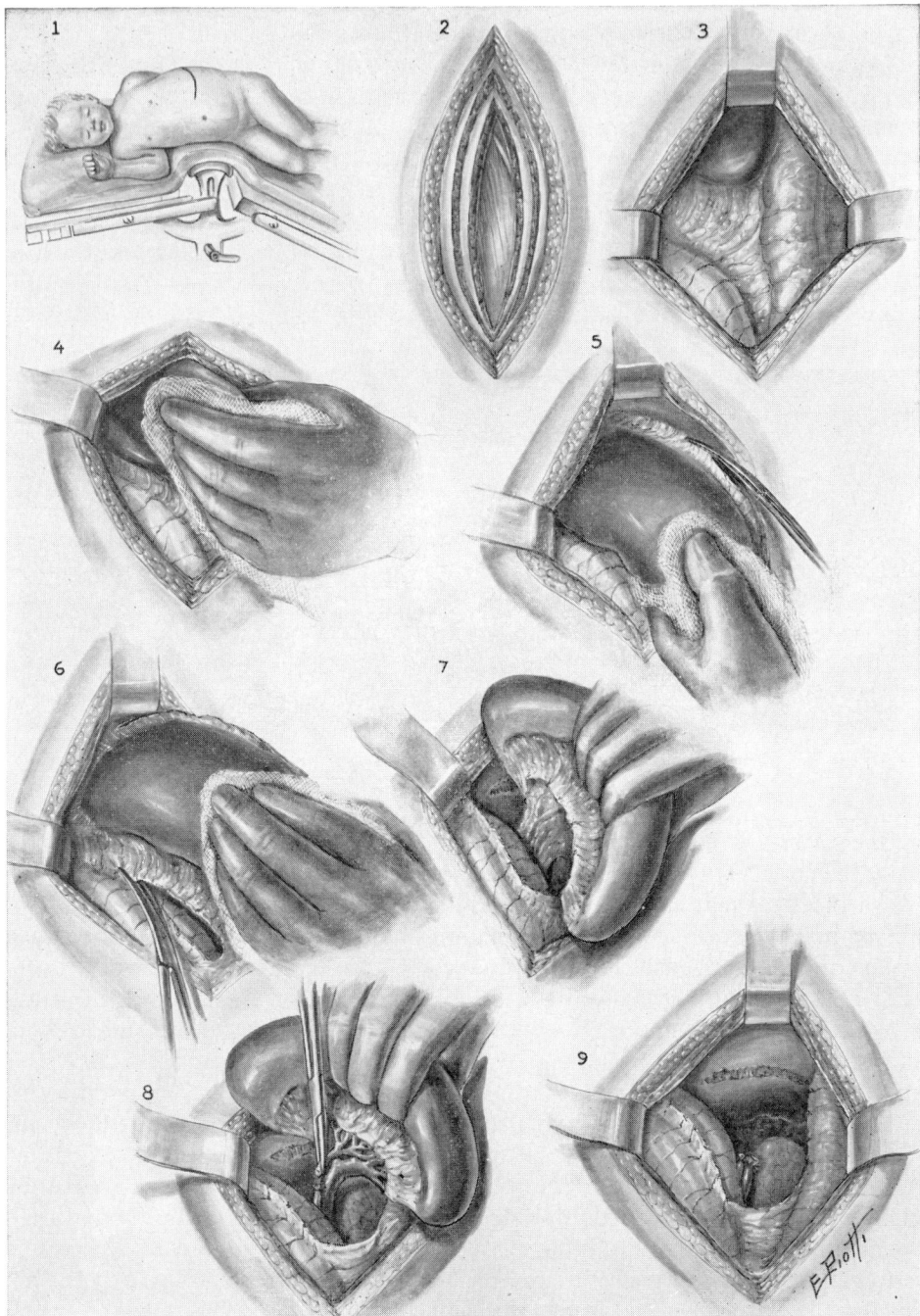

Fig. 313. Technique of splenectomy. 1. Child in position on the table. Kidney bench raised under flank. Body rolled back slightly. Position of incision shown. 2. External oblique and internal oblique muscles divided, carrying the incision to the outer border of the rectus sheath. Nerve lying on the transversalis will be saved. 3. Wound opened. Intestines rarely enter the field. Tip of spleen visible. 4. With a single layer of gauze, spleen is grasped and pulled downward and forward as far as possible. 5. While assistant maintains constant tension, pulling spleen out and down from its bed, the lieno-renal ligament is divided. This rarely has any vessels in it which need ligation. 6. Spleen pulled downward and somewhat posteriorly to allow separation of spleen from stomach. Short gastric vessels generally

is very high at the time. Prior to the present series of splenectomy cases, we had one child who developed excessive platelet concentrations and died from portal thrombosis, proved at autopsy. We have therefore felt that any child who, in the two or three weeks after splenectomy, develops very high platelet counts should be protected temporarily by giving anticoagulant therapy.

It is difficult to state the point beyond which a further rise is to be regarded as dangerous. As a working rule, we have arbitrarily chosen 1 million as the level, above which the child will be treated by administration of anticoagulants. The *time* when a high platelet count is found is of some importance; if it is beyond the tenth or twelfth postoperative day, possibly little concern need be felt because from this date onward the counts will probably be falling. Conversely, if a count over 1 million is found

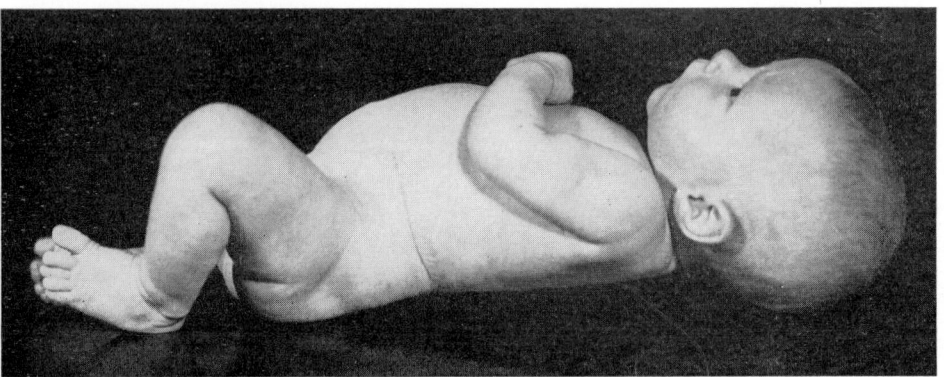

Fig. 314. Photograph of baby one month after splenectomy, showing position of the wound and excellent healing thereof.

before the seventh or eighth day, there is considerable reason for alarm because almost certainly the counts will be higher in the subsequent few days.

As a practical matter, to avoid unnecessary laboratory examinations, it is never helpful to make platelet count determinations before the sixth or seventh day after operation; rises to dangerous levels never occur before this time.

For *anticoagulant therapy* we have found heparinization the most useful. It can be given by constant intravenous drip, a method which is generally troublesome in children. It can also be given by intravenous injections every four hours, which is likewise not very practical in very young patients who have small veins. It has been found relatively easy to maintain satisfactory anticoagulant therapy by use of Depo-Heparin* (without vasoconstrictors). It is impossible to determine beforehand what a suitable dosage will be. As a trial figure, about 100 mg. for each 50 pounds of body weight is given intramuscularly each twelve hours (double this amount for the *first* dose). During the first twelve hours, the clotting time† of venous blood is determined each three or four hours to get an estimate of whether the heparin dose has been too large or too small. Ideally the clotting time should not get below fifteen to twenty minutes at any time. After this first twelve-hour trial, the second dose can be scaled upward or downward as indicated. It is necessary to repeat the clotting time determination only once just *before* each subsequent twelve-hour dose is given; such clotting time will represent the

---

* The Upjohn Company. This is for deep subcutaneous or intramuscular injection. It is sold in ampules containing 200 mg.

† By the Lee-White method.

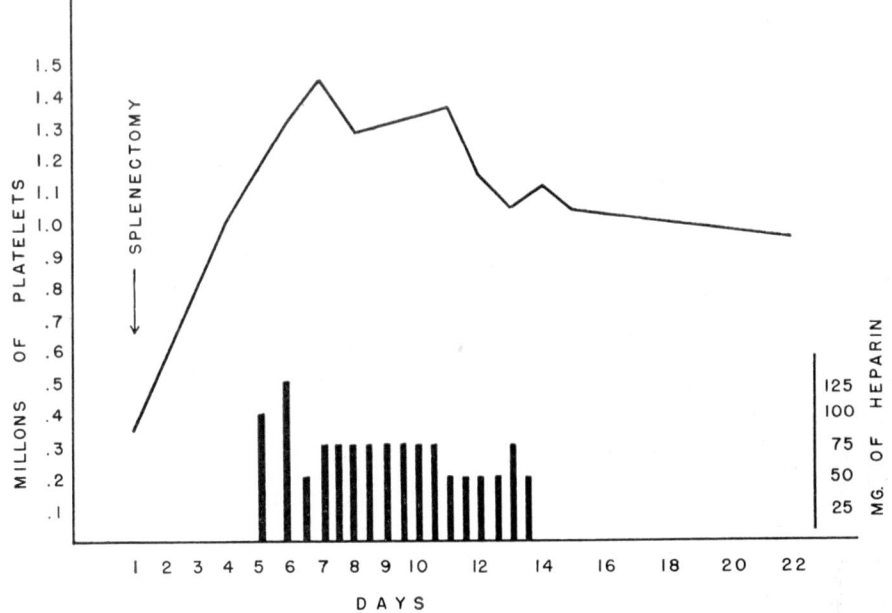

Fig. 315. Graph showing number of circulating blood platelets before and after splenectomy; from a six-month-old child with congenital hemolytic anemia. In the second week after operation there was a dangerous rise above 1 million, during which time heparin was given to prevent intra-vascular clotting.

lowest figure during the twelve-hour stretch; it should be kept above fifteen to twenty minutes. On the basis of the clotting time which is found, determinations are made for the amount of Depo-Heparin which next will be given. Thus it is possible to carry the patient along in a reasonably satisfactory way with but two injections and two clotting time determinations each twenty-four hours. It is seldom necessary to keep up the heparinization for more than three to five days, at the end of which time the danger of thrombosis will have passed. (We are willing to admit that most, and maybe all, of the patients to whom we give anticoagulant therapy might survive without this adjunct; we feel on safer ground by giving it.)

REFERENCES

CONGENITAL HEMOLYTIC ANEMIA

1. Coller, F. A., Blain, A. and Andrews, G.: Indications for and Results of Splenectomy. Am. Lect. Series. Charles C Thomas, Springfield, Illinois, 1950.
2. Diamond, L. K.: Indications for Splenectomy in Childhood. Results in 52 Operated Cases. Am. J. Surg., 39:400, 1938.

ACQUIRED HEMOLYTIC ANEMIA

3. Dameshek, W., Rosenthal, M. C. and Schwartz, L. I.: The Treatment of Acquired Hemolytic Anemia with Adrenocorticotrophic Hormone (ACTH). New England J. Med., 244:117, 1951.
4. Gardner, F. H., McElfresh, A. E., Harris,

J. W. and Diamond, L. K.: The Effect of Adrenocorticotrophic Hormone (ACTH) in Idiopathic Acquired Hemolytic Anemia as Related to the Hemolytic Mechanisms. J. Lab. & Clin. Med., 37:444, 1951.

THROMBOCYTOPENIC PURPURA

5. Bethell, F. H., Miller, S. and Myers, M. C.: Administration of ACTH and Cortisone in Hypersplenic Syndromes. Proceedings of the Second Clinical ACTH Conference, Edited by J. R. Mote. Vol. 2. Therapeutics. The Blakiston Co., Philadelphia, 1951, pp. 173–181.
6. Elliot, R. H. E., Jr., and Turner, J. C.: Sple

ectomy for Purpura Hemorrhagica. Surg., Gynec. & Obst., *92:*539, 1951.

7. Epstein, R. D., Lozner, E. L., Cobbey, T. S., Jr., and Davidson, C. S.: Congenital Thrombocytopenic Purpura. Am. J. Med., *9:*44, 1950.

8. Jacobson, B. M. and Sohier, W. D.: The Effects of ACTH and of Cortisone on the Platelets in Idiopathic Thrombocytopenic Purpura. New England J. Med., *246:*247, 1952.

9. Newton, W. A. and Zuelzer, W. W.: Idiopathic Thrombocytopenic Purpura in Childhood. New England J. Med., *245:* 879, 1951.

10. Stefanini, M., Santiago, E. P., Chatterjea, J. B., Dameshek, W. and Solomon, L.: Corticotropin (ACTH) and Cortisone in Idiopathic Thrombocytopenic Purpura. J.A.M.A., *149:*647, 1952.

11. Troland, C. E. and Lee, F. C.: Thrombocytopen: A Substance in the Extract from the Spleen of Patients with Idiopathic Thrombocytopenic Purpura That Reduces the Number of Blood Platelets. J.A.M.A., *111:* 221, 1938.

12. Whipple, A. O.: Splenectomy as a Therapeutic Measure in Thrombocytopenic Purpura Hemorrhagica. Surg., Gynec. & Obst., *42:* 329, 1926.

PORTAL HYPERTENSION

13. Baronofsky, I. D.: Portal Hypertension: with Special Reference to the Acid-peptic Factor in the Causation of Hemorrhage and Extensive Gastric Resection in Its Treatment. Surgery, *25:*135, 1949.

14. Blakemore, A. H. and Fitzpatrick, H. F.: The Surgical Management of the Post-splenectomy Bleeder with Extrahepatic Portal Hypertension. Ann. Surg., *134:*420, 1951.

15. Chalmers, T. C. and Davidson, C. S.: A Survey of Recent Therapeutic Measures in Cirrhosis of the Liver. New England J. Med., *240:*449, 1949.

16. Linton, R. R.: The Selection of Patients for Portacaval Shunts. Ann. Surg., *134:*433, 1951.

17. Rousselot, L. M.: The Late Phase of Congestive Splenomegaly (Banti's Syndrome) with Hematemesis but without Cirrhosis of the Liver. Surgery, *8:*34, 1940.

18. Sengstaken, R. W. and Blakemore, A. H.: Balloon Tamponage for Control of Hemorrhage from Esophageal Varices. Ann. Surg., *131:*781 1950.

19. Smith, R. M. and Farber, S.: Splenomegaly in Children with Early Hematemesis. J. Pediat., *7:*585, 1935.

20. Taylor, F. W. and Egbert, H. L.: Portal Tension. Surg., Gynec. & Obst., *92:*64, 1951.

21. Warthin, A. S.: The Relation of Thrombophlebitis of the Portal and Splenic Veins to Splenic Anemia and Banti's Disease. Internat. Clin., *4:*189, 1910.

22. Whipple, A. O.: The Problem of Portal Hypertension in Relation to Hepatosplenopathies. Ann. Surg., *122:*449, 1945.

HYPERSPLENISM

23. Dameshek, W. and Estren, S.: The Spleen and Hypersplenism. Grune and Stratton, New York, 1947.

24. Doan, C. A. and Wright, C. S.: Primary Congenital and Secondary Acquired Splenic Panhematopenia. Blood, *1:*10, 1946.

25. Wiseman, B. K. and Doan, C. A.: A Newly Recognized Granulopenic Syndrome Caused by Excessive Splenic Leukolysis and Successfully Treated by Splenectomy. J. Clin. Investigation, *18:*473, 1939.

26. Zollinger, R. M., Martin, M. M. and Williams, R. D.: Surgical Aspects of Hypersplenism. J.A.M.A., *149:*24, 1952.

SPLENIC TRAUMA

27. Anderson, N. A.: Traumatic Rupture of Spleen in Children, With Special Reference to Left Shoulder Pain. J. Pediat., *15:*535, 1939.

28. O'Neil, J. F. and Rousseau, J. P.: Roentgenologic Examination of the Abdomen as an Aid in the Early Diagnosis of Splenic Injury. Ann. Surg., *121:*111, 1945.

29. Scott, H. W., Jr., and Bowman, J. R.: Traumatic Rupture of the Spleen in Childhood. J.A.M.A., *130:*270, 1946.

30. Solis-Cohen, L. and Levine, S.: Roentgen Diagnosis of Lacerated Spleen. Radiology, *39:*707, 1942.

CYSTS AND TUMORS

31. Fowler, R. H.: Cystic Tumors of the Spleen. Internat. Abstr. Surg., *70:*213, 1940.

32. Montgomery, A. H., McEnery, E. T., and Frank, A. A.: Epidermoid Cysts of Spleen. Ann. Surg., *108:*877, 1938.

33. Sherwin, B., Brown, C. R. and Liber, A. F.: Cystic Disease of Spleen. Ann. Surg., *109:* 615, 1939.

MISCELLANEOUS REFERENCES

34. Blackfan, K. D. and Diamond, L. K.: Atlas of the Blood in Children. Oxford University Press, London, 1944.

35. Blain, A. W. and Blain, A., III.: Ligation of the Splenic Artery, the Operation of Choice

in Selected Cases of Portal Hypertension and Banti's Syndrome. Ann. Surg., *131*:92, 1950.

36. Bruschi, M. and Howe, J. S.: Classification of the Hematologic Variations and Abnormalities Associated with Boeck's Sarcoid. Blood, *5*:478, 1950.

37. Carter, B. N.: Combined Thoracico-abdominal Approach with Particular Reference to its Employment in Splenectomy. Surg., Gynec. & Obst., *84*:1019, 1947.

38. Cole, W. H., Walter, L. and Limarzi, L. R.: Indications and Results of Splenectomy. Ann. Surg., *129*:702, 1949.

39. Crile, G., Jr.: Transesophageal Ligation of Bleeding Esophageal Varices. Arch. Surg., *61*:654, 1950.

40. Curtis, G. M. and Movitz, D.: Surgical Significance of Accessory Spleen. Ann. Surg., *123*:276, 1946.

41. Davis, H. H. and Sharpe, J. C.: Splenic Vein Thrombosis Following Splenectomy. Surg., Gynec. & Obst., *67*:678, 1938.

42. King, H. and Shumacker, H. B., Jr.: Splenic Studies. 1. Susceptibility to Infection after Splenectomy Performed in Infancy. Ann. Surg., *136*:239, 1952.

43. Lahey, F. H. and Norcross, J. W.: Splenectomy: When Is It Indicated? Ann. Surg. *128*:363, 1948.

44. Pemberton, J. deJ. and Kiernan, P.: Surgery of the Spleen. S. Clin. North America, *25*:880, 1945.

45. Vogt, E. C. and Diamond, L. K.: Congenital Anemias, Roentgenologically Considered. Am. J. Roentgenol., *23*:625, 1930.

CHAPTER 44

Hypoglycemia

Hypoglycemia in infancy and childhood is a condition which it is important to recognize, because if left untreated it almost certainly leads to extensive damage of the brain, mental deterioration, and disintegration of the personality. Fortunately, these catastrophes can be avoided if hypoglycemia is detected early and is appropriately treated by medical or surgical means. Most of the literature which has accumulated concerning hypoglycemia and its surgical therapy has been descriptive of adult patients. While not so common in childhood or infancy, the condition is even more important to detect because the sequelae in an untreated child are more disastrous and irreversible than are those in adults.

There is no sharp dividing line below which a blood sugar level can be regarded as abnormal, but it has been generally accepted that fasting levels below 50 mg. per 100 cc., if consistently or repeatedly present, represent a situation of great seriousness. Patients vary somewhat in regard to the level of the blood sugar below which they begin to have symptoms. Some children and babies tolerate depressions down to 60 to 70 mg. per cent without distress, whereas others show definite abnormalities when the blood levels are in this range; almost without exception, all subjects have difficulties of one sort or another when the levels are below 50 to 55 mg. per cent.

Without doubt, severe hypoglycemia can occur in infancy and childhood to a degree incompatible with normal development or even maintenance of life. The condition may be uncontrollable by medical means and may require surgical resection of a pancreatic islet adenoma or pancreatic islet tissue to restore the blood sugar to normal levels and thereby abolish the central nervous symptoms. It is important to give effective therapy in time to prevent permanent damage of the brain.

PATHOLOGY. ETIOLOGIC FACTORS

There are a number of conditions which can give rise to hypoglycemia in the young individual. Among these must be included: (1) Any mechanism which interferes with absorption of products from the alimentary tract. (2) Diseases of the liver which interfere with the storage of glycogen, or with its proper mobilization. (3) Diseases of the adrenal cortex (Addisonian states) or of the anterior pituitary (hypopituitarism) which interfere with normal gluconeogenesis. (4) Tumors (benign or malignant) of the pancreatic islands, producing hyperinsulinism. (5) Hyperplasia of pancreatic islands, producing hyperinsulinism. (6) Instability of the carbohydrate metabolism of the body, the causation of which cannot be found by any physiologic test or pathologic examination (surgical or autopsy).

When dealing with hypoglycemia in infancy and childhood, the first three of the above listed conditions have to be thought of and ruled out, but on the whole they are quite rare. Most of the patients with hypoglycemia will have one of the last three conditions.

Nicholls reported the first islet-cell tumor in 1902, but gave no clinical history of the case. Wilder et al.[16] made the first surgical proof of hyperinsulinism by operation (W. J. Mayo) on a patient (a physician) with hypoglycemic symptoms which were found to come from an insulin-secreting, metastasizing carcinoma of the pancreas. Two years later the first surgical cure was accomplished by Roscoe Graham (Howland et al.[10]) by removal of an islet-cell (suspiciously malignant) tumor. Subsequently, descriptions began to appear of islet-cell tumors with hypoglycemia in adults and also in childhood (Sherman,[12] six-week-old baby; Wolf et al.,[18] ten-year-old boy). Reports have been made of patients (including children) who had hypoglycemia and were found to have extensive hyperplasia of pancreatic islands (Dannenberg et al.,[4] three-year-old child; Calloway,[2] eight-year-old girl; Greenlee et al.,[8] five-month-old baby). Furthermore, patients (including children) have been found to have hypoglycemic states and (even though partial pancreatectomy has been curative) no pathology has been detected in the pancreas (Graham and Hartman,[7] year-old baby).

Whipple[15] has made valuable contributions to the surgery of hyperinsulinism; in 1944 he studied from the literature 160 cases of hyperinsulinism and added 32 of his own. Howard, Moss, and Rhoads[9] were able to collect and analyze data from 398 cases of hyperinsulinism; 14 were in children under fifteen years of age. Of these 14 children, 9 were found to have islet adenomas, 2 were found to have hyperplasia of the pancreatic islet cells, and 3 were found to have a normal pancreas. It appears that in infancy and childhood, hypoglycemia is much less commonly on the basis of islet tumor than are the findings in adults.

Islet tumors can appear on the surface of the pancreas and therefore are identifiable at the operating table, but many of them are small and lie completely buried in the substance of the gland so that they cannot be detected by external inspection or by palpation. While there have been many earlier reports giving the impression that islet tumors are largely found in the tail of the pancreas, it is now evident that they can be found in any part of the organ.

CLINICAL FINDINGS

Regardless of the cause for a low level of circulating blood sugar, there are certain pictures which are commonly found and which—while not diagnostic—are certainly suggestive of the underlying physiologic abnormality. Weakness, stupor, and drowsiness are most commonly observed. Pallor, sweating, disorientation, and restlessness are frequently seen. In the more severe cases, twitches and convulsions (without a localizing pattern) are found. All of the symptoms are more apt to appear in the morning (after a long night without food). Most cases on admission to the hospital are deemed to be neurologic or neurosurgical problems. Electroencephalographic studies show slowing of the waves (which can be speeded up temporarily by the administration of glucose).

The finding of low blood sugar levels during an attack (below 50 to 60 mg. per cent) certainly suggests a causal relationship between the two. A single blood sugar determination which is low should not be used as a sufficient basis to establish a diagnosis of hypoglycemia, but repeated low values are of prime significance. (In our patient 4 (Table 65) 11 fasting blood sugars were taken before operation; 8 of them had a value under 50 mg. per cent and 3 were between 50 and 61 mg. per cent.) The symptoms can be quickly alleviated by the ingestion of food (sugars are most rapidly assimilated) or by the intravenous injection of glucose.

It is well recognized that functional hypoglycemia is not rare during the first few days or weeks of life; at such times the blood sugar level may be considerably depressed while producing no clinical symptoms or only transient ones in the newborn. As a rule the blood sugar level becomes stabilized and normal about fourteen days after birth without complications.

DIFFERENTIAL DIAGNOSIS. ESTABLISHMENT OF THE DIAGNOSIS

Any child who has periods of weakness, excessive fatigue, stupor, drowsiness, or convulsions should be studied from the viewpoint of determining whether hypoglycemia is an etiologic factor. Such study almost certainly requires a period of hospitalization for observation and performance of certain laboratory tests. Little is accomplished when it is merely determined that an individual has "hypoglycemia," for indeed some children tolerate relatively low levels of blood sugar extraordinarily well, with little or no symptomatology therefrom. In the study of a patient who has symptoms which might possibly arise from hypoglycemia, it is important to prove beyond doubt two relationships: *First*, that during periods of the symptoms, tests actually show low levels of blood sugar. *Second*, that symptoms can be promptly and fully relieved by the administration of glucose (either by oral or intravenous route). To become convinced that these relationships actually do exist in a given patient, generally requires study during several of the attacks.

Once having established the fact that a patient's symptoms are dependent upon a hypoglycemic state, there are certain considerations which help in recognition of the causes of the hypoglycemia. Fraser, Albright, and Smith[6] have presented a comprehensive discussion of carbohydrate metabolism and the methods for detection of its various abnormalities.

1. Abnormal Alimentation

Any disorder of absorption from the intestinal tract is almost always overshadowed by other symptoms indicating intestinal obstruction, abdominal neoplasm, collection of ascitic fluid, or abnormalities by gastro-intestinal roentgenologic examination so that one's attention is almost certainly drawn to the intestine as the seat of primary pathology. Therefore, it is relatively easy to rule out conditions of the alimentary tract or mesentery as the cause of a hypoglycemia.

2. Hepatic Disease

Certain conditions of the liver, notably hepatitis and von Gierke's disease, may interfere with the proper storage of glycogen or may hinder its mobilization by the normal mechanisms of glyconeogenesis. In von Gierke's disease there is abundant glycogen in the liver but it fails to serve as a proper source of glucose. The various liver function tests (including cephalin flocculation, Bromsulphalein, thymol turbidity, and a measurement of the serum albumin) give some evaluation of the general state of the liver. Of particular importance is an epinephrine tolerance test; normally epinephrine mobilizes glucose. If the injection of a standard dose of epinephrine is not followed by an appropriate rise in the blood sugar level, this can be assumed to be evidence that glycogen is not present in proper concentration in the liver (and other depots) or else it cannot be mobilized adequately. A normal epinephrine curve suggests that liver disease is not the cause for an existing hypoglycemia (Fig. 316).

3. Pituitary or Adrenal-Cortical Disease

Blood sugar levels are kept up by glucose arriving from the intestinal tract and by glucose which is converted from glycogen (gluconeogenesis). This second source is under the control of hormones from the adrenal cortex. The reduction in these hormones by disease of the adrenal cortex, or by disease of the pituitary gland (which activates the adrenals), can depress the blood sugar levels by cutting down that portion of the glucose which comes from gluconeogenesis.

Serious lesions of the adrenal gland are almost always accompanied by other obvious androgen disturbances or by evidence of Addison's disease, so that one's attention is easily directed to the adrenals as the primary cause of the complaints.

EPINEPHRINE TEST

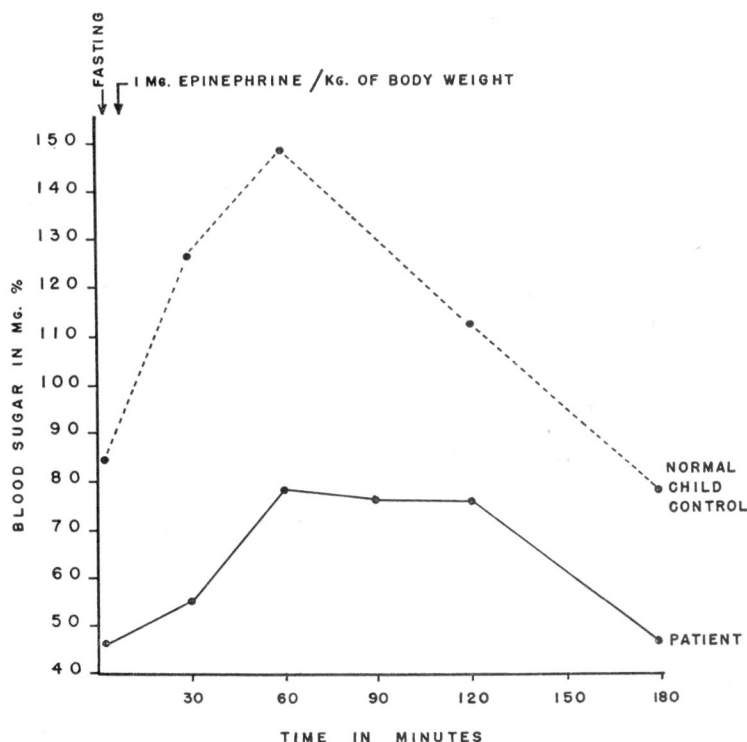

Fig. 316. Case 4. Preoperative epinephrine test. The striking rise in the patient's blood glucose level would indicate that glycogen is adequately stored (in the liver and other depots) and can be mobilized in the form of glucose. Therefore the liver is presumably normal and hepatic disease is not the cause of the patient's hypoglycemia.

Any abnormality of the anterior pituitary gland (e.g., Simmond's disease) sufficient to give a hypoglycemic state is almost certainly accompanied by evidence of a serious neurologic disorder, by visual disturbances or defects in the visual fields, and by x-ray findings of an expanding lesion (cyst or tumor) within the sella or in the supra-sellar region.

Serious disorders of the pituitary gland or adrenal cortex can be recognized (or excluded) by an epinephrine-eosinophil test, devised by Crain and Thorn.[3] The principle involved is that epinephrine stimulates the anterior pituitary gland to secrete adrenocorticotropic hormone (ACTH), which in turn will stimulate the adrenal cortex. Compounds from the adrenal cortex will depress the eosinophils. Therefore, changes in the eosinophil count act as an indicator of pituitary ACTH secretion followed by adrenal cortical activation and secretion. For conducting the test, breakfast is held and a fasting eosinophil count is made. Then 0.3 cc. of 1:1000 epinephrine (adult dose) is injected

Table 65

Children with Hypoglycemia Treated by Pancreatectomy
(Children's Hospital Series)

Case Number Sex Year of Operation	Essence of History	Age at Operation	Duration of Illness Prior to Surgery	Effect of Medical Therapy
1 M 1939	Onset of severe coma and convulsions at 2 months. Prolonged coma. Severe brain damage before first operation	12 weeks 13 weeks 22 weeks	4 weeks 5 weeks 14 weeks	Hypoglycemic status intractable to intermittent therapy
2 F 1941	Sudden onset of drowsiness and fits of staring. No loss of consciousness	6 mos.	7 weeks in hospital, experiencing several mild "seizures"	Seizures recurring in spite of dietary changes
3 F 1942	Sudden onset of seizures which ceased spontaneously, to recur 4 mos. later. They continued sporadically while in hospital under observation	21 mos.	5 mos. of sporadic seizures	Always temporary relief from glucose. Prolonged medical therapy not attempted
4 F 1943	Recurring stupor and drowsiness, particularly in mornings. Sudden onset of 5 short convulsive seizures	18 mos.	7 mos.	Temporary relief by glucose in hospital. Diet of no help
5 M 1947	Intermittent seizures whenever feedings were delayed. Stupor but no prolonged periods of coma	11 mos.	5 mos. Progressively more frequent seizures	Temporary relief by glucose. Diet changes of no help. ACTH shown to be of temporary benefit
6 F 1950	Sporadic seizures of stupor and brief loss of consciousness	6 mos.	10 weeks of recurrent seizures	Seizures somewhat reduced but not abolished by dietary measures

Table 65 (continued)

Operation	Pathology	Remarks	Over-all Result
2/3 pancreatectomy. 1/6 more excised. Complete pancreatectomy	No tumor or hyperplasia in specimens 1 and 2. 3rd specimen lost	Hypoglycemia unrelieved by first 2 operations. After 3rd op., diabetes for 2 mos., then normal blood sugars	Patient decerebrate by time 3rd op. performed. Institutionalized. Died 7 mos. later of bronchopneumonia. A few nubbins of pancreas regenerating along duodenum. Marked cerebral atrophy found
4/5 pancreatectomy. Liver biopsy	Normal pancreas	No diabetes. 2 days after op. blood sugar became normal	For $1\frac{1}{2}$ years followed, child completely well. No G.I. disturbances
4/5 pancreatectomy.	Normal pancreas	No diabetes. Blood sugar became normal after op. Patient much improved	Completely well until 2 years after op. when infectious encephalitis developed. (No carbohydrate disturbance at time.) 9 yrs. postoperative carbohydrate metabolism normal. Marked mental and physical retardation, almost certainly on basis of the encephalitis
4/5 pancreatectomy.	Normal pancreas	No diabetes. Blood sugar became normal on 3rd day. Patient much improved	Reevaluation on several occasions showed normal carbohydrate metabolism. Child alert and completely well. Excellent condition 9 yrs. later
3/4 pancreatectomy.	Normal pancreas	No diabetes. Only slow improvement in low sugars and seizures. After 3 mos. completely well	Marked improvement. Last seen at 5 yrs., completely well and normal
3/4 pancreatectomy.	Marked hyperplasia of pancreatic islands	No diabetes. Child promptly recovered normal carbohydrate metabolism. Abolition of seizures	Normal carbohydrate metabolism when restudied at 3 and 6 mos. Completely well remainder of life. Suddenly died of overwhelming infection 8 mos. after op. Pancreas normal at autopsy

subcutaneously. The patient may eat after the injection. Lunch is held until four hours later, at which time the final eosinophil count is obtained. Normal levels of circulating eosinophils are 125 to 300 per cubic millimeter. A fall of 50 per cent or more in circulating eosinophils excludes serious anterior pituitary or adrenal cortical insufficiency as a cause of the hypoglycemia. An insignificant fall would indicate that the pituitary gland or the adrenals are at fault.

Patients with serious disease of the pituitary gland or adrenal cortex are extremely sensitive to insulin; they do not have sufficient gluconeogenesis to replace sugar which is burned by insulin. Therefore the injection of insulin in such patients gives a precipitous and dangerous fall in the blood sugar level; indeed so great can be the reaction, that one should not perform an insulin-tolerance test if disease of the pituitary gland or adrenal cortices is suspected.

4. States of Hyperinsulinism

Whether they be caused by adenoma of islets, by hyperplasia of pancreatic islet cells, or by poorly understood hormone imbalances in which the pancreatic islet cells are normal, there are certain features by which these states can generally be recognized. First, one finds no other pathologic states, such as disease of the intestine, liver, pituitary, or adrenal cortex, the exclusion of which have been discussed above. Second, there is the possibility of demonstrating that the individual has an increased tolerance for insulin, presumably because he already has a high level of this circulating hormone. With an insulin-tolerance test, there is less depression than normal of the blood sugar levels (Fig. 317). For the insulin-tolerance test there is injected intravenously 0.05 unit of regular insulin per kilogram of body weight. Normally the blood sugar usually falls to 50 per cent of the fasting level (in twenty or thirty minutes) but it should return to normal in ninety to one hundred and twenty minutes. (Whenever insulin is injected, the investigator should be prepared to terminate the test immediately by the injection of glucose if a severe hypoglycemic reaction results.)

All of the blood-sugar level tests (epinephrine response, insulin tolerance, glucose tolerance, insulin-glucose tolerance) have serious shortcomings. Each of them can give equivocal results and indeed can give widely different values and impressions when conducted on different days or under different conditions of food intake, recent exercise, et cetera. Sometimes the various tests are helpful, oftentimes they are not. Minor variations cannot be regarded as significant; important deviations from the normal can probably be accepted as indicating which mechanism is at fault in causing a hypoglycemia. We have come to feel that there is some merit in making both the epinephrine response and insulin-tolerance tests, but we have usually found that glucose-tolerance tests or combined insulin-glucose tolerance tests are valueless and even confusing.

TREATMENT

Any infant or child with hypoglycemia, stupor, and lassitude will almost certainly fail to develop properly because his sensoria are dimmed; he will not have all those sensations and experiences which are necessary for the process of education and maturation. Furthermore, any child who has convulsive disorders will sustain increased and progressive damage of the brain, eventuating in mental deterioration, progressing to the point where permanent institutionalization mya become necessary. With this grim outlook, it becomes highly important to treat all children who have neurologic symptoms from a hypoglycemic state.

Attention must not be focused merely on treating a child who has a low blood sugar. The emphasis must be on the treatment of all those individuals who have *stupor, lassitude, convulsions*, et cetera, which are known to be on a basis of hypoglycemia. A program of therapy should not merely be directed toward trying to raise a blood-sugar level; the emphasis should be on providing a medical or surgical therapy which is effective in keeping the child continually alert and also free of convulsions. Regardless of what the blood-sugar determinations happen to show, any therapy is ineffective and

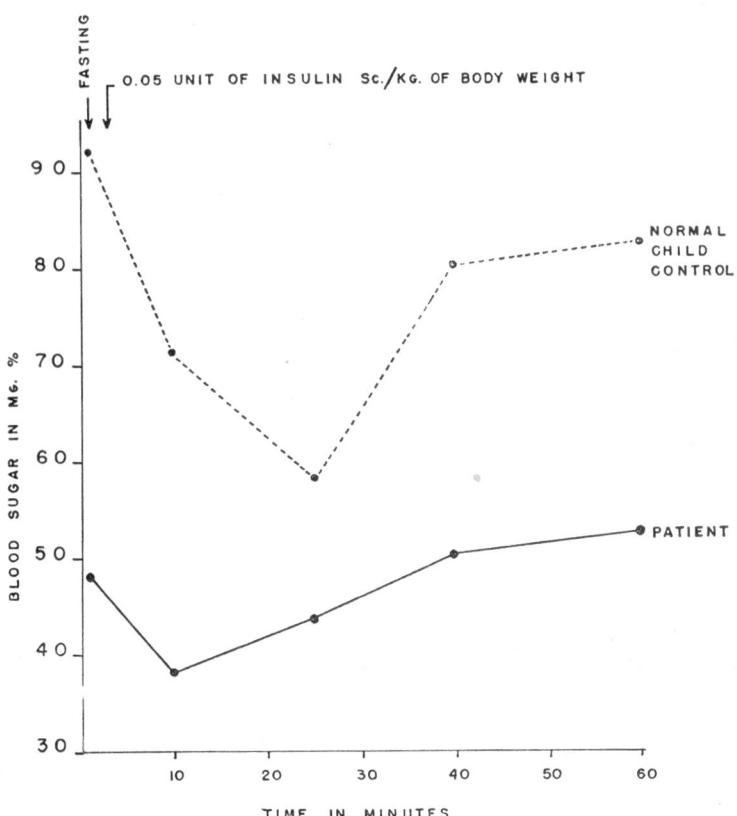

Fig. 317. Case 4. Preoperative insulin-tolerance test. Note the marked fall in blood glucose level in the normal control child. In comparison, the patient had little change, probably indicating that a high concentration of insulin was already present and that the addition of small amounts of insulin by subcutaneous injection would not appreciably change the situation. Furthermore, the rather flat insulin-tolerance curve of the patient excludes lesions of the anterior pituitary and the adrenal cortex as a cause of the patient's hypoglycemia, because in both of these there is a marked hypersensitivity to insulin and there would be a precipitous and dangerous decline in the curve.

insufficient which does not keep the child free of all neurologic and psychologic mani-festations of the condition. Four general methods of attack on the problem have been used:

1. *Alloxan Therapy* has been suggested and has been tried by Talbot et al.[13] This drug has a necrotizing action on pancreatic islets and therefore theoretically would be of value in the treatment of any individual who has hyperinsulinism. Unfortunately, it is difficult to control the extent of the action of the drug; its use is therefore dangerous and is not recommended.

2. *Dietary Management* should be offered, the essentials of the regimen being the

use of frequent feedings, the avoidance of long intervals without feeding, and particularly the employment of a high-protein diet. While carbohydrates give an early and high rise in blood sugar, it has been shown by Thorn et al.[14] that high protein in the diet gives a later and more sustained rise and elevation in blood-sugar values.

3. *The Use of ACTH* has been tried in the treatment of hypoglycemia of early life with beneficial effects. The stimulation of the adrenal cortex increases gluconeogenesis and tends to correct any low blood-sugar levels. ACTH therapy is not effective for some infants or children; it has been shown by McQuarrie et al.[11] to be very useful and sufficient in others. The disadvantage of the therapy is that injections are only of temporary value and that generally they must be continued over a long period of time. However, it appears that if some children (presumably the ones who have no pathology in the pancreas and whose hypoglycemia depends on an ephemeral imbalance) can be tided over for a few months, the underlying imbalance tends to correct itself and no further therapy is necessary. Under such circumstances, a limited period of treatment by ACTH may be all that is necessary.

McQuarrie has shown that, at least in some patients, the ACTH does not have to be continued at frequent intervals. He described one case in which it was used at first each six hours, later every twelve hours, then lengthening the intervals up to twenty-four and forty-eight hours and even to four days, eventually stopping the drug at one year when the child's imbalance apparently had disappeared.

While the observations to date have been made with the use of ACTH injections, doubtless the same desirable effects could be obtained more easily and more cheaply by the use of cortisone, given by mouth.

An important consideration against the use of ACTH or cortisone would be the fact that in occasional patients (particularly those beyond infancy) use of the drugs would divert attention from a neoplasm of the pancreas which should be removed surgically.

4. *Surgical Removal of a Portion of the Pancreas* should certainly be undertaken for any individual who cannot be controlled by the above measures. Excision of a tumor, or (in patients who have no adenoma) the removal of a considerable part of the pancreas will reduce the amount of insulin which is poured into the circulation. These operations can be performed in a child of any age. The risk of operation should be low. The possibility of effecting a permanent cure is high.

Technique of Pancreatectomy

During these operations, a drip of glucose solution should be given continuously into a vein to keep the patient in the best possible state. The optimum exposure for exploring and resecting the pancreas is by a transverse incision above the navel, running across both rectus muscle bellies and extending the incision farther to the right or the left as becomes necessary. After division of the gastro-colic omentum, an excellent view is obtained of the pancreas and surrounding structures. The organ can be inspected and palpated for an adenoma but there is relatively little chance of finding one, particularly if the subject is a baby. If no tumor is found, the decision must be made of how much of the pancreas to remove. It has been a contention of some that total pancreatectomy should be done, but we are strongly opposed to this view, because it will certainly throw the child into a severe and permanent diabetes and might possibly introduce disturbances from the lack of certain enzymes in the intestinal juices. We believe that the best policy is to remove 75 to 80 per cent of the pancreas since, in the limited experience so far, this seems to be highly effective in ablating enough islet tissue to combat hypoglycemia, and yet it does not produce permanent diabetes or cause important alterations of alimentation.

Beginning with the spleen which is mobilized from its bed, the dissection of the pancreas is carried from left to right, raising and isolating the tail and then the body, all of which can be done very quickly and easily. The liberation can be continued over to the superior mesenteric vessels, which must be identified with care and left undisturbed as the pancreas is separated from them. When 75 or 80 per cent of the pancreas has been mobilized, it is transected. The remaining head will have an adequate blood

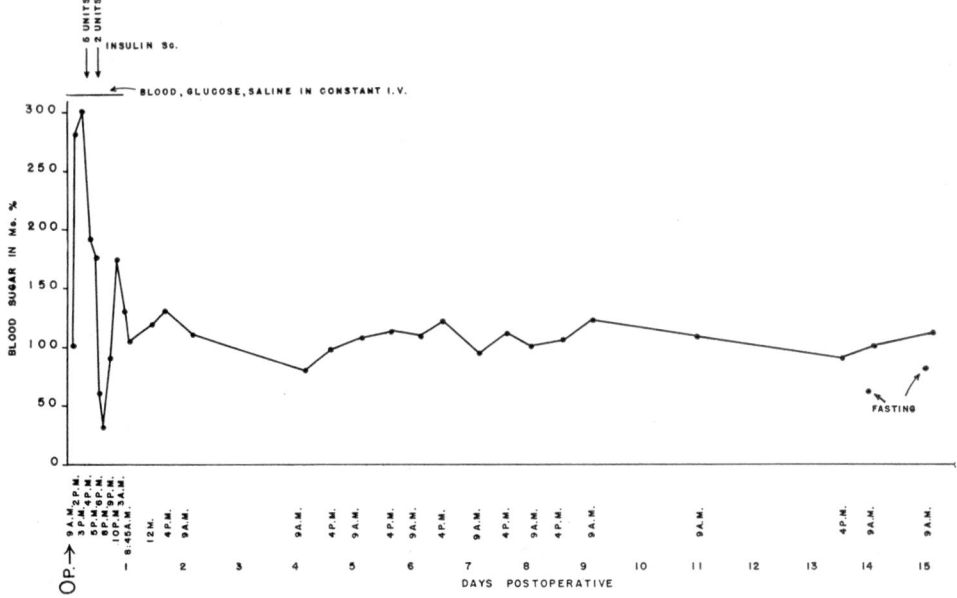

Fig. 318. Case 4. Blood glucose curve for fifteen days following subtotal pancreatectomy. For twenty-four hours following operation there was a temporary diabetes with rises in the glucose levels which required administration of insulin. After this first day there was no further diabetes, nor was there hypoglycemia.

supply from the pancreatic-duodenal vessels. It is generally possible to identify the stump of pancreatic duct and ligate it. It is best to cut across the pancreas in a wedge-shaped manner so that the remaining anterior and posterior edges of pancreatic substance can be brought together and opposed to one another with a series of fine, interrupted silk sutures to completely close over the pancreatic end and to minimize the chance of leakage of pancreatic fluid.

Following removal of a major portion of the pancreas, it is essential to be prepared for very close observation and support of the patient for the following twenty-four or forty-eight hours, during which there may be great instability in the sugar metabolism. A cannula or polyethylene tube should be kept in a vein, so that fluids can be constantly dripped in, varying the constituents as indicated from time to time. One cannot predict whether the patient will continue in hypoglycemia (because of some lesion which might conceivably have been left in the remaining head of the pancreas) or whether he will be thrown immediately into diabetes of some degree. Rather than run the risk of any hypoglycemic shock, it is best to continually infuse dilute glucose solution, to follow the levels of the blood sugar by frequent glucose determinations, and to administer insulin if blood levels rise above 200 or 250 mg. per cent.

In a few individuals it is found that some degree of diabetes is introduced which will require either dietary control or insulin administration for its control. If the patient has been thrown over into a diabetic state in the early postoperative period, it does not necessarily imply that diabetes will be permanent. In one of our children (in whom a total pancreatectomy had been performed) there was severe diabetes which required intensive insulin therapy; by the end of two months all evidence of diabetes has disappeared. Apparently, pin-head, minute nubbins of pancreatic substance along the curve

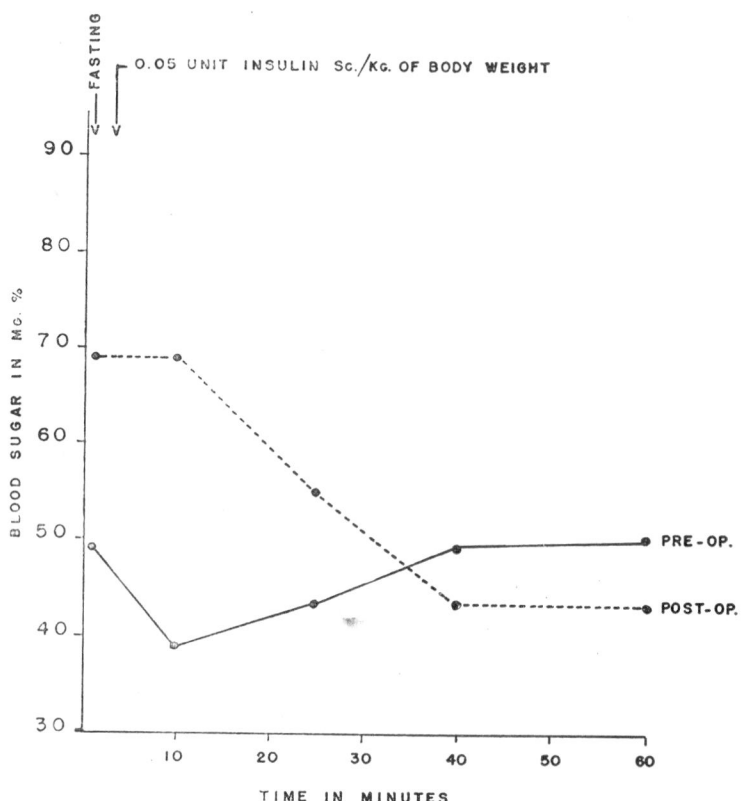

Fig. 319. Case 4. Postoperative insulin-tolerance test. The greater fall in the curve after operation (compared to the preoperative one) indicates a greater sensitivity to insulin after operation (presumably there is a reduction of circulating blood insulin).

of the duodenum had regenerated in such a way that sufficient islet tissue was reestablished to spontaneously correct the diabetes.

For most patients who have had a 70 to 80 per cent pancreatectomy, the carbohydrate fluctuations generally disappear after a few days, after which one can gain a fairly clear idea of the level at which the carbohydrate metabolism will become stabilized. If the correct amount of pancreatic substance has been removed to restore a proper balance, the blood-sugar level will be found in normal or low-normal ranges (Fig. 318).

RESULTS OF THERAPY

In the Children's Hospital material there have been 11 patients who were known to have convulsive seizures on the basis of hypoglycemia. The ages of these at the time of first symptoms were: 2 days, 4 weeks, 4 months, 5 months, 6 months, 6 months, 16 months, 16 months, 19 months, 3 years, and 3 years. Severity and duration of symptoms prior to hospitalization for institution of specific therapy varied from a few attacks in a few days to repeated and intensive seizures over a span of 6 or 7 months.

It was possible to treat 5 of these patients under medical management alone in a reasonably satisfactory way, with the employment of frequent feedings, high-protein diet, and in one instance by the use of ACTH. On the whole, these 5 subjects had had but few attacks, less impressive symptoms, and shorter durations of illness than was the average for those other patients who were subjected to surgery.

Six children were treated by surgical means after it was felt that medical therapy was insufficient to control the hypoglycemic disorder. Some data concerning these are

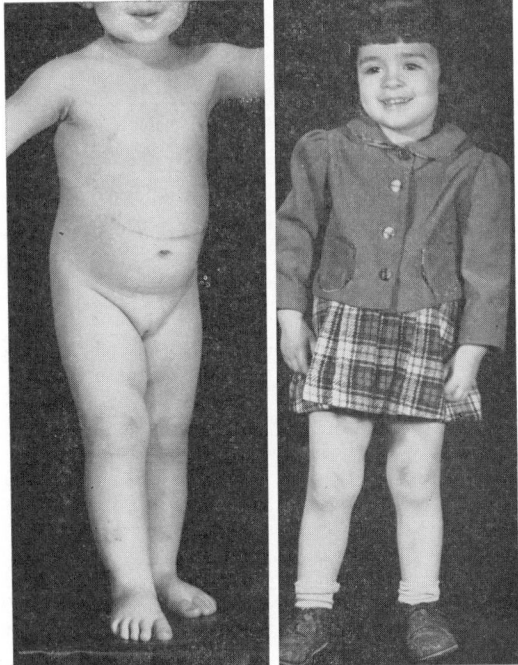

Fig. 320. Case 4. *Left,* Photograph showing position of the transverse wound which gave an excellent exposure of the pancreas. *Right,* Photograph of patient one year after operation. Before operation she had been lethargic and slow; now note the alertness of her expression.

summarized in Table 65. There was no fatality from pancreatectomy. The electroencephalograms, which showed slowing of the waves before operation, had these changes reversed thereafter. No steatorrhea or intestinal disturbances were noted in any case, but fat studies on the stools have not been made. In the first of these patients, operation was carried out in three stages, removing first the tail, then the body, each of which had little effect on the general picture. Finally, the entire head was removed, following which there was immediate supplantation of the hypoglycemia by a diabetes (which required therapy for two months and then spontaneously disappeared). By pathologic examination no tumor or hyperplasia was present in the first two specimens; unfortunately, the third specimen was lost and was not examined pathologically. This child had severe cerebral damage prior to the undertaking of surgery; by the time of the third operation he was almost decerebrate and had to be institutionalized permanently thereafter. He died from bronchopneumonia seven months after the third operation. There were a few little nodules of regenerating pancreas in the curve of the duodenum.

Each of the patients, 2, 3, 4, 5, and 6, had 75 to 80 per cent of the pancreas removed in a one-stage procedure. In one of these, pathologic examination showed marked hyperplasia of the islands, whereas the pancreas was histologically normal in all others. One of the children (case 5) showed only slow improvement over the next three months but was entirely normal thereafter. The other 4 patients recovered from hypoglycemia within a few days after operation. All of these patients had great benefit from their operative procedure as far as the abolition of stupor and convulsions were concerned.

Two years after operation, patient 3 developed encephalitis which almost certainly had nothing to do with the previous disease; she received extensive cerebral damage from this infectious process. Patient 6 died suddenly of an overwhelming infection eight months after operation.

The over-all salvage from surgery might seem to be poor, but the 2 deaths (patients 1 and 6) were unrelated to carbohydrate disturbances, and the retardation in case 3 was almost certainly on the basis of an intercurrent infectious encephalitis. The 3 remaining patients are in excellent health and are quite stable.

We have had no patient who was recognized as having a pancreatic-islet adenoma (patient 1 might possibly have had one). However, adenomas have been removed from babies and children (listed in Table G of Howard et al.[9]). Our cases have been similar to those of Greenlee et al.[8] (five-month-old child, subtotal pancreatectomy, hyperplasia of islands), and Graham and Hartmann[7] (a year-old baby, 80 to 90 per cent pancreatic removal, no abnormality of islets).

From the observations at hand there would seem to be little doubt that children who have cerebral and neurologic disturbances from hypoglycemia should promptly be given therapy to prevent permanent damage of the brain. If medical therapy is not quickly and completely curative, surgery should be proceeded with because 80 per cent pancreatectomy seems to be relatively safe and yet gives a high promise of preventing further hypoglycemic attacks and their devastating effects on the central nervous system.

REFERENCES

1. Boone, J. A.: A Case of Hyperinsulinism without Demonstrable Pancreatic Changes in an Eleven Year Old Child. New England J. Med., *211*:49, 1934.
2. Callaway, E.: Subtotal Resection of the Pancreas of an Eight-Year-Old Girl for Hyperglycemia. J.M.A. Georgia, *35*:164, 1946.
3. Crain, E. L., Jr., and Thorn, G. W.: Functioning Pancreatic Islet Cell Adenomas. A Review of the Literature and Presentation of Two New Differential Tests. Medicine, *28*:427, 1949.
4. Dannenberg, A. M., Bell, M. A. and Gouley, B.: Spontaneous Hypoglycemia due to Hyperinsulinism in a Child. J. Pediat., *7*:44, 1935.
5. Frantz, V. K.: Adenomatosis of Islet Cells, With Hyperinsulinism. Ann. Surg., *119*: 824, 1944.
6. Fraser, R., Albright, F. and Smith, P. H.: The Value of the Glucose Tolerance Test, the Insulin Tolerance Test, and the Glu-

cose-Insulin Tolerance Test in the Diagnosis of Endocrinologic Disorders of Glucose Metabolism. J. Clin. Endocrinology, *1*:297, 1941.
7. Graham, E. A. and Hartmann, A. F.: Subtotal Resection of the Pancreas for Hypoglycemia. Surg., Gynec. & Obst., *59*:474, 1934.
8. Greenlee, R. G., White, R. R. and Phillips, C.: Chronic Hypoglycemia in an Infant Treated by Subtotal Pancreatectomy. J.A.M.A., *149*:272, 1952.
9. Howard, J. M., Moss, N. H. and Rhoads, J. E.: Hyperinsulism and Islet Cell Tumors of the Pancreas. With 398 Recorded Tumors. Surg., Gynec. & Obst. (Internat. Abstr. Surg.), *90*:417, 1950.
10. Howland, G., Campbell, W. R., Maltby, E. J. and Robinson, W. L.: Dysinsulinism. Convulsions and Coma due to Islet Cell Tumor of the Pancreas, with Operation and Cure. J.A.M.A., *93*:674, 1929.

11. McQuarrie, I., Ziegler, M. R., Wright, W. S., Bauer, E. G. and Ulstrom, R. A.: Further Studies on the Effects of ACTH on Spontaneous Hypoglycemia. Mote, J. R., Editor: Proc. of Second Clinical ACTH Conference. Vol. II. Therapeutics. The Blakiston Co., Philadelphia, 1951, p. 69.

12. Sherman, H.: Islet Cell Tumor of Pancreas in a Newborn Infant (Nesidioblastoma). Am. J. Dis. Child., 74:58, 1947.

13. Talbot, N. B., Crawford, J. D. and Bailey, C. C.: Use of Mesoxalyl Urea (Alloxan) in Treatment of an Infant with Convulsions Due to Idiopathic Hypoglycemia. Pediatrics, 1:337, 1948.

14. Thorn, G. W., Quinby, J. T. and Clinton, M. J.: A Comparison of the Metabolic Effects of Isocaloric Meals of Varying Composition with Special Reference to the Prevention of Post-Prandial Hypoglycemic Reactions. Ann. Int. Med., 18:913, 1943.

15. Whipple, A. O.: Hyperinsulinism in Relation to Pancreatic Tumors. Surgery, 16:289, 1944.

16. Wilder, R. M., Allan, F. N., Power, M. H. and Robertson, H. E.: Carcinoma of the Islands of the Pancreas. Hyperinsulinism and Hypoglycemia. J.A.M.A., 89:348, 1927.

17. Wilkins, L.: The Diagnosis and Treatment of Endocrine Disorders in Childhood and Adolescence. Chap. 19. Charles C Thomas, Springfield, Ill., 1950.

18. Wolf, A., Hare, C. C. and Riggs, H. W.: Neurological Manifestations in Two Patients with Spontaneous Hypoglycemia. Bull. Neurol. Inst. New York, 3:232, 1933-34.

CHAPTER 45

Embryoma of the Kidney
(Wilms' Tumor)

Embryoma of the kidney is the most common tumor of the abdomen in childhood. The neoplasm is a highly malignant one and has been variously called "renal carcinoma," "sarcoma," "rhabdomyosarcoma," "angiosarcoma," and so on, depending upon the predominating type of tissue. While any given tumor may be largely comprised of one histologic substance, an adequate microscopic examination of blocks from different parts of the specimen almost always shows a mixed structure. Hence, it is preferable to designate these lesions as *embryomas* or *mixed tumors* of the kidney.

Considerable pessimism has sprung up regarding the prognosis for children with this neoplasm, and while it is still true that the mortality rate is high, the outlook is not as hopeless as many textbooks and reports would suggest. A review of the Children's Hospital material indicates that about a half of patients can be permanently cured, and indeed the survivals are as high as 75 or 80 per cent when dealing with the neoplasm in infancy.

PATHOLOGY

For more than two decades the Children's Hospital pathologic material on Wilms' tumor of the kidney has been carefully preserved and studied by Dr. Sidney Farber. His records have been used liberally in summarizing data for previous reports and for the following section.

Gross Pathology

An embryoma always arises within the renal substance, and as it grows, the kidney capsule is expanded around the neoplasm for a considerable period of time before it ruptures. Embryomas vary greatly in size; a few are as small as a fist; many are as large as a grapefruit; some have the proportions of a football. The growth tends to be spherical or oblong. The external surface is smoothly rounded or slightly lobulated. For the most part the neoplasms are solid, though cystic spaces and areas of degeneration are common. The color is gray to grayish red, but some zones may have a pinkish or yellowish tint. The tissue may be quite firm, or else highly cellular and rather soft. On the whole, the vascularity is poor, but the surface vessels can be quite large. The neoplasm tends to be sharply demarcated from the compressed kidney by a narrow band of connective tissue, but it is impossible to dissect the neoplasm away at such a septum. The kidney may retain a more or less normal contour, but it is more apt to be squeezed into a distorted shape. Likewise, the kidney pelvis may be narrowed, elongated, or otherwise deformed. Tumor tissue may project into the renal pelvis, but in the great majority of cases it does not do so. The tumor metastasizes through the retroperitoneal lymphatics, and especially by invasion of the renal veins and the blood stream.

years of age, are seldom seen beyond eight or ten years of age, and are very rare in adult life; in our series the youngest was two months and the oldest was nine years. Females and males are affected in about equal numbers. Embryoma appears with about equal frequency on the two sides, while in 4 of our cases each kidney was the site of a separate neoplasm.

ROENTGENOLOGIC EXAMINATION

Films of the abdomen without contrast media almost always show an opaque mass with displacement of intestines to the middle or opposite side of the abdomen. *Intravenous pyelography* gives additional information; such studies should be made in all cases. The pelvis of the kidney may be compressed, greatly elongated, or completely normal. It can remain in its customary position, but it often rides at the upper or lower pole of the tumor shadow. Hence, the dye-filled pelvis can be found well up toward the diaphragm or quite low in the iliac fossa. The kidney pelvis and ureter are almost never displaced laterally, but they are frequently pushed medially to a considerable degree. Lateral films may show the kidney pelvis displaced forward or backward in relation to the shadow of the neoplasm. Evidence of dye excretion is almost always seen on the involved side; it is quite rare that no dye appears. It has been our practice to obtain an *intravenous* pyelogram in all patients, but whenever these leave the diagnosis in doubt, *retrograde* studies have been resorted to. We have found it necessary to perform cystoscopy and retrograde pyelography in only a small minority of cases.

It is possible to recognize an embryoma of the kidney with a rather high degree of accuracy without roentgenologic studies, but such investigation should always be carried out because occasionally the clinician is misled by a neuroblastoma or even a hydronephrosis. Furthermore, roentgenologic visualization of the kidney aids the surgeon because it gives preoperative data regarding the position of the renal pedicle and blood vessels.

DIFFERENTIAL DIAGNOSIS

In infancy and childhood, embryoma of the kidney must be differentiated from several other masses which may occur in the region.

Neuroblastoma Sympatheticum

These tumors (see Chapter 46) arise from adrenal gland medulla or from other neural tissues in the retroperitoneal spaces. They are almost as common as renal embryomas. They are highly malignant lesions and are found in the same age groups. In general, these neoplasms are not apt to be as large as some of the embryomas. They metastasize early, and even when the primary tumor is small there may be widespread secondary growths in the liver and particularly in the skeleton. The primary neoplasm is firm or hard and generally has a pebbly or finely nodular surface, in contrast to the more smoothly rounded or gently lobulated contour of an embryoma. The neuroblastoma usually has an irregular outline, poorly defined borders, and possibly an extension far across the midline of the abdomen, whereas an embryoma has a spherical or oblong shape, better delineated borders, and less tendency to reach beyond the vertebral column.

Since a neuroblastoma can invade the adjacent kidney and distort its pelvis, pyelographic study is usually of little aid in differentiating the two conditions.

The metastases of these two growths appear in quite different places. Embryomas spread to regional lymph nodes and to the lungs. Neuroblastoma metastases are more widely scattered to the liver, kidneys, brain, orbits, and particularly to the skeleton which is peppered with small destructive lesions; the lungs are involved only late in the

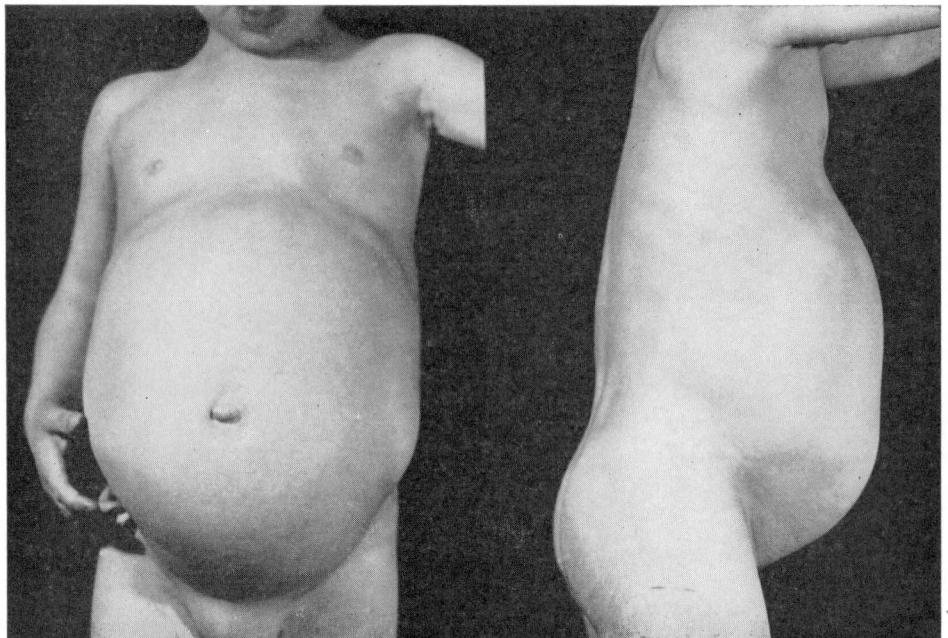

Fig. 322. Child with huge embryomas of both kidneys. This photograph was taken in 1940. Right tumor removed; left one treated by x-ray therapy. The child is alive, well, and free of neoplastic disease in 1952.

disorder. The roentgenologic characteristics and distribution of the metastases (when they exist) will often make a clear differentiation between the two forms of neoplasm.

Hypernephroma of the Kidney

Hypernephroma, or the *Grawitz tumor,* is a solid neoplasm arising within the kidney and composed of cells with clear, foamy cytoplasms resembling those of an adrenal cortex. It is believed that such growths arise from rests of adrenal cortical tissue which are not infrequently found in otherwise normal kidneys. The Grawitz tumor is one which appears in middle or late adult life. It is exceedingly rare in childhood and we have not encountered a single specimen during the last thirty years at the Children's Hospital. It is important to recognize the difference between these two entirely distinct neoplasms of the kidney; it is scarcely necessary to mention the hypernephroma, except to clarify the hazy impressions which some physicians still hold concerning the two conditions. The extreme rarity of hypernephroma in childhood makes it rather superfluous to consider the lesion in a differential diagnosis.

Unattached Retroperitoneal Embryoma or Teratoma

This term has been employed to describe a solid or partially cystic, mixed tumor which may appear anywhere along the posterior abdominal (or thoracic) wall. The adjective "unattached" is meant to imply that it is not connected with the kidney in spite of the fact that histologic resemblance to renal embryoma may be close. This neoplasm is believed to arise from remnants of the primitive pronephros or mesonephros and hence may be found on either side of the vertebral column from the fourth cervical segment downward as far as the internal genitalia. It often attains a very large size

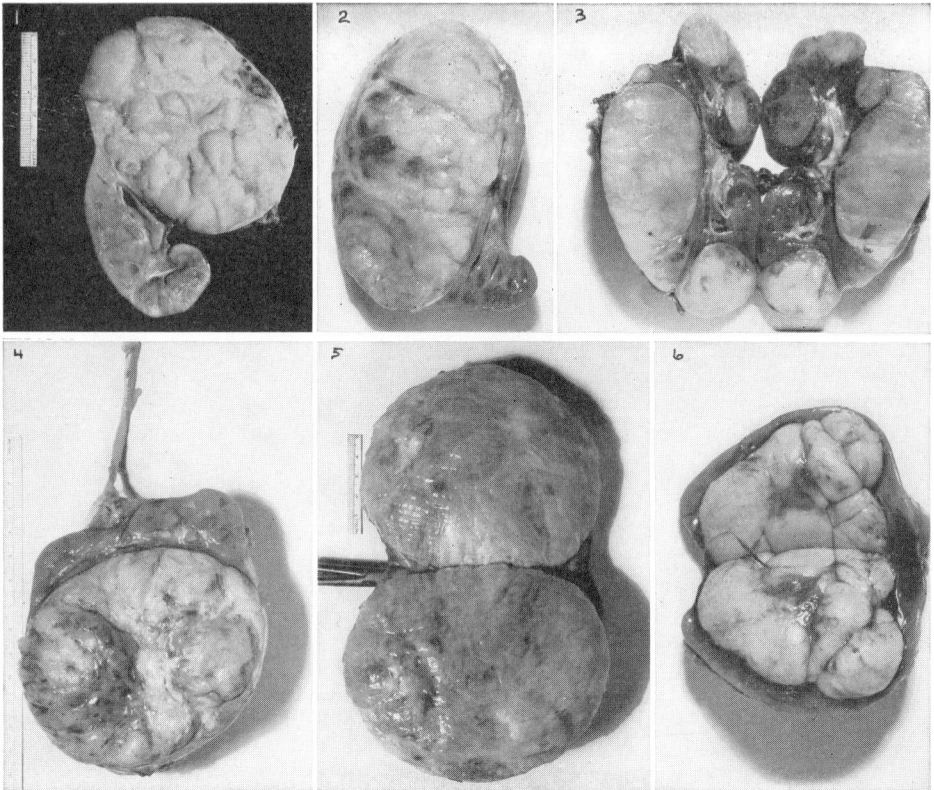

Fig. 323. Surgical specimens, embryoma of the kidney. 1. Eleventh-month-old child. Tumor arising from top of kidney. 2. Ten-month-old baby. Kidney substance compressed to one side by the tumor. 3. Tumor apparently of multicentric origin in kidney. 4. Four-year-old child. Spherical tumor, around which the renal capsule is expanded. 5. Ten-month-old baby. Very little renal tissue remaining. 6. Eight-month-old baby. Tumor entirely within renal substance.

before attracting attention. The prognosis is somewhat dependent upon the degree of malignancy and upon the promptness with which the lesion is recognized and removed; some of them have a rather well differentiated structure and hence carry an excellent outlook in spite of their large size. If a massive unattached retroperitoneal embryoma has a high position, it is usually impossible to distinguish it before operation from an embryoma of the kidney. If it should arise in the lower abdomen, embryoma of the kidney can be excluded because the mass does not extend into the renal fossa. Retroperitoneal embryomas are rare; most of them are found in adult life. During a period of years in which we have encountered 96 embryomas of the kidney, only 11 retroperitoneal teratomas have been seen.

Hydronephrosis

Hydronephrosis is relatively common in this age group; it follows some congenital obstruction either at the ureteropelvic junction or at the ureterovesical valve. Usually it is accompanied by pain, fever, or pyuria. In an occasional instance a kidney pelvis can attain enormous proportions and fill a large part of the abdomen, may be unaccompanied by urinary infection and may be attended by very little pain. Under these circumstances, it might be virtually impossible by physical examination alone to differen-

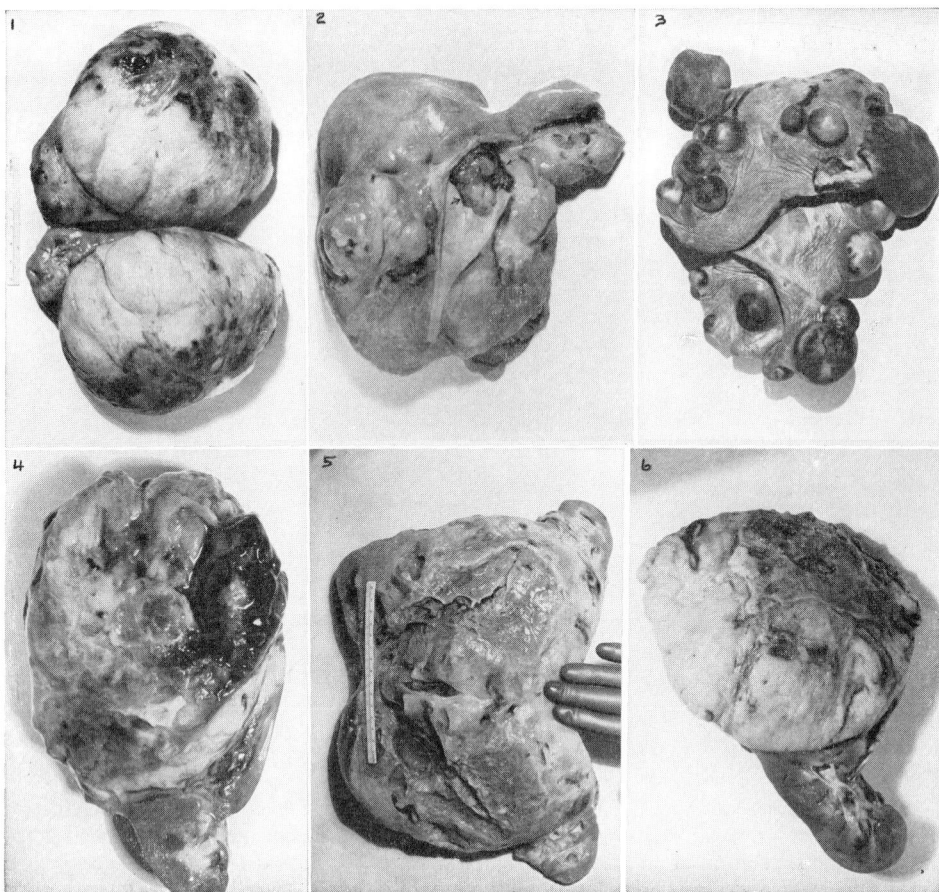

Fig. 324. Embryomas of the kidney. 1. One-year-old child. Specimen weighed 744 gm. Some hemorrhage in tumor. 2. Nine-year-old boy. Large embryoma, growing into pelvis (arrows). 3. Multilobular mass. 4. Very large tumor; recent hemorrhage into its substance. 5. Massive tumor, weighing 2870 gm., from a ten-year-old boy. Much necrosis and dissolution in the tumor. 6. Nine-year-old girl. Tumor arising from one pole; it had broken through its capsule, at right upper border.

tiate it from an embryoma of the kidney. Generally, the fluid nature of a hydronephrosis is evident by palpation, but a tensely distended hydronephrotic sac has not infrequently been mistaken for a solid tumor! If physical findings leave the physician in doubt, intravenous or retrograde pyelograms will quickly settle this differential diagnosis.

TREATMENT

When a diagnosis of embryoma of the kidney has been made, the course of therapy must be decided upon. If left untreated, these individuals rapidly develop metastases in the retroperitoneal lymph nodes or lungs, and possibly in the liver or brain. If no metastases are demonstrable, the primary growth should be removed in all cases no matter how large it might be. While the size of the abdominal swelling may make the prognosis seem dubious, *surgical excision* holds almost the only hope of cure.

Preoperative Irradiation

There can be little argument about the fact that many of these tumors are quite radio-sensitive. Some clinicians, notably Kerr,[7] Kretschmer,[8] Wharton,[15] Priestley and

Broders,[11] and Prather and Friedman,[10] have advocated the use of preoperative irradiation over the growth with two thoughts in mind: (1) To reduce the size of the local mass so that it will be easier to remove. (2) To kill off the more malignant cells and possibly prevent their escape into the blood stream during the manipulations of operation.

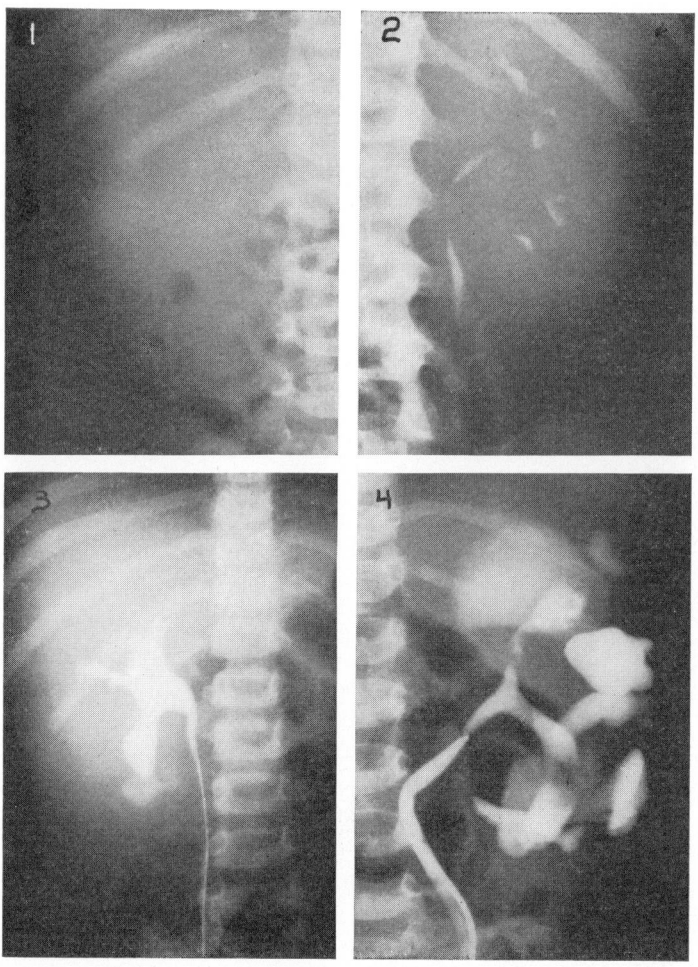

Fig. 325. Roentgenograms from four children with embryomas of the kidney. 1. Large shadow of a mass in right upper quadrant of abdomen. 2. Compression and separation of calyces by tumor which surrounds them. 3. Attenuation and distortion of pelvis and calyces in a renal mass. 4. Marked distortion of drainage system by kidney tumor.

While these arguments presumably are valid there are also strong theoretical reasons against the employment of preoperative irradiation: (1) It puts off operation for one to several weeks, and thereby increases the time during which metastases can occur. (2) It can soften or even liquefy tumor and thereby increase the chances of tumor cells breaking out into the blood stream. After due consideration of the pros and cons of this dispute, I am quite convinced that preoperative x-ray therapy has been employed too widely. The decision to use preoperative irradiation should never be made because of the ease it might afford the surgeon; it should be employed only when it can be shown to increase the chances of permanent cure of this malignant disease. Thus far, no one has published reasonable evidence that preoperative irradiation has actually improved cure rates. Indeed, it cuts down the percentage of survivors.

By personal communications, various surgeons and urologists have informed us of children who had preoperative x-ray therapy and who have been cured. Usually these have been only a few successful cases in the hands of any one man; when compared to the number of deaths following the same combination, these isolated cures become

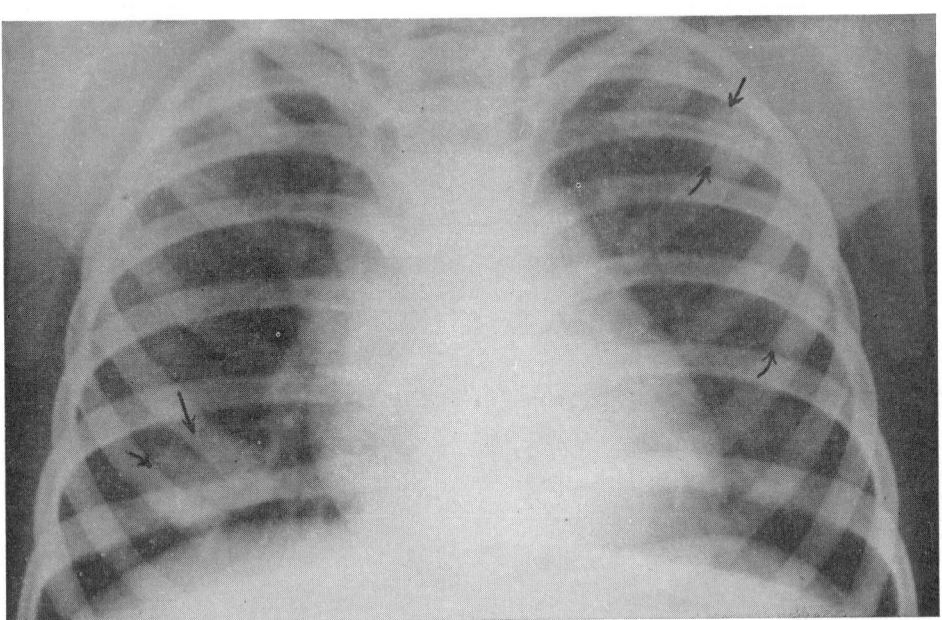

Fig. 326. Chest film from a child with renal embryoma; several metastases are seen in the lung fields.

very unimpressive. Unfortunately, no convincing information is available in the literature which gives factual evidence regarding the value or the harmfulness of preoperative x-ray therapy. To settle this point, we began in 1949 to *give such irradiation to every other patient* who entered our service. Two to three thousand roentgens were given over the presenting mass, in divided doses extending over a period of ten to fifteen days. *Within a year it became so evident that the fatality rate was skyrocketing above former figures that we felt completely sure that such irradiation before operation was very detrimental;* we have therefore completely abandoned it. It is our strong conviction that immediate surgery (combined with postoperative irradiation) gives the highest possibility of a permanent cure.

Immediate Excision of Tumor

During the last twenty years at the Children's Hospital the large size of a tumor has never been considered a contraindication to operation. Since 1932 there has been no operative fatality in any case (we define operative mortality as any death from any cause which takes place while the child is in the hospital). This record refutes the statement, so often made, that preoperative irradiation is necessary to obtain a low operative mortality.

Preoperative Preparations. If anemia is present, preoperative *transfusion* is indicated. Arrangements must always be made to administer blood during and immediately after operation, because the extent of the dissection often produces considerable shock which can be combated adequately only by transfusion. It is quite important to place a cannula or a plastic tube into an ankle vein before starting the laparotomy so that intravenous fluids and blood can be given at a moment's notice if the need arises.

It is firmly believed that these subjects *should be operated upon very promptly.* There is little excuse for having them lie in a hospital for several days or more before surgery is undertaken. While we do not regard such operations in the category of emer-

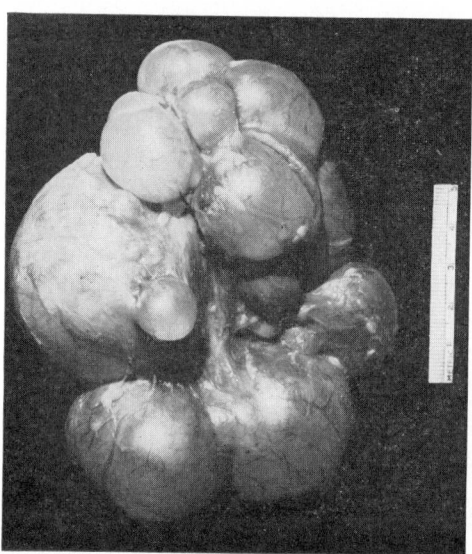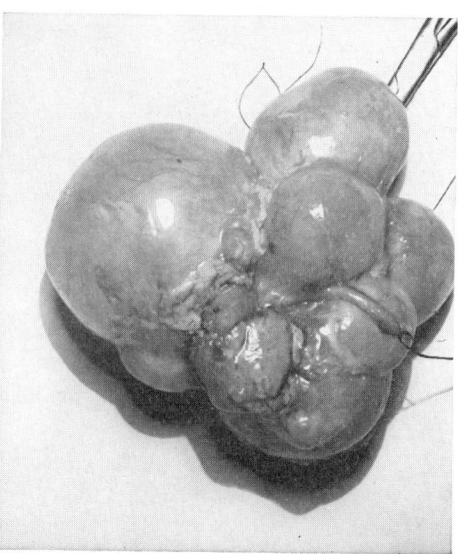

Fig. 327. For comparison of renal fossa masses, two specimens of unilateral polycystic kidneys, removed from two infants. *Left*, From a nineteen-day-old baby. *Right*, From a nine-month-old child; specimen weighed 375 gm.

aencies, we have found that it is generally possible to admit the patient, gather the important data, and surgically remove the neoplasm within four or five hours. These pbdominal masses are apt to create considerable interest on the part of physicians, nurses, and students; repeated palpation and handling theoretically increases the likelihood of releasing tumor cells into the blood stream. It is our feeling that the mass should be handled gently, should be palpated only by those who are directly concerned with the case, and that the sooner the tumor is removed the better are the chances of cure.

Transabaominal Exposure. It is unwise to attack one of these lesions through an oblique postero-lateral incision in the flank, because this gives too small an opening between the ribs and iliac crest of a child. An oblique, thoraco-abdominal exposure is preferred by some; it gives an excellent view of small or medium-size tumors, but is less desirable than an anterior, transperitoneal approach for the very large masses. For all cases we much prefer an anterior, transperitoneal opening because it allows ligation and division of the renal vessels before the tumor is disturbed. It is highly important to close the renal vein early in the operation to diminish the dangers of liberating tumor cells into the blood stream.

The incision should run from the costal margin downward as far as the circumstances of the case dictate (Fig. 328); not infrequently it must be carried to the pubsi. The rectus muscle can be split, but it is preferable to retract it laterally and thus gain a stronger wound postoperatively. In some cases we have used a transverse wound. The ascending or descending colon, according to whether the tumor is right- or left-sided, is

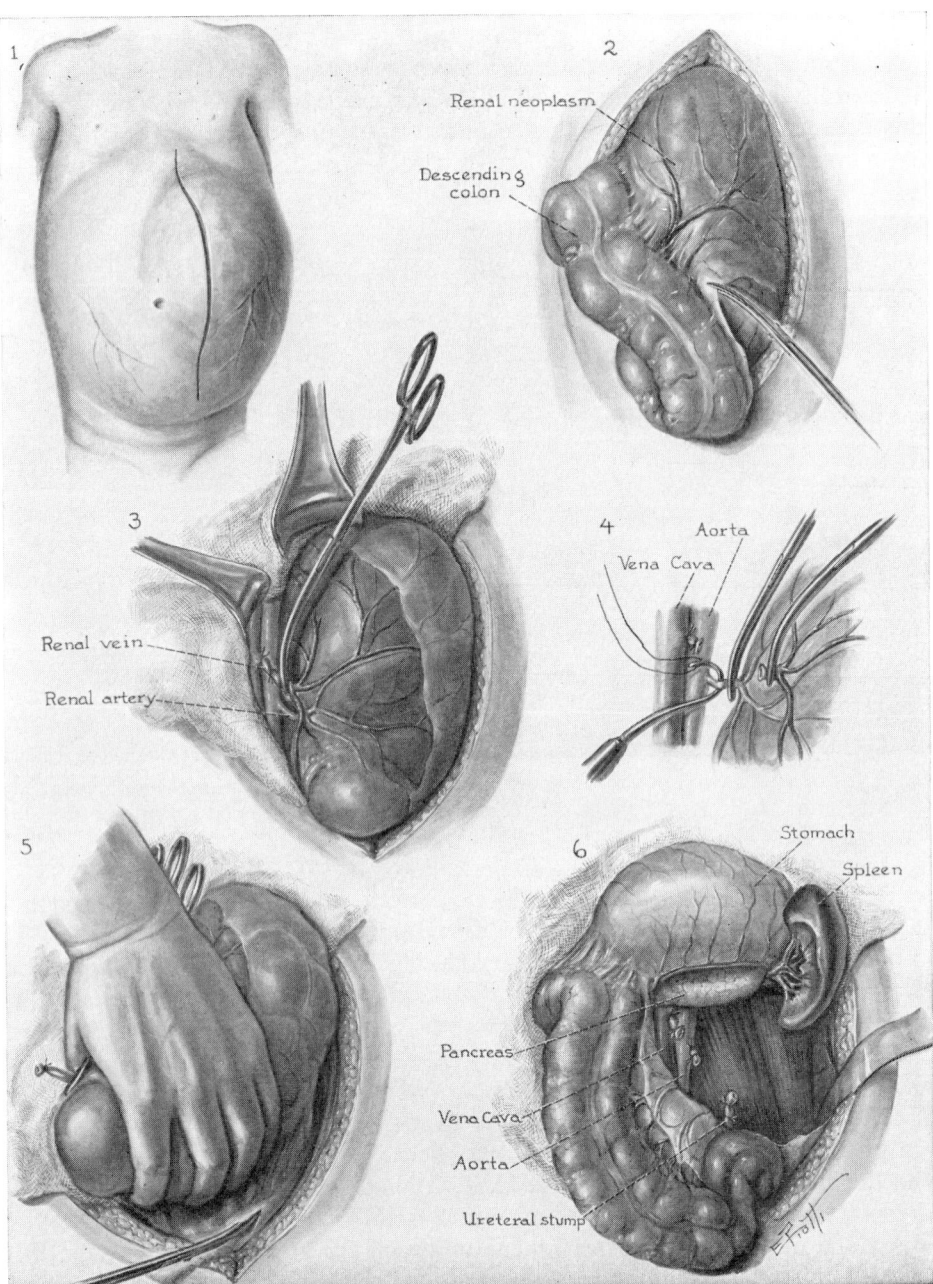

Fig. 328. Operative excision of an embryoma of the left kidney. 1. Position of the bulging mass and the long, left rectus incision. 2. Colon displaced downward and medially by tumor. Peritoneum will be cut to mobilize the colon and expose the neoplasm. 3. Colon pulled medially. Renal pedicle treated before the tumor is disturbed. Vein being tied and clamped. 4. Renal vein divided. Renal artery clamped; ligature being passed around it. 5. Renal vein, artery, and ureter all divided. Inferior and posterior dissection of mass being carried out. 6. Tumor removed from renal fossa. The colon will be dropped back into this raw space.

a few isolated metastases in the lungs, it is probably desirable to treat these intensively and repeatedly, as long as there is no evidence of important spread to other parts of the lungs.

RESULTS OF TREATMENT

It is necessary to dispel the feeling of gloom and hopelessness which has long been expressed by many who have handled these cases. While disappointments and failures are frequent, there is a brighter side to the picture when we see increasing percentages of cures following early and thorough attack on the problem.

When summing up the results in a series from any one institution, authors should feel obliged to include *all* cases they have encountered; only against such a background can the cures be presented to calculate the true percentage of survivors. There has been a widespread tendency to report series of the more hopeful cases (patients who have been operated upon or otherwise treated) and to use this number when calculating the percentage of cures which result therefrom. The figure thus obtained indicates the results in the treated cases, but it certainly does not tell what is happening to the entire group of patients encountered in a given institution. Such considerations should be taken into account when scrutinizing published reports.

Weisel, Dockerty and Priestley[14] in 1943 reported 7 cures in 44 patients, in 42 of whom the treatment included nephrectomy—a cure-rate of 16 per cent. For some of their patients irradiation was employed postoperatively; in others such treatment was given both before and after operation. While their material gives convincing evidence of the power of roentgen rays to shrink many of these neoplasms and thus make easier their operative removal, the data are not presented in any way which proves that radiation increases the number of cures over that which can be obtained by surgery alone.

Dean[2] in 1945 summarized his findings in the treatment of 20 patients by irradiation only, of whom 5 were still alive without evidence of disease for more than five years. In none of these was a positive diagnosis established by biopsy; this raises the slight possibility that some of these youngsters might actually have had other types of neoplasm. While his series is open to some criticism regarding diagnostic accuracy, the material does give considerable evidence regarding the destructive effects of roentgen rays on some of these growths.

In 1946, Nesbit and Adams[9] presented a series of 16 children with Wilms' tumors; 12 of these had nephrectomies (a few with postoperative radiation) with 7 cures, a survival rate of 58.4 per cent. Another was treated by biopsy and irradiation, with cure. The survival of 8 patients out of 16 in whom the diagnosis of embryoma was positively made gives a combined cure-rate of 50 per cent. In the same ten-year period they observed 11 other patients in whom a presumptive diagnosis of embryoma was made but for various reasons was never confirmed by pathologic examination. It is possible that some of these children did not have an embryoma, but the evidence recorded by these experienced men would suggest that most of these subjects actually did have embryomas; 7 (possibly 9) are known to have died subsequently. Thus, if one considers the entire group of 27 patients with proved or probable embryomas of the kidney, the over-all cure percentage would be somewhere in the middle or upper thirties.

Silver,[13] in a series of 18 cases reported in 1947, had 10 survivals, a figure of 55 per cent (Table 66). A closer inspection of his material shows inclusion of two adults (twenty-one and twenty-seven years), so that if one is considering only the problem in childhood ages, there were 16 cases and 8 survivals, a cure of 50 per cent. No uniform treatment was employed. While the small number of cases with each type of therapy might possibly lead to erroneous conclusions, the valuable data reported are certainly worthy of study and can be summarized as follows. The last group, while small, is noteworthy.

Table 66

Therapeutic Statistics from Silver's Series

Treatment	Outcome	
	Alive	Dead
No therapy...	0	2
Irradiation alone..	0	3
Nephrectomy alone..	3	1
Nephrectomy plus postoperative irradiation......................................	3	2
Preoperative irradiation, nephrectomy, and postoperative irradiation..............	4	0

Dickey and Chandler[3] in 1949 reported 12 cases of Wilms' tumor in which the diagnosis was confirmed by examination of the gross or microscopic tissue; 4 patients survived (33 per cent). The treatment had been transperitoneal nephrectomy, followed (in some instances) by postoperative irradiation.

A brief review of our own material from the Children's Hospital of Boston provides the basis for some comments and conclusions. We have counted *all* patients who have been seen in the hospital who have had an embryoma of the kidney, whether treated or not; therefore the series includes some who had metastatic disease when first seen, and for whom only palliative treatment and terminal care could be offered. We have studied patients treated up through 1947, because it is now five years since treatment in all these cases and it is possible to make reasonably accurate statements regarding the cures and the failures. The data are summarized in Table 67, the material being divided into three groups, 1914–1930, 1931–1939, and 1940–1947, because the methods of treatment varied in these three periods.

Table 67

Statistics from All Cases in Boston Children's Hospital Series

Period of Study	Percentage of Cures		
	Patients Below 12 Months of Age	Patients Above 12 Months of Age	All Patients of All Ages
1914–1930 inclusive 27 cases (4 cures)	42.8	5.0	14.9
1931–1939 inclusive 31 cases (10 cures)	71.4	20.8	32.2
1940–1947 inclusive 38 cases (18 cures)	80.0	43.3	47.3

From 1914 through 1930 there were 27 cases, with 4 cures, a survival of 14.9 per cent. During this time no special attention was paid to the condition; patients were operated upon by a number of visiting surgeons. The operative mortality alone was 23 per cent. It is not surprising to find that the haphazard methods then employed were followed by few long-term survivors.

From 1931 through 1939 there were 31 patients and a sharp rise in the cures to 32.2 per cent. This great improvement can be attributed entirely to the efforts of Dr. William Ladd, who became interested in the problem and promptly introduced changes in the technical aspects of the surgery to eliminate the hazards previously associated with such surgical undertakings. Proper anesthesia was developed, intravenous fluids and blood were given to prevent shock, a transabdominal approach was universally employed to facilitate removal of the larger growths and to allow early division of the renal vessels. Attention to the technical details quickly led to elimination of deaths on the table and in the immediate postoperative period; *after 1932 there were no deaths from operation in spite of the fact that all tumors were removed, regardless of their size.* Many of these neoplasms were enormous; in one instance, the weight of the growth was one-quarter that of the child. Improving the operative technique was richly rewarded by cure rates which were higher than any that appeared in the medical literature of that time.

From 1940 through 1947, there were 38 patients and 18 apparent cures, a survival of 47.3 per cent. Essentially, the surgical procedures have been the same as those developed in the 1931–1939 period; there have been no operative fatalities. Preoperative irradiation has not been employed, and tumors have been excised irrespective of the great size of many of them. It is quite possible that neoplasms were being seen earlier for operation because of the increasing interest of pediatricians and practitioners in this area; this factor is very difficult to evaluate, but we must recognize that prompt detection certainly contributes to a higher probability of cure. However, all of the cases could not be regarded particularly as favorable ones, since some of the tumors greatly distended the abdomen. This 1940–1947 group differs from the 1931–1939 series primarily by the fact that *postoperative x-ray irradiation was given in all (except two) cases.* The rise in cures to 47 per cent we attribute largely to this routine use of x-ray treatments over the renal fossa.

The presence of *embryomas in both kidneys* (in the absence of metastases to the chest) does not necessarily present an insuperable problem (Fig. 322). Of the 4 such patients who have come to our attention, 3 have died of widespread metastases, but 1 is apparently cured. This surviving patient was first seen in 1940 at which time there was a very large mass in each kidney area, the right one being somewhat bigger than the left. At transabdominal exploration each renal fossa was found to be filled with a massive tumor which had all the gross characteristics of embryoma in each kidney. A biopsy of the right one showed microscopic evidence of such a mixed tumor. Following this exploration, roentgen irradiation was given to the abdomen (2650 r) which had a remarkable effect in reducing the size of the masses—only to be followed some months later by return to their original size. Seven months after the first exploration, a second operation was undertaken at which time a right nephrectomy was performed and the left kidney was palpated and inspected through the open abdomen. On the left was a mass, somewhat irregular in shape, but having a volume larger than a grapefruit. It had all the external gross characteristics of an embryoma of the left kidney; unfortunately no biopsy of it was taken. Following operation irradiation was given; 750 r over the right renal fossa, 1350 r over the left-sided mass, and 600 r over the lung fields. Subsequent palpations showed that the left renal mass slowly shrank. Twelve years later this child is alive and presents no evidence of neoplastic disease.

Various *chemical agents* or radioactive compounds are known to have destructive effects on Wilms' tumors that have extended through the abdomen, or have metastasized to various parts of the body; no cures have been obtained by these methods. It is highly probable that considerable progress will be made in this direction in the future.

It is important to add a note regarding *prognosis in relation to the age of patients* when first treated. A study of our cases has consistently shown that *babies in the first 12 months of life have a far better outlook than do older subjects.* This is particularly emphasized in the last group (1940–1947) wherein the cures in patients of all ages have been 47 per cent, while in the portion below twelve months of age the cures have been 80 per cent. The reason for this striking difference is unknown. Repeated review of pathologic material does not show any essential difference in the histologic make-up of tumors in the younger and older groups. It is quite possible that the better outlook for a baby is related to the fact that the young child is examined more often by physicians and that it is handled more frequently by the mother who bathes, changes, and otherwise cares for it; these factors probably lead to earlier detection of intra-abdominal masses.

Symptoms of Recurrence

If recurrence is found after operation, a firm irregular mass is usually felt in the renal fossa, in the liver, or in some other portion of the abdomen. The first evidence of recurrence is sometimes detected by respiratory distress or by roentgenologic examination of the chest. Development of pulmonary metastases heralds the onset of a rapidly downhill course. Extreme emaciation, intestinal obstruction, or superimposed pulmonary infection usually precedes exitus.

Parents are always anxious to know how long it will be before they can feel that their treated child is free from the danger of recurrence. A review of our material shows that *if recurrence was to take place, it was always evident within nine months* (by palpation of a mass within the abdomen or by discovery of metastases in a chest roentgenogram), except in two instances when it was first manifest at twenty months and at five years. The vast majority of deaths from recurrent disease occurred within one year. These observations indicate that *if a patient survives operation for a year and a half without evidence of recurrence, it is probable that a permanent cure has been attained.*

REFERENCES

1. Bradley, J. E. and Pincoffs, M. C.: Association of Adeno-myo-sarcoma of Kidney (Wilms' Tumor) with Arterial Hypertension. Ann. Int. Med., *11*:1613, 1938.

2. Dean, A. L.: Wilms' Tumors. New York State J. Med., *45*:1213, 1945.

3. Dickey, L. B. and Chandler, L. R.: Embryoma of Kidney (Wilms' Tumor) in Children. Pediatrics, *4*:197, 1949.

4. Hansmann, G. H. and Budd, J. W.: Massive Unattached Retroperitoneal Tumors; Explanation of Unattached Retroperitoneal Tumors Based on Remnants of Embryonic Urogenital Apparatus. J.A.M.A., *98*:6, 1932.

5. Horton, B. T.: The Relationship of Hypertension to Renal Neoplasm. Proc. Staff Meet., Mayo Clin., *15*:472, 1940.

6. Hughes, J. C., Rosenblum, H. and Horn, L. G.: Hypertension in Embryoma (Wilms' Tumor). Pediatrics, *3*:201, 1949.

7. Kerr, H. D.: Treatment of Malignant Tumors of Kidney in Children. J.A.M.A., *112*:408, 1939.

8. Kretschmer, H. L.: Malignant Tumors of Kidney in Children. J. Urol., *39*:250, 1938.

9. Nesbit, R. M. and Adams, F. M.: Wilms' Tumor. A Review of Sixteen Cases. J. Pediat., *29*:295, 1946.

10. Prather, G. C. and Friedman, H. F.: The Immediate Effect of Preoperative Radiation in Cortical Tumors of the Kidney. New England J. Med., *215*:655, 1936.

11. Priestley, J. T. and Broders, A. C.: Wilms. Tumor; Clinical and Pathological Study' J. Urol., *33*:544, 1935.

12. Priestley, J. T. and Schulte, T. L.: The Treatment of Wilms' Tumor. J. Urol., *47*:7, 1942.

13. Silver, H. K.: Wilms' Tumor (Embryoma of the Kidney). J. Pediat., *31*:643, 1947.

14. Weisel, W., Dockerty, M. B. and Priestley, J. T.: Wilms' Tumor of the Kidney: Clinicopathologic Study of 44 Proved Cases. J. Urol., *50*:399, 1943.

15. Wharton, L. R.: Preoperative Irradiation of Massive Tumors of the Kidney. Arch. Surg., *30*:35, 1935.

16. Wharton, L. R.: Transperitoneal Nephrectomy for Malignant Tumors of the Kidney. Surg., Gynec. & Obst., *60*:689, 1935.

17. Wilms, M.: Die Mischgeschwulste. A. Georgi, Leipzig, 1899, Heft 1.

CHAPTER 46

Neuroblastoma Sympatheticum

Neuroblastomas have been described under various names, including "sympathico-blastoma," "sarcoma of the adrenal gland," and "neuroblastoma sympatheticum." Excepting leukemia, they are the most frequently encountered neoplasms of infancy and childhood. When occurring within the abdomen, they are about half as common as the embryoma of the kidney. Neuroblastomas should be classified with the neurologic tumors, for they originate from tissue which gives rise to the adrenal medulla or other portions of the sympathetic system. They are highly malignant, they metastasize early and widely, and they have a serious but by no means uniformly fatal prognosis. The curability of neuroblastoma was pointed out by Lehman[10] in 1932. A hopeful attitude was expressed by Farber[5] in 1940 after a study of the Children's Hospital material.

Sites of Origin of Neuroblastomas

Though most commonly derived from the adrenal medulla, these tumors can arise from sympathetic tissue anywhere in the body. They can develop in the brain, but are more common in structures outside of the central nervous system. They can appear from the sympathetic chains in the neck, the thorax, or the abdomen. In a group of 96 cases studied to determine origins, the following distributions were found:

	%
Abdomen	57
Central nervous system	23
Pelvis	7
Thorax	5
Neck	2
Origin unknown	6

Types of Tumors Arising from Adrenals

An adrenal gland can give rise to four different types of neoplasm, the first two of which give endocrine disturbances and the latter two of which do not. Of these four neoplasms, the neuroblastoma is by far the most common:

1. From the cortex can come tumors, either benign or malignant, which give masculinizing changes of the genitalia, deepening of the voice, increase in the skeletal development, physical precocity, acne, hypertension, and increase in the excretion of urinary androgens.

2. From the medulla can come a pheochromocytoma which by liberation of epinephrine-like substances has striking effects in the formation of intermittent or continuous hypertension. These tumors are unilateral or bilateral. They are much more common in adult life, but have been found in early childhood.

3. From the medulla can develop the rare ganglioneuroma, which is an entirely benign growth, with no endocrine disturbance.

4. From the medulla can come the neuroblastoma, which arises from neural tissue, is highly malignant, has no endocrine disturbance, and is found in infancy and childhood.

PATHOLOGY

Gross Pathology

The neuroblastoma grows with considerable rapidity. While it may remain encapsulated for a short period, it has a marked tendency to break out, spread along tissue planes, invade surrounding organs, and metastasize by way of lymphatics and especially by blood stream dissemination. Specimens vary greatly in size. Some are so small that they cannot be felt and yet they give off widespread metastases; others are

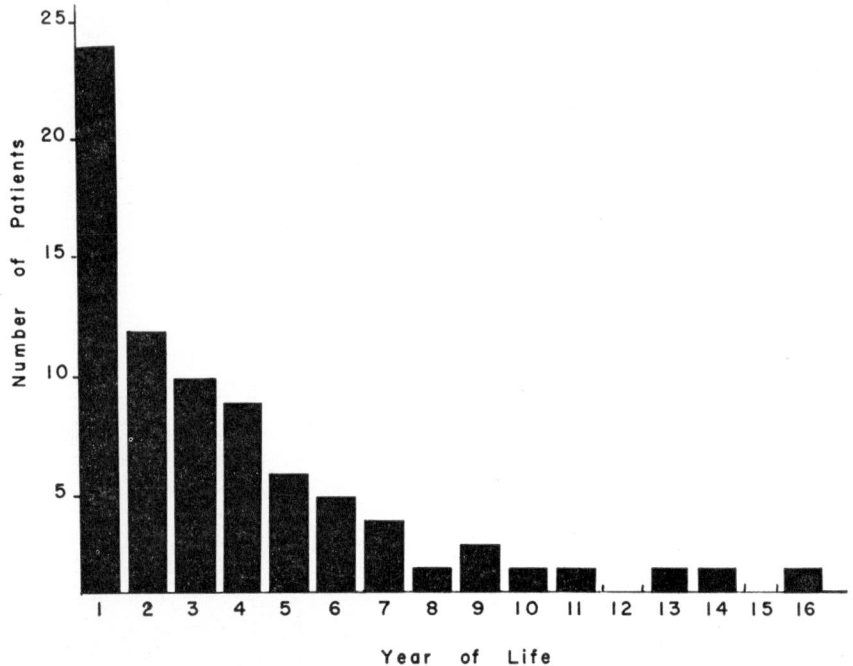

Fig. 330. Age incidence in a series of patients with neuroblastoma.

so large that they greatly distend one side of the abdomen or they compress a lung. When small and encapsulated, the tumors are smooth and rounded, but more often they are large and attain a finely lobulated or nubby surface. This nodularity frequently enables the physician to distinguish by abdominal palpation the lesion from an embryoma of the kidney, which tends to have a smooth or lobulated surface even when of enormous size.

Neuroblastomas arise on either side of the vertebral column, but they have a strong tendency to extend far across the midline. Furthermore, they are apt to spread retroperitoneally and even invade the retropleural tissues. The growth may involve vertebral bodies or pedicles and in a few instances has extended into the spinal canal. The tumor surface is extremely vascular; the vessels are rather small and appear as a fine network. The external surface therefore has a distinct reddish or grayish red color when viewed during life. While some of the growths can be dissected away cleanly from surrounding organs, the more advanced lesions infiltrate and directly invade adjacent kidney, renal pelvis, regional veins, root of the mesentery, body of the pancreas, lymph nodes, etc. It

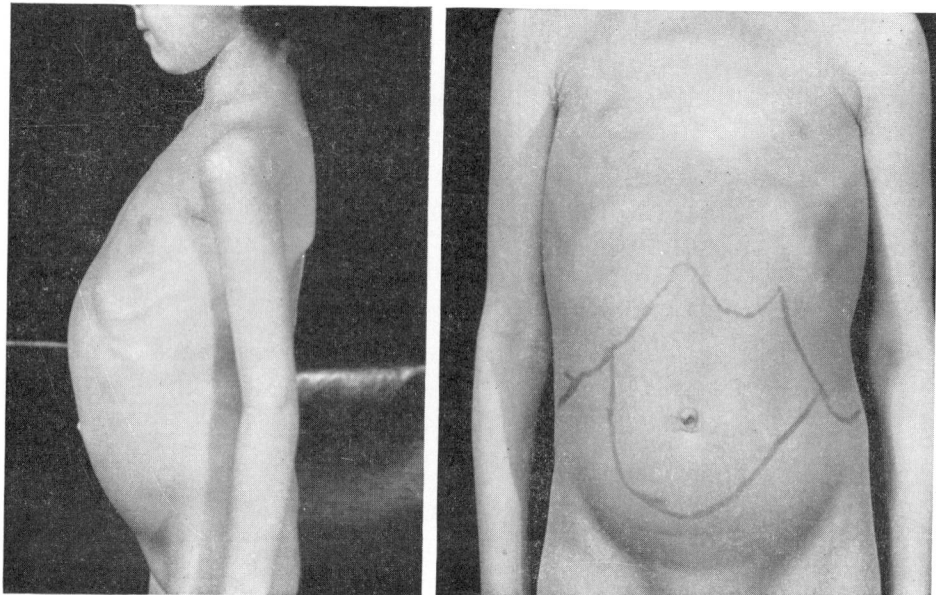

Fig. 331. Girl with extensive neuroblastoma of the upper abdomen.

can be extremely difficult to identify the pancreas, lymph nodes, retroperitoneal vessels, or other structures when they are permeated by neoplasm.

The cut surface of a tumor is soft, grayish or reddish gray, highly cellular, and possesses little supporting stroma. Some of the tumors have a mushy consistency and bits of substance will extrude or ooze out when the specimen is cut open. Blood vessels

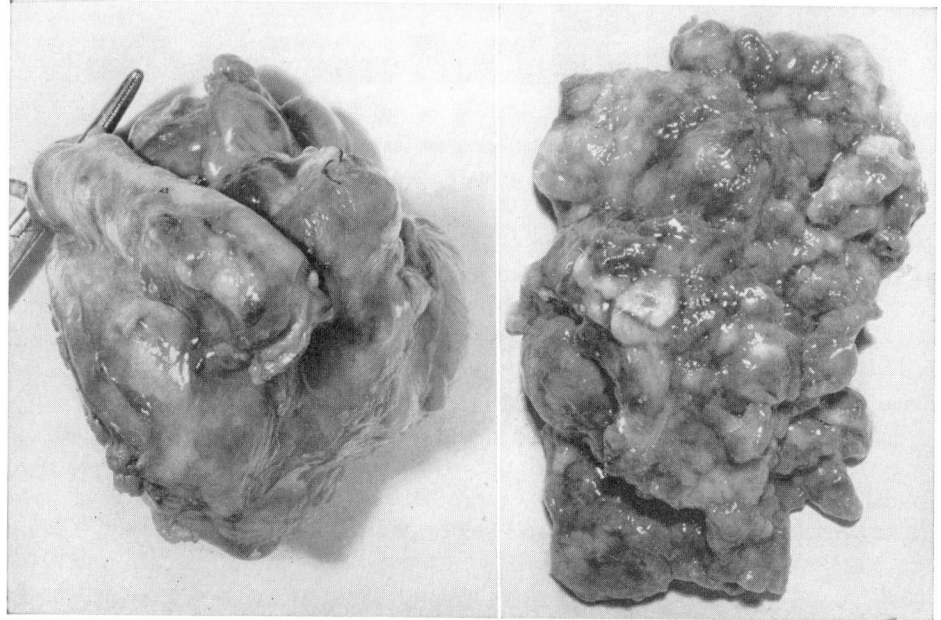

Fig. 332. Two surgical specimens of neuroblastomas removed from the abdomen. *Left,* Showing irregular contour of the mass, with a portion of splenic flexure of colon which was removed with the neoplasm. *Right,* Showing the nubby surface which these tumors are apt to have.

are numerous but small. Necrosis and hemorrhage are common; fine scattered calcification is occasionally seen.

Metastases

Metastases take place by way of both lymphatic and especially blood stream invasion. In a minority of cases they are limited to regional lymph nodes or massive invasion of the liver. More frequently they are widely disseminated through the kidneys, orbits, brain, and other organs, with a special predilection for the skeletal system. The bone marrow may be widely replaced, even before roentgenographic changes are seen in skeletal films, a finding which should be suspected if there is any important anemia. The tumor tends to avoid the lungs until very late in the course of the disease. Pepper (in 1901) called attention to "sarcoma of the adrenal" and involvement of the liver, and for many years this combination was spoken of as the *Pepper syndrome*. In 1907 Hutchinson described primary adrenal tumors with metastases to the skull and orbits, producing unilateral or bilateral exophthalmos. This group of findings has been referred to as the *Hutchinson syndrome*. There is no need for perpetuation of these designations since the pathology in either instance is the same and the clinical manifestations are merely dependent upon what part of the body is invaded by tumor.

In 60 per cent of our cases, the tumor had already metastasized by the time patients were hospitalized. Study of 44 patients with metastases showed the following distribution of these:

Skeleton only	22
Liver only	7
Mediastinum only	4
Skeleton and mediastinum	3
Liver and mediastinum	3
Liver and skeleton	2
Liver, skeleton, and mediastinum	1
Liver and skin	1
Skin, skeleton, and mediastinum	1

Of particular interest is that group of patients in whom extensive liver metastases are found by physical examination and proved by abdominal exploration. We have encountered 7 of these, 9 days, 11 days, 3 months, 4 months, 3 months, 6 months, and 4 months old respectively. It would appear that the tendency to development of metastases which are limited to the abdomen and liver is a peculiarity of very young infants and is seldom seen in older neuroblastoma patients.

Histologic Features

Microscopic examination shows a highly cellular, rapidly growing neoplasm with great invasive qualities. The supporting stroma is quite scanty. Blood vessels are usually of rather small caliber. The tumor cells occur in broad sheets and clusters. They have somewhat the appearance of lymphocytes but are a little larger than such cells. Because of this feature, the tumors were often described in the past as sarcomas or lymphoblastomas. In general, the cell nuclei are polygonal or have a spherical contour. There is a moderate amount of chromatin which has either a fairly even distribution or a peripheral arrangement. One to several nucleoli are often seen. The cystoplasms are amphophilic. Since these stain poorly in improperly preserved specimens, the microscopic appearance is that of a syncytial mass. Mitotic figures are numerous. In only a few areas do the cells take on an elongated or spindle form. Invasion of blood vessels is often seen.

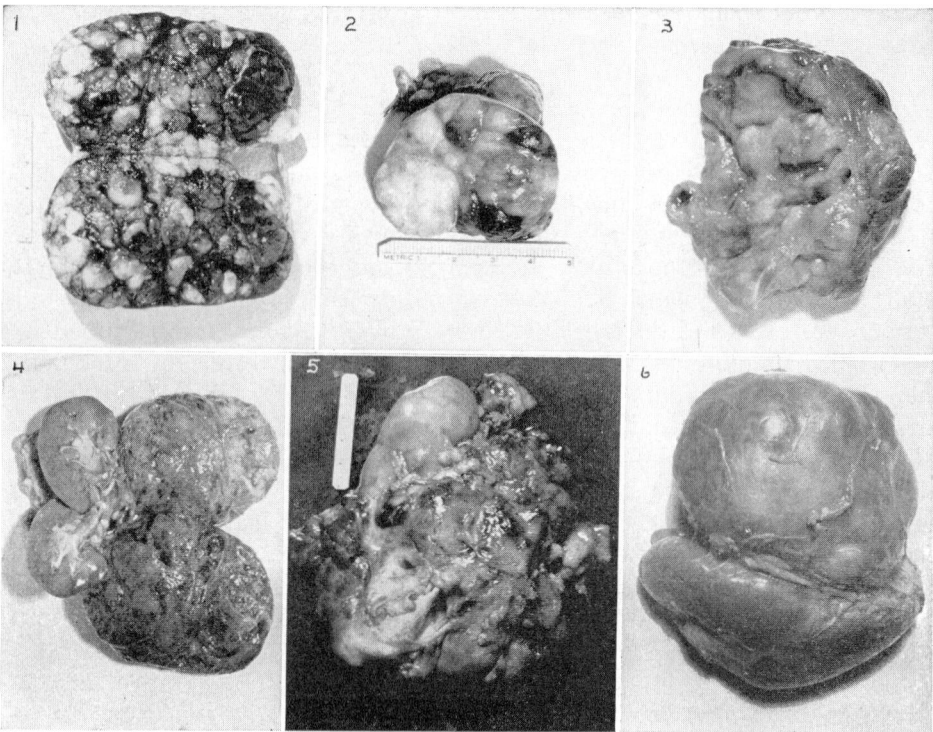

Fig. 333. Six surgical specimens showing some of the characteristics of neuroblastoma. 1. From four-month-old baby with adrenal tumor. Shows very well the islands of well preserved neoplasm, interspersed between which are extensive areas of necrosis. 2. Well encapsulated adrenal tumor from an eleven-month-old baby. 3. A neuroblastoma from the organ of Zuckerkandl. 4. A well encapsulated tumor adjacent to kidney. 5. Neuroblastoma extensively surrounding kidney, from a three-year-old girl. 6. A nicely encapsulated neuroblastoma alongside of kidney; seventeen-month-old girl.

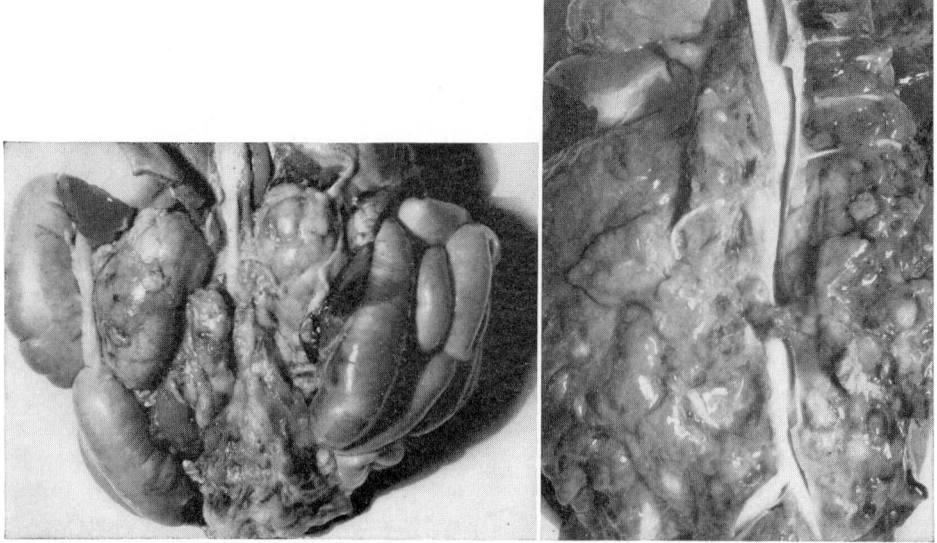

Fig.334. From two cases, autopsy specimens to show the infiltrative nature of neuroblastoma. After exenteration, the viscera are viewed from behind. In each there is a diffuse pannus of nodular tumor embedding the great vessels and abdominal organs.

There are two characteristics which positively identify the neuroblastoma. The first is the occasional arrangement of a score or more of cells into a *rosette* with peripheral distribution of nuclei and a central concentration of the cell cytoplasms. The second is the development of *neurofibrils* which can be seen with the phosphotungstic acid-hematoxylin stain. These delicate fibrils may appear anywhere through the tumor, but they are particularly apt to be found in the central portions of the rosettes, since they arise from the tail processes of cells in these formations.

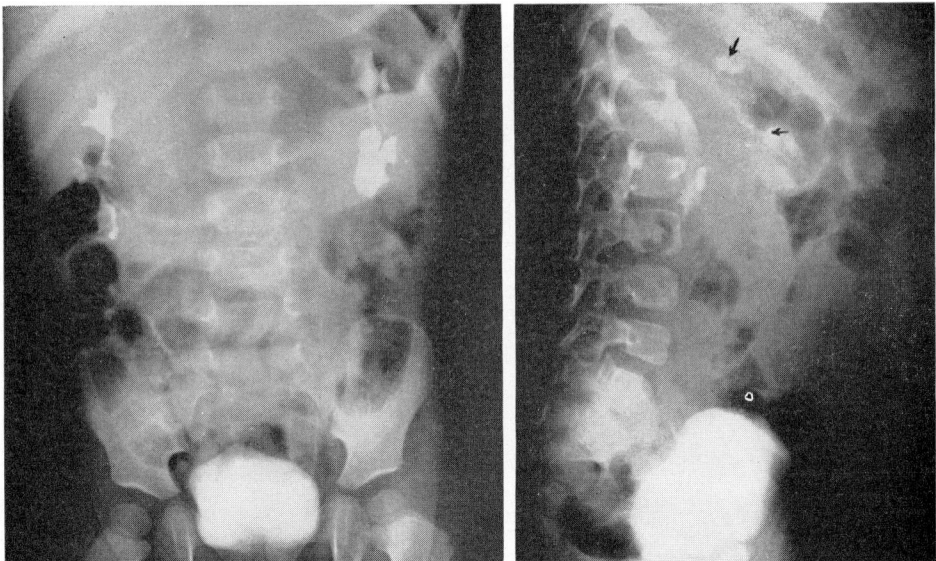

Fig. 335. Pyelograms from a child who had an extensive retroperitoneal neuroblastoma. In the *left* film, both kidneys can be seen displaced outward, rotated, and distorted. In the *right* film, some flecks of calcium (arrows) are found in the mass which extends far in front of the kidneys.

While the histologic features already enumerated are typical of the common run of neuroblastomas, occasionally one finds a more malignant growth in which the cells are a little smaller and in which no rosettes or fibrils can be identified. This more embryonic type of neoplasm is classified as a "sympathogonioma" or "sympathicoblastoma." Conversely, a tumor with many of the features of a neuroblastoma may show some areas differentiating into ganglion cells; to indicate a more favorable prognosis it can be designated as a "neuroblastoma-ganglioneuroma" or "neuroblastoma differentiating into ganglioneuroma."

CLINICAL FINDINGS

Neuroblastomas are encountered in any childhood age, but they are largely tumors of the first few years of life (Fig. 330). About 30 per cent occur in the first year, 80 per cent within the first five years, and only 20 per cent beyond that age. The tumor is very rare in adult life. Our youngest patient was one day of age, and the oldest was fifteen years. The frequency of occurrence is about equal in the two sexes.

Symptoms

In the abdominal growths, the most common initial complaint is related to a *swelling* which is generally painless. The appearance of *pain* is somewhat suggestive of neoplastic involvement of retroperitoneal nerves or invasion and obstruction of a ureter or the intestine. The history usually indicates that there has been *pallor*, increasing *fatigue*, and possibly *weight loss* for several months. *Loss of appetite* is common. If metastases have occurred there may be discomfort from an enlarged liver, headache or vomiting from expanding nodules in the brain, ecchymosis or protrusion of an eyeball from an orbital growth, swelling of the head from a lesion of the calvarium, and possibly pain in an extremity from pathologic fracture or slipping of an epiphysis at a site of skeletal destruction.

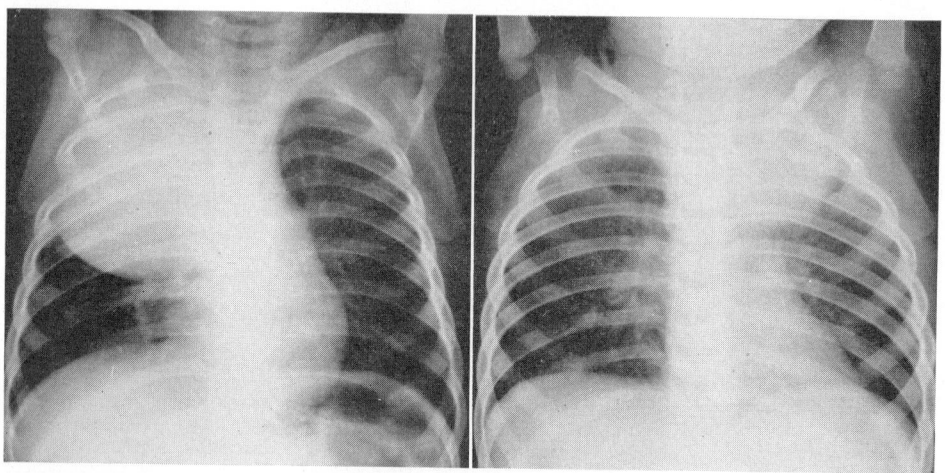

Fig. 336. Films showing neuroblastoma primary in the thorax, originating from the paravertebral sympathetic chains. *Left*, From a thirteen-month-old girl. *Right*, From a twenty-two-month-old female.

When originating in the thorax, the tumors can give rise to weight loss, cough, or bizarre symptoms of pulmonary involvement.

Physical Findings

In the great majority of the abdominal cases, examination discloses a *firm, nodular mass* in one side of the abdomen which may have spread across the midline and which might even be connected with a smaller lump on the opposite side. Such a mass can be located anywhere from the adrenal region down to the promontory of the sacrum, according to the site of origin. It is non-tender, is obviously fixed to posterior abdominal structures, and does not move during inspiration. The *liver* may be nodular and enormously enlarged if it contains metastases. In advanced cases, evidence of secondary lesions may be found elsewhere in the body, such as proptosis of an eye, a raised mass on the scalp, a Macewen sign (in young individuals), palpable left cervical lymph nodes (extensions by way of the thoracic duct), or tenderness over bones of the extremities. In a few cases there are neurologic changes which have resulted from compression of the spinal cord. Fever may appear whenever there is necrosis of a considerable amount of tumor tissue.

For those growths which are primary in the neck there may be a single firm and fixed mass on either side, or there may be scattered involvement of many nodes to which the tumor tends to extend while the primary lesion is still very small.

For those neoplasms which are primary in the thorax, examination shows dullness or flatness over the area, diminution or absence of breath sounds, and possibly dyspnea.

Laboratory Data

The urinary sediment rarely is abnormal; the finding of red cells suggests that a kidney or renal pelvis has been invaded. A mild degree of *anemia* is present in the vast majority of cases. This does not necessarily mean that bone marrow has been replaced by metastatic growth, nor does it necessarily imply that blood has been lost by way of the urinary or intestinal tract. Indeed, it is hard to explain the cause for anemia in many of these children. However, marked anemia should arouse suspicion regarding the possibility of widespread metastases to the hematopoietic system, and should be studied by aspiration or biopsy of the sternal marrow.

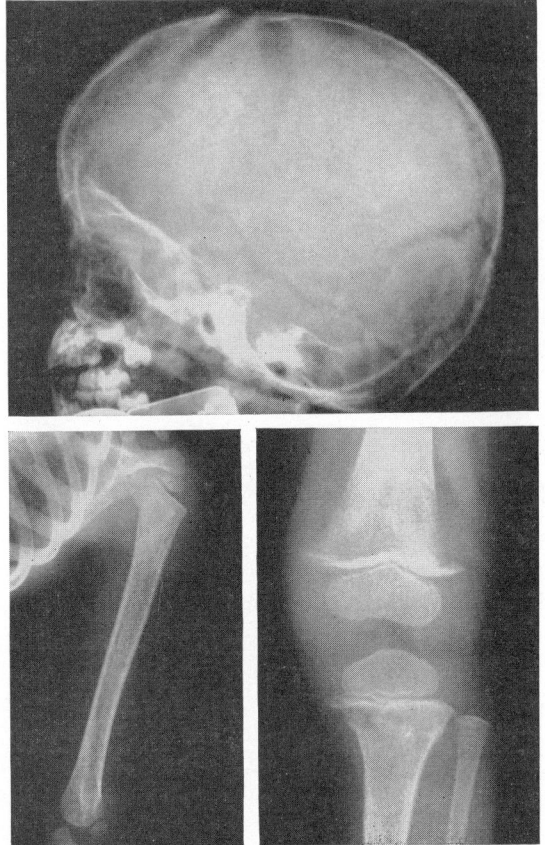

Fig. 337. Roentgenograms from a child with skeletal metastases from abdominal neuroblastoma. *Above,* Mottled appearance of tables of skull, indicating bony metastases. Sutures separated because of metastases in brain. *Below,* Destructive lesions in humerus, femur, tibia, and fibula.

Roentgenologic Examination

In the abdominal growths roentgenograms show an opaque mass which has nothing outstanding whereby the type of tumor can be positively identified. Small deposits of calcium appear in some neuroblastomas, but these are also found in occasional embryomas of the kidney and are especially common in organizing hematomas of the adrenal gland. Pyelograms by intravenous or retrograde routes seldom give important additional information. They may visualize a kidney pelvis which is normal, distorted, or displaced. Generally it is impossible by *plain films* or *pyelograms* to differentite roentgenologically between neuroblastoma, embryoma of the kidney, and "unattached" retroperitoneal teratoma.

While the roentgenographic changes of the primary abdominal lesion are not characteristic, *metastases*, when present, will usually indicate the type of malignancy, particularly if they are found in association with an abdominal mass. The cranial bones (in patients under two years of age) may be separated and the sutures widened, indicating the presence of an expanding intracranial lesion. In early invasion of the marrow cavities, the bones may only appear to be decalcified, and not yet show any punched-out lesions. In more advanced cases the skull, spine, ribs, pelvis, and the long bones of the extremities may be extensively peppered with small destructive lesions which have a moth-eaten appearance. The lesions tend to be symmetrically distributed on the two sides of the skeleton. The distal third of the arms and legs are rarely involved (in contradistinction to leukemic infiltrations). Proliferative bone lesions are sometimes found, and in rare cases the sclerosing appearance in the spine and pelvis is somewhat similar to that seen in Paget's disease. Metastases seldom appear in lungs until very late in the course of the disease.

Neuroblastomas which are primary in the chest give opaque shadows of marked density and clearly defined peripheral borders. They are close to the spine, and appear especially at either apex of the chest. The presence of tumor between ribs generally shows roentgenographic separation of the posterior portion of ribs, with some narrowing and erosion of the same. These thoracic neuroblastomas are more extensively described in Chapter 58.

DIFFERENTIAL DIAGNOSIS

A few of the conditions from which neuroblastoma must be differentiated are:

Embryoma of the Kidney

This occurs in children of about the same age distribution. By palpation it is usually well circumscribed and has a smooth contour which is limited to one side of the abdomen. In contrast, the neuroblastoma has borders which are less well defined, a surface which is apt to be nodular or pebbly, and possibly an extension in front of and beyond the vertebral column. In the majority of cases careful palpation will rather clearly indicate which of the two neoplasms is present, but in some instances it is impossible to make the differential diagnosis by physical examination or indeed by any means other than surgical exploration. X-ray studies of the abdomen give little differential information. If roentgenograms show metastases to lungs, the primary tumor is more apt to be renal embryoma, while the wider distribution of metastases to brain, and particularly the skeleton, is almost diagnostic of neuroblastoma.

Unattached Retroperitoneal Teratoma

This term has been used to designate cystic or solid, mixed growths which arise on either side of the vertebral column anywhere along the posterior abdominal or thoracic wall. They are believed to originate from remnants of the pronephros or mesonephros. They are benign or malignant. They may reach an extremely large size. The description, "unattached," implies that they are not derived from the kidney, even though the histology is often similar to that of a renal embryoma. It is usually difficult to differentiate these retroperitoneal neoplasms from a neuroblastoma except by operation or autopsy. They are quite rare, compared to the relatively common neuroblastomas.

Other Tumors of the Adrenal Gland

1. The *ganglioneuroma* is a benign, slowly growing, encapsulated neurologic tumor which does not metastasize and which does not reduce any endocrinologic dysfunction. It is impossible to differentiate it accurately except by direct pathologic examination.

2. The *chromaffinoma* is a benign (occasionally malignant) tumor[6] producing profound circulatory disturbances because of the release of excessive amounts of epinephrine or nor-epinephrine into the blood stream. Such patients have periods in which the blood pressure is elevated to as much as 200 mm. or more of mercury. The attacks appear at irregular intervals, and as often as several times a day. They are characterized by epigastric distress, excitability, sweating, headache, rapid pulse, and subsequent exhaustion. The individual may die from cardiac failure or a hypertensive vascular accident. The growths usually are circumscribed, can often but not always be felt in the adrenal region, and extirpation of them brings complete relief of symptoms.

3. An *adrenal cortical neoplasm* is a malignant or benign tumor[6] producing structural and functional changes by the formation and liberation of androgenic substances. It can be small and well encapsulated but it is often large, irregular, and fixed to adjacent structures. It gives striking endocrinologic alteration, characterized by a hypermasculinization and enlargement of the penis in the male, masculinization with enlargement of the clitoris in the female, a deepening of the voice in either sex, acne of the skin, enhancement of the somatic growth beyond the expected normal, mild to moderate hypertension, advancement of the bony development (by roentgenologic examination of the wrists and epiphyses), and a greatly increased excretion of androgens in the urine. In most instances death results from local extension or pulmonary metastases. The obvious endocrinologic alterations serve to differentiate sharply the adrenal cortical tumors from the neuroblastomas.

TREATMENT

If there are widespread metastases through the skeleton, probably little can be accomplished other than giving terminal care of the child to make him as comfortable and happy as possible during his declining days; in some cases it may be desirable to perform a biopsy to make sure of the diagnosis, and to bring, if available, some chemotherapeutic attack on the tumor, even though no cures have yet been reported by such methods.

Operation

In those children with no demonstrable metastases operation should be undertaken in all instances, with three things in mind. First, if it is possible to completely remove the mass, this should certainly be done because it gives the highest chance of producing a cure. Second, if the entire mass cannot be excised, as much as feasible should be cut away, reducing the size of the mass which must be treated by x-ray therapy, for this still gives a reasonable chance of cure. Third, if it is utterly impossible to remove any of the mass, at least a biopsy should be taken so that the diagnosis can be established with certainty and the subsequent roentgen therapy can be directed most intelligently.

Operations for removal of a neuroblastoma from the abdomen or chest can be most difficult; it is important to be adequately prepared by inserting a cannula or plastic catheter into a vein prior to operation, so that blood or supportive fluids can be given during operation without delay.

Excision of the Tumor. For attack on an abdominal tumor it is best to employ an anterior transabdominal approach, because only in this way can the operator study the boundaries of the lesion and determine whether or not there are metastases in the liver or other abdominal viscera. Removal of a primary growth should not be started until reasonably thorough inspection and palpation of its posterior and medial attachments have been made. All too frequently one begins dissection, only to find that the entire mass cannot be removed and that tumor tissue must be cut across which sets up bleeding

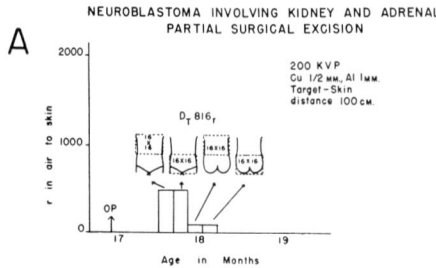

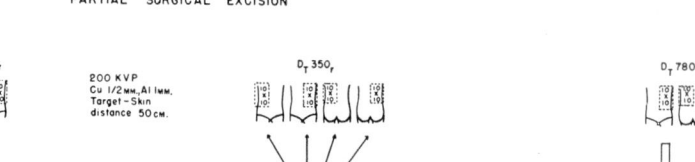

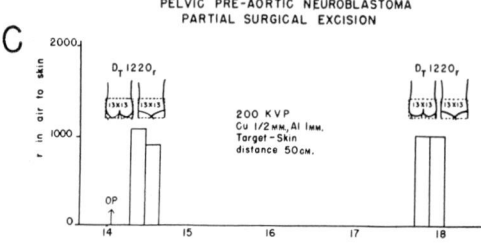

Fig. 338. Examples of postoperative roentgen technique employed for three patients with localized abdominal neuroblastoma when it was impossible to excise the mass completely. In each of the three charts, ordinates represent "r in air to the skin," but on the portal sketches the estimated tumor dose (D_t) is noted. A, Data from Case 11, Table 68. B, Data from Case 13, Table 68. C, Data from Case 18, Table 68. (From Wittenborg: Radiology, vol. 54.)

that is difficult to control. Of course, every effort should be made to remove the lesion, but in some instances a judicious withdrawal from the abdomen is a wiser choice. After evaluating the findings, it often appears that the neoplasm can be totally removed, but subsequent stages of the operation dismally show that tumor tissue has been cut across. While it is most desirable to enucleate a mass without breaking into it, disruption of tumor certainly does not remove all hope for a permanent cure. In many of our patients there was distressing spillage of neoplastic material in the field, but with subsequent x-ray therapy a permanent cure has been obtained.

If a first-rate surgical team is in attendance, and the general condition of the child is reasonably good, there should be no hesitation about embarking on a very radical excision when it is required. Figure 341 is a photograph of a child from whom was removed a large mass which included a tremendous left adrenal neuroblastoma, the engulfed left kidney, the left descending mesocolon, a portion of the descending colon, and a segment of the abdominal aorta. For some weeks we were apprehensive about the pallor of the legs but at no time was there ischemia of serious degree. Postoperative irradiation was given. The boy subsequently has been normally active and at the end of eight years shows no evidence of recurrent neoplasm. The case indicates that extensive and radical surgery has a definite place under certain circumstances and can lead to permanent cure even though there has been invasion of regional organs and tissues.

In one of our patients there were symptoms and signs primarily related to spinal cord compression. Dr. Franc D. Ingraham removed tumor tissue from the spinal canal which had extended in a collar-button fashion from a neuroblastoma of the right adrenal area. At a second operation the abdominal portion of this neoplasm was excised. Fortunately, the histology was one of a neuroblastoma differentiating into ganglioneuroma. Local x-ray therapy was given and apparently a cure has been achieved (Case 8, Table 68). A somewhat similar case has been reported by Cushing and Wolbach.[4]

Roentgen Therapy of Widespread Metastases

Widespread metastases to the skeleton should not be treated by x-ray irradiation. If pain is severe in some particular area, this might possibly be relieved by palliative therapy. There has never been a cure in a patient who has had skeletal metastases, hence it is useless to give intensive therapy with a hope of effecting one. The fact that neuroblastoma is a very radio-sensitive tumor and can be destroyed by x-ray irradiation has led to the thought that irradiation of major portions of the body and extremities might kill off all metastatic tumor cells. Unfortunately, "spray" treatments have serious depressing effects on the bone marrow and can produce an aplastic anemia. Therefore, while widespread metastases in the skeleton can be rather effectively treated by x-rays, the destruction of hematopoietic tissue is of serious and fatal consequence. Likewise, heavy irradiation over *both* the abdomen and the thorax of a baby or child can lead to uncontrollable anemia, as has been found in two of our cases. It is felt that heavy irradiation can be given over *either* the thorax *or* the abdomen in any given case, but that it is extremely dangerous to give it to both of these areas.

Postoperative Roentgen Therapy

For those patients without evidence of skeletal metastases, a neuroblastoma, even though apparently completely excised, should have local postoperative irradiation to kill off any cells or bits of tissue which might have been left unwittingly. A neuroblastoma with extensions or metastases limited to the abdomen, whether these be in lymph nodes, retroperitoneal tissues, or in the liver, should not be regarded as a hopeless situation because x-ray irradiation can still effect a cure in many instances.

In the Children's Medical Center of Boston the x-ray therapy of these tumors has been directed by Dr. George Wyatt and more recently by Dr. Edward B. D. Neuhauser and Dr. Martin H. Wittenborg. Their experiences are admirably summarized in the publication of Dr. Wittenborg,[16] from which all of the following statements have been drawn. The techniques of administration have varied greatly over the years, but some examples of successful forms of therapy are graphically summarized in Figure 338. In these diagrams the abscissas represent time (in months) and the ordinates represent roentgens in air delivered to the skin, each column indicating a separate port as shown by the sketch above it. The width of each column gives the extent of time during which the irradiation lasted. In all cases single daily doses, using one port daily, were given, with alternation of ports daily. Figure 338, A, represents Case 11, Table 68; there was a neuroblastoma of the left adrenal and kidney, surgical excision of 50 per cent of the mass followed by irradiation as summarized; the girl is alive and perfectly well twelve years

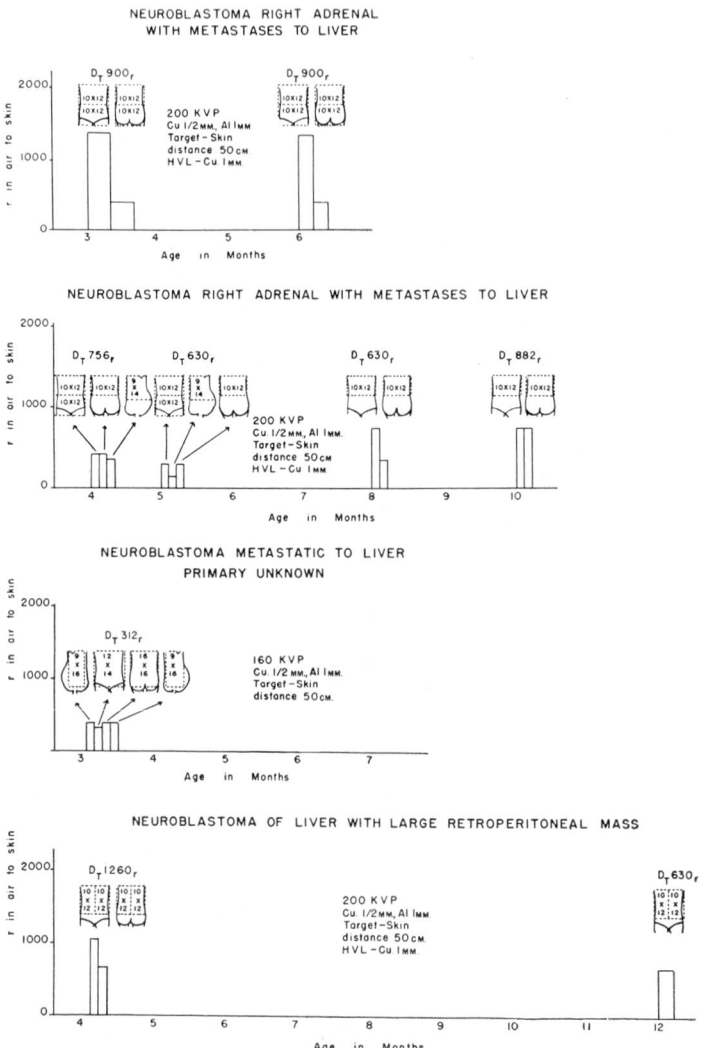

Fig. 339. Examples of roentgen therapy for 4 babies with abdominal neuroblastoma and widespread metastases to the liver (proved by abdominal exploration and biopsy). The patients are all living and well and are apparently cured of their neoplasms. On each chart the ordinates represent "r in air to the skin," but on the portal sketch the estimated tumor dose (D_t) is noted. (From Wittenborg: Radiology, vol. 54.)

later. Figure 338, B, represents Case 13, Table 68; in spite of very radical surgery some tumor was probably left behind; irradiation was given as summarized; the boy is living and well eight years later (Fig. 341). Figure 338, C, represents Case 18, Table 68; a large amount of tumor was known to be left in the pelvis; irradiation was given as indicated; the child is quite well three and a half years later.

Of special interest has been the group of patients with massive metastases to the liver, but with no extension of disease outside the abdomen. We have encountered 7 cases of this sort; there was death in the first a few days after surgical exploration. In the other 6, abdominal exploration and liver biopsy was followed by roentgen irradiation with cure in all instances; these children are alive and in excellent health and with normal-sized livers 14, 13, 7, 5, 5, and $3\frac{1}{2}$ years later (see Figs. 343 and 344). Programs of x-ray therapy in four of these cases are summarized in Figure 339.

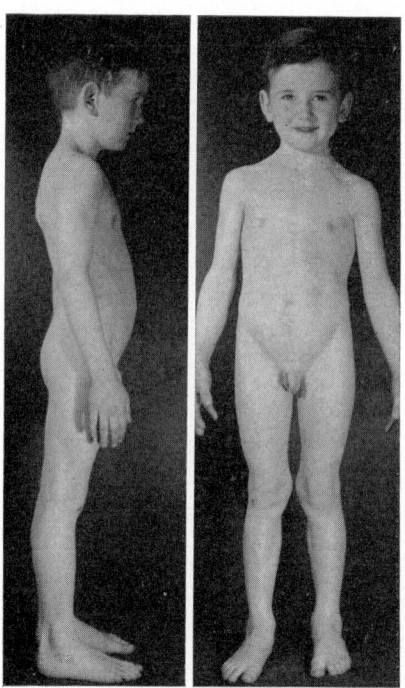

Fig. 340. Case indicating the potentiality of neuroblastoma to disappear spontaneously (which we have witnessed in 3 patients). At six weeks of age abdominal exploration disclosed an extensive and widely attached pelvic tumor which was thought to be inoperable and hopeless; a biopsy proved the diagnosis of neuroblastoma. The above photograph shows the excellent condition of the child at six years, at which time no abdominal mass was palpable. (The boy is in excellent health at nineteen years.)

After reviewing the therapy of patients who failed to recover, as well as all those who are apparently cured, it is felt on the basis of the information available, that one cannot be dogmatic about the technique of x-ray administration or the dosage which is optimum. However, *certain empirical statements may be made:*

1. On the premise that the tumor dose and time factors are the most important elements in the response of an individual tumor, it should be emphasized that complete regression of tumor with cure has been achieved with as small a tumor dose as 400 r in sixteen days. Conversely, viable tumor has been found post mortem at the site of a primary growth following a tumor dose of 600 r in ten days, repeated again one month later (total D_t 1200 r).

2. It should be pointed out that almost all of our patients who survived without complications of treatment received initial tumor doses of 800 to 1200 r in ten to fourteen days, usually followed by a second comparable series in three months.

3. The practice of earlier therapists of initiating treatment with very small doses of 50 to 75 r, with gradual increases, has not been followed in the past ten years. The fear

that larger initial doses might initiate fatal hemorrhage has not proved to be well founded in recent experience.

4. It has been our practice in recent years to give postoperative irradiation as soon after surgery as possible and not wait until the surgical incision is healed. Patients are taken directly from the operating room to the x-ray therapy department and *treatment is begun on the day of operation.* An initial dose (200 r in air delivered to the skin) is usually given through a port opposite the surgical incision (which is the exit port).

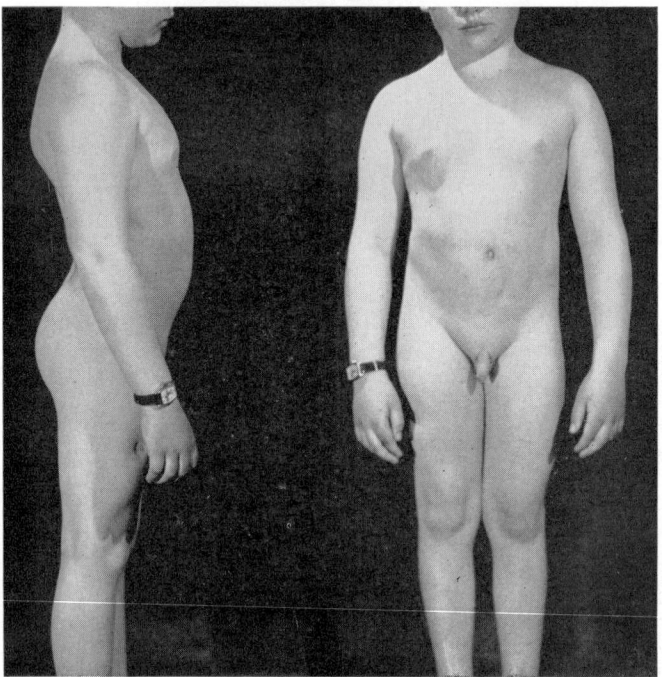

Fig. 341. Child, following extensive surgery and subsequent x-ray therapy for neuroblastoma. At fourteen months, operation disclosed a large tumor originating in and spreading from the left adrenal. To cleanly remove all visible tumor it was necessary to excise the neoplasm along with the left adrenal, the left kidney, a segment of the descending colon, and a portion of the abdominal aorta (operation by Dr. William E. Ladd). This photograph is taken eight years later; the boy has no evidence of recurrence.

Dosages of this magnitude are repeated daily until the incision is healed; thereafter the ports are alternated. It is believed that if wounds are carefully closed in layers and no adhesive tape is applied, there need be no fear of wound complications from postoperative irradiation with air doses to the skin of 1400 to 1800 r in seven to ten days. *Complete absence of wound complications in our series confirms this statement.*

5. The limiting dosage factor in the treatment of infants and small children is not the skin, but the destruction of hematopoietic tissue. Postmortem examination of vertebrae which were within the direct field of therapy showed evidence of bone marrow depression, at times amounting to complete hematopoietic suppression and to fibrous replacement of marrow. This was true for calculated tumor dosages of as little as 600 r in ten days, repeated twice, one month apart. Marrow specimens distant from the field of irradiation showed evidence of hyperplasia, presumably compensatory. It is axiomatic that the total amount of hematopoietic tissue irradiated and the dosage to which it is subjected are the decisive factors in determining the recovery of the infant or small child

from radiation effects. Two patients in our series died with clinical pancytopenia and extensive bone marrow suppression, confirmed at autopsy. Both had received roentgen therapy to the chest and abdomen and thus had the major portion of their hematopoietic tissue exposed to deep irradiation. *Conversely*, in the group of patients who survived, none had received irradiation to *both* chest and abdomen. Although statistically we are dealing with small groups, the experience would seem to indicate that deep x-ray therapy directed to the mediastinum and abdomen in tissue dosages above 600 r, if justifiable at all, should be undertaken with considerable reservation.

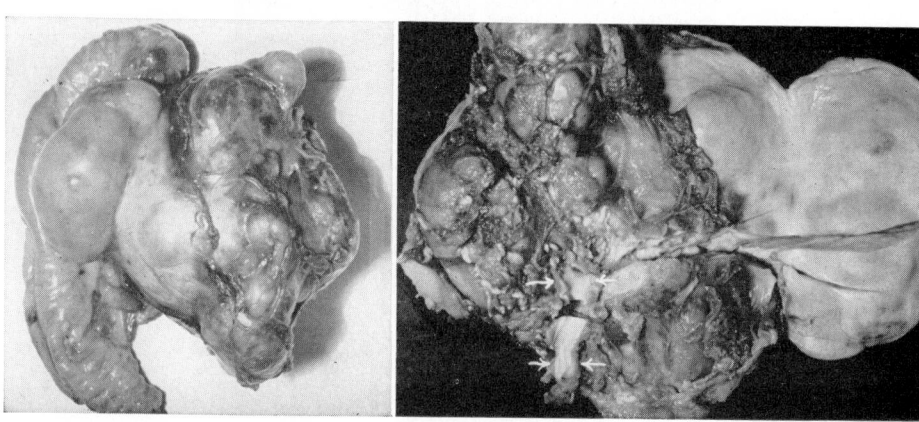

Fig. 342. Specimen removed from the child shown in Figure 341. *Left*, The view shows neoplastic mass, kidney, and segment of colon. *Right*, A view of the posterior aspect of the specimen, showing segment of aorta (arrows) which was removed.

6. Preoperative x-ray therapy has not been used in the patients of this series. Reduction in the size of a mass has not been considered a valid indication for such therapy because the size of a tumor has not proved to be a limiting factor in the surgical attack. The argument that reduction of incidence of metastases might be achieved by preoperative x-ray therapy is still a theoretical one to be evaluated in the light of necessary delay of operation and the hyperemia produced by the irradiation. Our material sheds no light on this problem.

7. Growth disturbances in the spine, though observed, have not proved to be a decisive factor in selecting x-ray therapy. One child who had abdominal and intraspinal tumor, with a two-stage transabdominal and intraspinal removal of this, followed by x-ray therapy, has a considerable scoliosis. Eradication of the tumor has left a moderate deformity which may have resulted from neoplastic destruction of bone, surgical trauma, or irradiation effects—or a combination of all of these. Scoliosis and kyphosis have not been observed as complications in any case in which x-ray therapy was given for tumor which was limited to the abdomen.

RESULTS OF TREATMENT

In the majority of children with untreated neuroblastoma, metastases develop and there is a rapid downhill course leading to death within a few months. It is not possible to set a definite time limit, beyond which a surviving patient can be said to be cured. However, the extremely rapid proliferation of this neoplasm has made us feel that an individual who is well for a year after treatment and has no recurrence by physical examination or x-ray study can probably be regarded as a permanent cure; it is very rare for recurrence or metastases to appear at a later date.

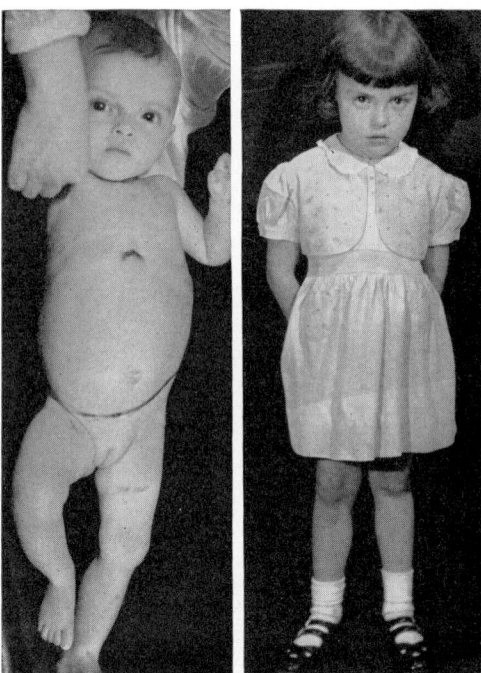

Fig. 343. Photographs of child with abdominal neuroblastoma and massive metastases to liver treated by x-ray irradiation. *Left*, Preoperative picture at six months; the lower edge of the huge liver is outlined by pencil. (Abdominal exploration for diagnostic purposes and biopsy of liver metastases.) *Right*, Picture five years later showing excellent general health. (The liver edge has receded to the costal margin.)

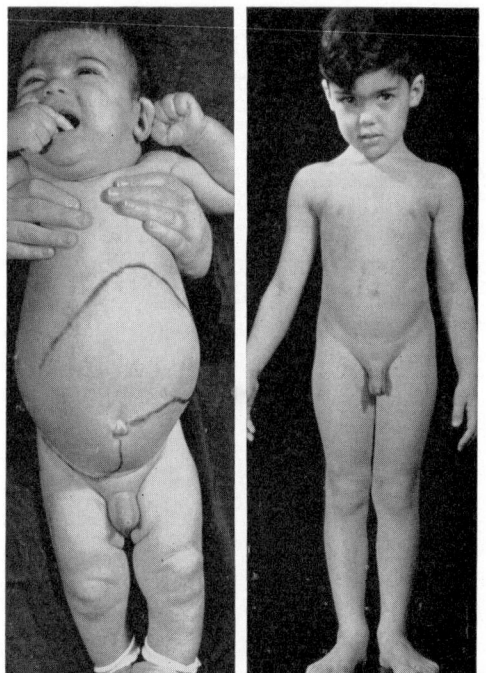

Fig. 344. Photographs of boy with right adrenal neuroblastoma, massive metastases to the liver, and therapy by x-ray irradiation. *Left*, Picture at four months, just before abdominal exploration. Diagnosis proved by biopsy of one of the hepatic metastases. Outline of the enormous liver shown by pencil marks. *Right*, Excellent status seven years later. (The liver is barely palpable.)

Table 68
List of Favorable Cases of Neuroblastoma

Case	Year	Age and Sex	Pathology	Treatment	Follow-up
1	1921	10 yrs. F	Spread through posterior abdomen	Biopsy only!	Died 3½ yrs. later.
2	1932	6 wks. M	Large pelvic tumor. Thought hopeless at exploration	Biopsy only!	Perfectly well 19 yrs. later.
3	1933	4 days F	Encapsulated mass in left flank, extra-adrenal	Clean removal.	Perfectly well 16 yrs. later.
4	1935	6 mos. M	Cervical neuroblastoma	Partial removal plus x-ray.	Perfectly well 14 yrs. later.
5	1935	5 yrs. F	Left adrenal and peri-adrenal mass	Removal and nephrectomy. X-ray.	Perfectly well 15 yrs. later.
6	1935	2 yrs. F	In right adrenal (differentiating into ganglioneuroma)	Removal.	Perfectly well 15 yrs. later.
7	1936	11 mos. F	Origin in thorax. Thought to be hopeless at exploration.	Biopsy only!	Completely well and no tumor in chest by x-ray 10 yrs. later.
8	1937	2 yrs. F	Right retroperitoneal mass and extension into spinal canal	Laminectomy and laparotomy, each with partial excision of tumor. X-ray.	No evidence of neoplasm 8 yrs. later. Some scoliosis.
9	1937	11 days F	Origin in right adrenal. Widespread metastases to liver.	Removal of right adrenal mass. Biopsy of liver tumor. X-ray.	Perfectly well 12 yrs. later.
10	1938	3 mos. F	Abdominal origin, and extensive metastases to liver.	Biopsy. X-ray.	Perfectly well 13 yrs. later.
11	1939	17 mos. F	Left adrenal mass	Partial removal and nephrectomy. X-ray.	Perfectly well 12 yrs. later.
12	1941	4 yrs. F	Left lumbar mass	Clean removal.	Completely well 8 yrs. later.
13	1944	14 mos. M	Left adrenal. Involving kidney, base of mesocolon and abdominal aorta.	Removal of mass, kidney, portion of colon and part of aorta. X-ray.	Perfectly well 7 yrs. later.
14	1944	4 mos. M	Right adrenal tumor with metastases to liver.	Liver tumor biopsy. X-ray.	Completely well 7 yrs. later.
15	1945	3 mos. M	? origin. Liver full of metastases.	Biopsy of liver tumor. X-ray.	Perfectly well 5 yrs. later.
16	1945	21 mos. F	Origin in organ of Zuckerkandl	Completely enucleated.	Perfectly well 4 yrs. later.
17	1946	6 mos. F	Massive metastases to liver	Biopsy. X-ray.	Completely well 5 yrs. later.
18	1947	14 mos. M	Large intra-pelvic mass	Partial excision. X-ray. Nitrogen mustard.	Alive and well 3½ yrs. later.
19	1947	4 mos. F	Retroperitoneal tumor with widespread liver metastases	Biopsy. X-ray.	Perfectly well 3½ yrs. later.
20	1947	7 mos. M	Left adrenal tumor	Excision. X-ray.	Completely well 3 yrs. later.
21	1947	15 yrs. F	Large retroperitoneal tumor. Differentiating into ganglioneuroma.	Excision of about 75% of mass. X-ray.	Entirely well 3 yrs. later.
22	1947	14 mos. M	Left adrenal tumor	Excision. X-ray.	Completely well 3 yrs. later.

Table 69

Results in Treatment of Neuroblastomas

Up through 1940	57 Cases 11 Surviving more than 3 years without recurrence 19% Cures
From 1940 through 1947	38 Cases 11 Surviving more than 3 years without recurrence 29% Cures

When evaluating the final results in a series of patients with neuroblastoma, one cannot conclusively attribute a success in any instance to surgery alone, to x-ray irradiation alone, or even to a combination of these therapeutic procedures. It is known that a neuroblastoma can undergo spontaneous hemorrhage and necrosis and completely disappear without any treatment whatever. We have seen three examples of this (Fig. 340).

In rare cases a neuroblastoma sympatheticum develops into a more slowly growing lesion, the ganglioneuroma. The rapidly growing neuroblastoma part may burn itself out or may be destroyed by x-ray irradiation and leave the benign ganglioneuroma portion which can be subsequently excised. This happy sequence of events was observed by Cushing and Wolbach[4] and it occurred in several of our patients.

In the handling of neuroblastoma cases in which there are no skeletal metastases, it has been our general policy to proceed with operation, to remove the mass in its entirety if possible, but failing this, to remove as much of the tumor as feasible, following in either instance by x-ray irradiation. When the mass is obviously inoperable, at least a biopsy is obtained, and x-ray irradiation instituted. Therapy failures are numerous and are disappointing, death usually coming within a year. In spite of these discouragements, the fact remains that considerable salvage can be obtained. Table 68 lists all of our patients who have been apparently cured for three or more years. These favorable results emphasize that this highly malignant neoplasm can be brought under control in an appreciable number of instances. Of these 22 patients, 3 had biopsy but no therapy (a spontaneous disappearance of neoplasm), 5 had only surgical excision, 8 had surgical excision (complete or incomplete) plus x-ray irradiation, and 6 had biopsy and only x-ray therapy.

A breakdown of our material into two groups (Table 69), one before 1940 and the other into a more recent period, 1940 through 1947, shows an encouraging rise in the

Table 70

Age of Patient in Relation to Prognosis
(1940 through 1947)

Under 2 years of age	20 Cases 9 Survivors 45% Cures
Over 24 months of age	18 Cases 2 Survivors 11% Cures

three-year cures from 19 per cent to 29 per cent, an increase which is attributed to improved operative techniques and more intensive use of x-ray irradiation.

An analysis of material according to age of the patients shows an important difference in prognosis, a vague dividing line occurring at about two years (Table 70), While those children above twenty-four months of age had but 11 per cent cures, the subjects under twenty-four months of age had a cure rate of 45 per cent.

REFERENCES

1. Bielschowsky, M.: Neuroblastic Tumors of Sympathetic Nervous System. In Cytology and Cellular Pathology of the Nervous System, Wilder Penfield. New York: Hoeber, 1932, page 1085.
2. Blacklock, J. W. S.: Neurogenic Tumors of the Sympathetic System in Children. J. Path. & Bact., 39:27, 1934.
3. Chandler, F. A. and Norcross, J. R.: Sympathicoblastoma. J.A.M.A., 114:112, 1940.
4. Cushing, H. and Wolbach, S. B.: The Transformation of a Malignant Paravertebral Sympathicoblastoma into a Benign Ganglioneuroma. Am. J. Path., 3:203, 1927.
5. Farber, S.: Neuroblastoma. Abstract in Am. J. Dis. Child., 60:749, 1940.
6. Gross, R. E.: Neoplasms Producing Endocrine Disturbances in Childhood. Am. J. Dis. Child., 59:579, 1940.
7. Hartung, A. and Rubert, S. R.: Roentgen Aspects of Sympathetic Neuroblastoma. Radiology, 24:607, 1935.
8. Hauser, H.: Radiosensitive Neuroblastoma. Am. J. Roentgenol., 31:234, 1934.
9. Holmes, G. and Dresser, R.: Roentgenologic Observations in Neuroblastoma. J.A.M.A., 91:1246, 1928.
10. Lehman, E. P.: Adrenal Neuroblastoma in Infancy—15 Year Survival. Ann. Surg., 95: 473, 1932.
11. Redman, J. L., Agerty, H. A., Barthmaier, O. F. and Fisher, H. R.: Adrenal Neuroblastoma—Report of a Case and Review of the Literature. Am. J. Dis. Child., 56:1097, 1938.
12. Rypins, E. L.: The Roentgen Diagnosis of Neuroblastoma in Children. Am. J. Roentgenol., 37:325, 1937.
13. Schrager, V. L.: Surgical Aspects of Neurogenic Tumors of the Abdomen. Surg., Gynec. & Obst., 68:1085, 1939.
14. Tileston, W. and Wolbach, S. B.: Primary Tumors of the Adrenal Gland in Children. Am. J. M. Sc., 135:871, 1908.
15. Wahl, H. R. and Craig, P. E.: Multiple Tumors of the Sympathetic Nervous System; Report of a Case Showing a Distinct Ganglioneuroma, Neuroblastoma, and a Cystic Calcifying Ganglioneuroblastoma. Am. J. Path., 14:797, 1938.
16. Wittenborg, M. H.: Roentgen Therapy in Neuroblastoma. Radiology, 54:679, 1950.
17. Wyatt, G. M. and Farber, S.: Neuroblastoma Sympatheticum. Roentgenological Appearances and Radiation Treatment. Am. J. Roentgen., 46:485, 1941.
18. Zuelzer, W. W., Palmer, H. D. and Newton, W. A., Jr.: Unusual Glomerulonephritis in Young Children, Probably Radiation Nephritis. Am. J. Path., 26:1019, 1950.

CHAPTER 47

Retroperitoneal Teratoma

Tumors of the retroperitoneal area constitute a most important group of neoplasms in infancy and childhood. The two most common ones in this region are embryoma of the kidney (Wilms' tumor) and neuroblastoma sympatheticum; teratomas are third, and are much less frequently encountered.

Several excellent papers on the subject of retroperitoneal teratomas have been published. Hansmann and Budd[6] drew attention to them in 1932, with an excellent description of "massive unattached retroperitoneal tumors." By "unattached" they meant that the growths did not arise from the kidney or the adrenal gland. According to Palumbo and his associates,[9] there were 58 "bona fide" cases (listed in a table) of primary retroperitoneal teratomas reported in the literature up to the time of their publication in 1949; cases in children and adults were studied. Arnheim[1] has made a very informative summary of the subject as it refers to infancy and childhood; he lists data from 39 patients. The following section has largely been gleaned from Arnheim's paper, supplemented by experiences from cases which have been observed at the Children's Hospital in Boston.

PATHOLOGIC FEATURES

In the development of the human there can be a division and segregation of tissue or a group of cells at any time, particularly during the very early period of embryonic life. The splitting-off of substance in the blastula stage, in such a way that the separated tissue stays incorporated within the host, gives rise to an included twin which can attain an extraordinary degree of development, leading to a *fetus in fetu*. If the tissue becomes segregated at a somewhat later time, cells are involved which still have totipotent potentialities and can give rise to structures representing all three germ layers, so-called teratomas. In the latter, the derivatives of the ectoderm, mesoderm, and endoderm may appear in rather undifferentiated form (so-called teratoid growths) or they may progress to well differentiated organs which can be recognized grossly or microscopically. Thus, there can appear within a child a wide range of secondary subordinate growths which vary from a well formed fetus to solid teratomas or even cystic structures. On the whole, retroperitoneal teratomas are highly differentiated, but a minority have definitely taken on malignant characteristics. While it is best to group together all cysts and teratomas arising behind the peritoneum, and to consider that they might have an origin from totipotent cells very early in embryonic life, there are some of these growths which probably have had an origin from the urogenital ridge, the mesonephros, or from the degenerating Wolffian and Müllerian systems.

Teratomas can appear in many parts of the body. They are most common in the sacrococcygeal area; they are next most frequently seen in the paravertebral gutter, behind the posterior peritoneum. Almost all teratomas are tridermal, for they frequently contain skin, teeth, or nerve tissue (ectoderm), respiratory or alimentary epithelia (endoderm), and connective and vascular tissue (mesoderm). The most benign teratomas consist entirely of mature substance, with no signs of proliferative activity; the malignant ones contain abundant, wildly growing neoplasm which may represent all or only a segment of the specimen. Teratomas may be predominantly cystic or entirely solid; usually both types are intermixed. Cysts are usually multiple and may contain either clear fluid or sebaceous material.

Retroperitoneal tumors generally arise rather high in the abdomen, close to the pancreas and kidneys. They may lie entirely to one side of the midline, though many specimens bulge far beyond the spinal column. The tumors are somewhat more common on the left than on the right side. As a rule, they have a fairly well defined capsule, or at least they can be dissected away easily from surrounding normal structures. Their blood supply is usually from vessels of small size.

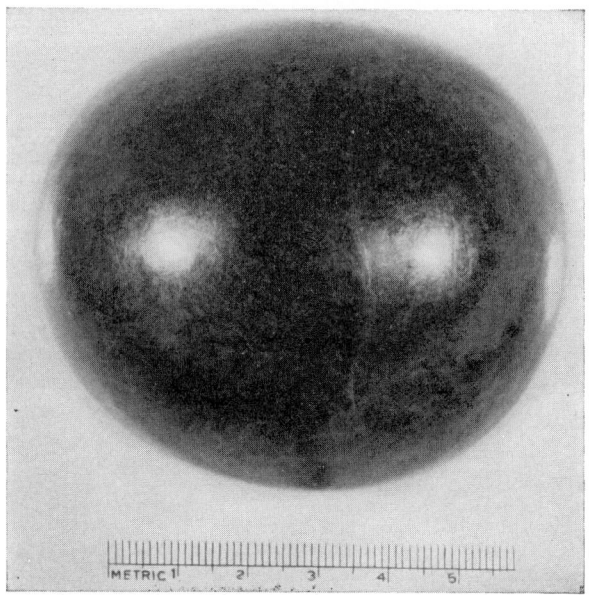

Fig. 345. Case 4, Table 71. Retroperitoneal cyst 7.5 cm. in diameter, removed from a five-month-old child.

CLINICAL FINDINGS

Retroperitoneal teratomas are predominantly lesions of young individuals. They are particularly apt to be detected within the first few months of life. Slightly more than half of them have appeared within the first year; about two-thirds have appeared in the first two years. The few remaining ones are scattered through childhood. Females are somewhat more affected than males.

The presenting complaints are usually related to a rather silent and progressive swelling on one side of the abdomen. Palpation reveals a mass of variable size, frequently distending a small abdomen. The masses are usually rather firm, with fairly defined borders (though on the right side they might merge with the liver), and they tend to be slightly lobulated or irregular. Dilated veins are frequently seen over the abdominal wall.

Late in some cases, fever, vomiting, loss of weight, anorexia, and constipation are occasionally noticed. Although the mass usually lies against the kidney or ureter and may produce dislocation, distortion, or moderate obstruction of these, urinary symptoms are rarely seen.

Roentgenographic examination shows a shadow, generally in one side of the abdomen, but sometimes having a more central position, with air-filled loops of bowel pushed away from this region. A very high proportion of cases show some irregular calcification within the tumor. This may be spotty and not suggestive of any well developed bones or teeth, but in many patients there is more mature osseous formation or a considerable portion of a fetal skeleton. By intravenous pyelography, the kidney on the ipsilateral side is generally displaced, possibly somewhat compressed, and at times shows evidence of mild hydronephrosis because of ureteral blockage. One does not see the extensive distortion of the renal pelvis which is so commonly found with Wilms' tumors. Visualization of the gastro-intestinal tract can show great distortion and displacement of the stomach or other hollow viscera, depending upon the position of the new growth and which viscera are pushed away.

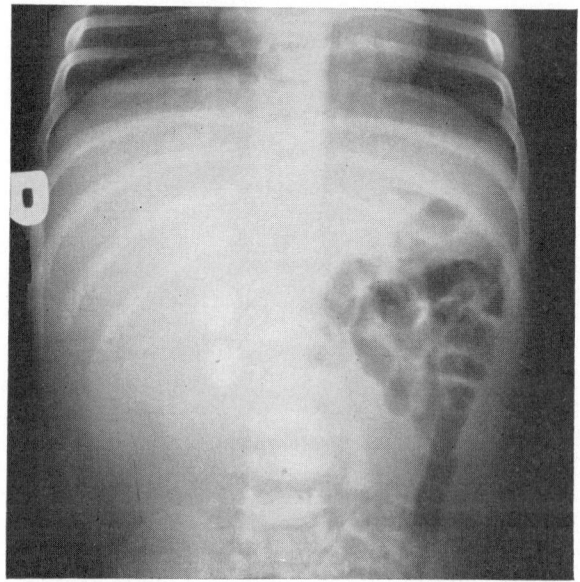

Fig. 346. Case 7, Table 71. Retroperitoneal teratoma. Roentgenogram showing blunting of right renal pelvis. Opacity of the neoplasm below right kidney.

DIFFERENTIAL DIAGNOSIS

A mass in the posterior portion of the abdomen, particularly lying toward one side and rather high, suggests a neuroblastoma sympatheticum, embryoma of the kidney, or retroperitoneal teratoma. Often, it is impossible to tell before operation which of these neoplasms exists but in many instances there are certain features which will point to the correct diagnosis before surgical exploration.

First of all, on a statistical basis, neuroblastomas and Wilms' tumors are much more common than are retroperitoneal teratomas.

On the basis of age, neuroblastoma and embryoma of the kidney are more apt to be encountered towards the end of the first year or beyond this, with a peak of incidence somewhere between the second and fourth years; retroperitoneal teratomas are most common in the first year, particularly in the early months of life.

A neuroblastoma generally has finely nodular surfaces and poorly defined borders, findings which are less frequent with the teratomas.

Plain x-ray films of the abdomen rarely show ossification in Wilms' tumors. Calci-

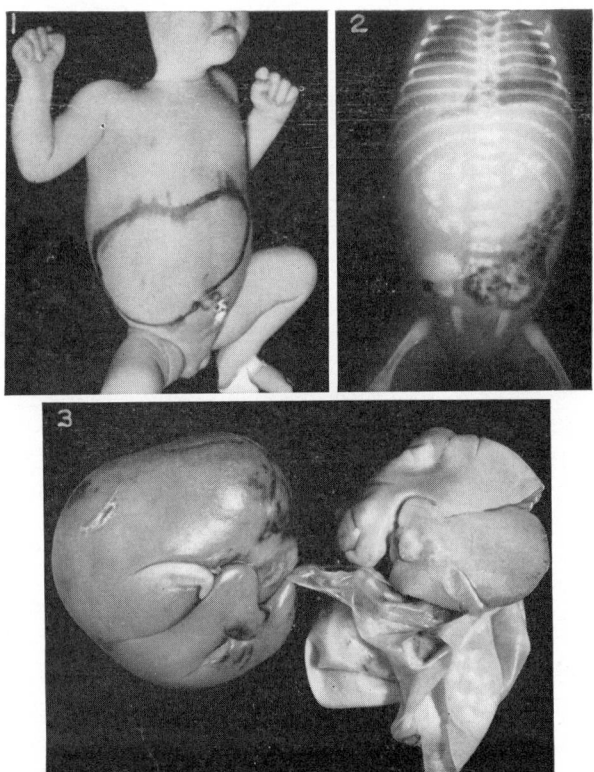

Fig. 347. Case 8, Table 71. Two-day-old baby with twin fetuses in fetu. 1. Photograph, showing the intra-abdominal mass outlined by pencil. 2. Roentgenograms, showing calcification in various parts of the mass. (Well defined long bones, skull, and spinal structures could be identified on the original film.) 3. Photograph of the surgical specimen. The structure had been surrounded by a tough and unbroken membrane, here opened and turned down to the right. On the left is a well formed fetus, with its flexed head and limbs. At the upper right is a less perfectly formed fetus, with its head and a limb-bud.

fication can be found in both teratomas and neuroblastomas, but certainly any structure with a conformation of tooth or bone will rule out a neuroblastoma and will make a positive diagnosis of teratoma (among which *fetus in fetu* is classified). By retrograde pyelography or excretory visualization of the urinary tract, great distortions of the renal pelvis and calyces are more suggestive of a Wilms' tumor. Should any metastases be found in other parts of the body, multiple destructive lesions in the skull and long bones are quite characteristic of a neuroblastoma, whereas metastases limited largely to the lungs are more suggestive of an embryoma of the kidney.

TREATMENT

The treatment of retroperitoneal teratomas is surgical removal, in spite of the huge size which some of them attain. The incision should always be a transperitoneal approach. It is far better to make the wound in a transverse manner, because the size and the extent of many of these lesions require an incision running from the flank well around the anterior abdominal wall, sometimes extending over beyond the midline. Maximum freedom in the operative field is an extremely important consideration; the operator must have liberal exposure for excising a neoplasm which has attachments to the kidney, the duodenum, the aorta, the vena cava, the pancreas, et cetera. It might appear that the growth is extensively fixed to one of these structures, but pathologic and surgical observations have generally shown that it is possible to peel away the mass from the normal vessels or organs in the vast majority of cases. Obviously, the magnitude of these operations implies that a cannula (or plastic tubing) must be placed in an ankle vein prior to operation so that blood can be administered for support during the laparotomy.

Our difficulties with these growths at the operating table have been great, but to date our experiences make it fully evident that the outlook is almost hopeless if radical attack is not performed; conversely, heroic surgery can generally be followed by survival of the child and a cure thereafter. Hence, every effort should be made to persist and remove the growth in its entirety. In one of these children (Case 9, Table 71), an exploration of the baby allowed only partial mobilization of the mass, which seemed to have such wide and dense anchorage along the vertebral column that its removal appeared impossible. Particularly distressing was the fact that the vena cava had been stretched out as a ribbon-like structure over the anterior bulge of the mass, with distortion and dislocation of the renal veins upward and to the left, making it difficult to identify them with certainty; operation was abandoned. A second attempt was made six weeks later and at this time a very lengthy wound was employed, running from the right flank across the right upper quadrant of the abdomen and extending far over through the left upper quadrant. Through this great aperture, better visualization allowed us to see the entry of both renal veins into the vena cava. To inspect these areas, the base of the mesentery had to be dissected away from the mass and pushed to the left. The growth so involved the right kidney (by compression) that the kidney had to be removed along with the tumor. The vena cava was so attenuated over the neoplasm that it was not possible to dissect it free and save it; the vessel was transected just above the junction of

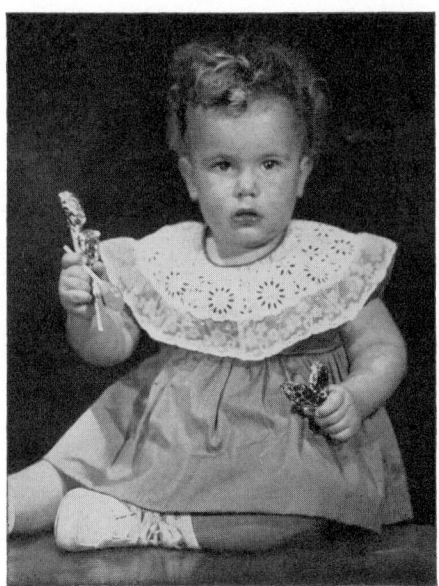

Fig. 348. Case 9, Table 71. Photograph of patient one year after removal of a solid, very large retroperitoneal teratoma, which contained malignant elements. The child is in excellent health three years after operation.

the common iliac veins and also at a point just below the entry of the left renal vein, and was removed along with the tumor to which it was adherent. It was finally possible to sweep around the entire mass and lift it out cleanly. This most extensive dissection was quite worth-while because, in spite of the fact that the teratoma had some malignant components, the child is alive and is in excellent health three years later without evidence of recurrence (Fig. 348).

In another patient (Case 8, Table 71), the teratomatous development took the form of twin fetuses, one of which was quite well developed and the second one imperfectly so (Fig. 347). Both of them were encased in a thick common membrane, which had broad attachments to the base of the mesentery and anterior aspect of the pancreas, deriving most of the blood supply from the superior mesenteric vessels. It was possible to cleanly remove the sac with the enclosed "twins."

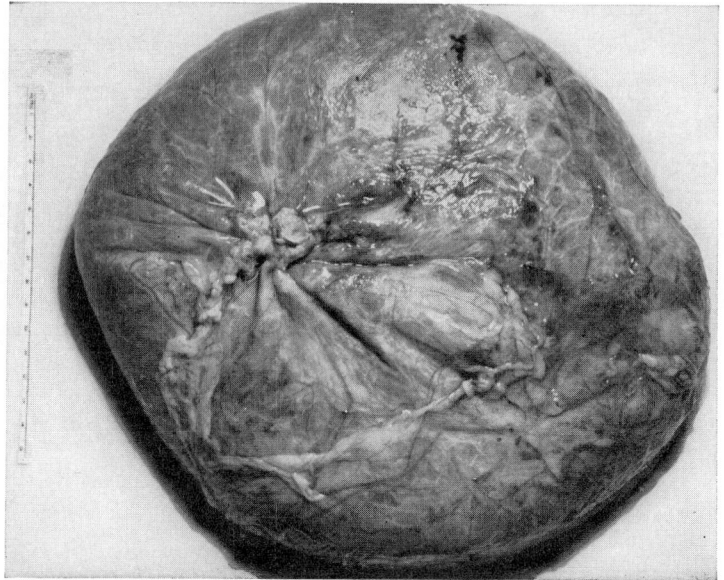

Fig. 349. Case 10, Table 71. Huge retroperitoneal cyst, weighing 3845 gm., removed from a ten-year-old girl. Several tiny cysts were found surrounding this.

In Case 11, Table 71, there was an upper abdominal mass (Fig. 350) presenting more towards the right than to the left, with rather well-demarcated borders which lay behind the gastro-colic omentum, the division of which clearly disclosed the underlying teratoma. Around its anterior two-thirds it could be easily separated from the surrounding structures; posteriorly it was broadly attached over the head of the pancreas from which it had to be cut away by sharp dissection. The teratoma was completely removed. Postoperatively, there was leakage of pancreatic fluid into the general peritoneal cavity, producing a marked distention of the abdomen with murky pancreatic fluid and giving extensive fat necroses over the visceral and parietal peritoneal surfaces; a month later a secondary operation was required for removal of this fluid and for the placement of a drain down to the site of leakage. The pancreatic fistula closed off spontaneously during the ensuing weeks. The child has had excellent recovery thereafter.

In Case 7, Table 71, a three-month-old baby was found to have a functioning kidney only on the right side and a retroperitoneal teratoma below this kidney, the mass being hemorrhagic and largely cystic. At exploration all fluid and blood clot were evacuated;

biopsy of the remaining shaggy wall showed malignant growth. Because of the obliteration of tissue planes and structures by the hemorrhagic changes, no attempt was made
to identify and dissect any remaining tumor, most of which seemed to be impossible to
remove. The child was given x-ray irradiation through an anterior and a posterior port
(total 1800 r), which was purposely given in only moderate intensity because of the
possible damage to the sole kidney. Seven years later the child has no demonstrable
evidence of neoplasm.

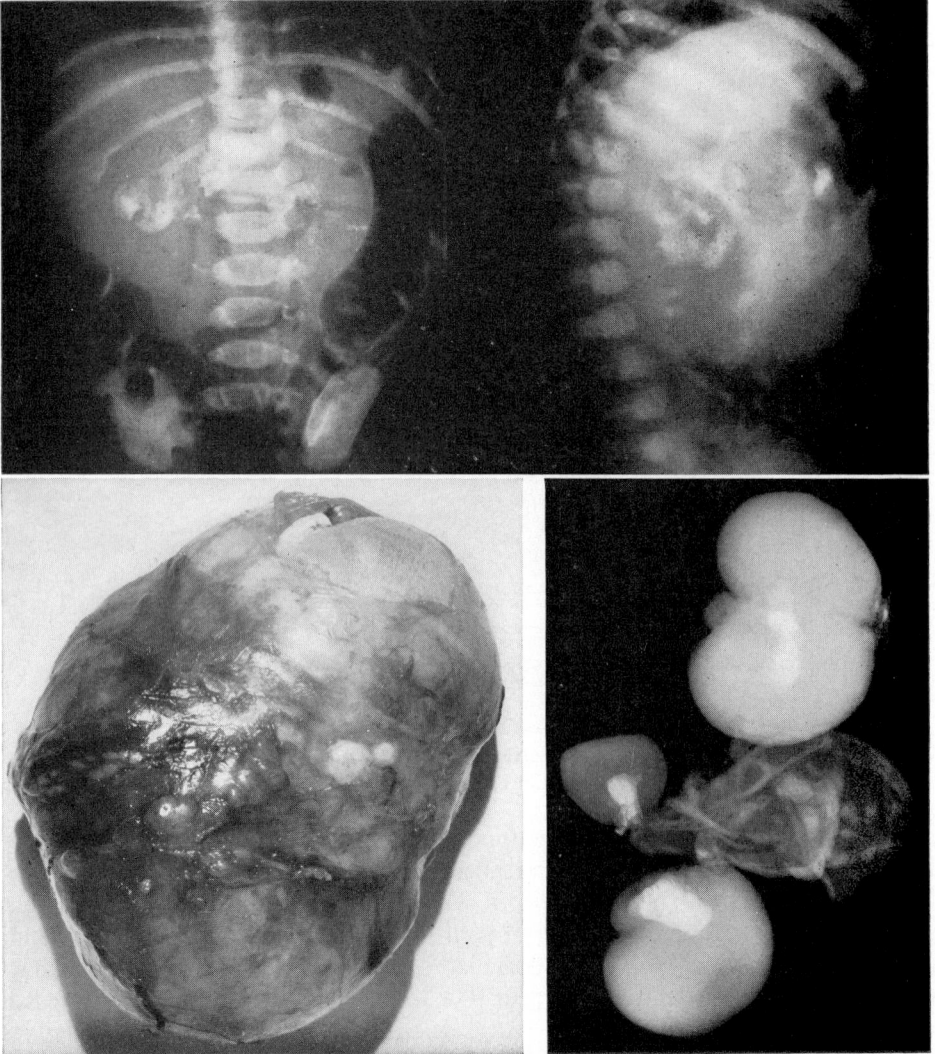

Fig. 350. Case 11, Table 71. Teratoma in a baby. *Above,* X-rays of abdomen showing calcification in
the mass. *Below,* Photograph of surgical specimen, and roentgenogram of the specimen.

RESULTS OF THERAPY

Arnheim has stressed the necessity for removal of these tumors, because in the
reported cases all untreated patients have died. Surgical mortality rates have been high
(29 per cent in those studied), the causes of death being largely attributable to hemorrhage and shock. In the past two decades operative recoveries have increased, particu-

larly because of the benefits of intravenous infusion of glucose or blood during and after the surgical procedures.

From Arnheim's study, of the 19 children discharged from the hospital after removal of a benign retroperitoneal teratoma, 4 had no follow-up observations, 2 died within the first year after operation; 3 were well under one year, 6 from one to two years, and 1 each at two, four, five, and eight years respectively after operation. Three children with malignant retroperitoneal teratomas survived operation, but 2 died of recurrences and metastases later; follow-up data were not available for the remaining case.

In the Children's Hospital material there have been 11 patients with retroperitoneal cysts or teratomas, concerning whom various data are listed in Table 71. Three of the lesions were cysts, removal of which has been followed by cure. Two of the tumors were only biopsied, x-ray therapy being given subsequently; one of these children is known

Table 71

Retroperitoneal Cysts and Teratomas

Case	Age Sex	Year	Tumor	Treatment	Result
1	6 mos. F	1929	Right huge retroperitoneal myxomatous cyst, 840 gm.	Removal	Well 6 years later
2	6 yrs. F	1930	Left. Huge. Inoperable. Malignant.	Biopsy only	Died 2 mos. later
3	18 mos. M	1934	Left, extending up into thorax. Metastases. Papillary adenocarcinoma.	Biopsy	Died
4	5 mos. F	1935	Right. Cyst 7.5 cm. diameter.	Excision	Cured
5	6 mos. M	1938	Left. Huge. Inoperable. Malignant.	Biopsy	Died
6	8 mos. M	1944	Left. Large. Inoperable. Malignant epithelial tumor.	Biopsy. Irradiation (1600 r)	Died
7	3 mos. M	1945	Below right kidney. Cystic and hemorrhagic degeneration. By biopsy a malignant, rapidly growing tumor, probably largely fibrous tissue elements.	Evacuation of clot. Biopsy. X-ray therapy (1800 r)	Well 7 years later
8	2 days F	1947	Twin fetuses in fetu in upper abdomen.	Complete excision	Well 5 years later
9	5 mos. F	1949	Distended entire right side of abdomen. 335 gm. 8 x 12.5 x 5 cm. Contained some malignant neural components.	Complete excision	Well 3 years later
10	10 yrs. F	1950	Left. Several small cysts and one huge one 24 cm. in diameter weighing 3845 gm.	Excision	Cured
11	5 mos. M	1952	Larger than a fist. Lay in front of head of pancreas. Largely dermoid.	Complete excision	Well 8 mos. later.

to be alive and well seven years later, the other died of extending neoplasm. All 3 of those who had biopsy (no x-ray therapy) are known to have died. The 3 teratomas which were removed (2 of them were found to contain malignant tissue) have apparently been followed by cure.

REFERENCES

1. Arnheim, E. E.: Retroperitoneal Teratomas in Infancy and Childhood. Pediatrics, *8:* 309, 1951.
2. Baker, W. J. and Ragins, A. B.: Pararenal Teratoma. Case Report. J. Urol., *63:*982, 1950.
3. Cohen, H. J., Marcus, M. and Sherwin, B.: Retroperitoneal Teratoma in Infancy. Am. J. Dis. Child., *80:*75, 1950.
4. Cole, J. W. and Gerrish, E. W.: Removal of a Primary Lateral Retroperitoneal Teratoma with Survival in a Fifteen-Hour-Old Infant. Surgery, *30:*371, 1951.
5. Gross, R. E. and Clatworthy, H. W.: Twin Fetuses in Fetu. J. Ped., *38:*502, 1951.
6. Hansmann, G. H. and Budd, J. W.: Massive Unattached Retroperitoneal Tumors. J.A. M.A., *98:*6, 1932.
7. Langley, G. F.: Pararenal Teratoma. Brit. J. Urol., *22:*217, 1950.
8. Large, H. L., Jr., Williams, M. and Neel, J. B.: Gastric Tridermal Teratoma in Infancy. J.A.M.A., *149:*824, 1952.
9. Palumbo, L. T., Cross, K. R., Smith, A. N. and Baronas, A. A.: Primary Teratomas of the Lateral Retroperitoneal Spaces. Surgery, *26:*149, 1949.
10. Lightwood, Q.: Abdominal Foetal Implantation. Retroperitoneal Teratoma. Proc. Roy. Soc. Med., *25:*1736, 1932.

CHAPTER 48

Uretero-Pelvic Obstruction

Among the most common abnormalities of the urinary tract are congenital obstructions at or near the uretero-pelvic junction. They can be devastating because of the renal destruction which follows them. All pediatricians and surgeons who deal with children should be mindful of these malformations, the early recognition and treatment of which give the best assurance for saving as much as possible of the renal parenchyma and function. There is a very extensive literature concerning these anomalies; our experience with them has been based upon observations and treatment of 156 obstructive lesions (in 145 patients) at the Boston Children's Hospital from 1926 through 1950.

PATHOLOGY

Type of Anomaly

Several forms of anatomic abnormality must be considered when studying or treating a child with uretero-pelvic obstruction. In our series, the block has come from a lesion which was intrinsic in the drainage system in 44 per cent of instances and it has risen from some external factor in 48 per cent; there has been a combination of the two in 8 per cent. At least six forms of conditions have been encountered, all with sufficient frequency to warrant consideration (Fig. 351). (1) There may be an aberrant or accessory renal vessel passing to the lower pole of the kidney, giving uretero-pelvic (or high ureteral) obstruction. (2) There may be intrinsic stenosis at the uretero-pelvic junction, with little more than a pin-point opening at this level. (3) There may be a flap of mucosa forming an internal valve-like structure at the uretero-pelvic zone. (4) There may be a kinking and distortion of the upper end of the ureter, the structure being held in this unusual shape by veil-like bands which cover it and bind it to the posterior abdominal wall. (5) The upper few centimeters of ureter may have a very narrow lumen and a zig-zag or convoluted pathway, a persistence of the fetal form. (6) In rare cases there is an adynamic obstruction because of absence (or diminution) in the musculature of the upper part of the ureter, the tube being little more than a translucent structure with interference of its peristaltic activity.

Side Involved. Sex

Such obstructions can occur on either side, but they are distinctly more common on the left. In our series there were:

Left............................... 87
Right.............................. 47
Bilateral........................... 11

In 3 patients, the obstruction was in a solitary kidney. Males are possibly a little more affected than females, the proportion being 83 to 62 in our series.

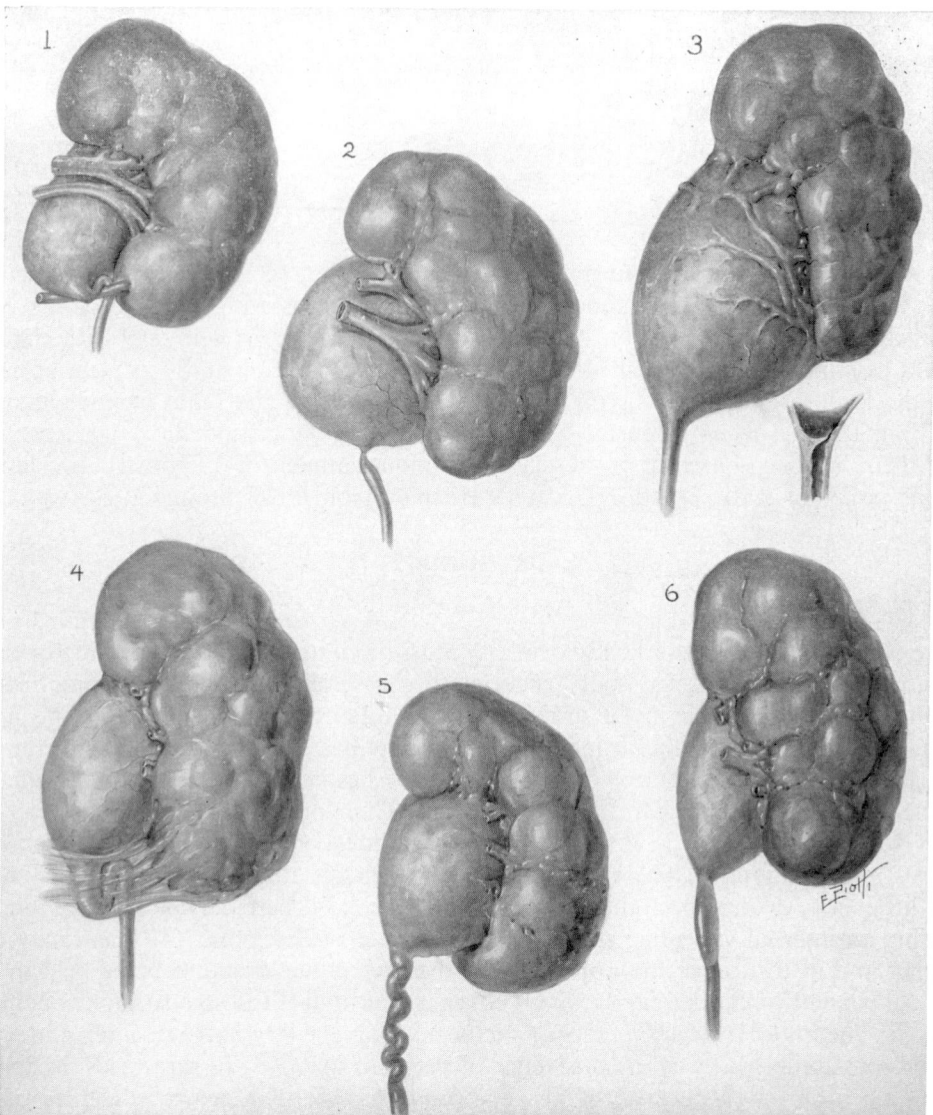

Fig. 351: Types of pathologic disturbances producing obstruction at the uretero-pelvic junction. 1. Accessory renal vessels supplying lower pole of the kidney. These vessels can branch from the main renal artery and vein, or they can individually connect with the aorta and vena cava. 2. Obstruction from intrinsic stricture of the uretero-pelvic junction. 3. The external surface shows no apparent local abnormality, but internally there is a small mucosal flap-valve producing obstruction. 4. The upper end of the ureter is held in a kinked position by overlying bands or veils of fibrous tissue. 5. The upper end of the ureter has a persistence of the fetal form in which there are multiple coils or convolutions. 6. There is obstruction because of segmental lack of ureteral musculature. There is interference with propagation of ureteral peristaltic waves.

Renal Damage

With each of the forms of obstruction, hydronephrosis can occur in any degree from mild to severe. With increasing or long-continued back-pressure, there is dilatation of the pelvis and calyces, as well as an atrophy and thinning of the renal substance. In some patients, the kidney is largely destroyed and is little more than an enormous sac filling the flank. Superimposed infection often adds to the ravages of the kidney damage; pyelonephritis is common. In an occasional case there may be perforation of the renal capsule and development of a peri-renal abscess, which, however, is almost always limited by the surrounding Gerota's fascia. While the ureter below a block is generally small or normal in size, superimposed infection can give a hypotonia which allows it to dilate.

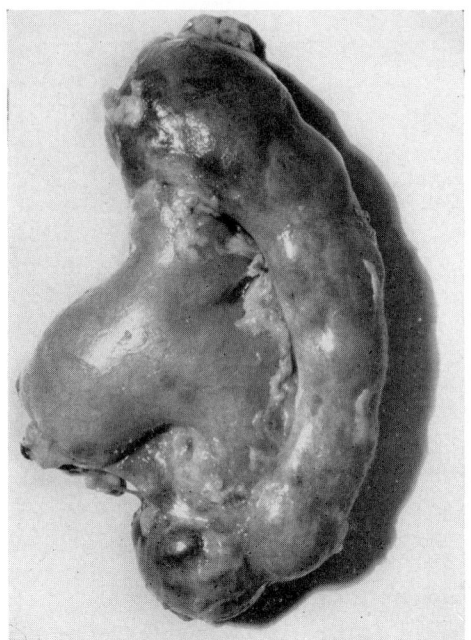 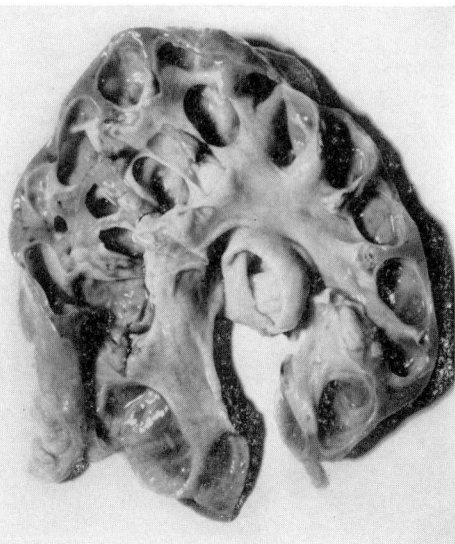

Fig. 352. Nephrectomy specimen. There had been advanced hydronephrosis and destruction of renal tissue because of ureteral obstruction from an aberrant renal vessel.

CLINICAL FINDINGS

Symptoms. There are a wide variety of complaints in these babies and children; there is no clear-cut picture which is diagnostic of uretero-pelvic obstruction. Abdominal pain, nausea, and vomiting are the most common complaints (68 per cent of our cases). In older children the pain might be well localized toward one flank or one side of the abdomen, but the vast majority of youngsters are unable to describe symptoms which indicate on which side the pathology exists. A large number of these urinary tract abnormalities are detected when, in the course of study of a child who has abdominal pain, an intravenous pyelogram discloses the condition.

Urinary Injection. Superimposed infection is rather common but is by no means universal. Pyuria, chills, or fever (39 per cent of our cases) accompany bacterial invasion of the urinary system. It is not uncommon to have a child with absolutely no complaints, but who on routine examination is found to have pyuria, search for the cause of which brings the anomaly to light.

Hematuria. Oddly enough, hematuria is occasionally seen (14 per cent) and, indeed, might be the only complaint or finding. Presumably, mucosal vessels in or near the obstruction become engorged and one of them ruptures, giving gross or microscopic amounts of blood in the urine.

Injury. In several of our patients there had been some manner of abdominal injury, such as occurred from a fall or from an automobile accident; during examination of the child an abdominal flank mass has been found. Presumably, hydronephrosis had been present before the time of the accident but had been entirely silent.

Age. Evidence of uretero-pelvic obstruction can appear at any time in early life. The average age of our patients was slightly under five years; the youngest was one month and the oldest was fourteen years. A large proportion of them had had symptoms for a long time prior to the discovery of their urinary tract abnormality; the average

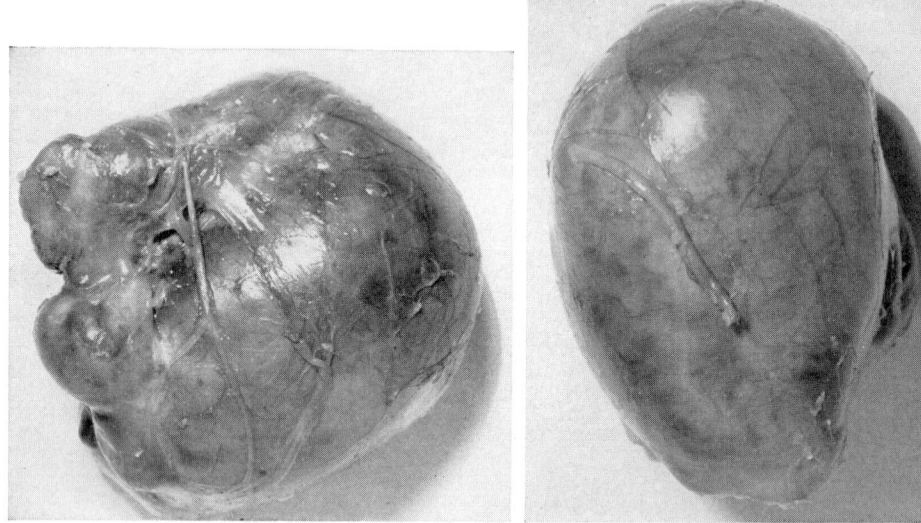

Fig. 353. Advanced hydronephrosis from intrinsic uretero-pelvic stricture.

duration of symptoms before treatment was about eighteen months. Many of these youngsters had difficulties which probably should have alerted their physicians to the possibility of a urinary tract lesion at a much earlier date.

Physical Examination. Whether or not a dilated kidney can be palpated depends upon the extent of the hydronephrosis, the thickness of the abdominal wall musculature, the relaxation of the child at the time of examination, et cetera. In 20 per cent of our patients the renal swelling could be felt during physical examination. Indeed, in a few cases it was the only finding that the child had; subsequent pyelography showed the hydronephrosis.

Hypertension. Hypertension is rare but does occur in some forms of renal damage and ischemia; it was found in 1 per cent of our cases.

ROENTGENOGRAPHIC FEATURES
Excretory Urography

Intravenous pyelography should be carried out in all cases where these anomalies are suspected. In some instances, uretero-pelvic obstruction is of such high degree that kidney secretion is poor, or else the dye is markedly diluted in a great hydronephrotic sac; in either instance, little or no visualization is obtained by this method. In the vast majority of infants and children, it is possible to see the excretory tract in a satisfactory way. One can observe dilatation of the pelves and calyces, the dye appearing in sufficient concentration to show these conditions very well. Oftentimes a sharp cut-off can be identified at the uretero-pelvic zone, or there may be an angulation of the ureter, suggesting a looping of the structure over an aberrant renal vessel or the anchorage of

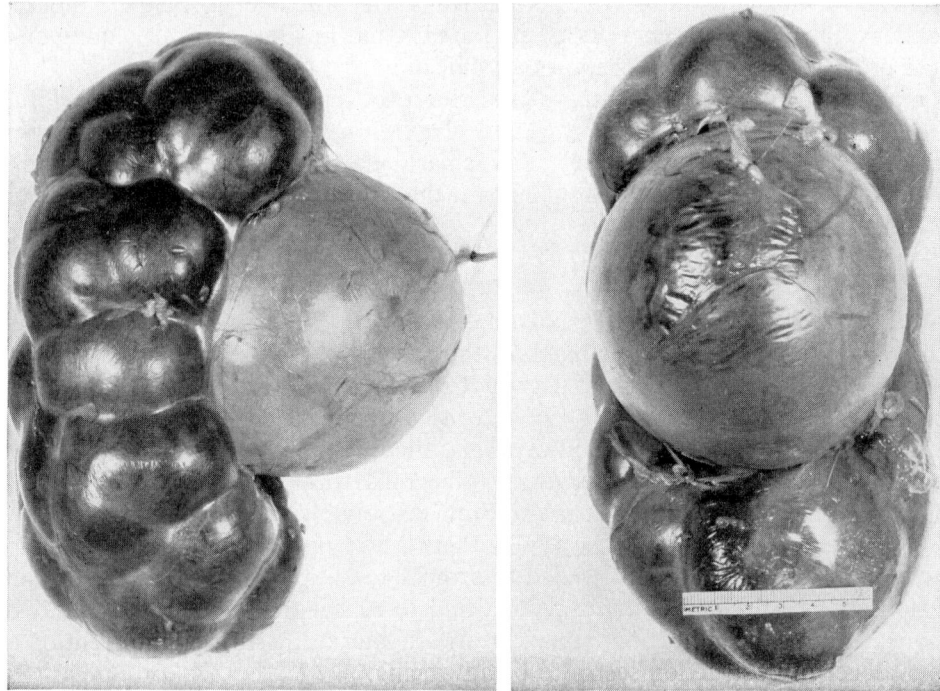

Fig. 354. Advanced hydronephrosis because of uretero-pelvic stricture. The calyces are greatly dilated, leaving only a shell of renal substance.

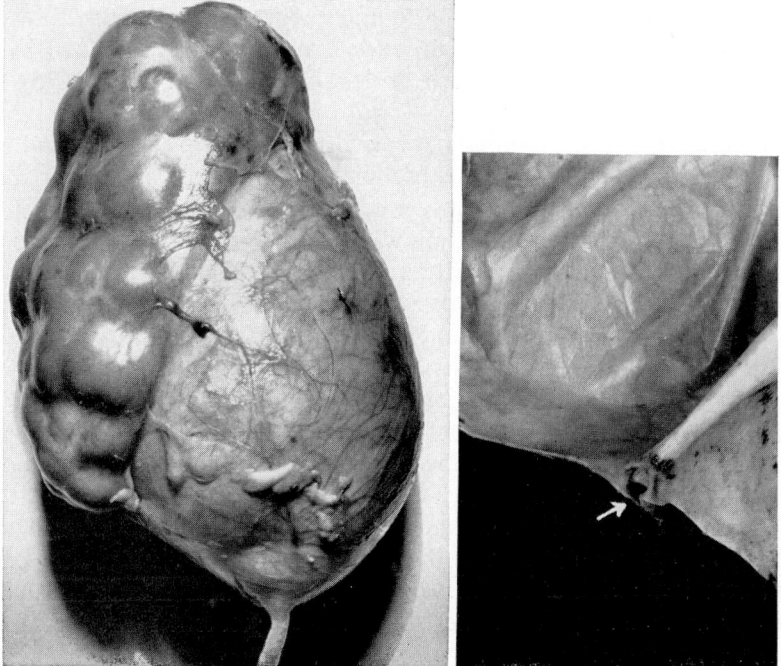

Fig. 355. *Left*, Marked hydronephrosis from obstruction. *Right*, Specimen opened; the obstruction was due to mucosal folds (arrow) acting as valves at uretero-pelvic junction.

the ureter in a kinked position by external bands which lie over it. Below a block, the remainder of the ureter is generally normal in size, but in some cases it is quite dilated because of atony from a coexisting urinary infection.

In addition to the routine antero-posterior exposures, it is sometimes helpful to take views in the oblique direction since they give information concerning the alignment of the ureter in relation to the kidney. This is particularly helpful when there is kinking or angulation of a ureter which might suggest that it is draped over an accessory renal vessel.

Borderline Cases

In those cases in which there is marked obstruction, there can be no doubt concerning the presence of an important block at the uretero-pelvic area. However, there are many children who have a minimal degree of stasis from an apparent narrowing which might be due either to a very mild stricture or to a spasm at the uretero-pelvic junction. Such cases with equivocal findings always raise the question of whether further investigation and operative therapy are required. Generally speaking, it is best to avoid any surgical procedure if the kidney seems to drain reasonably well (in pyelograms 30, 60, and 90 minutes after injection of the dye), if there is no pyuria, and if there are no important symptoms which can be attributed to a renal condition. It is justifiable to handle such subjects by conservative management and to repeat the pyelographic study at a subsequent date as the indications seem to warrant, later using surgical intervention only if the evidence of obstruction seems to be advancing.

Cystoscopy. Retrograde Pyelography

In some cases it is possible to get all of the evidence which is desired by intravenous pyelography alone, but in the vast majority of subjects in whom there is obstructive uropathy, it is desirable to gather more complete data by cystoscopy and retrograde pyelography. Indeed, in some patients no visualization at all is obtained by the intravenous method, and all of the important observations have to be made by retrograde methods.

While it is possible in most adults to perform cystoscopy under local anesthesia, it has been our custom to make all cystoscopic examinations on infants and children under general anesthesia. This is certainly much easier for the patient as well as for the cystoscopist. Furthermore, it generally allows the maximum amount of information to be gained from the investigative procedure.

The plan of approach in any cystoscopic examination must always be individualized. There is little point in using a standard or complicated procedure for all children in whom cystoscopy is undertaken. There should be clearly in mind all the facts which are to be gathered so that the information desired is obtained without making the study unnecessarily long or intricate. In some patients the most important step to be considered is microscopic examination of the sediment from one or both ureters, or a study of divided kidney function. In others, visualization of the ureter as it enters the bladder is a point of greatest importance. In most instances, the passage of catheters up the ureters and the retrograde injection of dye for inspection of kidneys and ureters gives the main information which is sought. In a high proportion of cases, visualization of only one ureter and renal pelvis is necessary to complement what has been learned already by intravenous pyelography.

When retrograde studies show a high degree of obstruction at a uretero-pelvic junction, this is probably all the information which is desired at the moment. In some

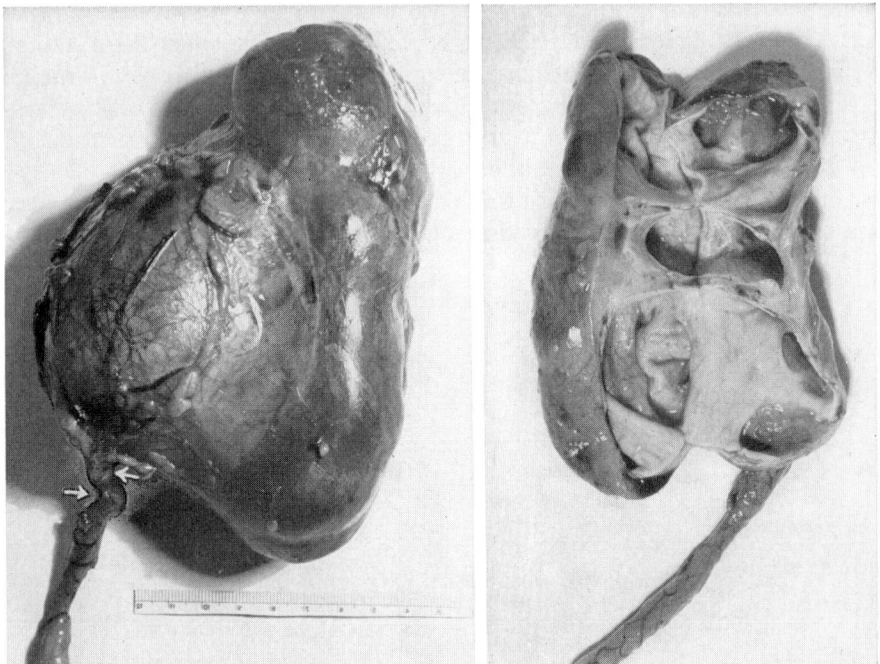

Fig. 356. Hydronephrosis and destruction of kidney by obstruction which resulted from persistence of fetal tortuosity in upper end of ureter (arrows). (The lumen of the upper 2 or 3 cm. of ureter was tiny and convoluted.)

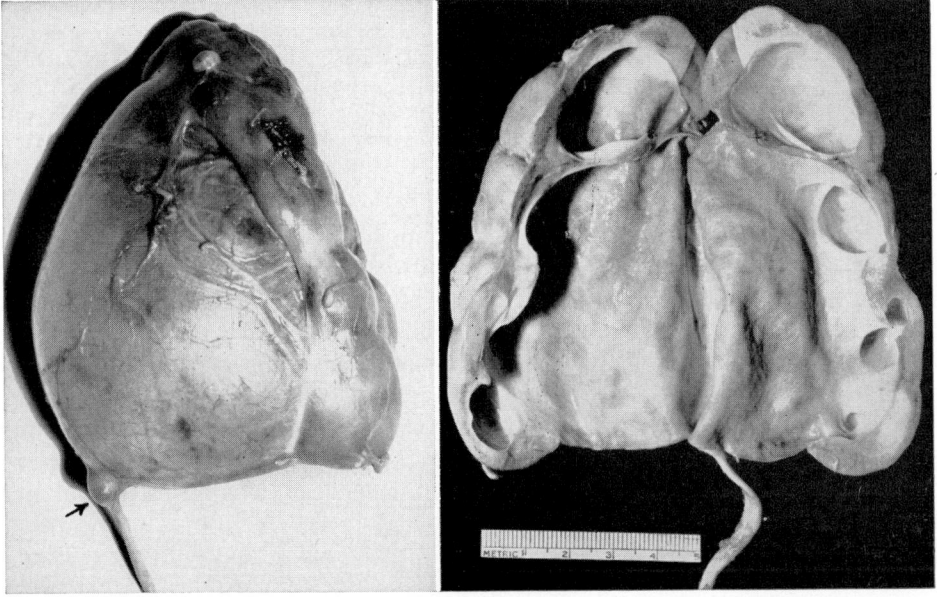

Fig. 357. Destruction of kidney from functional obstruction due to lack of musculature in upper 7 or 8 mm. of ureter (arrow).

cases, good visualization of the uretero-pelvic area can give a fairly clear idea of the pathology which will be encountered; this is particularly true when there is angulation over an aberrant renal vessel or a sharp cut-off of a stricture. However, in the majority of cases it is impossible to predict before operation the exact type of obstruction which will be found. In those patients who have only a mild degree of obstruction, it is very helpful to take several films during fifteen or twenty minutes while the patient is held in a semi-sitting position (the table being tilted appropriately), so that an impression can be gained concerning the freedom of drainage from the affected pelvis.

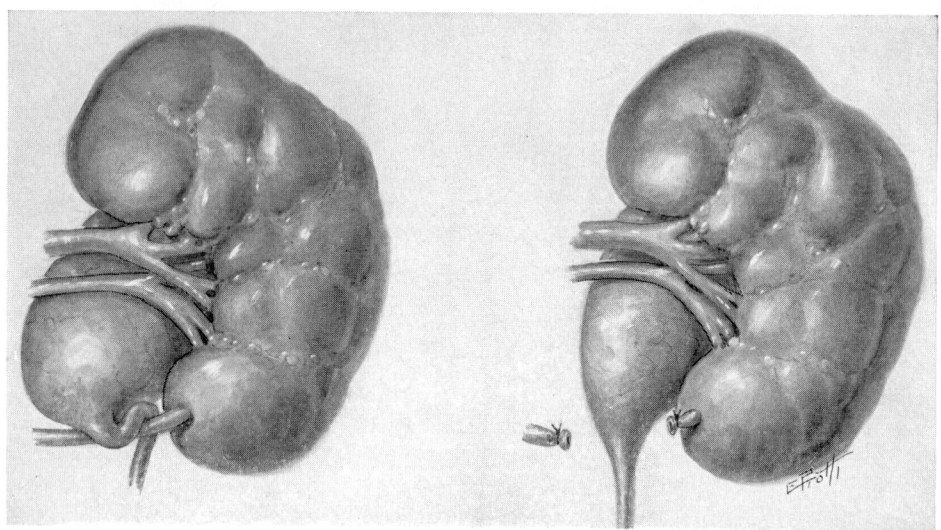

Fig. 358. Surgical correction of uretero-pelvic obstruction which has been caused by accessory or aberrant renal vessels to lower pole of the kidney. *Left,* The hydronephrosis and kinking or angulation of the upper end of ureter over the accessory vessel. *Right,* Double ligation and division of the accessory renal vessel, completely freeing the ureter. In all cases in which this operation is done, the pelvis should now be opened and the interior of the uretero-pelvic zone examined, to rule out the possibility of associated intrinsic uretero-pelvic blockage, which is not infrequently found.

LABORATORY DATA

The urine might be clear; indeed it was so in the majority of our patients. Pyuria, however, is a common finding. Culture of the urine and identification of the offending organism frequently has little practical value, but in some cases in which there is a stubborn infection, bacteriologic study might lead to the shift to some other chemotherapeutic or antibiotic agent which is more effective in combating the organism which is present.

The level of the blood non-protein nitrogen (or urea nitrogen) should be determined to estimate the effectiveness of the excretory tract in clearing the blood stream of waste products, a point of particular importance when one is dealing with obstruction in both kidneys or involvement of a sole kidney.

TREATMENT

Preoperative Measures

In those children who have obstructive uropathy, who do not have high fever, and whose general condition is good, operation can be proceeded with immediately. However, when there is fever of important degree, the child is critically ill, or there is excessive retention of nitrogen products (as determined by non-protein nitrogen or urea nitrogen), surgery might be tolerated poorly and it is quite important to prepare and support the child before a major operation is undertaken. Much can be accomplished by the urging of fluids to wash out the urinary system; if the child does not drink well, it may be neces-

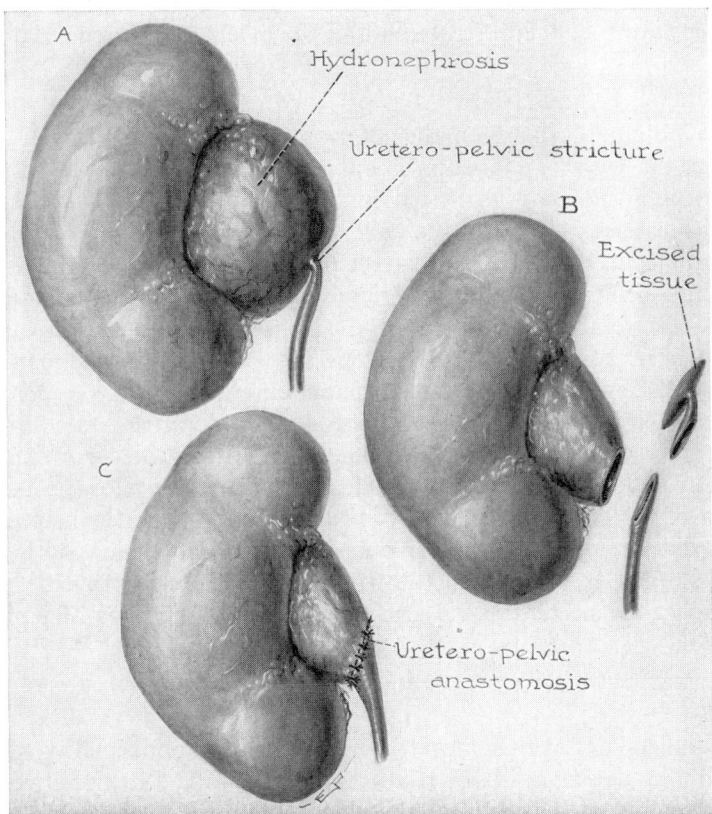

Fig. 359. Method for removal of a uretero-pelvic stricture with reestablishment of the continuity by anastomosis of pelvis to ureter. A, The pathology which is found, showing moderate hydronephrosis but fairly well preserved renal parenchyma and a fibrous constriction at the uretero-pelvic junction. B, Complete excision of the narrowed area. The ureter has been slit along one side for at least 1 cm., to give an adequate opening. C, Reconstruction by direct suture with interrupted 0000 chromic catgut stitches which pass through the entire thickness of the wall, excepting the mucosa. It is sometimes possible to bring together a little areolar tissue outside of this with a few interrupted silk stitches to support the anastomosis. A polyethylene tube should now be placed as an internal strut. It has several holes cut in the part which will lie in the pelvis. (See Fig. 360.) The tube pierces renal substance and is brought out through the flank wound. A single tube therefore serves as a strut and also provides for pelvic drainage for twelve to fourteen days.

sary to give intravenous solutions. Antibiotic therapy is of help in combating any pyelonephritis; bacterial infection of the urinary tract can be reduced by such measures, but no hope for complete relief or even for important diminution in pyuria should be entertained until the obstruction can be removed surgically. Generally, it is not difficult to make ready for operation a child who has a unilateral lesion; when there is bilateral obstruction and serious reduction of renal reserve, it is essential to put the child in the best possible state before undertaking surgery. In complicated cases, the operative risks are high and the optimum moment for a major procedure must be carefully chosen.

Type of Operation

The finding of uretero-pelvic obstruction which is beyond a minimal grade always demands operative intervention. When hydronephrosis and kidney destruction are marked, nephrectomy can be contemplated before operation; in most cases, the decision regarding the type of therapy to be employed can be made only after surgical exploration shows the exact nature of the obstruction and the extent of the renal damage.

Operative Approach

The space obtainable between the inferior border of the thoracic cage and the superior part of the wing of the ileum is apt to be rather narrow in babies and small children, therefore positioning of the patient on the table merits attention in obtaining the widest exposure possible. With the child on his side, the mid-portion of the trunk is arched up by placing beneath it a blanket roll, or preferably raising a kidney bench under the flank to bend the body appropriately. Running the oblique flank incision far up into the costovertebral angle posteriorly, and well forward and downward beyond the anterior superior spine of the pelvis, generally provides an adequate wound. The peri-renal capsule (Gerota's fascia) should be cut carefully so that its borders are clean and its edges can be approximated at the end of the operative procedure. The kidney and upper part of the ureter must be stripped bluntly from the surrounding fibro-fatty tissues so that structures are mobilized to a degree sufficient to allow proper observation and evaluation of the pathology which is at hand. Sometimes it is helpful to pass two linen tapes around the upper and lower poles of the kidney which aid in gently lifting the kidney out as far as possible in the wound to give an improved view. It is now possible to inspect the uretero-pelvic area and ascertain the type of pathology which exists.

Double Lesions

It is essential to realize that more than one form of abnormality can be present. We have seen many errors and poor results from assuming that there was but a single anomaly, only to find at a later date that incomplete relief of obstruction had been afforded. Thus, one sometimes finds that an aberrant renal vessel can be divided and seemingly matters appear to have been thoroughly corrected, only to learn later that there is an advancing hydronephrosis because of a stenosis at the uretero-vesical junction (Fig. 366). We therefore feel strongly that in all cases in which aberrant renal vessels have been divided, the pelvis should be opened and the interior of the uretero-vesical junction be inspected and probed.

Nephrectomy

The first decision to be made relates to whether the kidney should be removed or whether an attempt should be made to save it. There is no clearly defined line separating those situations in which an immediate nephrectomy seems desirable from those in which conservative methods of treatment are preferable. Certainly, there can be no doubt that in the presence of an advanced hydronephrosis, great thinning of the renal parenchyma, and extensive pyelonephritis, the child is better off to have the kidney resected at once (assuming that the opposite kidney is in good condition). On the other hand, kidneys with lesser degrees of damage have an enormous capacity for repair (or at least return of reasonable function) if they are relieved of obstruction. Therefore, with mild or moderate obstruction, even though there has been some destruction of

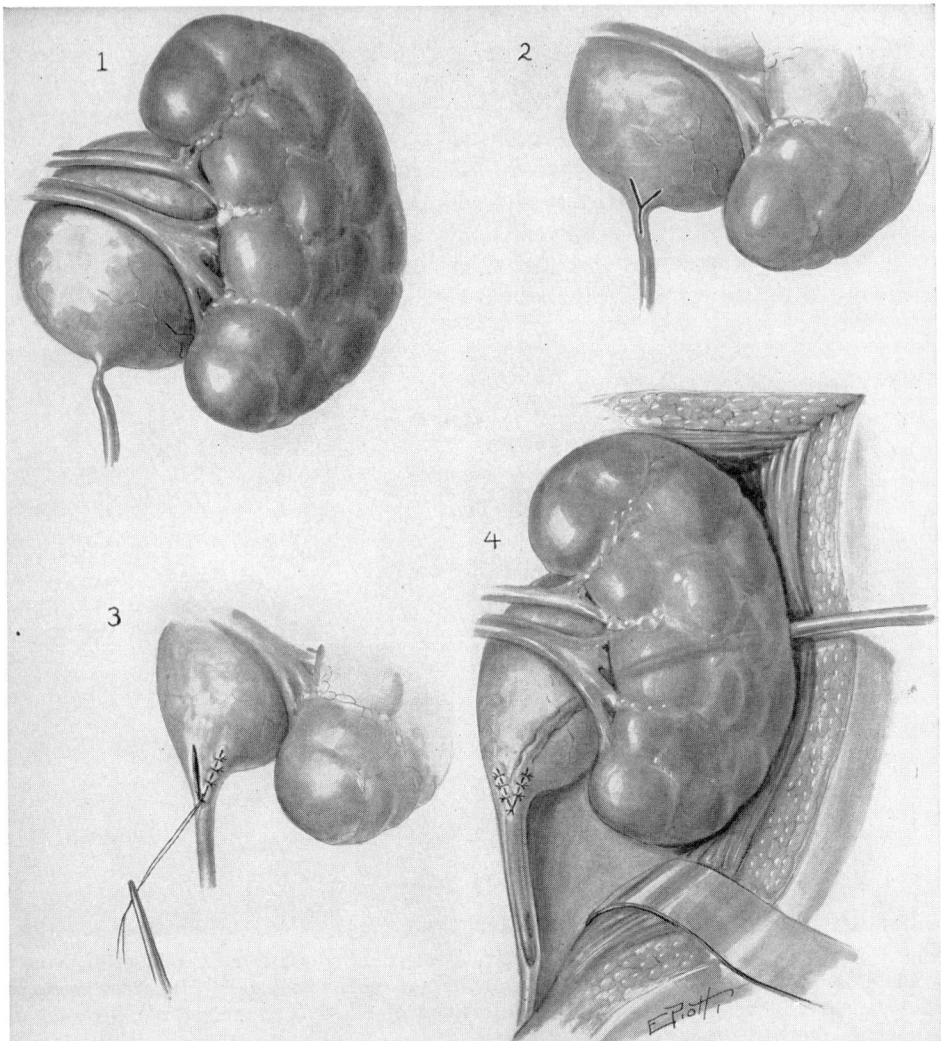

Fig. 360. Method of treatment of uretero-pelvic stricture by a Y-V plastic procedure. 1. The pathology found, with some thinning of the renal parenchyma, with marked hydronephrosis, and a marked uretero-pelvic stricture. 2. Position of the incisions. The upper limbs of the Y run up onto the renal pelvis; the lower leg of the Y extends down for 8 to 10 mm. into normal ureteral substance below the stricture. 3. The Y is converted to a V by bringing the apex of tissue down to the lower end of the ureteral incision and anchoring it there with a stitch as shown. The traction suture helps to maintain alignment of the adjacent tissues while the stitches are being placed. The repair is with interrupted 0000 chromic catgut stitches which run through all layers except the mucosa. 4. Completion of the V union. A polyethylene tube inserted for use as an internal strut and also to provide pelvic drainage during the early postoperative period. The tube extends down the ureter for 5 or 6 cm. That portion of the tube which lies in the pelvis contains several holes. The tube is left in place for twelve to fourteen days, and is then withdrawn.

renal parenchyma, it is best to take a conservative attitude and spare the kidney by removing the uretero-pelvic block. Such a plan is generally rewarded by successful issue, but in a small proportion of cases it is followed by a poor result which requires nephrectomy at a subsequent date.

The treatment of uretero-vesical obstruction depends entirely upon what type of abnormality is encountered.

Division of Aberrant Renal Vessel

Aberrant renal vessels can be recognized instantly as artery or vein, or both, which run to the lower pole of the kidney from the vena cava or aorta; sometimes they branch downward from the main renal artery and vein. The vessel can lie in such a position that the uretero-pelvic area (or the upper end of the ureter) is compressed by or is angulated over the structure; sometimes this takes the form of a pronounced S kinking of the ureter as it is draped over the vessel which runs in front of it. In some cases, there is a

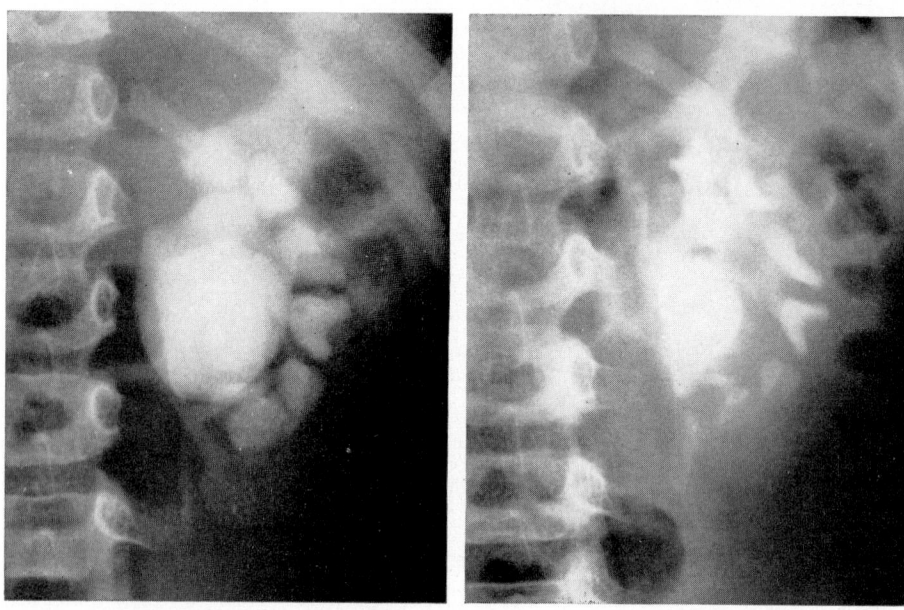

Fig. 361. Two-year-old boy with uretero-pelvic obstruction and a considerable left hydronephrosis; at operation this was found to be due to an aberrant renal vessel. *Left,* Pyelogram made before operation at which aberrant renal vessels were divided. *Right,* Pyelogram five months after operation, showing improvement in the kidney picture.

definite hydronephrosis and yet the ureter does not seem to be particularly constricted by the vessel; presumably, the artery lies against the ureter, interferes with its peristalsis, and thereby gives a functional obstruction.

Three general methods are available for correction of the situation. (1) The kidney can be mobilized and raised or turned in such a way that the ureter is led away from the vessel, a technique which has very little merit. (2) There are some urologists who feel that severance of the polar artery gives sufficient renal ischemia to produce hypertension; they have preferred to save the vessel and to sever the ureter, bringing it in front of the vessel for an anastomosis, which gives it good alignment. We do not favor this procedure. (3) The aberrant vessel can be severed, to provide a clear and unobstructed path for the ureter.

Division of an aberrant renal artery can produce some paleness in the lower pole of the kidney, but this is seldom of importance. We have never seen sloughing or necrosis of renal tissue because of this step; it is possible that some of the renal substance atrophies, but in most cases there is sufficient cross circulation from the remainder of

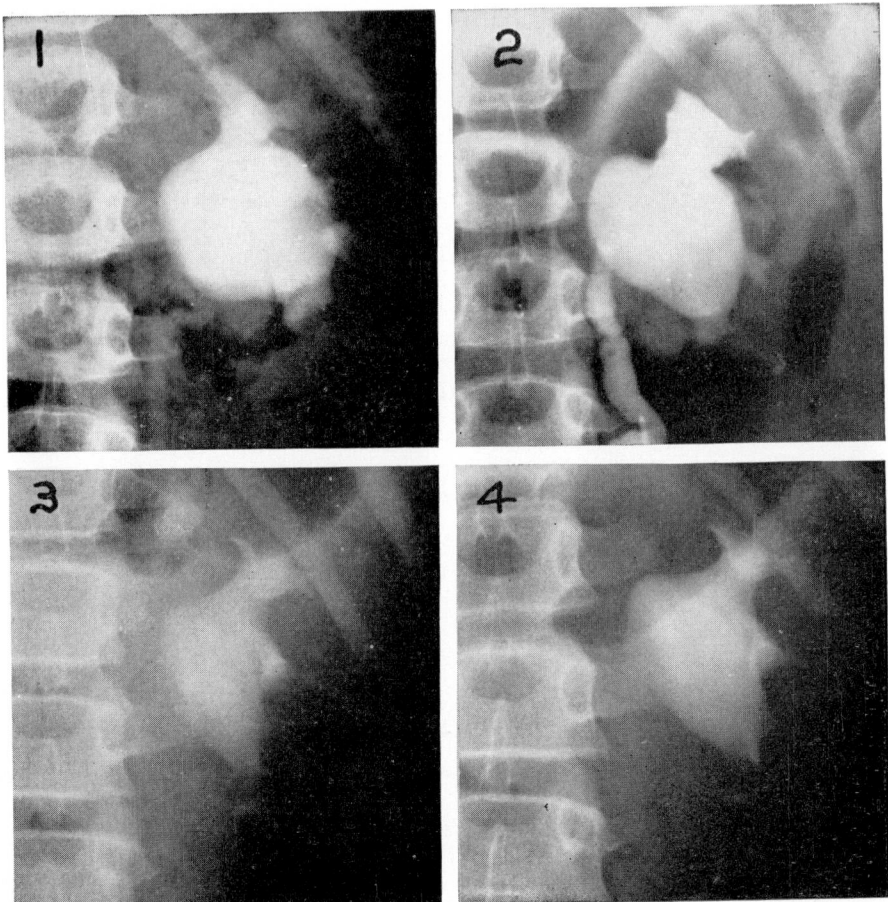

Fig. 362. Six-year-old girl with left hydronephrosis of considerable degree, which was found to be due to aberrant renal vessels. Treatment by division of the accessory renal artery and vein. 1. Pyelogram before operation showing hydronephrosis and also enlargement and blunting of the calyces. 2. Condition three months after operation, with relatively little change. 3. One year after operation, with some improvement and sharpening of the calyces. 4. Condition two years after operation, with fairly sharp calyces but with some hydronephrosis remaining. The child is completely asymptomatic and has clear urine eight years after operation.

the kidney to provide an adequate blood flow. In only one case have we seen postoperative hypertension which was thought to be due to renal ischemia and which required subsequent removal of a kidney. In general, it is possible to divide the offending vessel with impunity.

After cutting aberrant vessels, the operator is all too apt to believe that everything necessary has been done to relieve the obstruction. While in the majority of cases this is true, there are some who continue to have difficulties because an intrinsic obstruction has been overlooked. It is sometimes impossible to recognize this intrinsic obstruction by external inspection and palpation; we therefore feel that in all cases it is imperative to open the renal pelvis and to inspect or probe down into the uretero-pelvic area to make sure that no intrinsic lesion exists. If such is found, it must be treated appropriately; if no intrinsic obstruction is encountered, this small pyelotomy wound can be closed tightly with a running fine catgut suture which should be reenforced by a few fine silk stitches to the adventitial structures.

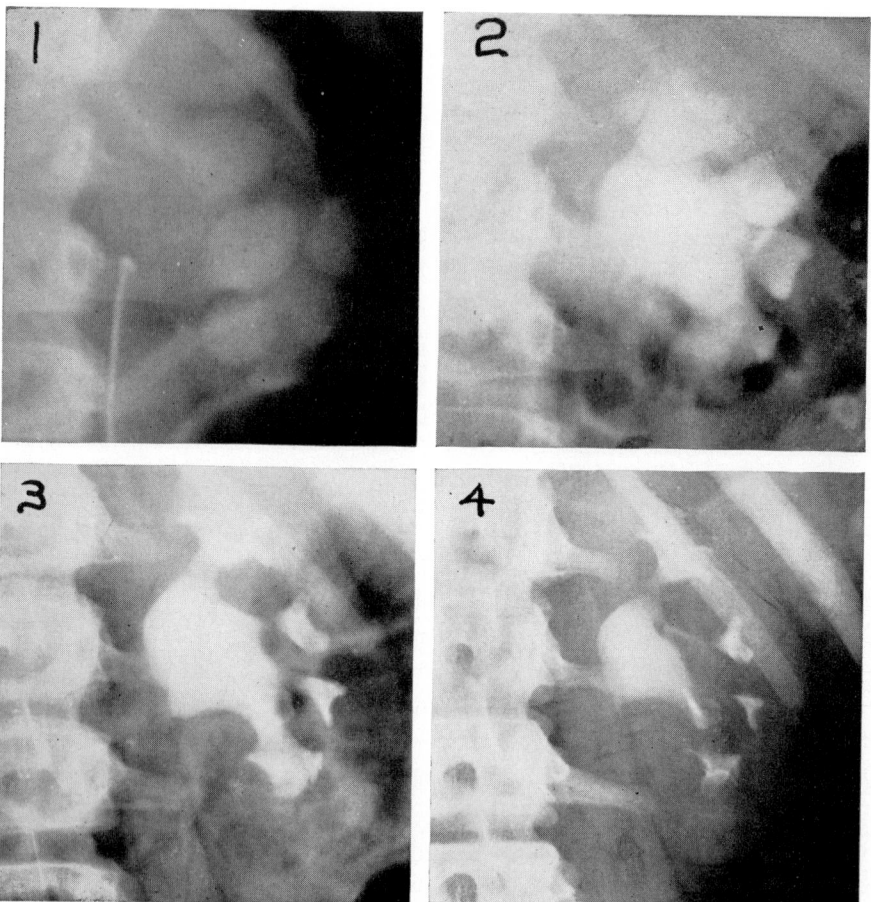

Fig. 363. Seven-year-old boy with left hydronephrosis, the kidney being obstructed by an accessory renal vessel. 1. Preoperative appearance, showing the marked blunting and dilatation of the calyces. 2. Two weeks after division of the accessory vessel, showing rather good excretion of the dye. Calyces are slightly smaller than preoperatively. 3. Appearance four years after operation, showing marked improvement. 4. Appearance seven years after operation, showing essentially normal configuration. The kidney has shown an extraordinary capacity for return of function and form towards normal after the obstruction has been removed.

Treatment of Uretero-Pelvic Stricture

We are quite convinced that any efforts to dilate uretero-pelvic strictures are generally insufficient in relieving obstruction. We have had no luck in attempting to dilate mild strictures by the passage of catheters or dilators in a retrograde manner by cystoscopic manipulation. Furthermore, even under direct vision at a flank operation, the introduction of dilators through a pyelotomy wound, passing these down through the strictured site, might seem to be reasonably effective in stretching the area, but we have been so disappointed by follow-up observations in cases in which this has been done that we believe it should be abandoned completely in favor of some cutting procedure which is done to enlarge the opening between the pelvis and ureter.

Two general methods are available for the treatment of strictures. The narrowed zone can be cut out and a new stoma made between ureter and pelvis, or else it can be enlarged by some plastic rearrangement of tissues. The complete excision of a stricture and the establishment of an anastomosis is thought by some to be unduly radical, because, while a large opening can thereby be established, there might possibly be some interference with progression of the peristaltic wave from pelvis to ureter, thereby setting up a "functional" obstruction. To obviate this possibility, plastic procedures have been devised which enlarge the pathway but leave intact a portion of the wall (and presumably thereby facilitate the passage of the peristaltic wave). Much can be accomplished by these plastic procedures, but generally the opening obtained is not as large as that which

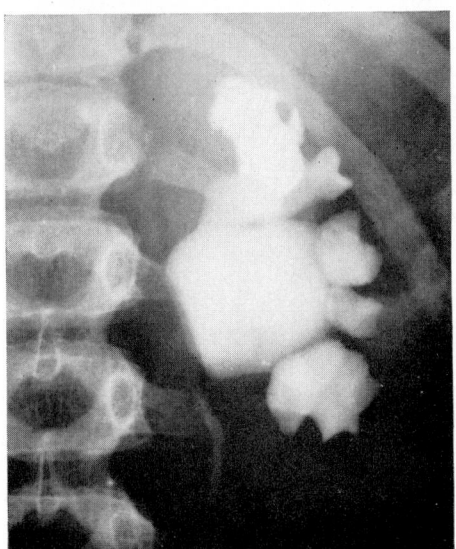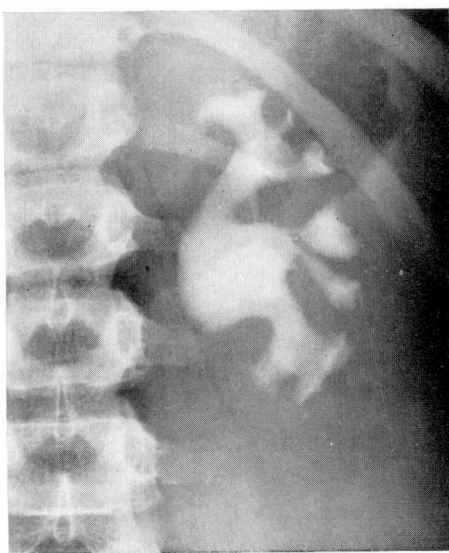

Fig. 364. Nine-year-old boy with left renal obstruction from an aberrant renal vessel to the lower pole of the kidney, treated by division of the vessel. *Left*, The preoperative picture, showing moderate hydronephrosis as well as dilatation and blunting of the calyces. *Right*, The appearance four months after operation, indicating diminution in size of the pelvis and a sharpening of the calyces.

can be produced by excision of a stricture and establishment of a uretero-neopyelostomy. There is a real need for further study to determine which of these methods gives the better long-term result. We have used both, have achieved excellent results with both, and have had failures with both. In general, if the stricture is a short one, and there is a soft, rather normal tissue immediately above and below it, we prefer to perform a plastic procedure; if the stricture is a long one, or the nearby tissues are scarred and thickened, we prefer to excise as much of this abnormal substance as possible, and establish an anastomosis.

Complete Excision of Stricture. In completely excising a stricture, the following steps are carried out (Fig. 359). After elimination of the narrowed zone, the remaining ureter should be slit down one side for a distance of at least a centimeter, to provide a long stoma so that subsequent shrinking at the anastomotic site will not give rise to a secondary obstruction. On a number of occasions we have attempted to determine what sort of suturing at the union is apt to give the best results, but have been unable to reach any final conclusions in favor of any one method. Certainly, silk should not be used in the repair in any way which allows it to protrude into the lumen and thereby give a foreign body on which calculi might form. It is best to make the anastomoses with 0000 or 00000 chromic catgut, on an atraumatic needle. We have made many of these in a continuous fashion, but believe that it is probably better to use interrupted sutures. Whether the ureteral and pelvic ends should be turned inward, should be brought in direct apposition of edge to edge, or should be turned outward is a matter for debate; there seems to be no conclusive study to show which is preferable. Currently, we favor a type of union in which no attempt is made to turn the edges either inward or outward; taking very small bites, the sutures pass through the entire thickness of

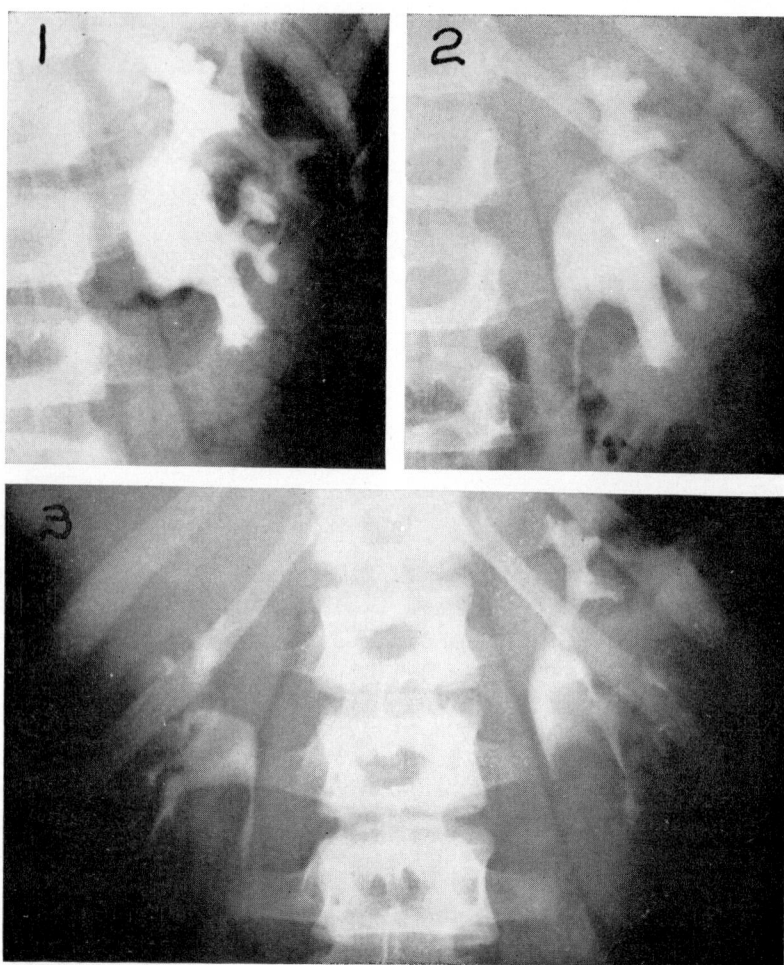

Fig. 365. Six-year-old girl with left hydronephrosis, caused by an aberrant renal vessel, which was divided at operation. 1. Preoperative appearance, showing medium grade of hydronephrosis as well as dilatation and blunting of the calyces. 2. The appearance four months after operation, with some improvement in the picture. 3. Intravenous pyelogram seven years after operation, showing the return practically to normal. (When last seen ten years after operation, the child was completely asymptomatic and had clear urine.)

the ureteral and pelvic walls, excepting the mucosa. There might be some fear that catgut sutures would disintegrate too early, and thereby allow total or partial disruption to occur at the anastomotic site. To avoid this catastrophy, we have generally been able (after the anastomosis is completed) to bring together some light areolar tissue over the anastomotic line, joining these with a few interrupted fine silk stitches (00000 Deknatel) placed appropriately around the anastomosis and in this way have relieved any strain or pull on the anastomosis itself.

Plastic Procedure for Stricture. Of the various plastic operations devised for uretero-pelvic stricture, the Y-V rearrangement is the one which has attained the widest use (Fig. 360). To make this revision, the Y is placed in such a manner that the two upper limbs of the Y extend up onto the pelvis, the crotch of the Y comes just at the level of

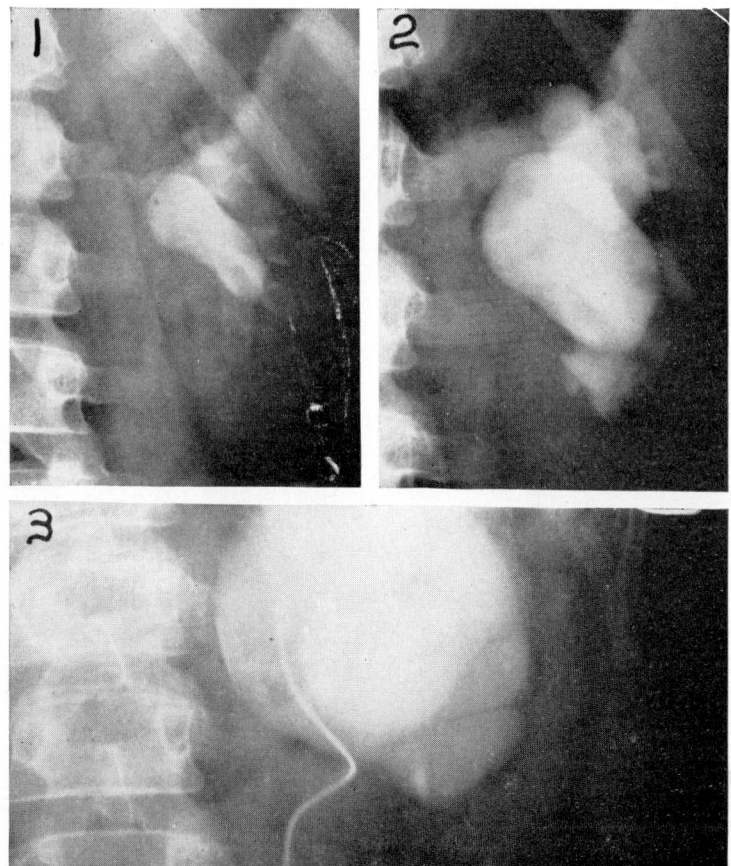

Fig. 366. Twelve-year-old boy with advanced hydronephrosis. There was a marked degree of pyelonephritis. 1. Preoperative roentgenogram, showing only slight hydronephrosis before operation at which time an accessory renal artery was severed. 2. One month after operation, showing considerable advancement in the obstructive picture. 3. Situation ten months following operation, indicating a great advance in the hydronephrosis. Note that a catheter could be inserted up the ureter and readily into the pelvis. The child continually ran a pyuria and a moderately elevated blood pressure. Because of the advancing symptoms, a left nephrectomy was subsequently performed. There was a valve of mucosal tissue at the uretero-pelvic junction, which allowed upward passage of a catheter but which prevented the satisfactory egress of urine. At the first operation, the pelvis had not been opened to inspect its interior. This case emphasizes that whenever an aberrant renal vessel is divided, a pyelotomy should also be performed, so that any intrinsic obstruction can be detected and treated.

the stricture, and the lower limb of the Y extends down onto the normal part of the ureter. After this Y incision has been made through the entire thickness of the pelvis and ureter, the upper flap is brought down to the lowest point of the incision in the ureter and is sutured into this new position (thus transforming the Y into a V). This lowest stitch is used as a traction suture; by keeping it taut, the sides of the V will be brought into proper juxtaposition so they can be sewed most easily. The sides of the V are now closed with interrupted sutures; it appears to be best to make these with 0000 chromic catgut, and to pass the stitches through all layers of the wall, excepting the mucosa. It is generally possible to support this reconstruction with a few fine silk sutures taken in the surrounding areolar tissue.

Whenever there has been excision of a stricture and establishment of a uretero-pelvic anastomosis (or when there has been a plastic procedure to a uretero-pelvic stricture), a catheter (or polyethylene tube) should be used as an internal strut for at least

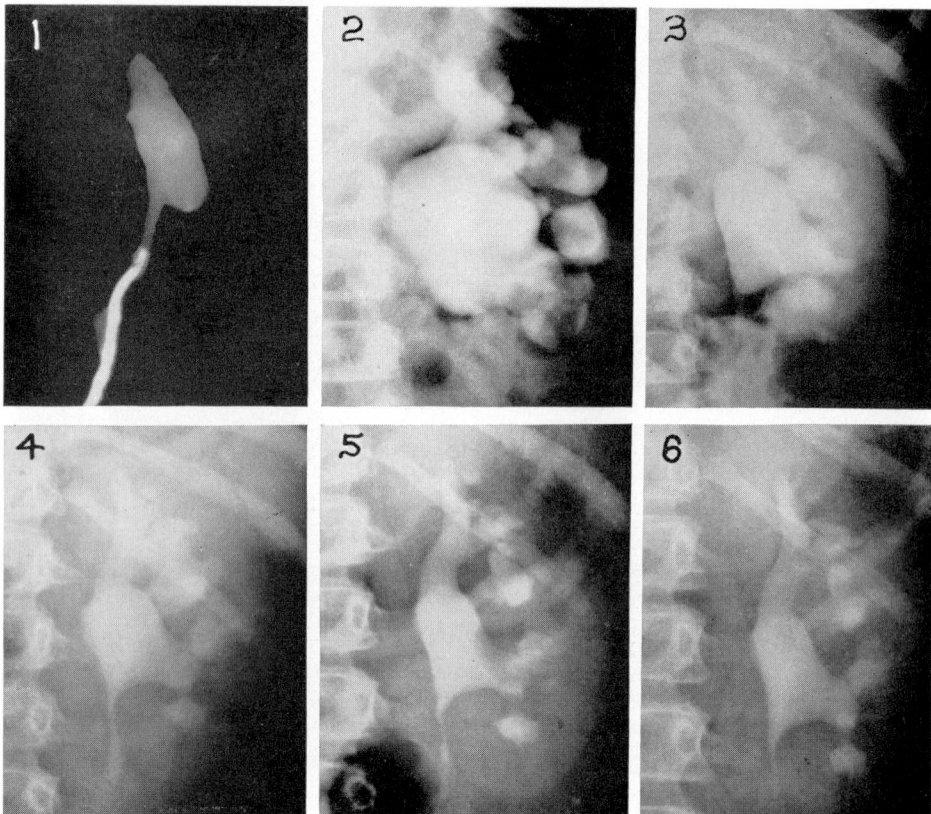

Fig. 367. Five-year-old child with hypoplastic right kidney and a high degree of obstruction of the left kidney which was caused by a short segment just at the uretero-pelvic area which had a deficient musculature. 1. Roentgenogram of the hypoplastic right kidney specimen which was removed because of poor function and extensive pyelonephritis. 2. Preoperative appearance of the left kidney, showing marked hydronephrosis and obstruction. The anomalous zone at the uretero-pelvic junction was excised and the ureter brought to the pelvis for uretero-pelvic anastomosis (Fig. 359). 3. Appearance one month after operation, showing some improvement. 4. Two years after operation, showing good function of the kidney, considerable diminution in the hydronephrosis, and excellent drainage into the ureter. 5. Intravenous urogram three years after operation, showing an excellent renal picture. 6. Check-up examination six years after operation (the child being completely asymptomatic and having clear urine); note the excellent appearance of the kidney.

ten days to two weeks following operation. This insures that the lumen remains open, that the mucosa can reform in a smooth manner with an ample diameter, and that the alignment of the pelvis and ureter are maintained as they become fixed to surrounding structures during the process of healing. Several holes should be cut in that portion of the catheter which lies in the kidney pelvis so that the single tube also functions as a drain to carry off urine from the kidney during the time that it is in place. A No. 8 or 10 urethral catheter can be used for this purpose, but we favor the use of a polyethylene tube because it probably sets up less reaction in the ureter. This tube can be led out of a pyelotomy wound, but when placed in this way it sometimes does not lie in a very satisfactory direction or it is difficult to pull out subsequently. We much prefer to pierce the lateral border of renal substance and lead the catheter directly out through the kidney and then through the flank wound.

Treatment of Mucosal Flap-Valve

In those cases in which there is a hydronephrosis and yet one finds no visible evidence of obstruction by external inspection and palpation of the uretero-pelvic zone, a pyelotomy and examination of the interior of this area oftentimes shows a tiny flap of membrane which has a valve-like action and which can greatly impede the downward flow of urine. Sometimes it is possible, through a fairly low pyelotomy wound, to excise cleanly this flap and to establish a satisfactory pathway. In other cases, the redundancy is so marked that it seems best to excise the entire segment and to bring the ureter to the pelvis by a clean anastomosis (Fig. 359), giving a lumen of appropriate dimension.

Treatment of External Veils or Bands

In those cases in which the ureter is kinked upon itself and is held in this position by bands or folds which encase and hold it against the posterior abdominal wall, it is not difficult to free up and cut away all of the bands; these are quite avascular. Such dissection frees the ureter and allows it to be straightened out in a satisfactory way. In addition, it might be necessary to perform a nephropexy, raising the kidney to a position which will attenuate and straighten out the ureter. Such elevation can be accomplished by fixation of the kidney to the periosteum of the twelfth rib or by bringing together Gerota's fascia underneath the lower pole of the kidney as a sling to keep the kidney supported in an elevated position. All of these patients should have a pyelotomy for inspection or probing of the lumen of the upper ureter, to make sure that some intrinsic obstruction does not coexist. Furthermore, it is always best for a week or ten days to leave an internal strut running through the ureter, the pelvis, out through the kidney substance, and out through the flank wound, to keep the ureter and pelvis in proper alignment as they heal with the surrounding structures in the postoperative period.

Treatment of Convoluted Ureter

We have occasionally encountered these lesions, and for some it has been possible to make a pyelotomy opening in the pelvis above, to insert instruments of increasing size down the ureter, which seem to straighten out the folds and give a fair lumen to the ureter. In most instances it is advisable to excise entirely an area of this sort (which is generally not more than a centimeter or two in length) and then bring the remaining ureteral stump to the pelvis for an anastomosis (Fig. 359).

Treatment for Deficiency of Ureteral Musculature

In those cases in which deficiency of the ureteral musculature is extensive, little or nothing can be accomplished by operative means. However, in some cases the anomalous segment is only a centimeter or two in length; it is possible to excise it, and bring good ureteral substance upward to join with the pelvis for an anastomosis

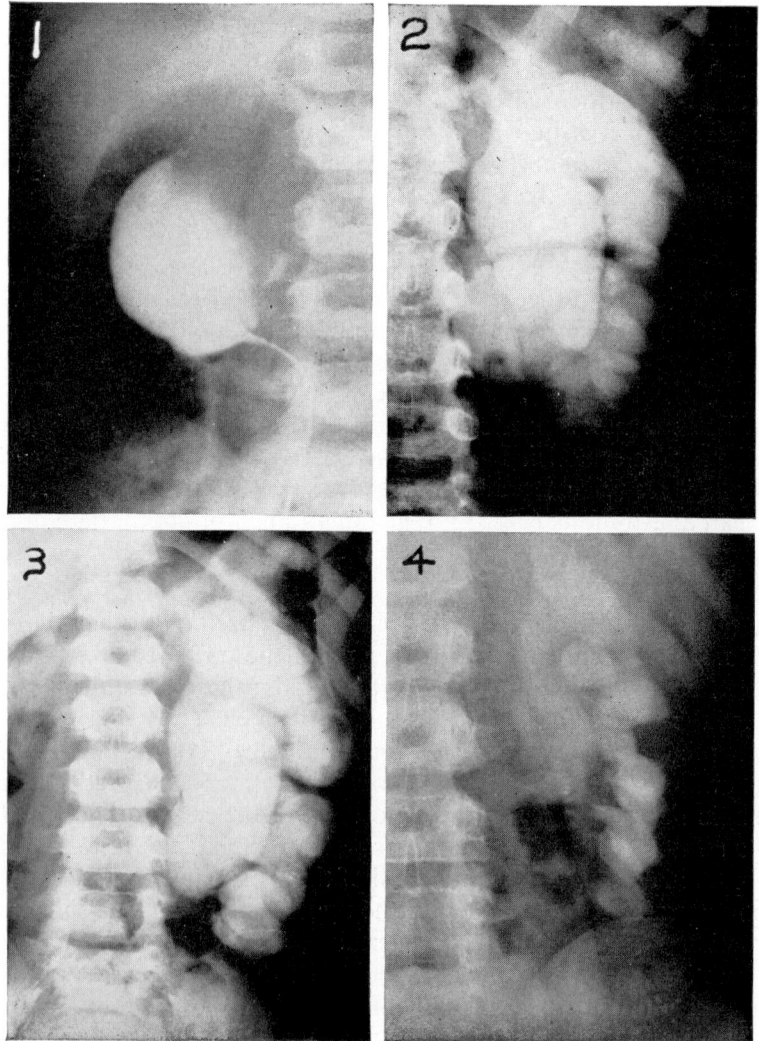

Fig. 368. Five-year-old boy with marked bilateral hydronephrosis and pyelonephritis. 1. The right kidney was a pus-filled sac, with very little excretion of urine. A right nephrectomy was performed. 2. Appearance of the left kidney, showing advanced hydronephrosis which was due to a uretero-pelvic stricture and which was treated by complete excision of the strictured zone, followed by anastomosis between pelvis and ureter (Fig. 359). 3. Intravenous urogram three weeks after operation, showing excellent excretion by the kidney, but no important diminution in size of the pelvis and calyces. 4. Intravenous urogram five years after operation, showing some reduction in size of the pelvis and calyces. The child was completely asymptomatic at this time. (Ten years after operation the child is in excellent health, has no symptoms, and has a clear urine.)

Flank Drainage

Following operation, drainage of the kidney fossa is seldom necessary when nephrectomy has been performed. However, in any case in which a ureter or pelvis has been opened, a soft rubber drain should be left running out the flank wound, to permit escape of urine if any should occur at the operative site. In those cases in which a catheter (or polyethylene tube) has been inserted as a ureteral strut and has been brought out the flank wound, we do not use in addition another drain, since any fluid can leak out around this tube.

Postoperative Measures

Postoperatively, chemotherapy or antibiotic therapy should be maintained for the combating of any infection which persists in the urinary tract; the intensity and duration of such therapy can be guided best by examination of the urinary sediment from time to time. Just how long such treatment will have to be maintained depends entirely upon the circumstances in any case. Generally, it can be stopped after a few weeks, but in some it might have to be continued for several months. Needless to say, any chemotherapy will probably be ineffective in controlling residual infection if obstruction has not been adequately relieved.

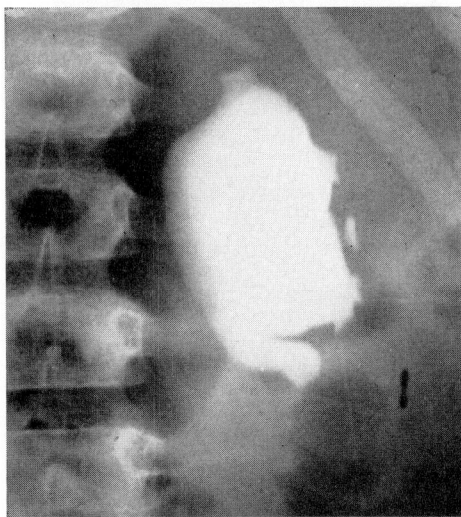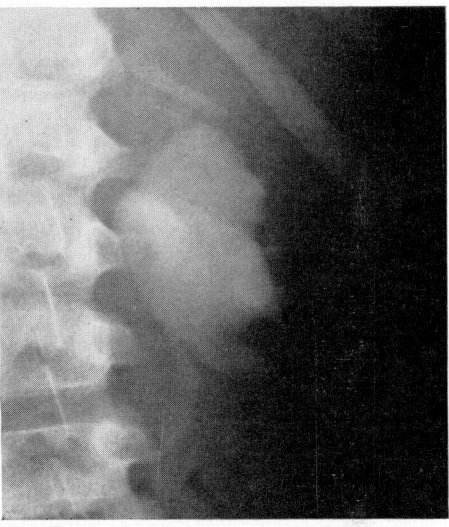

Fig. 369. Eight-year-old boy with left hydronephrosis on the basis of a uretero-pelvic stricture. *Left*, Retrograde pyelogram before operation, showing considerable hydronephrosis. Treatment by revision of strictured area with a Y-V plastic procedure. *Right*, Intravenous urogram eight months after operation; there is beginning diminution in the size of the pelvis. The child was completely asymptomatic at this time (and is completely well three years later).

Patients who have been operated upon for relief of uretero-pelvic obstruction (the kidney being saved) should have x-ray visualization of the urinary tract at subsequent times, to determine what has been accomplished and whether the situation is improving or deteriorating. Such examination might require cystoscopy and retrograde study, but in most instances the necessary information can be gathered by intravenous pyelography which, in addition to visualization of the region, gives a fair impression of the function of the kidney by the amount and concentration of the dye which is excreted. Little is learned by performing urographic examination within the early weeks or months after operation, unless there are some complications which warrant such a step; generally, there is not sufficient change during this period to justify the expense and trouble of making such a test. However, urography six months after surgery is of great interest and begins to give a fairly good idea whether the renal situation is getting better or worse. Depending upon the observations, such reevaluation should probably be repeated at intervals of six to twelve months for the subsequent few years.

RESULTS OF THERAPY

In our series of 145 patients there were 156 uretero-pelvic obstructions. In 7 instances no surgery was performed; in all of the remaining there was some operative correction, there being no operative fatality in any case.

Sixty-five obstructions were of an intrinsic type; in 23 of these therapy was by a primary nephrectomy, in 23 there was a resection of the stenotic area, with establishment of an anastomosis, in 10 there was a Y-V plastic to the strictured area, and in 9 there was dilation of the stricture through a pyelotomy wound.

For the 71 lesions in which there was extrinsic obstruction, there was a primary nephrectomy in 5, division of an aberrant vessel in 44, lysis of adhesive bands in 20

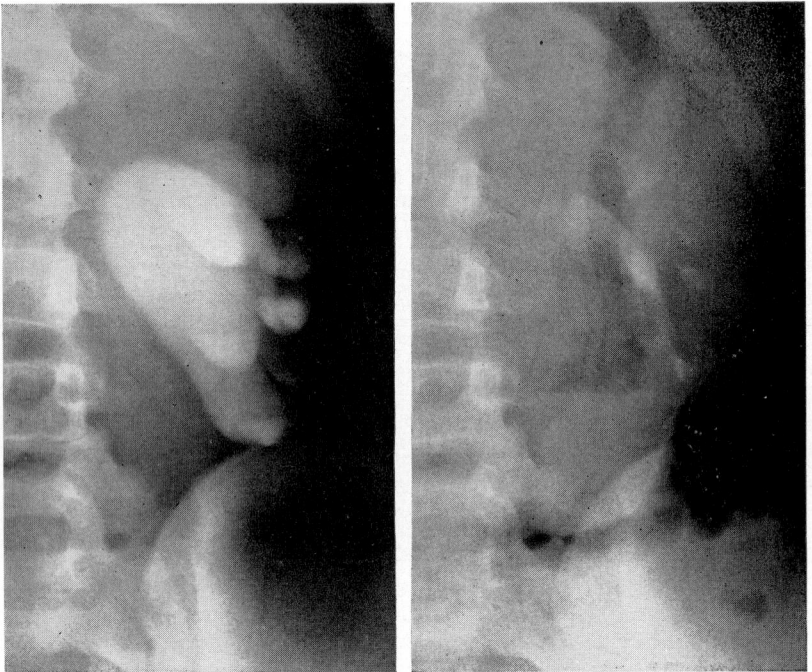

Fig. 370. Ten-year-old boy with marked left hydronephrosis, due to a uretero-pelvic stricture, which was treated by a Y-V plastic procedure (Fig. 360). *Left*, Appearance before operation. *Right*, Intravenous urogram two years after operation, showing marked improvement in the renal picture. The child is completely asymptomatic at this time.

(5 of these also had nephropexy), resection of a ureteral kink in one, removal of an overlying double ureter in one.

In 13 instances in which there were combined intrinsic and extrinsic lesions, there was primary nephrectomy in 5, a resection of the uretero-pelvic area in one, division of an aberrant vessel and treatment of an intrinsic stenosis in 7.

Of the 33 patients who had a primary nephrectomy, the opposite kidney being normal, all have remained free of any urinary trouble and appear to be in excellent health. This is distinctly in contrast to some of the patients who have been treated by "conservative" operative measures and who have had continuing symptoms and recurring urinary infection over a period of many years (some of whom have required secondary nephrectomy). This state of affairs makes us believe that in a few instances we have probably been too conservative; when we have made efforts to save a badly damaged kidney, it might have been better to perform a primary nephrectomy and thus give prompt and permanent relief of the child's difficulties.

To sum up the results after all types of operation in which the kidney was saved (116 instances), a rather extensive follow-up study was carried out in 1951; certain features were clear-cut and easily defined, whereas others were not. Three general evaluations could be made: these related to: (1) Relief of preexisting symptoms. (2) Correction of the urographic picture by intravenous or retrograde pyelography. (3) Control of urinary infection. Fulfillment of all three of these criteria has been listed as an "excellent" result. When there has been complete relief of symptoms and any preexisting infection, and there has been reasonably satisfactory reduction in the size of the renal pelvis (the kidney might drain well, but still have some hydronephrosis remaining), the result has been termed "good." When there has been persistence of pyuria, or progressing hydronephrosis, the result has been classified as "poor" or "failure."

An "excellent" result has been obtained in 48 per cent of the cases. A "good" result has been gained in an additional 25 per cent of the patients. A "poor" result has appeared in 27 per cent. In this latter group of 32 patients, 10 subsequently required secondary nephrectomy (one of these died a year later in uremia). In summary: of the 116 operations, 73 per cent made a satisfactory recovery ("excellent" and "good" group) and 27 per cent did not.

More detailed findings with reference to some of the particular procedures were as follows: (1) Of those who had division of an aberrant renal vessel, there was an "excellent" result in 50 per cent, a "good" result in 22 per cent, and a "poor" result in 28 per cent. (2) Of those who had division of an aberrant renal vessel plus dilation of an intrinsic stenosis, there was an "excellent" result in 60 per cent, a "good" result in 20 per cent, and a "poor" result in 20 per cent. (3) Of the cases treated by resection of a stenosis, there was an "excellent" result in 53 per cent, a "good" result in 19 per cent, and a "poor" result in 28 per cent. (4) Of those who had a plastic procedure to a strictured area, there was an "excellent" result in 33 per cent, a "good" result in 44 per cent, and a "poor" result in 23 per cent. (5) Of those who had dilation of a stenosis (through a pyelotomy) there was an "excellent" result in 22 per cent, a "good" result in 11 per cent, and a "poor" result in 67 per cent.

When conservative measures were employed for treatment of a uretero-pelvic obstruction (the kidney being saved), it was usually quite evident within a few months whether pyuria and symptomatology would be completely and permanently relieved, or whether one was faced with a long continued course in which close supervision (or secondary operation) would be required to combat pyelonephritis.

REFERENCES

1. Davis, D. M.: Intubated Ureterotomy. A New Operation for Ureteral and Ureteropelvic Stricture. Surg., Gynec. & Obst., 76: 513, 1943.
2. Deming, C. L.: Ureteropelvic Obstruction due to Extrinsic and Intrinsic Lesions of the Ureter as a Clinical Entity and Its Treatment. J. Urol., 50:420, 1943.
3. Foley, F. E. B.: A New Plastic Operation for Stricture at the Uretero-Pelvic Junction. J. Urol., 38:643, 1937.
4. Geraghty, J. T. and Frontz, W. A.: A Study

of Primary Hydronephrosis. J. Urol., 2: 161, 1918.
5. Gibson, T. E.: Hydronephrosis. Classification and Plastic Repair of Ureteropelvic Obstructions. Surg., Gynec. & Obst., 80: 485, 1945.
6. Henline, R. B. and Menning, J. H.: The Management of Hydronephrosis due to Ureteropelvic Obstruction: Preliminary Report. J. Urol., 50:1, 1943.
7. Lubash, S. and Madrid, A.: Ureteropyeloneostomy for Hydronephrosis with Case and

Experimental Reports. J. Urol., *38*:634, 1937.

8. Quinby, W. C.: Factors Influencing the Operative Procedure in Hydronephrosis. J. Urol., *38*:673, 1937.

9. Schreiber, M.: Ureteral Stricture, Its Anatomical and Pathological Background. Surg., Gynec. & Obst., *45*:423, 1927.

10. Soley, P. J.: Ureteropelvic Obstruction in Children. Incidence and Etiology. J. Urol., *55*:46, 1946.

11. Walters, W., Cabot, H., and Priestley, J. T.: Operative Results in Non-Calculus Hydronephrosis. Results in 71 Plastic Operations. J. Urol., *38*:688, 1937.

12. White, R. R. and Wyatt, G. M.: Surgical Importance of the Aberrant Renal Vessel in Infants and Children. Am. J. Surg., *58*:48, 1942.

CHAPTER 49

Double Ureters

Duplications of kidneys and ureters are common anomalies of the urinary tract. Ureters may be doubled throughout their entire length, having separate openings into the bladder, or they may have an incomplete fission (Y-shaped ureter), the lower part of the system having but a single orifice in the bladder. Duplications may appear on either side; they may be bilateral. A vast literature has grown up concerning observations on, and therapy for, persons with these various anomalies. The following remarks are made largely from a study of 145 infants and children at the Boston Children's Hospital (1926 through 1950) who were found to have duplication of the ureter either when investigated during life (109 cases) or when examined at the autopsy table (36 specimens). Some data on the anatomic findings in these are listed in Table 72.

Table 72

Anatomic Varieties of Ureteral Duplication in 145 Infants and Children
(From 109 Patients and 36 Autopsies)

Anatomic Configuration	Male	Female
Left double ureter	12	46
Right double ureter	14	27
Bilateral double ureters	4	15
Left Y-shaped ureter	1	6
Right Y-shaped ureter	7	4
Bilateral Y-shaped ureters	0	3
Double ureters on left, Y-shaped on right	2	1
Double ureters on right, Y-shaped on left	0	1
Right double ureter, upper ureter ectopic in vagina or urethra	0	2
Totals	40 (22%)	105 (78%)

PATHOLOGIC OBSERVATIONS

Renal Structure. A kidney may have a double appearance, with a marked constriction between its two segments, or the renal substance may appear to be a single unit, emptied by two drainage systems. The two pelves may drain equal amounts of renal tissue, but in general the upper one is a much smaller system and represents only 15 to 30 per cent of the renal mass. Intercommunication between duplicated pelves is exceedingly rare.

Ureteral Conformation. In about 85 per cent of cases, the ureters which drain double renal pelves run as completely separate structures all the way to the bladder, into which they open independently. With but very rare exceptions, the ureter draining the upper renal pelvis enters the trigone in a position lower than its mate. In about 15 per cent of cases, the two ureters have a Y configuration, only one ureter entering the bladder. Double ureters are held together closely by virtue of the fact that they are within the confines of the long, narrow, and tubular Gerota's fascia which encompasses them down to the bladder.

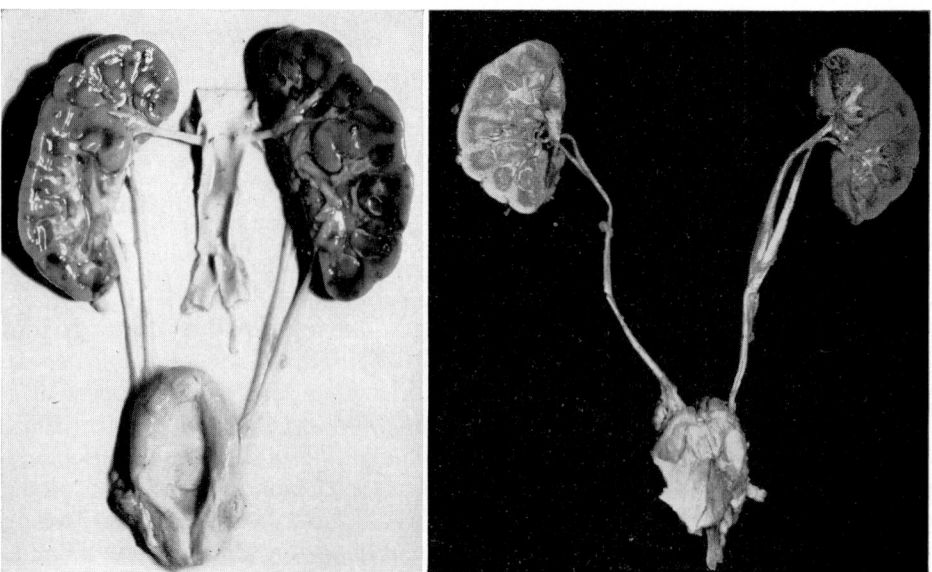

Fig. 371. *Left*, Photograph of double ureters, showing complete duplication of ureter on either side. Eight-month-old child who had extensive pyelonephritis, myriads of punctate renal abscesses, and bacteremia. *Right*, Y-shaped ureters, viewed from behind; the branches join at different levels on the two sides.

Obstruction. With complete doubling of ureters on one side, it is quite common to have mild obstruction of the ureter which runs from the larger, lower pelvis because the other ureter is curved and angulated around it. The compression might not be great, but the fact that one ureter lies against the other is believed by some to interfere with peristaltic activity. Hydronephrosis from such a mechanism is seldom more than mild or moderate degree. When marked distention of a pelvis (or pelves) is seen in conjunction with double ureters, there is almost always some other obstructive factor such as an aberrant renal vessel, an intrinsic uretero-pelvic block, or a ureterocele at the lower end of the ureter.

Pyelonephritis. While double ureters, whether complete or incomplete, can be tolerated through a long life without complications, a considerable number of them give rise to difficulties, generally in the form of superimposed infection. There may be varying degrees of pyelitis or pyelonephritis, involving either segment of the kidney and its drainage tract. Generally speaking, incomplete divisions are far less apt to be accompanied by infection than are the complete duplications of a ureter.

Other Anomalies. Double ureters are apt to be accompanied by other malformations in the urinary tract, a finding in nearly 20 per cent of our patients.

It is not uncommon to have formation of a ureterocele in conjunction with a double ureter. When this association occurs, the uterocele is almost always of that ureter which empties lowest in the trigone (and is therefore connected to the upper pole of the kidney on this side).

In an occasional case, one of double ureters may open in an ectopic position beyond the bladder outlet, in the urethra, in the vestibule, or in the vagina; when this occurs, it is almost always the ureter draining the upper renal pole which drains ectopically. (Whenever an ectopic ureteral opening is found outside of the bladder, it almost always implies that there are double ureters on one side.)

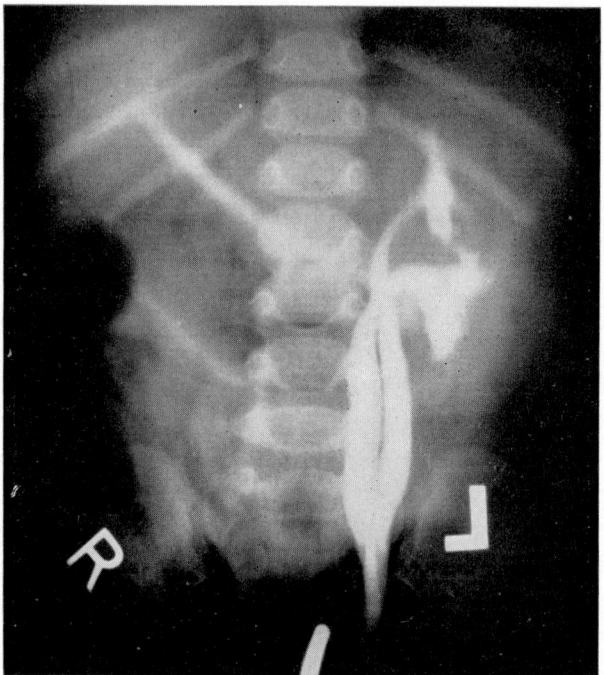

Fig. 372. Roentgenogram of Y-shaped ureter on left side. The two ureteral limbs join and make a single ureter entering the bladder (there being one ureteral orifice in a normal position on the left side of the trigone).

Side Involved. Sex. These anomalies are somewhat more common on the left side than on the right; there is a bilateral abnormality in nearly 20 per cent of cases. The malformations are far more frequent in females than males.

CLINICAL FINDINGS

Symptoms

Duplication of ureters is often completely asymptomatic and is discovered only during some routine study of a patient, or is incidentally found at autopsy examination. Not uncommonly, however, the anomaly gives rise to important symptomatology, among which urinary infection, pyuria, and fever are outstanding. In study of our patients who had symptoms from the urinary malformations, the following findings occurred in the percentages indicated:

	%
Pyuria	63
Pyrexia	45
Abdominal pain	39
Loss of urinary control	31
Elevated NPN	18
Weight loss	12
Flank pain	10
Hematuria	10
Elevated blood pressure	5

The most common picture is that of a child who, because of abdominal pain, fever, dysuria, or frequency, is studied and is found to have pus in the urine and who, on in-

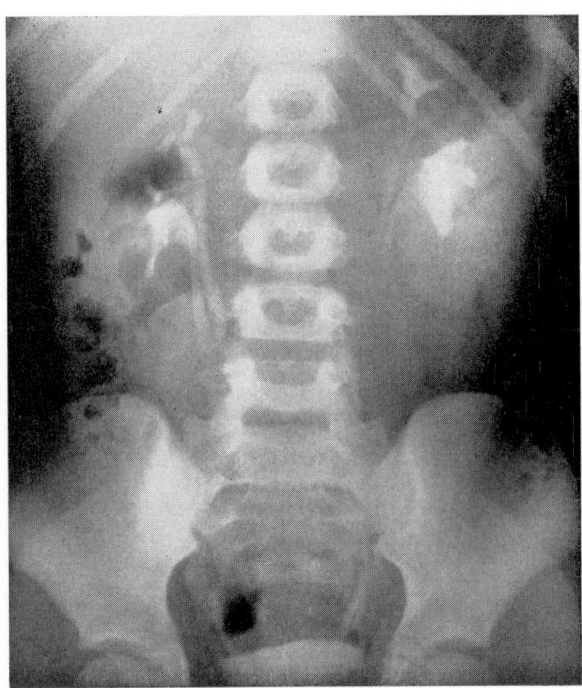

Fig. 373. Bilateral double ureters in a six-year-old girl. Incidental urographic findings. Child had no pyuria and no complaints which could be attributed to the urinary tract abnormality. No therapy necessary.

vestigation by intravenous urography, is found to have duplication of a kidney pelvis or ureter. Whenever there has been pain, the localization of it to the side of the pathology has generally been quite poor.

The average age of our patients when first studied was 5.1 years. The average duration of symptoms was 6 to 8 months. There was a frequent finding of weight loss or failure to gain weight. Because of hydronephrosis, an enlarged kidney occasionally could be palpated through the abdominal wall; giant hydronephrosis was very rare. Elevation of the non-protein nitrogen of the plasma was found only when there was bilateral abnormality or when there were other associated anomalies in the urinary system. With stasis in some part of the urinary system, stones may appear; they were found in two of our patients.

Ureteral Ectopia

In occasional cases, duplications of the ureter are combined with an ectopia of one of them; it empties into the urethra beyond the bladder sphincter or else opens in some area outside of the urinary tract; a discussion of this subject is given in Chapter 50. The anomalous opening might be in the urethra, anywhere in the vulva (particularly to one side of the urethral meatus), in the vagina, or in the uterus. Under any of these circumstances there will be a constant dribbling of urine day and night. This perpetual wetness of the perineum is in spite of the fact that the child does at normal intervals empty the bladder of urine; investigation of the bladder shows it to be of normal capacity and function. While it is possible for a single ureter to empty in an ectopic position outside of the bladder, the presence of an ectopic ureteral orifice generally implies that there are double ureters on the involved side.

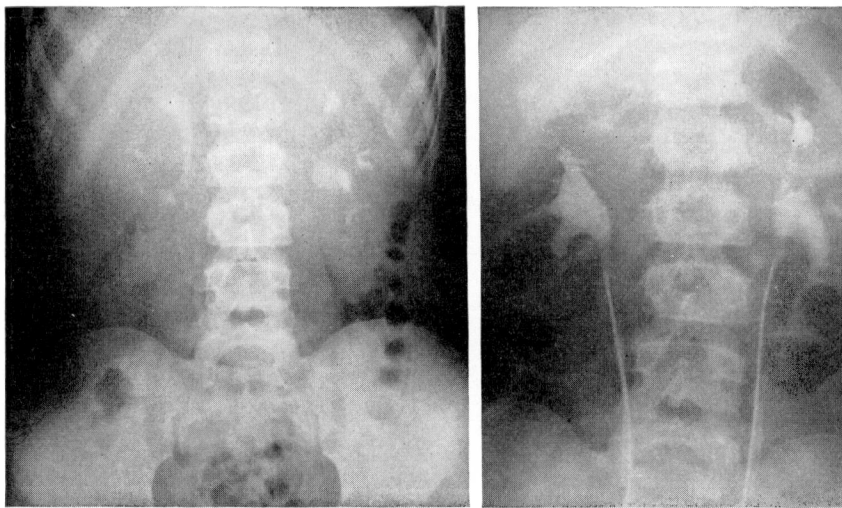

Fig. 374. Urograms from a child who had a single ureter on the left side and double pelves and complete duplication of ureters on her right. *Left*, Intravenous urogram with a suggestion of a duplication on both sides. *Right*, Retrograde pyelogram; catheterization and injection of the ureteric orifice which lay in a normal position on the right side of the trigone filled only the lower three-quarters of the kidney (compared to the intravenous urographic picture). Completed studies showed that there are double pelves and ureters on patient's right, one ureter of which opened in the vestibule. On patient's left there is a single pelvis with an elongated upper calyx.

Recognition of the Anomaly

Generally, double ureters can be suspected or can be accurately diagnosed by the findings of intravenous pyelography. By this method it may be possible to visualize very well and in their entirety the double pelves and also the ureters which are draining them. There may be dilatation of one or the other incomplete pelvis; generally, if there is any hydronephrosis it is of the lower portion. It is not uncommon to obtain visualization of only a part of the system, and one does not gain a complete picture of the extent of the malformation. There might be good concentration of dye in one pelvis and its ureter, but because of the smallness of this pelvis (in relation to the size of the renal mass) it leaves one with the suggestion that there might be another pelvis which has not shown up. Under these circumstances, cystoscopy and retrograde studies are in order.

Cystoscopy

Study by cystoscopic means is often necessary to gain complete knowledge about the position and character of the ureteral openings in the bladder and to delineate accurately the size of the ureters and their relation to one another. Furthermore, there may be other types of abnormality in the urinary tract which can be discovered by such investigation. If there is any concurrent pyuria, the sampling of urine from various parts of the drainage system will give information regarding the focus of the infection. Divided excretion of phenolsulfonphthalein from the different parts of a kidney might give a clue regarding the functional status of each, but generally, such an examination is not too satisfactory. One can more accurately gain an idea of the size of the renal segment which is drained by each ureter by visualizing each individual pelvis and thereby estimating what proportion of the total renal mass it represents.

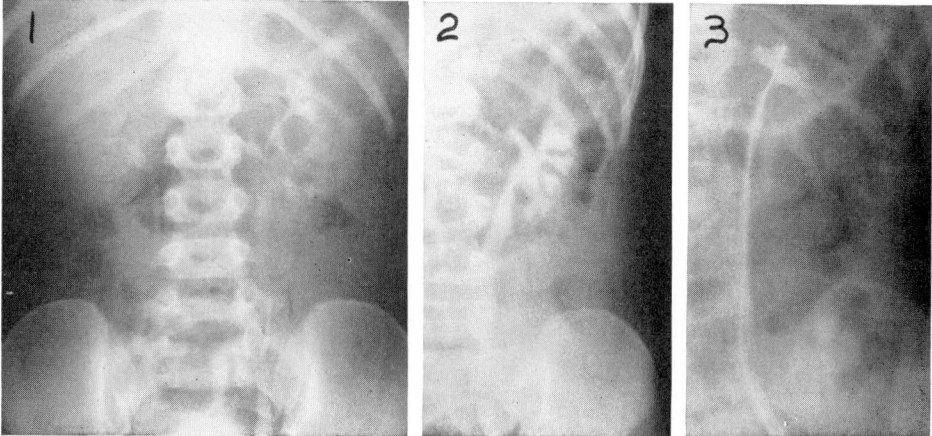

Fig. 375. Films from a girl who had persistent pyuria. 1. Intravenous urogram faintly suggesting duplication of pelvis and possibly of the ureter on the patient's left. 2. Retrograde injection of *upper* ureteric orifice on patient's left, visualizing a ureter and the lower portion of the kidney. 3. Injection of *lower* ureteric orifice, visualizing the upper segment of kidney on patient's left. Subsequently treated by a heminephrectomy, removing the lower portion of the kidney from which the pus had come.

TREATMENT

No Therapy

Many patients with double ureters will never require any specific therapy; slightly more than half of our patients have not needed surgery during the periods they have been followed. If there are no complaints which can be related to the urologic abnormality, if there is no important obstruction, and if there is no pyuria, nothing need be done. It is not uncommon to see patients with double ureters go through a long life with absolutely no symptoms therefrom.

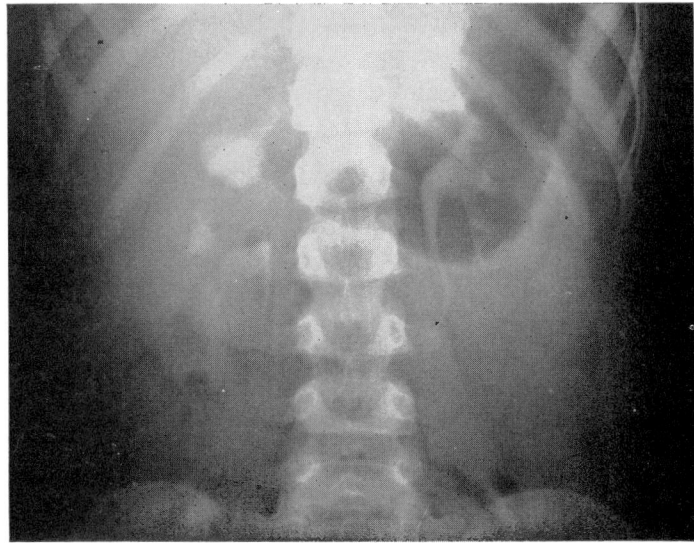

Fig. 376. Roentgenogram from a girl who had a normal renal architecture on her left and double pelves with complete duplication of ureter on her right. Exudate came from the upper segment of renal substance. Subsequently treated by right upper heminephrectomy.

Antibiotics

If there is pyuria, and no significant degree of obstruction, it is permissible, and generally successful, to treat the patient with chemotherapy or antibiotics. A drug with a broad spectrum of antibacterial activity is desirable, such as aureomycin or terramycin. If these are not effective in bringing infection under control in a reasonable time, a urine culture might probably show a type of organism calling for some other agent which is more potent against the particular bacterium. While an intense course of aureomycin or terramycin may be necessary to bring a pyuria under control, small doses of Gantrisin, continued over periods of weeks or months, are often desirable to avoid recrudecsence of infection.

Heminephrectomy

For those patients whose pyuria cannot be brought under control by drug therapy, or in whom there are symptoms or x-ray findings indicative of obstruction, the operation which has been found to be most useful is that of partial nephrectomy. It is possible to remove a portion of the renal substance (Fig. 377), leaving a part which is essentially normal and which can function in a satisfactory manner. Either the upper or the lower segment of a kidney can be excised, but as a rule the superior is the smaller of the two, has the poorest urinary flow, and is the one which should be sacrificed. Even if the lower (and larger) part of the kidney is the one whose pelvis is dilated and which has been demonstrated to be the source of the pyuria, it is still generally advisable to excise the upper segment, as the removal of this ureter will allow the ureter of the lower kidney pole to lie in a better position and to be relieved of its obstruction.

The ureter which is to be excised (usually the one from the upper renal pole) is severed at a very low level, a point of great significance, because only in this way can the *remaining* ureter be given a free and unobstructed course. Gerota's fascia should be split open along the ureters as far down as can be reached, and the ureter to be removed then cut off quite close to the bladder.

Blood vessels for the two units of a kidney often connect directly to the aorta and vena cava, a situation which simplifies removal of one renal segment. More commonly, the blood supply to the smaller pole branches off of the main renal vessels; even so, they can be dissected out and can be divided while sparing the vascular supply of the part of the kidney which is to be left. The main renal artery should always be isolated so it can be clamped temporarily during the cutting apart of the two portions of kidney, in this way minimizing bleeding from the cut surfaces.

It is always well to strip back the renal capsule from the part to be removed, leaving it attached to the segment which is to remain. This flap will be of use later in the closure of the transected renal surface.

Severance of the two parts of a kidney is facilitated by distending with fluid the pelvis of the part which is to be removed. This clearly defines its borders; dissection can then be carried from the renal hilus outward, staying close to this distended pelvis, making a sharp dissection out through the renal parenchyma. If possible, the cuts through the renal tissue should be made in a wedge-shaped manner, which will facilitate closure of the renal stump which remains. It is generally possible to cut apart the two renal masses without entering either pelvis. With a serrefine clamp temporarily on the renal artery, there is little or no bleeding during the renal division; any tiny vessels projecting up from the cut renal surface should be sutured with figure-of-eight fine chromic catgut stitches. It does not appear to do harm to leave a serrefine clamp on the renal artery for fifteen to thirty minutes; an occasional patient will develop a transient hyper-

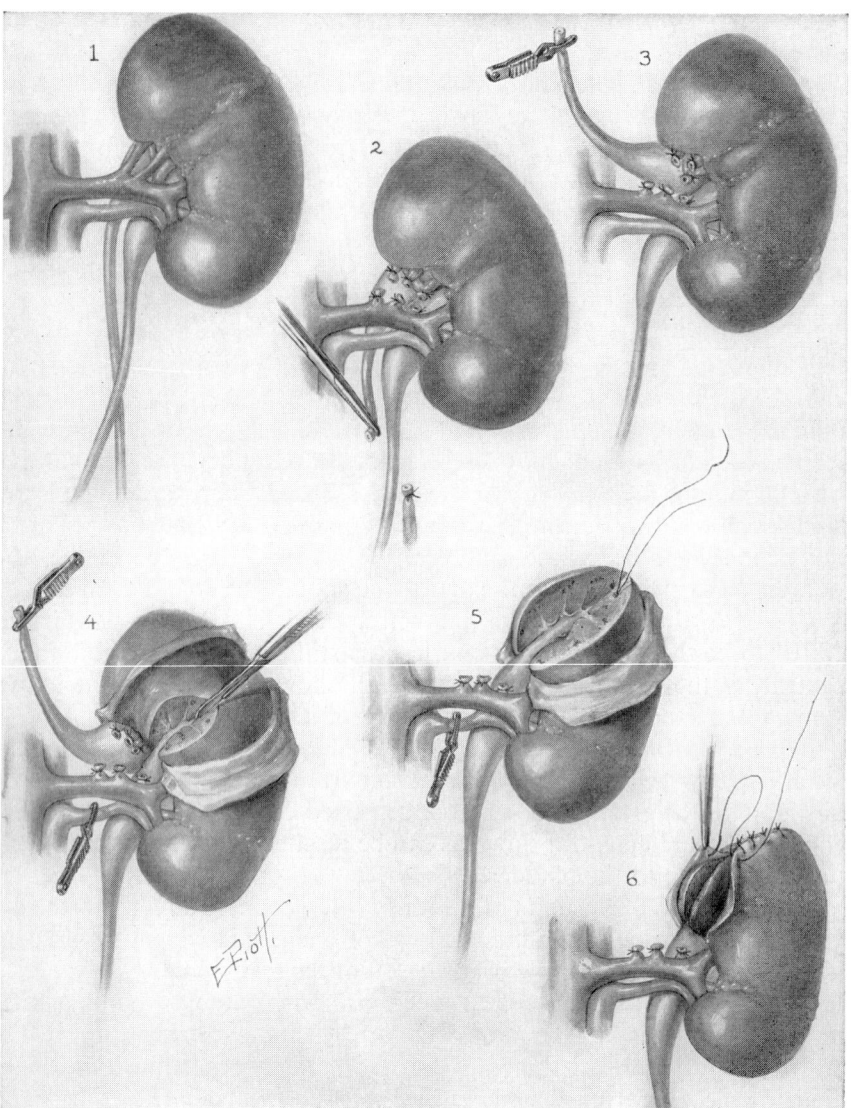

Fig. 377. Operative steps for heminephrectomy in cases in which there is a double pelvis. 1. The pathologic anatomy, showing duplication of pelves and ureters. The ureters cross one another, which often gives an obstruction of the ureter which drains the lower pelvis. 2. Severance of ureter draining upper pole of the kidney, making sure that this division is done below the point where the ureters cross one another. Gerota's fascia must be slit open enough so that the remaining ureter will not be constricted or angulated in any way. Division of artery and vein which supply rudimentary upper pole of the kidney. Generally, these branches come off of the main renal artery and vein, though in some instances they have a separate supply from the aorta and vena cava. 3. Ureter draining the upper renal pole has been pulled upward and also has been distended with saline so that the margins of the upper pelvis can thereby be identified clearly during subsequent dissection. 4. A small serrefine clamp is placed temporarily on the main renal artery. The renal capsule is incised along a line superior to that where the renal substance will be cut. This flap of capsule is turned backward and is saved for the subsequent closure of the raw end of the kidney. Dissection is begun through renal substance, carrying this outward between the two renal pelves. The dissection is made very close to the upper pelvis, so that the lower one can be left uninjured and unopened. 5. The upper pole of the kidney and its drainage apparatus have been completely cut away. The pelvis of the lower portion of the kidney is left

tension during the first postoperative day, but it always disappears within twenty-four to forty-eight hours.

The raw end of the remaining portion of kidney is now closed by bringing together with silk stitches the flaps of renal capsule. This maneuver folds inward the kidney substance and makes a substantial closure.

Leakage is rare but it is well to place a soft rubber drain from the kidney bed out through the flank wound; it can be withdrawn in two or three days.

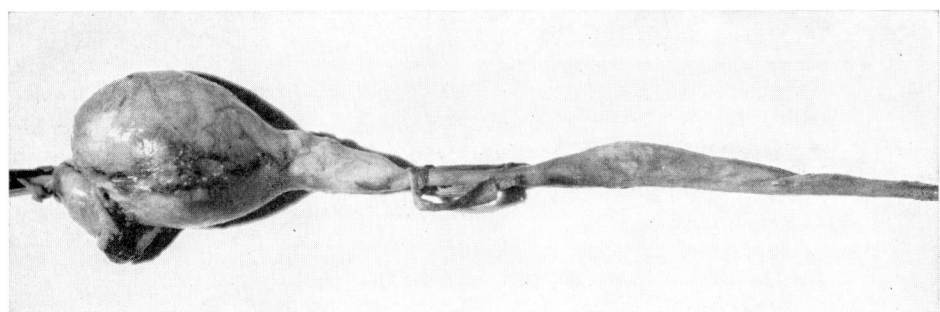

Fig. 378. Photograph of specimen removed at upper pole heminephrectomy. The dilated pelvis can be seen. Very little renal substance has supplied this portion of the drainage system, in which there has been extensive infection.

Uretero-Ureterostomy

Theoretically, such an operation would have some merit in saving all of the renal parenchyma. The ureter from the upper segment can be severed and its end implanted into the ureter (or the pelvis) of the lower system, thereby creating a more active flow through the remaining ureter. While this operation has at times been successful, it is probably better therapy to perform a heminephrectomy, removing the small segment which is functioning poorly, which is generally infected, which has a poor urinary flow, and which is seldom worth saving.

Nephrectomy

When the entire kidney is seriously diseased from the outset, or when there has been a failure after a previous conservative operation such as heminephrectomy, the kidney must be excised, removing as well as much of the ureter as can be reached through the flank wound.

Treatment of Ureterocele

While a ureterocele can exist at the lower end of a single ureter, not uncommonly it is found at the base of a ureter which is part of a duplicate system. The ureterocele must be treated by some procedure which opens it up and allows it to drain adequately. In older children, a ureterocele can be managed by cystoscopic manipulation, enlarging the ureteral opening with cystoscopic scissors or with an endothermy cutting instrument.

---

uninjured. The cut across the renal substance has been made in a V-shaped manner, which will facilitate later closure of the raw end of the kidney. With a momentary release of the serrefine clamp from the renal pedicle, any major vessels can be identified. These are now closed with fine chromic catgut sutures. 6. Closure of the raw end of the kidney. It is generally best to avoid sutures in the friable renal substance. It is wholly satisfactory to coapt the ends of the kidney by sutures through the renal capsule. No wad of fat, absorbable oxidized gauze, or other hemostatic mass is necessary. The field is completely dry.

Table 73

Therapy and Results of Treatment for 109 Patients with Duplicated Ureters
(1926 through 1950)

A. Unilateral Complete Double Ureters.................................... 70 patients
    1. No operation.. 45
        Good result............................. 38
        Poor result.............................. 6
        Dead..................................... 1
    2. Nephrectomy.. 6
        Good result.............................. 6
    3. Upper heminephrectomy............................. 13
        Good result.............................. 9
        Poor result.............................. 3
        Nephrectomy later........................ 1
    4. Lower heminephrectomy............................. 3
        Good result.............................. 3
    5. Uretero-ureterostomy............................... 1
        Good result.............................. 1
    6. Retrograde dilation of ureters....................... 2
        Good result.............................. 1
        Died..................................... 1
B. Bilateral Complete Double Ureters.. 14 patients
    1. No operation.. 9
        Good result.............................. 7
        Poor result.............................. 2
    2. Unilateral heminephrectomy......................... 2
        Good result.............................. 1
        Poor result.............................. 1
    3. Bilateral heminephrectomy.......................... 1
        Poor result.............................. 1
    4. Retrograde dilation of ureters....................... 1
        Poor result.............................. 1
    5. Nephrolithotomy................................... 1
        Good result.............................. 1
C. Unilateral Y-shaped Ureters... 3 patients
    1. No operation.. 3
        Good result.............................. 3
D. Double Ureters on One Side, Y-shaped Ureters on Other Side.................. 2 patients
    1. No operation.. 1
        Poor result.............................. 1
    2. Bilateral heminephrectomy.......................... 1
        Good result.............................. 1
E. Unilateral Complete Double Ureters, with Other Anomalies.................... 15 patients
    Posterior Urethral Valve
    1. Suprapubic cystostomy............................. 1
        Died..................................... 1
    2. Cystostomy and Nephrectomy........................ 1
        Poor result.............................. 1
    Ipsilateral Ureterocele
    1. Incision of Ureterocele............................. 8
        Poor result.............................. 1
        Died..................................... 1
        Heminephrectomy later................... 3
        Nephrectomy later........................ 3
    Contralateral Ureterocele
    1. Incision of ureterocele.............................
        Poor result.............................. 1

Table 73 (continued)

Uretero-pelvic Obstruction
    1. Division aberrant vessel............................... 2
        Good result............................... 1
        Poor result............................... 1
Upper Ureter Ending Ectopic in Vagina or Urethra
    1. Heminephrectomy...................................... 2
        Good result............................... 2
F. Bilateral Complete Double Ureters, with Other Anomalies...................... 5 patients
Unilateral Ureteroceles
    1. Incision of ureterocele................................. 3
        Poor result............................... 1
        Dead....................................... 1
        Heminephrectomy later...................... 1
Bilateral Ureteroceles
    1. Incision of ureteroceles.............................. 1
        Poor result............................... 1
Uretero-pelvic Obstruction, Unilateral
    1. Uretero-pyelostomy.................................. 1
        Good result............................... 1

We believe it is safer and better in all babies and small children to open a ureterocele under direct vision through a suprapubic cystotomy. The slit should be made 3 to 5 mm. in length.

It has been our experience that ureteroceles which arise from a single ureter (where there is no duplication) can be treated with a high degree of success by simple incision of the uterocele; following this there is a good flow of urine and a rapid subsidence of any infection. In contrast, incision of a ureterocele which is from one of double ureters is followed by failure in the vast majority of cases. Presumably, the ureter subsequently has only a small flow of urine through it, drains only a rudimentary upper pole of a kidney, and does not have a sufficient flushing of urine to clear the stream of infection. Therefore, if prompt relief does not follow the local treatment of a ureterocele (which is part of a double system), heminephrectomy should be undertaken as a secondary operation.

Treatment of Other Urologic Anomalies

It is well to remember that in about one-fifth of patients with double ureters there are other anomalies in the urinary tract which demand surgical attack. For instance, there might be some obstruction at the bladder outlet requiring specific therapy or there might be uretero-pelvic obstruction from stricture or aberrant vessel, the treatment of which will allow the kidney to be spared.

RESULTS OF THERAPY

A detailed analysis of therapy for our 109 patients is listed in Table 73; this indicates the types of conditions treated, the form of operations undertaken, and the end results which have been achieved. Some summarizing statements regarding the over-all picture follow.

In the 109 patients who were known to have some form of double ureters, the condition did not require any therapy (or could be handled satisfactorily by medical measures) in 58. In the entire group of 109 patients, 4 died either in the hospital or in the subsequent few years from the ravages of urinary tract disease. Of the 51 who required surgery, one kidney was so damaged from the outset that primary nephrectomy was performed in 6.

The most common operation utilized was that of heminephrectomy, which was performed on 28 kidneys (26 patients, 2 of whom had bilateral heminephrectomies). Of the 28 heminephrectomies, 3 were for removal of a lower pole and 25 for excision of the smaller upper segment. In the patients who had heminephrectomy, there was generally a temporary occlusion of the main renal artery for fifteen to twenty minutes during operation; in a few of these a mild hypertension was noted in the ensuing twenty-four to thirty-six hours, but in no case did it last more than two days. Of the 28 heminephrectomies, 21 had a completely satisfactory postoperative course, 6 had a poor result (some persistence or recurrence of complaints or pyuria), and 1 subsequently required a nephrectomy.

Of the 109 patients with duplication of the ureter, 20 had other serious malformations in the urinary tract requiring therapy; among these, ureterocele was the most common anomaly. When occurring on the side where there were double ureters (as was the finding in most instances), the ureterocele was always at the site of the *lower* ureteric orifice (which was supplied by the upper segment of kidney on that side). While it has been our experience (Chapter 51) that incision of a ureterocele which arises in conjunction with a solitary ureter has generally given an excellent result, similar treatment of ureteroceles which are in conjunction with double ureters has been most disappointing. Presumably, the opening up of this latter type of ureterocele is followed by only a small flow of urine (since it is fed by only a tiny segment of kidney) and there is insufficient flushing to rid this part of the system of infection. Therefore, the incision of a ureterocele (which arises from one of double ureters) has generally been followed by a bad result and has had to be followed by a heminephrectomy or nephrectomy.

In the 109 patients with some form of duplication of the ureters, there were 2 in whom one of the ureters opened in an ectopic position outside the bladder trigone. They were treated successfully by heminephrectomy; because of the special interests and problems presented by this small group of cases, they are separately described in the following chapter.

Many of the patients included in this series of 109 cases were treated before chemotherapy or antibiotic agents were available and therefore the over-all picture of results is probably not as good as those which can be attained today when these potent drugs are widely employed.

REFERENCES

1. Adams, P. S.: Ureterocele: Treatment by Transurethral Resection. Am. J. Surg., *50:* 249, 1940.
2. Beer, E. and Mencher, W. H.: Heminephrectomy in Disease of the Double Kidney. Ann. Surg., *108:*705, 1938.
3. Burstein, H. J.: Double Kidney with Y-Shaped Ureter and Ureteral Calculus in an Infant. Urol. & Cut. Rev., *42:*575, 1938.
4. Campbell, M. F.: Uretero-heminephrectomy in Infancy. J. Urol., *26:*433, 1931.
5. Campbell, M. F.: Hemipyonephrosis in Infants and Children. Treatment by Heminephrectomy. Am. J. Surg., *21:*85, 1933.
6. Cornwell, P. M.: Giant Hydronephrosis in a Duplicated Kidney. J. Urol., *55:*238, 1946.
7. Gibson, T. E.: Hydronephrosis. Classification and Plastic Repair of Ureteropelvic Obstruction. Surg., Gynec. & Obst., *80:*485, 1945.
8. Goyanna, R. and Greene, L. F.: The Pathologic and Anomalous Conditions Associated with Duplication of the Renal Pelvis and Ureter. J. Urol., *54:*1, 1945.
9. Greene, L. F.: Duplication of the Renal Pelvis and Ureter. S. Clin. North America, *24:* 910, 1944.
10. Gutierrez, R.: Double Kidney as a Source of

Impaired Dynamism. Its Surgical Treatment by Heminephrectomy. Am. J. Surg., 65:256, 1944.

11. Hanley, H. G.: Blind-Ending Duplication of the Ureter. Brit. J. Urol., 17:50, 1945.

12. Hanley, H. G.: Discussion on Partial Nephrectomy. Proc. Royal Soc. Med., 43:1027, 1950.

13. Hawthorne, A. B.: The Embryologic and Clinical Aspect of Double Ureter. J.A.M.A., 106:189, 1936.

14. Hess, E.: Heminephrectomy; Its Indications and Limitations. J. Urol. 38:43, 1937.

15. Higgins, T. T.: Anomalies of Ureter in Childhood. Brit. J. Urol., 22:145, 1950.

16. Lowsley, O. S. and Kirwin, T. J.: Clinical Urology. Vol. 2, Chapter 38. Operative and Non-Operative Treatment of the Kidney. Heminephrectomy. Williams and Wilkins Company, Baltimore, 1944.

17. Lund, A. J.: Uncrossed Double Ureter with Rare Intravesical Orifice Relationship. J. Urol., 62:22, 1949.

18. Meyer, R.: Normal and Abnormal Development of the Ureter in the Human Embryo —A Mechanistic Consideration. Anat. Rec., 96:355, 1946.

19. Nation, E. F.: Duplication of the Kidney and Ureter: A Statistical Study of 230 New Cases. J. Urol., 51:456, 1944.

20. Smith, E. C. and Lazarus, A. O.: A Clinical and Statistical Study of 471 Congenital Anomalies of the Kidney and Ureter. J. Urol., 53:11, 1946.

21. Smith, I.: Triplicate Ureter. Brit. J. Surg., 34:182, 1946.

22. Wehrbein, H. L.: Double Kidney, Double Ureter, and Bilocular Bladder in a Child. J. Urol., 43:804, 1940.

23. Young, H. H. and Davis, E. G.: Double Ureter and Kidney with Calculous Pyonephrosis of One Half: Cure by Resection. The Embryology and Surgery of Double Ureter and Kidney. J. Urol., 1:17, 1917.

CHAPTER 50

Ectopic Ureter

Instead of its terminus being placed normally in the trigone of the bladder, a ureter may end in an ectopic position, either within the bladder, beyond the bladder sphincters, or in other portions of the genito-urinary tract. While ureteral ectopia is rather uncommon, it is very important to recognize this abnormality because much can be accomplished by surgical means for the child who is so afflicted. Our observations come from 8 patients with ureteral ectopia who were treated up to September 1, 1952.

PATHOLOGIC CONSIDERATIONS

When there is a single ureter on one side, this structure can open in an ectopic position. However, it is generally found that when there is an ectopic ureteral orifice outside of the bladder, this comes from a ureter which is one of a pair on this side of the body. The ectopic ureteral orifice almost invariably drains the upper pole of the kidney on the same side. Since the ureter involved usually drains only a small upper segment of kidney, the flow of fluid from it is generally of only small amount.

Low Opening in Bladder

An ectopic ureteral orifice can be situated very low in the trigone of the bladder, in which case there will be no dribbling, but since the terminal portion of the ureter becomes compressed by the contracting bladder sphincters, that portion of the urinary system which is drained by the ureter becomes blocked; pyuria can supervene and pyelonephritis can develop in the obstructed portion of the kidney.

Ureteral Opening Beyond Bladder Sphincter or Elsewhere

Ectopic ureteral orifices are far more common in females than they are in males. All of our patients were girls; Campbell's experience has been similar to this. In the male, an ectopic ureter can drain into a seminal vesicle, a vas deferens, or into the posterior urethra. Urinary incontinence is generally absent in the male since the ectopic orifice is almost always situated above the competent external urinary sphincter. The predominating clinical picture is urinary infection, which on investigation is found to reside in the upper urinary tract. In the female, the most common location for an accessory orifice is in the introitus immediately alongside of the external urethral meatus. Almost as commonly, they open directly into the urethra. Occasional ones have emptied into the vagina or even into the uterus. With great rarity, the accessory ureter can discharge into the rectum.

Presence of Obstruction

The ectopic ureteral orifice usually drains a system which is unobstructed. However, in an occasional case the orifice may be so tiny and contracted that this portion of the

Page 672

urinary tract is obstructed, giving a mild or moderate hydronephrosis or a superimposed infection in that part of the kidney which is involved.

Cases Found in Literature

According to Abeshouse,[1] a review of the reported cases discloses that an ectopic ureter occurs as often on the right side as on the left, regardless of whether the ureter is of the single or of the supernumerary variety. He reported the anomalous opening of a ureter into the uterus and cited 4 other such cases from the previous literature.

In 1949 Burford et al.[3] made an extensive review of the subject of ectopic ureter and collected 404 cases on which statistics were available; rare patients had two ectopic openings. The distributions of the anomalous orifices were as follows:

Males—104 cases

Bladder	5
Posterior urethra	49
Prostatic utricle	13
Seminal vesicle	26
Ejaculatory ducts	7
Vas deferens	6
Rectum	1
	107 sites

Females—300 cases

Bladder	21
Urethra	100
Vestibule	107
Vagina	68
Cervix or uterus	11
Gartner's duct	2
Rectum	2
	311 sites

In classifying ectopic ureters from a standpoint depending upon the type of kidney drained by the anomalous ureter, Burford et al. make the following summary of published material (418 ectopic openings in 404 cases):

1. Unilateral single ureter (normal kidney) with ectopic opening ... 66 instances
2. Bilateral single ureter (normal kidney) with bilateral ectopic openings ... 13
3. Unilateral complete duplication of the pelvis and ureter (double kidney) with ectopic opening of one or both ureters ... 256
   a. Ureter from upper pelvis ... 164
   b. Ureter from lower pelvis ... 6
   c. Both ureters ... 5
   d. Type not stated ... 81
4. Bilateral complete duplication of pelvis and ureter ... 60
   a. With unilateral ectopic opening ... 39
   b. With bilateral ectopic opening ... 21
5. Congenital solitary kidney with ectopic opening ... 10
6. Congenital ectopic kidney (pelvic dystopia) with ectopic ureteral opening ... 2
7. Horseshoe kidney with ectopic opening of one ureter ... 2
8. Unilateral complete triplication of pelvis and ureter with ectopic opening of one or more ureters ... 2
   a. With single ectopic opening ... 1
   b. With two ectopic openings ... 1
9. Type not stated ... 7

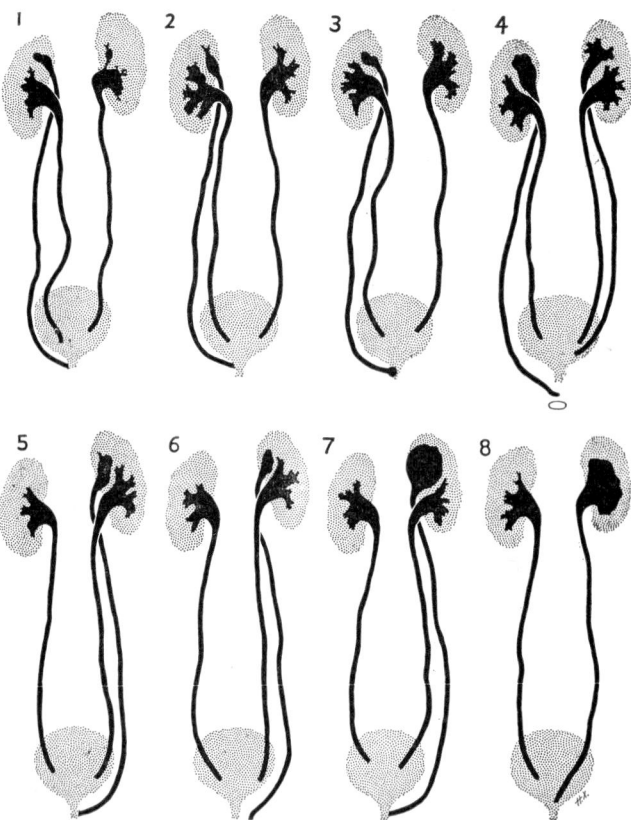

Fig. 379. Conditions found in 8 patients from the Boston Children's Hospital who had ectopic ureteral openings; all were females. In Case 8 there was persistent pyuria because of obstruction of the ureter at the bladder neck; in the other 7 patients there was continual wetting of the perineum. 1. Bifid left kidney (of no significance). Small upper pole of right kidney draining into urethra. 2. Small upper pole of right kidney draining into urethra. 3. The extra ureter ends in the urethra; ureterocele at its lower end. 4. Bilateral double ureters. The ectopic ureter opens in the midline of the vestibule, between the urethral meatus and the vaginal orifice. 5. Upper pole of the left kidney draining into urethra. 6. Upper pole of the left kidney draining into vestibule, to left of urethral meatus. 7. Upper half of left kidney draining by pin-point opening into urethra; obstruction of this entire system. 8. The sole ureter on the left enters bladder at its neck, giving partial obstruction and pyelonephritis on this side.

CLINICAL FINDINGS

The main complaint is that of constant *wetting* of the vulva and perineum. In some patients, the wetting is only during the day, when the child is in the upright position. In a few cases, the wetting has been only at night, presumably when the structures of the perineum are relaxed and allow the ectopic ureter to discharge its fluid. Generally, there is wetting both day and night. This is accompanied by a discharge of bladder urine from time to time in a completely normal and satisfactory way. This combination of constant perineal wetting and normal bladder function should at once suggest that there is an accessory ureter with an orifice in some ectopic position which demands thorough investigation.

It is a very common story to hear that these children have been thought to have a variety of conditions, while the correct diagnosis is not made for many years. Not infrequently the girl is thought to have "enuresis" and attempts at management varying

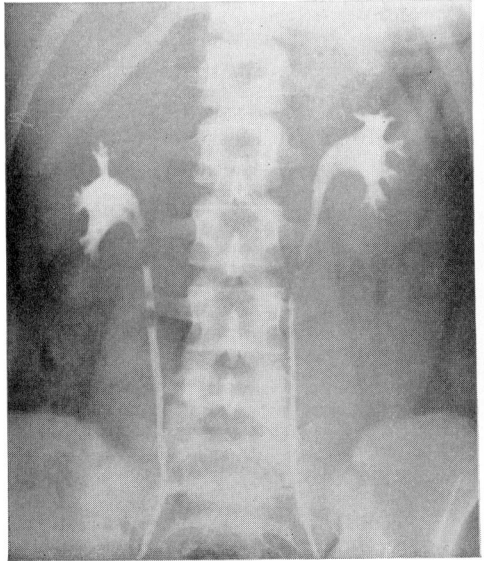 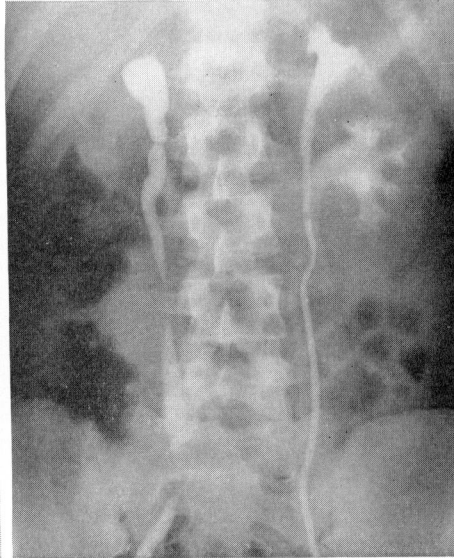

Fig. 380. Roentgenograms from a girl who had had continuous wetting of the perineum since birth (No. 4 on Figure 379). *Left*, Retrograde injection of ureteral openings which were in normal position at either upper tip of the bladder trigone, visualizing lower portion of each kidney. *Right*, Retrograde injections showing upper portion of each kidney. On the child's left the accessory ureter opened at a low point on the left side of the bladder trigone; on her right side, the accessory ureter opened in the midline of the vestibule, between the urethral meatus and the vaginal orifice.

from psychiatric attack to scolding have been made in the effort to get her to stop the annoying bed-wetting. Those girls who have constant wetting of the perineum and clothes during the day are often thought to have dribbling from the urinary bladder, either from a local disturbance at its outlet or from some neurologic condition in the spine. These children are miserable, and it is amazing to find how many of them have gone five, ten, fifteen or more years before the underlying pathologic anatomy is discovered and is treated adequately.

When the diagnosis of ureteral ectopia is suspected, a complete study in the form of intravenous urography, cystoscopy, retrograde pyelography, and a thorough examination of the introitus and genital tract are in order to identify any accessory ureteral orifice which might be present.

Intravenous pyelography is very apt to be misleading, because it shows all of the calyces in both kidneys and if there does not happen to be visualization of the ureters, one might assume that a normal kidney on each side is drained by a single ureter. By cystoscopy and retrograde injection of the ureteral orifices which are found in the bladder, it is evident that only a portion of kidney is visualized on one side (compared to the intravenous urographic picture). The segment thus visualized by retrograde method is almost always the lower two-thirds or three-quarters of the renal system. Such a finding immediately indicates the side on which there is duplication of kidney and ureter and it thus gives a lead regarding which side of the labia, introitus, vagina, or urethra must be carefully inspected in an attempt to find the anomalous ureteral opening.

To make a careful search, the patient must be put up on an examining table in the lithotomy position. The membranes of the external genitalia are exceedingly sensitive; probing and manipulations are apt to be painful and disagreeable. Therefore, to carry out a completely satisfactory search usually implies that the child must be under general anesthesia, a measure which makes the study much easier for the patient, and makes the inspection more satisfactory for the doctor. As the labia are spread apart, one might quickly see a drop or two of urine exude from some part of the introitus, generally just to one side of the urethral meatus. In most cases it is exceedingly difficult to locate the point of emission of urine from the accessory tract; the utmost patience

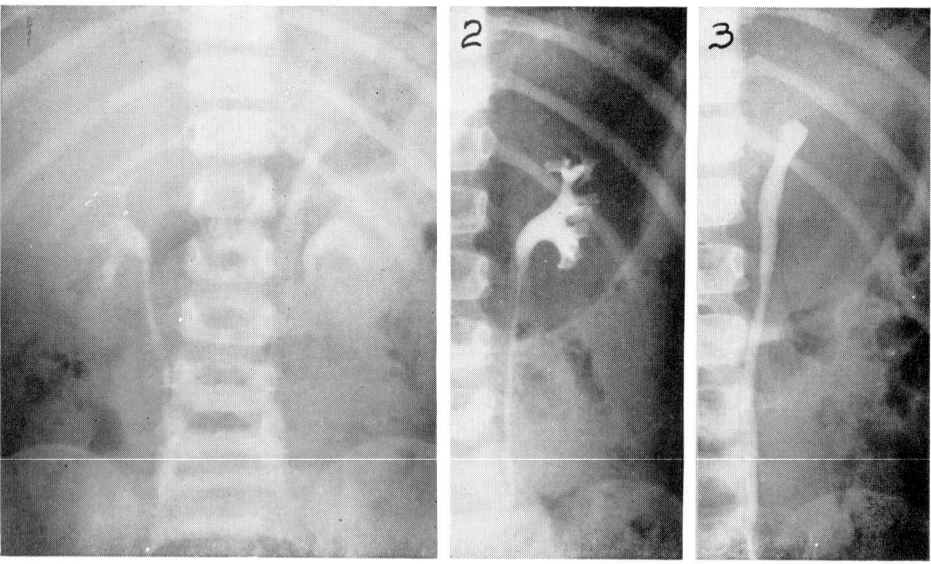

Fig. 381. Roentgenograms from female who had had constant wetting of genitalia all her life because of ectopic ureter draining into the urethra beyond the bladder sphincter (No. 5 on Figure 379). 1. Excretory pyelogram shows a normal pelvis on child's right and double pelvis on her left. 2. Retrograde injection of the ureter which entered the left side of the bladder trigone. Observed by itself, this has the appearance of representing the entire renal structure on this side. 3. Retrograde injection of the ureter which opened into the distal urethra, visualizing an accessory upper pole of the left kidney.

is required in the hunt for the opening which can be exceedingly tiny and which may barely admit the smallest of probes. Manual pressure on the abdomen, placed over the side suspected, to massage urine downward, may help in expressing fluid in the perineum so that its point of exit can be seen. Intravenous injection of a dye such as indigo carmine is helpful in identifying urine which comes from such an ectopic orifice. Particularly difficult to find are those accessory ureters which empty into the urethra itself; as fluid seeps out of the urethral meatus one might gain the impression that there is bladder incontinence. It is sometimes possible to spread open the urethra with the jaws of a right-angle clamp (or a small nasal retractor), so that as the membranes are stretched out urine can be seen running from some part of its wall.

When an ectopic ureteral opening is finally identified, a small ureteral catheter should be inserted into it and retrograde visualization made. Almost invariably this will show that the orifice drains a ureter coming from an upper pole of the kidney on the same side of the body.

TREATMENT

Ligation of Ureter

In one patient we dissected out the ureter for a centimeter or two in the perineum (just above its orifice) and tightly ligated the ureter with silk ties. Subsequently, there was atrophy of the upper segment of kidney which had been drained by this ureter; there was complete relief from the wetting. It was known beforehand that this child had no infection of the urine; the procedure was simple and was highly effective. In general, this type of therapy is not to be recommended because it is too apt to be followed by suppuration in that portion of the excretory tract which has been obstructed.

Partial Nephrectomy

The best method of therapy for a ureter which has an ectopic orifice (which opens externally and gives wetting) is by partial nephrectomy. The small segment of the kidney can be sacrificed with impunity; it is removed, along with its pelvis and ureter (Fig. 377). In this operation as much of the accessory ureter is removed as can be reached down through the flank wound. It is not harmful to leave a ureteral stump remaining below this, provided its lower orifice is freely open. (If there is a stricture at the lower end of the ureter, the entire ureter must be removed.)

Before excising a portion of kidney, it must be perfectly clear (by intravenous urography and retrograde pyelography) just what is the nature of the pathologic anatomy which is being dealt with. It is generally possible to gather all such information before operation, but in two of our children we were unable to identify the accessory orifice in female urethras; however this was known to exist because intravenous pyelography had shown a double pelvis on one side, and retrograde injection (through the ureteral opening in the bladder trigone) had visualized only the lower three-quarters of the kidney on this side. We therefore felt reasonably certain that there must be an accessory upper pole of kidney which was draining through a separate ureteral system into the urethra beyond the bladder sphincter. When the kidney was exposed at the operating table, a double pelvis was found. The upper pelvis was opened and a ureteral catheter then threaded down the entire length of the ureter; it came out the urethra where, by inspection, an assistant could now identify the emergence of the ureter a few millimeters inside of the external urethral meatus. After this positive demonstration of the pathologic anatomy, upper-pole heminephrectomy and ureterectomy were done.

Uretero-Neocystostomy

For those cases in which there is obstruction of an entire kidney because its single ureter inserts very low in the bladder trigone, the transplantation of this ureter into a higher position in the bladder wall is a very satisfactory procedure which conserves renal tissue. However, when dealing with an ectopic ureter which is one in a duplicate system, it is not worth while attempting to save the small amount of renal tissue in the rudimentary upper segment of the double kidney by reimplantation of the ureter into the bladder or by attempting to anastomose the two ureters or the two pelves. It is far better to remove completely the accessory ureter and the rudimentary portion of kidney which it drains (heminephrectomy-ureterectomy).

RESULTS OF THERAPY

In our 8 cases (all females) of ectopic ureteral opening, one drained the entire kidney on the left side and entered the bladder just at its outlet, giving rise to mild hydronephrosis and recurrent pyelonephritis. The lower end of the ureter was transplanted upward into a normal position on the trigone; there was good kidney drainage and complete cessation of pyuria thereafter. In the other 7 patients, the anomalous opening was part of duplicate ureteral system and always connected with the upper pole of a kidney; there was dribbling in each case. The ectopic opening was in the urethra in 5 (in one case it terminated in a ureterocele, bulging from the urethra); in the other 2 it was in the vestibule, just to one side or just posterior to the urethral meatus. One of these was treated by firm ligation of the accessory ureter, while the other 6 were subjected to heminephrectomy. In all 7 children there was cessation of the wetting which before had been so troublesome and annoying.

There are few conditions which are more satisfactory to treat than the constant dribbling which comes from an ectopic ureteral orifice. The patients are extremely grateful when operation makes them dry and comfortable.

REFERENCES

1. Abeshouse, B. S.: Ureteral Ectopia: Report of a Rare Case of Ectopic Ureter Opening in the Uterus and a Review of the Literature. Urol. & Cutan. Rev., 47:447, 1943.
2. Alldred, A. J. and Higgins, T. T.: The Ectopic Ureter in Childhood with an Account of Four Personal Cases. Brit. J. Surg., 38:460, 1951.
3. Burford, C. E., Glenn, J. E. and Burford, E. H.: Ureteral Ectopia: A Review of the Literature and 2 Case Reports. J. Urol., 62: 211, 1949.
4. Deming, C. L.: Ectopic Vaginal Ureter. Surg., Gynec. & Obst., 62:843, 1936.
5. Goldstein, A. E. and Klotz, B.: Ligation of a Supernumerary Ureter. Am. J. Surg., 70:13, 1945.
6. Hepler, A. B.: Bilateral Pelvic and Ureteral Duplication with Uterine Ectopic Ureter. J. Urol., 57:94, 1947.
7. Honke, E. M.: Ectopic Ureter. J. Urol., 55: 460, 1946.
8. Meads, A. M.: Ectopic Ureter. J. Urol., 59: 390, 1948.
9. Torres, L. F., Jr.: Double Kidney Pelves and Double Ureters, Upper Ureter Ending Ectopically at Vestibule of Vagina. Case Report. J. Urol., 58:171, 1947.

CHAPTER 51

Ureterocele

Of the various types of obstruction in the urinary tract, blocks at the uretero-vesical junction with formation of a ureterocele are relatively few in number, but they can lead to a high degree of renal damage. It is important to recognize them because they can be treated by relatively simple means with a high degree of success.

Obstruction of a ureteral orifice inevitably leads to ureterectasia and hydronephrosis but it does not always produce a ureterocele. When stenosis of the ureteric orifice is accompanied by a congenital weakness or thinning of Waldeyer's sheath (the fibrous envelope of the lower end of the ureter), there is a ballooning out of that portion of the ureter which passes through the bladder, which results in the formation of a "cystic" structure, one to several centimeters in diameter, protruding into the bladder lumen (Fig. 382). Ureteroceles are lined with the transitional, mucosal epithelium of the ureter and are covered externally by the mucosa of the bladder. In their wall is a thinned-out, interstitial mesenchymal layer of fibrous tissue and smooth muscle.

The following remarks are drawn largely from observations on 32 infants and children who have been seen at the Children's Hospital with this condition.

PATHOLOGIC FINDINGS

The pathologic changes associated with ureteroceles can be separated into two phases. The first are those which are directly attributable to *obstruction* of the urinary tract and the second are those related to *superimposed infection* which occurs with great frequency. In none of our patients was there a ureteral calculus, but such complications have been observed by other surgeons. In its early stages there may be little or no dilatation of the renal pelvis or upper part of the ureter, but blockage of long standing is accompanied by severe degrees of dilatation and destruction of renal parenchyma. Added to this can be all the ravages of bacterial invasion, which is so likely to occur when there is stasis of urinary flow.

In 15 of our 32 cases there were double ureters on one or both sides. When a ureterocele occurred on that side where there were double ureters, the ureterocele always arose from the lower ureteric orifice. In no instance with ipsilateral duplication of ureters did the ureterocele arise from the upper ureteric opening (which, of course, drains the lower pole of the kidney on the affected side). Ignorance of this fact can often lead to confusion at cystoscopy or at the operating table. When an ipsilateral duplication of ureters exists, the ureterocele mass may bulge upward and partially block the second ureter by compression, so that both ureters on that side will be found dilated.

A ureterocele may be large enough so that it bulges over beyond the midline and obstructs the ureteric orifice of the opposite side. If a ureterocele is of sufficient size, it can flop over and plug the bladder outlet and thereby produce obstruction of the bladder and the entire urinary tract. In rare instances a ureterocele may actually prolapse through the urethra of a female and present itself externally.

The left side is most frequently involved. In our series, 19 ureteroceles were on the left, and 9 on the right; in 4 cases there were bilateral abnormalities. Campbell found them equally distributed as to side, with 15 per cent bilateral.

It is apparent that cases can be placed into one of five groups: (1) Those with obstruction of the involved ureter (14 of our cases). (2) Those with ipsilateral obstruction of the involved and adjacent (double) ureter (9 cases). (3) Those with obstruction of the

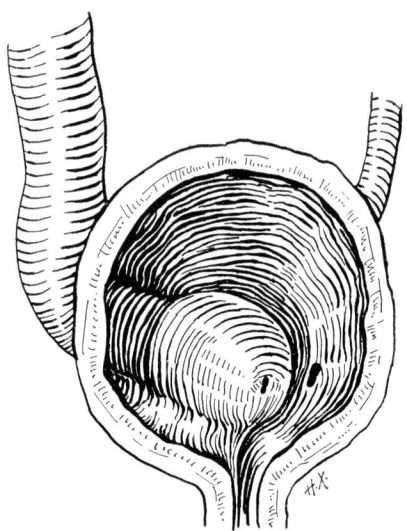

Fig. 382. Typical ureterocele. Ureteric orifice on right is tiny. That portion of ureter which courses through bladder wall has become dilated and forms a mass which balloons into lumen of bladder.

entire urinary tract by a single ureterocele which blocks the vesical outlet (4 cases). (4) Those with obstruction of both upper urinary tracts, from bilateral ureteroceles (4 cases). (5) Those with a double ureter, one ureter entering the urethra where it forms a ureterocele bulging out through the urethral meatus (1 case). The wide variety of combinations are shown graphically in Figures 383 and 384. Some of the patients also have other anomalies in the urinary tract. Since there can be varying degrees of obstruction and different combinations of obstructions, it is imperative to investigate the entire urinary tract so that a clear picture of the situation is gained before surgical attack is made on an isolated part of the system.

CLINICAL PICTURE

History

As with most congenital anomalies of the genito-urinary tract in infants and children, evidence of pyuria is the most common complaint (Table 74). In about half of the cases, the finding of a cloudy urine led to the seeking of medical advice. In about a quarter of the subjects, pus was found on microscopic examination of the urine during routine studies. In only two cases was the urine clear. Secondary changes from superimposed infection are found in a very high percentage of patients. Fever, malaise, loss of weight, anorexia or vomiting, leukocytosis and urinary frequency are commonly found. Hematuria is occasionally seen.

Fairly prominent in the picture are those symptoms suggesting irritation of the bladder. Dysuria, frequency, enuresis, and hesitancy in starting the urinary stream are found in about half of the patients. Urgency, dribbling and inability to void, and a

Table 74

Symptoms and Signs in 32 Patients with Ureteroceles

Findings	Present in	Chief complaint in
Cloudy urine (pyuria)	27	17
Vesical irritation	11	7
Fever	12	0
Recurrent abdominal pain	7	1
Vomiting	6	0
Urgency and hesitancy suggesting bladderneck obstruction	6	2
Failure to gain weight	4	2
Hematuria	3	2
"Cyst" presenting from urethra (in female)	2	1

palpably enlarged bladder (suggesting intermittent or continuous bladder-outlet obstruction) are observed in a few.

These children seem to have less pain than is often the case with obstructions high in the urinary tract. It appears to be present in less than a third of them. Of course, the young age of many of these subjects makes it impossible to give any accurate statement regarding the actual frequency with which abdominal pain occurs.

With few exceptions, ureteroceles have a congenital origin though they may be asymptomatic and unrecognized in early life. The lesions may be unnoticed for years until symptoms appear which are referable to superimposed infection, bladder irritation, or advancing urinary tract obstruction. Various authors have indicated that ureteroceles may not be discovered until adult life; the average age of the patients in our series at the onset of the presenting illness was 21 months; the youngest was 2 days of age, the oldest was 10 years; fourteen were less than 1 year (Fig. 385). The average duration of symptoms was nine months, with a range from six days to several years.

The sex incidence is noteworthy, since the abnormality is somewhat more common in females; 19 of our subjects were females and 13 were males.

Physical Examination is usually of little help in establishing the correct diagnosis, except when there is flank tenderness from an active pyelonephrosis or when there is a palpable mass in the lower abdomen which represents a distended bladder as a result of vesical-neck obstruction. In only rare instances is it possible by rectal examination to palpate a mass in the region of the bladder floor, which may be either a distended ureter or a ureterocele itself.

Examination of the Urine shows varying degrees of pyuria and albuminuria in most instances. Casts are rarely found. The non-protein nitrogen level in the blood is significantly elevated in only rare instances, but in occasional cases there may be a severe uremia. Cultures of the urine almost always show a bacilluria, with a variety of organisms which can be identified.

Roentgenologic Findings

Several simple procedures are available for aid in recognition of a ureterocele. *Excretory pyelography* is diagnostic in only about a third of the cases, but it usually can give evidence which is strongly suggestive of a ureterocele. Obstruction is found in some portion or all parts of the upper urinary system. There may be visualization of an entire ureter, particularly in its lower quarter (indicating delay of urinary flow). In some instances, the ballooned-out and dye-filled ureterocele is more opaque than the bladder shadow (wherein the dye is more dilute); this with the intense and continued opacification of a ureter on the same side, particularly when this is dilated, should make one suspect obstruction at the ureteric orifice. A translucent, filling defect, shown by pyelography or by cystography (with 4 per cent sodium iodide) is almost certainly caused by a ureterocele (only rarely by neoplasm in this age group).

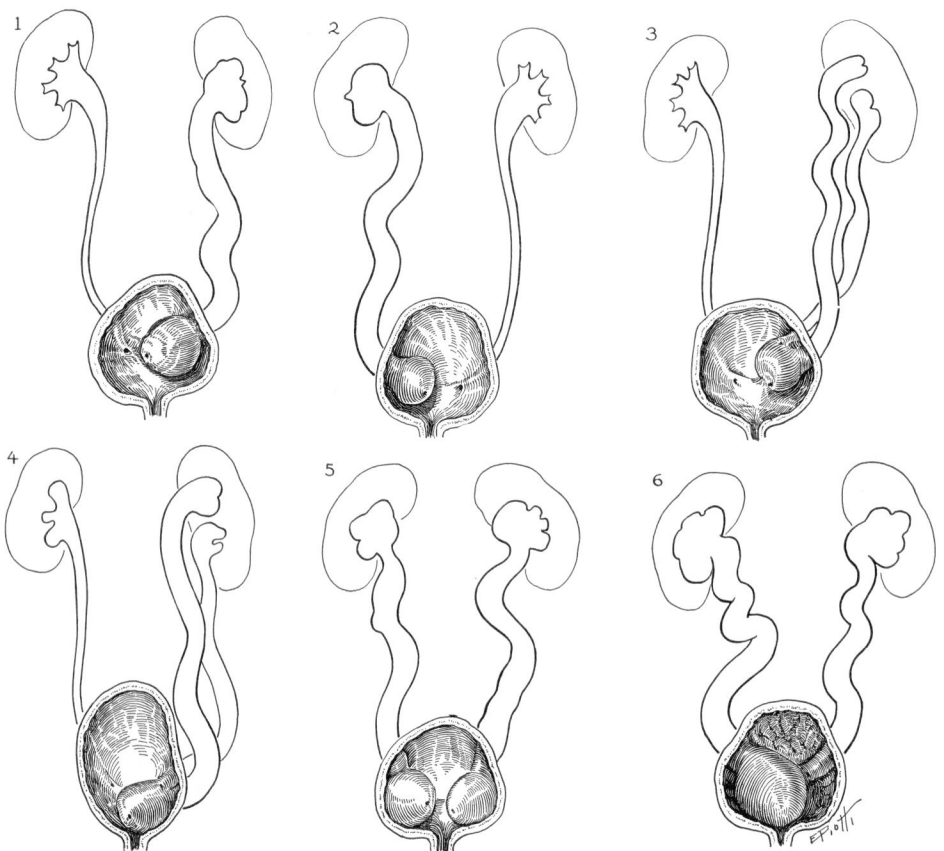

Fig. 383. Ureteroceles and associated pathology which were encountered in our series. 1. Left ureterocele with left hydro-ureter and hydronephrosis. 2. Right ureterocele with right hydro-ureter and hydronephrosis. 3. Ureterocele from left lower ureteric orifice, partially compressing upper orifice on left side of trigone. 4. Same as 3, but ureterocele is larger and partially blocks bladder outlet and produces mild hydronephrosis on right, and more extensive hydronephrosis on left. 5. Bilateral ureteroceles with bilateral marked hydronephrosis. 6. Ureterocele blocks bladder outlet, gives obstructed trabeculated bladder and bilateral hydronephrosis.

Cystoscopy is not required in all cases, but generally it is desirable to confirm the diagnosis which has been already made by roentgenographic means or to establish the diagnosis when other types of examination have failed to indicate clearly the nature of the pathology which is present. When a ureterocele is large, it may press directly against the cystoscope and thereby shut off a view of the bladder interior. Ureteroceles of small or moderate size can be seen as dome-shaped swellings replacing one side of the bladder trigone, the mass projecting into the bladder and being surmounted by a stenotic ureteral orifice. The tiny opening will rarely allow a catheter to be passed up the ureter. Occasionally, the "cyst" appears to vary in size and tension as some urine escapes from it or as the sac has transmitted to it the rhythmic peristaltic contractions of the ureteral system.

TREATMENT

Salvage of Renal Substance. As with most obstructive uropathies in infants and children, a conservative attitude toward definitive treatment is preferable. One is loath to deprive a growing child of renal tissue which is not irreparably damaged; for this

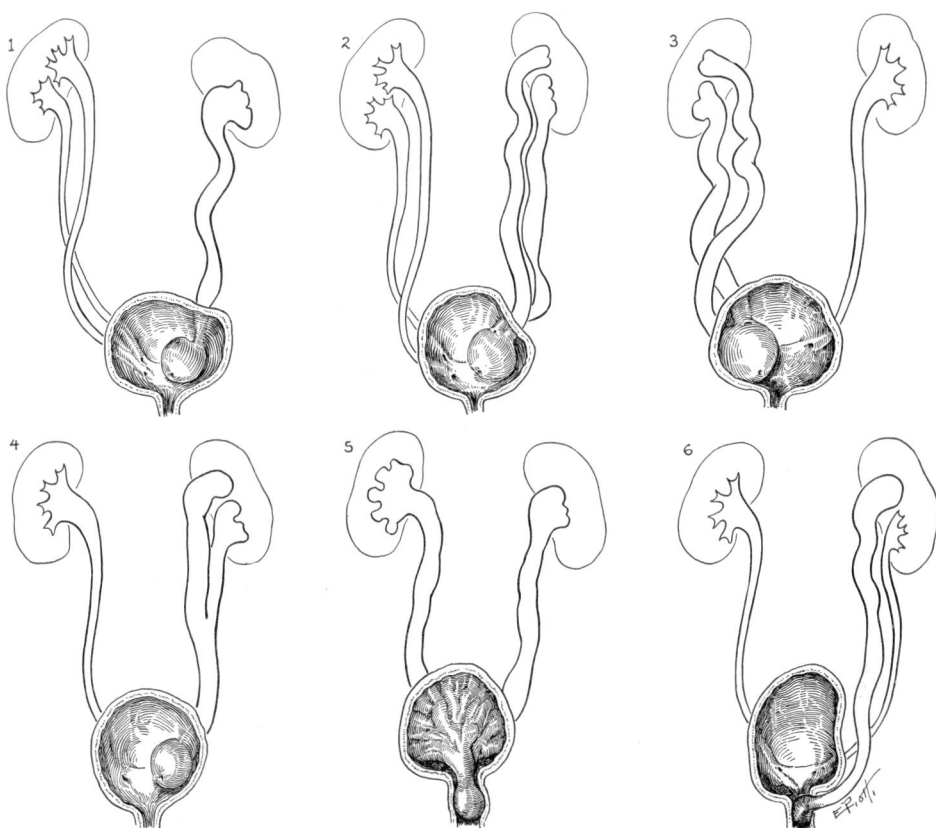

Fig. 384. Continuation of sketches of ureterocele and associated pathology which we have encountered. 1. Left ureterocele and hydronephrosis. Right double, unobstructed ureters. 2. Double ureters both sides, unobstructed on right. On left, ureterocele arises from lower ureteric orifice and by compression it blocks upper ureteric orifice, giving obstruction of both ureters on patient's left. 3. Double ureter, right, with ureterocele at lower orifice, partially compressing superior ureteric orifice, giving dilatation of both ureters on right. 4. Bifid ureter on left, with ureterocele at lower end of same. 5. Right ureterocele prolapsed through female urethra, giving bladder obstruction and trabeculation, with bilateral hydronephrosis. 6. Double ureter on left, one ureter entering urethra and giving rise to ureterocele there.

reason nephrectomy (or heminephrectomy) is necessary only occasionally. The vast majority of patients can be handled by some direct attack on the ureterocele, the incision of which allows an adequate flow of urine, gives a reasonable chance of combating infection (with or without chemotherapy), and at the same time makes it possible to save whatever kidney substance is present.

Method of Approach. In choosing a method of operative approach to a ureterocele.

one should be guided by the age and sex of the patient, the availability of specialized instruments, and the ability of the surgeon. While urologists have been eminently successtul in treating ureteroceles in older children or adults by transurethral approach and incision of the lesion with cystoscopic scissors or by puncturing it with an endothermy instrument, it is our firm conviction that for infants and small children it is far safer and more effective to treat them through a suprapubic opening of the bladder. Under direct vision and handling, the ureterocele can be treated quickly and easily. It is believed that in intants and small children, particularly males, this is the approach of choice, and for most surgeons it is less hazardous than cystoscopic manipulation.

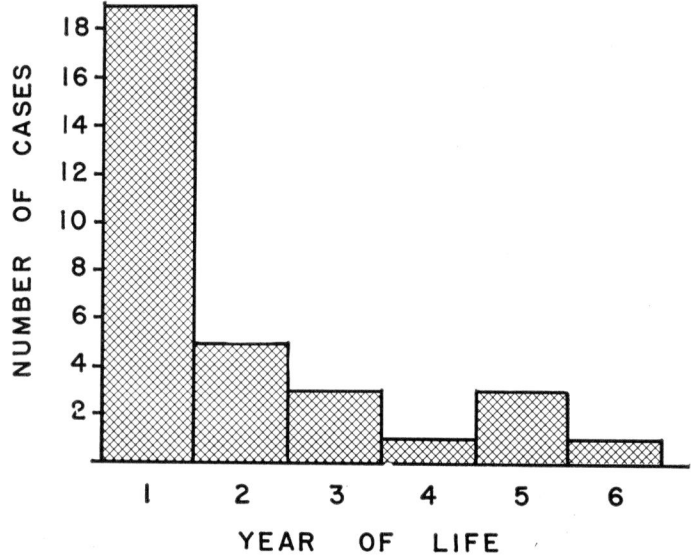

Fig. 385. Age of ureterocele patients at beginning of symptoms.

Inadequacy of Dilation. While theoretically it might seem to be adequate, simple dilation of a ureterocele orifice, even when it is done under direct vision through an open bladder, gives disappointing end results; we have always had to follow it with some other form of treatment and have therefore abandoned this mode of therapy.

Excision To Be Avoided. Great stress must be given to the fact that excision of a ureterocele—in part or in toto—is not only unnecessary but is distinctly harmful. Obviously, the removal of tissue will relieve existing ureteral obstruction, but it is quite apt to produce an incompetence of the uretero-vesical valve mechanism. It allows a reflux of bladder urine up into the ureter, gives rise to an increasing hydronephrosis and a continuing pyonephrosis, all of which contribute to progressive renal damage. In the past, we have performed operations for "uncapping" or "removing" ureteroceles; *follow-up studies give indubitable evidence* that the over-all results have been extremely poor. Visualizations (by cystogram) some months or years later have shown reflux of urine on the operated side; the urine has long continued to be filled with pus; there has been progressive loss of renal function on the affected side. In 2 instances, secondary operations have been performed to reimplant the ureter through the bladder wall to reestablish some valve-like action, with a modicum of success. Our studies have led us to the conclusion that "excision" of ureteroceles should be abandoned.

Incision of Ureterocele. Without question, the treatment of choice is the simple vertical incision of the dome of the ureterocele, making a slit-like enlargement of the existing ureteric orifice. Such incision should vary from 3 to 5 mm. in length, depending upon the over-all size of the ureterocele, having in mind that the larger masses will shrink more as they collapse and hence any slit in them will shorten more than is the case with small ureteroceles. No attempt should be made to suture the membrane of the ureter to that of the bladder. To promote a thorough flushing out of the urinary tract, a mushroom suprapubic catheter should be left in place and kept open for a week

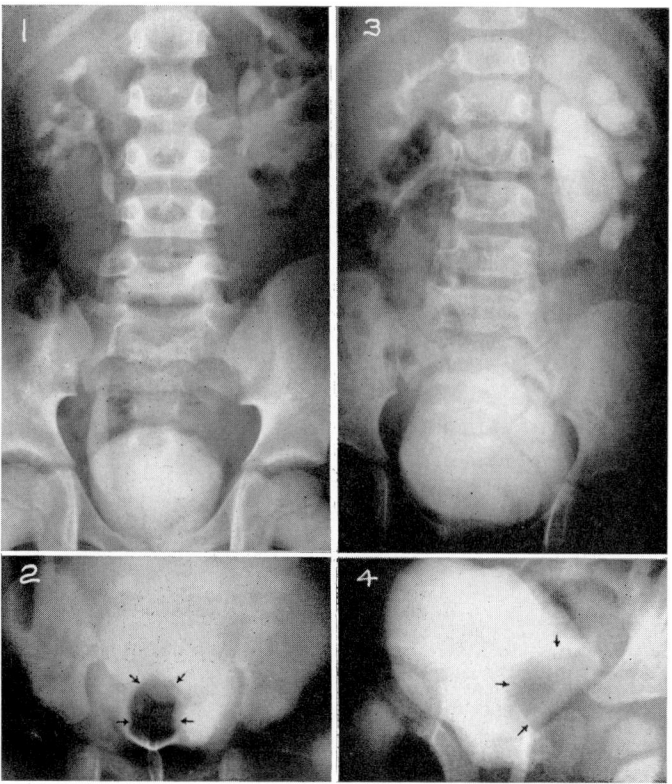

Fig. 386. Films from patients with ureteroceles. 1. Intravenous pyelogram from boy with right ureterocele. There is only slight blunting of calyces of right kidney. Note how dye is delayed in entire right ureter. Furthermore, right ureter is moderately dilated, particularly in its lower half. 2. Cystogram from a baby with bladder outlet obstruction. Filling defect is made by ureterocele (indicated by arrows). 3. Intravenous pyelogram from child with left-sided ureterocele and resultant marked hydronephrosis on same side. 4. Cystogram from same patient showing large filling defect (indicated by arrows) made by ureterocele which projects into bladder lumen.

or two, in some cases longer. The bulbous end of this catheter should be placed high in the bladder so that it does not rest against the trigone and cause undue discomfort. Furthermore, the catheter should be led obliquely upward through the abdominal wall, a direction which facilitates rapid and spontaneous closure of the sinus when the catheter is withdrawn.

Chemotherapy. As an adjunct to the surgical treatment of each patient, pyuria should be intensively treated with the best available chemotherapeutic agent. After determining the type of organism which is present in the urine, that drug is selected which is most apt to achieve sterilization. Aureomycin and terramycin are the two drugs with a wide range of antibacterial activity which are found to be most useful.

They are given in appropriate doses and are kept up until a few days after withdrawal of the suprapubic tube; it is rarely necessary to continue them for a longer period. It is hardly necessary to point out that infection cannot be satisfactorily or permanently eradicated unless the mechanical obstruction has been completely relieved.

<h2 style="text-align:center">RESULTS OF TREATMENT</h2>

Upon reviewing cases and tabulating the success or failure which has followed various surgical procedures, it becomes quite clear that achievement of uniformly satisfactory results depends upon the accomplishment of three things: (1) relief of the obstruction; (2) control of the infection; (3) avoidance of any operative procedure which destroys the uretero-vesical valve and permits urinary reflux. Remarkable restorative powers in the ureters and kidneys of children have been observed provided stasis, obstruction, and infection are controlled and provided reflux does not occur. The simplest possible correction—that of making a small slit in the wall of the ureterocele—will relieve the obstruction and will permit a satisfactory flow of urine but will not jeopardize the chances of a successful result since it does not incur a loss of the uretero-vesical valve. In infants and most children, this incision of a ureterocele is best made under direct vision, working through a suprapubic cystotomy. It has sometimes been impossible to predict the exact outcome of operation. We have seen apparently adequate slits in a ureterocele followed by scarring and subsequent recurrence of the obstruction. We have also seen a small slit followed by loss of uretero-vesical valve action, leading to increasing hydronephrosis. It is quite evident that, while most of these patients respond nicely and recover very promptly, others have a long-drawn out course so that one becomes dubious about what has been accomplished, only to find that after a year or two the entire picture and the renal function change distinctly for the better. Particularly troublesome are those cases in which there are other lesions in the urinary tract, making combinations which seem almost hopeless to treat. While the majority of ureterocele patients recover in a satisfactory and prompt manner, there are a few who must be followed and reevaluated for many years, using, if necessary, additional operative steps to improve the situation.

In our series of 32 cases the over-all results have been as follows: In one child there was a fatality; this three-month-old baby had advanced uremia and died on the operating table. There have been no other fatalities either during hospitalization or subsequent thereto. In one child, a hypoplastic kidney was removed. In 3, a nephrectomy or heminephrectomy was done because of advanced or increasing renal damage. In the early part of the series there were 14 patients who had "excision" or "uncapping" of ureteroceles in which the end results were very dismal; only 3 were cured of hydronephrosis and infection. In the remaining cases, wherein a simple incision of a ureterocele had been performed, the follow-up studies have shown a satisfactory result; in most the situation has been brought under control in a month or two, but in a few who preoperatively had severe damage or complications from other anomalies, supervision during a period of one or two years has been required.

It has become quite clear that results of therapy for ureterocele depend a great deal upon whether there are one or two ureters on the side occupied by the ureterocele. In the former instance, opening the ureterocele gives a good flow of urine, an adequate flushing, and a very promising result. In the latter instance, when a ureterocele is at the lower end of a duplicated ureter, opening the structure is apt to be followed by only a small flow of urine (it drains only the tiny upper pole of the kidney) and there is apt to be continuing infection and pyuria. In this latter type of case, our experience with conservative treatment of ureteroceles (by incising them) has been most disappointing; we have generally had to follow it by a heminephrectomy.

REFERENCES

1. Adams, P. S.: Ureterocele: Treatment by Transurethral Resection. Am. J. Surg., *50:* 249, 1940.
2. Campbell, M. F.: Ureterocele. J. Urol., *45:* 598, 1941.
3. Campbell, M.: Ureterocele. A Study of 94 Instances in 80 Infants and Children. Surg., Gynec. & Obst., *93:*705, 1951.
4. Emmett, J. L. and Logan, G. B.: Ureterocele with Prolapse through Urethra. J. Urol., *51:*19, 1944.
5. Gottlieb, J.: Zur Arbeit über die Frage der "Pathogenese und Therapie der Ureterocele." Ztschr. f. urol. Chir., *20:*1, 1926.
6. Goyanna, R. and Greene, L. F.: Pathologic and Anomalous Conditions Associated with Duplication of Renal Pelvis and Ureter. J. Urol., *54:*1, 1945.
7. Kickham, C. J. E.: Ureterocele with Extrusion through Urethra. J. Urol., *52:*235, 1944.
8. Martius, H.: Zur Behandlung der Ureterocele Vesicalis. Zentralbl. f. Gynäk., *51:*327, 1927.
9. Patch, F. S.: Ureterocele, with Report of Case. J. Urol., *16:*125, 1926.
10. Smith, E. C. and Orkin, L. A.: Clinical and Statistical Study of 471 Congenital Anomalies of Kidney and Ureter. J. Urol., *53:* 11, 1945.
11. Thompson, G. J. and Greene, L. F.: Ureterocele: Clinical Study and Report of 37 Cases. J. Urol., *47:*800, 1942.

CHAPTER 52

Exstrophy of the Bladder

Exstrophy of the bladder is one of the most distressing congenital malformations which the surgeon must treat. The bladder, opening as it does on the anterior abdominal wall, allows a continual escape of urine which produces *malodor and a disagreeable wetting of the clothing.* The everted and *exposed mucous membrane is very sensitive* and is easily irritated by any overlying pad or dressing. The deformity is accompanied by a *wide separation of the pubic bones*, so that there is a *waddling and unstable gait.* These individuals rapidly beome socially ostracized because of the uriniferous odor which always attends them; furthermore, they are quite apt to become introspective and retiring because of the physical deformity which they possess.

The therapeutic problems are fourfold: (1) To provide an adequate receptacle which can receive and discharge urine at suitable intervals. (2) To remove the discomfort caused by the exposed mucous membranes. (3) To improve the appearance and structure of the genitalia. (4) In the male, to construct a urethral tube which will permit reproductive activity.

CLINICAL FINDINGS

In our series of 80 patients with exstrophy of the bladder, 62 were males and 18 were females. Exstrophy in either sex is a deformity in which the entire lower urinary tract from the apex of the bladder to the external urethral meatus is opened (as if by an anterior midline cut) and lies exposed and everted. The bladder mucosa is thrown into folds and has a bright cherry-red color, in contrast to the surrounding skin (Figs. 387 and 388). The trigone and its ureteral orifices can be viewed in the lower part of the mass. The membrane about the ureteric orifices tends to become heaped up and cauliflower-like. The ureters intermittently discharge droplets of urine. Below is the verumontanum (in the male) and in both sexes there is usually a complete epispadias. The membranous lining of the urethra is smooth, red, and moist. Touching any portion of these various surfaces will make the child wince and cry with discomfort and pain. This hypersensitivity diminishes somewhat in a year or two because squamous epithelium replaces a portion, but not all, of the bladder mucosa. As much as a half or two-thirds of the bladder may be thus converted and rendered less irritable. In occasional cases there may be double ureters (or Y-shaped ureters) on one or both sides. A considerable number of these individuals have bilateral indirect *inguinal hernias;* in the males *undescended testicles* are not infrequently found.

Such a forward dislocation of the bladder and urethra is always accompanied by a *complete separation of the pubic bones* (Fig. 389), the ends of which are bridged by a flattened, fibrous cord. By palpating the lower abdominal wall, to either side of the bulging bladder, the rounded ends of the pubic bones can be felt. The two sides may be separated from each other by as much as 2 or 3 inches. This part of the deformity is associated with a wide *diastasis recti* below the umbilicus.

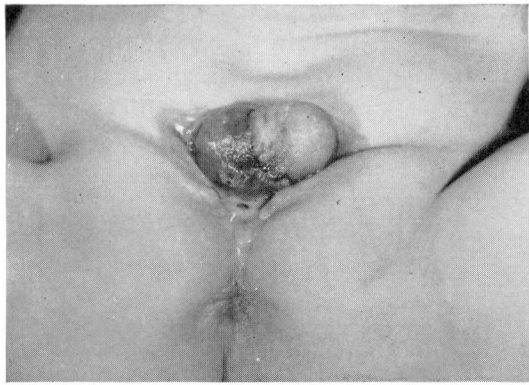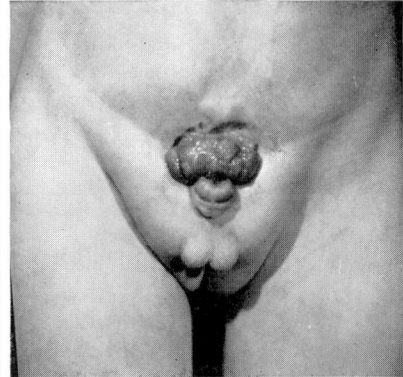

Fig. 387. *Left*, Exstrophy of bladder in two-year-old girl. Note cleft condition of vulva, also bifid clitoris with vaginal orifice in full view. Squamous epithelium is replacing transitional epithelium on some of the exposed bladder surface. *Right*, A four-year-old boy with exstrophy of the bladder and complete epispadias.

The external exposure of the ureters might lead one to believe that ascending infection is common, yet it is quite rare to find an important ureteritis or pyelitis. Numerous observations on untreated children have shown little microscopic change in the urine. It is with great rarity that one finds dilatation of the pelves or ureters by retrograde or intravenous pyelography.

TREATMENT

Historical

Some of the earliest efforts to treat this malformation were directed toward anatomic restoration of the bladder and urethra. The bladder was turned in, closed, and was given an intra-abdominal position, but these operations were never successful, because it was impossible to reconstruct a suitable vesical outlet and sphincter muscle. Young[17] reported one success with such a reconstruction in a female.

Many early surgical attempts were confined to excision of the bladder and transplantation of the ureters to the loin, groin, or onto the penis itself. With the ureters in such positions, various types of rubber apparatus could be strapped to the body or thigh to collect urine. Such attachments were very cumbersome and this form of treatment has completely fallen into disuse.

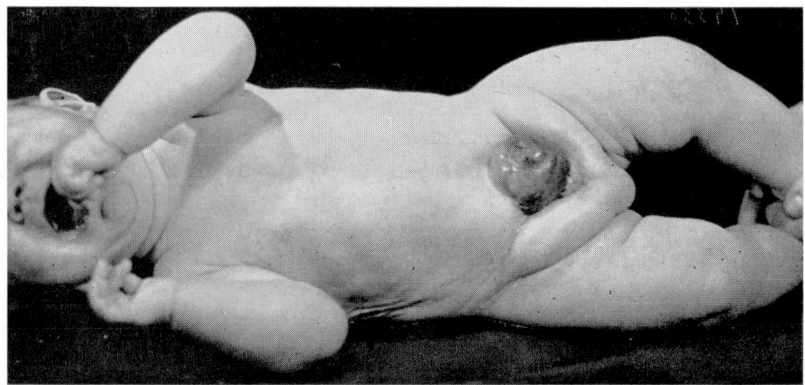

Fig. 388. Five-month-old patient with exstrophy of the bladder. There are also bilateral indirect inguinal hernias; the association is common.

Uretero-Colonic Anastomoses. For nearly sixty years the rectum has been employed as a urinary reservoir, but the methods for anastomosing the ureters to the sigmoid have passed through many modifications. In 1894 *Maydl* accomplished this by excising and discarding most of the bladder, and then implanting the trigone (with the attached ureters) into the colonic wall. In this way he hoped to save the valve-like action of the uretero-vesical junctions. Unfortunately, the blood supply was so seriously reduced that often the trigone sloughed. In 1901 *Peters* improved upon this technique by implanting the ureters separately, carrying along only a narrow rim of trigonal tissue around each ureteric end. This procedure was followed by many successes; some individuals are still alive and in good health twenty to thirty years after such operations.

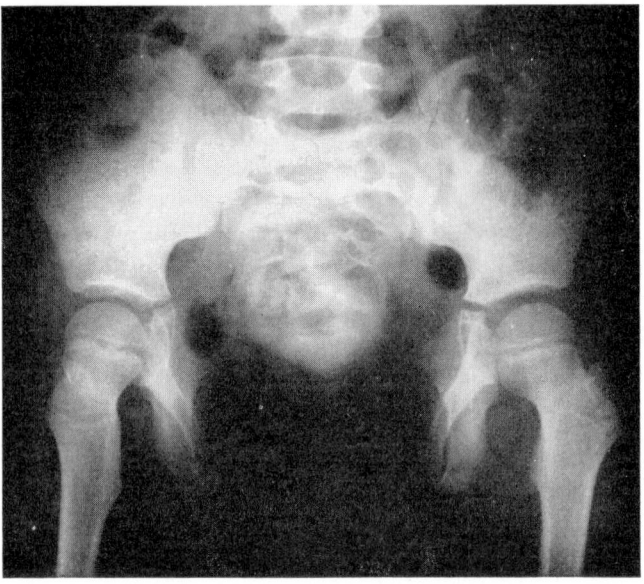

Fig. 389. Pelvis of a girl with exstrophy of the bladder, showing the wide separation of the pubic bones.

In 1909 *Coffey* suggested that a valve-like structure could be obtained if ureters were run along a sufficient distance between the coats of the colonic wall. The first operations employing this principle were done in the next few years at the Mayo Clinic. During the following two decades Coffey made numerous studies of the methods for best performing uretero-colonic anastomoses. The *Coffey No. 1 technique* was quite elaborate; it involved an extensive preparation of the bowel, and implantation of the ureters into the sigmoid, using inlying ureteral catheters which were led down through the rectum and anus for external drainage for a week or ten days. In this way a continuous flow of urine could be maintained; postoperative edema and swelling at the anastomotic site could not shut off the flow of urine. The *Coffey No. 2 technique* was similar, but in addition a sleeve of rubber tubing was placed over that segment of the catheter whch passed through the implanted part of the ureter. This was done to insure making a sufficiently large tunnel through the bowel wall, and thus avoid constriction of the ureter after the catheters were removed. In the *Coffey No. 3 technique* no ureteral catheters were used. Only one ureter was transplanted at a time, and the lower end of it was temporarily closed by an obstructing suture which sloughed through in a few days and established a communication between the ureteral and colonic lumina. In all three of his procedures Coffey used the oblique, submuscular position of the ureter to obtain a valve-like action, which is his important contribution to this field of surgery.

Since Coffey's publications there have been numerous experimental studies and modifications for ureteral transplantations. In many of these the ureter has been purposely obstructed by a catgut stitch, silk suture, a dress snap, or other contrivance which spontaneously sloughs through in a few days' time. This has been done in the hope of avoiding early bacterial contamination along the ureteral lumen or the periureteral lymphatics. I am completely opposed to all these *occlusive types* of anastomosis because they are unnecessary and are unduly complicated. There are adequate clinical observations to show that the simplest anastomotic methods are more apt to give uniform and satisfactory results.

Present Concepts

In recent years there has been some tendency to place less emphasis on the oblique form of anastomosis and any valve-like action which it might possess. Greater attention has been paid to an accurate mucosa-to-mucosa union, feeling that such a junction gives the best chance of avoiding stricture-formation in this area. To make a membrane-to-membrane union, the ureter must join the bowel at nearly a right angle; it is almost impossible to run it along in any submuscular channel. With mucosa-to-mucosa anastomosis there is undoubtedly some reflux of fecal material up the ureter, and yet the kidney has a high chance of remaining free of suppurative infection. These facts emphasize that ureteral peristalsis can keep the tube swept clear, provided its lower end is not obstructed.

In viewing the merits and deficiencies of the two types of union, the excellent results which have been obtained by a submuscular implantation (with particular attention to avoiding stricture) would seem to make this much the preferable one. We prefer it for routine operations, and have used the open, mucosa-to-mucosa union only in those rare cases when the ureter has been much larger than normal, and hence could not be placed in a tunnel in the bowel wall.

We do not believe that an extraperitoneal operation for implantation of ureters into the bowel is logical or necessary. There is great objection to this approach because it carries considerable danger of unknowingly angulating the bowel or ureters at the site of anastomosis.

There are some who advise and practice transplantation of the ureters within the first year of life, a management which is selected in the hope of preventing infection from entering the exposed ureteral orifices. There is very little to support this view because ascending infection in one of these exteriorized ureters is almost unknown; it has not occurred in a single one of our patients. Furthermore, shifting a ureteral opening from a relatively clean abdominal wall to the bacteria-filled colon can hardly be a satisfactory way of minimizing renal contamination.

There is a second point of importance in the choice of time for ureteral transplantation. It is technically possible to join the ureters to the colon in a small baby, but the filling of the rectum with fluid material does not give the child a good chance of learning bowel control. We believe it is far better to have the child develop rectal control *first*, and *then* turn the fluid material into the rectum; in this way the youngster has the best possibility of maintaining continence. With these thoughts in mind, the optimum age for ureteral transplantation seems to lie near three or four years of age. The removal of the bladder and repair of the epispadias can be done six months to a year later.

Technique of Uretero-Sigmoidostomy

During the decade prior to 1930 the operative results in the Children's Hospital cases were not good. Most of the patients had been treated by the elaborate Coffey No. 1 technique, and in some an extraperitoneal approach had been used. Mortality rates from peritonitis were high. The methods employed were poorly suited to children, because they were too time-consuming and complicated. The inlying catheter often set up a severe traumatic ureteritis which paved the way for a superimposed and chronic infection. Because of these unsatisfactory results, animal experimentation was performed by Lanman and Colby, and it is largely from this work that the Children's Hospital methods of uretero-sigmoidostomy (since 1930) have been evolved.

Principles of the Operation. The principles which are regarded as of fundamental importance are: (1) simplification of technique; (2) a transabdominal exposure; (3) establishment of a long, intramural, submuscular implantation of the ureter; (4) the projection into the lumen of the bowel of only a very short segment of ureter, to minimize subsequent scarring and obstruction; (5) adequate anchorage of the ureter in its tunnel so that it cannot withdraw and give leakage or obstruction; (6) leaving a small urethral catheter in the ureter during establishment of the anastomosis, so that the tunnel cannot be made too tightly; (7) omission of inlying ureteral catheters after operation, so that the incidence of ureteritis is diminished. Pyelitis and pyelonephritis seldom come from ascending infection alone; they usually follow ureteric obstruction. It is therefore highly important to make sure the operation is carried out in such a way that there will be no subsequent delay in the flow of urine.

While it was formerly our policy to transplant only one ureter at a time, during the last decade we have customarily transferred both ureters at once; in no instance have we regretted this. Since this method seems to be safe, it is preferred because it reduces the number of operations and the length of hospital stay.

Details of Ureteral Transplantation. The child should have a low-residue diet and a daily enema for several days prior to operation. In this way fecal material in the rectum can be kept at a minimum during and shortly after operation. The use of antibiotics, such as Sulfasuxidine, to reduce the bacterial flora of the bowel seems to be of little consequence. We have had perfectly satisfactory results without them, and ordinarily do not prescribe them before operation. It is much more important to perform a careful and suitable anastomosis than it is to make a careless union and hope that antibiotics will prevent disaster.

A rectal tube is inserted so that fluid can escape from the bowel. The exstrophied bladder and abdominal wall are suitably cleansed with a soft cloth and liquid soap, following by aqueous Zephiran solution. The bladder is walled off from the operative field (Fig. 390) which is made through a long, low, left rectus incision; the muscle belly is retracted laterally. On either side, the ureter is identified at the pelvic brim and from this point downward the posterior, parietal peritoneum is opened so that the ureter can be dissected from its bed. It is freed almost to the bladder, where it is divided. The lower end is ligated and allowed to retract down behind the peritoneum. A No. 8 or 10 soft rubber catheter is now inserted into the upper end of each ureter. Three or 4 inches of catheter are fed up the ureter, and the remainder is allowed to hang free. This catheter keeps the ureter slightly distended while it is being implanted into the bowel; it thus insures that a large enough tunnel will be formed in the colonic wall. Since it is a little more difficult to deal with the left ureter, this one is implanted first. A proper point is selected on the sigmoid so that the ureter may be directed into it without angulation.

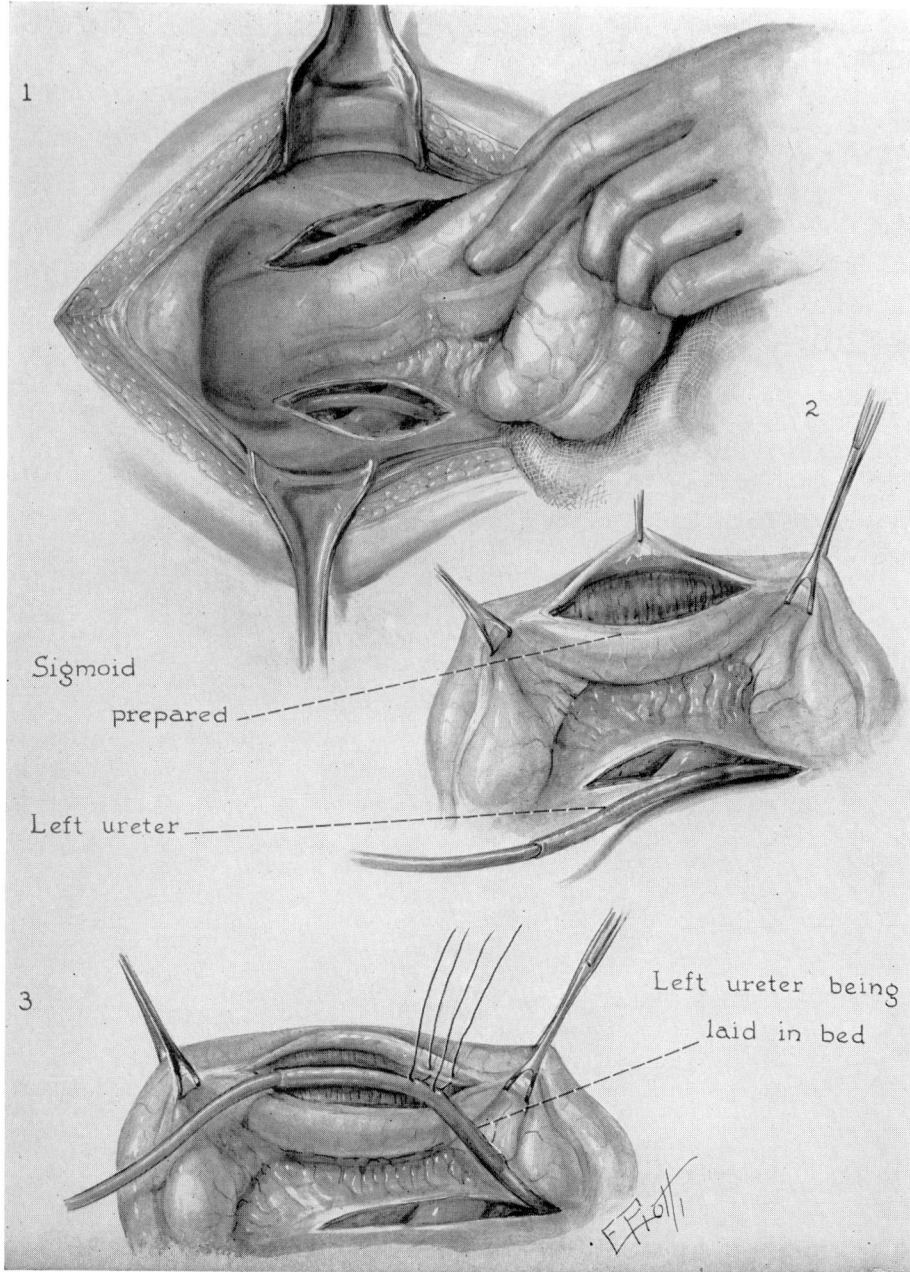

Sigmoid

prepared

Left ureter

Left ureter being
laid in bed

Fig. 390. Transplantation of both ureters into sigmoid in one stage. 1. Transperitoneal approach to sigmoid which is drawn upward. The posterior pelvic peritoneum has been opened on either side to isolate each ureter. 2. Sigmoid held up with Babcock clamps. Flaps of muscularis freed up, the dissection being carried down to the submucosa. Small rubber catheter has been inserted into either ureter. 3. The ureter is anchored in the upper portion of the colonic bed with two silk stitches, so that it cannot move upward or downward in the channel which will be formed.

Furthermore, there must be no torsion or kinking of the colon. The first ureter must be united at a low enough level so that sufficient room is left higher up in the bowel for the other one. A single implantation can be made through a taenia; it is seldom possible to insert both through them.

The selected portion of colon is held up with Babcock clamps at either end of the

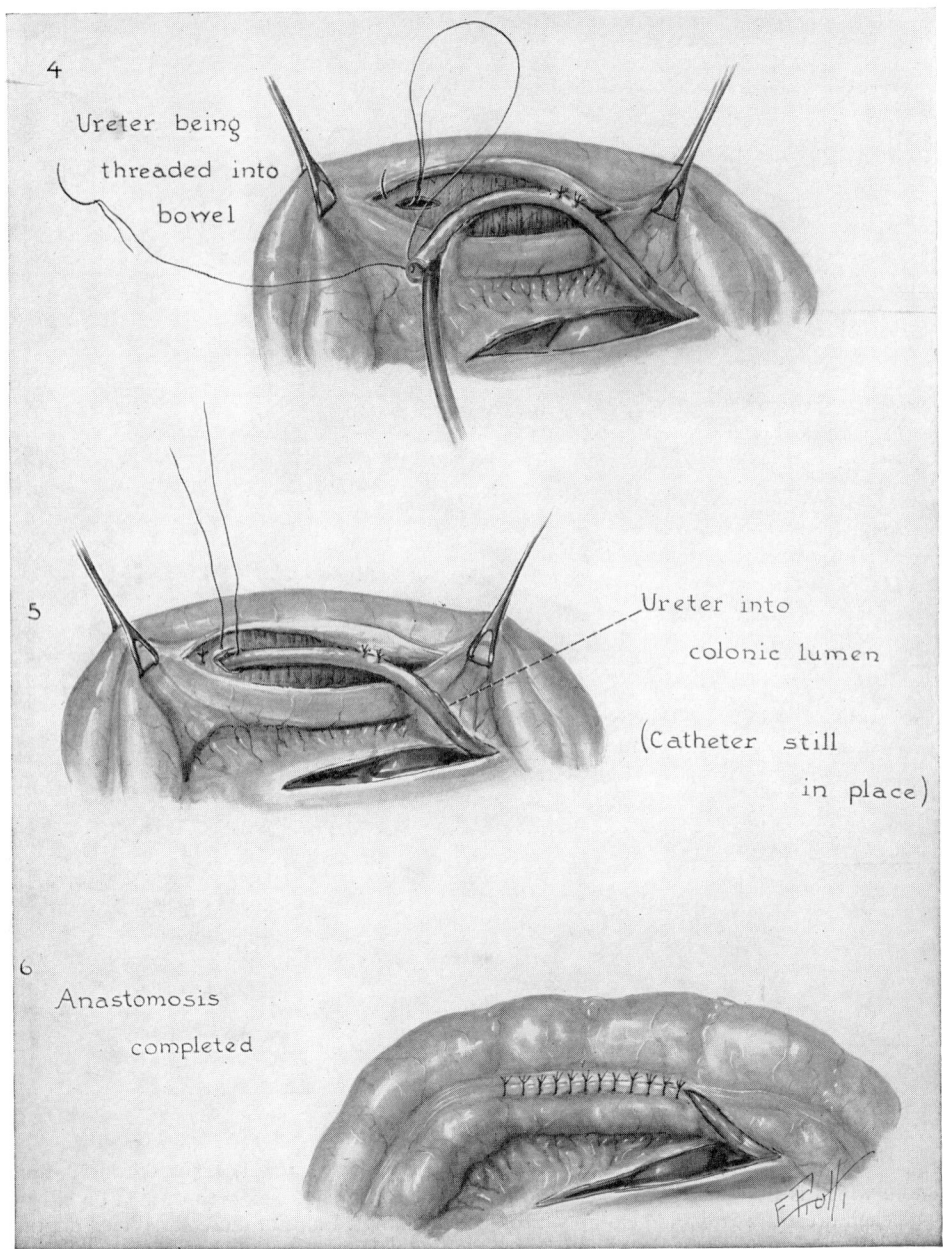

Fig. 390 (*continued*). 4. Opening made through mucosa of bowel. Ureteral end has a short slit to flair open its end. Ureter threaded with fine catgut suture, with double needles which will be led into bowel as shown. 5. Catheter and ureteral end thrust into sigmoid. Anchoring stitch at end of ureter tied. The colonic membrane is now anchored to the ureteral wall. 6. Muscularis brought together with a single row of interrupted fine silk stitches.

segment. A longitudinal incision about $2\frac{1}{2}$ inches in length is made by sharp dissection through the serosa and muscularis; on either side a flap is freed from the underlying submucosa. The ureter is now laid onto this bared submucosa, and at the upper end of the bowel wound the ureter is anchored to the sigmoid with one or two fine silk sutures so that the ureter cannot move upward or downward in the tunnel which is to be formed The end of the ureter is slit longitudinally for about $\frac{1}{4}$ inch to flare open its orifice.

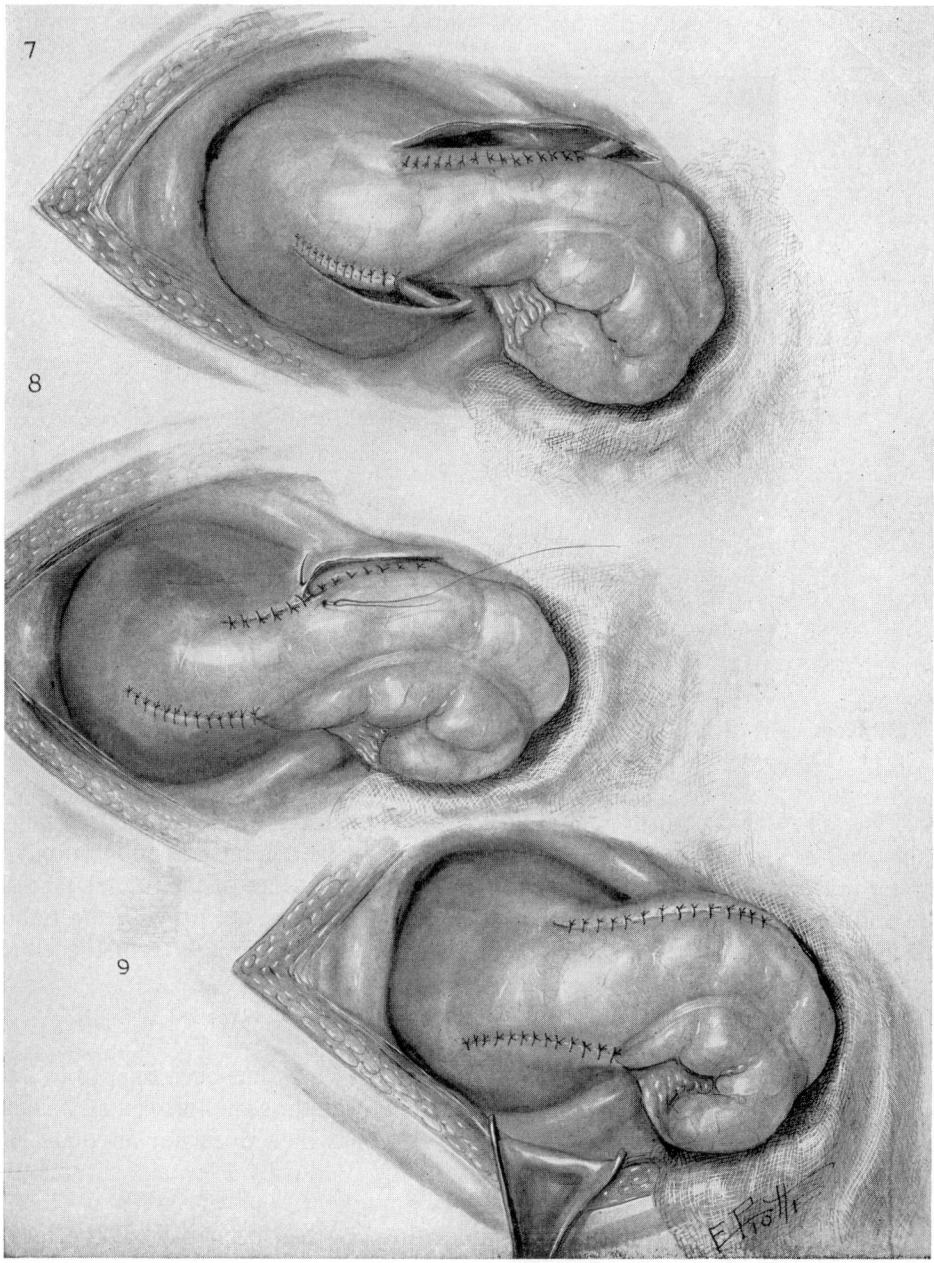

Fig. 390 (*continued*). 7. Right and left ureteral transplantations completed. 8. Lateral flap of posterior pelvic peritoneum being brought over to the sigmoid, to anchor the latter and to cover over the anastomosis. 9. Coverage completed on both sides.

Opposite this slit the ureter is pierced with a double-needled, fine catgut suture, the needles passing from within outward. Toward the lower end of the prepared colonic bed, the mucosa is opened and the catheter (carrying along with it the ureter) is pushed into the bowel. The catgut suture is passed from the interior of the bowel lumen outward so that tying of it will anchor the ureteral orifice not more than an eighth of an inch beyond the mucosal hole. If desired, an additional stitch can be taken between the edge of the mucosa and the areolar tissue of the ureter to further fix it. The flaps of muscularis are now brought together loosely over the ureter with a single row of inter-

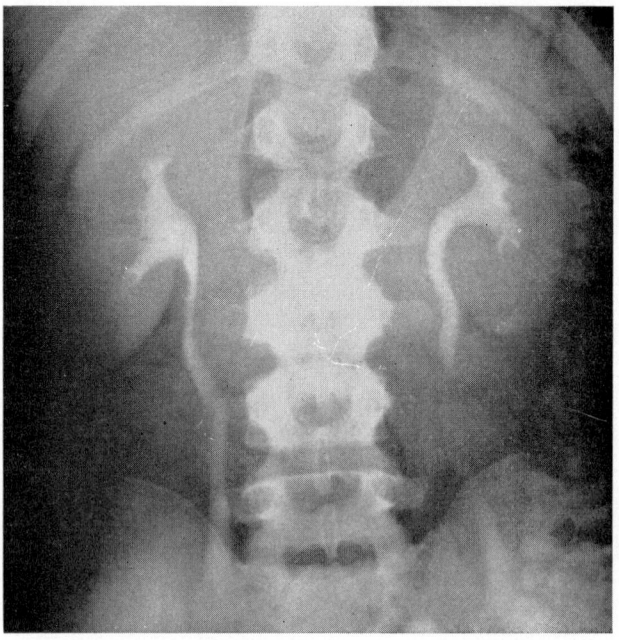

Fig. 391. Pyelogram from a girl, one year after transplantation of ureters to sigmoid. There is excellent preservation of architecture; there is very little dilatation of the ureters.

rupted, fine silk (00000) sutures, taking great care to have these flaps lax enough so that they will not press tightly on the ureter. It cannot be emphasized too strongly that the ureter must not be constricted by overconscientious closure of the tunnel. (If during these various steps of implantation the assistant holds the bowel up with the Babcock clamps, there will be no soiling of the field—only gas can escape from the elevated sigmoid loop.)

The second ureter is now implanted at a slightly higher level on the opposite side of the bowel.

The lateral flap of posterior, parietal peritoneum (which has been opened to isolate the ureter) is now brought over and attached to the bowel, thus anchoring it and covering the anastomosis. The sigmoid must lie in a position which does not angulate either ureter; it may be necessary to adjust its position and hold it by a few silk sutures to the posterior abdominal wall to maintain correct alignment. The abdomen is closed in layers without drainage. After the abdominal dressing has been placed, the legs are drawn up, and through a proctoscope the urethral catheters are identified in the rectum, are grasped, and are gently withdrawn.

Following operation it is easier to care for the child if he is placed on a Bradford frame, with the buttocks resting over a hole in the supporting canvas. With the frame positioned 6 or 8 inches above the mattress, it is easy for the nurse to insert a bed-pan under the child whenever necessary. Urinary discharge into the rectum usually begins immediately but it may be delayed for some hours. Following operation a high fluid intake should be urged for several days, to maintain an adequate flow of urine. If the child does not drink well, supplemental fluid should be given by parenteral routes.

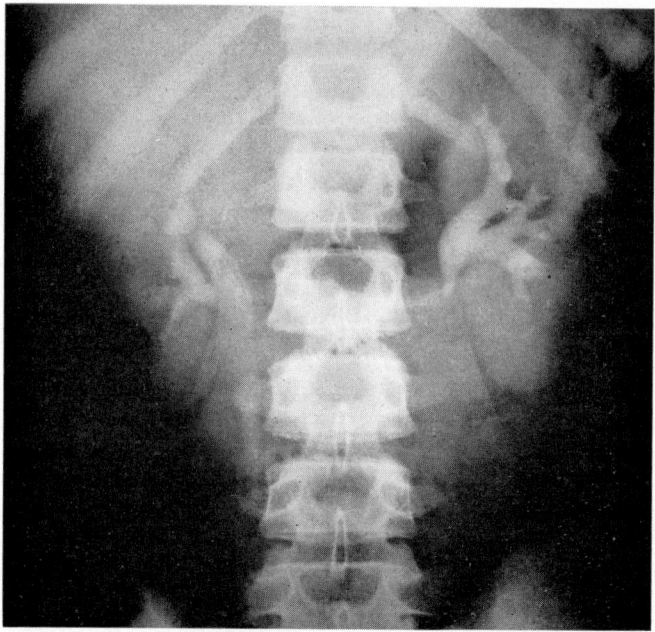

Fig. 392. Intravenous pyelogram of thirteen-year-old girl, eight years after bilateral ureterosigmoidostomy. Patient has bilateral bifid renal pelves. There is excellent preservation of architecture of the pelves and calyces.

Removal of Bladder and Repair of Abdominal-Wall Hernia and Epispadias

After both ureters have been transplanted, the next surgical problem is concerned with: (1) removal of the bladder; (2) repair of the abdominal-wall hernia; (3) correction of the epispadias. If the child is in good condition this may be undertaken during the same hospitalization, but it is preferable in most cases to defer it for some months until there has been full recuperation from the first operation.

The best method for accomplishing these three steps is removal of most of the bladder membrane, appropriate closure of the abdominal-wall fascia, and repair of the epispadias by a modified Young's procedure. The details of these steps are illustrated in Figure 393, but a few general comments are in order here. The bladder mucous membrane can be dissected free from the underlying vesical musculature; it is not necessary to remove the latter. In stripping away that portion of bladder membrane which is to be discarded, it is sometimes difficult to accomplish this without opening into the peritoneal cavity. If the peritoneum is accidentally nicked, it should be stitched closed immediately. At the junction of bladder and posterior urethra, a flap of bladder membrane, about 1.5 cm. in diameter, while raised from its bed, is left attached to the depths of the urethra so that a bulbous end can later be formed and an ejaculatory apparatus constructed. The hernia between the widely separated rectus muscles can be repaired by poking the mass of bladder muscle inward and then bringing in front of it

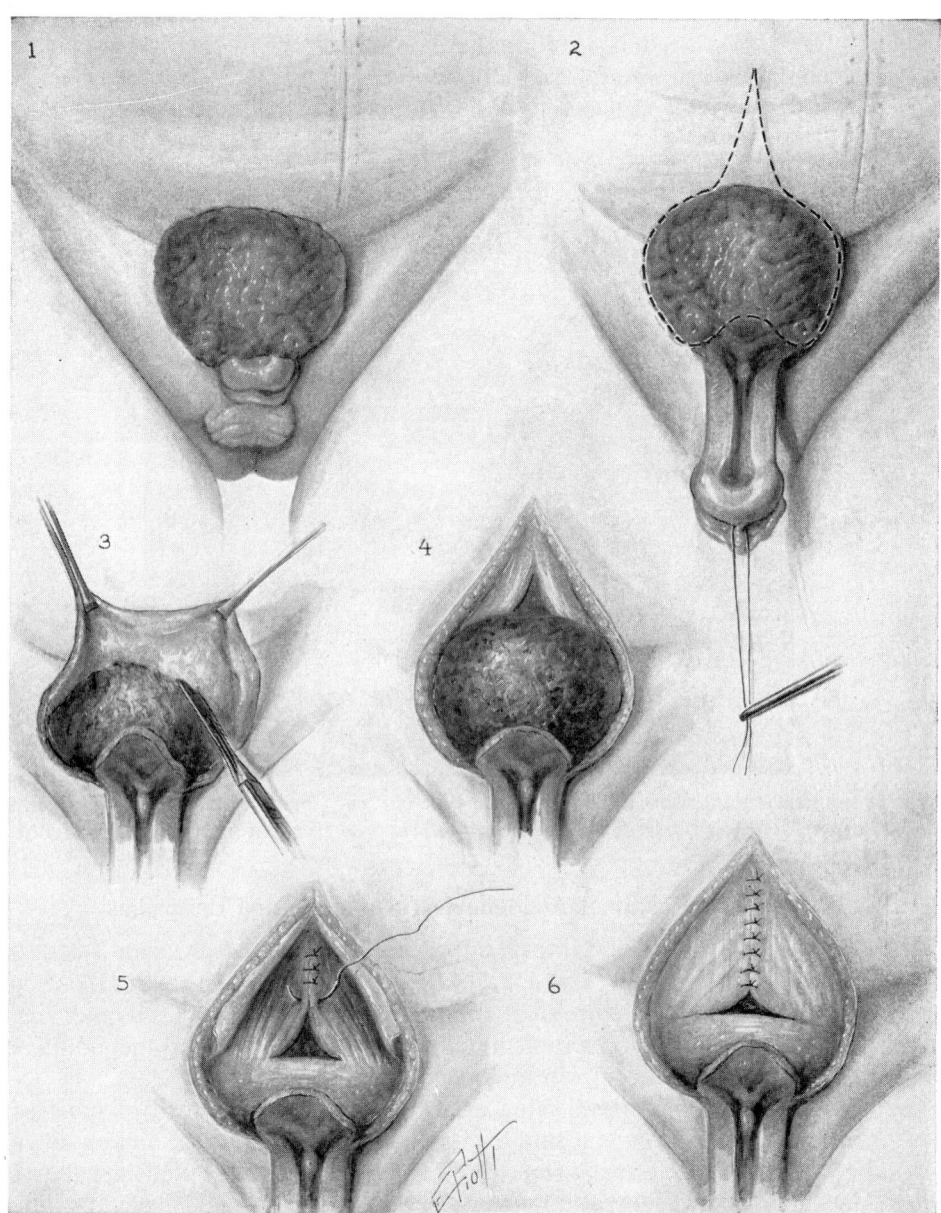

Fig. 393. Removal of exstrophied bladder mucous membrane, repair of abdominal wall defect, and repair of epispadias. 1. View of bladder and complete epispadias. 2. Outline of incisions for removal of bladder membrane. A small portion of membrane is left at the base of the penis. 3. Bladder membrane being stripped from bladder musculature. 4. Bladder membrane excised. The bladder musculature is left in place. 5. Bladder muscle pushed inward. Rectus sheath split to liberate muscle bellies. Muscles are being brought together at the midline. 6. Closure of fascia with interrupted silk stitches. Lower edges of the fasciae are sutured transversely to the fibrous symphysis pubis.

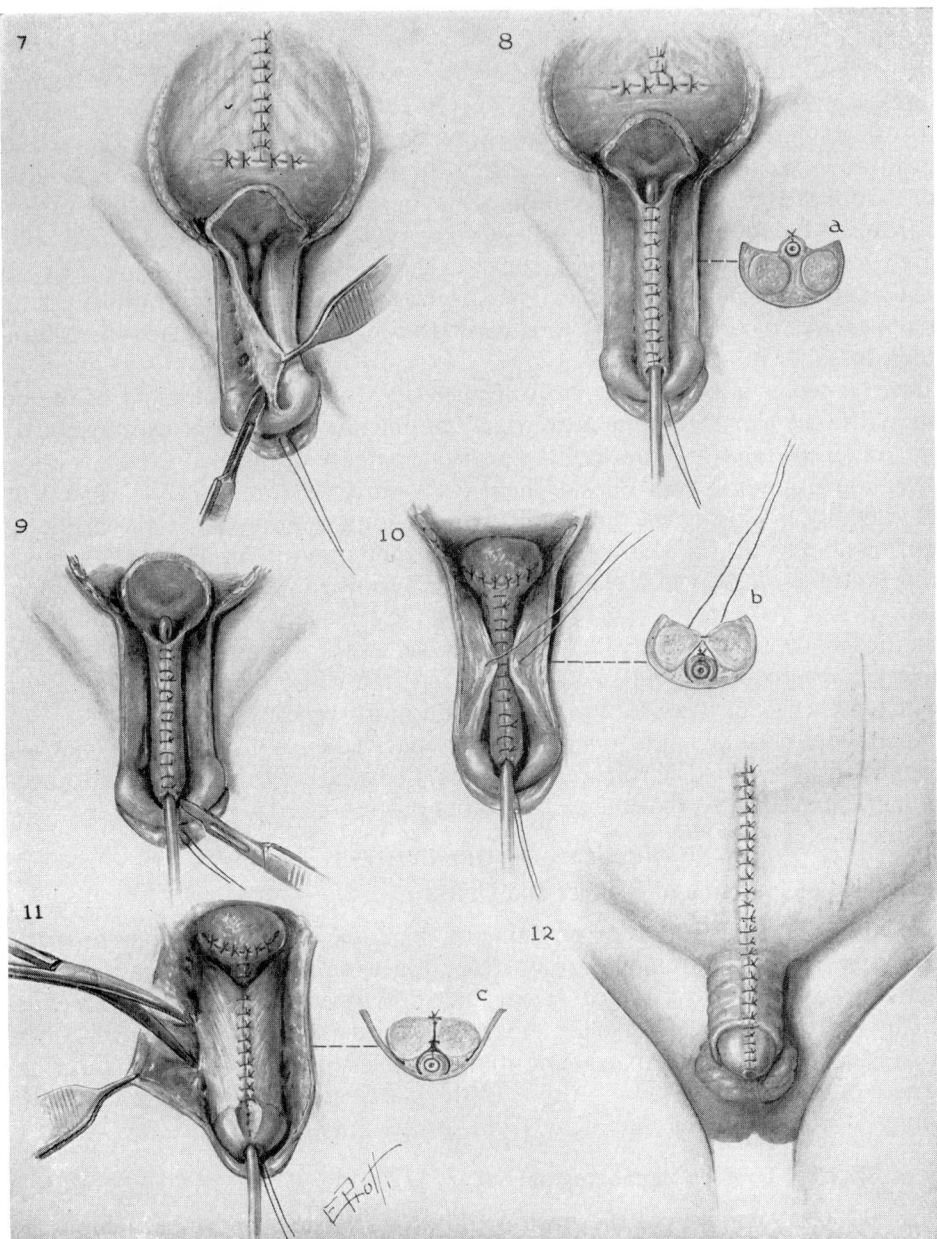

Fig. 393 (*continued*). 7. Abdominal wall repair completed. Urethral membrane being freed from its bed. 8. Urethral membrane turned inward with fine interrupted catgut stitches, making the repair over a small catheter. 9. Urethra being further freed from its bed, so that it can be displaced toward under side of penis. 10. Receptacle formed at base of urethra by turning the remnant of bladder membrane inward, connecting it to the urethral tube. Corpora being brought together over urethra. 11. Corpora completely brought together in midline. Glans being reconstructed over the urethra. Skin is widely freed from sides and under surface of penis. 12. Cutaneous closure of abdominal wall and dorsum of penis.

the rectus muscles or fasciae. If any gap remains it can be closed by raising a flap of one anterior rectus fascia, turning this over the midline like a book-flap, and suturing it to the fascia of the opposite side.

A urethral tube can be constructed by freeing the lateral edges of this membrane and bringing them together, over a No. 8 or 10 French urethral catheter, infolding the edges, using interrupted 00000 chromic catgut for this line of sutures. The tube thus built can now be further freed on either side by sharp dissection, so that it is virtually isolated from the two corpora cavernosa of the penis. There need be no fear of cutting it off from its blood supply, for it will subsequently be deeply imbedded and will live as a free graft. It is very important to separate the urethra extensively from the corpora and the sides of the glans, so that it can be *dislocated and pushed* down toward the under (inferior) surface of the penis, and thus allow the corpora and the glans to be brought together dorsal to it.

Often it seems impossible to get sufficient skin to cover the dorsum of the penis. Additional tissue can be obtained by widely mobilizing the glob of excess skin which always lies on the inferior surface of the penis at the base of the glans, thereby allowing this to rotate around on both sides of the penis toward the dorsum of the same. If there is still difficulty in closing the cutaneous wound along the dorsum of the penile shaft, it is permissible to slit the skin in the midline on the inferior surface of the penis, and sew this up transversely, which has the effect of allowing more skin to slip around to the dorsum.

In the female, the entire bladder mucosa as well as the open urethra can be removed, the defect in the abdominal wall suitably repaired, and without much trouble the tissues brought together from the sides to reconstruct a mons veneris.

No attempt need be made to stabilize the separated ends of the pubic bones, which are connected by a broad fibrous cord. In time, the wings of the pelvis tend to become somewhat less mobile, so that the gait becomes more normal.

RESULTS OF OPERATION

Ineffectiveness of Inversion of Bladder and Urethra

We have treated 3 patients by inverting the bladder, infolding and reconstructing a urethral tube, and attempting to reconstruct the external sphincter muscles of the bladder. Two of these had wholly unsatisfactory urinary control, and were subsequently treated by uretero-sigmoid transplantations. The third boy has a good urinary stream and a considerable bladder capacity; however, he does have some dribbling during the day. These disappointing results—in spite of the one favorable report of such treatment by Young[17]—completely discourage us from further attempts in this direction.

Safety of Bilateral Uretero-Sigmoidostomy

Since 1930, 54 children at the Boston Children's Hospital have been subjected to bilateral uretero-sigmoidostomy, according to the general principles above described. There have been no deaths either during the postoperative period or subsequent thereto. In the very early part of the series, two patients developed abdominal abscesses and peritonitis following a ureteral transplant, but both of these recovered after surgical drainage of the peritoneal cavity. These infections resulted either from contamination of the peritoneum at the time of operation, or from a temporary leak at the site of anastomosis. The comparative rarity of peritonitis (two instances in 54 cases) makes it evident that the transperitoneal approach is a relatively safe one. In the last decade there has been no such complication.

Obstructive Symptoms after Operation

A slight or moderate degree of hydronephrosis is found in most cases, but minimal dilatation will not impair the individual's health if there is no superimposed infection. In an occasional patient the urinary tract is quite dilated for several months after operation, but then is smaller in size when visualized a few years later. Presumably, edema or low-grade infection at the anastomosis can partially obstruct a ureter for weeks or months, but when this reaction subsides the ureter obtains a free drainage and shrinks to more normal proportions. In many patients there is no dilatation of the ureters or pelves at any time.

In one girl a very large ureter (which had been previously obstructed by another congenital anomaly) was unwisely implanted into the colon and subsequently this kidney and ureter had to be removed because of poor function and infection. In a second child a non-functioning, obstructed kidney was removed. In two other children, recurrent flank pain and evidence of malfunctioning kidney by pyelographic studies led to reexploration of the abdomen and inspection of the ureteral anastomoses; in one there was a ureteral angulation and in the other there was a stricture. The correction of each obstruction was followed by relief of symptoms and return of satisfactory kidney function. None of these complications has been encountered in the last decade.

Postoperative Pyelitis

While the Coffey principle of establishing a valve at the junction of ureter and sigmoid has undoubtedly been one of the greatest advances in the treatment of these cases, there is little question that bacteria from the colon often get into and ascend the ureters. It is important to grasp the concept that *pyelitis and ureteritis are not often due to reflux, but are more apt to follow obstruction in the excretory system.* During the last decade, when particular attention has been paid to the implantation of ureters into the colon in a manner free of any constriction or angulation, subsequent pyelitis has been extremely rare; the vast majority of patients have been entirely free of it. When it has occurred it has responded promptly within a few days to chemotherapy, using preferably sulfadiazine, aureomycin or some such antibiotic which has a wide range of effectiveness and a particularly high activity against gram-negative bacilli.

Sphincter Control after Operation

Patients with discharge of urine into the rectum can gain an adequate control of the anal sphincter, if cooperation is good and adequate training is provided. These considerations emphasize that the best age for performing ureteral transplantation lies between three and five years. During the day these children can go as long as two, three, or four hours without emptying the rectum, and without soiling themselves between times. They may have to get up once at night but some sleep through the entire night without defecation or soiling. Some patients develop a mild proctitis and have an urgency to void; giving them sodium bicarbonate three or four times a day tends to alkalinize the rectal fluid and reduce the irritation.

Physical Appearance

The postoperative appearance of two of these patients is shown in Figures 394 and 395. While an anatomic repair is not entirely obtained, all of the previously exposed mucous membrane is either removed or covered, the genital canal of the penis is completed, and the local region in male or female is considerably improved from the cosmetic standpoint. The penis is apt to be somewhat short, but has erectile power.

Stabilization of Bony Pelvis

To date no one has attempted to restore the anterior continuity of the bony pelvis. It would be technically possible to inlay a graft of bone to stabilize the two sides of the pubic structures, but such extensive operation is seldom justified. While children have a waddling gait, the pelvis becomes more rigid in later years. Walking improves as the child grows older and, indeed, some of our patients have indulged in athletics, including football.

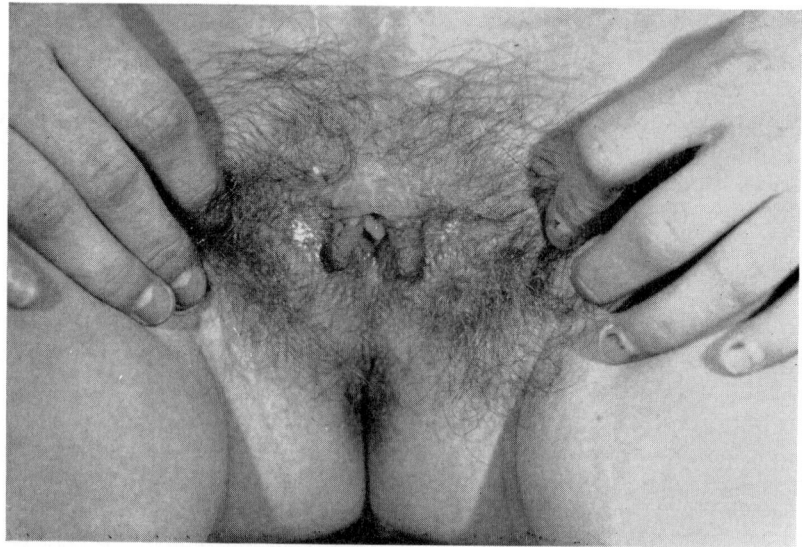

Fig. 394. Exstrophy of bladder in a female. Photograph ten years after transplantation of ureters into sigmoid and removal of bladder and urethra.

Double Bladder, One of Which Is Exstrophied

In addition to the above 80 patients, 54 of whom were treated by ureteral transplantation and 3 of whom were treated by infolding the bladder and urethra, we have seen 3 cases of double urinary bladder, (one within the abdomen and drained by a normal urethra, the others being exstrophied). In each case the exstrophied bladder did not receive a ureter; it was excised and each patient has done well.

Electrolyte Disturbances

Insidious and marked disturbances in electrolyte balance can appear in occasional patients, complications which are much more apt to appear in adults than in children. There may be varying degrees of hyperchloremic acidosis and even hypopotassemia. It has been suggested that these states are caused by the excessive burden placed on the kidneys by reabsorption of urinary solutes from the bowel, but it is now generally agreed that they do not appear unless, in addition, there is a considerable pyelonephritis which interferes with the selective excretion of electrolytes by the kidneys and also disturbs its capacity to synthesize ammonium. The picture is characterized by excessive weakness or even muscle paresis. It can be relieved by urging the patient to empty the bowel

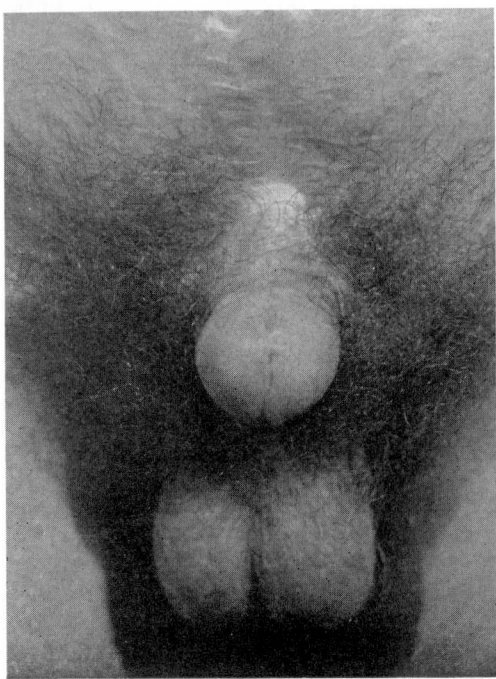

Fig. 395. Exstrophy of bladder in a male. Photograph nine years following transplantation of ureters, removal of bladder, and reconstruction of urethra and penis.

frequently (thereby reducing reabsorption) and by oral administration of sodium bicarbonate.

Over-all Results

The results of surgical treatment of exstrophy of the bladder have been very satisfactory. These individuals who were previously ostracized are now able to play with other children, to attend school, and to have an improved cosmetic appearance. Without doubt there are some psychologic problems which must be considered. In the female these are of little concern, but in the male—who must sit down to urinate—considerable mental readjustment is sometimes necessary. Understanding parents and teachers can do much to rehabilitate these youngsters. It is possible for the males to reproduce. Cases have been reported in which females have borne children. While the life expectancy of patients with ureteral transplants will be undoubtedly diminished below normal it is important to note that there are published accounts of patients who are in very satisfactory health twenty-five to thirty years or more after ureteral transplantations.

REFERENCES

1. Coffey, R. C.: Transplantation of the Ureters into the Large Intestine in the Absence of a Functioning Urinary Bladder. Surg., Gynec. & Obst., *32:*383, 1921.
2. Coffey, R. C.: Transplantation of the Ureters into the Large Intestine. Surg., Gynec. & Obst., *47:*593, 1928.
3. Coffey, R. C.: Further Studies and Experiences with Transfixion Suture Technic (Technic 3) for Transplantation of Ureters

into Large Intestine. Northwest Med., *32:* 31, 1933.
4. Cordonnier, J. J.: Ureterosigmoid Anastomosis. J. Urol., *63:*276, 1950.
5. Creevy, C. D. and Reiser, M. P.: Observations upon the Absorption of Urinary Constituents after Ureterosigmoidostomy: The Importance of Renal Damage. Surg., Gynec. & Obst., *95:*589, 1952.
6. Estes, W. L.: Exstrophy of the Urinary Blad-

der: Implantation of Both Ureters into Rectum; Prolongation of Life Twenty-Four Years. Ann. Surg., *99:*223, 1934.

7. Ferris, D. O. and Odel, H. M.: Electrolyte Pattern of the Blood after Bilateral Ureterosigmoidostomy. J.A.M.A., *142:*634, 1950.

8. Higgins, C. C.: Exstrophy of the Bladder: Review of Seventy Cases. J. Urol., *63:*852, 1950.

9. Hinman, F. and Weyruch, H. M.: A Critical Study of the Different Principles of Surgery Which Have Been Used in Uretero-Intestinal Implantation. Tr. Am. A. Genito-Urin. Surg., *29:*15, 1936.

10. Ladd, W. E. and Lanman, T. H.: Exstrophy of the Bladder. New England J. Med., *216:*637, 1937.

11. Lanman, T. H.: Treatment of Exstrophy of the Bladder. Postgrad. Med., *7:*129, 1950.

12. Peters, G. A.: Transplantation of Ureters into Rectum by an Extraperitoneal Method for Exstrophy of Bladder. Brit. Med. J., *1:*1538, 1901.

13. Randall, L. M. and Hardwick, R. S.: Pregnancy and Parturition Following Bilateral Ureteral Transplantation for Congenital Exstrophy of the Bladder. Surg., Gynec. & Obst., *58:*1018, 1934.

14. Turner, G. G.: The Treatment of Congenital Defects of the Bladder and Urethra by Implantation of the Ureters into the Bowel: With a Record of 17 Personal Cases. Brit. J. Surg., *17:*114, 1929.

15. Von Geldern, C. E.: The Etiology of Exstrophy of the Bladder. Arch. Surg., *8:*61, 1924.

16. Walters, W. and Braasch, W. F.: Ureteral Transplantation to Rectosigmoid for Exstrophy of Bladder, Complete Epispadias, and Other Urethral Abnormalities with Total Urinary Incontinence: Study of 85 Operative Cases. Am. J. Surg., *23:*255, 1934.

17. Young, H. H.: Exstrophy of the Bladder. First Case in Which a Normal Bladder and Urinary Control Have Been Obtained by Plastic Operations. Surg., Gynec. & Obst., *74:*729, 1942.

CHAPTER 53

Epispadias

Epispadias is one of the rarest of congenital anomalies, but it can lead to tragic results if not suitably repaired. This cleft on the upper side of the urethra occurs both in the male and female. Dees,[6] in 1949, studied its incidence from a review of files from eight large hospitals and found a ratio of one in 117,604 males and one in 481,110 females. This incidence of about 5 to 1 corresponds with our series of 18 patients, of whom 15 were males and 3 were females.

Much has appeared in the surgical literature during the past seventy-five years regarding the surgical therapy of this condition. The multiplicity of operative attacks would seem to indicate that no one has been outstandingly successful, but a review of our material strongly emphasizes that this malformation can be suitably corrected in most instances. It is possible to give a good cosmetic appearance to the genitalia and to provide bladder continence when this has been lacking.

CLINICAL PICTURE

In the male there are three general forms of epispadias, these being descriptive of the extent of the cleft. The *balanitic type* is the most uncommon of the three, the defect involving only a slit in the glans, in the base of which the distal part of the urethra lies open and exposed. There is no associated incontinence. The *penile type* is that in which the shaft of the penis and the glans are open superiorly along their entire length; the urethra is displaced dorsally and forms a gutter between the two corpora. The urethral tube emits urine at the base of the penis; incontinence may or may not be present, depending upon the degree of deficiency or development of the bladder-neck sphincters. In the *penopubic type* there is an opening along the entire length of the penis and extending a short distance up the lower abdominal wall. In all such cases the bladder sphincter muscles are deficient and there is a constant dribbling of urine, at least when the child is in a standing position. With this laxness of the bladder outlet some patients show an eversion or a herniation of a portion of the bladder out through the relaxed orifice during periods of coughing, straining, or other activity which increases the intra-abdominal pressure. The pubic bones may be joined by a short symphysis in the balanitic and penile types of epispadias, but in the more extensive penopubic form there is always a separation of the bones, which may be joined only by a fibrous cord.

In the balanitic form of epispadias, coitus and insemination are possible, but in the more extensive deformities the seminal fluid is discharged at the base of the penis. While there can be a good urinary stream in the balanitic type, this is not possible with the longer clefts; the necessity of assuming a sitting position during evacuation of the bladder is usually a great embarrassment to older boys and to adult patients.

In the female three general forms are also found. In the first there is merely a *bifid clitoris* and a urethral opening which is slightly enlarged on its upper aspect. In the *intermediary type* the cleft extends along the entire urethra but does not include the

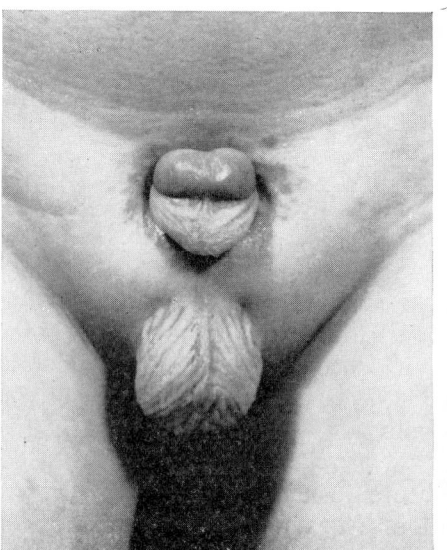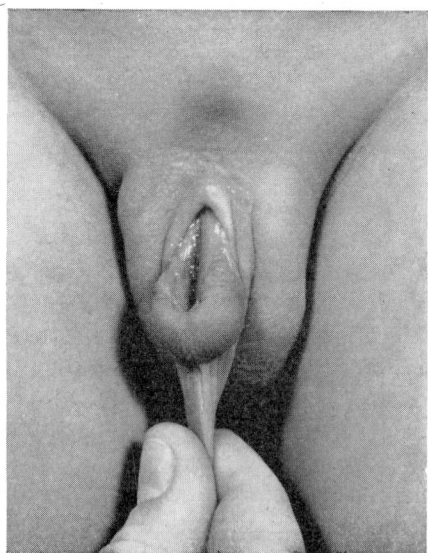

Fig. 396. Complete penile epispadias in a male child. The bladder sphincter was intact and there was no dribbling.

bladder sphincter; there is no incontinence. In the *complete type* the ventral split involves the entire urethra and the bladder sphincter, so that incontinence is a distressing part of the picture. In the female, there is very apt to be a depression of the mons veneris, giving the region a flattened or grooved appearance. There may or may not be separation of the pubic bones, but this is generally found in all cases with the more extensive malformations. In the female, the lesser forms of the anomaly may go unrecognized for long periods of time, and indeed, the deformity may be so mild that nothing need be done about it because, when older, there will be coverage of the area by enlarging labia and pubic hair. The reproductive organs are not involved and the individual can reproduce normally.

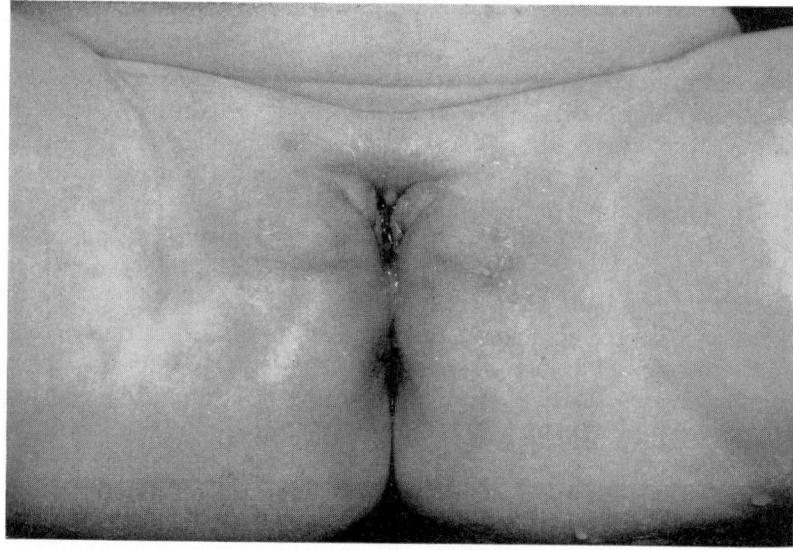

Fig. 397. Epispadias in a female child. There was some incontinence.

muscles at the bladder neck must be thorough and extensive, for only by the liberation of these and placement of them in a saddle fashion over the bladder neck can continence be attained.

To promote healing, a large suprapubic tube, of a self-retaining type, must be employed and kept open at all times for about ten days, so that the operative field is constantly kept dry.

We have not attempted to stabilize the pubic bones by any shortening of the symphysis ligaments (though these may be several inches in length). It has been our experience that the pelvis subsequently tends to become reasonably stable and nothing need be done in an operative way to facilitate this.

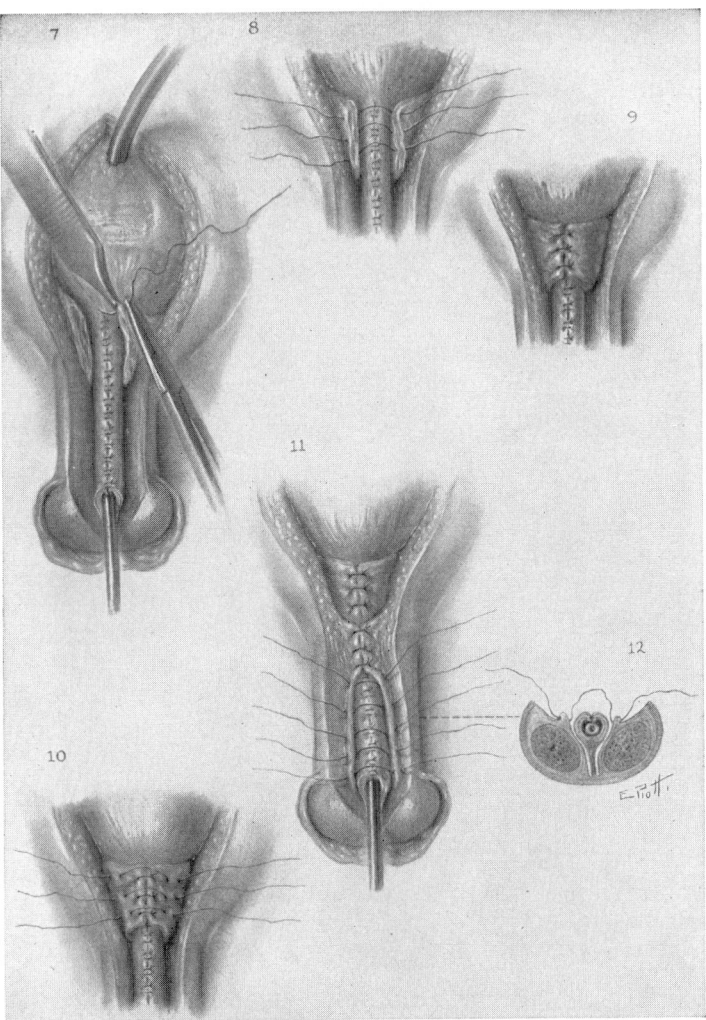

Fig. 398 (*continued*). 7. Over a small catheter, urethral membrane turned inward with interrupted 00000 chromic catgut sutures. Muscular tissue of bladder outlet being brought together with interrupted silk stitches. 8. Silk stitches in external sphincter muscle. 9. Muscular tissue approximated. 10. If the urethral catheter is not tightly snugged by the first muscular approximation, additional compression can be gained by a second layer of stitches to tighten the muscle. 11. Edges of corpora being brought together over urethra with 00000 Deknatel silk, as indicated. 12. Cross-section as indicated.

It is not known whether the maintenance of the penis in an extended position during the healing phase improves the ultimate outcome, but it has been our practice to employ such a traction apparatus for a week or ten days following operation (Fig. 399). A silk stitch is put through the frenulum, close to the glans, and is attached by a rubber band to an overlying, semi-curved, metal bar which is supported by the lower part of the abdomen and upper thighs. This tends to keep the penis attenuated, though there is no real evidence to prove conclusively that this treatment increases the length of the organ subsequently.

RESULTS OF THERAPY

During the past twenty years, 18 patients with epispadias have been treated surgically at the Children's Hospital. In this series there were 3 cases of balanitic epispadias.

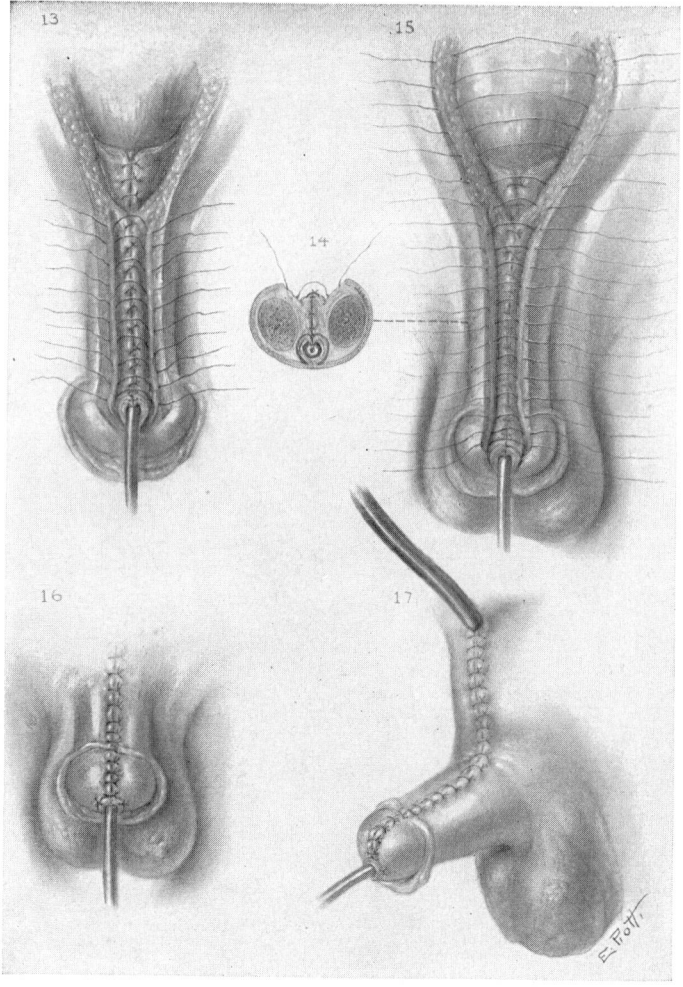

Fig. 398 (*continued*). 13. Second layer of silk sutures approximating anterior edges of corpora. 14. Placement of subcutaneous, fine silk sutures, as shown in 15, throughout length of glans, penile shaft, and suprapubic wound. 16. Cutaneous closure throughout entire length of wound. Urethral end appropriately stitched to edges of glans. 17. Repair completed. Large suprapubic drainage tube in place. The urethral reconstruction has been made over a small catheter, which can now be pulled out.

4 of the penile variety, and 11 of the penopubic or complete form. Fifteen of these were male and 3 were female, all of the latter having complete epispadias.

In the early part of the series 2 patients with penoscrotal epispadias were treated by bilateral uretero-sigmoidostomy. One of these died of peritonitis; the other has good

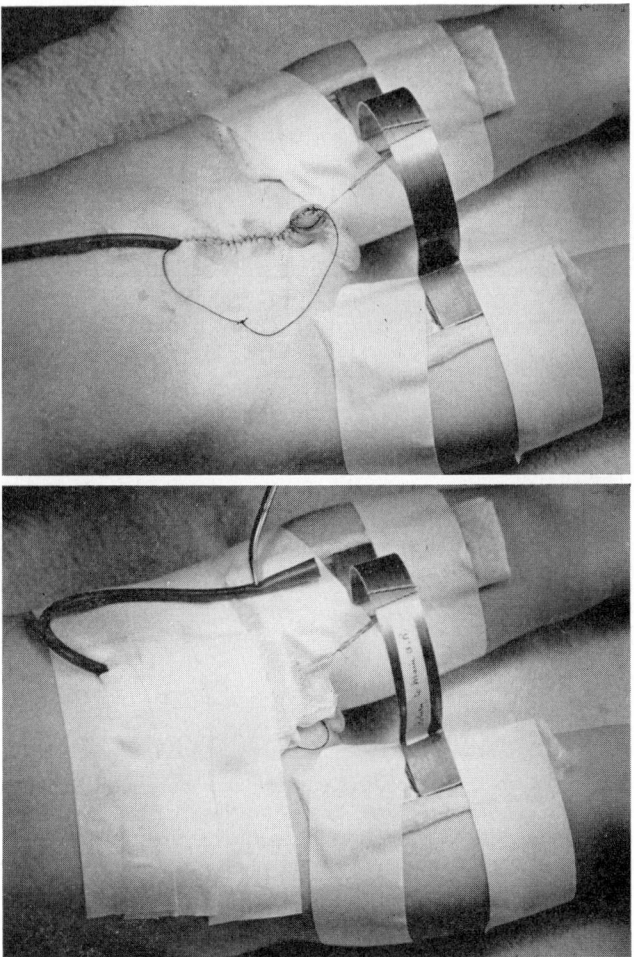

Fig. 399. Apparatus employed for eight to ten days following surgical repair, to give traction on penis. *Above*, There is a heavy silk string through the urethra and emerging from the suprapubic wound. This can be used subsequently for leading a dilator through the urethra. The silk traction stitch through the frenulum is attached by a light rubber band to the curved metal bar. *Below*, Dressing in place.

rectal control of urinary and fecal discharge. We now feel quite strongly that uretero-sigmoidostomy is seldom justified for the treatment of this condition, and certainly would not now propose it unless local plastic repair has been tried and has failed.

Of the remaining 16 patients, 13 were incontinent before operation. In this group of 13, there have been 9 with perfect urinary control and 4 with occasional dribbling. This wetness is inconstant and occurs only during times of forceful activity or great physical stress. Two of these youngsters had a secondary operation, at which time sphincters at the neck of the bladder were further tightened. These have been followed

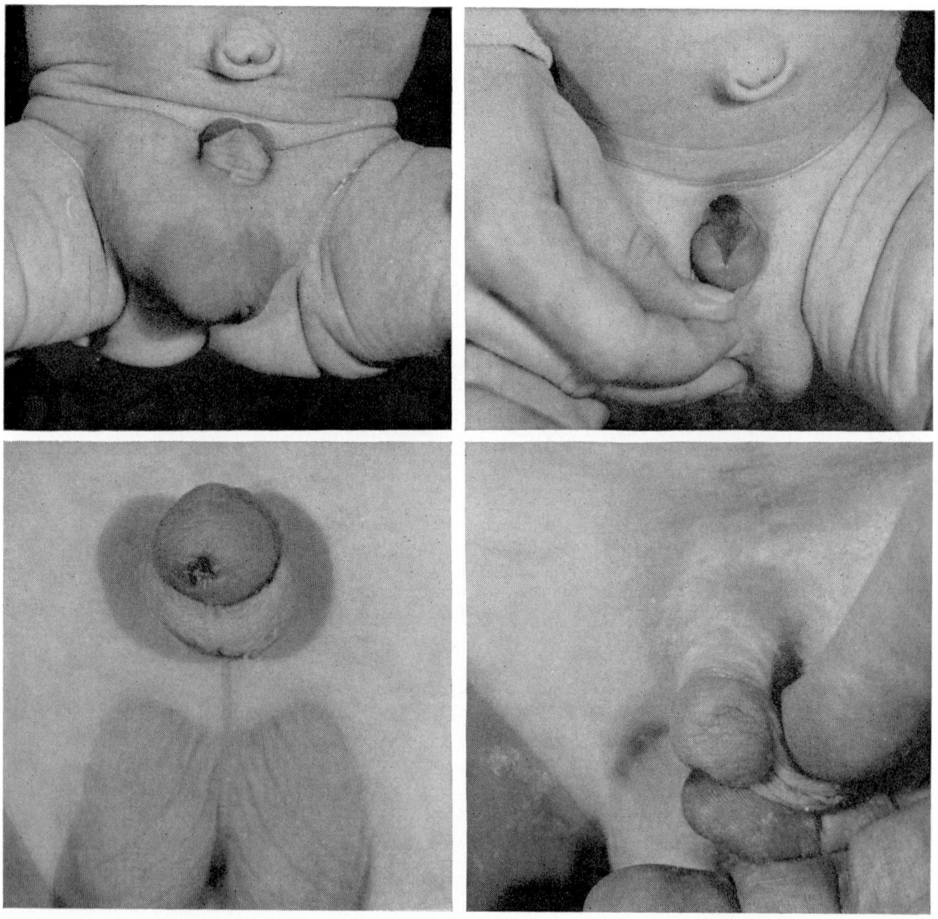

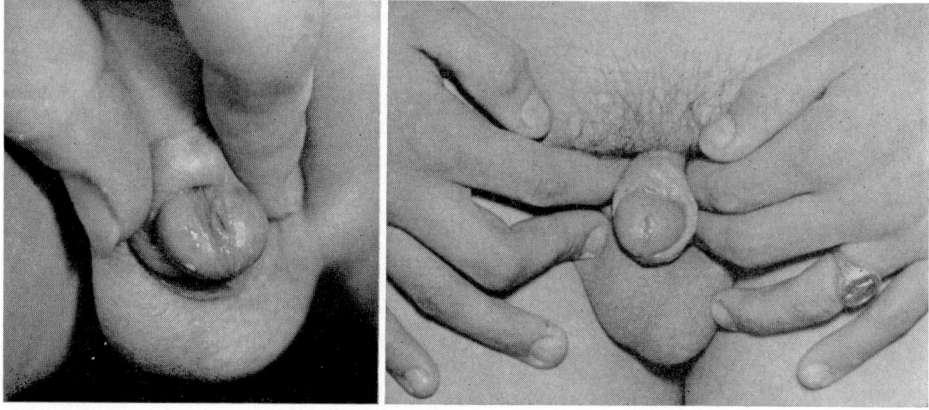

Fig. 400. Photographs of child with complete epispadias who had urinary incontinence *Above*, Preoperative pictures. There is a large inguinal hernia on the child's right. When the penis is drawn downward, its dorsal defect is visible. *Below*, Postoperative pictures. The left photograph shows the normal position of the urethral meatus. The right photograph shows the excellent repair of the dorsal surface. (The child is completely continent.)

Fig. 401. *Left*, Preoperative state, showing epispadias of glans and shaft. *Right*, Photograph ten years after operative repair, showing satisfactory appearance of penis and urethral orifice.

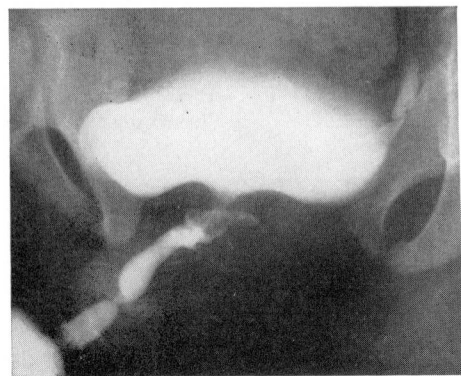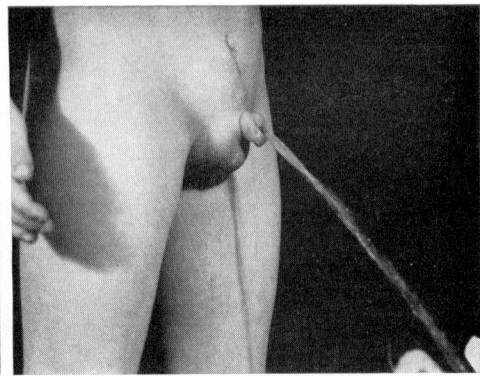

Fig. 402. *Left*, Postoperative urethro-cystogram in a boy who previously had complete epispadias and total urinary incontinence. The bladder now has good capacity and has a well supported and constricted outlet. (There is now complete urinary continence.) *Right*, Same patient. Now, following surgical repair, there is a good urinary stream and a satisfactory bladder capacity.

by complete continence, so that in our end results there are now 11 with urinary control and only 2 with some dribbling.

Our studies have shown conclusively that in those youngsters who have marked incontinence before operation (and hence have a small and collapsed bladder), there is an excellent possibility of distending the organ in the postoperative period so that it will attain a reasonable capacity. A cystogram on such a subject is reproduced in Figure 402, which shows an organ of suitable size and with a rather sharp cut-off at the bladder outlet.

From the cosmetic viewpoint, the reconstruction has been quite satisfactory, as illustrated in Figures 400 and 401.

REFERENCES

1. Ballantyne, J. W.: So-called Epispadias in Woman; with an Illustrative Case. Edinburgh Hospital Reports, 4:249, 1896.
2. Barney, J. D.: An Operation for the Relief of Epispadias in the Male. Surg., Gynec. & Obst., 23:594, 1916.
3. Bremer, J. L.: Hypospadias and Epispadias: A Philological Note. New England J. Med., 207:537, 1932.
4. Cantwell, F. V.: Operative Treatment of Epispadias by Transplantation of the Urethra. Ann. Surg., 22:689, 1895.
5. Cecil, A. B.: A Further Report on the Cure of Hypospadias and Epispadias. J. Urol., 34:278, 1935.
6. Dees, J. E.: Congenital Epispadias with Incontinence. J. Urol., 62:513, 1949.
7. Stiles, H. J.: Epispadias in the Female, and Its Surgical Treatment. Surg., Gynec. & Obst., 13:127, 1911.
8. Thompson, A. R.: A Case of Epispadias Associated with Complete Incontinence Treated by Rectus Transplantation. Brit. J. Child. Dis., 20:146, 1923.
9. Young, H. H.: An Operation for Cure of Incontinence Associated with Epispadias. J. Urol., 7:1, 1922.

CHAPTER 54

Hypospadias

Hypospadias is an abnormality which is encountered quite commonly. The urethra terminates in an abnormal position in the area of the frenulum, along the ventral surface of the penis, at the peno-scrotal angle, or even in the perineum. The malformation is apt to be associated with some degree of chordee, giving downward contraction and bowing of the penis. With the more severe form of hypospadias, the entire phallus is sometimes underdeveloped. With all types there is a hooding of the foreskin, giving redundancy of preputial skin on the dorsal and lateral aspects, but a paucity of it toward the ventral area.

Literally scores of reconstructive operations have been proposed or have been employed in the treatment of hypospadias. Many of these have now fallen into disuse. In recent years there has been a greatly renewed interest in the repair of these urethral abnormalities. Sound principles in the surgical repair of the deformity have crystallized a great deal since 1940. The following sections have been prepared largely on the basis of an experience with observation on, or the treatment of, 392 patients at the Boston Children's Hospital from 1931 to 1951.

CLINICAL FEATURES

Position of Urethral Opening

In our series of patients with hypospadias, the following positions of the urethral meatus have been observed:

Frenular..............................	260 cases
In shaft of penis.........................	32 "
Peno-scrotal or perineal...................	100 "

In the minimal types of deformity, the urethral orifice is at the level of the corona, situated but a few millimeters back from its normal position, thereby replacing the frenulum. In a few instances the orifice is tiny and may give obstruction to the urinary flow; generally, such is not the case. The foreskin is invariably hooded. There is seldom any chordee of the penis.

In those cases in which the opening appears along the penile shaft, the foreskin is hooded, and there may or may not be some degree of chordee. If the orifice is toward the distal end of the penis, the individual is able to direct the urinary stream while in a standing position; insemination during coitus is possible. With the openings which are more proximally located on the shaft, urination in a standing position is unsatisfactory, and insemination during coitus cannot be accomplished.

When the urethral meatus appears at the peno-scrotal angle or in the perineum (the latter generally being associated with a bifid scrotum), the patient must sit down to urinate; insemination is impossible. There is generally some degree of chordee.

Page 714

Chordee

Degrees of chordee can vary within wide limits. In many cases it is negligible or is a minimal consideration. In a large proportion of cases with the more serious abnormalities (peno-scrotal and perineal types) chordee may be marked; the penis is drawn downward in a sharp angulation, such deformity becoming more pronounced as the genitalia grow beyond the second or third year of life. This is an item of special importance in later childhood after puberty when penile erections may be disagreeable or even painful.

Rudimentary Penis

When there is failure of development of the penile urethra, the corpus spongiosum may be rudimentary and the entire phallus can be diminutive in size, a factor particularly prominent prior to the time when hormonal stimulation appears at puberty.

Other Anomalies of Urinary Tract

It has not been our policy to perform intravenous pyelography on patients with frenular types of hypospadias, but we have usually made such studies on boys who have had penile, peno-scrotal, or perineal types of hypospadias. Whenever such investigations have been carried out, the finding of other congenital abnormalities in the urinary tract did not seem to be any more frequent than would be the incidence in an average run of children (who do not have urethral abnormality).

Determination of Sex

When dealing with an individual with a peno-scrotal or perineal hypospadias, there must be particular care to make sure that the subject does not have other reproductive abnormalities and is not in fact a eunuch or a female. In those subjects in whom the scrotum is intact and contains two structures which are apparently normal testes, there need be little apprehension, but when there is "cryptorchidism" or when there are other regional abnormalities of the scrotum and external genitalia, there is a reasonably high chance that one is dealing with some profound sexual malformation.

Additional important information can be gained in several ways: (1) Rectal examination will generally permit identification (by palpation) of a uterus if one exists. (2) Roentgenographic visualization, by injection of the "urethral" meatus with radiopaque material (such as Diodrast), can give clear-cut information as to whether one is dealing with a urethra which connects to the bladder or whether the external orifice is actually the termination of a urogenital sinus, which receives both a urethra and a female genital tract. For such studies, lateral or oblique views are the most helpful. (3) Determinations of the level of urinary excretion of 17-ketosteroids can give pertinent data. If the value is greatly elevated, it suggests the presence of an adreno-genital syndrome which has produced masculinization and enlargement of the phallus of a female subject. (4) If the above investigations leave any doubt concerning the identification of the sex, pelvic laparotomy should be done to gain accurate information about the internal genitalia. Frequently, this procedure is most illuminating. Inspection of the gonads and pelvic organs occasionally shows structures of the female sex, or of both sexes. The procedure should include not only inspection of those structures which lie free within the pelvis, but also examination of gonads which may be in the upper part of the inguinal canal; this can be accomplished either by withdrawing them into the abdomen or by dissecting (from the central wound) a tunnel toward the inguinal regions through the superficial layers of the abdominal wall. Gonads, regardless of whether they appear externally to be typical testes, or typical ovaries, should always be biopsied for micro-scopic examination, so that positive identification of the tissue can be made; some of these turn out to be ovo-testis.

In our series of 100 patients with severe hypospadias (peno-scrotal or perineal), 32 had some degree of cryptorchidism or had anorchism. Of these, 13 have been ex-plored surgically; 8 were found to have female internal genitalia and a ninth was found to be a true hermaphrodite. Obviously, the discovery of such anomalies of the internal genitalia has called for management which may partially or completely overshadow any therapy for "hypospadias" for which the patient was initially hospitalized. Dealing with the manifold physical and psychologic problems related to handling a female (who was previously known as a male) can be most troublesome and disturbing. The earlier in life that the profound readjustments have to be made, the easier it is on the subject and his family. We therefore feel very strongly that any child who has a severe hypo-spadias (peno-scrotal or perineal in type), about whom there is any question regarding the sex, should have pelvic laparotomy in the early weeks or months of life to determine beyond a shadow of a doubt the actual sex of the individual.

Symptoms

A coronal or glandular type of hypospadias seldom gives rise to symptoms except-ing those rare cases in which constriction at the meatal opening produces urinary ob-struction. Generally, attention has been drawn to the anomaly by the hooded appear-ance of the foreskin; closer examination of the penis shows the retrocessed position of the urethral opening. When the orifice is in the mid-shaft of the penis, the condition not infrequently goes undetected in infancy; later in life it is noted that, during attempts to void in the standing position, there is wetting of the surrounding floor, clothes, and shoes during the act of urination. With the peno-scrotal or perineal types of hypospadias, the magnitude of the deformity is generally great enough so that the anomaly is noted very shortly after birth. In the perineal, peno-scrotal, and in some of the more prox-imally located shaft hypospadiases, the boy must sit down to void, a situation which generally does not disturb him very much until four to six years of age when other chil-dren take cognizance of the fact that he does not stand up to urinate like other boys. Taunted and harassed a great deal by his comrades, this consideration becomes of special importance during the early years of schooling. During this time the psychologic reactions are the most important parts of the problems which have to be dealt with.

TREATMENT

In the management of a patient with hypospadias there are three main considera-tions. The functions of both micturition and procreation are foremost. Not inconsider-able is the fact that there might be a great deal of psychologic trauma to the child's parents, and also to the youngster himself, after he attains the age of five or six years. The latter can generally be handled satisfactorily with patience and understanding on the part of the physician.

Mild Hypospadias

Those openings of the urethra which are situated but a few millimeters back from the normal area should never be treated with any idea of moving the orifice out to a normal position. The Beck operation, mobilizing the meatus and terminal portion of urethra, so that these can be moved distally, is very apt to be followed by sloughing, regional infection and scarring, and a magnification of the deformity; the whole situation is made worse than it was before. We believe that this is a meddlesome procedure and should never be undertaken; we have seen many disastrous results following it. Generally, the management of such a case is concerned wholly with the alleviation of the parents' apprehension. It is quite easy to assure them that the child will be able to micturate normally and in later life will be able to procreate in a completely satisfactory manner. Therefore, since the *function* of the organ will be normal, no operative correction of the minimal deformity should be entertained. In an occasional case there is a tiny orifice at the urethral meatus which gives mild obstruction. Under these circumstances, the opening should be dilated or else should be enlarged by introducing one blade of a small pair of scissors into the urethra and slitting open the meatus somewhat. In all of these cases the appearance of the penis can be made more acceptable by removal of the hooded foreskin; circumcision is advisable for cosmetic reasons.

Severe Hypospadias

In all cases of hypospadias in which the orifice is in the shaft, in the peno-scrotal angle, or in the perineum, certain principles of surgical care have now become quite clear. In all of these situations, a circumcision must be avoided because the foreskin may later be an important source of integument when rearranging cutaneous flaps or shifting skin to the under surface of the penis in correction of the urethral abnormality.

Evaluation of Operation. Many types of operations have been used for the correction of severe hypospadias. No attempt will be made here to summarize, evaluate, or criticize the various procedures which have had varying degrees of success or failure in the hands of those who have proposed or have used them. An excellent critique on the repair of hypospadias has been made by Smith and Blackfield,[22] to which reference may be made by those who would like to make a study of the different operative methods. A few comments are in order, since they form the basis for selection of the procedure which we currently routinely employ for the treatment of hypospadias.

OMBRÉDANNE OPERATION. By the Ombrédanne procedure, a large funnel-shaped sac is fashioned by raising skin from the ventral surface of the penis and from the scrotum, leaving the urethral meatus at the base of this funnel, puckering the flaps to form an orifice at the distal end of the penis, covering over raw surfaces by rearrangement and transportation of skin from the hooded area. A small series of such repairs was done in this hospital in the early 1930's; in spite of the fact that the procedures were undertaken by men with a great deal of experience in plastic surgery, the results were exceedingly disappointing. A great glob of tissue presents on the under surface of the penis; during times of erection the shaft extends beyond this underslung mass; the general appearance has little resemblance to a normal human penis. Any construction of a urethra which utilizes skin from the proximal half of the penis or from the scrotum, can form a channel which is elastic, has the potentialities of growth with the individual but always has the very disagreeable feature of producing a pathway which contains hair. This becomes particularly troublesome if concretions and calculi form on these hidden hairs; the treatment of such complications can be extraordinarily difficult. The Ombrédanne operation has absolutely nothing to recommend it!

DENIS BROWNE OPERATION. Repair by the so-called Denis Browne technique, which is a resurrection in all respects of the procedure described by Duplay in 1880, has received wide trial and comment, but we are very skeptical about it for several reasons: (1) A urethra is not formed in its entirety, since a catheter is merely laid along the pathway where the urethral tube is to be constructed, leaving a strip of skin along the dorsal aspect of this catheter, while covering over its ventral part with the raw under-surfaces of skin flaps which are drawn over it from the sides of the penis. Without doubt a smooth urethral tube will subsequently develop around the catheter, either by formation of fibrous tissue or by proliferation of epithelium from the dorsal strip of skin. We believe that a good deal of scarring will almost certainly lead to a longitudinal contraction of the penis in later years. (2) There have been many reports of the development of fistulas, a complication which might be expected because the longitudinal junction of skin edges along the ventral surface of the penis immediately overlies the urethra which is being formed; these frequently require secondary operative closure. (3) This operation necessitates a good deal of shifting of skin from the dorsum and lateral sides of the penis to cover the ventral surface of the penis. To relieve tension, a long dorsal incision is made, this wound being allowed to separate and to granulate in subsequently. We cannot see how this can fail to produce contractions which are undesirable. (4) The operation has been recommended for all forms of hypospadias, but it is obvious that in employment of it for perineal, for peno-scrotal, or for those with openings in the proximal half of the penis, the newly formed tube will be hair-bearing and therefore troublesome.

Recommended Method for Hypospadias Repair

Over a period of many years, we have come to rely on the technique of repair indicated in Figures 403, 404, and 405. This is essentially the operation devised by Nové-Josserand and later revised by McIndoe and others. In our clinic, this work has all been done under the direction of Dr. Donald W. MacCollum, whose experience and suggestions are summarized herewith and whose clinical material forms the basis of this chapter. The therapy consists of procedures in three stages: (1) Relief of the chordee in early childhood. (2) Construction of a urethral channel by tunneling through the substance of the penis and lining this with a Thiersch graft, usually performing this step near the age of puberty. (3) Six months later, joining of the newly formed penile urethra with whatever normal urethra is available proximal to it. (Young and Benjamin anastomose the inlaid graft to the hypospadiac opening at the second operation, thereby eliminating one stage.)

First Stage. Treatment of Chordee. For this preliminary step (Fig. 403) the child is usually admitted to the hospital at two or three years of age, though in some instances when there is delayed onset of chordee, it is necessary to make the operative correction at a later time according to the indications in the case. A catheter is inserted into the bladder through the presenting urethral opening so that the penis can be kept dry post-operatively. The prepuce can be sewed on either side to the anterior abdominal wall for purposes of traction and anchorage during operation. An inverted V-shaped incision is made just distal to the presenting urethral opening. This is extended distally toward the glans, preferably making it in a zigzag or W shape. All fibrous tissues producing the downward deformity of the penis are removed. Constant traction is maintained on the glans penis, so that any taut bands in the substance of the penis can be identified and cut out. The tight structures not only lie distal to the site of the urethral meatus, but oftentimes are situated proximal to it. It is therefore frequently necessary to free some portion of the existing urethra from surrounding structures; during such liberation, the urethral meatus generally retracts considerably toward the perineum. When all limiting bands have been excised, the penis will lie in an elongated form on the lower abdominal wall. Considerable freeing and shifting of skin can be accomplished by wide undermining of the integument around both sides of the penis, carrying this dissection up into the hooded area of the foreskin on the dorsum of the penis if necessary. Mobilized skin can

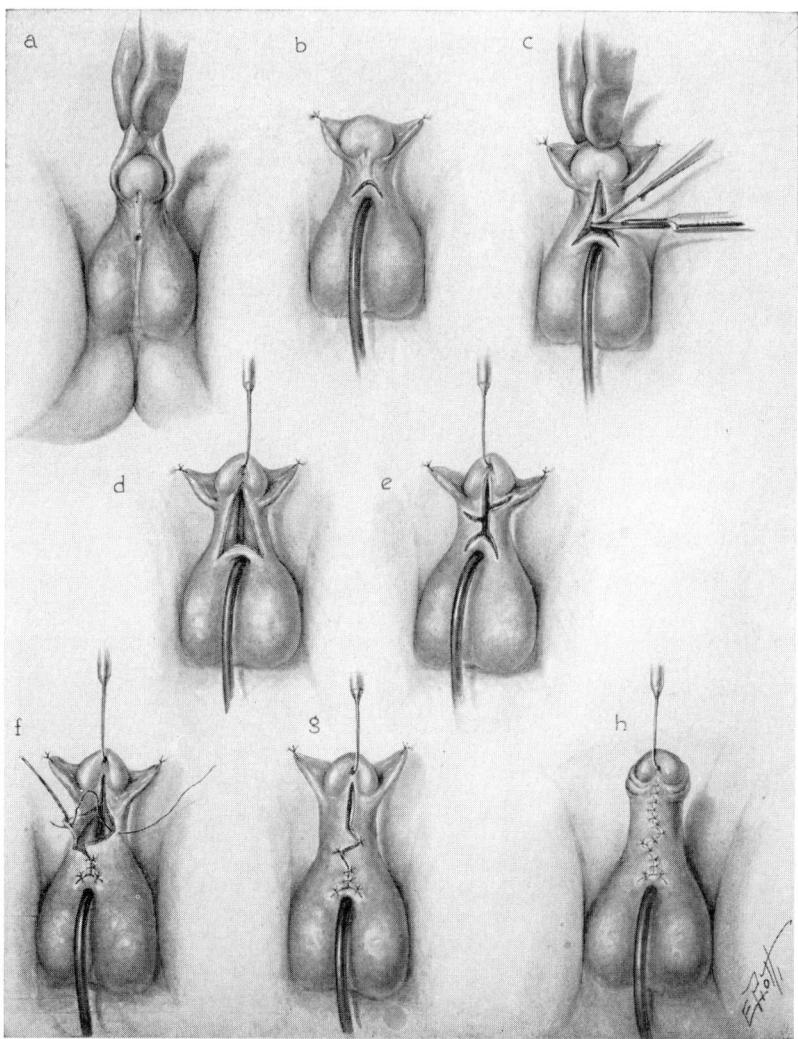

Fig. 403. Operative correction of penile chordee. a, Hypospadias of a peno-scrotal type. Hooded foreskin. b, The prepuce anchored to the abdominal wall. Catheter inserted through urethra into bladder, for postoperative drainage. Inverted V-shaped incision distal to urethral meatus. c, Longitudinal incision along ventral surface of penis to expose any fibrous bands which are then sharply dissected out. d, Penis attenuated. e, Lateral incisions facilitate undermining flaps of skin and dissection around the hooded foreskin. f, Flaps of skin being closed in a zigzag fashion, to give maximum length to the underside of penis and to minimize subsequent contracture. g, Interdigitation of flaps being continued. h, Closure of undersurface of penis completed.

be shifted toward the ventral side of the penis without making a dorsal slit or relaxing incision.

Along the underside of the penis, subcutaneous tissues are now closed with interrupted 00000 plain catgut sutures and the skin is brought together with interrupted 00000 plain catgut mattress stitches, interspersed with single sutures of the same material. If this closure is made in a zigzag fashion, there will be a minimizing of any tendency to subsequent scar-contracture. A soft and resilient pressure dressing is placed in a manner to give compression of the penis against the lower abdominal wall. The catheter is left in the bladder for about a week and is then withdrawn. Every attention to detail should

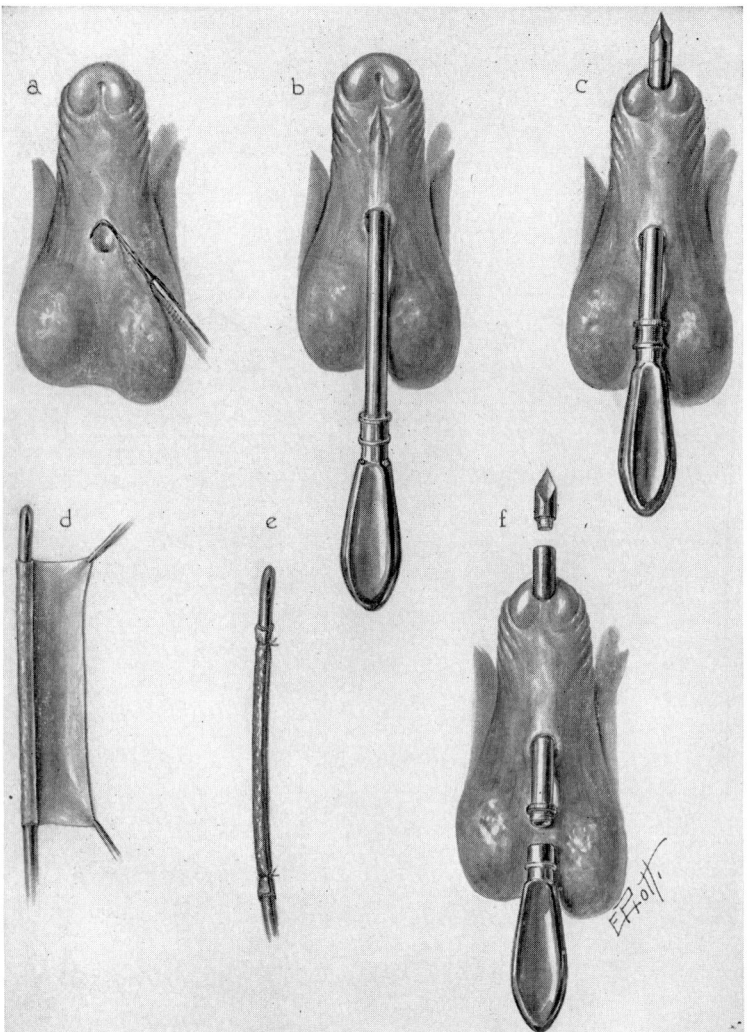

Fig. 404. Second stage of treatment of hypospadias; construction of penile urethra. a, Inverted V-shaped incision just distal to urethral opening. b, Trocar being thrust through substance of penis, carrying this near the ventral surface of the organ. c, Instrument passed through length of penis, emerging at tip of glans. d, Thiersch graft being wrapped around catheter, the epidermal side inward. e, Ligature around either end of graft, to keep it from unrolling. f, Bladed point and handle being unscrewed from trocar.

be made in the treatment of chordee because the elimination of this part of the deformity is essential for any reconstruction of the urethra which will be undertaken later.

Second Stage. Construction of Urethra. Following correction of a chordee, parents frequently ask for immediate construction of the urethra so that all correction of the anomaly can be completed by the time the child attends school. While freely admitting that early completion of surgery has desirable features, it has been our feeling that if urethral construction can be deferred until the penis has grown and has approached the mature size and form, the surgeon is given the best chance of making a urethral tube which will be most satisfactory through the remainder of the individual's life. When the facts and the ultimate goal are carefully explained to parents, we have had no difficulties

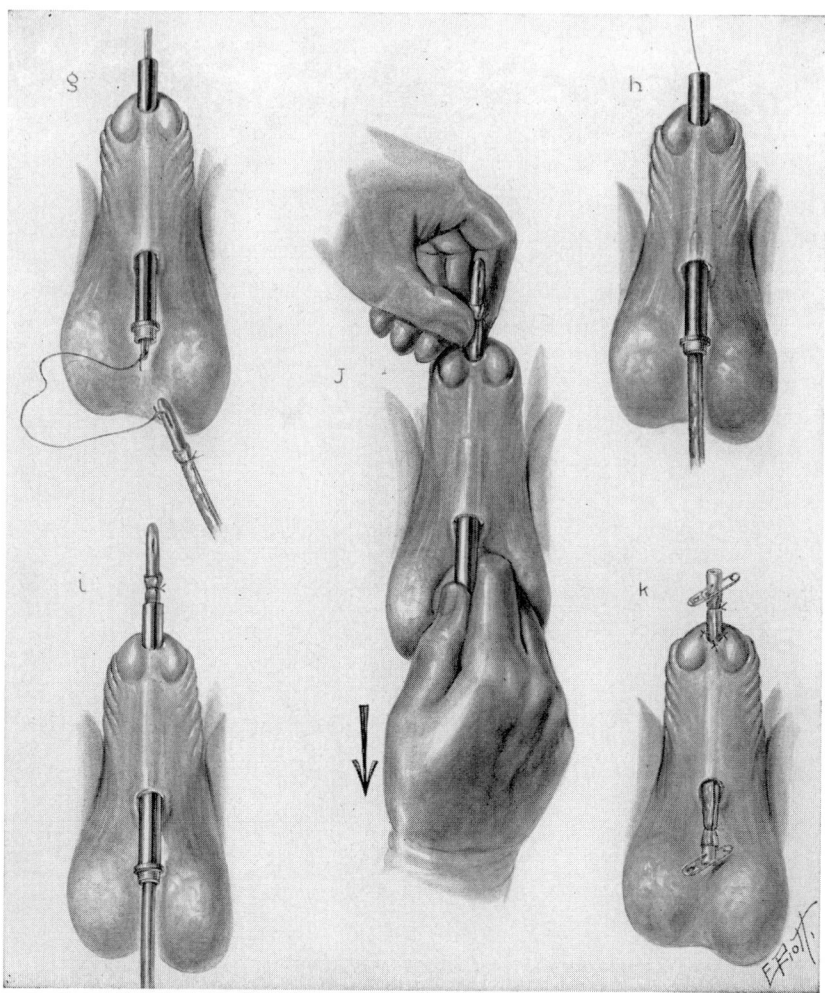

Fig. 404 (*continued*). g, Leader-needle passed through penile instrument, the following thread attached to the catheter. h, Thread being pulled through the penile tube, bringing the catheter and graft into place. i, Catheter, carrying the graft, in suitable position. j, Catheter and graft held with left hand; instrument being withdrawn with right hand. k, Piece of catheter, carrying the graft, in place.

with the proposal to defer operation until late childhood or the pubertal years. We believe that the advantages of delaying the construction of the urethra until such time so outweigh the disadvantages, that we have found it quite worth-while to carry these children along during the years until the surgery is to be undertaken. Without doubt, some of these boys are embarrassed by always having to use a sitting position for the passing of urine. However, this psychologic hurdle, which at first seems to be great, can always be overcome. Generally, the patient can respond to any queries from his confreres by merely stating that he is in the habit of moving his bowels when he urinates— a not uncommon physiologic phenomenon in an entirely normal individual. Thus, with very little prevarication, these youngsters are able to mask their urination as an act of defecation and thereby avoid further embarrassing questions.

In later childhood, or approaching puberty, after the penis has become considerably enlarged, thereby providing the best opportunity for working upon it, the construction

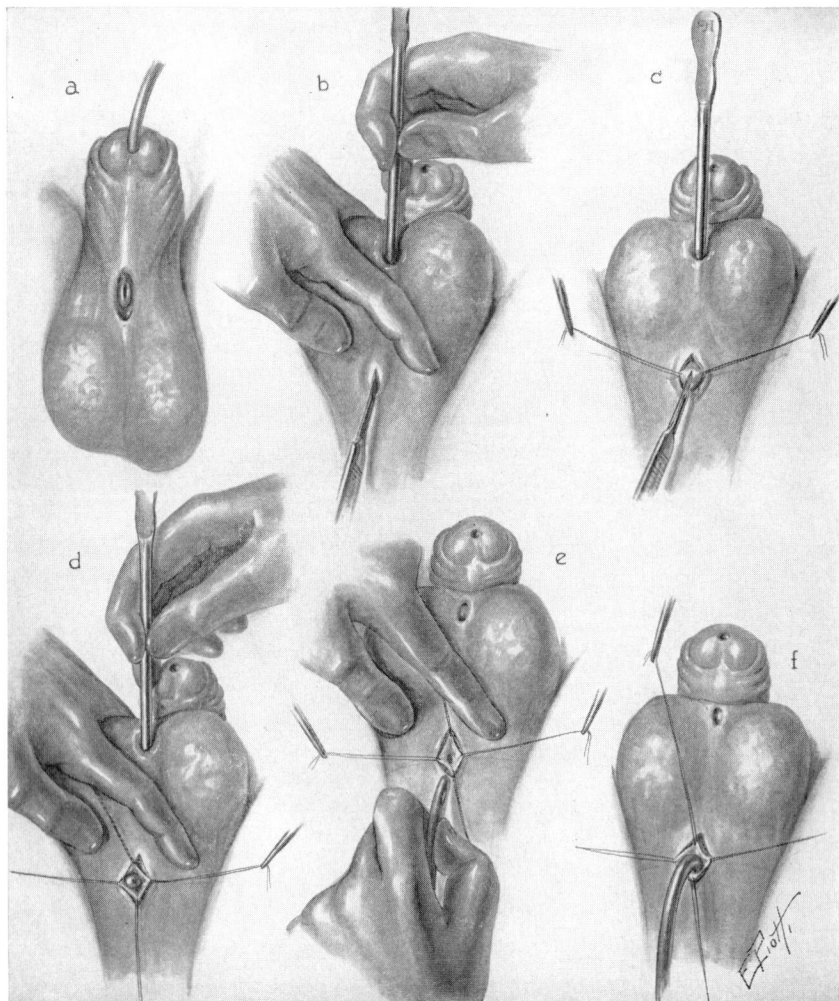

Fig. 405. Third stage of hypospadias operation; joining the penile urethra to previously existing urethra. a, Catheter inserted through the newly constructed urethra, demonstrating its patency. b, Urethral sound passed in toward bladder; perineal urethrostomy being established. c, Opening perineal urethra. d, Urethra opened. e, Catheter being inserted proximally toward bladder. f, Perineal catheter placed.

of the urethra is carried out (Fig. 404). This entails the use of a free inlay Thiersch graft to line a urethral pathway which has been made by a piercing instrument. The formation of a urethral tube in this way has the enormous advantage of eliminating any ventral union of skin, thereby practically eliminating the problem of fistula formation. Of less importance, but yet a desirable feature, the new urethra will emerge at the apex of the glans. In one stage, a urethral pathway can be made from the existing urethral meatus all the way to the tip of the penis.

To keep the field dry, a Foley catheter is inserted through the existing urethral meatus and run into the bladder, so that all urine is diverted for a week or ten days after operation. With an appropriate trocar, a channel is pierced through the penis, toward its under-surface, coming out at the tip of the glans. This instrument is constructed in such a way that its hollow shaft carries a pointed blade at one end and a handle at the

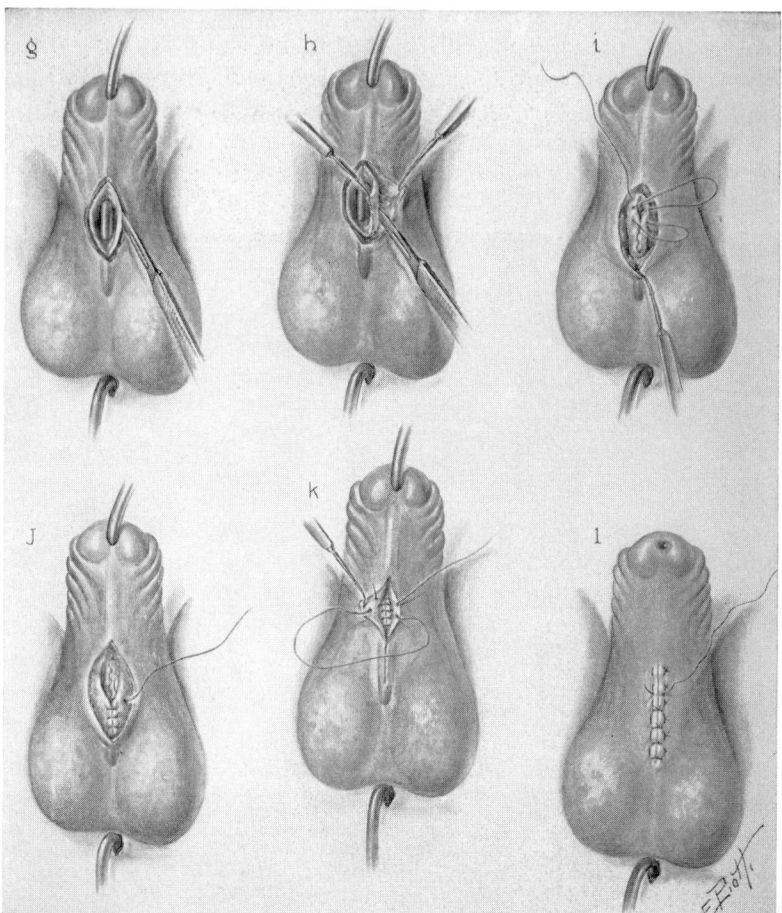

Fig. 405 (*continued*). g, Perineal catheter (draining bladder) in place. The second catheter is placed through anterior urethra. The skin is incised around urethral orifice. h, Freeing of cutaneous flaps around urethral orifice. i, Inversion of cutaneous flaps with running catgut suture. j, Buttressing of urethral closure with interrupted silk stitches. k, Interrupted catgut sutures to subcutaneous tissues. l, Closure of skin.

other, both of which can now be unscrewed and removed, leaving the hollow, metal tube through the substance of the penis. A catheter, which should be 50 per cent larger than the size of the urethra which is desired, is now wrapped with a split-thickness graft which has been obtained from a non-hair-bearing part of the body. The catheter is covered with this sheet of graft so that there is considerable overlay as the skin is wound around the catheter. The skin is lightly tied at either end to keep it in place while being introduced into the penis. As shown, this catheter, carrying the skin, is then introduced through the hollow tube, which is now withdrawn, leaving the skin-surrounded tube in place. The tubular graft thus lies against a rich vascular bed, insuring an adequate "take." This operative step is a rather short and simple procedure. It has a tremendous advantage in that its success does not depend upon perfect healing of any long or complicated lines of suture, such as are necessary when a urethral tube is made by swinging and rearrangement of cutaneous flaps.

Postoperatively, the penis is immobilized and held upward against the pubic arch and lower part of the abdominal wall with a soft compression dressing, leaving all of this undisturbed for seven to ten days. The catheter draining the bladder can then be removed. At this time, the patient is discharged home, but a No. 16 catheter is left in place at all times through the newly made urethral channel. There is very little sensation, and certainly no pain, with this catheter in place. It acts as a strut and prevents any narrowing of the urethra during the subsequent months. This short piece of catheter should be changed about once a day; the boy can do this himself.

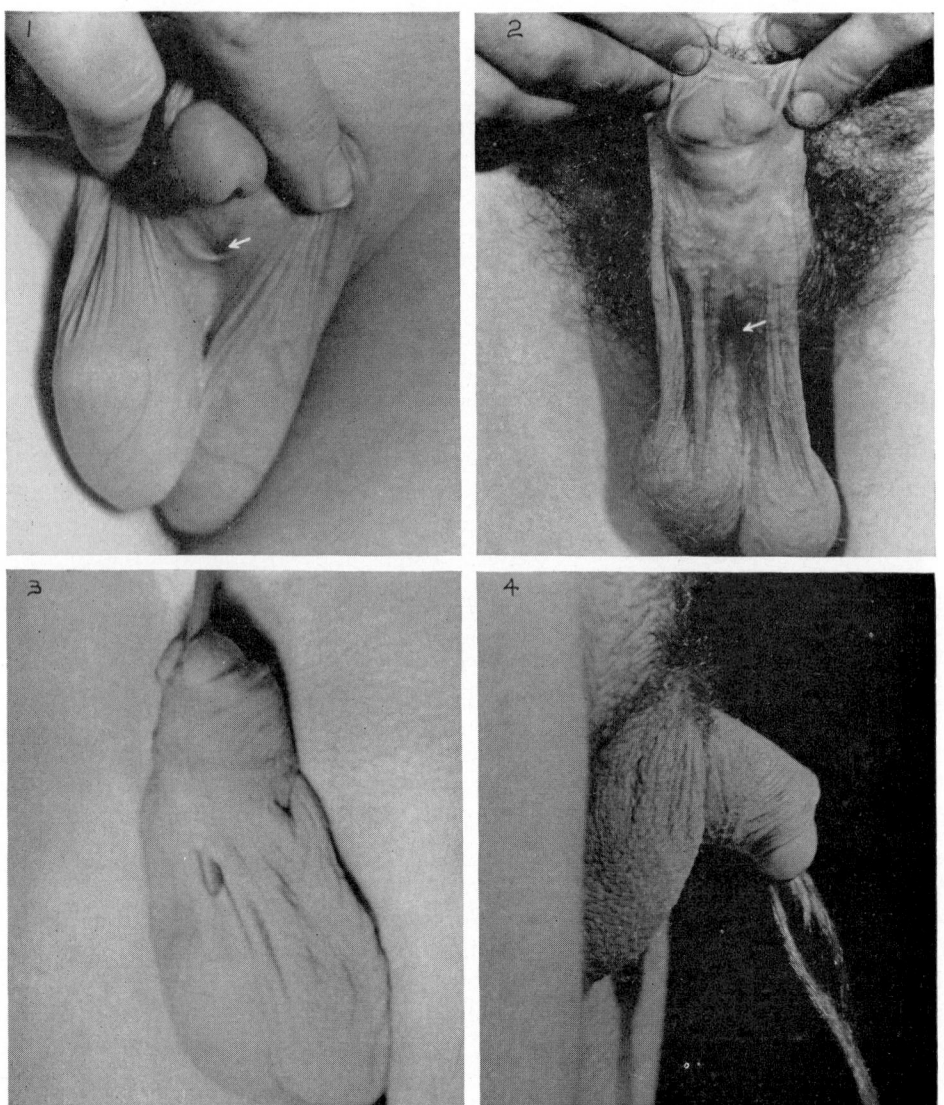

Fig. 406. Stages in treatment of hypospadias; construction by method shown in Figures 403–405. 1. Patient twelve years of age. Note the marked ventral chordee and the urethral opening at the peno-scrotal angle. 2. Patient at fourteen years, after correction of chordee. Note that the penis is straight and that the distance between the glans and the urethral opening has been greatly increased. 3. Patient at fifteen years. following construction of a penile urethra by an inlay graft. A catheter is inserted through the length of this tunnel, to demonstrate its patency. Note that there is no ventral contracture from the graft. 4. Patient following the third-stage procedure in which the urethral continuity is established. There is a normal caliber and force of urinary stream as it emerges from the tip of the penis.

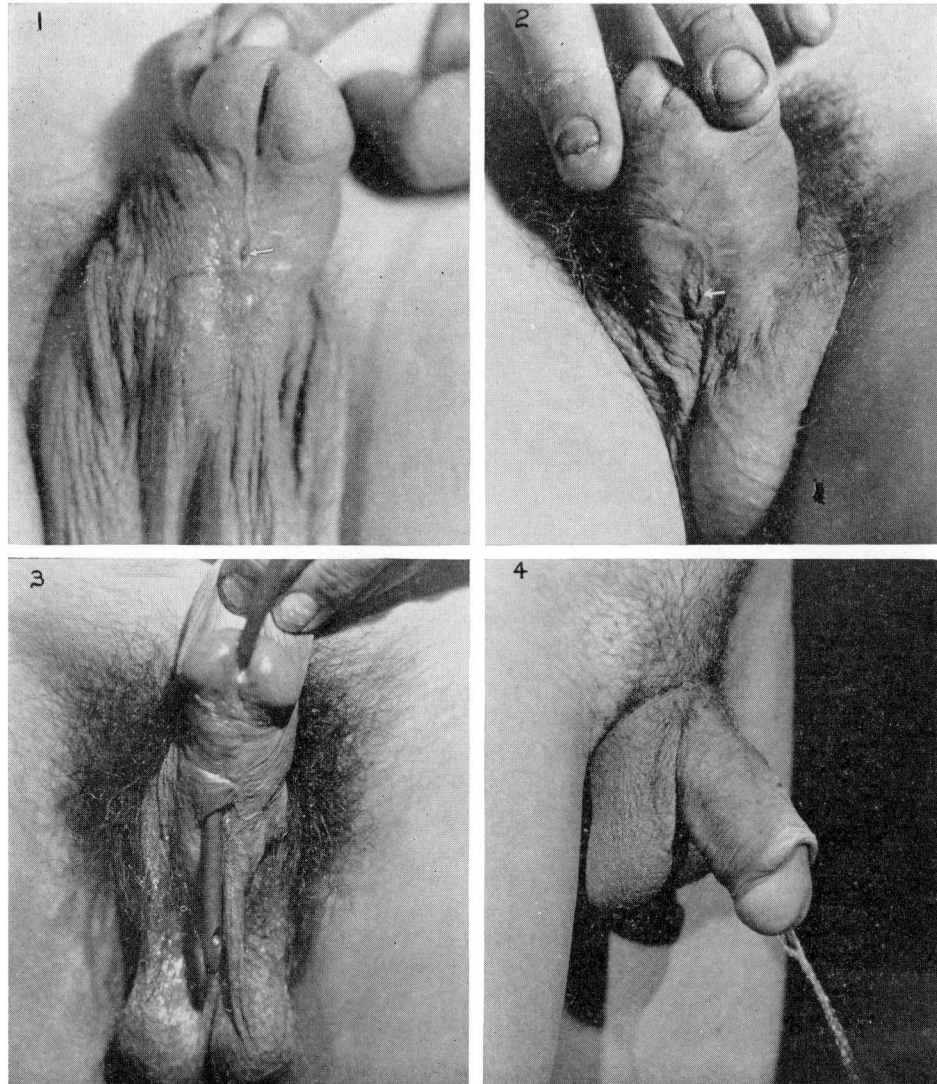

Fig. 409. Stages in treatment of a mid-shaft hypospadias. 1. Patient at fifteen years of age. The urethral meatus is in the mid-shaft, some ventral chordee extending from this point to the penile tip. 2. One year later, following correction of the chordee and straightening of the penis. Note the rather indistinct Z-shaped scar on the ventral surface. 3. Photograph following construction of the penile tube. The urethral graft has been in place for one year. 4. Patient six months after completion of the third stage of the repair, showing excellent length and straightness of the penis and a good urinary stream.

(or the scrotum) so that these can be brought to cover the underlying repair. To accomplish this, subcutaneous tissues are approximated with interrupted (or continuous) 00000 plain catgut stitches. The skin is united with interrupted mattress sutures of 0000 plain catgut, interspersed with single stitches to give accurate closure of the cutaneous margins. The use of four layers of closure is good insurance against formation of any fistula; we have not had this complication in any case.

Following operation, the catheter which had been left in place for urinary drainage (through a perineal urethrostomy, or through the entire length of the urethra) is withdrawn in ten days. A perineal urethrostomy will close spontaneously within a few days. The patient now voids through the urethral pathway.

RESULTS OF THERAPY

The three-stage procedure which has been outlined in the preceding paragraphs has proved to be a safe, simple, and a very effective method of correction of severe degrees of hypospadias. The repair does not require the use of greatly complicated or delicate reconstructive steps. Furthermore, the formation of a penile urethra does not depend for its success on the meticulous approximation of long suture lines, or the bringing together of widely undermined flaps of tissue on the under surface of the penis. Scarring along the operative site is minimal. There has been no trouble repairing a urethra in any case.

Possibly the same operative steps could be undertaken in childhood during the pre-school years, an approach advocated by Young and Benjamin, but we are fearful that the long-term results following such early surgery will not be as good as those we have been able to obtain when the corrections have been deferred until the pre-pubertal or pubertal years. It seems a lot to ask for skin grafts to keep pace with the growth which appears during and after puberty and also to have enough laxity to permit an erection in adult years without ventral curvature. With these beliefs in mind, we feel that the deferment of operation until the penis has attained adequate size will give the individual a penis which is most nearly normal in adult life.

The constructions which have been made by the method described have provided excellent urethral tubes which are free of stricture, are devoid of hair, and are lacking in calculus formation. These operations give a penis of reasonable appearance, and with a minimum of lumpy or scarred tissue, which attributes can seldom be accorded to other types of repair. The cosmetic results are very good. The functions of micturition and coitus are completely cared for after the construction is completed. There is no interference with erection or copulation because of persistent chordee or longitudinal contraction along the pathway which has been established.

To date, 40 patients have had their chordee relieved in a very satisfactory manner. Of these, 18 have had completion of the urethral construction by the methods described. The results have been exceedingly satisfactory and we see little need for improvement or change in the operative technique, with the possible exception that earlier repair might have been desirable for some of these boys, a consideration which we did not find to be of great importance in many instances.

REFERENCES

1. Blair, V. P. and Byars, L. T.: Hypospadias and Epispadias. J. Urol., *40*:814, 1938.
2. Browne, D.: Hypospadias. Post-Grad. M. J., *25*:367, 1949.
3. Browne, D.: An Operation for Hypospadias. Proc. Roy. Soc. Med., *42*:466, 1949.
4. Burns, E.: The Denis Browne Operation for Hypospadias. J. Urol., *64*:382, 1950.
5. Byars, L. T.: Functional Restoration of Hypospadias Deformities. Surg., Gynec. & Obst., *92*:149, 1951.
6. Cecil, A. B.: Surgery of Hypospadias and

Epispadias in the Male. J. Urol., *27*:507, 1932.
7. Cecil, A. B.: Repair of Hypospadias and Urethral Fistula. J. Urol., *56*:237, 1946.
8. Charnock, D. A. and Kiskadden, W. S.: Hypospadias. J. Urol., *49*:444, 1943.
9. Creevy, C. D.: The Operative Treatment of Hypospadias. Surgery, *3*:719, 1938.
10. Culp, O. S.: Early Correction of Congenital Chordee and Hypospadias. J. Urol., *65*:264, 1951.
11. Davis, D. M.: The Surgical Treatment of Hy-

pospadias, Especially Scrotal and Perineal. Plast. & Reconstruct. Surg., *5*:373, 1950.

12. Duplay, S.: De l'hypospadias périnéo-scrotal et de son traitement chirurgical. Arch. Gén. de Méd., *133*:513, 657, 1874.

13. Duplay, S.: Sur le traitement chirurgical de l'hypospadias et de l'epispadias. Arch. Gén. de Méd., *145*:257, 1880.

14. Havens, F. Z. and Black, A. S.: The Treatment of Hypospadias. J. Urol., *61*:1053, 1949.

15. Loughran, A. M.: Observations on Hypospadias, including Late Results of Ombrédanne's Urethroplastic Operation. Brit. J. Plast. Surg., *1*:147, 1948.

16. Marion, G. and Pérard, J.: Technique des opérations plastiques sur la vessie et sur l'urètre. Masson and Cie, Paris, 1942.

17. McIndoe, A.: Deformities of the Male Urethra. Brit. J. Plast. Surg., *1*:29, 1948.

18. Nesbit, R. M.: Plastic Procedure for Correction of Hypospadias. J. Urol., *45*:699, 1941.

19. Nesbit, R. M., Butler, W. J. and Whitaker, W.: Production of Epithelial Lined Tubes from Buried Strips of Intact Skin. J. Urol., *64*:387, 1950.

20. Schaefer, A. A. and Erbes, J.: Hypospadias. Am. J. Surg., *80*:183, 1950.

21. Smith, C. K.: Surgical Procedure for Correction of Hypospadias. J. Urol., *40*:239, 1938.

22. Smith, D. R. and Blackfield, H. M.: A Critique on the Repair of Hypospadias. Surgery, *31*:885, 1952.

23. Spence, H. M. and Baird, S. S.: Surgical Correction of Hypospadias. South. M. J., *43*:392, 1950.

24. Walters, W.: Successful Operations for Hypospadias. Ann. Surg., *103*:949, 1936.

25. Wehrbein, H. L.: Hypospadias. J. Urol., *50*:335, 1943.

26. Young, F. and Benjamin, J. A.: Preschool Age Repair of Hypospadias with Free Inlay Skin Graft. Surgery, *26*:384, 1949.

27. Young, F. and Benjamin, J. A.: Repair of Hypospadias with Free Inlay Graft. Surg., Gynec. & Obst., *86*:439, 1948.

CHAPTER 55

Urinary Obstruction from Posterior Urethral Valves

Blockage of the urinary tract from congenital valves in the posterior urethra is one of the most devastating abnormalities which can be found in the urinary system. These tiny flap-valves can produce high degrees of obstruction and extensive damage to the kidneys; they are generally accompanied by superimposed infection, and they lead to urinary stasis, uremia, and fatality in a very high percentage of cases. The outlook has always been exceedingly poor for these boys. We have taken a very dismal view of what can be accomplished for these children until the recent development of a technique for removal of valves under direct vision, a procedure which now gives considerable hope for the treatment of the condition.

PATHOLOGY AND CLINICAL PICTURE

Posterior urethral valves can be of many forms, but most commonly they are paired flaps arising from the verumontanum which flare outward and are attached to the anterior and lateral walls of the urethra (Fig. 410). These valves are situated in such a manner that it is always possible to pass an instrument *inward* through them, whereas any *outward* flow of urine makes the leaflets flop together and impede or completely shut off the stream of urine. The bladder becomes greatly distended, markedly thickened, and trabeculated, in its efforts to squeeze urine past the urethral obstruction. The back pressure is transmitted up the ureters and into the renal pelves, giving ureterectasia and hydronephrosis of advanced degree. With this obstructive uropathy, the competence of the uretero-vesical valves is maintained for a short time, but generally there comes a stage wherein the uretero-vesical junction completely loses its valve-like action and the great pressure exerted by the hypertrophied bladder is transmitted up the urinary tracts, thereby increasing the renal damage. Superimposed on this stasis, bacterial invasion almost always occurs, except when the condition is detected very early in infancy. Destruction of renal parenchyma (from increased pressure and from bacterial infection) gives high degrees of renal insufficiency and increasing uremia, leading in the vast majority of subjects to fatality in infancy or early childhood.

It is very easy to detect posterior urethral obstruction if the physician thinks of the condition and performs a few simple tests for confirmation of his suspicions. These males all have difficulties in voiding from the earliest days of life. Urinary dribbling may be overlooked during the ages when a baby is wearing diapers and wets himself at frequent intervals. There are, however, straining and discomfort during attempts at the act of voiding; in between these the child is reasonably comfortable. Efforts to void are possibly more frequent than normal. As the baby or boy is observed during urination, there is marked diminution in volume and force of the urinary stream; only a small quantity or a few driblets may appear from the external meatus. These observations are particularly significant if simultaneous palpation of the abdomen reveals that the bladder is distended and obviously contains urine. If the child is fussy and the bladder cannot be suitably palpated through the anterior abdominal wall, bimanual examination, with one finger in the rectum, will almost certainly disclose a greatly enlarged urinary vesicle.

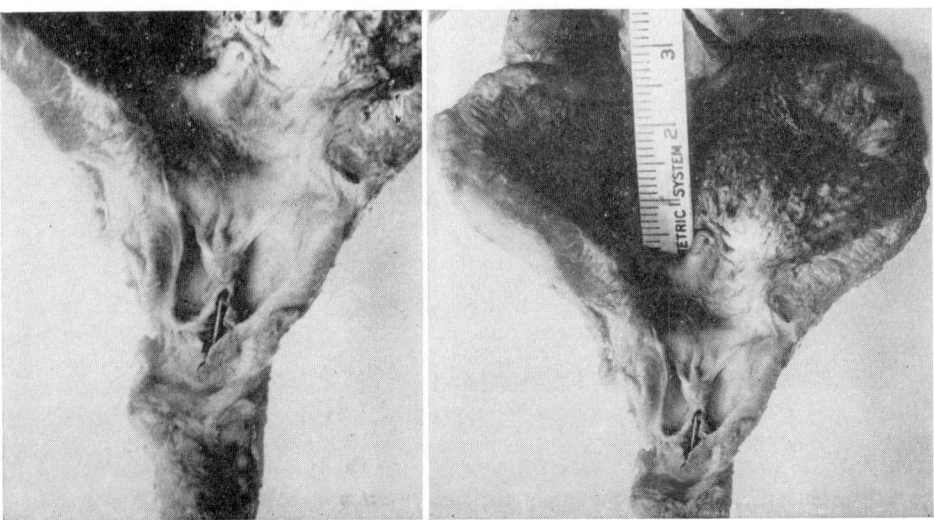

Fig. 410. Autopsy photographs from two boys who died of uremia and pyelonephritis which were caused by obstruction from posterior urethral valves. The valve flaps can be seen running from either side of the anterior end of the verumontanum. The bladders are greatly hypertrophied.

Not uncommonly, irregular masses (which might appear to be firm) are found in either lateral side of the abdomen and in the flanks, these being tremendously and tensely distended ureters and renal pelves. There is apt to be *fever* from superimposed infection, and indeed in many instances this is the primary complaint for which the child is brought to the physician. Examination of the urine in small infants may show no pus, but beyond a few months of age urinary infection is the rule. The child may exhibit drowsiness, poor weight gain, vomiting, or any of the other manifestations of marked uremia, a point which can be accurately determined by measurement of the blood urea nitrogen or non-protein nitrogen.

When one suspects that a baby (or boy) is suffering from urethral obstruction and inability to pass urine properly, the diagnosis may be established, and the child temporarily helped, by passing a catheter in through the urethra to drain urine from the bladder. A No. 8 or No. 10 urethral catheter generally can be inserted through the urethra and beyond the valves without difficulty, entering the bladder from which a large amount of urine gushes forth. (In infants it is generally undesirable to attempt to pass stiff ureteral catheters through a urethra because they are too apt to perforate it and produce urethral damage which further complicates the whole picture.)

ROENTGENOGRAPHIC FINDINGS

The most important observations can be made from a cysto-urethrogram. With a small catheter introduced through the urethra into the bladder, the latter can be filled with opaque solution such as Diodrast or 12 per cent sodium iodide. The bladder may

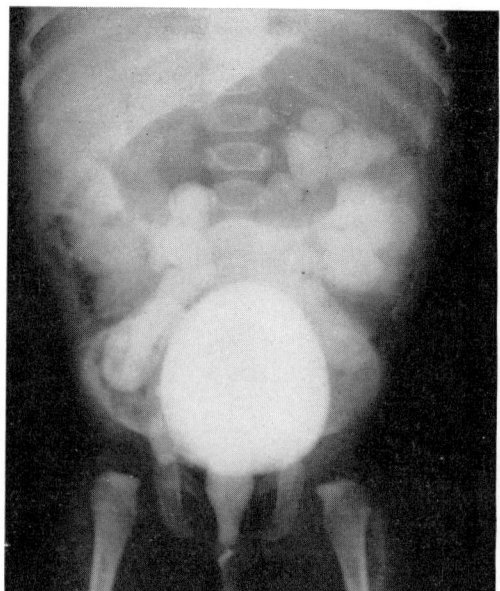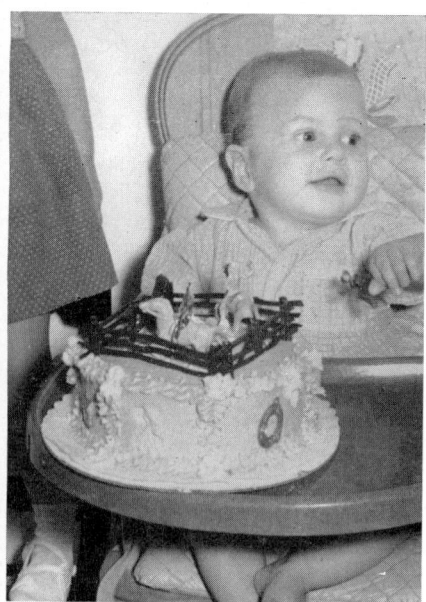

Fig. 411. *Left*, Cystogram from a three-month-old baby who had advanced uremia from posterior urethral obstruction. The large bladder can be seen; the posterior urethra is greatly dilated to the point where valves are present. From back-pressure and dilatation, the uretero-vesical valves have become incompetent, producing marked dilatation of the ureters and destruction of the kidneys; the dye readily flows up into the enormously distended pelves and ureters. *Right*, This child was treated by resection of the urethral valves (Fig. 414) and prolonged suprapubic drainage. Photograph shows his excellent status on his first birthday. The child voids a good stream; a cystogram shows no reflux up the ureters; the kidney function has greatly improved and uremia has disappeared.

be found quite capacious. It generally has a serrated inner surface indicating trabeculation (marked increase in the muscular structure of the wall) indicative of long-standing obstruction at or beyond the bladder outlet. If there has not yet been destruction of the valvular action of the uretero-vesical junction, there will be no reflux of dye up the ureters. Conversely, if there is incompetence of these valves, dye will flow up either, or both, ureters and visualize them and the renal pelves which almost always show extensive ureterectasia and pyelectasia. The observations of greatest importance are those at the bladder outlet and posterior urethra. Visualization of these in the anterior, lateral, and particularly the oblique views are essential to give a complete picture of the pathologic configurations which are present. Visualization of the bladder outlet and the urethra might not give all the available information if the exposures are taken while the child is in a relaxed state. It is very important to withdraw the urethral catheter, make the child attempt to void (or in a small baby suprapubic pressure can be made over the bladder with a fist), and to take the x-ray exposures at such time. These give the best view of the dilated posterior urethra out to that point where valves exist, and a normal, or apparently small, stream beyond this (Figs. 411, 412, and 413). If there is particular luck in taking the film, and if the patient happens to be in exactly the right position, the thin flap-like valve can actually be identified as a filling defect in the opaque urinary stream.

If it is impossible to get a catheter through the urethra into the bladder, dye can be injected into the urethra and bladder from a syringe which carries a rubber acorn tip which is pressed snugly into the external meatus.

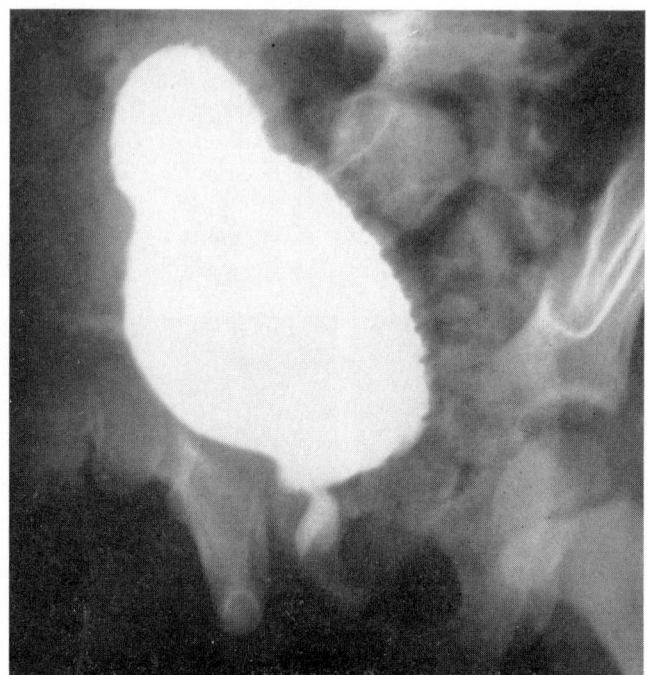

Fig. 412. Voiding cysto-urethrogram from a four-year-old boy with posterior urethral valves. The bladder is trabeculated. The posterior urethra is slightly dilated and the dye is cut off at the site of the valves.

If visualization of the bladder by cystogram examination does not show a reflux of dye up into the ureters, the upper urinary tract should be visualized by intravenous pyelography. In some instances when there is marked urinary retention and poor kidney function, it is necessary to decompress the urinary tract appropriately before intravenous pyelography is safe and is effective in showing up the kidneys.

TREATMENT
Decompression of Bladder

If in a given case it is determined that there is urinary obstruction from posterior urethral valves, and a catheter has been passed into the bladder so that urine escapes, it is highly important to avoid withdrawal of all of the urine at one time; a sudden decompression of a chronically obstructed urinary system often leads to renal shut-down and fatality. *It is important to decompress the urinary tract slowly*, which can be accomplished by connecting the catheter with a piece of tubing, the distal end of which is elevated to a point far above the level of the bladder and at which height urine will barely escape. From time to time during the following twenty-four or forty-eight hours, the distal end of this tube can be gradually and progressively lowered so that the pressure within the urinary tract is accordingly reduced slowly.

With babies or children who have advanced uremia, marked renal damage, and especially if there is superimposed infection, it is poor judgment to make an early attempt at definitive removal of the urethral obstruction. *As a preliminary step, it is highly important to drain effectively the urinary system over a long period of time so that it can become flushed out*, the kidneys can regain some competence, the blood stream can be cleared of the excess waste nitrogenous products, and the general condition of the patient can be improved. This will generally require a period of several weeks or more. It should never be done by leaving a urethral catheter in place. While such a catheter can be used for a day or two while initially decompressing the urinary tract, to leave it in place for a longer period sets up a marked urethritis and causes such severe local changes that the verumontanum and the valves become greatly thickened, edematous, and congested; the regional anatomy becomes obscured and greatly increases the operator's difficulties when a subsequent attempt is made to remove the valves. After any preliminary urethral drainage of a day or two, more prolonged flushing of the urinary system should be accomplished by the use of a suprapubic tube.

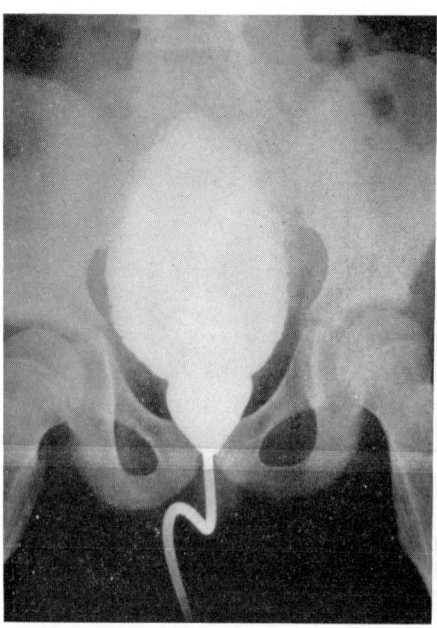 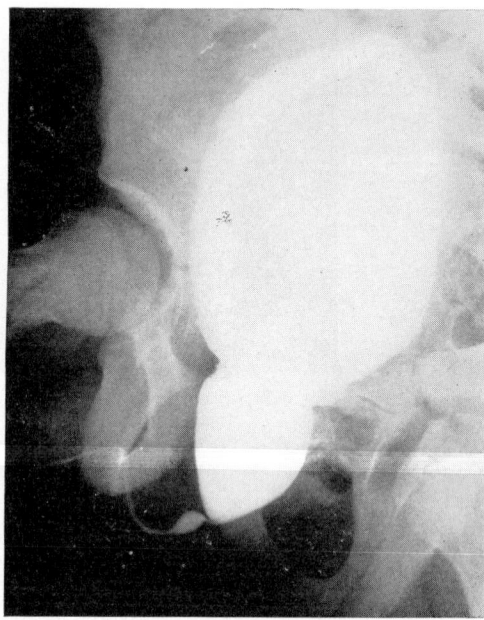

Fig. 413. Cysto-urethrograms from a twelve-year-old boy who had a constantly distended bladder, urinary dribbling, and difficulty in voiding. The child had obstruction from posterior urethral valves. *Left,* There is no difficulty running a catheter *in* to the bladder. Visualization with dye shows great dilatation and trabeculation of bladder, and an enormously dilated posterior urethra. *Right,* Oblique view after withdrawing the catheter and making a roentgenogram *while the child was attempting to void.* There is tremendous distention of the posterior urethra down to the point where the valves are located; beyond this only a very fine stream of urine passes out the urethra. (Child subsequently treated successfully by resection of valves under direct vision as shown in Figure 414.)

Suprapubic Drainage

For the institution of suprapubic catheter drainage, two methods are available. In older children, it is possible under light general anesthesia or under local procaine infiltration to insert a punch-trocar through the abdominal wall into the bladder, passing a catheter into the bladder through this, and then withdrawing the trocar over the tube. This is simple, quick, and very effective in large subjects. We have had great difficulty in employing it in babies in whom it is sometimes found to be dangerous; the trocar slips off to one side of the bladder or might actually enter the peritoneal cavity and damage viscera within it. Therefore, for small children, and certainly for all babies, suprapubic drainage is most safely accomplished by incision-cystotomy, and the insertion of a mushroom catheter through this opening. It is not necessary to make an opening in the skin and deeper layers of the anterior abdominal wall more than a centimeter in length, using two small finger retractors to withdraw the wound edges down to the point where the bladder is brought into view; the bladder is then opened and a catheter inserted. This can be done under light general anesthesia or even under procaine infiltration in those subjects who are particularly ill.

A suprapubic tube must be of large size and must be left constantly open so that there is the best possible chance of flushing out the urinary tract. It is impossible to make any statements regarding the length of time during which suprapubic drainage should be carried out before definitive procedures are undertaken for removal of the urethral valves. The drainage must be long enough so that uremia is brought under reasonable control. The best guide for determining how much has been accomplished in this regard is the examination of the blood non-protein nitrogen from time to time. If there is associated pyuria, which is found in the vast majority of cases, appropriate antibiotic therapy of wide antibacterial activity must be intensively employed. If, in the occasional case, no pyuria is present, it is still important to use chemotherapy on a prophylactic basis.

Removal of Valves

To remove posterior urethral valves, three general methods have been previously employed, all of which have serious drawbacks and which have proved, on the whole, to be relatively ineffective. First, it is possible to introduce through the anterior urethra a Young's punch, engage the verumontanum and the valves in the side orifice of the instrument, and then, by running in the internal cutting sleeve, to shear off these structures. This is a completely blind procedure and our attempts with it, even when the instrument was directed into place while the bladder was opened so that the bladder outlet could be viewed, always left a great deal to be desired. It is impossible to know how much is being excised. Not infrequently large portions of the urethral wall are torn away, producing unnecessary damage and subsequent scar formations. The procedure cuts off the verumontanum, which obviously is unnecessary and undesirable. Second, more modern resectoscopes can be introduced into the urethra, cutting away (with the endothermy current) tissue which comes into the field. Theoretically, such a resection might be satisfactory, but from a practical viewpoint this seldom has proved to be true. The method might be a reasonably good one in older boys where the urethra is large and will permit the introduction and manipulation of the instrument; it is of practically no value in a small child or baby. Third, it is possible to open the bladder widely and hope to be able to look down through the bladder outlet and posterior urethra to see the valves, to cut them away with a ring-punch or some instrument which is introduced through the open bladder. Our attempts at this have always been exceedingly disappointing. One can look quite a way through the dilated bladder outlet, but it is almost impossible to see quite far enough to that point where exact operative manipulations and excisions are to be done.

Open Operation for Excision of Valves. Our results for the treatment of posterior urethral valve obstruction were so poor through all the years up through 1950 that it was decided to attempt some other method of therapy which might possibly be more effective. An operative procedure was devised, which is illustrated in Figure 414. The essentials of this are an anterior approach to the urethra, so that the urethra can be opened, valves brought clearly into view and then cleanly excised. In babies, up to a year or two of age, the exposure is greatly enhanced by cutting the symphysis and separating the pubic rami so that one has a direct approach to the area. In older children very little is accomplished by dividing the symphysis, since it is impossible to separate the bones very much without unjustifiable damage to the sacro-iliac joints; in older subjects the avenue of approach is made directly above the symphysis, mobilizing the bladder and attenuating this upward so that one can see fairly well the anterior aspect of the bladder outlet and the posterior urethra. Fortunately, when there has been long standing posterior urethral obstruction, the distended posterior urethra distorts and displaces upward the bladder outlet, thereby bringing it out somewhat from under the shadow of the pubic arch.

The bladder outlet and the posterior urethra are cleared on their anterior and

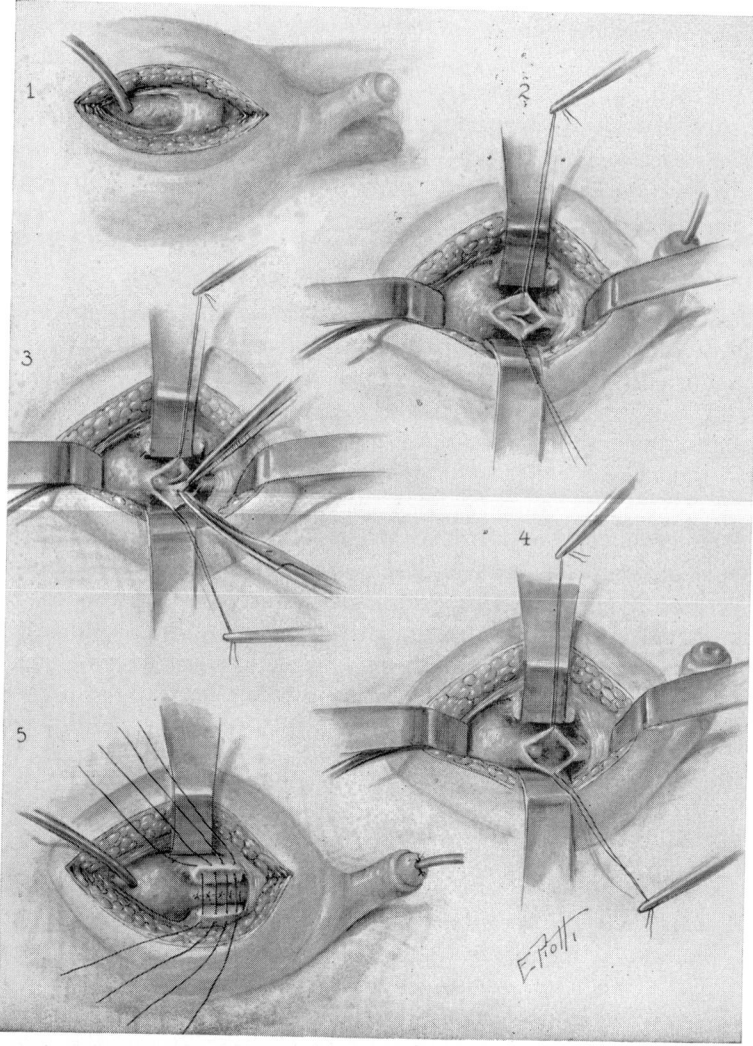

Fig. 414. Method for surgical excision of posterior urethral valves under direct vision. 1. Midline incision in front of bladder and pubes. Pubes exposed. (The bladder catheter has been in place for several weeks to allow free drainage of the urinary tract and treatment of uremia.) 2. Symphysis pubis divided, giving direct view of bladder outlet and posterior urethra. The urethra has been opened, its edges being retracted by sutures. Clearly brought into view is the verumontanum and from its anterior end the two valve flaps which flare outward. 3. The flaps of valves are picked up with fine forceps and cut off with small scissors. 4. The valve flaps have been cleanly cut out. 5. A urethral catheter has been run into the bladder, and the urethra closed while the catheter is in place. Beginning the repair of the pubic symphysis with silk sutures.

lateral aspects out to and slightly beyond the point of narrowing. It is now very advantageous to make the operative field completely dry and free of fluid or blood, so that one can obtain the clearest view after the urethra is opened. It is difficult to ligate bleeders in this deep wound, but oozing points can be coagulated with the endothermy, can be compressed for a few moments with a hot wet pack, or can be held for a few minutes by pledgets of epinephrine-soaked cotton. When the field has been made quite dry, a midline incision is made in the urethra, the edges of which are held upward and outward with a traction suture on either side. One can now look directly at the interior of the posterior urethra and the thin valve flaps which reside in it. (A sucker should not be used against the urethral membranes, because this is too apt to stir up bleeding which obscures the view.) With delicate, non-toothed forceps, each valve flap can be grasped and held up so that it can be nicely cut away from the urethral wall, a step which requires but a few moments. The verumontanum is left undamaged.

A urethral catheter is now run in through the penis, through the operative site, and into the bladder; while this is in place the longitudinal opening in the urethra is repaired by bringing its edges together with 00000 chromic catgut sutures. No silk should be used at this step for fear that some of it might protrude into the urethral lumen and subsequently set up a foreign-body reaction or become a structure on which encrustations accumulate. No attempt should be made to bring together the edges of the membrane itself; it is much better merely to close the tissues immediately outside the membrane, allowing the membrane to re-form itself as a smooth lining over the rubber catheter which serves as a strut and which should therefore be left in place for twelve to fourteen days. If the symphysis has been divided, it is repaired with silk sutures of appropriate size.

Postoperative Drainage

Postoperatively, suprapubic drainage must be prolonged, to give the urinary system the best possible chance to return toward normal. This does not necessarily imply that hospitalization need be more than a few weeks. After the child is discharged from the hospital, the suprapubic catheter of a baby can be connected by a rubber tube to a bottle placed at the side of the crib. Older children can be allowed to be ambulatory, employing a flat rubber bag strapped to the thigh, into which the suprapubic tube is left open at all times.

There should be no hurry about removal of the suprapubic tube; it certainly should be left in place for several months, and for much longer periods of time when there has been extensive renal destruction. Prolonged and free drainage accomplishes two things. *First*, it allows the kidneys to regain reasonable function. How much has been accomplished in this regard can be evaluated from time to time by measurement of the urine concentration, and by determining the level of the blood non-protein nitrogen. These two factors might appear to be fixed for many months, and only after a long siege begin to show signs of improvement, but the kidneys have an enormous restorative capacity if patience and long-continued wide-open bladder drainage are used. *Second*, constant drainage of the bladder permits it to shrink so that there will be a return of competence to the uretero-vesical valves. Drainage should never be discontinued when there is still incompetence of the valves. Information regarding this point can be determined quickly from time to time by cystographically visualizing the bladder, running in iodide solution and moderately distending the bladder. If any reflux is seen up either ureter, the uretero-vesical junctions are still incompetent.

Chemotherapy is required in all cases because urinary infection has been present in the vast majority, and it is certainly always present after operative manipulations and use of in-lying tubes. The bacteria generally change in type from time to time, and if pyuria cannot be brought under control and urinary pus kept at a minimum, the antibiotic agent should be shifted to one which is more effective against the particular organism which happens to be present at the moment.

RESULTS OF THERAPY

At the Children's Hospital, prior to 1950, 19 patients of varying ages were recognized as having posterior urethral valves, urethral obstruction, uremia, pyelonephritis, etc. Efforts to handle these babies and young children were most disappointing. In spite of all the measures which were employed, which included suprapubic drainage, attempts (in some) to remove valves by punch or cystoscopic means, supportive therapy, chemotherapy, and other means, 17 patients died while in the hospital. Only 2 survived, these being older boys with milder degrees of obstruction and renal damage who have gotten along in a fair manner after attempts at punch removal of the valvular area and the use of prolonged suprapubic drainage. In one of these there is considerable urinary dribbling, almost certainly brought about by the destructive removal of too much tissue at the bladder outlet from the blind procedure which was employed.

Particularly disappointing was the finding that many of the fatalities were in subjects only a few months of age; in spite of the fact that no attempt was made to attack the urethral anomaly directly, and that wide-open suprapubic drainage was given continuously to decompress the urinary tract and additional measures were given in the way of chemotherapy, intravenous infusions, and transfusions, the kidneys were already damaged to such an extent that prolonged hospitalization and supportive care was followed by fatality. These utter failures emphasize the point that the kidneys excrete urine during the early months of fetal life;[2] the urethral obstruction has brought about severe damage of the kidneys even before birth. This implies that if kidneys are to be saved, *it is imperative to recognize urethral obstruction in babies and to institute appropriate therapy promptly within the neonatal period.*

More recently, employing the methods of prolonged suprapubic drainage, and removal of posterior urethral valves under direct vision as shown in Figure 414, 4 patients have been operated upon with very gratifying results which make us feel that it might now be possible to treat this abnormality and stop its ravages. These 4 males have all survived the removal of valves and have had extraordinary recoveries, such as we have never seen with the older methods of therapy. These patients were aged 3 months, 4 years, 7 years, and 12 years, respectively. In each, it has been possible to relieve the obstruction and to gain a free urinary flow through the urethra. The suprapubic catheters have been left in place for periods from two months to one year. It has been possible to demonstrate (in the baby) that preexisting incompetence of the uretero-vesical valves could be completely reversed and that subsequently there was no reflux upward from the bladder. In this group of 4 patients, particularly pleasing was the result with the three-month-old child who was certainly at death's door, and for whom little or no hope of survival was given for several months, during which time the non-protein nitrogen remained elevated to high levels, the urine was extremely pale and of a low concentration, and there were extremely heavy amounts of pus in the urine. However, with suprapubic drainage over the course of the subsequent year, the kidneys showed a great capacity to regain reasonable function, the non-protein nitrogen returned to normal levels, and the urine regained a fair concentration; the general condition of the child has markedly improved (Fig. 411). The extremely hopeful aspects of these 4 patients certainly make us enthusiastic about attempting further use of these surgical methods in other subjects.

REFERENCES

1. Jorup, S. and Kjellberg, S. R.: Congenital Valvular Formations in the Urethra. Acta radiol., *30*:197, 1948.
2. Kjelberg, S. R. and Rudhe, U.: The Fetal Secretion and Its Significance in Congenital Deformities of the Ureters and Urethra. Acta radiol., *31*:243, 1949.

CHAPTER 56

Urinary and Fecal Incontinence
of Neurogenic Origin

One of the most perplexing problems confronting the surgical staff of a children's hospital is the care of those youngsters who have congenital abnormalities of the lumbosacral region, and consequent neuromuscular defects of the bladder and anal sphincters which give constant urinary and fecal soiling. Some of these individuals may have normal, or near-normal, sensation and motor power of the legs, but others have marked degrees of neuromuscular deficit in the lower extremities. In the latter, the problem of urinary or fecal soiling of the perineum and thighs is doubly troublesome and disagreeable because the subject must wear leg braces, use crutches, or be handicapped in his locomotion and thereby unable to cleanse and care for himself properly. These children are wet, smelly, uncomfortable, and rapidly become outcasts. Constantly soiled by their own excretions, they lead miserable lives, often are bed-ridden, and present such difficult and protracted nursing problems that home care is generally impossible, and institutionalization must become their lot.

The present review summarizes our experiences in attempting to help 21 of these children. It was fully realized that it would be impossible to restore any of them to normal, but yet it was felt that it would be worth-while trying to change their situation into something more tolerable.

CLINICAL DATA

These 21 children, ranging from four and one-half to ten years of age, all had congenital defects of the lumbosacral area (myelo-meningocele, sacral agenesis, myelo-dysplasia, et cetera) with obvious bony deformities of the lumbosacral spine, sacrum, or coccyx by roentgen examination and a wide variety of neurologic defects in the lower part of the trunk, the perineum, or the legs. Sixteen previously had had some form of neurosurgical operation for treatment of a meningocele or a myelo-meningocele, while 2 had had removal of lipomas from a deformed cauda equina. Seven of the children had had one or more orthopedic operations for improving the usefulness of the legs by tendon transplantation, tendon lengthening, stabilization of a foot, or correction of varus, valgus, or cavus deformity. Thirteen of the patients could walk reasonably well without braces or crutches; they had only slight neuromuscular deficiencies in the legs. Four required braces or crutches for ambulation. Two children had complete flaccid paralysis of the legs. Two patients had no weakness of the legs. Two children had moderate hydrocephalus but the process had been completely arrested. All of the children had severe incontinence of urine or feces, or both. While we have cared for other subjects with lesser degrees of incontinence, there was included in this

Table 75 (continued)

Patient	Operation	Follow-up
J. E. Female	1943 Loop colostomy, with ureters transplant- ed into distal, isolated sigmoid segment (Fig. 415, C)	1950 Bilateral hydronephrosis. Poor func- tion of right kidney. 1951 Colostomy situation is handled fairly well. Mental retardation.
B. H. Male	1944 Loop colostomy, with ureters transplant- ed into distal, isolated sigmoid segment (Fig. 415, C)	Wears one bag over both openings. Odor at first a problem, no longer so. 1951 Good adjustment. Goes to school. Has chronic urinary infection, requiring chemotherapy. Occasional bleeding from sigmoid bladder.
J. R. Female	1944 Loop colostomy, with ureters transplant- ed into distal, isolated, sigmoid segment (Fig. 415, C)	1945 Stone removed from sigmoid blad- der. 1952 Very well adjusted. Uses disposable colostomy bags. Well pleased. No odor, pain, or infection. Occasional bleeding from mucosa.
W. O. Male	1944 Loop colostomy, with ureters transplant- ed into distal, isolated sigmoid segment (Fig. 415, C) 1945 Closure of mesenteric defect following herniation of small intestine. 1950 Closure of perforation of sigmoid blad- der. 1951 Closure of perforation of sigmoid blad- der.	1952 Resides in state hospital-school. Occa- sional abdominal pain. Has hydronephro- sis on right. Bag emptied every four hours. Most of the urine removed by catheter in- serted into the sigmoid bladder every four hours. Good adjustment in school; mixes well. Has stones in the sigmoid pouch.
A. N. Female	1947 Sigmoid bladder constructed. Continuity of colon maintained (Fig. 415, D)	1951 General status excellent. Very well adjusted. Catheter fits snugly into sigmoid orifice. Catheter opened every three hours for release of urine.

Operations for Patients Who Have Both Urinary and Fecal Soiling

For 13 of our patients (Table 75) the urine was diverted into the colon (which ended as a colostomy) giving a wet colostomy, or else the urine was run into an artificial bladder which had been constructed from a segment of the sigmoid, one end of which had been brought as a stoma on the anterior abdominal wall. These various rearrangements of the urinary and colonic tracts are indicated in Figure 415. Rather than give the details of the individual operations, or the intricacies of care of the various patients, it is probably more informative to summarize the various experiences, pointing out what seemed to be helpful and what was undesirable in the various operative rearrangements.

The reconstruction depicted in Figure 415, A, is that which was tried for four patients who had both urinary and fecal incontinence. The lower sigmoid was divided, its distal end was closed, the proximal end of the sigmoid was brought out as a perma-nent colostomy, the ureters were transplanted into the upper sigmoid. This gave a "wet colostomy" through which both urine and feces were simultaneously discharged. With this rearrangement the patient was invariably and promptly improved by diverting all urine and fecal material from the perineal region, so that these areas could be kept clean, dry, and sanitary. All previously existing cutaneous inflammations and ulcerations of genitalia, perineum, or thighs healed very promptly. For such relief the patients and families were always very grateful.

However, the establishment of a wet colostomy brought problems of its own. The intermixture of urine and feces was generally difficult to handle, there being a constant emission from the colostomy stoma, producing a persistent mess, particularly in the older days when only a bag of rubber was available for the collection of such discharges. The rubber bags generally had a disagreeable odor in spite of repeated washings. More recently there have become available appliances which carry cheap, disposable, plastic bags, which when filled can be discarded. With these, the odor problem has now been almost completely eliminated. Our oldest patient with a wet colostomy is twenty years of age. This young woman went through an uneventful pregnancy and delivery of a baby in 1950. She currently works as a clerk in a department store. She is quite happy and is a well adjusted individual. She uses the disposable plastic colostomy bags; they cause little expense or inconvenience. The case illustrates what can be accomplished when the surgeon provides the patient with some sort of an arrangement which can be taken care of easily and when there is a patient who has a cheerful and realistic attitude towards her deformity.

Before the times when plastic colostomy bags became available, we had many tribulations from some of the wet colostomies because urea-splitting organisms acted on the urine and liberated ammonia. This disagreeable odor was impossible or difficult to mask. Because of this factor it seemed desirable to keep the bacteria out of the urine by separating the urinary and fecal streams (as indicated in Figure 415, B) in spite of the fact that this would give two orifices on the abdominal wall. This arrangement was tried for two patients. The lower sigmoid was divided and the upper end of the rectum was closed off. The sigmoid was used for construction of a pouch to receive urine. The lower part of the descending colon was brought out as an end-colostomy. In both patients in whom this arrangement was tried, there was immediate relief of the soiling of perineum, buttocks, and thighs, for which the patients were very grateful. While greatly diminishing or abolishing the odor problems, this arrangement was a little disturbing because there were two stomas on the abdominal wall to care for. In spite of its drawbacks, this general arrangement (when used in the early 1940's) appeared to be a distinct advance over the establishment of a wet colostomy. One of the patients cared for the sigmoid bladder by placement of a collecting bag over the presenting orifice. In the other case, the orifice could be made snug enough so that it acted as an obstructive mechanism, which, however, was large enough to allow the insertion of a catheter every few hours to withdraw urine which had collected in the pouch. Observing that the latter means was much more satisfactory and agreeable to the patient, we hoped to produce such a similar, narrow orifice in all subjects who were subsequently given sigmoid bladders, but we found it impossible to accomplish this with any regularity.

The arrangement shown in Figure 415, C, was used in six cases for treatment of patients who had both urinary and fecal incontinence. The lower sigmoid was divided and its distal end turned in. The upper sigmoid was brought out as a loop colostomy (subsequently converted into two separate but adjacent orifices), using the major portion of the sigmoid for an artificial bladder, into which the ureters were transplanted. This general arrangement was used in the hope that one colostomy bag could be employed to cover the two orifices which were quite close together, but yet there might be the advantage of keeping the urea-splitting organisms out of the urine (before they discharged into the bag) and in this way minimizing the ammoniacal odor. This over-all set-up initially appeared to be somewhat better than that shown in Figure 415, A, but we would now feel that it really has little or no advantage over it.

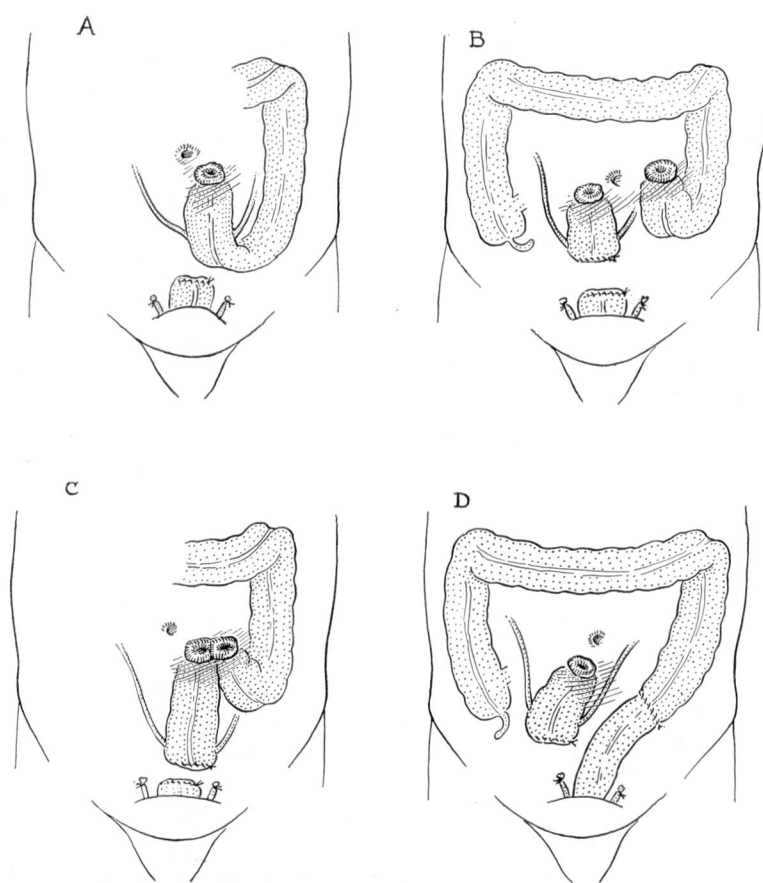

Fig. 415. Methods of therapy employed for patients listed in Table 75. A, For rectal and bladder incontinence. Lower sigmoid divided, turning in lower end. Establishment of end colostomy. Ureters transplanted into upper sigmoid, giving a wet colostomy. In some patients these steps were accomplished in multiple stages, in other cases all of the steps were done at one procedure. B, Treatment of fecal and urinary incontinence by division of lower sigmoid with closure of its lower end, establishment of a sigmoid bladder into which the ureters are transplanted, and establishment of an end colostomy. The two stomas are widely separated on the abdominal wall. C, Procedure rather similar to B, but colostomy opening and sigmoid bladder opening are close together so that a single bag can be fitted over them. D, Treatment employed in one case wherein there was urinary incontinence but fair anal control. A sigmoid bladder has been constructed. The continuity of the sigmoid has been reestablished.

Figure 415, D, depicts the operative procedure which was used for one child who had total urinary incontinence and a fair anal tone, but whose anus was not competent enough to allow transplantation of the ureters into the sigmoid and thereby give discharge of urinary and fecal material by rectum. A segment of the sigmoid was removed from the colonic circuit so that it could be employed as a sigmoid bladder after implanting the ureters into it; the continuity of the sigmoid was reestablished. This patient has gotten along very well during the five years that the sigmoid bladder has been used.

There is a snug orifice into which the child can pass a catheter each three or four hours for withdrawal of urine; between times there is no leak of urine from the opening. The whole picture has been extremely pleasing. However, we doubt if this arrangement is really much more satisfactory than that which could have been attained more simply by using the urinary bladder as a receptacle as is described in a subsequent section and as is indicated in Figure 416 (the urethra is closed off and a permanent cystostomy is established).

Sigmoid bladders (such as depicted in Figure 415, B, C, and D) brought certain risks and complications: (1) While the segment of sigmoid was usually a redundant, capacious receptacle and would receive much urine before discharging it to the exterior, in one instance there were recurring spasms of this pouch which were extremely difficult to treat. At unheralded intervals there would be a paroxysm of severe abdominal pain, and urine would shoot out under great pressure. It was impossible to control such activity in spite of local instillation of anesthetics, soothing solutions, or the administration of antispasmodics. (2) Some of the sigmoid bladders were frequently the site of collection of calcareous deposits, some of which would be free within the lumen, while others were in the form of encrustations adherent to the mucosal lining, the removal of which was sometimes very traumatizing to the bowel wall. (3) In many of the sigmoid bladders there was ulceration and bleeding, which at times was of severe degree. (4) The greatest hazard of a sigmoid bladder occurred in a boy who on two different occasions perforated the sac, requiring emergency surgical closure thereof. The escape of urine into the general abdominal cavity caused peritonitis, intestinal obstruction, and a near-fatality each time.

Having struggled through the building of sigmoid bladders and the tribulations in caring for the children thereafter, our experience with them now convinces us that they have certain advantages and also very real risks. A decade ago they appeared to be distinctly better than anything which was available at the time for the treatment of the child who had uncontrollable incontinence. We now feel that such surgical reconstruction should no longer be used. This change in policy has been brought about by the current availability of some such appliance, such as a Rutzen enterostomy bag, which can be cemented to the abdominal wall over a bowel stoma, and to which can be attached disposable plastic sacs. If properly fitted and used, such an apparatus can keep the patient clean and odorless. With this newer adjunct, we now feel that if urinary and fecal incontinence are so severe that it is necessary to divert both streams away from the perineum, it is simplest to establish a wet colostomy (Fig. 415, A) because this can be managed by the patient in a reasonably satisfactory way. In those patients in whom there is only urinary incontinence it seems best to handle the situation by surgical closure of the bladder outlet, accompanied by permanent suprapubic cystostomy.

Operation for Patients Who Have Only Urinary Incontinence

For all of the 8 patients listed in Table 76 there was severe urinary incontinence which required some drastic surgical relief, but it was felt that the fecal soilage could be handled, in spite of anal laxity, by giving a constipating diet, by properly cleansing the colon, and then washing out the colon once daily with an enema. It has been possible in all of these children to take care of the bowel in this way with fair satisfaction. This more recent experience in 1950, 1951, and 1952 makes us feel that probably some of the older patients who were listed in Table 75 might possibly have been treated without diverting their fecal streams out through a colostomy. It also leads us to hope that in the future it will rarely be necessary to establish a colostomy for any children with

Table 76

Division of Urethra and Establishment of Permanent Cystostomy for Urinary Incontinence

Patient	Operation	Follow-up
R. L. Male	1946 Cystostomy. Suprapubic closure of bladder outlet. Leakage recurred. 1946 Perineal closure of urethra. Leakage recurred. 1946 Perineal excision of segment of urethra.	1950 Because of greatly contracted bladder and difficulties in keeping catheter clean, bilateral ureterostomies done (elsewhere). Kidney condition greatly improved thereafter.
N. C. Female	1949 Cystostomy. Perineal division of urethra. Leakage recurred. 1949 Perineal division of urethra. Leakage recurred. 1949 Suprapubic division of urethra.	1951 Wears thigh rubber bag. Some urinary odor. Stones removed from bladder. Patient well adjusted. Mother pleased.
S. F. Female	1950 Cystostomy. Suprapubic division of urethra.	1951 Is in state hospital-school. Releases catheter every hour during day. On constant bladder drainage at night. No psychologic problems.
C. A. Female	1950 Cystostomy. Suprapubic division of urethra without anesthesia.	Mentally retarded. 1951 Wears rubber thigh bag. No infection, pain, or stones. Perineum dry. Mother pleased.
C. C. Female	1950 Cystostomy. Suprapubic division of urethra. Leakage recurred. 1951 Suprapubic division of urethra.	1952 Mild urinary infection. Controlled fairly well with Gantrisin. Wears rubber thigh bag. Perineum dry. Pleased with results.
C. D. Female	1950 Cystostomy. Suprapubic division of urethra.	1951 Does not wear bag. Releases catheter every 2 to 3 hours. No pain, infection, or stones. Perineum dry. Mother pleased.
M. C. Female	1950 Cystostomy. Suprapubic division of urethra. Leakage recurred. 1950 Suprapubic division of urethra.	1952 Does not wear bag. Releases catheter every 2 to 3 hours, perineum dry. Well adjusted. Mother pleased.
M. M. Female	1950 Cystostomy. Suprapubic division of urethra.	1952 Wears rubber thigh bag in day. When infection or plugging of catheter occurs, uses Ruppel irrigator at night. Perineum dry. Pleased with results.

neurologic deficits, since adequate dietary measures and daily cleansing of the colon seem to prevent fecal soiling if the regimen is diligently carried out by the family.

In all of the youngsters listed in Table 76 the severe urinary incontinence was treated by surgical closure of the urethra and by establishment of a permanent suprapubic cystostomy (Fig. 416). In this way the bladder itself could be used as a urinary reservoir, or at least it could act as a channel through which urine was diverted outward into some kind of an external appliance. Each of these children was markedly improved because the perineum, vulva, thighs, and buttocks have been kept dry and clean; much has thereby been gained in rehabilitation.

There have been difficulties in dividing the urethra in a manner which would give a permanent closure of the bladder outlet. In 4 patients it was necessary to repeat this two or even three times before permanent urethral closure could be attained. Thus, it becomes evident that interruption of the urethra is not a minor procedure which is to be taken lightly. We have now learned that it is always inadvisable to attempt division of a urethra in a female by the perineal approach, since it is almost impossible to get adequate exposure. The division should be done by the suprapubic route, completely severing the urethra just beyond the bladder and then turning the bladder orifice inward with a row of interrupted silk stitches. These are then reenforced by an additional layer of interrupted silk stitches which turn the bladder further inward. Only in this way can permanent closure be assured. In placing a small mushroom catheter in the bladder, we have attempted to put it in a very high position so that it might be kept away from the trigone and thereby reduce irritation.

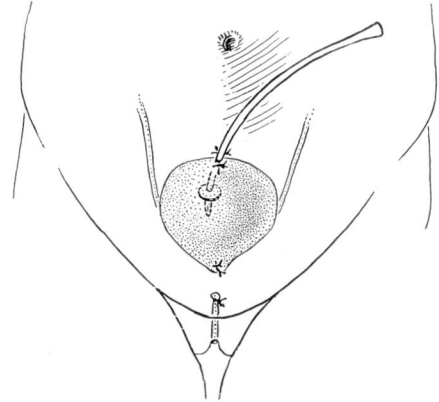

Fig. 416. Method of therapy employed for all patients listed in Table 76, all of whom had urinary incontinence but with fair anal tone (which, however, was insufficient to permit diversion of the urine into the rectosigmoid by uretero-sigmoidostomy). The urethra has been divided and the bladder outlet permanently closed. A permanent cystostomy has been made.

Usually, the bladder catheter should be changed about once a month. Any existing or recurring urinary infection should be appropriately treated by chemotherapeutic agents. If from time to time there is any important cystitis, a Ruppel irrigator can be connected with the catheter during the night so that the bladder can thereby be lavaged and cleansed.

The permanent cystotomy can be handled in one of two ways. The majority of our patients have had the suprapubic catheter connected to a rubber bag which is attached to a thigh, so the child could be ambulatory. In some children the urinary bladder has had a good capacity and no rubber bag has been used, the catheter merely being opened every few hours for release of urine. Whenever there is extensive kidney damage, incompetence of the uretero-vesical valves, or a bladder of a rather small capacity, it is best to leave the suprapubic catheter constantly open at all times and connected with a rubber receptacle so that the urinary tract might be given the best possible chance for function and for repair of damages which have already been sustained. Whenever the kidneys are in reasonably good condition, when there are competent uretero-vesical valves, and when the bladder has a fair capacity, it is permissible and more aesthetic to avoid the use of a rubber urinary bag and to merely open the catheter every few hours for the escape of urine.

All of these patients or their families have expressed great gratitude for what has been accomplished; the children are dry at all times. When a rubber receptacle has been necessary, it has not been troublesome or distasteful to manage. Two of the children are ardent swimmers; they merely clamp off the short catheter and tuck it under the bathing trunks when they take to the water. Needless to say, such transformation from a very miserable child into one who can enjoy life is a worth-while surgical attainment.

RECOMMENDATIONS

Summing up our various experiences of the past, it would be our policy at the present time to treat children with urinary and fecal incontinence (from lumbosacral neurologic disturbances) by the following general principles and procedures. It is realized fully that these attempts never end with entire satisfaction to the patient or the surgeon, but they seem to be about the best that can be accomplished in helping these miserable children out of the disagreeable urinary and fecal soiling to which they have been long subjected.

1. It should be made quite certain that everything possible has been gained by neurosurgical attack against the lumbosacral meningocele, spinal abnormality, or spinal cord tumor.

2. For those children who have only a mild urinary incontinence, and who are beyond three or four years of age, attempts should be made to strengthen the bladder sphincter by active exercises in which the urinary stream is started and stopped, started and stopped, so that the child can be made conscious of this shut-off mechanism and can frequently exercise it. Whenever there is *severe* laxity of the bladder outlet, such exercises are useless.

3. Whenever there is an "overflow" bladder, from excessive tone of the bladder sphincter, an attempt should be made to resect a portion of the bladder neck, hoping thereby to permit the detrusors to empty the bladder more efficiently. With or without such neck resection, prolonged drainage of a bladder (by cystostomy or by in-lying urethral catheter) permits a bladder to shrink, to gain an increased tone, and to empty itself more effectively after such drainage is stopped. Bladder-neck resections carry a variable outlook, which fact should be made known to the family beforehand. Some are quite successful in giving satisfactory bladder function; others make the situation worse by producing constant dribbling.

4. For the patient who has considerable laxity of the anal or bladder outlets (or both), there should be no radical surgical steps for local repairs or for diversion of urinary or fecal streams until the child is at least three or four years of age. In a few patients in whom there seems to be an almost hopeless soiling in the first few years of life, some neuromuscular control does subsequently appear; the situation is spontaneously ameliorated to a considerable degree. Hence, every chance for improvement should be given before any destructive or mutilating surgery is performed. If no important degree of neuromuscular improvement is evident by five or six years of age, there is almost no chance of having it appear at a later time.

5. Apparently, it will seldom be necessary to treat anal incontinence by establishment of a colostomy. While we have performed these in the past, more recent experience now makes us feel that this is probably seldom required. The bowel is usually sluggish and has a reduced tendency to spontaneous evacuation. A child who has a lax anal sphincter and severe soiling can generally be carried along reasonably well (beyond four or five years of age) by employing a constipating diet and a daily cleansing enema. If the colon is allowed to accumulate large and inspissated fecal masses, there is passage

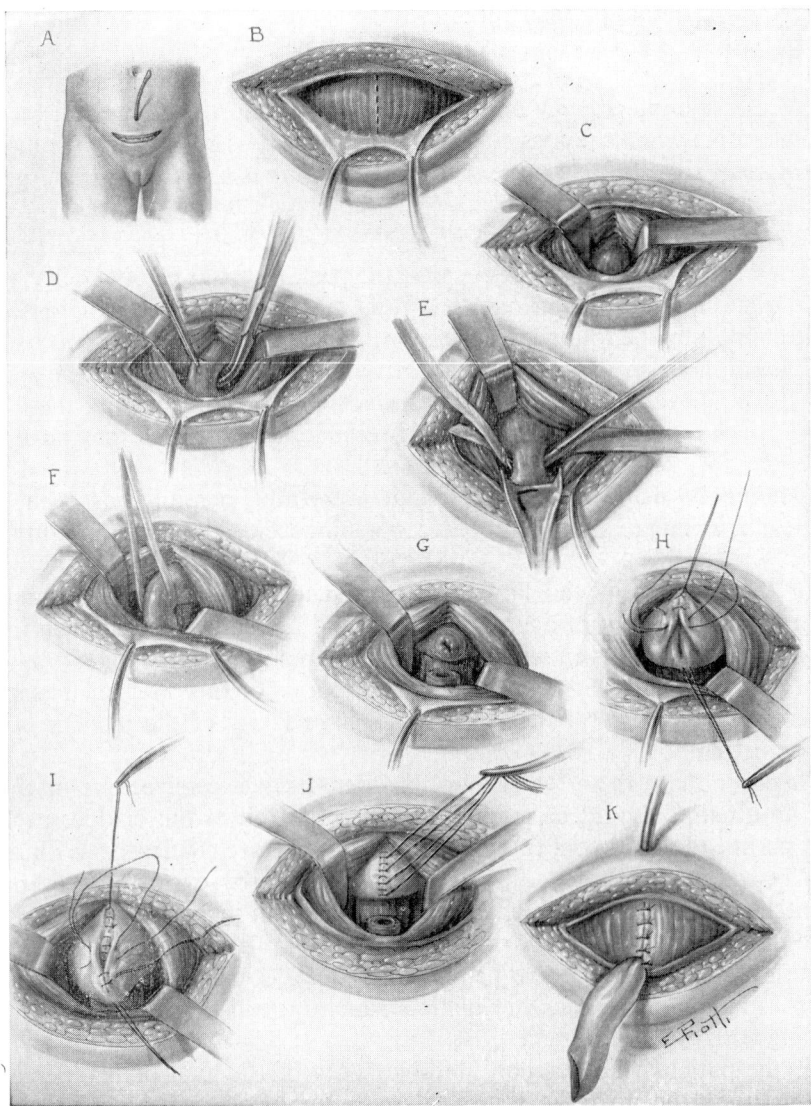

Fig. 417. Method for division and permanent closure of bladder outlet. A, Suprapubic catheter in place (having usually been placed there at a previous operation). Transverse incision above the pubes. B, Transverse opening of anterior rectus sheaths. Rectus muscles will be separated along the dotted line. C, Muscles retracted. D, Posterior urethra being dissected and circumvented. E, Tape being passed around bladder outlet. F, Raising urethra with a tape has facilitated extensive freeing of it. G, Urethra completely divided at bladder outlet. H, Bladder outlet being turned inward with interrupted silk sutures. I, Second layer of silk sutures to further invert bladder. J, Bladder closure completed. K, Rectus muscles approximated. Drain in pre-vesical space.

of fluid material around this which gives constant soiling. Conversely, if the bowel is kept free of accumulations by proper lavage, the colon usually moves only once a day (at the time of giving the enema), and there is little or no soiling between times. Certainly a long and concerted effort should be made at such conservative management before resorting to a colostomy. It is now our belief that a colostomy can be avoided in the vast majority of cases.

6. For the child who has great laxity of the bladder outlet and constant dribbling therefrom, it is generally desirable to attempt a plication of the bladder sphincters, using a retropubic approach and reefing in the dilated outlet by grasping muscular tissues at the sides and pulling them forward and sewing them in front of the bladder outlet to reduce the size of its lumen. While most of these plications have been ineffectual in accomplishing very much, in a few patients we have had urinary control established thereby. Certainly, in all cases in which there is mild laxity of the bladder outlet, plication of it should be tried before resorting to destructive surgery such as permanent drainage of the bladder, diversion of urine into a sigmoid bladder, or establishment of skin ureterostomies.

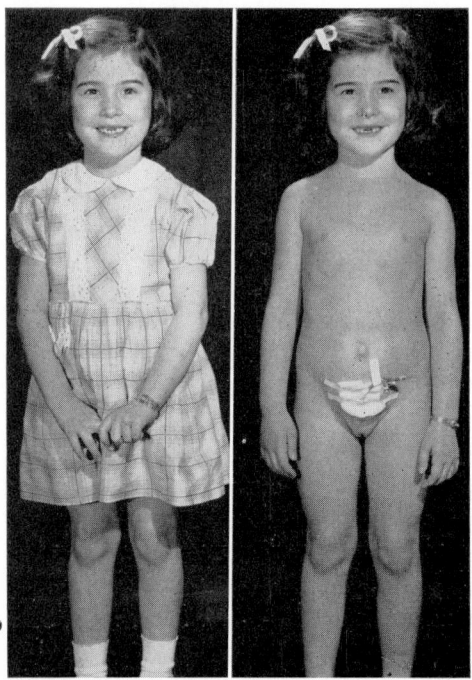

Fig. 418. Six-year-old girl (Case 7, Table 76) who had had fecal and urinary incontinence; a lumbosacral myelomeningocele had been removed in infancy. There was no anal tone. There was constant leakage of urine. Treated by constipating diet and daily colon lavage. Urinary problem handled by surgical closure of the bladder outlet and permanent suprapubic cystostomy. She opens the tube every three or four hours to allow escape of urine. The child is now dry, clean, odorless, and well adjusted to her abnormality.

7. In those cases in which it is fully evident that urinary incontinence is irreversible, the child should be provided with some means which will divert the urine so that the perineum and thighs can be kept dry. It is almost always impossible to transplant ureters into the sigmoid so that urine and fecal material can be discharged through the anus; the anus usually is too lax to give any satisfactory control over semi-fluid material. If both the urinary and fecal streams must be diverted away from the perineum, these can be done by establishment of a wet colostomy, which simultaneously discharges both fecal and urinary materials (Fig. 415, A). These can be collected in a colostomy bag made of disposable plastic sacs.

8. It is generally unnecessary, and indeed undesirable, to construct a sigmoid bladder (Fig. 415, B, C, or D). When there is no fecal soiling (this having been brought

under control by diet and by daily enemas) and when urine has to be diverted from the perineum to keep this dry, the situation can be handled by closure of the bladder outlet and establishment of a permanent suprapubic cystostomy (Fig. 416). When such permanent suprapubic drainage of the bladder has been established, the tube can be clamped most of the time but then opened every three or four hours if there is competence of the uretero-vesical valves and if there are fairly good kidneys. Conversely, the tube should be left open at all times and connected to a rubber bag on the thigh whenever there is incompetence of the uretero-vesical valves or there is marked damage of the kidneys.

9. Whatever method of therapy is outlined and given for these subjects, the patients must be indefinitely under the supervision of a physician or clinic staff who can guide them, alter the regimen, or care for those contingencies which almost certainly will arise from time to time.

REFERENCES

1. Bisgard, J. D.: Substitution of the Urinary Bladder with a Segment of Sigmoid; An Experimental Study. Ann. Surg., *117*:106, 1943.

2. Bisgard, J. D. and Kerr, H. H.: Substitution of Urinary Bladder with Isolated Segment of Sigmoid Colon. Arch. Surg., *59*:588, 1949.

3. Bricker, E. M.: Bladder Substitution with Isolated Small Intestine Segments. Am. Surgeon, *18*:654, 1952.

4. Chute, A. L.: The Relation between Spina Bifida Occulta and Certain Cases of Retention. J. Urol., *5*:317, 1921.

5. Elsberg, C. A.: Diagnosis and Treatment of Surgical Diseases of the Spinal Cord and Its Membranes. W. B. Saunders Co., Philadelphia, 1916.

6. Ewert, E. E. and Flint, L. D.: Rectus Muscle Sling for Neurogenic Incontinence. Surgery, *27*:688, 1950.

7. Gilchrist, R. K., Merricks, J. W., Hamlin, H. H. and Rieger, I. T.: Construction of a Substitute Bladder and Urethra. Surg., Gynec. & Obst., *90*:752, 1950.

8. Goebell, R.: Zur operativen Beseitigung der angeborenen Incontinentia vesicae. Ztschr. f. Gynäk. Urol., *2*:187, 1910.

9. Kelly, H. A.: Incontinence of Urine in Women. Urol. & Cutan. Rev., *17*:291, 1913.

10. Mertz, H. O. and Smith, L. A.: Posterior Spinal Fusion Defects and Nerve Dysfunction of the Urinary Tract. J. Urol., *24*:41, 1930.

11. Pickrell, K., Broadbent, R., Masters, F. and Metzger, J.: Construction of a Rectal Sphincter and Restoration of Anal Continence by Transplanting the Gracilis Muscle. Ann. Surg., *135*:853, 1952.

12. Rubin, S. W.: The Formation of an Artificial Urinary Bladder with Perfect Continence; an Experimental Study. J. Urol., *60*:874, 1948.

13. Smith, C. K. and Engel, L. P.: Neurogenic Vesical Dysfunction in Children. J. Urol., *28*:675, 1932.

14. Suby, H. I., Suby, R. M. and Albright, F.: Properties of Organic Solutions Which Determine Their Irritability to the Bladder Mucous Membrane. J. Urol., *48*:549, 1942.

15. Thompson, G. and Jacobson, C., Jr.: Neurogenic Vesical Dysfunction due to Spina Bifida and Myelodysplasia. Am. J. Surg., *61*:224, 1943.

CHAPTER 57

Pectus Excavatum (Funnel Chest)

Pectus excavatum, also known as funnel chest, *Trichterbrust*, or sunken sternum, is a condition in which there is a depression of a portion or all of the sternum and the adjacent cartilages. The deformity is present at birth or develops shortly thereafter, and generally becomes progressively more marked as the individual grows. The condition is not uncommon. Varying degrees of the abnormality are seen. The malformation occurs much more frequently in males than in females.

ETIOLOGY

The cause of pectus excavatum is obscure. Brown[1] has believed that there are unusually strong ligamentous attachments to the back of the sternum, providing a forceful pull from the diaphragm, a factor thought to be particularly significant in producing deformity during the development and growth of the sternum. While an excessive traction through the "substernal ligament" seems to be a factor of some importance in many cases, we doubt if it is the underlying cause for all sternal depressions. Occasionally tracheal obstruction, by increasing the negative pressure within the thorax during inspiration, seems to lead to development of sternal depression, but the vast majority of patients show no such blockage of the airway. Rickets seldom appears to play a part in the development of the deformity, but many of these youngsters do seem to have bones which are soft, springy, and less rigid than normal. A hereditary factor is sometimes evident in that the condition has been found in twins or in several members of one family. It has never been clearly established why a chest starts to have an anterior dishing, but it is clear that once it has started, the inward tilt of the costo-chondral areas compels the lengthening ribs to push the sternum inward still farther.

CLINICAL FINDINGS

Children who are affected by this anomaly are usually thin and rather asthenic in build. The rib cage is more compressible than normal; the ribs seem to be softer and more yielding. During respiratory movements there is usually a paradoxical movement, the sternum sucking in during inspiration. The extent of the sternal concavity varies from case to case. The degree of deformity may stay fixed through the childhood years, but in the more prominent examples of the abnormality, the depression becomes much more marked as the child grows. Once the costal cartilages and the costo-chondral junctions have become turned inward, all subsequent growth of ribs (at the costo-chondral epiphyses) pushes the cartilages and sternum in even more. In extreme cases, the depression is so severe that one side of the sternum slips from the midline and lies in the paravertebral gutter, actually posterior to the ventral surface of the vertebral body. The depression of the sternum and cartilages is generally symmetrical on the two sides of the midline; however, in some cases there is distinct irregularity, one side being more uneven or depressed than the other. As the lesion progresses, the child's head often

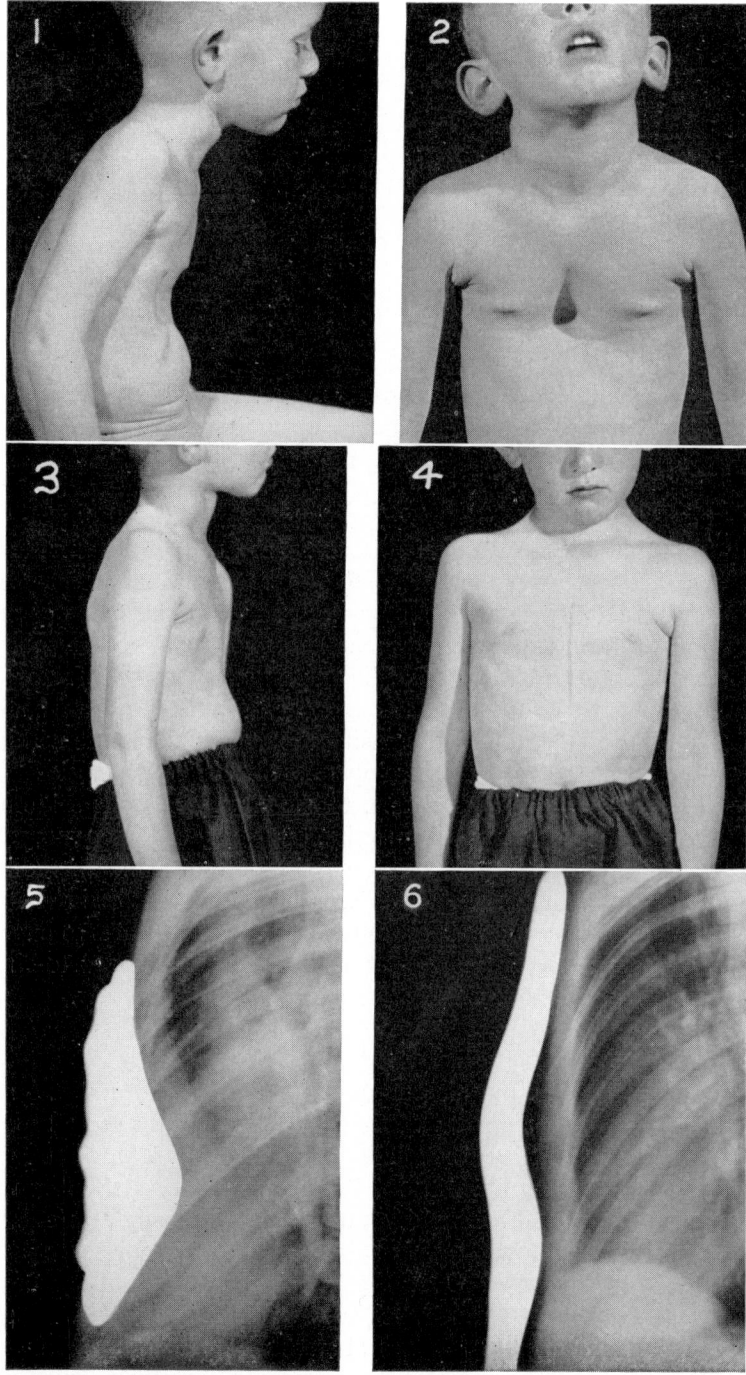

Fig. 419. Three-year-old boy who was treated for pectus excavatum. 1. and 2. Photographs before operation, showing the extent of the sternal depression. 3. and 4. Sixteen months after surgical repair of the pectus deformity, showing the very satisfactory cosmetic result. 5. Lateral roentgenogram before operation with a lead strip laid on the thoracic skin, to outline the marked sternal depression. 6. Similar roentgenogram, following operation, to show the correction of the sternal depression.

becomes thrust forward, and a mild dorsal kyphosis of the thoracic spine develops. While the deformity can generally be hidden by clothing, in the undressed state it frequently becomes a great source of embarrassment to the patient or his family.

The main complaints are usually related solely to the cosmetic abnormality of the chest, but aside from aesthetic considerations, a severe depression of the sternum can produce marked dislocation and possibly compression of some of the intrathoracic viscera. The heart can become pushed to one side and is apt to be displaced back into the left paravertebral gutter. Symptoms related to malfunction of intrathoracic viscera are extremely rare in childhood, but are occasionally encountered in adults. Shortness of breath, increased fatigue, cardiac irregularity, and even heart failure have all been described. Psychologic disturbances occur rather frequently. Playmates tease and torment the unfortunate child, who is therefore apt to become introverted, self-conscious, and shy.

Roentgen examination of the chest may show a displacement of the heart. Lateral views give an accurate and permanent record of the extent of sternal depression, and the relation of the sternum to the spine. The contour of the anterior surface of the thorax can be nicely shown in lateral films of the chest by applying barium paste or molding a strip of lead on the skin.

INDICATIONS FOR SURGERY

It is not necessary to repair all depressions of the sternum. Some are mild and the deformity is inconsequential; they are not of sufficient degree to warrant the use of a major corrective procedure. In the more advanced degrees of malformation, operation has much to offer. The risks of surgery can be made negligible. There is an excellent promise, but by no means a universal one, of restoring a normal, or reasonably normal, contour to the thoracic cage. The optimum age for surgical correction of a pectus excavatum lies somewhere between three and five years, thus providing correction of the deformity before the child attends school. Obviously, defects can be repaired in older youngsters; there is some question whether they should be corrected in infancy. Lester,[3,4,5] Brown,[1] and others have advised surgical procedures in babies, feeling that in the very young group it is necessary merely to divide the posterior sternal ligaments, the removal of which would theoretically allow the sternum to develop normally. We are somewhat opposed to this view because there are many babies in whom the deformity does not progress and in whom surgery can be avoided. Furthermore, we are not convinced that simple cutting of the substernal ligament is sufficient to arrest progress of the sternal deformity in the more serious cases; in some instances cutting of the ligament is followed by further advancement of the concavity. Therefore, while there are some favorable arguments for operating upon children in the first year or two of life, it has generally been our policy to defer surgery until three or four years of age to become more certain that operation is necessary and that following an extensive rearrangement of the bony structures, there will be enough rigidity of the bones to make less likely a recurrence of the deformity.

SURGICAL TREATMENT

Available Methods

Several therapeutic attacks are available. (1) Brown states that simple division of the "substernal ligament" in infants is all that is necessary to correct the condition. (2) It is possible to completely remove the dished sternum and its attached costal cartilages, to turn over this entire unit, and suture it in place as recommended by Hoff-

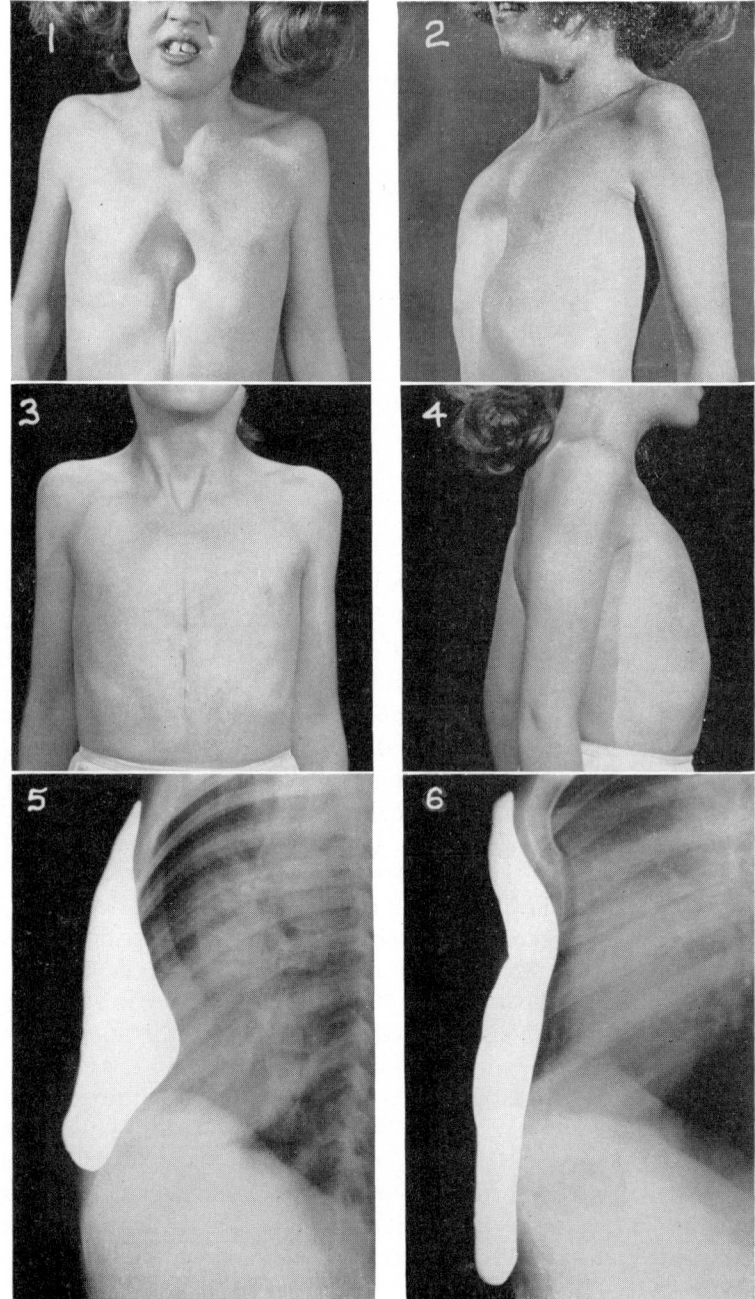

Fig. 420. Ten-year-old girl who was surgically treated for correction of a pectus excavatum. 1 and 2. Photographs before operation, showing the extent of the sternal depression. 3 and 4. Photographs six months after surgical correction of the deformity, showing the excellent cosmetic result. 5. Lateral roentgenogram before operation, with a strip of lead laid on the thoracic skin, to outline the bony depression. 6. Similar roentgenogram, following surgery, shows the satisfactory correction of the deformity.

meister;[2] this appears to be unnecessarily radical and risky. (3) Sweet[9] has raised the sternum somewhat, and excised medial portions of the depressed cartilages, sewing the remaining lateral ends of the cartilages to the borders of the sternum. We doubt if this method will be sufficient for treatment of the more severe lesions. (4) Ravitch has devised a method whereby the ensiform cartilage is cut away from the sternum, all of the depressed cartilages (with perichondrium) are excised and discarded, the sternum is transected at the upper end of the depression, and then pulled forward into a normal position. Ravitch has obtained excellent results with this, but many surgeons have hesitation in accepting a procedure which does not provide reasonable stability of the sternum until it becomes fixed again permanently. (5) We believe that the best results are probably accomplished by mobilization and realignment of the sternum and adjacent cartilages, anchoring all of these by appropriate stabilizing sutures, thus insuring considerable stability of the various parts until fibrosis and healing fixes them in their new positions. This operation is much more extensive than that devised and used by Ravitch, but we feel that the increased stability which is gained during the early postoperative period is well worth the additional surgical effort.

Recommended Procedure

Figure 421 indicates the steps which we have found to be quite satisfactory for the treatment of pectus excavatum. A few general remarks concerning the technique might be of value. This operation is by no means a small one and should not be undertaken lightly. Blood loss may be considerable; arrangements for transfusion should always be made ahead of time. One or both pleural sacs might be inadvertently opened during the dissection behind the sternum. An intratracheal tube should always be employed, so that positive pressure anesthesia can be given if necessary.

For positioning the patient on the table, a flattened sandbag or a folded sheet is placed under the patient's lower thoracic spine to thrust the chest forward. In making the various wedge-cuts in the cartilages, a scalpel is generally all that is required. Sometimes the apex of an anterior curve in the costo-chondral cage lies somewhat lateral to the costo-chondral junction; therefore the wedge-cut must be made in the rib itself, which will require a rib cutter or a saw. The transverse cut across the superior portion of the sternum is made at the very beginning of its depression; the transection must be quite high; it generally lies at a level between the first and second ribs. This transverse cut should be made in a wedge manner, carrying the apex back to the posterior table of bone. This can be done with an osteotome or gouge, but we prefer to use a Stryker electric saw for this step. Most depressed sternums are rather flat, but an occasional one has a longitudinal groove so that bringing the entire body forward will still leave a bony contour which is dished or furrowed. In such instances we have made a longitudinal cut throughout the length of the body of the sternum; this will allow breaking of the lateral halves of the sternum at the midline, and will bring them into a flatter alignment.

While it is generally possible to get good repair of the depressions which are symmetrical, some children have a marked irregularity, or asymmetry, of the two sides which taxes the operator's ingenuity in trying to bring them into proper position and satisfactory contour.

After the various osteotomies have been made properly, the sternum and the adjacent cartilages may be elevated into a more anterior and normal conformation. Indeed, when suitably released, they tend to spring out into this position. It is desirable to stabilize the structures in this corrected position by sutures placed appropriately at the various osteotomies and chondrotomies. For the transverse line across the upper end of the

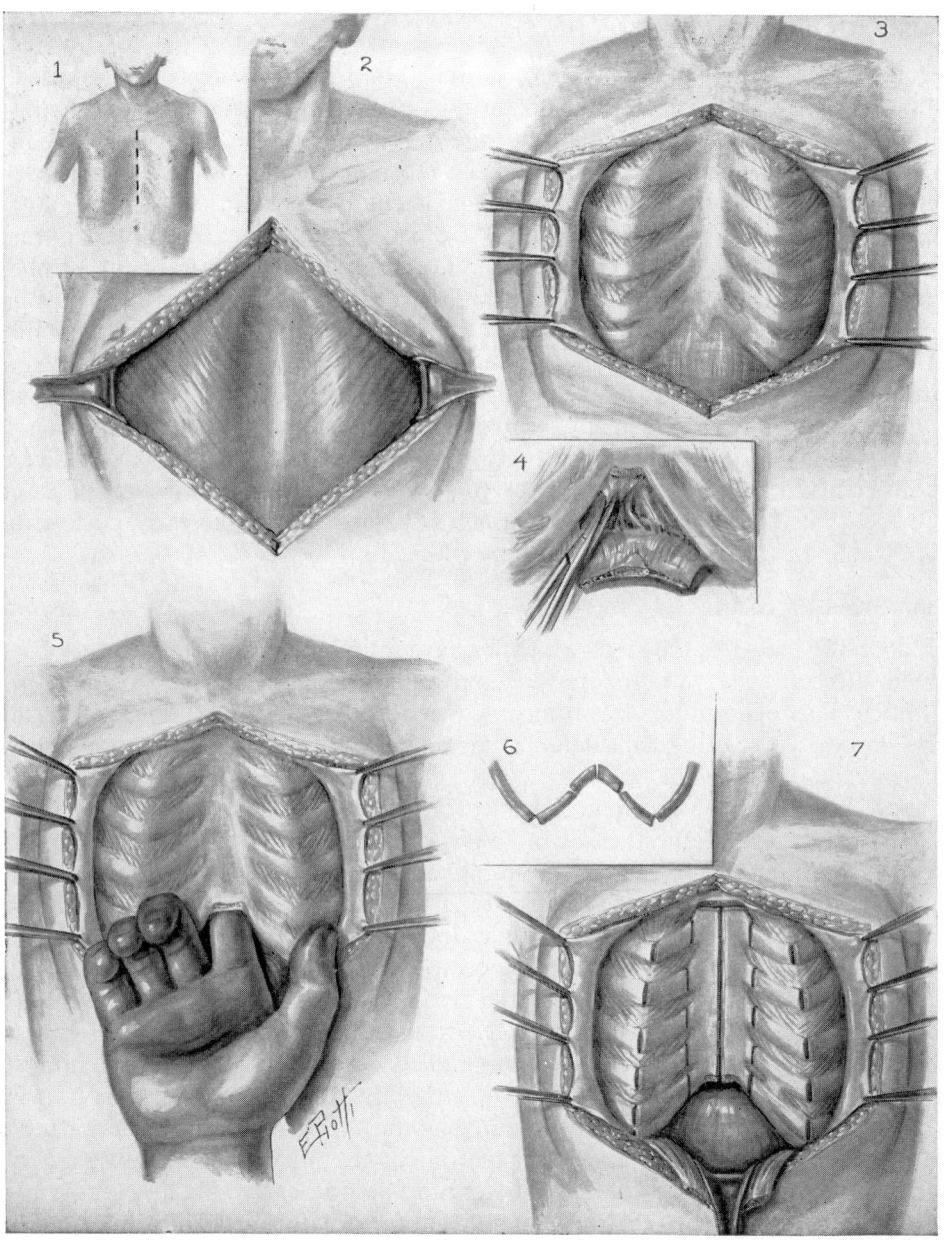

Fig. 421. Operative correction for pectus excavatum. 1. Position of the midline incision indicated.
2. Wide flaps of skin and subcutaneous tissue freed from the entire sternal area, running well out over
the pectoral muscles. 3. Incision of pectoral fascia in midline, and mobilization of pectoral muscles,
freeing them up widely from the underlying bony cage. 4. The ensiform process has been cut away
from the lower tip of the sternum. Ligamentous attachments between diaphragm and posterior surface
of sternum are now being completely severed. 5. By blunt and sharp dissection all structures are freed
from the back of the sternum and from the posterior aspects of the depressed portions of cartilages.
This wide dissection is carried well up to the manubrium. 6. Transverse schematic drawing of incisions
which will be made in the cartilages and in the sternum. On the anterior aspect of the lateral costal
bulge wedge-shaped portions of cartilages are removed, the wedge presenting anteriorly. At the attachments of cartilages to sternum the wedges are removed, the broad portion of wedge being toward
the posterior. The sternum is shown slit in the midline, a step which is sometimes necessary for correction of a sternum which has a longitudinal groove in it. If the sternum is relatively flat, this central
incision is not necessary. 7. Completion of the wedge-shaped incisions which were indicated in 6.
Wedges have been removed from the lateral portion of the cartilages and also from the inner portions
of cartilages where they join the sternum. A longitudinal incision has been made the length of the
sternal body. A wedge-shaped transection has been made across the upper end of the sternum.

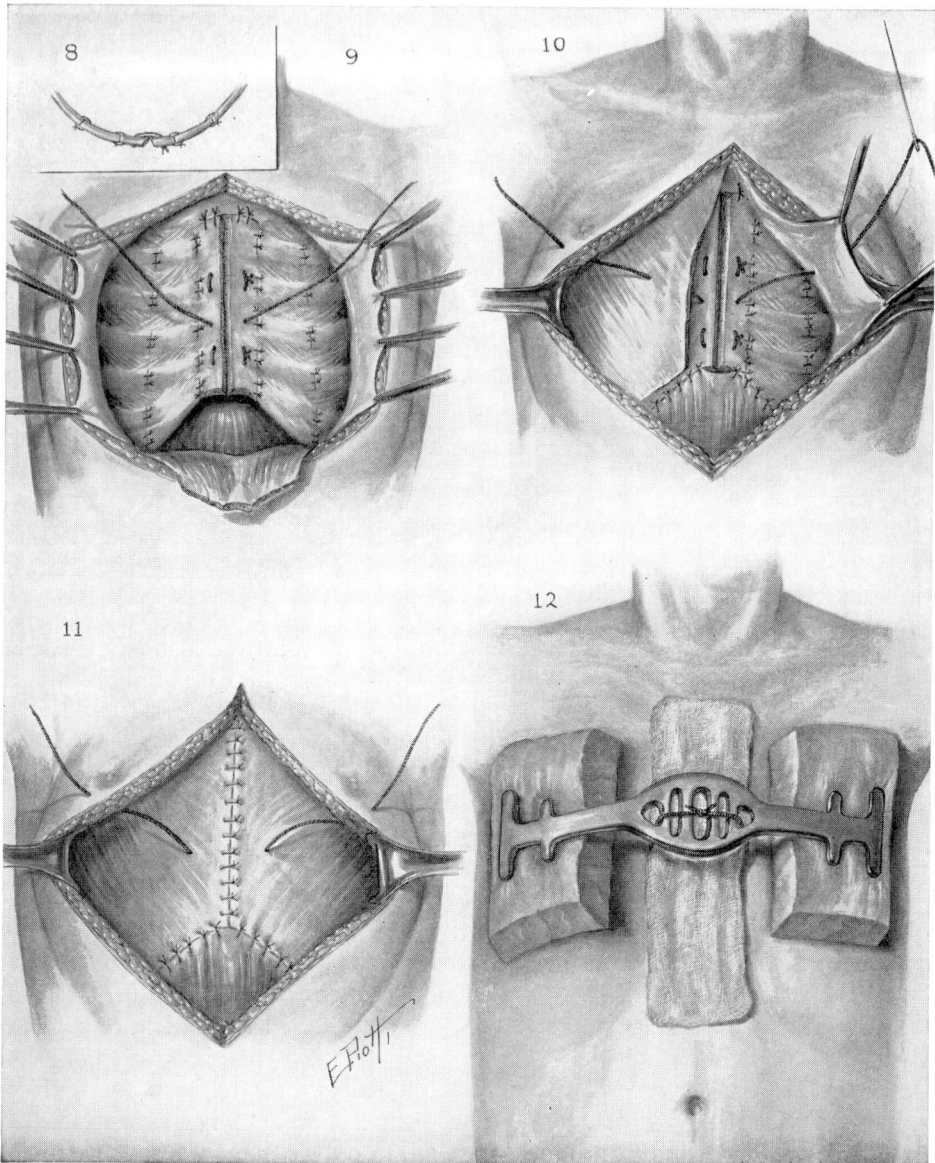

Fig. 421 (*continued*). 8. Schematic horizontal dissection through the chest, showing the manner in which sutures will bring into alignment the ribs, cartilages, and sternum. 9. Completion of sutures at lateral and medial ends of the various cartilages. The transverse incision across the superior end of the sternum has been repaired with silk stitches. The sternal cartilages have all been pulled into a normal contour. The placement and tying of the various stitches will maintain this contour. A heavy braided suture has been run through the body of the sternum, and will be used for postoperative traction. 10. The traction suture has been run out through the pectoral muscles and through the cutaneous layer. Rectus muscles have been appropriately anchored to inferior edge of the thoracic cage. 11. Pectoral fascia is brought together in midline, grasping the periosteum of the sternum. (It is believed that the pull of the pectoral muscles will help to keep the sternum pulled forward.) 12. Skin wound closed and covered with gauze. Over each antero-lateral border of the chest is placed a piece of sponge rubber about an inch thick. On this rests a transverse metal bar (after Lester) over which the traction suture is tied. The compressible sponge rubber provides a traction which is constant, of appropriate tension, but yet yields a little during respiratory excursions of the chest. This whole dressing and appliance will now be covered with adhesive tape.

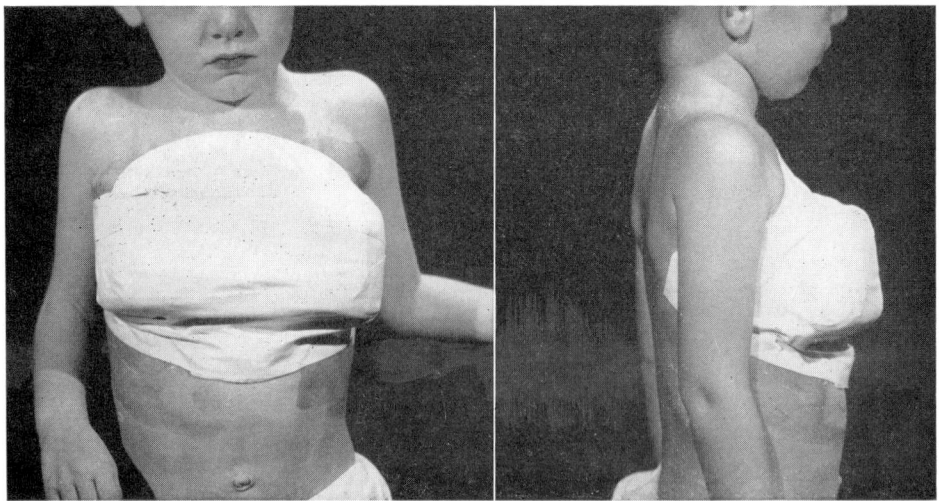

Fig. 422. Type of chest protection used for about a month following hospital discharge. The traction suture has been removed at the time of hospital discharge, but the rubber blocks and the transverse bar (Fig. 421, 12) are reapplied and covered with adhesive as shown. The child does not object to this dressing. We feel that it is probably desirable to use some such protection for the first month at home, until the bony cage becomes more fixed and stable.

sternum, heavy sutures of No. 1 Deknatel silk are used. For the repair of the cartilaginous junctions, 000 silk is employed. For the traction suture No. 3 Deknatel silk is suitable. It is not essential to employ a traction suture for the sternum during the postoperative period, but this adjunct is probably of some value and we have used it in most cases. This additional pull and stabilization for about two weeks after operation has been thought to be desirable. In such extensive work on cartilage and bone, utmost care must be used in the maintenance of sterility; we have not had infection in the wound or along the traction suture in any case. For a "bridge," to which the traction suture can be tied, a transverse bar of plastic material or metal is better than a plaster shell. We prefer to mount this bridge on blocks of sponge rubber, 1 inch thick, to cushion the pull exerted by the traction suture.

In the postoperative hospitalization it is probably best to keep the child from being partially propped up in bed at any time, since a slumped position with the thorax arched forward probably puts an unnecessary strain on the operative repair. It is much better for the child to lie flat in bed on his back, sit straight up in bed, or to get out of bed and stand or walk about. The skin sutures are removed on the sixth or seventh day, but the traction suture can be left twelve to fourteen days.

While a shield in front of the chest is not necessary after hospital discharge, we have usually employed some protective covering (Fig. 422) which will minimize the possibility of injury to the thorax while the child is with his playmates.

RESULTS OF OPERATION

While not uniformly perfect, the surgical repairs of pectus excavatum have been extremely satisfactory. One should not judge the postoperative results by the appearance of the chest at the time of hospital discharge, because in occasional cases there is a distinct tendency for the deformity to recur. We believe that this is usually evidence of an operation which has been incompletely or improperly performed. Conversely, when the parts have been brought into satisfactory alignment and have been held thus by adequate fixation for a long enough period of time during the healing process, the bones and cartilage become joined and they continue to grow in a normal contour.

When a preoperative deformity has been a symmetrical one, the postoperative result is generally quite good. When, before operation, there has been irregularity or asymmetry in the sternum, the final result may be somewhat disappointing. In the latter cases, fortunately a minority in any series, it may be impossible to correct completely all of the unevenness; the sternum and nearby cartilages have a bumpy contour, which may become more marked in subsequent years as the various osseous parts grow in an irregular and unpredictable fashion.

Table 77

Cases of Pectus Excavatum
Operated upon at Children's Hospital

Case	Age	Sex	Operation Date	Result
1	3 yrs.	F	4/4/47	Fair
2	7 yrs.	M	12/4/50	Poor
3	7 yrs.	M	11/21/50	Good
4	4 yrs.	M	1/24/51	Fair
5	3 yrs.	M	2/15/51	Good
6	3 yrs.	M	5/1/51	Good
7	5 yrs.	M	12/4/51	Good
8	10 yrs.	F	1/15/52	Good

At the Children's Hospital, 8 patients have been operated upon; 6 were males and 2 were females. They ranged in age from three to ten years. All wounds healed well and there has been no infection in any case. Three of the children had only a poor or fair result; in one there is moderate recurrence of the depression, whereas in the other two there is considerable irregularity which might subsequently require another procedure for cosmetic improvement. For the other 5 children, the reconstruction appears to be of permanent value; they have been classified cosmetically as very satisfactory. Two examples of these are shown in Figures 419 and 420. It has been amazing to find that several of the children, who previously were retiring and shy, have blossomed out after correction of their deformity, are smiling and are completely extrovert in their reactions.

REFERENCES

1. Brown, A. L.: Pectus Excavatum (Funnel Chest). J. Thoracic Surg., 9:164, 1939.
2. Hoffmeister, W.: Operation der angeborenen Trichterbrust. Beitr. z. Klin. Chir., 141:214, 1927.
3. Lester, C. W.: The Surgical Treatment of Funnel Chest. Ann. Surg., 123:1003, 1946.
4. Lester, C. W.: Funnel Chest and Allied Deformities of the Thoracic Cage. J. Thoracic Surg., 19:507, 1950.
5. Lester, C. W.: Funnel Chest: Its Cause, Effects and Treatment. J. Pediat., 37:224, 1950.
6. Ochsner, A. and DeBakey, M.: Chŏně-Chondrosternon. J. Thoracic Surg., 8:469, 1938.
7. Ravitch, M. M.: The Operative Treatment of Pectus Excavatum. Ann. Surg., 129:429, 1949.
8. Ravitch, M. M.: Pectus Excavatum and Heart Failure. Surgery, 30:178, 1951.
9. Sweet, R. H.: Pectus Excavatum. Ann. Surg., 119:922, 1944.

CHAPTER 58

Cysts and Primary Tumors of the Thorax

The literature contains many excellent treatises (Bradford et al.,[2] Heuer and Andrus[8]) on cysts and tumors of the mediastinum and other portions of the thorax; these comprehensively describe the pathologic types, the clinical manifestations, and the modes of therapy. Most of these reviews deal largely with the subject as it concerns adult patients; only a few of the general articles summarize the conditions as they appear in infancy and childhood. However, there have been a few reports dealing with individual types of cysts of neoplasms in the young. To gain a comprehensive view of the problem, it has seemed desirable in this chapter to include all of the forms of cysts, cystic tumors, and solid neoplasms which have been encountered in the early years of life. The following sections are based largely upon the experience of dealing with 49 such lesions (Table 78) in the thorax which have been treated at the Children's Hospital up to June 30, 1952. Because they are almost entirely of medical, and not surgical, significance, we have not included the many examples we have encountered of lymphoma (including Hodgkin's disease) which were primary in the mediastinum or which appeared as part of a generalized process.

GENERAL FINDINGS

Cysts and tumors of the mediastinum or other portions of the thorax can occur at any age, as a glance at the various data in Table 79 will show. About half of our patients were under two years; many were only a few weeks or a few months of age.

The *symptoms* included a wide variety of complaints. Frequently there was dyspnea or an increased respiratory rate. Not uncommonly there was a chronic cough. In a few there was fever or other evidence of infection, generally not from the lesion itself but more often from compression and infection of nearby lung substance. In some there was poor weight gain or retarded physical development; study of these led to physical or roentgenographic examination which disclosed the intrathoracic mass. In rare cases there was evidence of obstruction of the trachea or the superior vena cava. In a few there were no important symptoms, the abnormality being detected on a roentgenogram of the chest in a child who was thought to be well.

The *physical findings* have shown a wide variety of changes, the prominence of the features being related to the type of growth, the size of the lesion, and its position. Nonproductive cough was common. Dyspnea or tachypnea was found in a considerable number. Evidence of tracheal and superior vena caval obstruction has appeared with those lesions which are infiltrative in nature and are also situated in the superior mediastinum. Differences in movement of the two sides of the chest are apparent with some of the larger masses. Changes of the percussion note to either dullness or flatness, accompanied by diminution or absence of breath sounds, are found when there are lesions of moderate or large size. Hematemesis or hemoptysis has been seen with some of the duplications which give erosion of the adjacent esophagus or lung. Retardation in physical development occurs with some of the more slowly growing lesions; weight loss accompanies some of the more rapidly expanding conditions. With a few of the smaller cysts or tumors no important abnormality can be detected by physical examination.

Table 78

Intrathoracic Cysts and Primary Tumors*

Children's Hospital Material to July 1, 1952

Neuroblastoma	10 cases
Neuroblastoma and ganglioneuroma	3
Ganglioneuroma	2
Plexiform neuroma	1
Cystic hygroma	5
Malignant thymoma	2
Thymoma	1
Malignant teratoma	2
Teratoma	3
Osteochondroma	1
Hemangioma	1
Bronchogenic cyst	1
Neuro-enteric cyst	1
Duplications of alimentary tract (Chapter 17)	16
Total	49

* Does not include lymphomas, Hodgkin's disease, etc. Nor does it include intrapulmonary cysts (cystic disease of lungs).

Details of clinical course, complaints, physical findings, therapy, and results of treatment vary so widely from lesion to lesion that it is best to consider these individually for the various types of cysts and primary tumors.

NEUROGENIC TUMORS

Neurogenic tumors include a variety of growths, ranging from high malignancy to marked benignity. The group includes *neuroblastoma, neuroblastoma and ganglioneuroma, ganglioneuroma, neurofibroma.* Kent et al.[10] published an exhaustive review of the world literature up to 1944 and summarized surgical management of intrathoracic neurogenic tumors; they collected 105 cases and added 18 of their own. Only 3 of the patients were under ten years of age. About 40 per cent of the lesions were said to be malignant.

NEUROBLASTOMA

Neuroblastoma is the most common, primary neoplasm which is encountered in the thorax of a baby or child. In many of the neuroblastomas which originate in the abdomen (Chapter 46), one can find an extension of neoplasm behind and through the diaphragm so that secondary invasions of the posterior mediastinum are encountered. In the present chapter none of such lesions is listed. The discussion has to do only with those neuroblastomas which have appeared to arise initially within the chest.

Neuroblastoma is one of the most highly malignant neoplasms of early life. It comes from stem nerve cells of very young type. The neoplasms are exceedingly cellular, have little stroma, and are very rapidly growing. They can metastasize rapidly and widely to various parts of the skeleton and the brain; they have little tendency to metastasize to the lungs except very late in the course of their progression.

Neuroblastomas in the thorax almost always originate from the sympathetic apparatus, and therefore appear as masses in either paravertebral gutter. They occur with about equal frequency on the two sides and there is a distinct predilection for the upper third or quarter of the thorax. The symptoms have usually not lasted more than a few weeks or months. Generally there has been wheeze, cough, dyspnea, or some such respiratory complaint. In a few there has been fever, failure to gain, or even loss of weight. In two of our patients there has been a dumbbell-shaped tumor with extension through the vertebral foramina, masses presenting in the thoracic cavity and also in the dural canal; the spinal cord was compressed and there were neurologic disorders below the upper or mid-thoracic levels.

By physical examination it has usually been impossible to find very much of importance which could point directly to the neoplasm. In some there has been cough or evidence of weight loss. Occasionally there has been an ipsilateral Horner's syndrome. In two of the largest growths, alterations in percussion note or auscultatory sounds were evident, but in others the mass was not large enough to give such changes. In two there were neurologic disturbances related to compression of the spinal cord at a high thoracic level.

Roentgenologic examination always shows the mass and can give considerable evidence pointing to the correct diagnosis. The tumor is of variable size, is in either paravertebral gutter, and tends to be in the upper third or quarter of the thorax. Its medial border merges with the mediastinal shadow; its inferior and lateral edges are usually smooth and clearly defined from the adjacent lung against which it is silhouetted. It is unusual to find calcification in the mass, but some specimens do have a fine scattering of such material. It is common to see the growth insinuating itself between the necks of the ribs, separating or eroding them by expansion or by direct invasion. These latter two findings almost specifically indicate the presence of neurogenic tumors; to show them clearly it is necessary to take films of proper density which bring into focus the posterior portions of the ribs. In the occasional patient who has neurologic signs of cord compression, the visualization of the spinal canal by injection of radio-opaque material will clearly delineate the position and extent of the block. If metastases are present, it is rare to find them in the lung fields; they are more apt to appear in the spine, the long bones, and the skull.

When neuroblastoma is suspected, it is probably wise in all patients to perform a bone marrow biopsy, looking for seeding of the tumor into the marrow substance.

Therapeutic Considerations

Certain general statements are in order regarding therapy, fully realizing that knowledge in this field is limited and that any current policies might have to be changed as experience increases in the future. (1) Three of our patients were known to have metastases either to bones outside of thorax or to marrow (as shown by sternal biopsy). Regardless of any therapy which was given, all of these patients died very soon thereafter; we therefore feel that if metastases can be demonstrated, there is very little point in radical attack on the primary lesion by any method which is available to us at the present time. (2) When there are no demonstrable metastases (by marrow study or by roentgen examination of the skeleton), a concerted effort should be made to treat the growth by surgical removal and by x-ray irradiation. (3) While it is realized that the infiltrative nature of the tumor precludes its complete removal, excision of the major portion of the lesion seems to be of value because it reduces the mass of tissue which must be treated by irradiation. (4) Whether or not x-ray irradiation should be given before surgical removal is a moot question. We have used it in two subjects with rather promising results; we are inclined to feel that it deserves further trial and study. (5) X-ray therapy should be given in all cases following surgical excision, for almost cer-

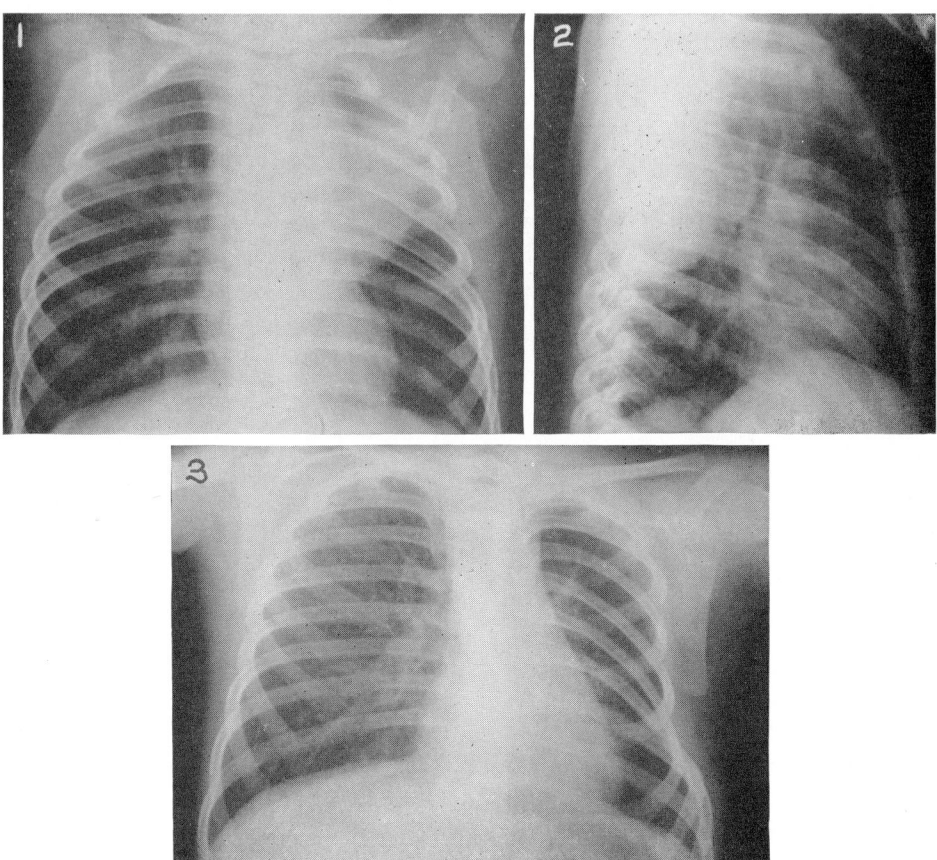

Fig. 423. Case 6. Films from an eleven-month-old child who had a dumbbell-shaped neuroblastoma which presented in the chest and also projected into the dural canal, giving compression of the spinal cord. 1 and 2. Preoperative films. Treatment by intraspinal and subsequently by intrathoracic removal of the tumor, followed by x-ray therapy. 3. Film three years after treatment. There is no evidence of neoplasm.

tainly bits of tumor have been left in the field which must be killed off. (6) Regarding the possibility of benefits from tumor chemotherapy, we have very little material from which definite statements can be made. Several agents have been tried in some of our patients, either for a localized process, or when metastases have been known to exist. While such chemotherapy has seemed to retard the growth of the tumor in some instances, in no case have we been able to attribute curative value to it (employing the substances which are available up to the present time).

Operative Treatment. It is felt that operation should be carried out in all cases (when no metastases can be demonstrated). This will allow histologic verification of the type of tumor which is being dealt with, and it also permits removal of a major portion of the mass. The attachment of the growth to the lateral surfaces of the vertebral column, to the necks of ribs, and to the intercostal muscles between ribs, makes it impossible to remove one of these growths entirely. They almost always present a smoothly rounded surface as they are approached through the pleural cavity. The parietal pleura can be peeled off, revealing a well defined capsule wherever the mass projects into the pleural cavity, or else the pleural coat can be left on the mass which is cut away. The mass can be liberated rather easily at first as its edges are freed, but as dissection is carried in more deeply along the vertebral column or along the necks of the ribs, it soon becomes evident that tumor tissue is being cut across in those regions where the neoplasm has invaded bone. At this point one raises the question whether a more thorough removal should be attempted by resection of the necks of involved ribs, or whether the main mass should merely be skimmed off the ribs, leaving some residual tumor tissue. Figure 425

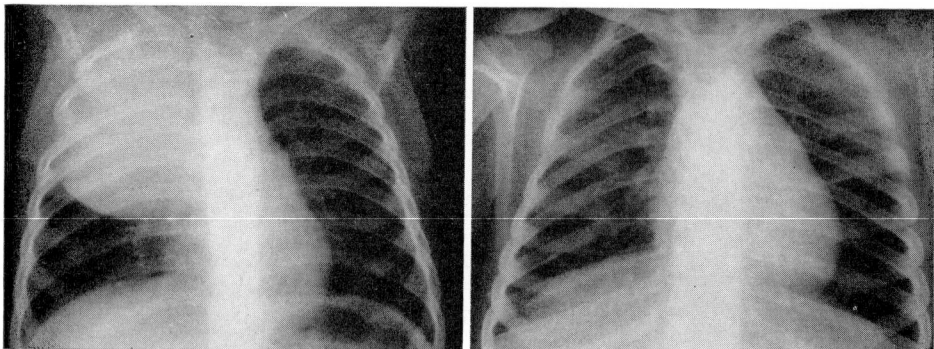

Fig. 424. Case 8. One-year-old child with neuroblastoma at the right apex of the chest. *Left*, Pre-operative film showing the mass. Treatment by surgical removal and by x-ray irradiation before and after operation. *Right*, Film two years following the therapy. There is no tumor remaining.

is from a child in whom portions of ribs were removed along with the tumor mass, feeling that this would give a more complete excision. While there has been subsequent deformity of the chest in this region, the apparent cure of the neoplasm raises some enthusiasm about further use of such an extended excision. However, Figure 424 is from a patient in whom the tumor was merely trimmed away from the ribs, not resecting any portions of the latter; there appears also to be a cure in this youngster. It is therefore impossible to make any definite statements whether or not the ribs should be resected. We are inclined to believe that if a tumor has no attachment to vertebral bodies, it is desirable to remove it without cutting into it; to accomplish this the involved portions of ribs are cut away with the neoplasm. However, when it is obvious that tumor invades vertebral bodies, there is little, if any, advantage in removing portions of rib necks, since it is impossible to completely excise the neoplasm anyway.

Postoperative Irradiation. In all patients, it is very important to give postoperative x-ray therapy over the operative site, preferably beginning this on the day of operation. Our enthusiasm for this adjunct is based upon the known value of x-ray therapy in the treatment of neuroblastoma (as long as it remains localized) when it has been primary within the abdomen. Further evidence for this optimism is given by the follow-up studies of a few of our patients with neuroblastoma of the thorax. In spite of the fact that tumor was known to have been left in the operative bed, 3 of the patients appear to be free of neoplasm for the two or three years that they have been followed.

End Results. The results of therapy for this neoplasm when primary in the thorax are most discouraging, but there is some hope in the over-all picture. Of the 10 patients we have seen, 5 are known to be dead. One had only a biopsy and in spite of this was known to be alive and in excellent health nine years later, though there was still roentgenologic evidence of a mass remaining in the chest; presumably the more malignant portions of the neuroblastoma had died off, while more slowly growing elements (ganglioneuroma) remained. There is one patient from whom only a biopsy was taken, who is receiving tumor chemotherapy; the lapse of time is too short to indicate as yet what the end result might be. In 3 patients there has been removal of as much of the mass as it was possible to excise by wide transpleural exposure, combining this with x-ray

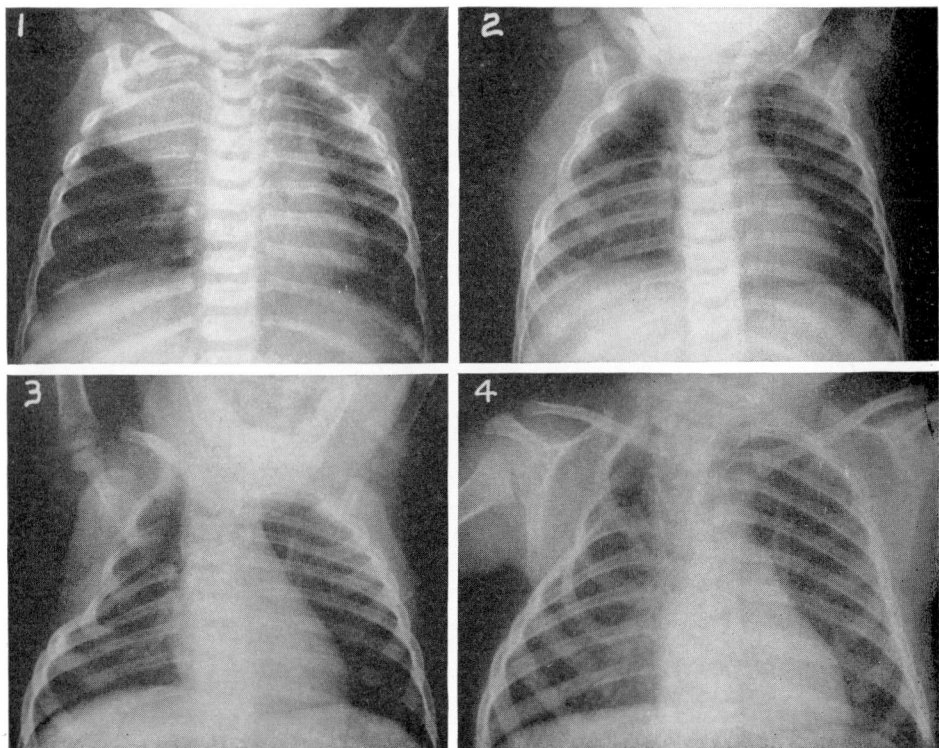

Fig. 425. Case 9. Eight-month-old baby with neuroblastoma at the right apex. 1. Film before therapy, showing the mass. 2. Film two months after surgical removal of the neoplasm and adjacent portions of three ribs. 3. Film six months after surgery showing the beginning collapse of the apical portion of the thorax. 4. Film two years after surgery. The apex is clear of tumor but there is considerable deformity of the thoracic cage.

therapy. These youngsters appear to be in excellent health without evidence of neoplasm two to three years later; we are hopeful that they might be permanently cured. It is of some importance to note that all of the patients who were more than two years of age when first seen are now dead. Conversely, the children who were seen in the early months of life, and certainly before two years of age, appear to have a much better outlook. The reason for a more favorable prognosis in very young subjects is unknown; it corresponds with the finding of a better outlook for children under two years of age who have a neuroblastoma within the abdomen (Chapter 46).

NEUROBLASTOMA DIFFERENTIATING INTO GANGLIONEUROMA

Some neurogenic tumors have a variable histologic composition; sections from most areas show a *neuroblastoma*, while other fields show the more highly differentiated *ganglioneuroma.* The tumors have a rapidity of growth which lies somewhere between the malignant neuroblastoma and the benign ganglioneuroma. They should always be regarded with considerable suspicion, because the neuroblastomatous element might predominate and produce a wildly growing or metastasizing lesion. However, it has been general experience that the finding of such an intermixture of neuroblastoma and ganglioneuroma gives some reason for adopting an optimistic outlook concerning the prognosis. We have therefore set these tumors apart from the neuroblastomas and from the ganglioneuromas.

The lesions arise from neural structures within the thorax, most commonly from the sympathetic chains or ganglia or from the first parts of the intercostal nerves. Therefore, they are always found in the paravertebral gutter on either side of the chest, particularly towards the apex. The symptoms are not unlike those that have been described for the neuroblastoma, except that in some cases there is an extremely long history of complaints. There may be a Horner's syndrome on the same side.

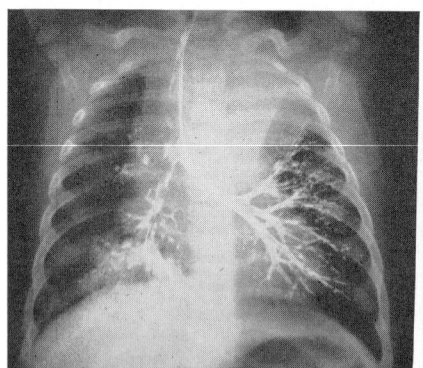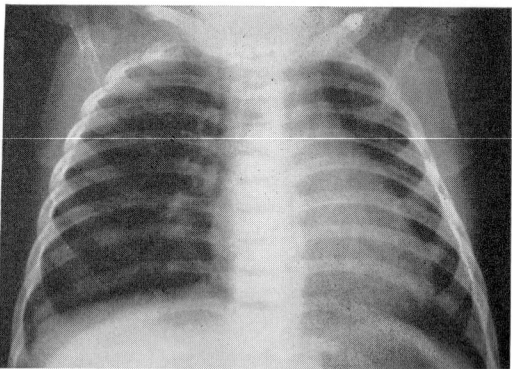

Fig. 426. Case 11. Three-month-old baby with neuroblastoma-ganglioneuroma at the left apex of the chest. *Left,* Preoperative film showing the mass and also the displacement of the trachea toward the patient's right. *Right,* Film six months following therapy. Apex clear. The child is entirely well three years after treatment.

While the neoplasms can reach considerable size and give local changes in percussion note and in auscultatory sounds, they tend to be small and show very little if any physical findings.

By roentgenographic examination a well circumscribed mass is found in either paravertebral gutter, generally in the apical region of the chest. Medially, the shadow is continuous with that of the mediastinal structures but laterally it is well rounded and clearly defined where it abuts against the lung. There is a common tendency for the postero-lateral parts of ribs to be spread apart or the necks to be eroded.

Treatment

For therapy a transpleural approach seems best, coming at the lesion as it projects into the pleural cavity. Either the overlying parietal pleura can be peeled away or this can be removed along with the mass, the latter probably being preferable. While the main portion of the tumor seems to be well circumscribed and can be circumvented easily, that part which lies against the spine and particularly against the necks of ribs is usually firmly adherent to these structures and cannot be clearly dissected away from them. After the main mass has been removed, all tissue which seemingly might contain tumor tissue should be cut away or curetted away from the rib necks or vertebral bodies. We believe that it is highly advisable to give x-ray therapy to all of these lesions after operation, preferring to start the irradiation on the day of operation.

Results of Therapy. Three patients have had lesions of this sort. They were all treated by removal (which was obviously somewhat incomplete) and all were given x-ray therapy subsequently. They are all doing exceedingly well from two to three years later; in this time none has shown evidence of recurrence or metastasis.

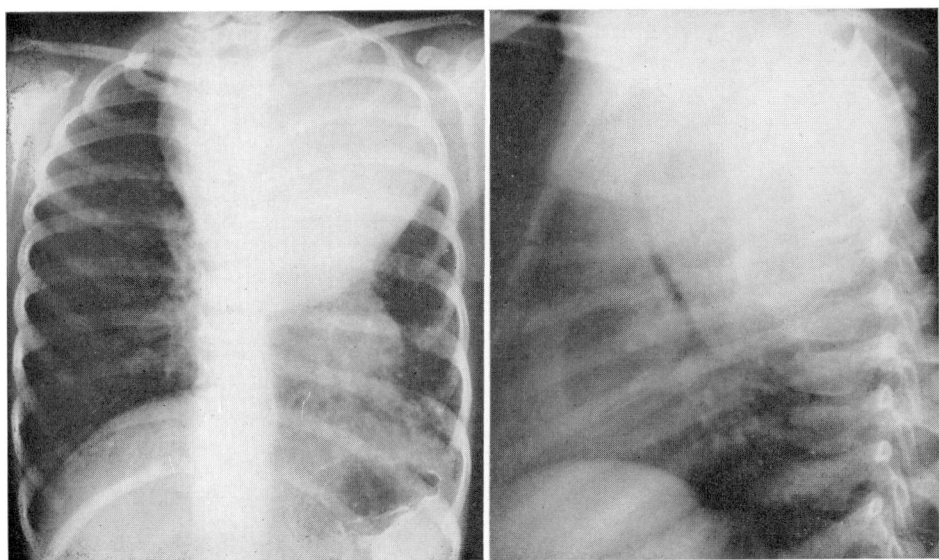

Fig. 427. Case 14. Roentgenograms from six-year-old girl with a large ganglioneuroma at the left apex. In the lateral view the shadow can be seen to reside in the posterior portion of the chest. The trachea is displaced forward.

GANGLIONEUROMA

Ganglioneuromas are exceedingly benign tumors of nerve cell origin. They are hard, well encapsulated, very slowly growing and carry an excellent prognosis. They arise from the sympathetic apparatus or from the first portions of the intercostal nerves. They are found in a paravertebral gutter or along the postero-lateral portions of the costal cage.

Jones and Effler[9] found ganglioneuromas in 4 patients, all under six years of age; they were all subjected to surgery and all recovered. We have had 2 patients with these tumors, both treated by operative removal of the ganglioneuroma, and without subsequent x-ray therapy. These children are in excellent health six months and two years later, respectively. With a neoplasm of this sort which grows slowly, it is advisable to follow the patient for several years, with x-ray film studies once or twice a year, to detect any recurrence which might require secondary excision.

PLEXIFORM NEUROMA

Neurofibromas are thought to arise from perineurial or endoneurial fibrous tissue and are distinguished from the tumors of the sheath of Schwann which are characterized by elongated fusiform cells and the palisading of nuclei. In some specimens of fibrous tumors of neural origin it is exceedingly difficult to ascertain which type of sheath might have given rise to the growth. Plexiform neuromas are irregular, elongated, slightly lobulated overgrowths of the fibrous tissue elements of nerve sheaths and occur along any nerve trunk of the body. They are occasionally seen within the thorax, springing from the phrenic, vagus, or the sympathetic trunks, but more commonly arising from the intercostal nerves or the various nerves which lie outside of the bony cage. They can be associated with overlying pigmented areas of skin, and in the more advanced forms have been known as von Recklinghausen's disease. They generally are benign, but later in life some of them do take on malignant characteristics. If a plexiform neuroma lies in an area where it can be completely excised, such therapy is relatively simple. However, many of the lesions appear in regions where they become intermixed with nearby im-

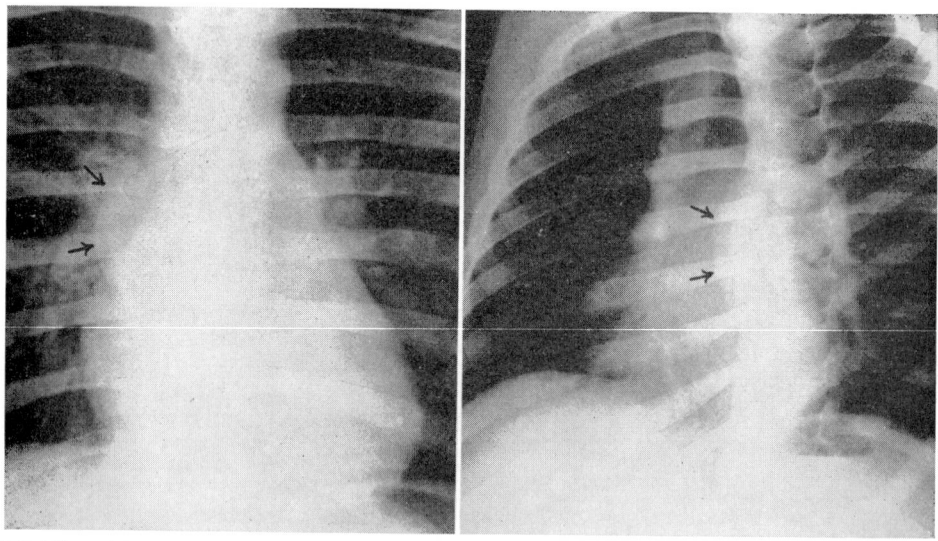

Fig. 428. Case 15. Mass in right postero-lateral portion of the thoracic cage in a six-year-old boy. Complete excision of the mass, which was found to be a ganglioneuroma.

portant anatomic structures, so that it is impossible to remove all of the neuromatous material without unwarranted destruction of adjacent organs or tissues. Therefore, the therapeutic handling is usually to remove the major portion of any such offending mass, fully realizing that there might be some regrowth years later which will require secondary removal.

Case 16, Table 79, is an example of a neuroma in the chest of a child. This nine-year-old boy, who for six years was known to have an external lump to one side of the scapula, was found by x-ray examination to have erosion of subjacent portions of ribs. Thoracotomy was performed for removal of the superficial part of the tumor and partial excision of the elongated neuromatous masses which lay between ribs. Thirteen years later this young man is in good health but by x-ray examination still has some small mass in the chest wall; it is very likely that this will require further excision at a future time.

CYSTIC HYGROMA

Lymphangiomas can be found in many parts of the body; they are particularly common about the shoulder girdle and especially in the neck (Chapter 68). A small number of them have been found in the thorax. Apparently they can arise anywhere in the mediastinum. They may be unilocular, but more uncommonly are multilocular affairs. They contain thin, clear fluid which is either colorless or slightly yellowish. They have thin walls and are lined by endothelial cells. Many excellent articles have been written describing celomic or pericardial cysts; Lillie et al.[12] collected 25 reports of such cysts (or pericardial diverticula) and added 12 of their own. These authors, like others, have believed that such cysts originate from misplaced portions of celomic or pericardial lining. Some of them have a stalk-like attachment to the pericardium or appear as a diverticular out-pocketing of the pericardium, thus suggesting a development which is

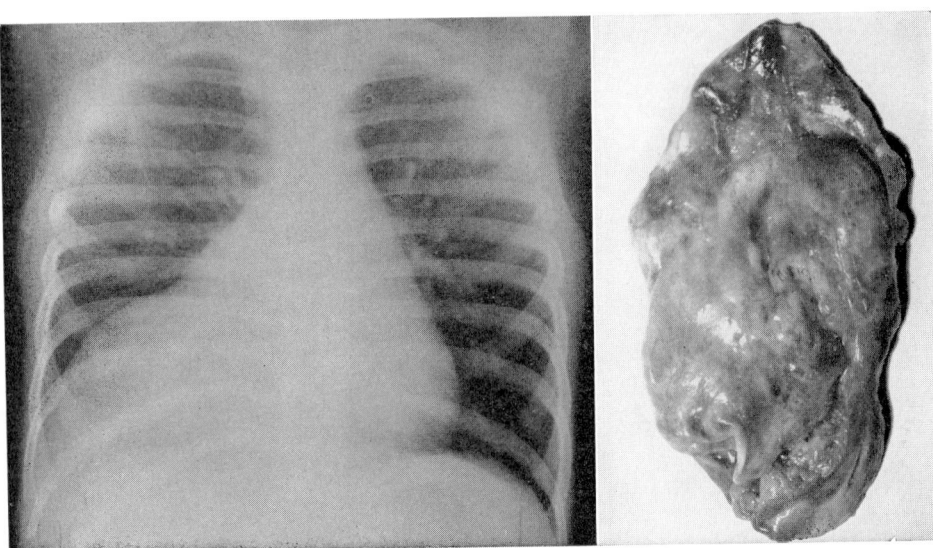

Fig. 429. Case 17. *Left*, Roentgenogram of a three-year-old boy with shadow in the right pericardiophrenic angle which at operation was found to be a multilocular hygroma. *Right*, Photograph of the hygroma which was removed.

closely related to that of the pericardium. However, the lesions have so many characteristics which are found in hygromas (cystic lymphangiomas) in other parts of the body that there seems to be little necessity for setting them apart as separate entities. We have therefore classified all cystic lesions which contain clear watery fluid and which are lined by endothelium as *hygromas*, regardless of where they might be found in the thorax.

Like cystic hygromas in other parts of the body, these lesions can be found in the mediastinum in the early months or years of life. If the mass reaches considerable size, it can press upon the bronchi or upon pulmonary tissue and give rise to chronic cough or other respiratory complaint. At times the smaller lesions may give relatively little difficulty and may only be discovered on routine chest plates. In two patients, wherein the primary complaints were related to hygromas of the neck, we found by x-ray investigation an extension down into the chest, projecting outward from the mediastinum and replacing a portion of the lung field. Such dumbbell-shaped hygromas, residing partially inside the thorax and partially above its apex, are apt to show variation in size of the cervical swelling from time to time, depending upon the pressure within the chest. When the child is at rest, the cervical growth has only moderate prominence, whereas during times of straining, crying, or coughing there is increased pressure on the intrathoracic portion which transfers fluid up into the cervical segment, temporarily making the neck lump much more prominent.

By x-ray examination it may be exceedingly difficult or impossible to differentiate a cystic hygroma in the mediastinum from other types of cysts or teratomas. The opaque shadow, with no calcium therein, can assume a variegated shape, can reach large size, and can project out from the mediastinum into the lung field on either side. In one of our patients there was a large flat lesion which lay between the right upper and middle lobes.

Treatment

All hygromas should be operated upon. There is an excellent chance of removing the entire cyst and thereby giving a very favorable outlook. Some of these lesions are mono-locular, or if multilocular they still have a well defined capsule, so that they can be dissected out and peeled away cleanly from surrounding structures. Some of them tend to insinuate themselves around important nerves or blood vessels, surrounding and engulfing these structures which then seem to run directly through the multilocular hygroma. Under such circumstances it is possible to remove only the major portion of

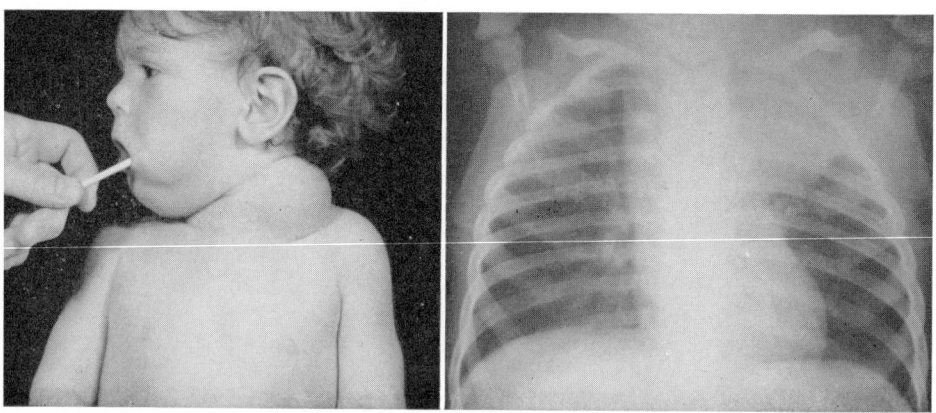

Fig. 430. Case 18. Fourteen-month-old girl who had a dumbbell-shaped cervico-thoracic hygroma. *Left*, The swelling at the base of the neck. *Right*, Roentgenogram of chest showing the hygroma in the upper portion of the left side of the chest.

the hygromatous tissue, leaving small bits of its substance around any important nerves or vessels. Generally, such operative attack will be followed by scarring over of any tiny remnants of hygromatous tissue which have been left in the wound. It is always well to remember that the treatment of cystic hygroma in any part of the body can be followed by some recurrence years later which might require secondary removal. Such secondary operations are generally of lesser magnitude and are followed by a high chance of permanent cure.

Results of Therapy. In our material there are 5 cases of cystic hygroma of the thorax. In patient 20 (Table 79) there was an extensive lesion between the upper and middle lobes of the right lung, the removal of which was followed by a broncho-pleural fistula and a chronic empyema, later requiring complete pneumonectomy. This child appears to be in good condition one year later. For patient 21, there was no difficulty in cleanly and completely removing the hygroma which projected out from the mediastinum into the right lung field; presumably the youngster is cured. In patient 17, x-ray study showed a mass lying between the pericardium and the right dome of the diaphragm. At opera-tion a multilocular but well circumscribed hygroma was excised from the pericardio-phrenic angle, the removal apparently being a complete one. The child has had no evidence of recurrence in the four years he has been followed. Patients 18 and 19 had cervico-mediastinal hygromas requiring operative removal of cervical as well as thoracic portions of the lesions. In the six and seven years that they have been followed there has been no recurrence of the mediastinal abnormality, but one of these patients subsequently required a secondary excision of a recurrent hygroma from the base of the neck.

THYMOMAS

During the past fifteen years there has grown up a considerable literature regarding the relationship between myasthenia gravis and tumors of the thymus; all of these discussions have dealt with adult patients. In some subjects with myasthenia a tumor of the thymus has been found, the removal of which apparently has improved the clinical picture of the debilitating disease. In contrast, other patients have not received benefit from surgical removal of thymic tumors. The majority of patients with myasthenia gravis have not been found to have neoplasms of the thymus. It is therefore difficult to establish any clear connection between the two conditions; during the last few years

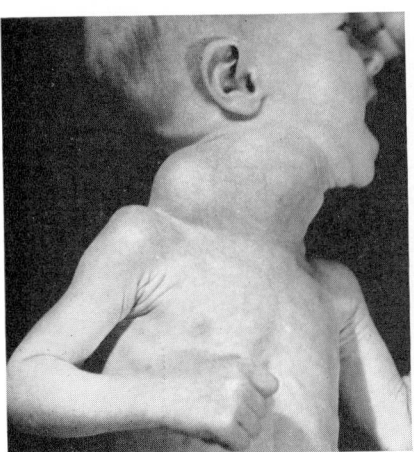 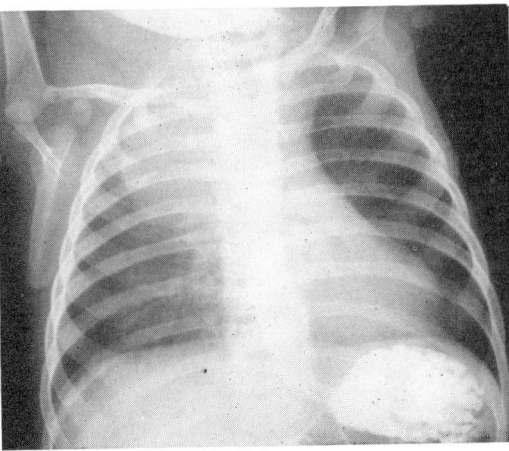

Fig. 431. Case 19. Seven-month-old girl with a dumbbell cervico-thoracic hygroma. *Left,* The mass at base of the neck was particularly prominent during crying. When the baby was relaxed most of this mass disappeared into the thorax. *Right,* Roentgenogram showing the hygroma in the upper portion of the right side of the chest.

there has been a diminishing tendency to try to establish a causal relationship. Certainly in the childhood ages, neoplasms of the thymus gland have not been known to cause any generalized or endocrine disturbance; their clinical and therapeutic considerations are concerned entirely with the treatment of a neoplasm, which, in a high percentage of cases, is a malignant one.

Malignant Thymomas

These are exceedingly rapidly growing tumors. They are generally derived from the lymphoid elements of the thymus gland, and they present most of the characteristics of a malignant lymphoma. Indeed, it may be histologically impossible to differentiate such a neoplasm from lymphomas originating in other portions of the body. Malignant thymomas are limited to the confines of the thymus or else they extend down as a sheet of tumor over the front and sides of the pericardium; they tend to surround and strangle the trachea and great vessels of the superior mediastinum. These lesions grow with great rapidity; they seem to spring up almost overnight, and generally the symptoms are not longer than a few weeks. They give distressing and agonizing symptoms very quickly because in the crowded superior mediastinum the advancing tumor circumvents and constricts the trachea and various blood vessels, particularly the superior vena cava.

The child has great difficulty in breathing, rapidly develops stridor, distress, hypoxia, and possibly cyanosis. The picture is made all the more striking and alarming by venous engorgement of the arms, the neck, and particularly the face; these become congested, suffused, and edematous.

X-ray examination (Fig. 433) shows a massive sheet of tumor extending from the thymus down into the anterior mediastinum in front of or on either side of the pericardium, reaching toward the hili of the lungs.

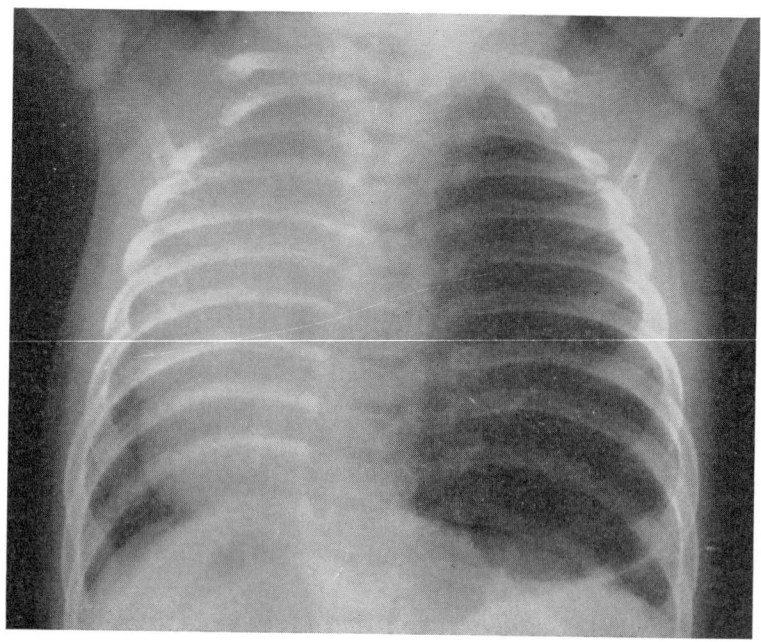

Fig. 432. Case 20. Four-month-old baby who had extensive lymphangioma (hygroma) between the right upper and middle lobes. There is obstruction of the right main bronchus, producing atelectasis of the right lung, and a displacement of the heart toward the patient's right.

Treatment and Results of Therapy. These tumors are overwhelming and they exact their toll very quickly. The two patients that we have encountered entered the hospital *in extremis.* In hopes of giving some relief, a tracheotomy was established, with the plan of bringing the localized thymic tumor under control by irradiation. Even with the improvement of the airway by the insertion of a tracheotomy tube, the vascular disturbances were such that death promptly followed and there was no chance in either case to give x-ray therapy.

Benign Thymomas

These tumors are occasionally seen. While histologically they may appear to be highly cellular tumors composed of lymphoid elements, it has been known that some of these remain as well circumscribed and encapsulated masses projecting out from the thymus gland, and can be followed by a relatively good outlook if appropriately treated.

Therapy. Our one experience with this type of growth was in a fourteen-year-old boy who had no symptoms and who was found to have a mediastinal mass on routine (tuberculosis survey) chest film (Fig. 434). To the left of the border of the heart was a well circumscribed mass which, because of its increased radio-lucency, was thought to be a lipoma. At operation this structure was proved to be a thymoma (composed of lymphoid elements and also containing considerable amounts of lipoid) extending down from the left lobe of the thymus as a pannus over the external surface of the pericardium. The mass could be cleanly removed. The child is in excellent condition six months later, but obviously must be followed further before making any statements regarding the ultimate prognosis.

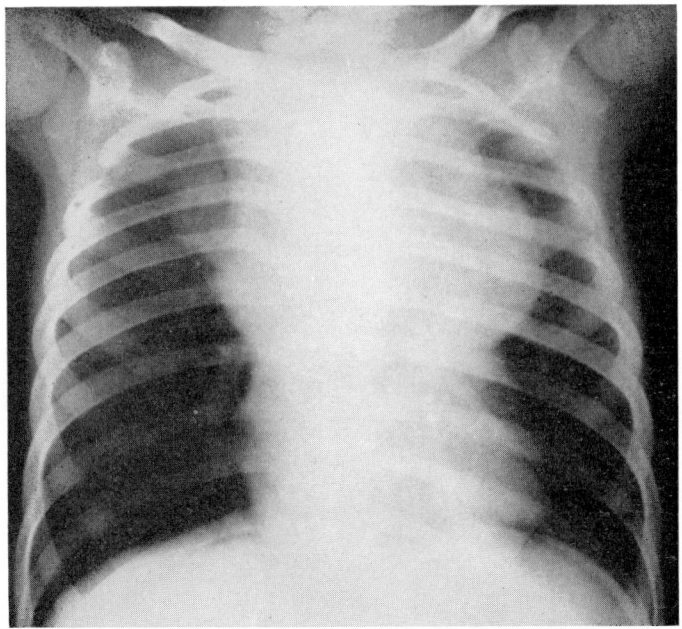

Fig. 433. Case 22. Roentgenogram of a five-year-old boy who had a malignant thymoma with compression of the trachea and superior vena cava. Rapid progression of neoplasm and death in spite of tracheotomy.

TERATOMA

Epidermoid cysts are structures with well defined capsule and with a lining of squamous epithelium which gives rise to soft or cheesy desquamated material within its cavity. *Dermoid cysts* are somewhat similar lesions but the lining has elements of the skin appendages, most striking of which is the formation of hair and sebaceous material which are accumulated within the cyst. *Teratomas*, while they may be largely filled by sebaceous substance, have elements from two or even three germ layers and therefore can contain any type of gross or histologic tissue. Teratomas may be solid but more often they are partially cystic and contain sebaceous material, hair, cartilage, or bone. Extensive examination of the wall or any solid portion will generally show elements which represent endoderm, mesoderm, and ectoderm. Frequently, what had first appeared to be a simple dermoid cyst on gross examination will prove, by extensive histologic investigation of representative parts of the specimen, to be a teratoma. Therefore, it is well to group all *epiaermoids* and *dermoids* in the class of *teratomas*.

Teratomas are most common in the superior and especially in the anterior mediastinum, though on rare occasions they can be found in the posterior part of the chest. In 1945 Laipply[11] collected 245 epidermoids, dermoids, and teratomas from the literature and added a dermoid of his own. Rusby[16] made an excellent summary of the pathology, clinical findings, and therapy in mediastinal dermoids and teratomas. There appears to be considerable justification for separating teratomas into malignant and benign groups because the former have invasive characteristics with a high chance of producing a fatality, whereas the latter (while they can assume a huge size) carry an excellent prognosis if they are completely enucleated.

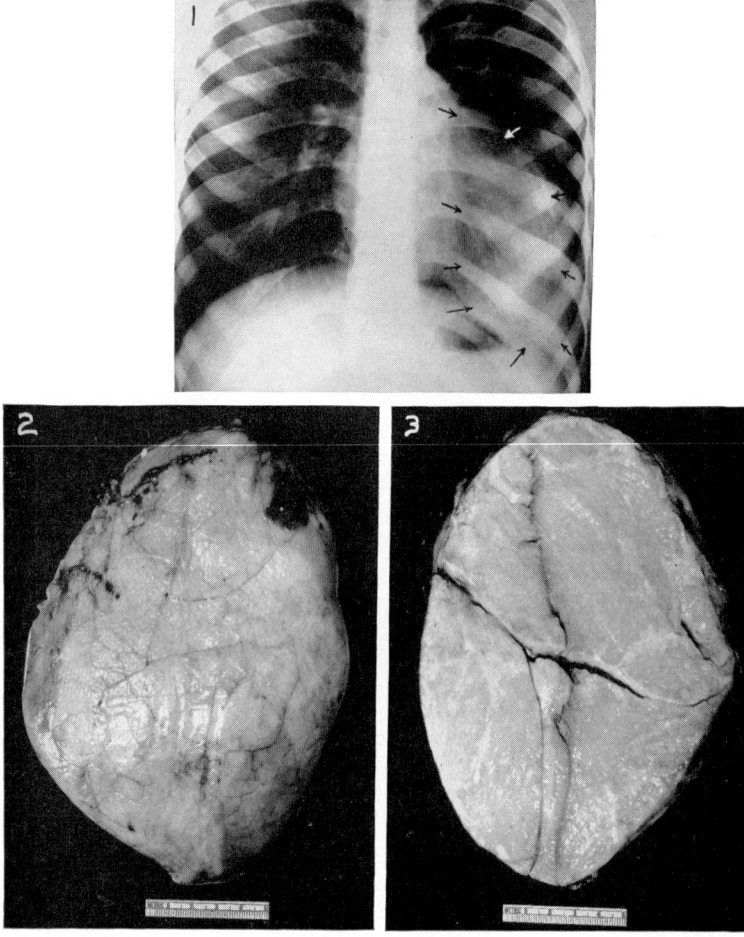

Fig. 434. Case 24. Fourteen-year-old boy with a thymoma extending over the left lateral surface of the pericardium. 1. Roentgenogram showing the tumor (which contained much fat) outlined by arrows. 2 and 3. Photographs of the specimen which weighed 490 gm. and measured 18.5 x 14 x 7.5 cm.

Malignant Teratomas

The two examples we have encountered were massive lesions extending out from the mediastinum and obliterating the pulmonary field on the left side. At exploration there was apparently extensive invasion into lung tissue. No clean plane of dissection could be made; only biopsy was performed. It is doubtful if the x-ray therapy given was of any great value; both these children died.

Benign Teratomas

These can attain great size (Fig. 436) and they produce their symptoms by compressing important anatomic structures within the confines of a rigid cage. They grow rather slowly and tend to produce symptoms over a long period of time. There can be increasing respiratory distress, dyspnea, failure to gain weight, or even loss of weight. As the tumors project out from the mediastinum, they are apt to give broadening of the mediastinal percussion note dullness and to cause diminution or absence of breath sounds at either side of the sternum. By roentgenographic examination, there is a dense structure within the anterior mediastinum, directly merging with other mediastinal

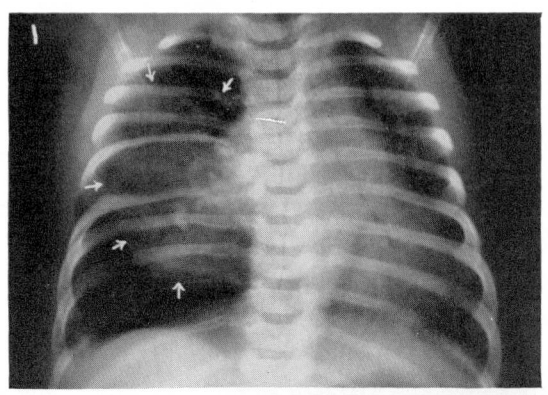

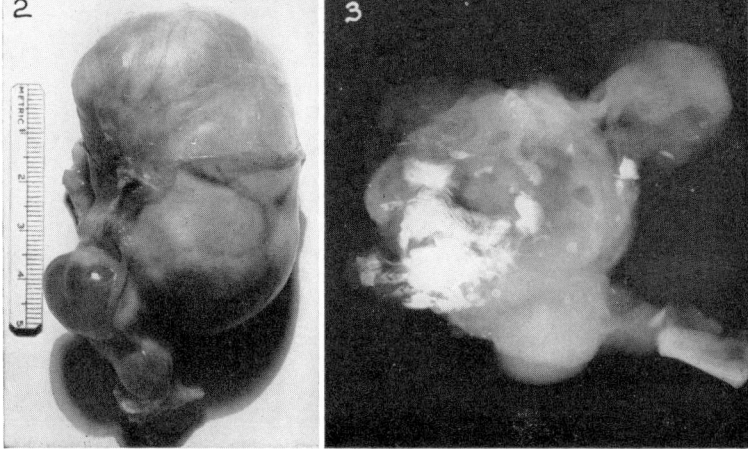

Fig. 435. Case 28. Two-month-old baby with mediastinal teratoma extending into right side of the chest. 1. Roentgenogram of teratoma of mediastinum extending out behind the right lung. Some calcification is seen in the mass. 2. Teratoma which was removed, measuring 7 x 5 x 4 cm. 3. Roentgenogram of the specimen showing the scattered calcification.

shadows, but generally having a well defined border on either side as the mass projects out against the lung. In some lesions there is scattered calcification representing abortive teeth or bones, which are conclusive evidence of the type of lesion which is being dealt with.

Treatment. The operative removal of a benign teratoma is not difficult. There is such a well defined capsule around the tumor that it is possible to approach it through either pleural cavity, to open the overlying parietal pleura, and to find a good plane of cleavage around which the dissection can be carried, generally having to extend this across the entire mediastinum and at times even into the opposite side of the chest. It is possible to follow the cleavage planes even in a small thorax and to remove the mass entirely. When this is done, the lungs can be immediately expanded to their full extent and the child's respiratory apparatus returned immediately to normal.

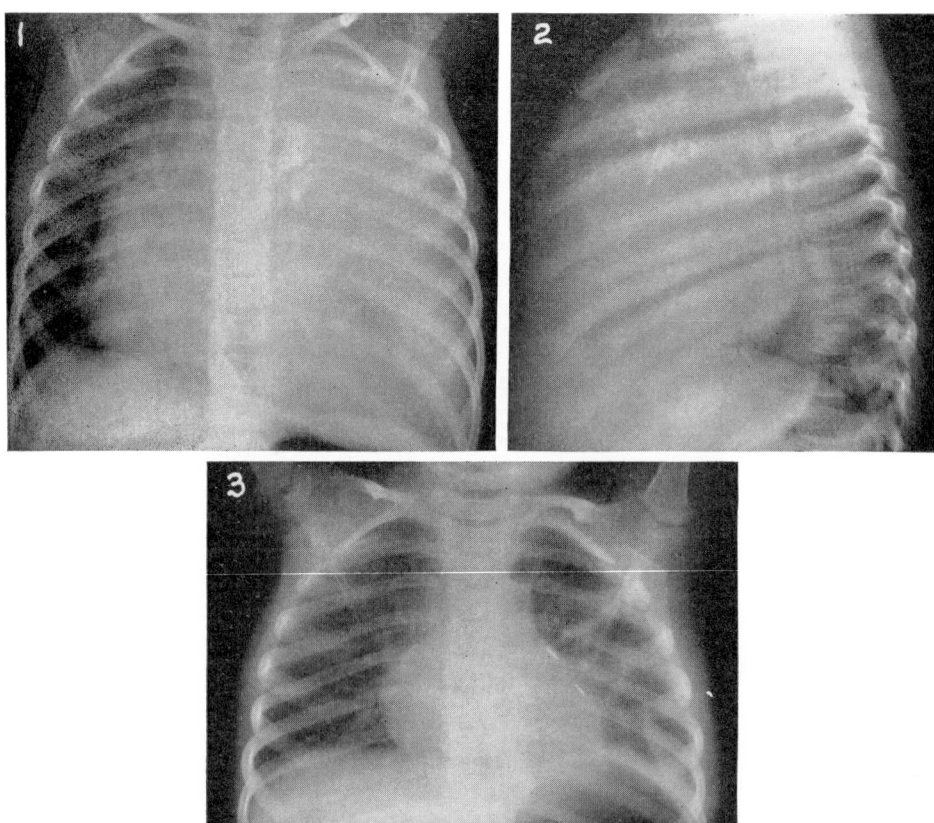

Fig. 436. Case 29. Nineteen-month-old child with a benign teratoma of the anterior mediastinum 1 and 2. Roentgenograms of the mediastinal mass which projected to both sides, particularly toward patient's left. Calcification can be seen in the tumor. 3. Roentgenogram of chest following surgical removal of the teratoma.

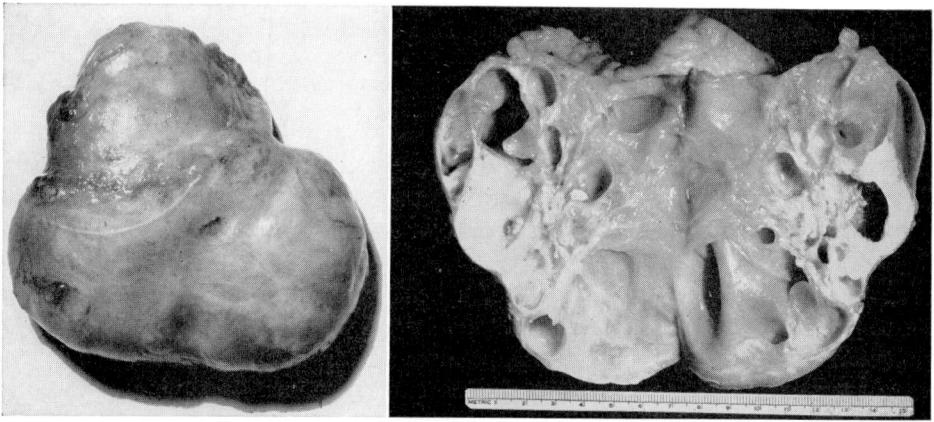

Fig. 437. Case 29. Teratoma removed from the anterior mediastinum of nineteen-month-old child. *Left*, External view. It measured 14 x 12.5 x 5.5 cm. *Right*, Teratoma cut open.

Results of Therapy. The clean removal of a mediastinal teratoma carries a very satisfactory outlook. Our three patients were twenty-one, two, and nineteen months of age respectively at the time of their operations. They have been followed eight, eleven, and nine years since their treatment and none has shown any evidence of recurrence.

OSTEOCHONDROMA

The complexity of the development of the thoracic cage gives rise to the possibility of displacement of bony or cartilaginous tissue which can lead to the development of neoplasms. These can be relatively benign but they have been known to reach huge size. Even though they tend to remain encapsulated, they can replace normal portions of the bony thorax, and can make large masses projecting out from or into the chest. The

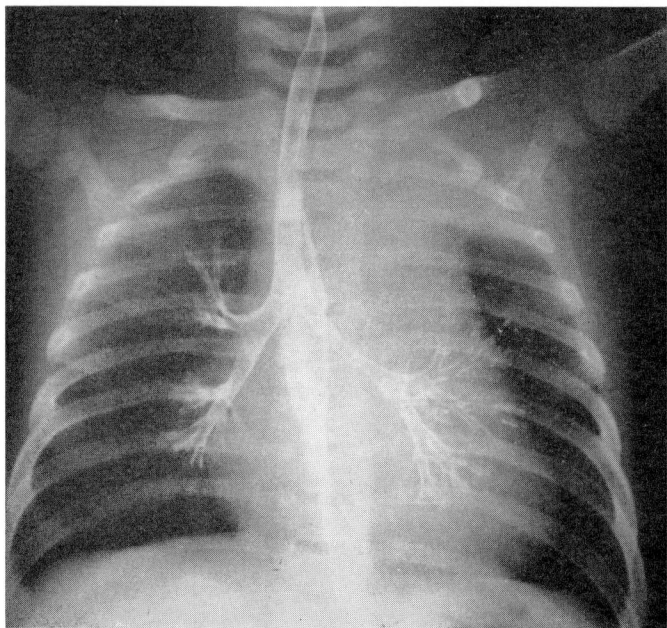

Fig. 438. Case 31. Hemangioma of the left apical region which was treated by biopsy and x-ray irradiation. There was subsequent complete disappearance of the mass.

smaller lesions tend to be well circumscribed and they should be attacked radically, removing them in their entirety, even though this implies that a large hole is left in the bony framework. Such destructive procedure can be followed at a later time by some appropriate reconstruction, by covering the area with tantalum mesh, flaps of muscle, or bony bridges which are made by swinging other ribs into the region. Our one experience with this type of growth was in a three-day-old baby who had an enormous mass which projected into and completely filled the right pleural cavity, even though it still retained a smooth parietal pleura over it. There was a dumbbell-shaped extension externally into the right axilla. The child entered the hospital *in extremis* and died shortly thereafter.

HEMANGIOMA

Hemangiomas can appear in either pleural cavity and are generally associated with angiomas within the abdomen. We have had two examples of such a combination wherein the growth was more extensive in the abdominal cavity. One of these, because of extensive bleeding from time to time, was followed by fatality. The other has apparently been brought under control by x-ray therapy over the abdomen and the thorax. It is possible to have an angioma primarily or solely within the chest (Fig. 438); the problems of therapy are quite similar to those of treatment of angiomas elsewhere in the body. Because of the difficulty, or the impossibility, of recognition of a hemangioma of the thorax without biopsy, operation should be performed in all cases at least to remove a portion of the tumor for histologic examination. When hemangioma is found by frozen section examination, and when the mass is of such a nature that it can be removed, excision should be proceeded with. However, it is acceptable therapy, once the diagnosis is established, to leave the mass and treat it by x-ray irradiation.

Our single patient with a primary hemangioma of the thorax was a three-month-old baby with a mass at the left apex of the chest, which was proved by biopsy. The baby has been treated by x-ray therapy and is apparently completely well one year later.

BRONCHOGENIC CYST

In the development of the lung bud from the foregut, portions of tissue can become sequestrated and give rise to cysts, which are recognizable by the fact that they form and retain mucoid material, that their lining is a ciliated columnar epithelium, and that their walls contain cartilage and smooth muscle. These bronchogenic cysts are of ectodermal and mesodermal origin. They are always in proximity to the lower part of the trachea or the main bronchi and generally lie behind them. Occasionally they may have a communication with the respiratory passages, but generally they do not. Reviews of the literature on bronchogenic cyst of the mediastinum reveal that about 90 cases have been reported, all but 4 or 5 of them being in adults. Meier[13] gives an excellent summary of his 8 patients who were treated by removal of bronchogenic cysts.

Our one experience with this lesion was in a six-month-old boy who for several months was noted to have harsh breathing, occasional fever, and by x-ray investigation was shown to have the lesion indicated in Figure 439. Through a right transpleural approach there was no difficulty in reaching the cyst, exposing it, and dissecting it away from the back of the trachea and bronchi. The child is in excellent health three years later with no evidence of recurrence.

NEURENTERIC CYST

In the early development of the embryo, tissues of the neurenteric canal can be displaced and give rise to structures which are subsequently found to have tissues representing both the nervous and alimentary systems. They are very apt to be associated with abnormalities of the vertebral bodies, and possibly a communication from the dural sheath to the cystic mass which lies in front of the spine. These lesions are extremely rare.

We have encountered but one example of this abnormality. The patient had multiple deformities of the upper thoracic spine and a communication from the spinal canal into a large cyst which lay in the upper part of the posterior mediastinum. As an initial procedure, a posterior approach was made through the spinal canal, attempting to close off the orifice in the dural sheath (we now doubt if this step accomplished much). At a second operation, a transpleural approach was made to the lemon-sized mass which lay behind the esophagus; this could be circumvented and removed in its entirety. We assumed that we were dealing with an anterior meningocele until histologic examination of the wall of the structure showed that it contained neural elements and also tissues representing portions of the gastro-intestinal tract.

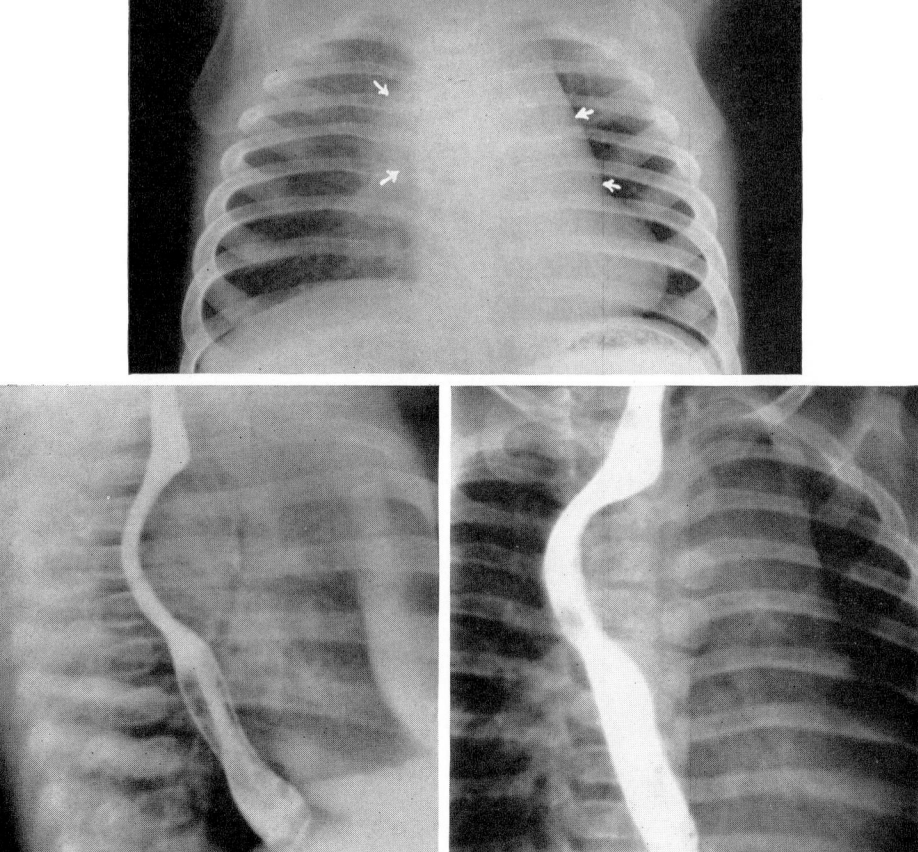

Fig. 439. Case 32. Six-month-old child who had a bronchogenic cyst of the mediastinum. This cyst lay behind the carina and in front of the esophagus. The esophagus was pushed to the patient's right. Surgical removal followed by cure.

DUPLICATIONS OF THE ALIMENTARY TRACT

There have been many excellent presentations regarding "gastrogenous cysts," "cysts of gastric origin," "gastric cysts of the esophagus," etc. All of these have possessed the characteristics of having a wall which is composed of one or several coats of smooth muscle, a lining which is similar to that of the stomach or some portion of the alimentary tube, and a position in contiguity to the esophagus. We prefer to call all of them *duplications*. Some of the lesions have been tubular, but more commonly they are round, cystic affairs. Most have no communication with the esophagus or alimentary tract but occasional ones do possess such an opening. The 16 examples of duplications of the alimentary tract we have encountered in the thorax need not be summarized here, since all of this material is presented as a portion of Chapter 17.

Table 79

Results of Therapy for Various Thoracic Cysts and Primary Tumors

Case	Sex Age	Year Initials	Treatment	Result
NEUROBLASTOMA				
1	F 10 mos.	1936 S. H.	Only biopsy!	1945 No mass in chest. Living and well.
2	M 4 yrs.	1937 E. P.	Removal (incomplete).	Died 12 hrs. later.
3	M 9 yrs.	1941 R. M.	Known metastases at time. Biopsy. X-ray Rx.	Died 6 mos. later.
4	M 6 yrs.	1946 W. C.	Known metastases at time. Biopsy.	Died 3 mos. later.
5	F 7 yrs.	1947 D. Y.	Removal (incomplete). X-ray Rx. Tumor chemotherapy.	Died with metastases Sept. 1949.
6	F 11 mos.	1949 D. C.	Transpinal and transthoracic removal of dumbbell tumor. X-ray Rx.	1952 Living without evidence of tumor but with slight neurologic weakness.
7	M 2 yrs.	1949 G. B.	Known metastases at time. Removal (incomplete). X-ray Rx. Tumor chemotherapy.	Died 5 mos. later.
8	F 1 yr.	1950 M. R.	Preop. x-ray Rx. Removal (incomplete). Postop. x-ray therapy.	Excellent condition 2 yrs. later. No evidence of tumor.
9	F 8 mos.	1950 C. M.	Preop. x-ray Rx. Removal (complete). Postop. x-ray therapy. Tumor chemotherapy.	Excellent condition 2½ yrs. later. No evidence of tumor.
10	F 20 mos.	1951 V. T.	Extending through into abdomen. Biopsy. Tumor chemotherapy.	6 mos. later still has extensive tumor.
NEUROBLASTOMA, with some areas of Ganglioneuroma				
11	M 3 mos.	1949 F. C.	Removal (incomplete). X-ray therapy.	Well 3 yrs. later.
12	F 10 yrs.	1949 J. H.	Removal (incomplete). X-ray Rx. Tumor chemotherapy.	Well 3 yrs. later.
13	F 2 yrs.	1950 J. A.	Removal. X-ray Rx. Tumor chemotherapy.	Well 2 yrs. later.
GANGLIONEUROMA				
14	F 6 yrs.	1935 D. W.	Removal (incomplete).	Well 2 yrs. later, but some tumor obviously remaining.
15	M 6 yrs.	1952 T. M.	Removal (complete).	Well 6 mos. later.
PLEXIFORM NEUROMA				
16	M 9 yrs.	1933 R. M.	Removal (partial).	13 yrs. later living, without complaints, but some mass still in chest.
CYSTIC HYGROMA				
17	M 3 yrs.	1944 F. S.	Removal.	4 yrs. later completely well.
18	F 14 mos.	1945 E. F.	Removal from neck and thorax.	7 yrs. later, completely well.

Table 79 (continued)

Case	Sex Age	Year Initials	Treatment	Result
CYSTIC HYGROMA *continued*				
19	F 7 mos.	1946 S. M.	Removal from neck and thorax.	6 yrs. later, excision of recurrent neck mass. Thorax normal.
20	F 4 mos.	1946 S. M.	Removal from between rt. upper and middle lobes. Fistula and lung damage later required pneumonectomy.	Well one year later.
21	M 5 yrs.	1952 J. A.	Removal.	6 mos. later, completely well.
MALIGNANT THYMOMA				
22	M 5 yrs.	1940 R. M.	Tracheotomy for respiratory obstruction.	Died next day.
23	M 7 yrs.	1947 R. B.	Tracheotomy for respiratory obstruction.	Died during op.
THYMOMA				
24	M 14 yrs.	1952 B. C.	Removal.	6 mos. later, no evidence of recurrence.
MALIGNANT TERATOMA				
25	F 2 yrs.	1932 D. E.	Post-mediastinal mass had invaded left lung. Biopsy. X-ray Rx.	No follow-up.
26	F 7 yrs.	1945 A. B. T.	Biopsy. X-ray Rx.	Died 4 yrs. later.
BENIGN TERATOMA				
27	M 21 mos.	1933 N. P.	Removal.	1941 Living and well.
28	F 2 mos.	1938 J. A.	Removal.	1949 Living and well.
29	F 19 mos.	1943 J. A.	Removal.	1952 Living and well.
OSTEOCHONDROMA				
30	F 3 days	1942 M. K.	Mass filled rt. chest. In extremis. No op.	Died.
HEMANGIOMA				
31	M 3 mos.	1951 F. C.	Biopsy. X-ray Rx.	Well one year later. Mass disappeared.
BRONCHOGENIC CYST				
32	M 6 mos.	1949 S. H.	Removal.	Well 3 yrs. later.
NEURENTERIC CYST				
33	M 4 yrs.	1952 P. M.	Removal.	6 mos. later, excellent condition.

DUPLICATIONS OF ALIMENTARY TRACT

16 cases, described in Chapter 17.

REFERENCES

1. Allbritten, F. F. and Templeton, J. Y.: Treatment of Giant Cysts of the Lung. J. Thor. Surg., *20*:749, 1950.

2. Bradford, M. L., Mahon, H. W. and Grow, J. B.: Mediastinal Cysts and Tumors. Surg., Gynec. & Obst., *85*:467, 1947.

3. Dugan, D. J. and Sampson, P. C.: The Surgical Treatment of Giant Emphysematous Blebs and Pulmonary Tension Cysts. J. Thor. Surg., *20*:729, 1950.

4. Gross, R. E. and Hurwitt, E. S.: Cervicomediastinal and Mediastinal Cystic Hygromas. Surg., Gynec. & Obst., *87*:599, 1948.

5. Hardy, L. M.: Bronchogenic Cysts of the Mediastinum. Pediat., *4*:108, 1949.

6. Harrington, S. W.: Surgical Treatment in Eleven Cases of Mediastinal and Intrathoracic Teratomas. J. Thor. Surg., *3*:50, 1933.

7. Heuer, G. J.: Thoracic Tumors. Arch. Surg., *18*:271, 1929.

8. Heuer, G. J. and Andrus, W. D.: The Surgery of Mediastinal Tumors. Am. J. Surg., *50*: 146, 1940.

9. Jones, J. C. and Effler, D. B.: Management of Intrathoracic Nerve Tumors in Young Children. Report of Four Cases. Pediat., *4*:342, 1949.

10. Kent, E. M., Blades, B., Valle, A. R. and Graham, E. A.: Intrathoracic Neurogenic Tumors. J. Thoracic Surg., *13*:116, 1944.

11. Laipply, T. C.: Cysts and Cystic Tumors of the Mediastinum. Arch. Path., *39*:153, 1945.

12. Lillie, W. I., McDonald, J. R. and Clagett, O. T.: Pericardial Celomic Cysts and Pericardial Diverticula. J. Thor. Surg., *20*:494, 1950.

13. Maier, H. C.: Bronchogenic Cysts of the Mediastinum. Ann. Surg., *127*:476, 1948.

14. Neale, A. E. and Menten, M. L.: Tumors of the Thymus in Children. Am. J. Dis. Child., *76*:102, 1948.

15. Ravitch, M. M. and Hardy, J. B.: Congenital Cystic Disease of the Lung in Infants and Children. Arch. Surg., *59*:1, 1949.

16. Rusby, N. L.: Dermoid Cysts and Teratomata of the Mediastinum. J. Thor. Surg., *13*:169, 1944.

17. Seybold, W. D., McDonald, J. R., Clagett, O. T. and Good, C. A.: Tumors of the Thymus. J. Thor. Surg., *20*:195, 1950.

18. Skinner, G. F. and Hobbs, M. E.: Intrathoracic Cystic Lymphangioma. J. Thor. Surg., *6*:98, 1936.

19. Sophian, L.: Mediastinal Ganglioneuroma. Ann. Surg., *101*:827, 1935.

20. Strode, J. E.: Cystic Disease of the Lung. J. Thor. Surg., *18*:404, 1949.

CHAPTER 59

Bronchiectasis

Pulmonary infection in childhood which requires surgical therapy or excision has undergone tremendous change in the last two decades; the types of lesions the surgeon was called upon to treat fifteen or twenty years ago were far different from those which he sees now. Formerly, the average case was one of "chronic pulmonary suppuration," with a lung riddled by acute and chronic inflammatory disease, its architecture largely destroyed, its substance filled with exudate; empyema or pyopneumothorax accompanied it with great frequency, and constitutional debilitation was usually marked. These children had extensive, stinking, necrotizing, pulmonary disease, which occasionally showed periods of temporary improvement, but which carried very high fatality rates regardless of the type of therapy which was instituted. Our medical students and house officers of today never see this picture. Now, "bronchiectasis" is the main suppurative process which comes to our attention; it is a relatively benign condition in its extent, in its ravages, and in its outlook, compared to the pulmonary lesions of bygone years. This tremendous change in surgical material has been brought about by improved living standards of our population and by the enormous influence of the widespread use of chemotherapy and antibiotics in aborting or combating infectious conditions. Without doubt, the techniques of surgical removal of pulmonary tissue have been greatly improved in the hands of all who have worked in the field, but the reduction in mortality figures and the virtual elimination of postoperative complications after removal of a lobe or lung should not be ascribed wholly to improved surgery; the type of material is vastly different from what it was in former years. These factors must constantly be kept in mind and no odious comparison should be made between the surgical statistics listed by pioneers in the 1930's and the figures which today are well-nigh perfect in so many medical centers.

There is little point in describing or discussing the "chronic pulmonary suppuration" which used to plague us, and which has now practically vanished. The following remarks all pertain to "bronchiectasis" as it is encountered today.

PATHOLOGIC AND ETIOLOGIC CONSIDERATIONS

Concepts of the Disease

The term "bronchiectasis" merely calls attention to one part of a destructive process which, after a variable period of time, causes tubular or saccular dilatation of the bronchial or bronchiolar lumen. Attention has been focused on this part of the picture because it can be visualized so well by roentgenographic means after instillation of radio-opaque material into the affected part. Actually, the mere enlargement of the lumen is probably the part which should concern us least. From the point of view of the patient's health, the processes which are most important are the extent and intensity of the inflammatory reaction in pulmonary tissues *around the bronchioles* and the prolificacy of the exudative process *within the bronchiolar pathways*. It is true that the three processes (formation of exudate within a lumen, dilatation of the bronchioles, and inflammation in surrounding lung tissue) can advance simultaneously, but they do not necessarily do so. Luminal suppuration can be marked and tissue reaction minimal, or conversely the bronchial exudate can be slight while the pulmonary tissue disease is

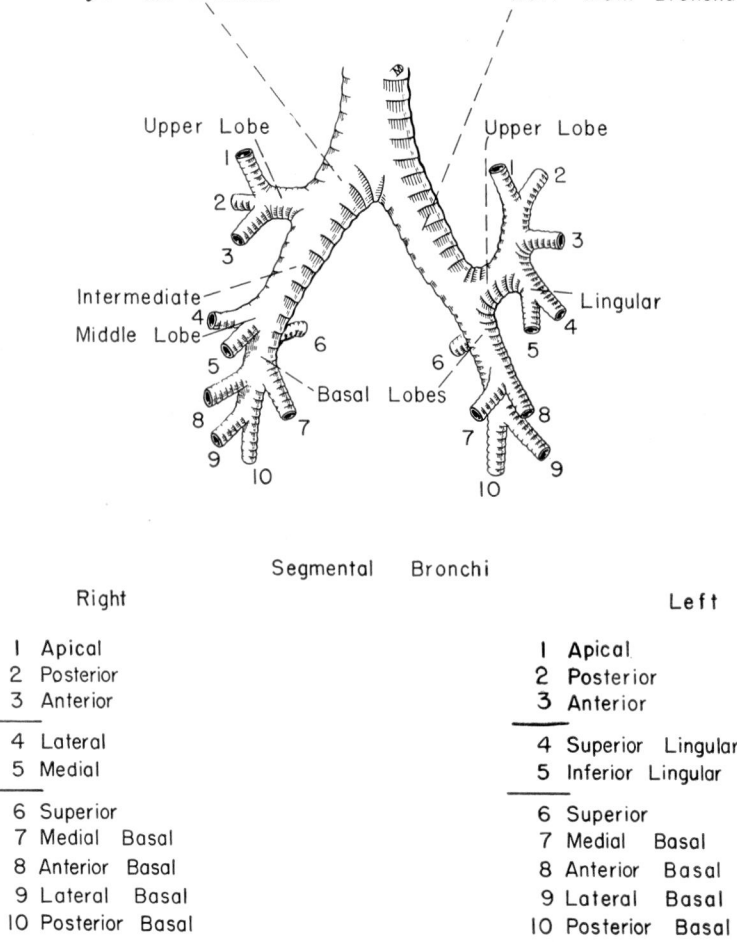

Fig. 440. Anatomy of the bronchial tree.

Segmental   Bronchi

Right

1	Apical
2	Posterior
3	Anterior
4	Lateral
5	Medial
6	Superior
7	Medial Basal
8	Anterior Basal
9	Lateral Basal
10	Posterior Basal

Left

1	Apical
2	Posterior
3	Anterior
4	Superior Lingular
5	Inferior Lingular
6	Superior
7	Medial Basal
8	Anterior Basal
9	Lateral Basal
10	Posterior Basal

extensive. It is possible to have great bronchiolar dilatation (which of course will persist) and yet reach a stage where there is little or no exudate in the bronchial tree and practically no consolidation of the pulmonary substance, but this is quite rare; the region is apt to be the seat of recurring inflammation.

Etiologic Background

In any series of children with bronchiectasis there are etiologic factors, some of which are quite obvious, others being very obscure. For our material, figures are listed in Table 80.

1. Foremost is that group in which there was a bronchopneumonia which did not resolve promptly, the lobe or segment of lung remaining collapsed, the poorly aerated

tissue becoming a nidus for invasion by secondary bacteria. Sometimes it is quite difficult to be sure whether the pneumonia and atelectasis have come in a lung which was previously entirely normal or whether these conditions represent complications after a minor bronchiectatic disease which was present previously but was unrecognized.

2. There is certainly a group of patients who from the etiologic point of view seem to have an important allergy. This is generally manifested by a chronic infection of the paranasal sinuses with continuous accumulation of muco-purulent exudate in the pharynx, some bits of which almost certainly get into the tracheo-bronchial tree and set up a disease process in the lung.

3. Clearly defined is that group in which aspiration of some foreign material has been the important etiologic factor. (While removal of a foreign body is generally followed by satisfactory healing in the lung, in a few instances the pulmonary disease continues to advance thereafter.)

4. Well recognized are those cases in which congenital abnormalities of the bronchial pathway have played an etiologic role. These include bronchial stenosis, deficiency of cartilage which allows the bronchus to collapse during the respiratory cycle, malformations which are called cystic disease, and finally those poorly understood conditions in which the bronchial epithelium produces a mucus which is extremely viscid (muco-viscidosis).

5. Finally, there is a residuum in which no clear-cut etiologic factor can be recognized by any method of study.

Table 80

Etiologic Factors in Development of Bronchiectasis

	No. of Cases
1. Unresolved Pneumonia and Atelectasis	27
2. Allergy or Chronic Sinusitis	18
3. Foreign Body	12
Timothy hay 4	
Post-tonsillectomy 3	
Aspiration of vomitus 2	
Peanut 1	
Tooth 1	
Nondescript 1	
4. Abnormalities of Bronchial Tree	8
Bronchial stenosis, or lack of cartilage 3	
Congenital cystic disease 4	
Anomaly of mucus (mucoviscidosis) 1	
5. Etiology Unknown	7

Bronchiectasis of Adults

Perry and King[28] reviewed 400 cases of bronchiectasis, largely concerned with adult material; their findings indicated that in 69 per cent of the series, bronchiectasis occurred before the twentieth year of life, and in 42 per cent it started before the tenth year. Their investigations emphasized the fact, also expressed by others, that bronchiectasis in adults commonly has had its origin as a childhood illness.

Reversibility

Without doubt, bronchiectatic inflammation, even in its most extensive form, can be influenced in the direction of either healing or recrudescence by certain factors. A good nutritional and economic background, and use of potent antibiotics, can do much toward improvement of the inflammatory picture. Conversely, poor nutrition, low vitamin intake, poor housing, and lack of medical care all tend to make the disease flare up and run a protracted advancing course.

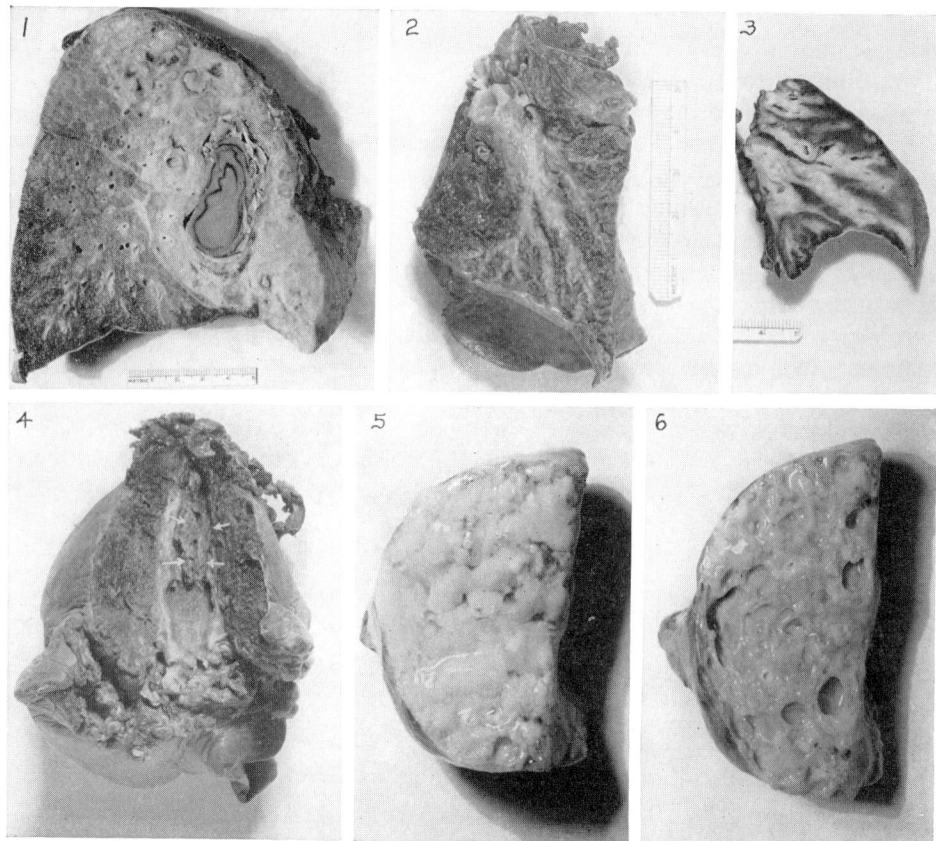

Fig. 441. Surgical specimens; pulmonary resection for bronchiectasis. 1. Right pneumonectomy, from an eight-year-old boy. Extensive bronchiectasis, peri-bronchial disease and fibrosis, particularly in upper-anterior two-thirds of lung. Note the large cavity, filled with a laminated plug of necrotic material. Possibly the lower lobe could have been spared? 2. Left upper lobectomy, from a nine-year-old boy. Thickening and reaction along bronchiolar tree. 3. Left lower lobectomy, from a seven-year-old girl. Marked bronchiectasis and peribronchial disease. 4. Right lower lobectomy, from a six-year-old girl. Marked dilatation of main lobe bronchus, which contains a tuft of timothy hay (arrows). 5. Left lower lobectomy, from a fifteen-month-old girl. Massive amounts of purulent exudate flow from the cut surface. 6. Same specimen as 5, after exudate has been allowed to run out, showing advanced bronchiectasis and destruction of pulmonary tissue.

Tendency toward Recurrence

Pathologic progression of bronchiectatic disease has certain relentless features. Even if bacterial invasion is largely overcome (by natural resistance or by use of antibiotics) there always remains some degree of scarring of lung parenchyma, some disruption of bronchiolar elastica, some dissolution of cartilage, and some permanent damage of the lining membrane; the mucosa is replaced by fibrous tissue or altered membrane which lacks the cleansing mechanism provided by a normal ciliated epithelium. The entire region has a lessened resistance to bacterial invasion; subsequent insults are very apt to extend further than the previous ones.

Tendency toward Spreading

The pathologic lesions of bronchiectasis have been frequently defined as more or less localized processes involving one or more lobes, but having a rather static quality. It is important to emphasize that the disease not infrequently has a dynamic quality and shows a marked tendency to become more severe or to extend to other portions of the same (or opposite) lung in spite of all therapeutic measures which are directed against it. This progressive feature is often seen in patients who have had no surgery, and at times it is all too evident in those for whom pulmonary resection has been performed. Of the cases that we have accepted for surgical ablation, nearly 20 per cent have subsequently shown, when followed over a period of many years, that bronchiectasis appeared in other parts of the lung (which were thought to be normal at the time of operation), or else minimal disease which was known to exist elsewhere has progressed in spite of all therapeutic attempts to abort it by modern medical management. In some of these patients, it is not difficult to understand why the condition involves new areas: (1) There may be a persisting purulent paranasal sinusitis which defies all efforts of medical and surgical therapy and continues to give pollution of the bronchial tree. (2) In spite of the fact that a considerable portion of diseased lung substance has been removed, residual inflammation which has been left near the base of such a lobe can extend to nearby bronchi and give cicatricial bronchial stenosis or bronchial compression, interfering with aeration and drainage of that adjacent lobe or segment. (3) Residual exudate can enter and block off neighboring passages, give rise to new areas of atelectasis, and thereby provide opportunity for development of additional bronchiectatic lesions. In any of these ways, virginal segments can become involved secondarily, and pulmonary disease can become so extensive that severe crippling or fatality ultimately results from diminution in the respiratory reserve.

CLINICAL PICTURE

Chronicity

Bronchiectasis rises slowly out of the smoldering ashes of some previous pulmonary insult or a long-continued pulmonary inflammation. Many months or indeed years may pass before the lung infection outwardly sickens the child or gives impressive enough symptoms to start an investigation. Whenever bronchiectasis is discovered, it is rather characteristic to find that a careful review of the history indicates that the lesion has been present for many years.

History in Relation to Etiology

Queries regarding the development of allergy, the occurrence of paranasal sinusitis, or the possibility of foreign body aspiration must be made when attempting to determine the etiologic background in any case. A family history is of importance in detecting Kartagener's syndrome (triad of chronic sinusitis, situs inversus, and bronchiectasis) or variants of this familial disease.

The detection of *mucoviscidosis* (pancreatic fibrosis) as a probable cause of bronchiectasis should not be overlooked, because with such a background it is almost always advisable to avoid surgical resection of bronchiectatic tissue; the disease will almost certainly extend postoperatively and involve other portions of the lungs. History of alimentary tract disturbances, a picture suggesting celiac disease, cough from early infancy, are all suggestive of this condition. Whenever this possibility presents itself, the pancreatic enzymes should be studied by duodenal intubation.

Cardinal Symptoms

Eventually, classic signs of broncho-pulmonary inflammation occur in all cases. *Bronchial irritation* is manifested by cough, wheezing, and productive sputum which may be frothy, purulent, or even blood-tinged. *Bronchial or peri-bronchial inflammation* is indicated by intermittent fever, coughing, general debility, weight loss, or failure to gain. *Peri-bronchial fibrosis* and replacement of pulmonary tissue is shown by dyspnea, exertional cyanosis, and possibly clubbing of the nails, but these appear only in the more severe and extensive cases. In some instances tuberculosis has been assumed to be present, and it is only after repeated negative bacteriologic data and the emerging picture of bronchiectatic disease that there is a change from the original opinion.

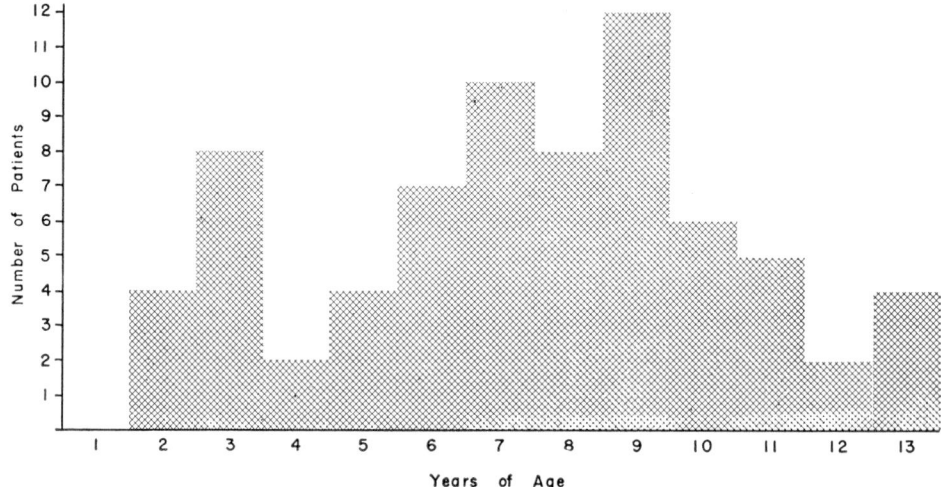

Fig. 442. Chart showing ages of patients at time they were subjected to resection of pulmonary substance.

Main Physical Findings

Except for cough and expectoration of sputum, examination of the patient often is remarkable only for the paucity of physical findings. The child's nutritional status might be excellent, but in the more advanced cases evidence of chronic debilitating disease is the rule. If the involved portion of lobe or lung is large enough, evidence of consolidation is elicited; generally, sticky rales can be heard. The absence of rales and productive cough does not necessarily mean that the bronchial passages are free of exudate; x-ray examination or bronchoscopy will sometimes show a considerable amount of material which has become pooled and sequestrated in a plugged-off bronchus. The pharynx, the nasal passages, and the paranasal sinuses should be thoroughly examined by appropriate means to detect any chronic infection which might exist there. In an occasional individual, detection of situs inversus, congenital heart disease, or evidence of pancreatic fibrosis (of which mucoviscidosis of the bronchial system is a part) is important in an evaluation.

Course

It is characteristic of bronchiectasis to undergo waves of improvement or recrudescence of infection, the process extending over exceedingly long periods of time. Inflam-

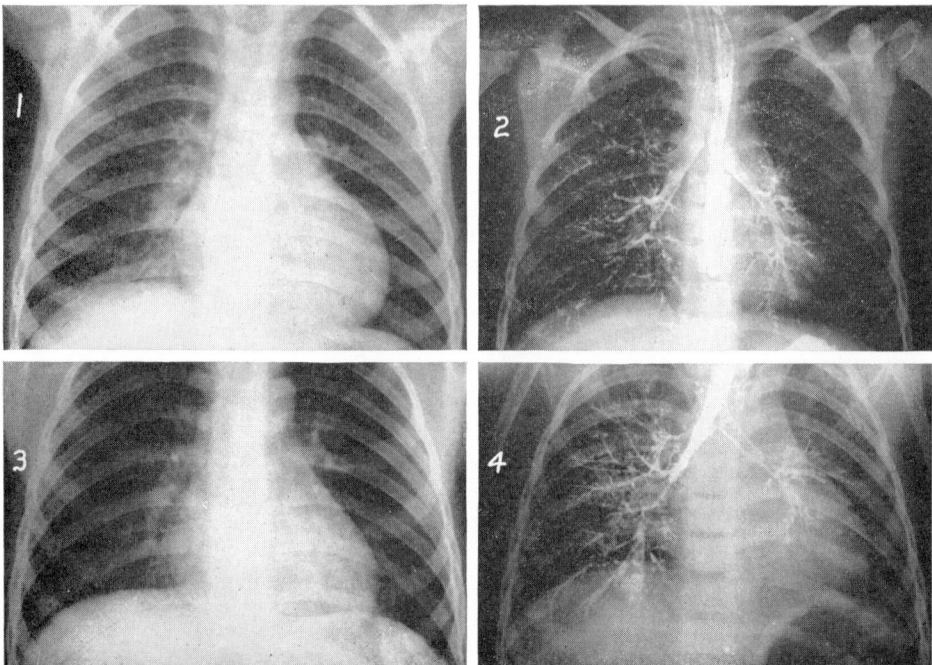

Fig. 443. 1. Plain film showing slight streaking at right base. 2. Bronchogram on same date showing no important abnormality in the bronchial structure. 3. Plain film, two months later, apparently indicating some clearing in the lung reaction. 4. Bronchogram on same date as 3, showing that there has actually been a definite advance in development of bronchiectasis.

mation can subside or the passages can be cleared by coughing up purulent material. The removal of such debris gives better aeration of the region and promotes healing within the lung tissue itself. In an unheralded way, the process can be lighted up by the accumulation of exudate which blocks a bronchus, produces regional atelectasis, and favors spread of bronchopneumonia in an area, segment, or lobe. The waning and waxing of pulmonary inflammation is generally reflected in improvement or setback in

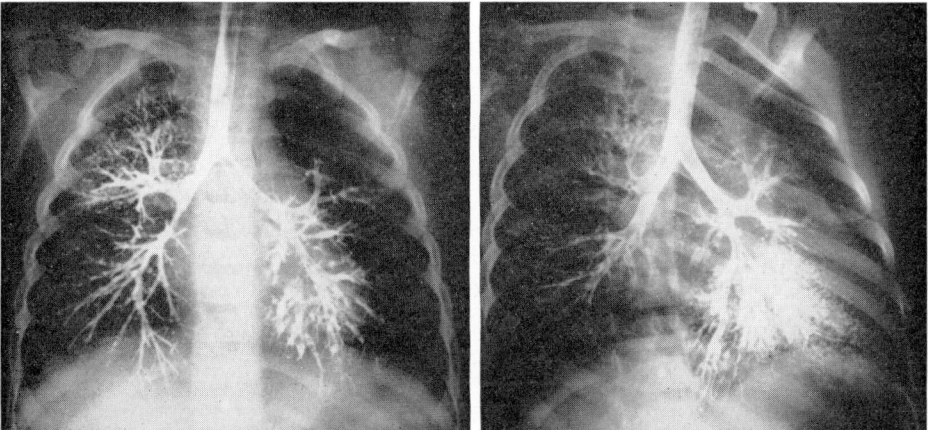

Fig. 444. *Left*, Bronchiectasis in left lower lobe. *Right*, Eight months later, following intensive medical treatment including continuous terramycin. Marked improvement in the clinical picture; some improvement in the roentgenographic findings.

the patient's general state of health. These waves can, of course, be influenced considerably by the medical management which is given.

DIAGNOSTIC STUDIES

If the history of the illness, with or without corroboration by physical findings, is suggestive of bronchiectasis, a detailed study of the child's bronchial tree should be made. Plain postero-anterior and lateral roentgenograms of the chest are, in a majority of cases, of help in showing peri-bronchial infiltration, segmental or patchy atelectasis,

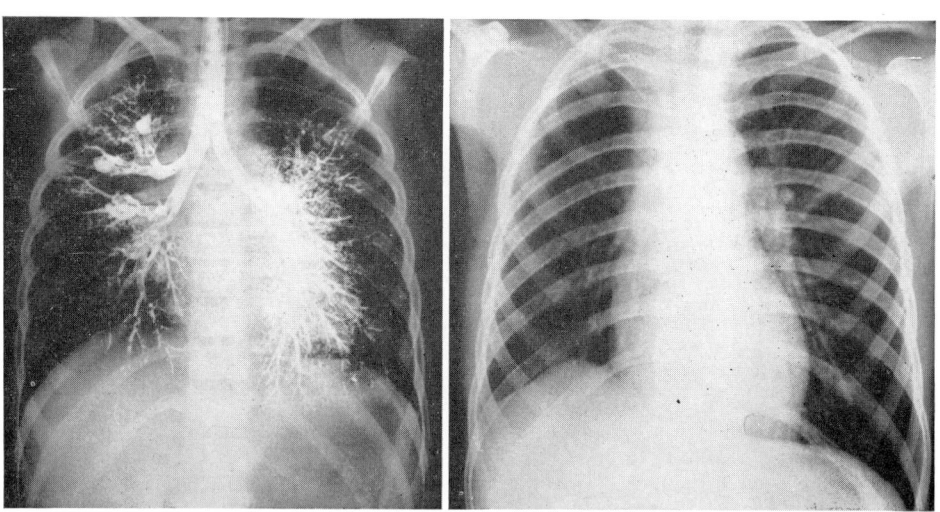

Fig. 445. *Left*, Ten-year-old girl with bronchiectasis in right upper and middle lobes. Symptoms for four years. Treated by removal of right upper and middle lobes. *Right*, Film two years after operation, showing that the lower lobe has filled the pleural space remarkably well.

pleural involvement, et cetera. While in former years empyema and complete lobar solidification were common findings, these are now seen with but great rarity. Even if plain roentgenograms show only minimal findings suggestive of a patch of consolidation or atelectasis which persists for a period of more than a few weeks, it is generally advisable to undertake bronchoscopic and bronchographic studies. Certainly, such investigation should always be performed when there has been long febrile illness or a persisting, productive cough. Such examinations in childhood should always be done under general anesthesia. By bronchoscopic means, one seeks to determine whether there is any foreign body, congenital abnormality of the bronchus, or inflammatory bronchial stenosis. Furthermore, it is possible to see accurately what part of a lung is involved, the nature and the amount of exudate, and possibly to secure some of this material for bacteriologic identification. Instillation of Lipiodol permits visualization of the bronchial tree on x-ray films. Bronchoscopy is not only investigative in nature, but clearing of the passages of exudate promotes better aeration and is a step in the therapeutic management.

TREATMENT

In the vast majority of childhood cases, the treatment of bronchiectasis is now being placed upon a rather satisfactory basis and has reached the point at which the disease should seldom be a crippling one and should rarely lead to fatality. These advances through the years have come about through a combination of factors: (1) Improvement in nutritional and living standards have markedly accelerated with the rise in the economic status of the population. (2) An awareness of bronchiectasis as a disease process now generally leads to earlier detection and institution of appropriate therapy. (3) Antibiotics have had a tremendous abortive or therapeutic effect in most cases. (4) Improved anesthesia has helped to lower the mortality rates of operation. (5) Refinements of surgical techniques as developed by Churchill, Graham, Blades, Overholt, and many others who have been active in this field, have reduced the risks of surgery and the incidence of postoperative complications.

From the outset, it must be realized that bronchiectasis is not necessarily a "surgical" disease. There are a large number of patients with minimal involvement who can be handled completely on a medical regimen. Even in the moderately advanced forms, medical therapy has much to offer by clearing somewhat the local pulmonary condition and by improving the patient's general health; at times these gains can be so dramatic

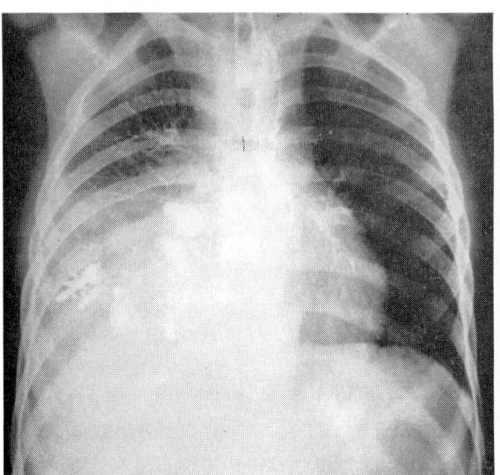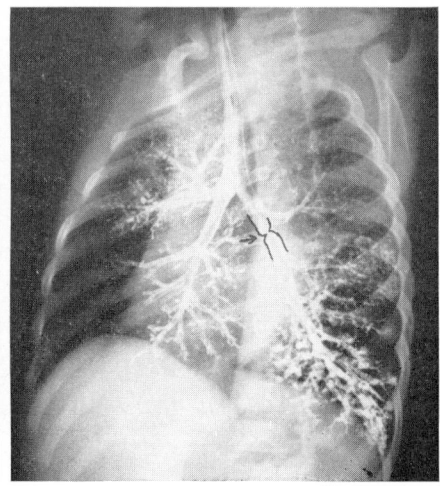

Fig. 446. *Left*, Ten-year-old girl with marked bronchiectasis and pulmonary suppuration of right middle and lower lobes. *Right*, Four-year-old boy who had chronic productive cough for more than two years. Only mild bronchiectasis of left lower lobe, but there is a stenosis, presumably congenital (arrow). Treated by left lower lobectomy.

that operation can be deferred more or less indefinitely. In cases in which the disease is advanced, but sufficient normal pulmonary tissue remains, surgery must almost certainly be employed. Attitudes in the selection of cases for surgery have changed markedly in recent years. Whereas formerly it was quite generally agreed that bronchiectasis in a localized form should always be treated by surgical ablation, it is now found that a majority of childhood cases can be treated very satisfactorily on medical measures and that it is only a minority (of a more refractory sort) which must come to surgical excision.

The evaluation of any patient with bronchiectasis should not rest primarily upon the roentgenographic demonstration of bronchiolar dilatation, unless this feature is marked. Evaluation is more correctly made upon the degree of suppuration (as shown by expectoration or by bronchoscopic aspiration), the extent of pulmonary infiltration (as shown by x-ray films), the ability of a patient to resolve inflammation in a reasonable length of time, the capacity of the individual to remain free of recrudescences, and the general status of the patient's health, as indicated by observations of temperature, weight, progress of growth, and ability to partake of reasonable exercise and activity.

Every patient with bronchiectasis should have therapy initiated by a proper and complete investigation, foremost in which is bronchoscopy under general anesthesia; this is both diagnostic and to some degree therapeutic. This step is of great importance to rule out a foreign body (or if such is found, to remove it), to make sure that there is no constriction or compression of bronchi leading to the involved area, to determine the extent of the process, to estimate the amount of exudate which is present, to obtain some of the material for bacteriologic study, and to remove by suction all of the purulent material which can be sucked away. In the hands of a competent bronchoscopist, these procedures disturb a child but little. Only by such examination can one make a proper evaluation of the condition and assemble base-line observations against which future comparisons can be made to determine the efficacy or the failure of therapeutic efforts in controlling the disease.

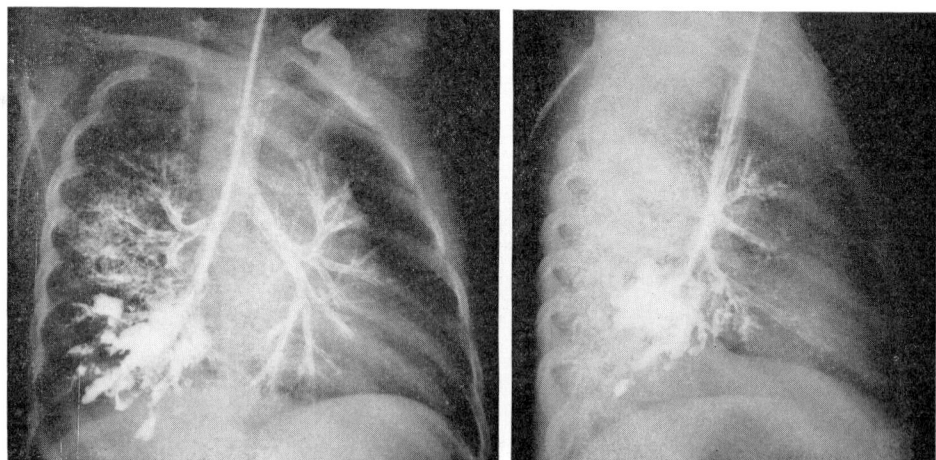

Fig. 447. Three-year-old girl who had had symptoms of pulmonary disease for one year. Extensive bronchiectasis of right middle and particularly the right lower lobe. Treated by right lower lobectomy.

Medical Measures

A vigorous, well supervised course of medical therapy can do much toward improving the child's general health and modifying the parenchymal inflammation of the lungs. In some cases, these simple measures are all that are required. Even in those children who will eventually come to surgery, these steps are of great importance in placing the patient in the best condition to withstand an operative procedure.

Postural Drainage. Much can be accomplished by postural drainage, placing the child over the soft edge of a mattress or inclining the bed and positioning the child's body in the optimum angle for promoting drainage from the diseased parts. To merely order "postural drainage" is generally useless; the child is made uncomfortable by lying over some hard edge or by assuming a head-down position which is too marked; he develops an aversion to the maneuver and subsequently refuses to do it, or else assumes the position for too short a time to be of any value. Conversely, it is helpful if the physician supervises the first attempts at postural drainage by making sure that the youngster is made as comfortable as possible, that the optimum position is attained, and that the child is encouraged to cough up sputum and clear the passageways. Postural drainage should be employed three or four times each day, paying particular attention to the early morning period, because at this time the lung is most apt to be filled with secretions which have accumulated during the night. If secretions are thick and sticky, the use of expectorants will help to thin the material and aid in its mobilization and removal. In some patients, postural drainage brings up a great deal of exudate and is therefore beneficial; in other patients, it brings up little more than that which is raised while the patient is in an erect position. If the former is true, postural drainage should be continued; if the latter is the case, there is little point in persisting with it.

Antibiotics. Antibiotics are of tremendous importance and should be employed intensively over long periods of time. In general, antibiotics with a wide range of effectiveness against gram-negative and gram-positive bacteria are the most efficacious. Amongst these aureomycin and particularly terramycin have become the favorites. While formerly we employed extensively the volatilization of antibiotics in nebulizers, feeling that the direct aspiration of these drugs into the air passages would give maximum effectiveness, we have now completely discarded this method of therapy anduse the drugs solely by oral ingestion.

General Measures. General supportive measures should not be overlooked. If the nutritional status is poor, a proper diet should be prescribed. An adequate vitamin intake, with particular stress on vitamins A and D, must be given. Reasonable housing and clothing should be provided; if, for the poorer strata of patients, these cannot be obtained at home, placement in a convalescent home or some such institution which can give adequate coverage at low cost is of tremendous benefit.

Change of Climate. There can be no doubt that removal of a patient from a damp, cold, and rugged climate to a region which is sunny, warm, and dry can be of inestimable value in treating pulmonary infection, but for the vast majority of patients such transplantation to a more beneficial climate involves economic factors which are insurmountable. We have seen more damage than good come from ill-considered advice to "move to a warmer climate." An outstanding example of this was a little girl who was transported from the rigors of New England to the balmy air of Arizona, a shift which necessitated moving her entire family. The child improved greatly but the family was thrown into economic disaster because the father had always earned his livelihood as a cook on fishing vessels! He and the whole family foundered badly when placed in a land-locked portion of the country.

Bronchoscopy. Bronchoscopy should be included under conservative measures. Just how often it should be used depends upon the findings in any particular case. If the child is able to clear the passages by coughing, bronchoscopy does not offer a great deal. However, there are some youngsters who simply refuse to cough, or who cannot get up the material by postural drainage. Exudate puddles in the bronchiectatic areas; under such circumstances bronchoscopy during the more severe periods of the disease can accomplish a great deal in clearing the passageways and giving the interstitial infection the best possible chance to subside. Furthermore, occasionally repeating the Lipiodol studies can give some indication of whether improvement or degeneration is taking place in the pulmonary picture.

Surgical Treatment

Although medical management has now been able to take care of the majority of children with bronchiectasis, there are some cases in which the lesion is advanced, does not respond adequately to conservative measures, or even advances in the face of medical therapy; removal of diseased tissue should be carried out. Even in those cases in which the process is not well localized, and involves many lobes, the ablation of that part where the process is most active can be of considerable benefit to the patient and can improve the chances of medical care being beneficial for the remaining parts where minimal disease remains.

Selection of Cases for Surgery. Just which patients should be operated upon and which should not, is a matter which cannot be settled by any pre-set rules. While marked dilatation of bronchi, even of a saccular variety, can occasionally be cleared of suppurative and surrounding inflammatory processes, and the individual can carry on in a reasonably good state of health for many years, the risks of surgery are so low that it is probably best to remove all those lesions wherein bronchiectasis is advanced. In the great bulk of cases, bronchiectasis is minimal or is only moderately advanced; whether

Table 81

Pulmonary Resections in Children's Hospital Cases

	No. of Cases
Left pneumonectomy..	8
Left lower lobectomy and lingulectomy........................	13
Of these, 1 was later subjected to left upper lobectomy.	
Left lower lobectomy.......................................	15
Of these, 3 were later subjected to left upper lobectomy.	
Right pneumonectomy......................................	5
Right upper and middle lobectomy...........................	1
Right middle lobectomy....................................	5
Right lower and middle lobectomy...........................	12
Of these, 1 was later subjected to left lower lobectomy.	
Right lower lobectomy.....................................	13
Of these, 1 was later subjected to right middle and upper lobectomy.	

or not these should have surgical excision depends entirely upon the findings in each case and the magnitude of the response which is obtained under medical care. If expectoration can be abolished or kept at a minimum, if lung tissues can be kept free of atelectasis, and if the pulmonary parenchyma can be cleared rather well, conservative measures probably should be continued and surgery avoided. Conversely, if the expectoration continues, atelectasis repeatedly recurs, or pulmonary consolidation persists in any important degree, it is preferable to undertake a surgical excision.

The ages of patients we have recently seen (in the 1946 through 1950 group), who required lobectomy or pneumonectomy, varied from fifteen months to fifteen years. While many of these subjects had symptoms from the first year of life, we seldom found it necessary to perform pulmonary resection within the first few years of life. However, a young age is, in itself, no contraindication to operation. Mendez, Leahy, and Butsch[24] have emphasized this point and have shown that surgery can be safe, their youngest patient being two and a half months of age at the time of lobectomy. (Resection of pulmonary disease for other conditions, such as a cystic lobe or lung, has been performed in much younger ages than this.)

Preparation for Operation. When, in any given case, surgical removal of bronchiectatic tissue is decided upon, the hazards of surgery can be greatly reduced by choosing the appropriate moment for the undertaking. A child who is very toxic is apt to withstand thoracic surgery poorly. If there is any marked degree of anemia and a considerable amount of blood is lost in freeing a very adherent lobe or lung, the result may be disastrous. Therefore, attention to the nutritional status, any important anemia, and rehabilitation in a convalescent or rest home are important factors in placing a patient in the best possible condition before surgery. The greatest single hazard of operation is the

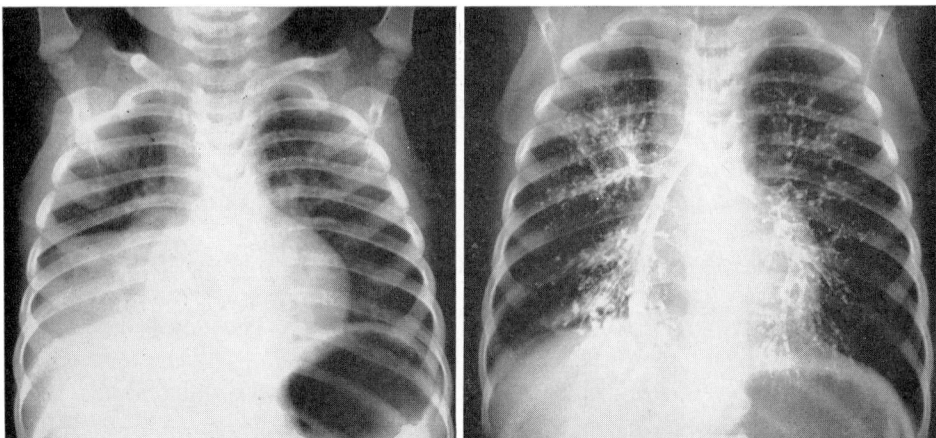

Fig. 448. Two-year-old boy with symptoms for nine months following aspiration of tuft of timothy hay. *Left*, Atelectasis and consolidation at the base of the right lung. *Right*, Bronchogram showing extensive bronchiectasis of right lower lobe. Treated by right lower lobectomy. Patient entirely well four years later.

spillover of bronchial exudate into adjacent lobe or the opposite lung. Therefore, everything possible should be done beforehand to clear out the airways by use of expectorants, encouragement of coughing, postural drainage, or in severe cases by repeated bronchoscopic aspiration. The time for operation should be selected when sputum is at a minimum. Furthermore, as soon as the patient has been anesthetized, bronchoscopy should be carried out and the bronchial tree sucked out before turning the subject up on one side for the thoracotomy, in this way minimizing any spillage.

Excision of Pulmonary Substance. As one views the procedures of pulmonary resection which have been widely employed by various surgeons in the treatment of bronchiectasis in childhood during the last fifteen or twenty years, it becomes quite clear that there is a change in view regarding the unit which should be removed. Whereas formerly a pneumonectomy was employed or attempted rather frequently, it is now a

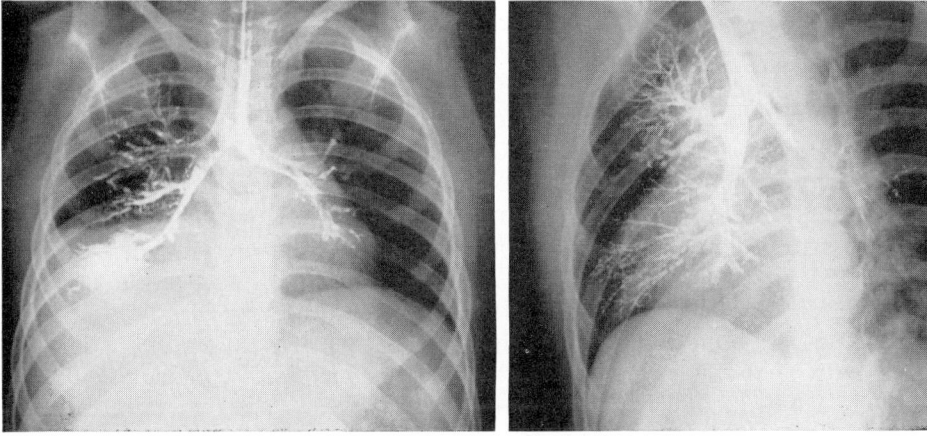

Fig. 449. *Left*, Six-year-old girl with productive cough and mild bronchiectasis of right middle and particularly the right lower lobe. Treated by right middle and lower lobectomy. *Right*, Another child with chronic and mildly productive cough. Bronchogram showing bronchiectasis of right middle lobe. Treated by right middle lobectomy.

procedure which is seldom necessary. There has been a gradual and progressive shift to emphasis upon lobectomy, and more recently toward a segmental resection. These changes in emphasis occur because patients with less extensive disease are now being operated upon, and because of the generally accepted principle of removing only diseased portion of lung and saving as much as possible of tissue which is normal or near-normal. Obviously, this shift to more conservative procedures is a desirable one, but there is room for some debate regarding just how far it should go. Lobectomy has become a well standardized procedure, the unit of tissue being well defined and circumscribable, such excision now being followed by complications but with great rarity. Conversely, in the segmental resection, the unit is sometimes difficult to define when there have been extensive inflammatory changes; the resection accomplished sometimes is better called a "wedge" removal; adjacent lung tissue which has been transected must now be compressed by sutures which are taken to close it, a step which almost certainly

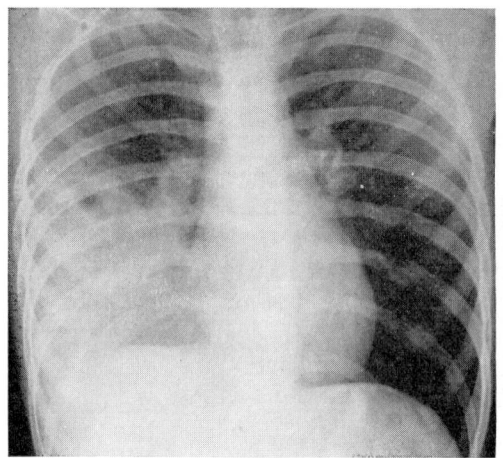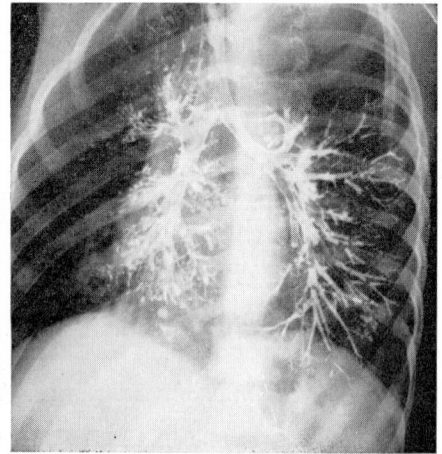

Fig. 450. Ten-year-old girl with rather short history of fever, debility, and productive cough. *Left*, Extensive consolidation in lower portion of lung. *Right*, Bronchogram showing moderate bronchiectasis of right middle and lower lobes. Treated by right lower lobectomy.

will keep it from expanding properly. Complications of empyema and broncho-pleural fistula are certainly much higher after segmental resection. Because of these various drawbacks, usually it has been our policy to perform lobectomy and to make very little use of segmental resection (excepting lingulectomy). It is fully realized that some of our patients might possibly have been treated by segmental resection, thereby sparing some normal tissue which was sacrificed by a lobectomy. However, the elimination of post-operative complications in our lobectomy series in the last ten years has led us to rely on this as the procedure of choice in the vast majority of cases.

Segmental Resection. Resection of anatomic subdivisions of the pulmonary lobe is one of the recent developments in thoracic surgery. It has become clear that the broncho-pulmonary segments are units with sufficiently distinctive anatomic boundaries to be removed individually and that certain lesions are sometimes confined to such units. The principal advantage of employing segmental resection is that only zones which include disease need be removed; nearby healthy and functioning pulmonary tissue is saved. In spite of these theoretical advantages, it must be emphasized that segmental resection is usually not an easy operation. A thorough knowledge of the anatomic relation of the tertiary hilar structures and of their anomalies is essential. Accurate identifi-

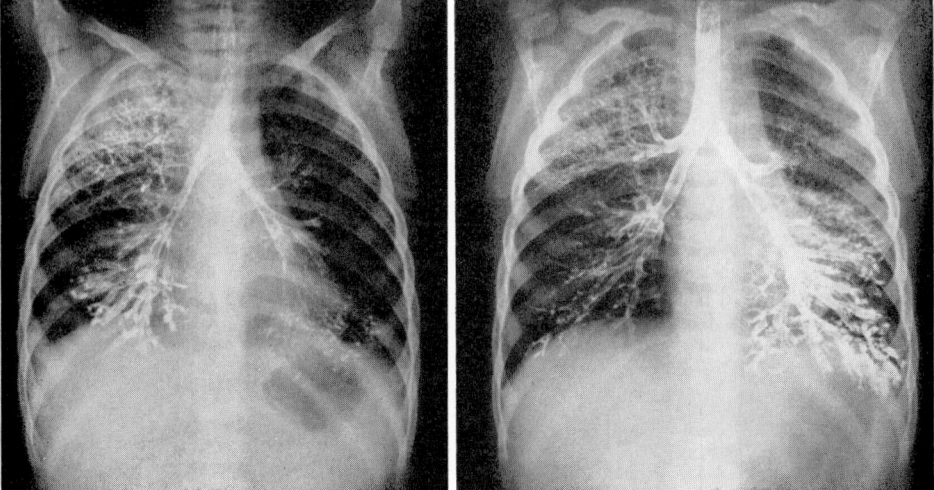

Fig. 451. *Left*, Rather advanced right lower lobe bronchiectasis. *Right*, Two years later, following conservative therapy, the right lower lobe cleared remarkably but there was extensive development and advancement of bronchiectasis in left lower lobe, which later required lobectomy.

cation of segmental vessels requires a most careful dissection. Separation of diseased segments from adjacent relatively normal tissue must be done precisely, if postoperative complications such as empyema and broncho-pleural fistula are to be kept at a minimum. Sometimes, what is commenced as a segmental resection leaves much to be desired because the natural boundaries of the segment have been obscured; dissection and removal of the unit is anything but satisfactory.

Whether segmental resection is preferable to lobectomy usually depends upon the extent of the bronchiectasis, the distribution of the disease, the cardio-respiratory reserve of the patient, and the experience of the surgeon. If all except one segment of a single lobe is diseased and the cardio-respiratory reserve is good, conservation of that single segment certainly does not justify the increased risk of segmental resection; a lobectomy

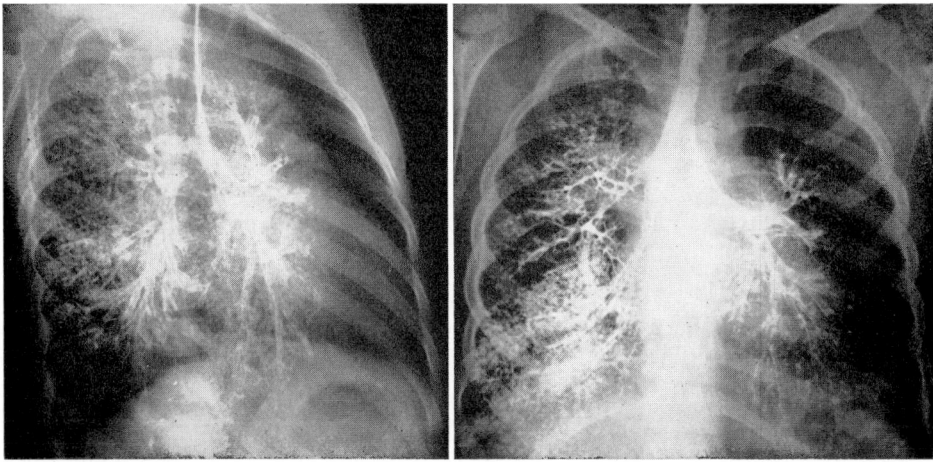

Fig. 452. *Left*, Diffuse bronchiectasis, most advanced in right lower lobe. Treated by right lower lobectomy, followed by intensive chemotherapy. *Right*, Three years later, showing the excellent expansion of remaining lobes to fill the thoracic cage on that side. Disease in remaining portions of the lung improved so that the patient became asymptomatic.

is far preferable. However, when multiple segments in different lobes become unilaterally or bilaterally involved and the cardio-respiratory reserve is limited, it becomes important to save as much undiseased substance as possible. While the value of segmental resection has been definitely established for adult patients (in spite of the slightly higher risk of postoperative complications), we are inclined to believe that it will have less usefulness in childhood.

Individual Division of Hilar Structures. Resection of a lung, or portion thereof, can be an operation which is exceedingly difficult or surprisingly easy. The main concerns are twofold: First, pleural adhesions can be very extensive and vascular; they can be time-consuming to deal with. Conversely, the absence of adhesions (or the presence of only a few minor ones) greatly simplifies the undertaking. Second, the degree of

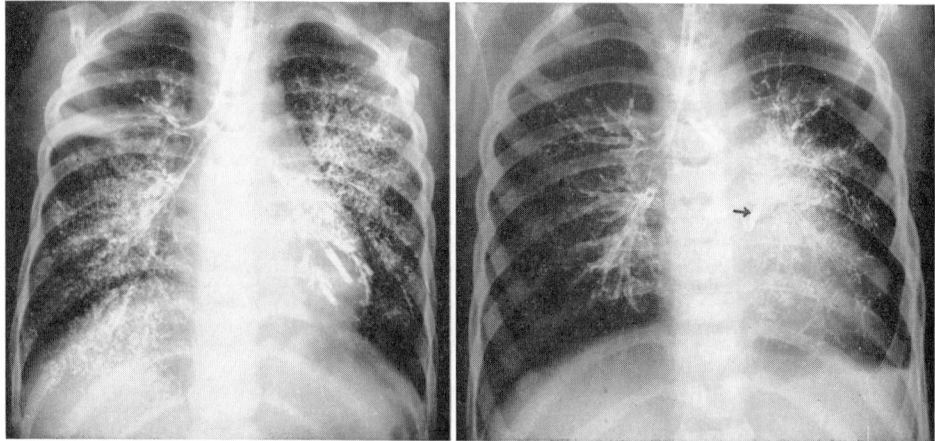

Fig. 453. *Left*, Severe bronchiectasis of left lower lobe, which was treated by lobectomy. *Right*, Bronchogram two years after operation, there being residual suppuration and persistent symptomatology. There has been incomplete removal of the lower lobe stump (arrow); this was a focus of infection.

reaction around the base of the lobe (or lung) has much to do with the ease or difficulty with which resection will be accomplished. The days of mass ligation and transection of pulmonary stump have long passed. The only acceptable way of removing a unit is by individual isolation, division, and closure of the vessels and the bronchus. If hilar inflammation is minimal, these steps go along rapidly and satisfactorily, but if structures are matted together, it can be exceedingly troublesome to isolate the various components, the dissection being tedious, bloody, and taxing of one's skill.

Handling of Bronchus. Regarding the severance of a bronchus, there are those who state that it should never be crushed, for fear of devitalizing the wall and leading to sloughing and establishment of a broncho-pleural fistula. We take no stock in these theoretical objections; we crush the bronchus in every case. After freeing it adequately, the bronchus is grasped by three Kocher clamps, and then cut across between the two distal instruments. This leaves two clamps on the bronchial stump, the distal one of which is removed, providing a cuff which can be closed with interrupted mattress stitches of silk, these sutures running through the entire thickness of the bronchial wall. After closure is completed, the remaining back clamp is removed. *It is now of fundamental importance to bring tissue of some sort to cover over and seal against this stump.* Usually this can be accomplished by swinging a flap of pleura over the raw area and completely burying the bronchial stump, the pleural flap being anchored around its periphery by fine silk sutures. These measures are so simple and effective that we see no need for changing them. In no case where they have been employed have we had postoperative broncho-pleural fistula.

Endotracheal Anesthesia. Endotracheal anesthesia should always be used because it gives the best possible control when positive pressure anesthesia is necessary; it also affords an avenue by which a catheter may be introduced at any time into the trachea or bronchi for removal of secretions which accumulate in the passageways. Clear airways are essential for safe surgery and for maintenance of a satisfactory anesthesia.

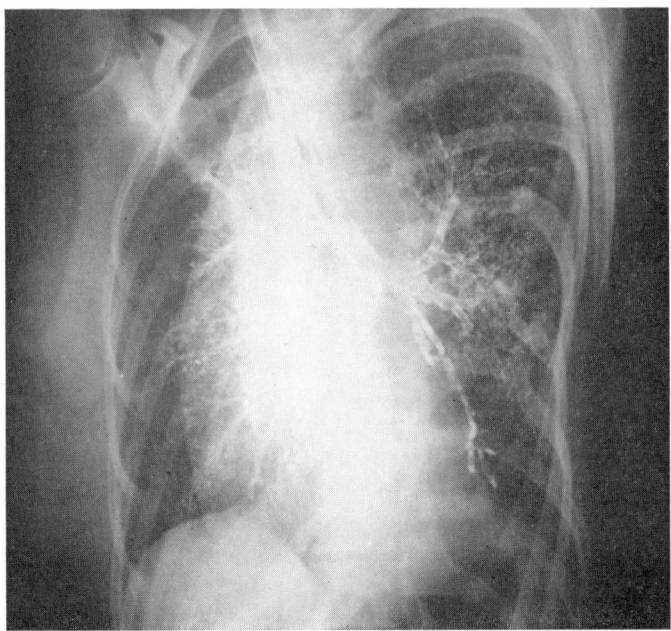

Fig. 454. Bronchiectasis in left lower lobe treated by lobectomy. Continuation of cough and expectoration postoperatively. This bronchogram three years after operation shows bronchiectasis in the lingula (which should have been removed at the original operation). Treated later by lingulectomy.

Pleural Drainage. Postoperatively, catheter drainage of the pleural cavity should always be provided for two reasons: First, all fluid should be carried out of the chest as soon as it is formed. While resection of pulmonary tissue can be kept relatively clean and neat, unavoidably there is some slight bacterial contamination of the pleural space; fluid should not be allowed to accumulate in the chest and provide a medium for the growth of bacteria. Constant drainage of the chest for several days is the most effective measure in avoiding development of empyema. Second, it is desirable to expand any remaining pulmonary tissue very promptly, and in this way prevent it from becoming adherent in an undesired position or becoming encased in a thickened visceral pleura which prevents its complete expansion and usefulness. The remaining pulmonary substance (after a lobectomy) can usually be made to expand and completely fill the pleural cavity within a few hours after operation. If this is attained, optimum results are assured.

RESULTS OF THERAPY

Table 82 summarizes statistics from the Children's Hospital material for surgical treatment of bronchiectasis. Certain features are worth emphasizing.

The need for pneumonectomy has almost completely disappeared. In the early part of this work, when pneumonectomy was indicated because of the extensiveness of the disease processes which had to be treated, this operation carried alarmingly high fatality rates. One of the deaths was caused by excessive bleeding during the freeing and dissec-

Table 82

Mortality in Surgical Treatment of Bronchiectasis*
(1934 through 1950)

Years	Operation	Number of Cases	Deaths†	Surgical Mortality, per cent	Late Deaths‡
1934	Lobectomy	7	0	0	2
through	Pneumonectomy	3	1	33	0
1937					
1938	Lobectomy	24	2	8	0
through	Pneumonectomy	8	4	50	0
1945					
1946	Lobectomy	28	0	0	0
through	Pneumonectomy	2	0	0	1
1950					

* The figures indicated are *patients*. The numbers for *operative procedures* were higher, some patients having had two lobectomy operations.

† Deaths, either during operation or in the postoperative course.

‡ These deaths all occurred subsequent to hospital discharge, varying from 4 months to 9 years thereafter, but all related to bronchiectasis spreading in remaining lobes, advancing pulmonary incapacitation, brain abscess, etc.

tion of a lung which was encased in massive vascular adhesions; the toxic and debilitated patient died from shock in spite of the fact that adequate transfusion was given throughout operation. Four of the deaths were due to drowning on the table; a lung containing much bronchial exudate allowed this material to spill over into the opposite lung, producing atelectasis and respiratory insufficiency. These catastrophes were in the days before chemotherapy was available. While one is seldom called upon to treat such cases today, the fundamental teaching must not be lost sight of that a lung should be made as dry as possible before bringing a patient to surgery.

Lobectomy has been placed on a very sound basis and is now an operation which carries a negligible risk. In the 54 lobectomies since 1942 we have had no fatalities, no empyema, and no broncho-pleural fistula.

Apparently the etiologic factor has had a great deal to do with the eventual outcome. When there was a bronchial obstruction (either from congenital stenosis or an inflammatory stricture), the bronchiectasis was almost always localized to the zone supplied by this bronchus; the surgical removal was followed by an excellent result. When bronchiectasis had developed on the basis of a foreign body, we have found in the vast majority of cases that the removal of the object generally has been followed by subsidence of the inflammatory reaction; those few subjects who eventually did come to lobectomy had a disease process which was localized, and which was always followed by an excellent result. When the etiologic factor seemed to be related to a chronic paranasal sinusitis, and repeated or continued pollution of the lung, the general outlook concerning the pulmonary picture was closely dependent upon what could be gained in controlling the sinusitis. If the sinuses could be cleared and existing bronchiectatic tissue could be excised, the patient generally did well. Conversely, pulmonary resection was apt to be followed by disease in other parts of the lungs if insults continued from naso-pharyngeal drippings. In those cases in which the etiologic factor was not clear, there constantly lurked the possibility that surgical excision for bronchiectasis might be followed by appearance of the condition in other lobes at subsequent times. These have not been seen often, but they can be disastrous. In spite of the fact that all diseased tissue was thought to have been removed, bronchiectasis appeared elsewhere and continued to advance in spite of all surgical and medical efforts to combat it, eventually producing over the course of years such inroads on the respiratory reserve that the patient succumbed.

A review of our material has emphasized the fact that if surgery is to be undertaken for the removal of a localized disease, every effort should be made to ablate it entirely. In at least 4 instances, too long a bronchial stump has been left, this error having been committed because surrounding regional inflammation made the operator hesitant to advance further, for fear of injuring the nearby bronchi. A stump which is long enough to accumulate fluid, but which does not have in it any to-and-fro excursion of air which by coughing could remove the fluid, has permitted a puddling of exudate and has given a continuation of symptoms which required secondary measures of treatment. Therefore, in spite of the fact that it might be a difficult dissection, every effort should be made to remove a bronchial stump back to a point closely approaching the next normal bronchus.

The over-all picture of surgical resection for bronchiectatic disease in childhood has been a very satisfactory one. The procedures now carry fatality rates which are almost nil, and in the vast majority of cases it is possible to remove completely the pulmonary disease. Only in a small minority of cases is there spread to other lobes, ending in pulmonary crippling or fatality.

Without doubt, many of the disagreeable and disappointing features in treatment of bronchiectasis in adult patients will be largely averted in the future because the disease is now being recognized and treated in childhood, when the physician and surgeon have the best chances of combating and arresting it before extensive pulmonary damage has been inflicted.

A long-term follow-up gives the following over-all findings: In those patients who survived pneumonectomy, 100 per cent have had a good or excellent result. The infection was clearly localized to one lung (generally on the basis of a congenital abnormality of the main bronchus). None of these patients has needed further therapy. In the lobectomy group, the mortality statistics and the incidence of postoperative complications not only improved tremendously through the years, but the surviving patients have progressively shown higher percentages of favorable courses after surgical therapy. Out of the 1934–1937 group, 40 per cent have now been found to be in good or excellent health. Of the 1938–1945 group, 50 per cent can now be regarded as having good or excellent health. From the last period, 1946 through 1950, 80 per cent of patients are in good or excellent condition. Possibly these figures might be interpreted as indicating that patients who have been followed longest after surgery are having more flare-ups of residual bronchiectasis and more time for deterioration (thereby cutting down the percentage of long-term favorable results). However, we do not believe that this is true to any extent. It is our conviction that the apparent improvement in results after surgery in recent years is due largely to the fact that we are now treating cases with more limited types of disease (which can be resected easily), and also to the fact that when residual disease does exist, it has been more appropriately and persistently treated by medical means following our surgical endeavors.

REFERENCES

1. Baker, J. M., Roettig, L. C. and Curtis, G. M.: The Prevention and Treatment of Atelectasis by the Control of Bronchial Secretions. Ann. Surg., *134*:641, 1951.
2. Berg, R. M., Boyden, E. A. and Smith, F. R.: An Analysis of Variations of the Segmental Bronchi of the Left Lower Lobe of 50 Dissected and 10 Injected Lungs. J. Thoracic Surg., *18*:216, 1949.
3. Bergstrom, W. H., Cook, C. D., Scannell, J. G. and Berenberg, W.: Situs Inversus, Bronchiectasis and Sinusitis. Report of a Family with Two Cases of Kartagener's Triad and Two Additional Cases of Bronchiectasis Among Six Siblings. Pediatrics, *6*:573, 1950.
4. Blades, B. and Dugan, D. J.: Pseudobronchiectasis. J. Thoracic Surg., *13*:40, 1944.
5. Boyden, E. A.: The Intrahilar and Related Segmental Anatomy of the Lung. Surgery, *18*:706, 1945.
6. Boyden, E. A.: A Synthesis of the Prevailing Patterns of the Broncho-Pulmonary Segments in the Light of Their Variations. Dis. of Chest, *15*:657, 1949.
7. Bremer, J. L.: The Fate of the Remaining Lung Tissue after Lobectomy or Pneumonectomy. J. Thoracic Surg., *6*:336, 1936.
8. Brock, R. C.: The Anatomy of the Bronchial Tree with Special Reference to the Surgery of Lung Abscess. Oxford University Press, London, 1946.
9. Carter, M. D. and Welch, K. J.: Bronchiectasis Following Aspiration of Timothy Grass. New England J. Med., *238*:832, 1948.
10. Churchill, E. D.: Lobectomy and Pneumonectomy in Bronchiectasis and Cystic Disease. J. Thoracic Surg., *6*:286, 1936.
11. Churchill, E. D. and Belsey, R.: Segmental Pneumonectomy in Bronchiectasis. The Lingula Segment of the Left Upper Lobe. Ann. Surg., *109*: 481, 1939.
12. Churchill, E. D.: The Segmental and Lobular Physiology and Pathology of the Lung. J. Thoracic Surg., *18*:279, 1949.
13. Clagett, O. T. and Deterling, R. A., Jr.: A Technique for Segmental Pulmonary Resection with Particular Reference to Lingulectomy. J. Thoracic Surg., *15*:227, 1946.
14. Dickson, J. A., Clagett, O. T. and McDonald, J. R.: Cystic Disease of the Lungs and its Relationship to Bronchiectatic Cavities. A Study of 22 Cases. J. Thoracic Surg., *15*: 196, 1946.
15. Edwards, A. T.: Modern Principles of Treatment in Bronchiectasis, Based upon 199 Cases Treated by Lobectomy or Pneumonectomy. Brit. M. J., *1*:809, 1939.
16. Field, C. E.: Bronchiectasis in Childhood. I. Clinical Survey of 160 Cases. Pediatrics, *4*: 21, 1949.
17. Field, C. E.: Bronchiectasis in Childhood. II. Etiology and Pathogenesis, Including a Survey of 272 Cases of Doubtful Irreversible Bronchiectasis. Pediatrics, *4*:231, 1949.
18. Field, C. E.: Bronchiectasis in Childhood. III. Prophylaxis, Treatment, and Progress with a Follow-up Study of 202 Cases of Established Bronchiectasis. Pediatrics, *4*: 355, 1949.
19. Findlay, C. W., Jr.: The Healing of Surgical Wounds of the Lung with Particular Reference to Segmental Lobectomy. J. Thoracic Surg., *20*:823, 1950.
20. Kay, E. B., Meade, R. H. and Hughes, F. A.: Surgical Treatment of Bronchiectasis. Ann. Int. Med., *26*:1, 1947.
21. Lanman, T. H.: The Surgical Treatment of Chronic Pulmonary Suppuration in Children with Special Reference to Bronchiectasis. Am. J. Surg., *39*:249, 1938.
22. Lindskog, G. E., Liebow, A. A. and Hales, M. R.: Bilobectomy—Surgical and Anatomic Considerations in Resection of Right, Middle and Lower Lobes through the Intermediate Bronchus. J. Thoracic Surg., *18*:616, 1949.
23. Mallory, T. B.: The Pathogenesis of Bronchiectasis. New England J. Med., *237*:795, 1947.
24. Mendez, F. L., Jr., Leahy, L. J. and Butsch, W. L.: Some Aspects of Bronchiectasis in Infants. J. Thoracic Surg., *24*:50, 1952.
25. Ochsner, A., DeBakey, M. and DeCamp, P. T.: Bronchiectasis. Its Curative Treatment by Pulmonary Resection. Surgery, *25*:518, 1949.
26. Overholt, R. H., Woods, F. M. and Betts, R. H.: An Improved Method of Resection of Pulmonary Segments. J. Thoracic Surg., *17*:464, 1948.
27. Paulson, D. L. and Shaw, R. R.: Chronic Atelectasis and Pneumonitis of the Middle Lobe. J. Thoracic Surg., *18*:747, 1949.
28. Perry, K. M. A. and King, D. S.: Bronchiectasis: Study of Prognosis based on Follow-up of 400 Patients. Am. Rev. Tuberc., *41*: 531, 1940.
29. Pryce, D. M., Sellers, T. H. and Blair, L. G.: Intralobar Sequestration of Lung Associated with an Abnormal Pulmonary Artery. Brit. J. Surg., *35*:18, 1947.

30. Ramsey, B. H.: The Anatomic Guide to the Intersegmental Plane. Surgery, *25*:533, 1949.
31. Royce, S. W.: Cor Pulmonale in Infancy and Early Childhood—Report on 34 Patients with Special Reference to the Occurrence of Pulmonary Heart Disease in Cystic Fibrosis of the Pancreas. Pediatrics, *8*:255, 1951.
32. Scannell, J. G.: Thoracic Surgery. Medical Progress. New England J. Med., *239*:924 and 961, 1948.
33. Scannell, J. G.: An Anatomic Approach to Segmental Resection. J. Thoracic Surg., *18*: 64, 1949.
34. Smith, F. R. and Boyden, E. A.: An Analysis of Variations of the Segmental Bronchi of the Right Lower Lobe of 50 Injected Lungs. J. Thoracic Surg., *18*:195, 1949.
35. Waddell, W. R., Sniffen, R. C. and Sweet, R. H.: Chronic Pneumonitis: Its Clinical and Pathologic Importance. J. Thoracic Surg., *18*:707, 1949.
36. Weinberg, J.: Experimental Production of Bronchiectasis. J. Thoracic Surg., *6*:402, 1936.

CHAPTER 60

The Patent Ductus Arteriosus

From a historical standpoint, surgical treatment of the patent ductus arteriosus is a fascinating chapter in modern therapeutics because it formed the opening wedge in the surgical attack on congenital cardiovascular anomalies. A treatise on the diagnosis and treatment of the persistent ductus is of considerable importance because it is now generally acknowledged that the abnormality can be detected with great accuracy and can be treated surgically with an extremely high degree of success. The following presentation is based upon a rather extensive experience with the condition during the last fifteen years, during which time 611 patients have been operated upon by myself, or by my associates and residents. Of this number, 85 per cent were in the childhood group.

CLINICAL FINDINGS

A patent ductus arteriosus is much more common in females (70 per cent in our series). Subjects with an open ductus may have little or no evidence of cardiac embarrassment or, conversely, they may have marked invalidism, depending upon the age of the person and the size of the leak which exists.

In general, the abnormality is tolerated well in childhood and decompensation is rare in that period. As a rule, youngsters have boundless energy, can indulge in strenuous sports, and are thought to be quite normal by their parents. In some instances, there is slight to moderate limitation of physical activity, or there may even be dyspnea, palpitation, and excessive fatigue after strenuous exercise.

Effect on Development

In an important percentage of childhood cases, but not in the majority of them, the general physical development is somewhat retarded. When compared with findings in normal children of the same age, the height and particularly the weight are distinctly less than the average; in some instances these findings are very striking. In no child have we seen lack of mental development which could be rightfully ascribed to the presence of an open ductus.

Cardiac Embarrassment

Patients in mid-life often have moderate cardiac embarrassment; less commonly they have the classic findings of failure. Adults frequently find that they cannot maintain former levels of work, that fatigue is marked, or that long periods of rest are required. There are a considerable number of individuals who present themselves in their thirties or forties, who have no frank symptoms or signs of cardiac failure, but who, nevertheless, have lost their pep and who drag about in their daily existence with no exuberance. While such people are by no means invalids in the common sense of the term, they are incapacitated and are limited in their effectiveness and usefulness.

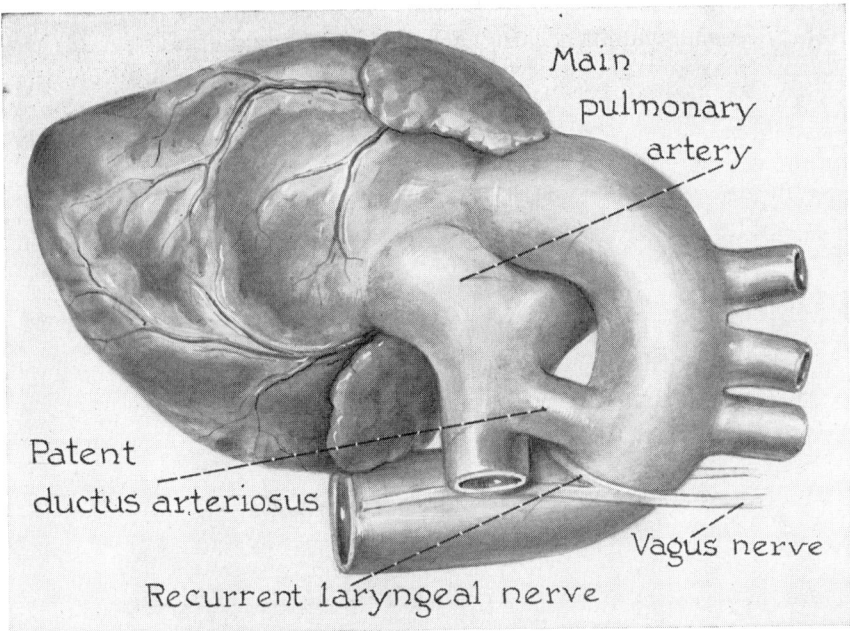

Fig 455. Drawing of heart and great arteries, showing relationship of aorta and pulmonary artery with a patent ductus arteriosus between them.

Physical Examination

The physical findings in a case of uncomplicated patent ductus arteriosus are clear-cut. It is important to emphasize that simple examination (with stress upon an intelligent auscultation) can lead to a rapid and accurate recognition of this congenital abnormality in more than 95 per cent of the cases.

The color of the skin and the mucous membranes is normal in most instances, but some pallor is present in others. Cyanosis is never found, unless there is frank cardiac failure and a reversal of blood flow through the ductus, a situation found only in terminal cases. The nails are not clubbed. The heart is normal or slightly increased in size; great enlargements are rare. The cardiac activity may be within normal limits, but if the ductus is large, there is an increased forcefulness of the impulse and there is a heaving pulsation over the neck vessels. These findings are more apparent in thin subjects than in those who are heavy-set.

Ductus patients usually have systolic blood pressures which are normal for their respective ages. The diastolic level is apt to be depressed, depending upon the size of the aortic leak. Small fistulas do not give any important change in the diastolic pressure, but large ones are accompanied by diminutions to 50 or 40 mm. of mercury. When the pulse pressure is high, there may be a Duroziez's sign or a visible capillary pulsation in the nail beds.

The femoral arterial pulsations are excellent, the pressures in the legs being above those of the arms; points of importance in ruling out a coarctation of the aorta.

Murmur. By auscultation a characteristic murmur is heard in the second or third intercostal space to the left of the sternum. (It is heard better and more intensely with a large flat (Bowles) chest-piece than with a cone-shaped (Bell) attachment.) It is continuous, is accentuated during systole, and dies off during diastole; it usually has a rumbling quality. The pulmonic sounds may be replaced by the murmur, or the second sound may be quite accentuated. The murmur has been well described as a "machinery" one, and the physician who has heard it several times should always be able to recognize it thereafter. It may be widely transmitted over the precordium, into the left axilla, up into the neck, or over the back, particularly to the left of the spine. While all of the murmur may be transmitted, it is more common to have only the louder, systolic portion carried to the cardiac apex, to the neck, or to the back.

Generally speaking, any loud systolic murmur (unaccompanied by a diastolic element) in acyanotic congenital heart disease comes from a septal defect or from a pure pulmonic stenosis. Rarely, it is possible for a tiny ductus to produce a murmur which is

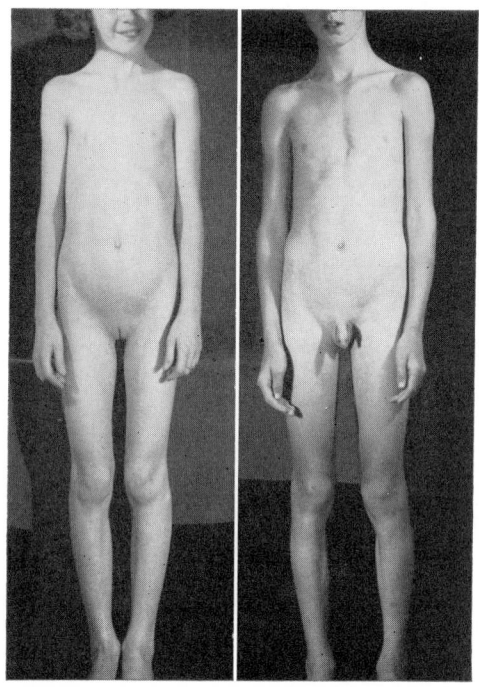

Fig. 456. Two children, subsequently proved to have patent ductuses, to show the slender habitus which a considerable portion of these patients possess. *Left*, Ten-year-old girl. *Right*, Eleven-year-old boy.

limited to systole; the murmur is of rather low intensity (roentgen study of the heart will show little or no variation from the normal). Also, in other rare cases, it is possible for an exceedingly large ductus to produce only a systolic murmur, because the pulmonary artery pressure mounts so high that there is a flow through the ductus only at the height of the systolic surge (such a patient almost certainly has considerable cardiac incapacitation and by roentgen study has a large heart and a very prominent pulmonary artery). In both of these situations with only a systolic murmur—of either a very tiny or a very large ductus—cardiac catheterization or aortography helps to clarify the diagnosis. It is well to emphasize that ductus patients with solely a systolic murmur constitute only a few per cent of any ductus series. Since more than 95 per cent of all ductuses give a continuous murmur, the diagnosis of an open ductus should not be made in the absence of such a murmur unless this can be supported by incontrovertible evidence from catheterization studies.

The classic sounds of an open ductus may not be found if one is examining a patient (usually an adult) during cardiac failure. At that time the pulmonary artery pressure may be exceedingly high, so that a near-equalization between it and the aortic tension gives a reduced ductus flow, no flow at all, or even a reversal of flow. Such conditions will give, respectively, a murmur limited to systole, no murmur, or a variable murmur associated with intermittent cyanosis. A good description of such a case has been presented by Johnson et al.[12]

A ductus murmur is generally one of considerable intensity, is indicative of a marked turbulence in the pulmonary artery, and hence is often accompanied by a thrill which can be felt in the precordium. About half the patients have a thrill. It may be continuous or it may be limited to systole; it is most intense over the pulmonic region, and it is seldom felt far from this area.

Streptococcus viridans infection, superimposed upon an open ductus, is rarely found in childhood, though we have seen it as early as four years. The peak incidence of endocarditis or pulmonary endarteritis comes in the third and fourth decades, following which time the frequency diminishes. The findings include fever, persistent sweating, anorexia, weight loss, chest pain, and phenomena in various parts of the body suggesting arterial embolism. The latter almost certainly indicate that vegetations are not limited to the ductus region, but that they have also developed on the mitral or aortic valves. Blood cultures provide positive proof of blood-stream infection, and they probably give some information regarding the severity of the invasion.

DIAGNOSIS

LABORATORY DATA

These patients do not have polycythemia.

Electrocardiogram

Electrocardiographic tracings are helpful in a surprisingly small percentage of cases. They are of no assistance in establishing the diagnosis of a patent ductus. However, they are an important part of the study of patients suspected of having a ductus. First, they might give evidence to indicate that the subject actually has some other form of cardiovascular anomaly. Second, if a ductus actually exists, the tracings can give some idea of the extent of any myocardial strain or damage.

In the vast majority of cases, particularly in children, electrocardiograms are normal and there is no axis deviation. In some tracings, particularly from adults, there may be a left-axis shift, especially in the presence of a shunt of moderate or large size. Fibrillation or indications of myocardial damage may be found in some of the older subjects when the cardiac strain has been excessive.

Electrocardiographic study is most valuable as a method of excluding cases with other cardiac lesions. Particular attention should be given to the presence of any right-axis deviation, the finding of which should make one strongly suspect some other anomaly such as a pulmonic stenosis or a tetralogy of Fallot. In only 6 patients have we found right preponderance when there was a pure patent ductus arteriosus; possibly the flow into the pulmonary circuit was very high or else there were secondary vascular changes in the lung bed, either of which could make the right ventricle hypertrophy as it pumps against an increased pressure.

Whenever a prolonged P-R interval is encountered, one should suspect that the auriculoventricular conduction apparatus is longer than normal and is probably stretched out around a septal defect.

Catheterization

Cardiac catheterization can give direct measurement of various blood flows, and can give a reasonably accurate idea of the size of a shunt. In the patient with a pure patent ductus, no arterial blood will be found flowing into the right side of the heart. In the pulmonary artery, blood samples from just beyond the valve will show degrees of unsaturation similar to those obtained in the right ventricle, but as the catheter is pushed along in the artery samples will show rising oxygen saturation which is proof of arterial blood flowing into this circuit through an open ductus. Sometimes, by a stroke of luck, it is possible to pass the catheter through a ductus into the aorta. Catheterization is not necessary as a routine study for average cases, but there are some patients with obscure abnormalities of the heart who should be studied in every way possible, including catheterization. It has been our experience that it is extremely rare to pick from the bizarre group a ductus which can come to operation which could not have been recognized by simpler means of roentgenography and cardiac auscultation.

Borderline Cases

More than 95 per cent of patent ductuses can be recognized with great facility and rapidity. If a characteristic murmur does not exist in a given patient, too much reliance should not be laid on laboratory or roentgenologic findings (other than catheterization) which might suggest the presence of a ductus, because thoracic exploration under such circumstances will generally lead to the finding of some other cardiovascular defect.

ROENTGENOLOGIC DATA

Roentgenologic studies often help in the recognition of a patent ductus arteriosus; film and fluoroscopic observations are also valuable in ruling out other cardiac abnormalities and rheumatic valvular disease. With a pure patent ductus the findings are those of a shunt from the aorta into the pulmonary circuit.[5] The heart is slightly or moderately enlarged, particularly in transverse dimension; marked enlargement is rare. While it may be difficult to tell whether there is hypertrophy (or dilatation) of one or both ventricles, generally it is possible to show that the left chamber is the predominant one. Often the pulmonary artery (sometimes incorrectly called the pulmonary conus) is fuller than normal and projects outward from the left border of the cardiac shadow. Likewise, vessels within the lung fields, particularly those of the hili, are apt to have increased fullness. In about half of the cases the central vessels of the lungs have a "hilar dance"; this may be quite difficult to observe, and too much stress should not be placed upon the presence or absence of this point. Right anterior-oblique and lateral views show left auricular enlargement in about half of the cases; this is best seen as an encroachment on the barium-filled esophagus. Such enlargement is dependent upon an increased flow through the left side of the heart; the left ventricle enlarges somewhat, whereas the thin-walled auricle dilates to a considerable degree. Fluoroscopic observation and kymographic tracings generally show increased expansion and contraction of the left ventricle as well as increased pulsations of the aortic knob and pulmonary artery.

Variation in X-ray Picture. If a ductus is small, the roentgenologic picture is normal or shows little change therefrom. Conversely, when a ductus is of moderate or large size, the roentgenologic findings are clear-cut and striking.

X-ray Findings Not Specific. The roentgenologic changes are not specific for a patent ductus arteriosus; they may be mimicked by certain other lesions. Septal defects are left-right shunts which give findings of an increased pulmonary flow. A fenestra between the first portions of the aorta and pulmonary artery gives roentgenologic pictures exactly like those of an open ductus. When the roentgenologist finds evidence of a left-right shunt, he is faced with the possibility of making several diagnoses. If, in addition to an augmented pulmonary flow, there is a right ventricular enlargement, he should lean toward a diagnosis of interventricular septal defect. If there is an associated right auricular enlargement, an interauricular septal defect is suggested. If there is no enlargement of the right side of the heart, he can be reasonably sure that the patient has a patent ductus arteriosus (or one of the rare defects between the first portions of the aorta and the pulmonary artery).

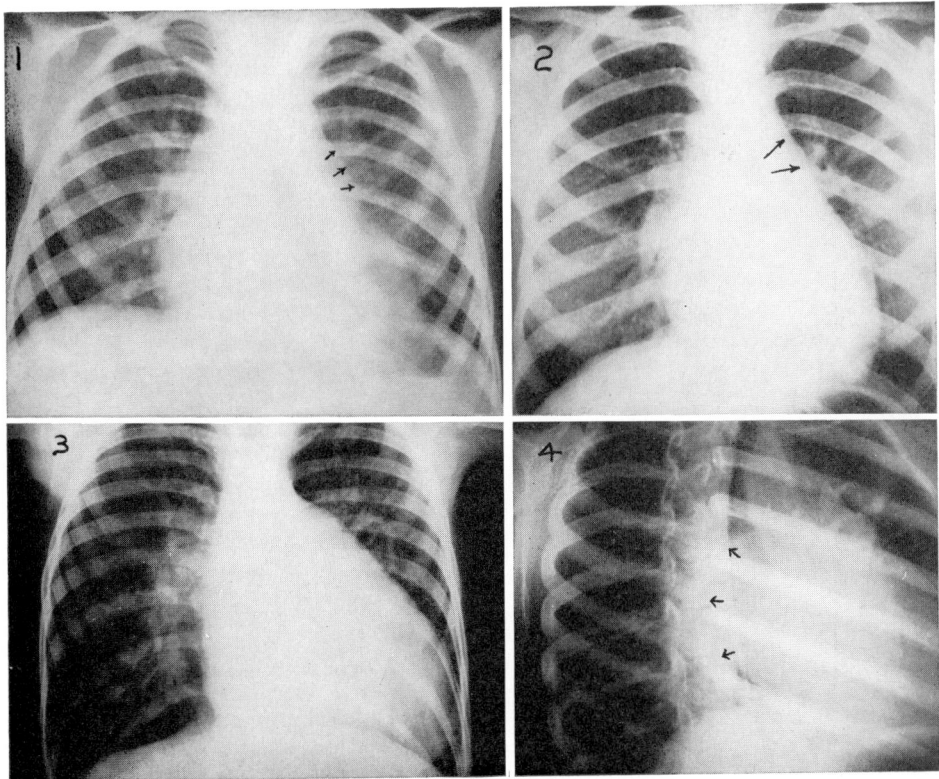

Fig. 457. Roentgenograms from children with patent ductuses, to illustrate various roentgen findings. 1. Slight enlargement of heart. Slight fullness of vessels in hilum of either lung. Slight fullness of pulmonary artery in region marked by arrows. 2. Only slight cardiac enlargement. Some increased fullness in pulmonary central vessels. Very slight fullness in pulmonary artery in region of arrows. 3. Marked enlargement of heart in a five-year-old girl (who weighed but 24 pounds). Marked fullness of left auricle and pulmonary artery. Increased pulmonary vascular markings. 4. Right anterior oblique view showing enlargement of left auricle, indicated by arrows.

DIFFICULTIES OF DETECTION IN INFANCY

Parents are often disturbed by the fact that a physician did not detect a cardiovascular abnormality in their child in the first few years of life. It is important to restore confidence in their doctor by pointing out that often it is utterly impossible to hear a murmur in infancy. While it is true that some babies with a patent ductus have a continuous and easily recognizable machinery murmur from birth, it is more common to find the following series of events: In the early months, the aortic pressure is low and the pulmonary pressure is normally high; there is no appreciable flow through the ductus and there is no murmur. In the subsequent year or so the aortic pressure rises and the pulmonary pressure falls; there is some ductus flow and a systolic murmur. By the third year the aortic pressure is high and the pulmonary pressure is low; there is now a considerable ductus flow and a typical continuous murmur. From these facts it is obvious that the best of physicians might not have been able to hear anything unusual in early life.

From the above considerations, it is clear that if one examines a child with congenital heart disease in the first year or two of life and hears only a systolic murmur, it is not possible to exclude a patent ductus; under such circumstances, it is important to examine the child again at three or four years, because if a ductus is present it will by that time produce a continuous type of murmur.

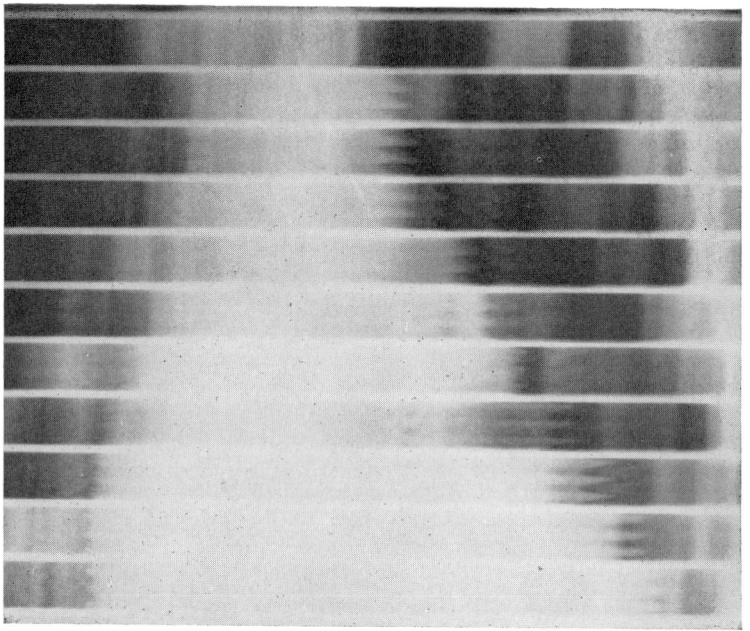

Fig. 458. Roentgen-kymographic tracing of activity of surface of heart and great vessels. Increased pulsation is shown along the left surface of the aortic arch and the pulmonary artery on the patient's left. Particularly prominent pulsations appear along the presenting border of the left ventricle.

PREDICTION OF THE SIZE OF A DUCTAL SHUNT

By cardiac catheterization it is, of course, possible to make a reasonably accurate estimate of the blood flow through an open ductus. Without catheterization it is still possible—in a rough way—to gain some impression of whether one is dealing with a ductus of small, medium, or large size. (1) If the heart is normal in size or is only slightly enlarged, if the beat is not overly vigorous, if the x-ray changes are minimal, and if the diastolic pressure is only slightly diminished, it is reasonable to assume that the shunt is a relatively small one. (2) If the heart is definitely enlarged, the murmur is intense and is possibly accompanied by a thrill, the diastolic pressure is moderately depressed, and the fluoroscopic findings indicate a considerable left-right shunt, one can assume that the ductus is of average size. (3) In rare cases (possibly one out of 30 or 40 patients) the heart is quite enlarged, there is a heaving beat which shakes the patient's chest or even the bed on which he lies, there are forceful pulsations in the neck, there are marked fluoroscopic changes, and the diastolic pressure is markedly depressed (though in a few instances the pulmonary pressure may be so high that the peripheral diastolic pressure is not particularly low); one can instantly predict that the shunt is of tremendous size. Under these latter circumstances one is apt to hear additional murmurs which are indicative of a greatly augmented flow through the left side of the heart; the large amount of blood (which may be two or two and a half times normal) will set up murmurs as it rushes through the orifice of a normal mitral or a normal aortic valve. Therefore, in addition to the continuous murmur of the ductus in the pulmonary zone, one can hear a separate diastolic murmur in the mitral area, or a separate systolic murmur in the aortic region. It is important to recognize these occasional cases with exceedingly large shunts so that the patient's family can be informed of the risks which are much higher than those of average cases, and so the surgeon can be adequately prepared to deal with a situation which will present technical difficulties enormously greater than those which are encountered in the common run of cases.

DIFFERENTIAL DIAGNOSIS

Aortic Septal Defect. On clinical grounds, it is extremely difficult to differentiate between an open ductus and a window between the first parts of the aorta and pulmonary aorta. Both are left-right shunts and give rise to quite similar murmurs and roentgenologic findings. It is virtually impossible to differentiate between the two conditions by angiocardiography (when the dye is injected by the venous route); it has been possible to visualize an aortic septal defect by retrograde arterial injection.[7] By catheterization, differentiation is impossible unless fortuitously the catheter can be passed through the existing shunt.[4] Aortic septal defects are about 1 or 2 per cent as common as open ductuses. They have been exposed at the operating table,[8] it being thought before operation that the patient actually had a patent ductus. In one patient we have been able to close such an opening.[11]

High Interventricular Septal Defect. It is worth describing a small group of patients who have high, interventricular septal defects which lie in such a position that the medial cusp of the aortic valve is incompletely supported, and hence collapses from time to time and gives aortic valve regurgitation. We have seen 12 such cases (about one to every 45 ductus patients). The murmur is most intense in the pulmonary area, but it does not have a truly continuous quality. It is more properly described as a "to-and-fro" murmur, which on occasions can be exceedingly difficult to differentiate from the continuous murmur of an open ductus. There is a marked tendency for the murmur to change in character from time to time. Patients with these high septal defects have a very low diastolic pressure (because of the aortic valve insufficiency), important A-V conduction defects by electrocardiographic tracings, and greatly increased pulsations of the aortic arch and pulmonary arteries by fluoroscopic study.

Septal Defects. Interventricular or interauricular septal defects can generally be readily differentiated from an open ductus by the fact that the murmur is more centrally located and is sharply limited to systole.

Pulmonary Stenosis. A pure pulmonary stenosis gives a murmur in the pulmonary area, but it is clearly limited to systole, is accompanied by marked right preponderance in the electrocardiograms, and has quite characteristic findings by roentgenographic study.

PROGNOSIS IN UNTREATED CASES

Whenever a ductus remains open beyond the neonatal period, the individual has a shunt which is somewhat similar to an arteriovenous fistula. The communication may be tolerated extremely well if the possessor is fortunate enough to escape superimposed infection and if the shunt is a small one so that the work of the heart is not greatly increased. In such favorable circumstances, persons have been known to live to advanced age, with little or no incapacitation, but such a happy outcome is not encountered very often. Certain hazards are apt to occur frequently in patients with an open ductus: (1) The shunt may divert so much blood from the aorta that the peripheral circulation is deficient; the individual has a retarded physical development. (This diminished arterial flow never causes mental deterioration; whenever mental retardation is seen in a ductus patient, the brain damage almost certainly is related to some other factor.) (2) The heart may increase its output, attempting to maintain the peripheral flow at a satisfactory level while simultaneously passing a large amount of blood back through the shunt; if these two things are accomplished, the heart is tremendously overworked. The individual may be well developed, but the heart will probably come to embarrassment or failure. (3) Bacterial infection may be superimposed upon the vascular abnormality, the causative organism commonly being the *Streptococcus viridans*. In patients who have been followed over sufficiently long periods of time, the incidence of this complication is probably 25 per cent. (4) There are rare complications such as aneurysmal dilatation or rupture of the ductus. The first of the above-named complications appears in childhood, whereas the others are more apt to be problems of adult life, particularly of the third and fourth decades.

While a patent ductus usually seems to be an innocuous affair in childhood, long-term observations show that commonly the outlook is serious because of the likelihood of late incapacitation and shortening of life. An excellent study of the prognosis for patients with an untreated ductus has been made by Keys and Shapiro.[13] They find that subjects who are alive at seventeen years of age with an open ductus have a subsequent life expectancy which averages only about half that of the general population.

SELECTION OF PATIENTS FOR OPERATION

Regarding the decision for or against operation, the following general policies have been developed and adopted:

Positive Indications for Operation

Certainly, there can be no disagreement with the recommendation that operation be undertaken for all children with retarded physical development which cannot be accounted for on some other basis. Likewise, it is generally agreed that cardiac fatigue or failure demands operative closure of the shunt regardless of age, so that the mechanical burden on the heart can be reduced. Operation is also desirable for those subjects—mostly in the third and fourth decades—who do not show ordinary signs of cardiac failure but who nevertheless drag about with fatigue, a reduced activity, and a definite knowledge that it is becoming increasingly difficult to carry on the job of life.

Infected Cases

Regarding the possible benefits of surgery for patients who have blood stream infection with *Streptococcus viridans*, opinion has taken several turns during the past decade. Prior to 1940 this serious malady could not be cured in more than 5 or 10 per cent of cases with the sulfonamides and other measures which were then available. In 1940 Touroff and Vesell[17] showed in a very dramatic way that such infection could be cured in about 75 per cent of the cases by surgical obliteration of the ductus, even without concomitant sulfonamide therapy. We corroborated this with 9 recoveries in 12 infected patients who were surgically treated in the pre-penicillin era. With the advent of penicillin in the mid-forties such recovery rates could be obtained, or even bettered, by penicillin therapy alone. This might seem to indicate that the infected patient should now be treated solely by penicillin, aureomycin, Chloromycetin or other antibiotics, but two important factors should be taken into account. First, it is known that subsequent attacks are not uncommon and it is possible that a second infection might come from an organism which is resistant to chemotherapy. Second, while it is possible to cure infection in a high percentage of cases by appropriate antibiotic therapy, this does not necessarily mean that the entire cardiac mechanism can be returned to normal. Patients whose infection has been dispelled are sometimes left as cardiac invalids by the scarring which remains in the heart muscle. Because infection always leaves some myocardial damage, it is highly desirable to reduce the mechanical load of the heart by surgically closing the open ductus.

It is our present opinion that: (1) Infected patients should be intensively treated by antibiotics for an appropriate length of time. If the blood stream cannot be sterilized by this alone, operation should be added during the active stage. (2) If it is possible to sterilize the blood stream by drugs alone—which can be accomplished in about four-fifths of the cases—operation can be deferred for several months. This delay in operation permits inflammatory reactions in the ductus wall to subside and thus lessens the technical difficulties of surgery. It also allows the patient to recover somewhat from the financial onslaught of an attenuated illness. It permits him to get out of the hospital for a period and to convalesce satisfactorily before undertaking a major operation. In summary, all infected cases should be treated by chemotherapy plus surgery, the latter being either early or delayed, depending upon the inadequacy or the efficacy of the drug treatment.

Asymptomatic Patients

After a consideration of the above three categories (the physically retarded youngster, the patient with cardiac failure or fatigue, and the subject with superimposed infection), one is left with a large number of patients—particularly in the childhood ages—who have no important symptomatology and who repeatedly raise the question of whether or not operation should be advised. The answer to this query depends almost entirely upon the fatality rates and the promise of a permanent ductus closure which can be offered by the surgeon. Obviously, if surgical complications or mortality rates are high in a given institution, it is preferable to leave these young asymptomatic subjects alone. However, in a large series of such patients we have been able to demonstrate that permanent closure can be assured by division of the ductus, that complications are almost nil, and that fatalities are distinctly less than 0.5 per cent. With this record, we feel fully justified in advising surgical closure of the ductus for all children and young adults, even though they are symptom-free at the moment. Without doubt, this approach will mean the subjection to operation of some individuals who admittedly might be fortunate enough to go through a long life with no important troubles from a small, open ductus. Yet when one considers the group as a whole, there can be no question about the fact that many future complications (such as cardiac fatigue and endarteritis) have been prevented by operating upon these subjects.

A few clinicians feel that it is preferable to avoid surgery for all who are asymptomatic, employing it only for those who develop complications in later years. This attitude certainly increases the surgeon's difficulties. Ductus operations in the young can be performed with relative ease, whereas those in older people give much anxiety because the cardiac reserve is reduced, the approach into the mediastinum is deeper, the regional vessels are more rigid and are much more difficult to deal with.

We are strongly impressed by the number of patients who had been entirely asymptomatic in childhood and in adolescence, but who then present themselves in middle life with symptoms which physicians would universally agree call for operative intervention. Operations on these men and women do not necessarily carry higher fatality rates but they certainly can tax the surgeon's ingenuity. A few experiences of this kind indicate that it is far wiser and easier to operate upon patients in childhood years when the cardiac reserve is greater, the operative exposure is simpler, and the regional vessels are softer, elastic, and much easier to work upon. In summary, we believe that it is good "prophylaxis," which can be obtained at a negligible mortality rate, to advise surgical closure of the ductus for all children and young adults even though they have no complaints at the moment.

Associated Cardiac Abnormalities

An associated *interventricular* or *interauricular septal defect* is not a contraindication to surgical closure of an open ductus. A ductus does not compensate for either of these anomalies; all three conditions are left-right types of shunts. Obviously, operation on a patient with an open ductus and a septal defect will not restore the cardiovascular apparatus entirely to normal, but at least the heart can be considerably improved by taking off some of its mechanical burden. We have operated upon 21 such patients, all of whom survived.

Rheumatic mitral stenosis is not a contraindication to operative closure of the ductus, provided there is no important rheumatic activity at the time operation is undertaken. Indeed, an associated rheumatic mitral stenosis is a clear-cut indication for surgical closure of the ductus, because such therapy will reduce the amount of blood which has to flow through the left side of the heart and the narrowed valve. Obviously, under these circumstances the cardiovascular apparatus cannot be made normal, but it can certainly be improved. We have operated upon 4 such individuals, all of whom survived.

The combination of *pulmonary stenosis* and a patent ductus is rare; it is not a contraindication to operation on the latter. A ductus in no way compensates for a bottleneck at the pulmonic valve (in contrast to the compensatory effects of a ductus on the tetralogy of Fallot). Operative closure of the ductus is a desirable procedure, even though it will not restore the cardiovascular apparatus to normal. We have operated upon 3 children with this combination of abnormalities; all survived. If in future years the pulmonary stenosis is of sufficient degree to produce important symptoms, the pulmonary orifice can be enlarged by the Brock technique.

Contraindications to Operation

A word of caution is necessary regarding children who have any cyanosis, and who also have the auscultatory sounds of a patent ductus arteriosus. With these findings, the ductus should never be closed surgically; either the patient is in terminal failure from a large ductus, or else there is a ductus which is acting as a compensatory mechanism for a complicated cardiovascular malformation.

Optimum Ages for Operation

A consideration of the indications for operation should include some comment regarding the ages during which it is preferable to undertake this surgery. In general, if there are pressing indications for operation such as stunting of physical growth, cardiac embarrassment, or superimposed infection, therapy should be undertaken with complete disregard for the age or size of the patient. We have operated upon an eleven-month-old baby who weighed but 13 pounds, who had marked physical retardation, and also had cardiac failure. This baby had a rapid recovery. Regarding operation on asymptomatic subjects, operation can be performed within a wide span of years. While it is quite possible to do so, there is seldom need for proposing such a step before three or four years. The surgeon still has excellent vessels to work upon until fifteen or twenty years of age, though this limit is by no means a sharp one. In short, for the elective cases, optimum ages run from three or four years up to fifteen or twenty years; the best chances for a smooth and relatively easy surgical procedure are generally provided between the ages of six and twelve.

TREATMENT

Anesthesia

Formerly we employed cyclopropane anesthesia for these cases, but since about half of our fatalities seemed to have been attributable to cardiac arrest or irregularity under this anesthetic, we have now completely abandoned cyclopropane and employ ether and oxygen as a routine choice. The anesthesia must be given with a closed system. An intralaryngeal tube should be used to insure an adequate airway at all times and to facilitate the suction-removal of any secretions from the lower respiratory tract. This gives the best chance for maintaining a quiet anesthesia and it reduces the incidence of postoperative pulmonary complications.

Surgical Approach

There are some who have employed a posterior thoracic approach, an exposure which seems to us to be unduly complicated and quite unnecessary for the average ductus case. It requires a more time-consuming exposure and closure. It certainly does not give the best view of the ductus. Its only possible superiority would be in the rare case with a huge ductus for which one might want to place a large Potts-Smith-Gibson

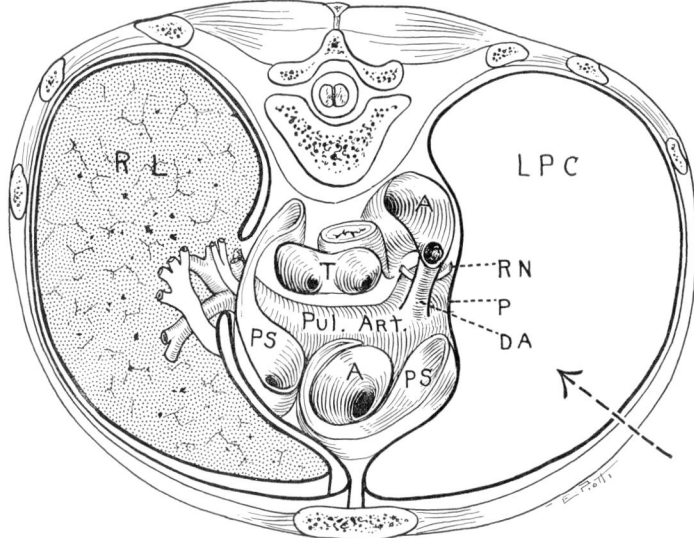

Fig. 459. Sketch of transection of human thorax at level of the fourth vertebral body, showing avenue of operative approach to patent ductus area, indicated by the arrow. The approach is through the left pleural cavity, anterolaterally. A, aorta. DA, ductus arteriosus. LPC, left pleural cavity. PS, pericardial sac. RL, right lung. T, trachea. RN, recurrent nerve.

or a Freeman clamp on the aorta to isolate the ductus area without completely occluding the aortic lumen; such an application is impossible or is awkward from the antero-lateral approach.

In all of our cases the chest opening (Fig. 459) has been through a left antero-lateral incision, made below the breast for cosmetic reasons, cutting the third intercostal muscles all the way around to the angle of the ribs. When dealing with patients with large ductuses in whom maximum exposure is desirable, the cutaneous and latissimus dorsi incisions should be carried as high in the axilla as possible and well around to the posterior axillary line. This exposure has been so satisfactory that we see little reason for changing it.

Mediastinal Dissection

When the mediastinum is entered in front of the lung root, it is essential to have a thorough knowledge of the local anatomy and of the congenital abnormalities which are apt to be encountered in this region. In so crowded a space, a single false step can lead to disaster. Probably the biggest cause of failure in this type of surgery has been the trepidity of those who feel unsure of the exact positions of the large vessels; being fearful of setting up an uncontrollable hemorrhage, they do not adequately free the ductus from its surrounding vestments. If the ductus has been incompletely liberated, it is subsequently almost impossible to work on it with any assurance of performing a satisfactory closure. Conversely, an accurate anatomic knowledge of the area will allow one to proceed rapidly and without risk, to free the ductus entirely of all its coats, to clean off the adjacent aorta, and to mobilize adequately the nearby pulmonary artery. Only by such an extensive and thorough freeing can one deal with the ductus in a proper manner.

Ductal Ligation Obsolete

In the earlier part of our work only ligation of the ductus was employed, using various types of material to accomplish this. In a series of 43 cases it was found that 80 per cent of the patients obtained a complete obliteration and a permanent closure of the shunt, 10 per cent had the ligatures cut through and some of the fistula reestablished, and the remaining 10 per cent had ligatures which were not put on tightly enough to close the vessel completely. While these over-all results might be considered satisfactory, it is obvious that they were not perfect. These observations are similar to those of Shapiro and Johnson[16] who (by personal communications with various physicians) accumulated data from 626 patients operated upon by 46 surgeons; the mortality rate in uninfected cases was 4.9 per cent and the incidence of recanalization was at least 8.7 per cent. Without doubt ligation is often a very satisfactory procedure, particularly if used on ductuses which are small and in those young patients in whom the vessels are soft and elastic. It is very risky and unsatisfactory for large ductuses and for those subjects where the vessels are firm and unyielding; under these circumstances, ligatures are very apt to cut through and either allow the fistula to reestablish itself or else by erosion lead to serious complications or even fatal hemorrhage. Blalock[2] has developed a method of "suture-ligation" which is distinctly better than all of the ligation techniques which we originally employed; it uses two encircling stitches at either end of the ductus, mattress sutures through the ductus, and an encircling tape of linen. Scott[15] has published a series of 161 closures of this type with excellent results. However, it has been widely recognized by vascular surgeons for many decades that *closure of any large artery or shunt is most satisfactorily accomplished by a complete severance of the vessel;* we believe that this fundamental principle also applies to the treatment of an open ductus. Complete division certainly seems to be the ideal method of therapy, and our experience shows that it can be accomplished without assuming a high risk.

Ductal Division Now Used Routinely

While complete severance of a ductus would seem to be fraught with dangers of uncontrollable bleeding, we have demonstrated to our own satisfaction that as a routine procedure the vessel can be cut in half and separate closures can be made of its pul-

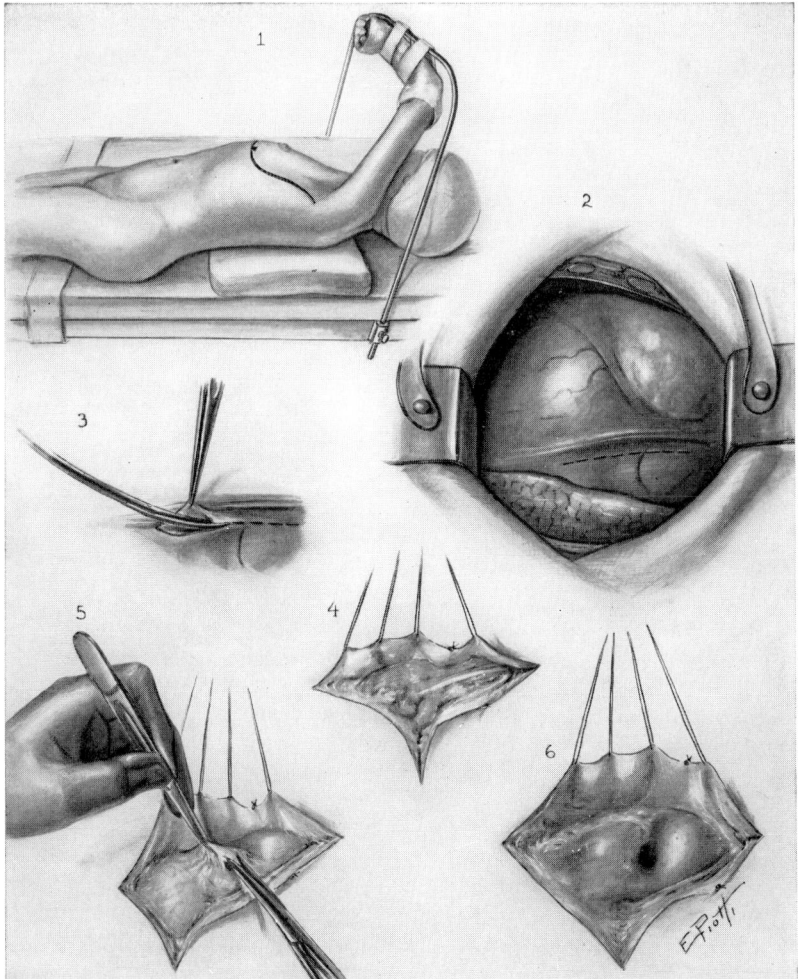

Fig. 460. Operation for complete division of a patent ductus arteriosus. 1. Position of patient on table with left side of chest and shoulder slightly elevated, and arm held up as shown. 2. Exposure through the third intercostal space, with division of the third and second costal cartilages. The third intercostal muscle has been divided well around to the angle of the rib. The phrenic nerve is a good landmark along the surface of the great vessels and heart. Behind it, along the dotted line, the parietal pleura will be opened. 3. The parietal pleura being opened posterior to the phrenic nerve. 4. The highest intercostal vein, which crosses the mediastinum, has been divided. The anterior flap of pleura has been held forward with silk retraction sutures. 5. Sharp dissection being made anteriorly between the aortic arch and pulmonary artery, anteromedial to the ductus. 6. The great vessels are coming into view after partial clearing of overlying fat and areolar tissue.

monic and aortic ends. We have now performed 568 complete divisions without the loss of a single patient from hemorrhage at the time of operation or subsequent thereto. The division technique requires a little more time and care at the operating table, yet we have found it possible to turn over a large number of these cases to assistant residents on the thoracic service who have performed a division in every instance without a single fatal hemorrhage.

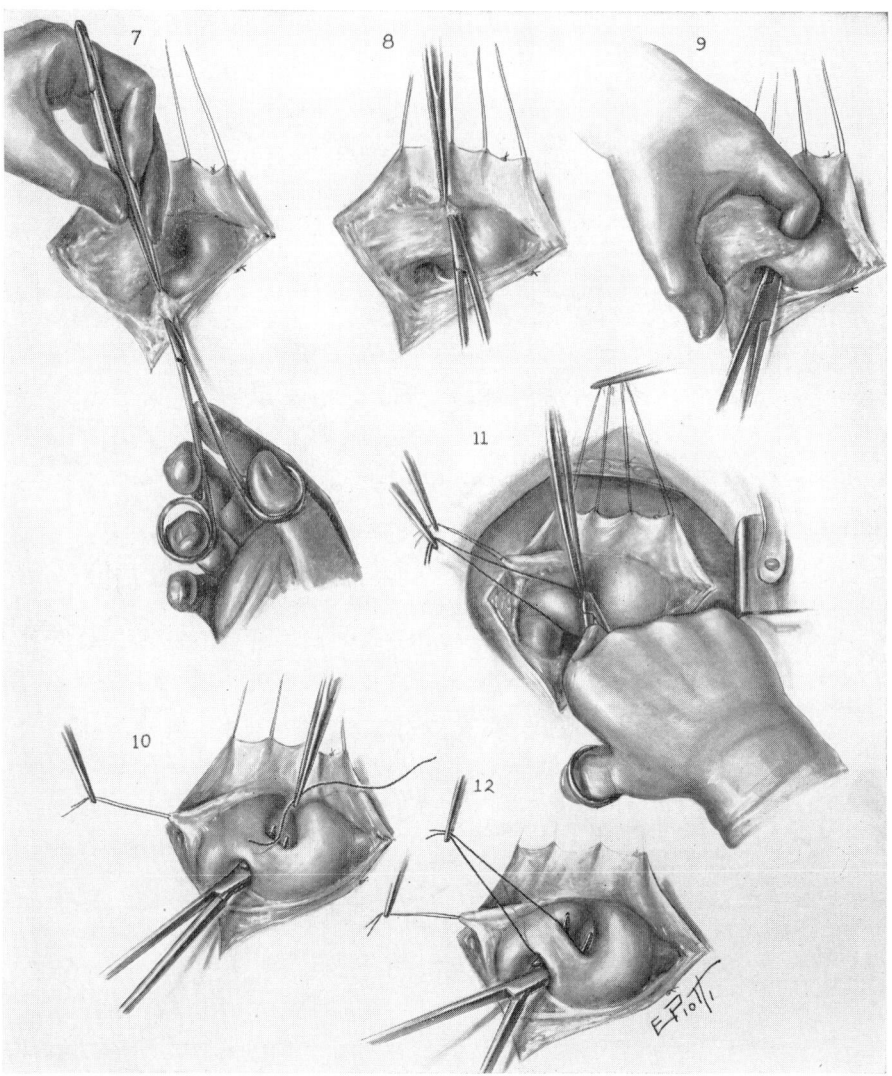

Fig. 460 (*continued*). 7. Dissection being started behind the ductus, clearing the underlying vagus nerve. 8. The vagus nerve identified. Recurrent laryngeal nerve seen coursing around behind the ductus. Further dissection being carried out medial to the ductus. 9. A right-angle clamp has been passed around behind the ductus and the tip of this is being approached bluntly with the tip of the left fore-finger inserted between the aorta and pulmonary artery. 10. The pericardial sac has been dissected upward and off of the front of the ductus and pulmonary artery, keeping the pericardial sac intact. A heavy braided silk thread is being passed around behind the ductus. 11. By means of the heavy braided silk, the ductus is pulled slightly outward so that the tissues behind and medial to it can now be adequately dissected. 12. Dissection behind the ductus has been completed, this being a most important part of the operation.

Excessively Large Shunts

We have explored (and withdrawn from) 4 patients who had enormous shunts (larger than 1.5 cm. in diameter); division seemed to be too formidable and risky; certainly any form of ligation or suture-ligation would have been ineffective and probably

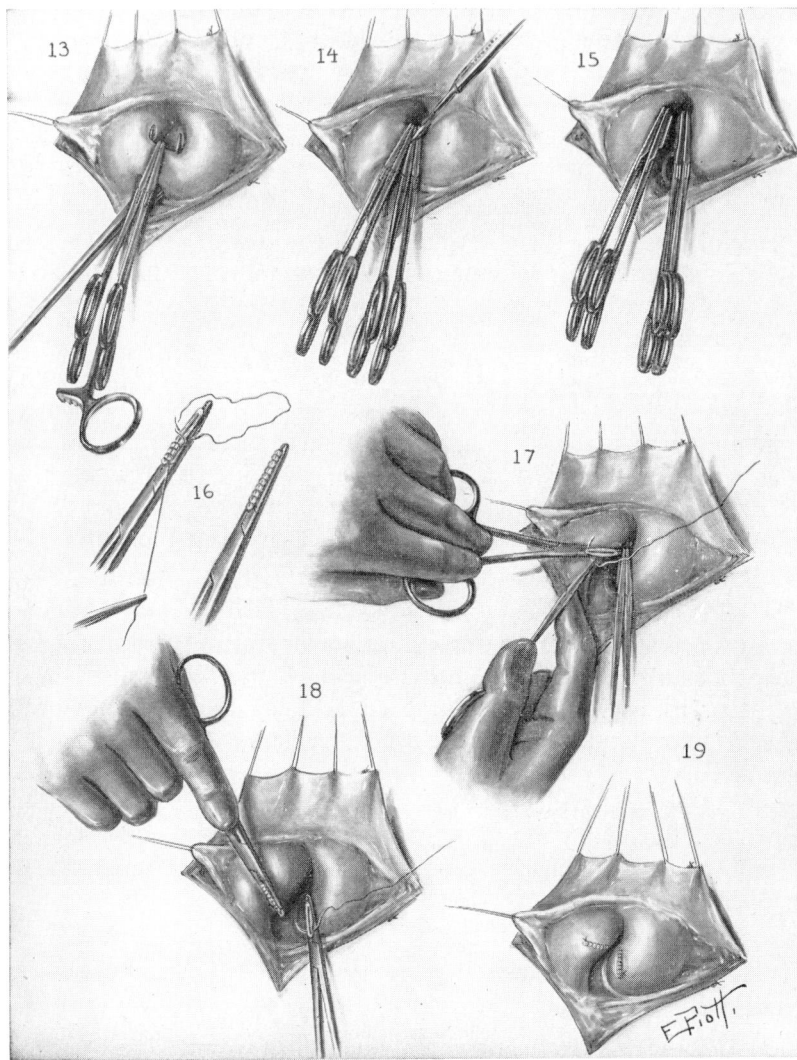

Fig. 460 (*continued*). 13. With a right-angle clamp spread behind the ductus, two hemostats are placed on the ductus. 14. Additional hemostats are placed so that four have been squeezed on to the ductus. The vessel is being cut between the two middle instruments. 15. The ductus has been completely severed, leaving two clamps on either end. 16. Enlarged view of treatment of an end of the ductus. The presenting clamp has been removed and the cuff thereby provided has been sewn over and over with a 00000 Deknatel silk stitch. 17. Closure of the pulmonary end of the ductus after removing one clamp and sewing the cuff with a silk suture. 18. The assistant pushes inward on the remaining pulmonary-end clamp, thereby giving increased room for suturing the aortic end. From the aortic end, one clamp has been removed and the tiny cuff is being closed with an over-and-over silk stitch. 19. After the closures have been completed, a pack is placed between the great vessels and the back clamps removed. After removal of the pack, the suture lines appear as shown. In only occasional cases is it necessary to place secondary stitches to bring adventitia over the suture line for reinforcement.

fatal because of vessel erosion and bleeding. For these rare shunts of great size (less than 1 per cent in our series) some special procedure must be developed, such as that suggested by Freeman and more recently by Conklin and Watkins.[3]

Thoracic Wall Anesthesia

The patient's postoperative course can be made quite comfortable by injection of a long-acting local anesthetic into the posterior portions of the upper four or five intercostal nerves while the chest is open. For the last twelve years we have routinely infiltrated Nupercaine (in oil) about these structures, producing a regional hypesthesia which lasts for a week or ten days.

Chest Closure

A very careful closure of the chest has much to do with a patient's postoperative comfort. Meticulous hemostasis minimizes the accumulation of fluid within the pleural cavity. In all cases some fluid does collect in the pleural sac, but in only a small percentage of subjects is this of sufficient degree to require postoperative tapping.

Chemotherapy

While chemotherapy is wholly unnecessary in most cases, there is some justification for using it as a routine prophylactic measure in the hope of avoiding postoperative pulmonary complications. It has long been our custom to give penicillin for twenty-four hours before operation and to continue it for four or five days thereafter.

Convalescence

Oxygen tents are not necessary during the postoperative period. If the left lung is completely expanded at the end of operation and if pleural fluid is kept at a minimum (by avoiding it or by aspirating any large collections), the respiratory apparatus is functionally satisfactory and an oxygen tent is a needless encumbrance.

Patients can be allowed out of bed on the fourth or fifth day and can be ambulatory shortly after that. Routinely they are discharged from the hospital on the eighth or ninth postoperative day. They are allowed increasing physical activity for the subsequent week or two, and ordinarily are back to complete and unrestricted activity one month after operation.

RESULTS OF SURGICAL TREATMENT

Mortality Statistics

Operation for surgical closure of a patent ductus has now become well standardized. It should seldom be followed by any serious complications; mortalities should not be more than a few per cent. In our series, 611 patients have been operated upon. Eighty-five per cent of these were under eighteen years of age; 70 per cent of them were under fourteen years. Forty-three of these had some form of ligation, an operative procedure which we now feel is obsolete; we have not ligated a ductus since 1944. Since that time, 568 patients have had complete division. In this latter group, there have been 10 fatalities, giving an over-all mortality rate of 1.7 per cent. Our series has included a considerable number of patients who had some degree of cardiac failure and also 12 who had active bacterial infection at the time of operation. In those patients who had no failure or infection prior to operation, the mortality rate has been less than 0.5 per cent.

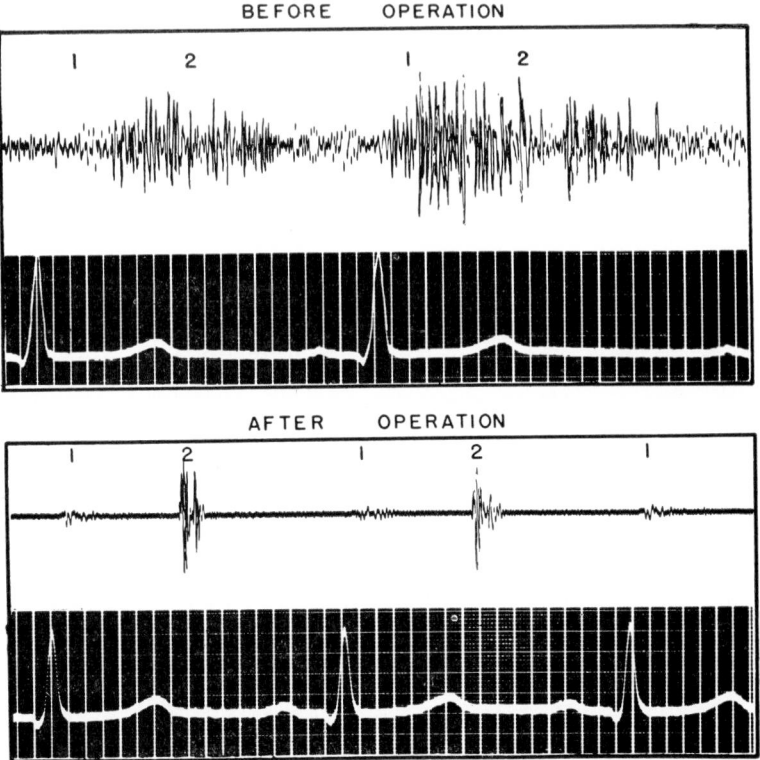

Fig. 461. Typical phonocardiograms from the third left interspace of a child with a patent ductus arteriosus, the tracing above being taken before operation, and the tracing below taken after operation. In the preoperative tracing there is a murmur which is continuous throughout the cardiac cycle. The figures 1 and 2 indicate the times when first and second heart sounds should be present. From 1 to 2 represents systole; from 2 to 1 represents diastole. There is a loud crescendo systolic murmur and there is a continuing diminuendo diastolic murmur. After operation there is only a pure first sound and second sound.

Postoperative Changes

In the surviving patients there have been certain changes which can be individually considered as follows:

The diastolic blood pressure rises immediately, the extent of rise varying with the depression which had existed prior to operation (Fig. 463).

Murmur. In all cases the continuous machinery murmur has disappeared following division of the ductus, and in more than 90 per cent of subjects no murmur of any kind can be heard after operation. In the remaining minority of cases there is a residual murmur, usually systolic in time, which in a few instances is believed to be functional, but which in 7 per cent almost certainly arises from such residual defects as a septal opening, a pure pulmonic stenosis, a bicuspid aortic valve, or a rheumatic mitral valvular deformity.

Cardiac Action. The activity of a heart strikingly diminishes after surgical closure of a ductus. This can be determined by inspection of the thorax, by noting reduced prominence in pulsations of the neck vessels, and by fluoroscopic or kymographic studies of the heart. A heart which before operation had a heaving, pounding, and forceful beat, will be found to have a postoperative activity which in comparison is quiet and much less vigorous. Diminution in cardiac action is not great if the ductus

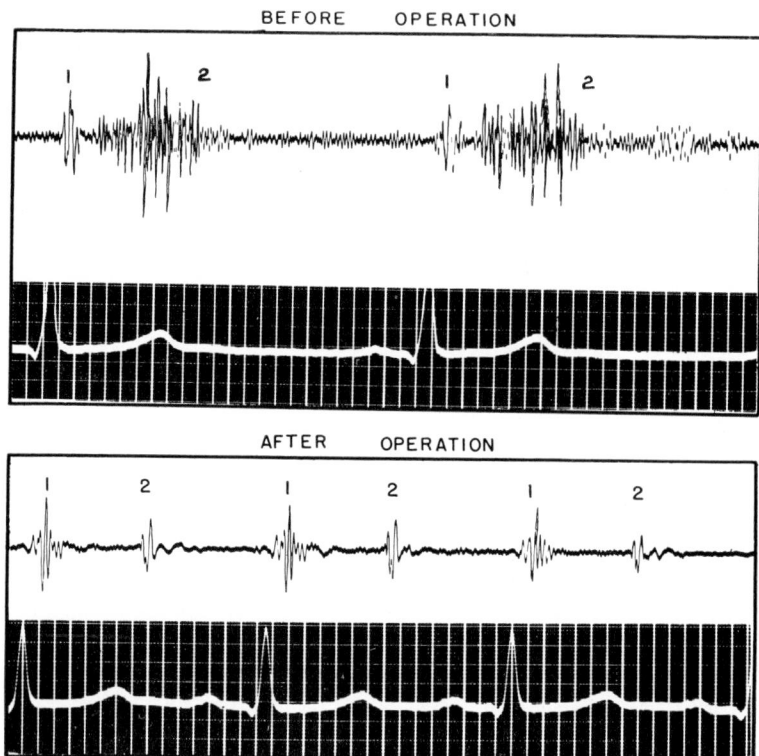

Fig. 462. Phonocardiogram from a child with a patent ductus arteriosus who had only a systolic murmur before operation. Following closure of the ductus, all murmur has disappeared.

had been a small one; in contrast, obliteration of a large shunt is followed by a decrease in forcefulness which is quite evident to both physician and patient.

Heart Size. Some change in the over-all size of the heart can generally be expected after closure of a shunt. Cardiac enlargement can be from hypertrophy or dilatation, but usually it is a combination of the two. If enlargement is due primarily to dilatation, this will disappear immediately following closure of the shunt (Fig. 464). If hypertrophy has existed, the heart apparently has little ability to shrink, but observations in a growing child will show that the thorax and other body measurements increase, whereas the heart grows very little for a period. After a year or two, a normal cardio-thoracic ratio becomes established. When a ductus shunt has been small, there is little diminution in the size of the heart following operation; when a fistula of large size has been closed, the over-all dimensions of the heart will decrease markedly. We have seen shrinkage in transverse diameters of as much as 1.5 cm.

Acceleration of Growth Rate. Individuals who had essentially normal physical development before operation show no important changes following surgery, but underweight children will generally exhibit a surprising and gratifying gain in weight during the year or two following surgery (Fig. 465). Apparently, closure of a shunt increases the peripheral flow of blood to the body and thereby improves the general physical state.

Cardiac Work. Data have been gathered relative to the changes in the circulation following closure of a patent ductus arteriosus. The figures all clearly indicate that obliteration of the shunt can greatly diminish the output of the left side of the heart (Fig. 466). Presumably, the cardiac reserve is accordingly improved.

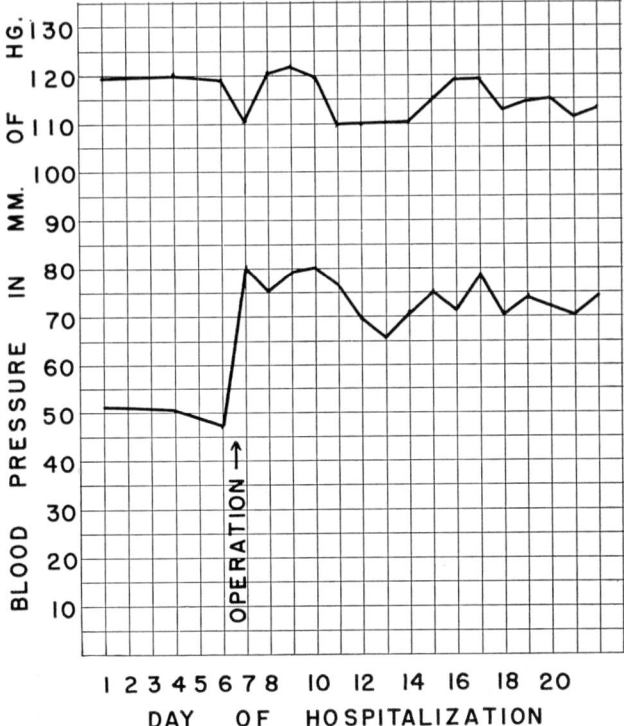

Fig. 463. Daily blood pressure chart from a ten-year-old child who had surgical closure of a patent ductus arteriosus of moderate size. Operation does not change the systolic pressure but it produces a marked rise in the diastolic pressure to normal level.

Infected Cases. In the pre-penicillin era 12 patients were operated upon during infection with *Streptococcus viridans*. Nine of these survived and were cured, whereas the others went on and eventually died of their infectious disease. Now that penicillin and chemotherapeutic agents are available, these should be used in conjunction with

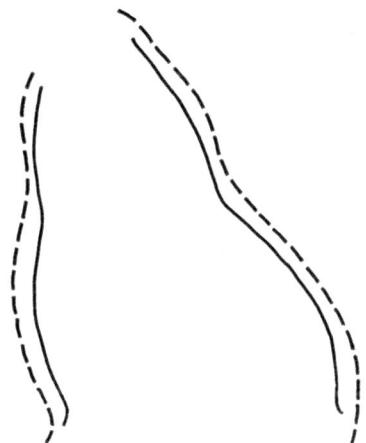

Fig. 464. Tracings taken from seven-foot roentgenograms of a heart of a nine-year-old child before surgical closure of a patent ductus (dotted line) and six weeks following operation (solid line).

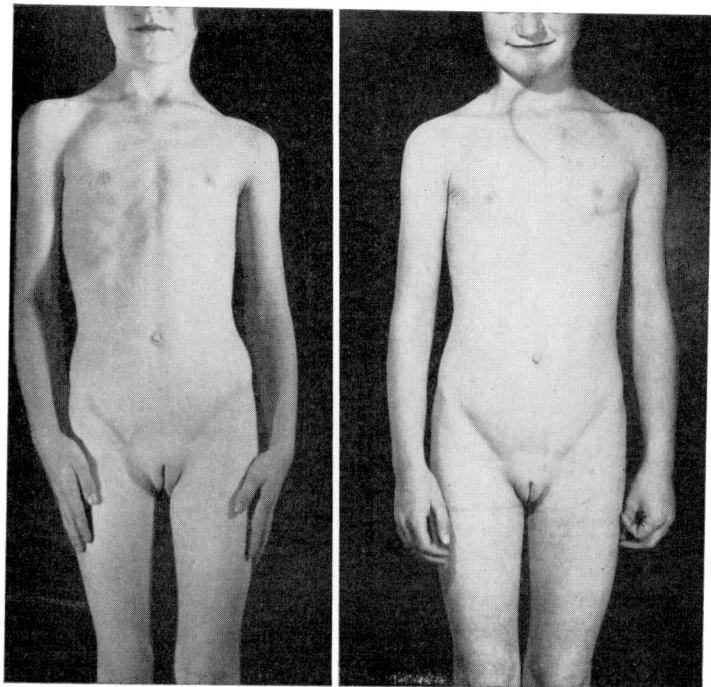

Fig. 465. Photographs of a seven-year-old girl who was operated upon for closure of a paten ductus, showing the gain in weight which is frequently observed in those children who were physically below par prior to operation. *Left,* Photograph a few days before operation. *Right,* Photograph six months following surgery.

surgery. We have employed surgery for 6 patients who already had been cured of their infection by antibiotics. All of them have survived, and it is believed that closure of the shunt was of value in their rehabilitation.

Prophylactic Operations. For those children and young adults who have been operated upon for "preventive" reasons there is general agreement that they, or their fam-

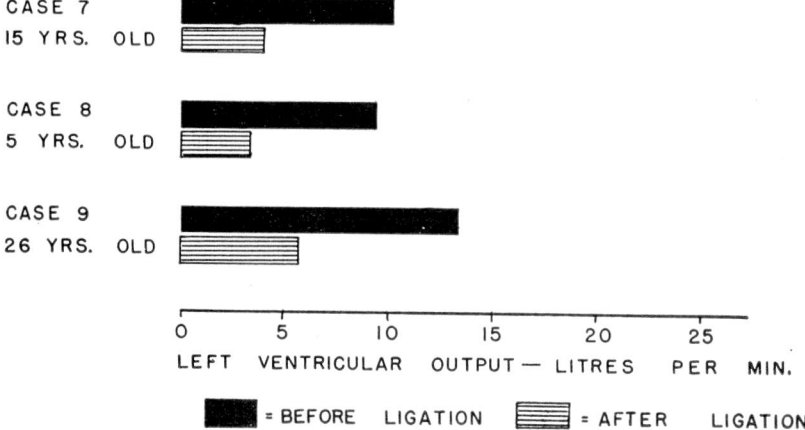

Fig. 466. Physiologic data from 3 patients, each of whom was subjected to surgical closure of a patent ductus, showing the left ventricular output of blood before and after closure the shunt. In each instance there is a marked diminution in the left ventricular output following surgical obliteration of the ductus.

ilies, feel better on psychologic grounds for having had the anomaly corrected. Many of these patients—or their families—had previously harbored a fear that something disastrous was hanging over their heads, and they were much relieved when this anxiety was removed—a consideration of no small significance.

It is quite reasonable to think that many of these individuals have been kept free of complications which might otherwise have developed. Our patients have been followed for periods as long as fifteen years after closure of open ductuses; none has yet developed bacterial endarteritis or cardiac failure. A considerable number of the females have subsequently gone through normal pregnancies and deliveries.

Studies on patients who have been operated upon leave no doubt about the benefits of closure of the congenital fistula. Experiences from many sources clearly indicate the effectiveness of surgical treatment when various complications have already developed. It is our firm conviction, based on low surgical fatality rates, that it is also advisable to operate upon all children and young adults who have an open ductus, believing that this prophylactic procedure is of considerable value in warding off cardiovascular complications in later years.

REFERENCES

1. Adams, F. H. and Forsyth, W. B.: The Effect of Surgery on the Growth of Patients with Patent Ductus Arteriosus. J. Pediat., *39:* 330, 1951.

2. Blalock, A.: Operative Closure of the Patent Ductus Arteriosus. Surg., Gynec. & Obst., *82:*113, 1946.

3. Conklin, W. S. and Watkins, E., Jr.: Use of the Potts-Smith-Gibson Clamp for Division of Patent Ductus Arteriosus. J. Thoracic Surg., *19:*361, 1950.

4. Dexter, L.: Catheterization of the Right Heart in Congenital Heart Disease. Mod. Med., *17.4:*92, 1949.

5. Donovan, M. S., Neuhauser, E. B. D. and Sosman, M. C.: The Roentgen Signs of Patent Ductus Arteriosus. A Summary of 50 Surgically Verified Cases. Am. J. Roentgenol., *50:*293, 1943.

6. Eppinger, E. C., Burwell, C. S. and Gross, R. E.: The Effects of Patent Ductus Arteriosus on the Circulation. J. Clin. Investigation, *20:*127, 1941.

7. Gasul, B. M., Fell, E. H. and Casas, R.: The Diagnosis of Aortic Septal Defect by Retrograde Aortography; Report of a Case. Circulation, *4:*251, 1951.

8. Gibson, S., Potts, W. J. and Langewisch, W. H.: Aortic-pulmonary Communication Due to Localized Congenital Defect of the Aortic Septum. Pediatrics, *6:*357, 1950.

9. Gross, R. E.: Complete Division for the Patent Ductus Arteriosus. J. Thoracic Surg., *16:*314, 1947.

10. Gross, R. E. and Longino, L. A.: The Patent Ductus Arteriosus. Observations from 412 Surgically Treated Cases. Circulation, *3:* 125, 1951.

11. Gross, R. E.: Surgical Closure of an Aortic Septal Defect. Circulation, 5:858, 1952.

12. Johnson, R. E., Wermer, P., Kuschner, M. and Cournand, A.: Intermittent Reversal of Flow in a Case of Patent Ductus Arteriosus. Circulation, *1:*1293, 1950.

13. Keys, A. and Shapiro, M. J.: Patency of the Ductus Arteriosus in Adults. Am. Heart J., *25:*158, 1943.

14. Potts, W. J., Gibson, S., Smith, S. and Riker, W. L.: Diagnosis and Surgical Treatment of Patent Ductus Arteriosus. Arch. Surg., *58:*612, 1949.

15. Scott, H. W., Jr.: Closure of the Patent Ductus by Suture-Ligation Technique. Surg., Gynec. & Obst., *90:*91, 1950.

16. Shapiro, M. J. and Johnson, E.: Results of Surgery in Patent Ductus Arteriosus. Am. Heart J., *33:*725, 1947.

17. Touroff, A. S. W. and Vesell, H.: Subacute Streptococcus Viridans Endarteritis Complicating Patent Ductus Arteriosus; Recovery Following Surgical Treatment. J.A.M.A., *115:*1270, 1940.

18. Wangensteen, O. H., Varco, R. L. and Baronofsky, I. D.: The Technique of Surgical Division of Patent Ductus Arteriosus. Surg., Gynec. & Obst., *88:*62, 1949.

CHAPTER 61

Coarctation of the Aorta

Constrictions can occur anywhere in the aorta from the mid-point of the arch down to the bifurcation of the vessel. A few are found in the abdomen or in the lower thorax, but fully 98 per cent of coarctations are located in the first part of the descending aorta, just beyond the arch (Fig. 467).

Infantile and Adult Forms

There has long been a tendency to regard coarctation of the aorta as having two somewhat distinct forms. The "infantile type" supposedly included those in which there was a very long segment of constriction, which generally involved the distal third or half of the aortic arch, was often associated with severe intracardiac abnormalities, and commonly led to death within the first year or two of life; because of this last factor the term "infantile" was affixed. In contrast, the "adult type" was supposed to have a blockage of only a short segment, was prone to involve the aorta beyond the origin of the left subclavian artery, and presumably was not accompanied by important intracardiac malformations; the prognosis was such that a large number of the subjects lived to adult years. It is now known that there is little point in classifying coarctations of the aorta into these two artificial groups, because a good deal of overlapping exists and makes such a classification useless. It is becoming clear that short aortic obstructions can be combined with intracardiac abnormalities or they can lead to cardiac decompensation or even fatality in the early months of life. Conversely, long aortic strictures can be found where there are no intracardiac anomalies and they can be found in adults. Such variations in combinations emphasize the desirability of abandoning separation into "infantile" and "adult" forms.

PROGNOSIS

The fact that most children with coarctation of the aorta do not have symptoms— indeed, in many the condition is not recognized—tends to make parents or physicians feel that coarctation is an innocuous affair. The fact that a few persons with aortic narrowing have lived to advanced old age has given a false impression that the prognosis is generally not serious. There is now increasing evidence to show that coarctation leads to crippling complications or even fatality in a very large percentage of cases.

It is not possible to obtain satisfactory estimates of the prognosis for coarctation patients by reviewing case reports from the literature, because there has been a widespread tendency to record those deaths which were caused by the abnormality and to leave unpublished those wherein exitus occurred because of some unrelated disease. A summary drawn from the existing reports would tend to show a prognosis which is more grave than is actually true.

In an effort to determine the outlook for patients with coarctation, Reifenstein, Levine, and Gross[26] reviewed postmortem material which had accumulated over several

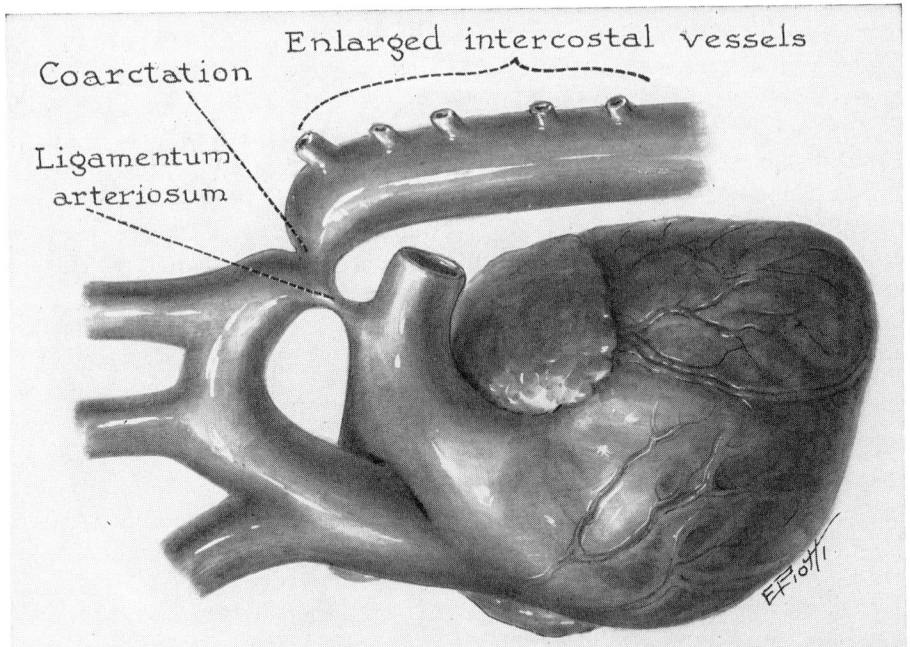

Fig. 467. Position where most coarctations of the aorta are found. They may appear in the abdomen or in the lower part of the chest, but 98 per cent of them are located in the first part of the descending aorta, generally in the region where the ligamentum arteriosum (or patent ductus) joins the aorta.

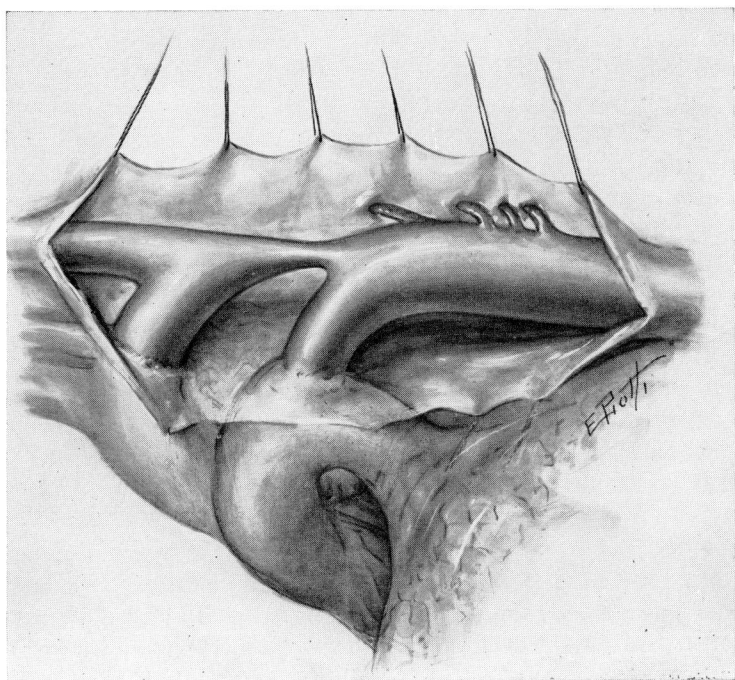

Fig. 468. Form of coarctation of the aorta, with high degree of obstruction (or complete block) beyond the aortic arch, the pulmonary artery widely communicating with the lower aortic segment. These patients have marked pulmonary hypertension, and possibly cyanosis in the lower part of the body and the legs. Fortunately this combination of abnormalities is rare; operative attack on it has been almost uniformly fatal.

decades, in the large hospitals of the Greater Boston area, and listed all cases of coarctation of the aorta. The review included those patients who had died of coarctation of the aorta or one of its complications and it likewise listed those who had succumbed to unrelated diseases and in whom the coarctation was an incidental clinical or pathologic finding. In this way it was hoped that a cross-sampling of the community could be obtained and that it would be possible to determine what was happening to people with coarctation of the aorta. From this survey certain general statements could be made which gave a fair idea of the prognosis. About 40 per cent of all the patients were found to have congenital bicuspid aortic valves. The subjects could be divided into four groups, each comprising about one quarter of the entire series.

1. About one-fourth (26 per cent) of the patients lived far into adult life—some to old age—with very little or no incapacitation. In this group, deaths were most common in the fifth decade of life, the average age at exitus being forty-seven years. Some of these patients had mild or moderate symptoms for which they had sought medical advice or help; the remainder had a lesion the presence of which was totally unsuspected until examination by a physician (for some other ailment) or until the time of autopsy. Taken as a whole, these patients had few difficulties and they enjoyed long and useful lives.

2. Approximately one-fourth (22 per cent) of the subjects died from bacterial endocarditis or aortitis, the causative organism of which was usually the *Streptococcus viridans*. Fatalities from bacterial endocarditis or aortitis occurred throughout the first five decades of life, but they were most common in the third; the average age at death was twenty-eight years. By the time death occurred, the widespread distribution of vegetations often made it difficult or impossible to determine whether the coarctation or some coexisting cardiovascular abnormality was the focus on which the bacterial invasion had started. There were a few septal defects, several examples of rheumatic valvular disease, and many congenitally deformed valves, which made one wonder whether the coarctation or the associated lesion was more responsible for promoting development of superimposed infection. Suffice it to say that *Streptococcus viridans* infections have been a real threat to those who possess an aortic obstruction; obviously this hazard is much lower today when the various antibiotic agents are available.

3. In about one-fourth (23 per cent) of the cases there was sudden death from rupture of the aorta. Such catastrophes usually occurred in the second or third decades of life, with an average at twenty-seven years. The aorta was most apt to rupture when there was preexisting hypertension, but fatal hemorrhage has been known to take place when the arterial pressures were relatively normal. Rupture occurred in the aortic arch, in the aorta just above the block, and in a considerable number of instances in the pathway below the obstruction. In some patients the rupture was sudden, and was fatal in a few moments. In others there was a dissecting aneurysm, leading to death within a few days. Fatality during pregnancy has been commented upon[13]; presumably the changes in blood-vessel connective tissue, or else the increased circulatory demands made by the gravid uterus, are factors in making the risk of rupture particularly great during pregnancy.

4. A little more than one-fourth (29 per cent) of the subjects died because of the hypertensive state. Deaths from cardiac failure were about twice as numerous as those from intracranial hemorrhage. Fatalities from congestive failure were most common in the fourth and fifth decades, the average age at death being thirty-nine years. Deaths from intracranial hemorrhage had peak incidences in the second and third decades, with an average at twenty-eight years. As has been pointed out before, pathologic studies often show that subjects with coarctation of the aorta also have congenital aneurysms of vessels

at the base of the brain; hence, the appearance of intracranial bleeding should not always be ascribed to hypertension alone. However, it is fair to assume that a congenital aneurysm of the brain is more apt to rupture when it is subjected to high arterial tensions.

Summary of Prognosis. As one summarizes material from all of the above four groups, several general statements can be made. The average age at death (including the patients who died from incidental causes) was about thirty-five years. In those who died from coarctation or one of its complications the average age at death was about thirty years. The seriousness of the prognosis can be indicated by pointing out that the general population is in excellent health between the ages of ten and thirty years and that deaths during this period are at a low ebb. In contrast, about 40 per cent of all humans with coarctation die between the ages of ten and thirty years. Sixty per cent of all coarctation patients apparently die by the fortieth year. It has become quite clear that, while some subjects may live a long and useful life with coarctation, the abnormality is one which brings great hazards to its possessor. It is this knowledge which prompts surgeons to attempt removal of aortic obstructions in the hope of bettering the outlook, particularly in alleviation of the hypertensive state.

CLINICAL PICTURE

Sex. Coarctation appears much more frequently in males than in females, the ratio being 2 to 1 in our series.

Ease of Recognition. With but rare exceptions, a coarctation of the aorta can be recognized quickly and with great accuracy by finding a few signs which are evident by physical examination. In these days, when there is an increasing tendency to employ expensive and complicated laboratory tests, it is appropriate to point out that coarctation can be accurately diagnosed—or certainly suspected—in a few moments by the intelligent use of one's finger tips, a stethoscope, and a sphygmomanometer.

Differences in Pulsation. Of greatest importance in detecting an aortic block is the disparity of pulsations (or blood pressures) in the arms and legs. Pulsations in the legs or lower part of the body are diminished or absent. If femoral pulsations appear to be reduced in intensity, the pressures in the popliteal artery should be checked with a sphygmomanometer. Normally, the systolic level in the legs is 20 to 40 mm. of mercury higher than that of the arms; in the presence of an aortic block the pressures in the legs are far below those in the upper part of the body.

Under normal circumstances the beats in the femoral and radial arteries come essentially at the same instant, but in the presence of a coarctation the femoral artery impulse starts at a slightly later time and there is a very slow rise in the pulse wave. The difference in timing can be recognized easily by simultaneous palpation of the radial and femoral arteries.

Hypertension. In young subjects with coarctation, the pressures in an arm may be normal or only slightly elevated, whereas in older persons one commonly finds a hypertension of moderate or marked degree. Certainly, in the majority of patients beyond the first decade, hypertension is the rule. The systolic pressure may be greatly elevated; the diastolic level can be raised to 80, 90, or 100 mm. of Hg, or even higher in advanced cases.

Variation with Activity. Blood pressure determinations made during an office visit or when a patient is at rest in bed do not necessarily indicate the state of affairs which exist when he is undergoing exercise or the physical strain of daily life. The value observed during rest is distinctly lower than that which exists during routine activity. It is well known that a normal person reacts to exercise by slight or moderate elevation in the blood pressure; in contrast, a patient with coarctation generally responds by extraordinary rises. The increased demands of the body raise the cardiac output, but the large quantity of blood cannot pass through an obstructed vascular bed; hence, there is a momentary and steep upswing of pressure in the head and arms.

Pressure Measurements in Both Arms. Arterial pressures should be measured in both arms because this might give a clue regarding the presence of an aortic constriction in the arch itself. Differences of 10, 20, or even 30 mm. of mercury between the two arms can be found in normal individuals and also in some who have an obstruction beyond the origin of the left subclavian artery. Conversely, a pressure which is more than 30 or 40 mm. of mercury lower in the left arm than in the right suggests that the aorta is narrowed in a place proximal to the origin of the left subclavian artery, an item of great significance when discussing the feasibility of surgery.

It is well to bear in mind that large differences in arm pressures can also be caused by an atresia (or hypoplasia) of the first part of the left subclavian artery, a finding in several of our patients. Furthermore, Stephens described a patient in whom the right subclavian artery did not originate from the innominate artery, but instead arose from the aorta below the obstruction; the arterial pressure in the right arm was distinctly lower than that in the left.

Collateral Arterial Channels. Collateral arterial circulation is by no means constantly observed, but when it is found it strongly favors the diagnosis of coarctation. It is rarely seen in children, but beyond the first decade it becomes noticeable, particularly in thin subjects in whom the vessels can be more easily detected by palpation and inspection. Pulsations may be seen and felt above and below the clavicles, in the axillae, along the intercostal spaces in the forward half of the chest, in the epigastrium, and particularly over the upper half of the back. When the establishment of collateral circulation is marked, pulsations may appear in the anterior abdominal wall and at times these can be traced downward to the inguinal regions.

Murmurs. There is nothing characteristic about the murmurs which are found. The most important thing to say about them is that they are extremely variable in form, in intensity, and in location. Most often, but by no means constantly, there is a systolic murmur of mild or moderate intensity over the precordium—especially toward the base—which is transmitted with slight diminution to the left side of the interscapular area. In some instances it may be louder in the back than it is in the front of the chest. Murmurs over the back do not, by their point of maximum loudness, give any indication of the actual level of the aortic anomaly. A few subjects with coarctation have absolutely no murmur; a small number have continuous ones.

We have little in the way of accurate information regarding the sources of murmurs which appear in patients with coarctation. It is tempting to think that blood rushing through a narrowed aortic segment sets up the vibration, but there is ample proof that this is not always true. While the systolic sound in some instances is known to come from the constricted area, in other cases it almost certainly originates from an angulated collateral channel, an associated septal defect, or a bicuspid aortic valve.

Particular attention must be paid to a diastolic murmur. If it is continuous with the systolic element, and is loudest in the pulmonary area, it may suggest the presence of a patent ductus arteriosus. If a continuous murmur is most prominent over the back, it may be indicative of blood rushing through large and tortuous collateral arteries. If the diastolic murmur is heard in the aortic area or to the left of the sternum, and especially if it has a to-and-fro quality in relation to the systolic component, one should strongly suspect aortic valve regurgitation. Slight regurgitations may not be accompanied by any depression in the diastolic level of blood pressure, but marked reflux is shown by a definite lowering.

Cardiac Failure. There is little need to comment on the picture of cardiac failure in adults which can follow longstanding hypertension. Myocardial weakness is one of the commonest causes of death in coarctation patients. In childhood, failure is rare but it does occur.

It is well to call attention to a small group of babies who apparently have cardiac embarrassment because of an aortic block. Presumably, these youngsters remain in fair health as long as a ductus arteriosus stays patent and blood can flow from the engorged upper portion of aorta back into the pulmonary bed. When the ductus closes and this relief mechanism is lost, the left ventricle must pump into a vascular system which has a high resistance and which has not yet developed many collateral channels. We have seen a dozen babies within the first year of life who had marked cardiac enlargement,

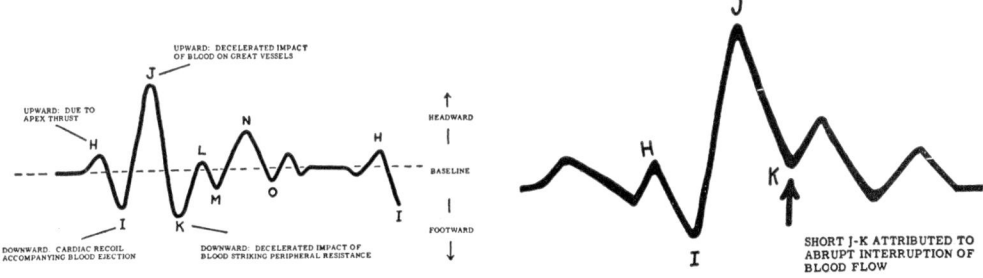

Fig. 469. Ballistocardiograms (from Brown, et al.). *Left,* Tracings from a human with a normal aorta. *Right,* Curve indicating the findings in the presence of an aortic obstruction (the downward J-K stroke is shortened).

dyspnea, cough, enlarged liver, and other signs of a failing heart. This decompensation was secondary to hypertension from an aortic block, the presence of which could be easily detected by physical signs. Two of these infants died from cardiac failure but the others could be tided over (by hospitalization, oxygen therapy, digitalization, and other measures) until they regained cardiac compensation. During this precarious interval of a month or two they probably developed collateral pathways which allowed an easier outflow of blood and which permitted the heart to regain stability.

DIAGNOSTIC AIDS

Ballistocardiogram

The diagnosis of coarctation of the aorta can apparently be made from ballisto-cardiographic tracings; there is a shortening of the J-K stroke (Fig. 469). While this phenomenon is an interesting observation, such investigation can hardly be classed as a method of practical, routine study.

Electrocardiogram

Electrocardiographic tracings are an important part of the examination, not because of help in recognition of coarctation, but because of the evidence that they might give regarding myocardial damage or of other cardiovascular anomalies. These studies are of the greatest value when attempting to determine whether a given patient will stand surgical correction of an aortic obstruction. Children generally show little or no change in electrocardiographic tracings; patients beyond childhood commonly show some degree of left axis deviation. Evidence of severe myocardial strain or bundle branch block must be regarded as strong warning that a patient might not stand operative removal of the coarctation; these are points of particular interest when dealing with subjects beyond twenty to thirty years of age.

Roentgenographic Findings

By roentgenographic study there may be certain findings in childhood to help support the diagnosis of coarctation, but in adult years the changes usually become more pronounced and clearly indicate the presence of this abnormality.

Cardiac Picture. In infancy one seldom finds more than generalized cardiac enlargement, unless there happens to be some evidence of circulatory failure. During the first eight or ten years of life there may be little variation from the normal except possibly for some left ventricular prominence and some diminution in the size of the aortic knob. In the teens and beyond, the roentgenologic findings are more numerous and more conclusive. The heart is apt to show mild or moderate increase in size, particularly of the left ventricle. Great enlargements should arouse suspicion regarding the possibility of some other abnormality, myocarditis, coexisting rheumatic disease, or cardiac failure.

Notching of Aorta. The base of the ascending arch is apt to be broadened. The left subclavian artery can usually be seen to be enlarged; it gives a widening of the left side of the superior mediastinum. The aortic knob or the distal part of the aortic arch lacks its normal prominence. Though it is by no means a constant finding, the descending aorta seems indented if the patient can be turned to an angle which will separate its shadow from the spine. In some cases it is impossible to see notching of the aorta.

Visualization of the Esophagus. With a swallow of barium in the esophagus some irregularity is usually found on its left side, below the level of the coarctation. Esophageal compression can come from that part of the aorta which is dilated just beyond the obstruction, or it can be made by enlarged right intercostal arteries which cross the mediastinum to enter the distal aorta. This configuration has been termed an "E sign" (Fig 471).

Rib Notching. Scalloping of the inferior edges of the postero-lateral portions of ribs is pathognomonic of an aortic block and compensatory collateral circulation. Such indentation is seldom found in the upper or the lower two or three ribs. It seldom appears before eight or ten years of age. It is generally present in teen-agers, and is rarely absent in adult patients.

Of rare occurrence, but of particular interest, is the case described by Bing and his associates[3] in which the left subclavian artery arose from the aorta below its block; there were few collateral channels on the left side of the chest and the rib notchings were confined to the right side. In this same category is the case of Stephens in which the right subclavian artery arose from the aorta below the obstruction; the rib notches were found only on the left side of the chest. We have seen a similar roentgenologic picture on a different basis in a twelve-year-old girl in whom the first portion of the left subclavian artery was atretic; chest film showed rib notches which were distinctly more marked on the right than on the left.

Though exceedingly rare, coarctation may appear in the lower portion of the thorax, or even in the abdominal aorta. Under these circumstances it is evident that the aortic knob would be normal in appearance and that the collateral channels should be over the abdomen and lower chest; rib notches appear only on the lowermost ribs.

Angiocardiography

Further information regarding the exact position of the stricture, the length of it, and allied data, are obtainable by angiocardiographic means. The dye can be injected

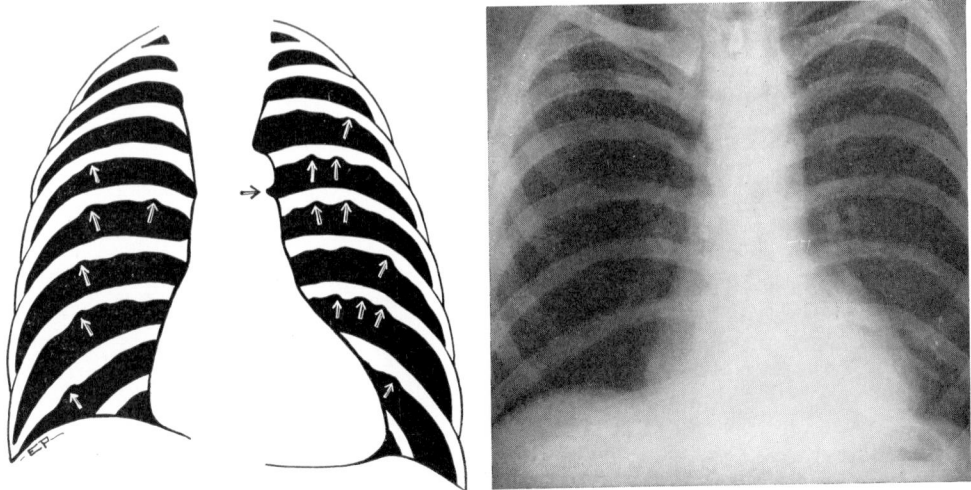

Fig. 470. Roentgenographic changes of patients with aortic obstruction. These might not be found before eight or ten years of age; they are nearly always seen in adults. *Left*, Sketch showing a notch in the descending aorta and also the multiple notches on the posterior-inferior portion of ribs which have been made by dilated, tortuous, intercostal arteries. *Right*, Film from a twelve-year-old child showing serrations along the inferior borders of some of the ribs.

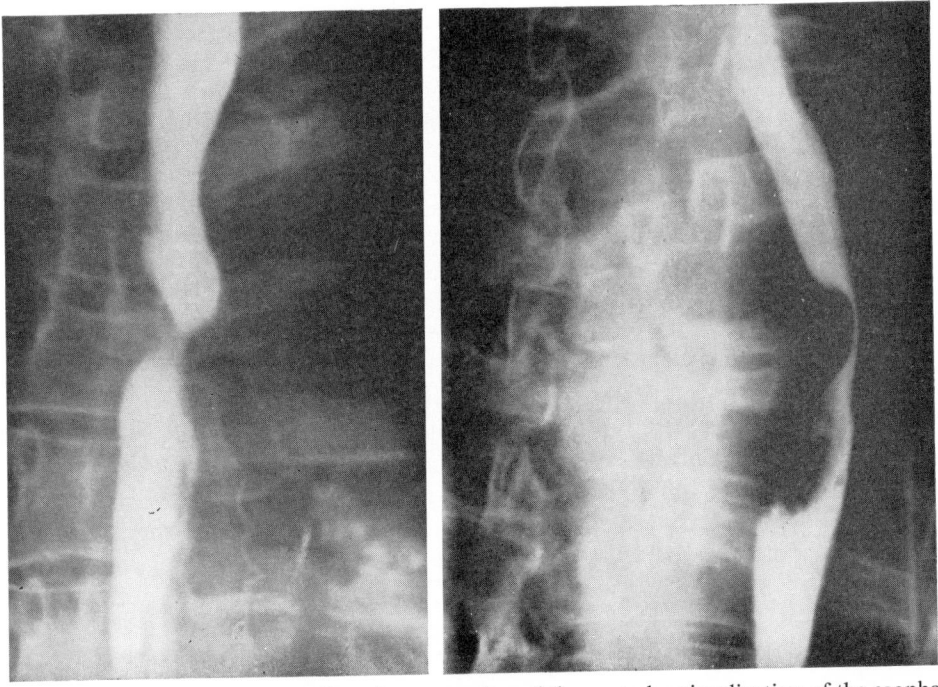

Fig. 471. Roentgenographic findings in coarctation of the aorta by visualization of the esophagus. *Left*, Showing the indentations (so-called "E sign") on the left side of the esophagus, caused by dilatation of the aorta beyond its block and also by large right intercostal arteries which come into the aorta below its constriction. *Right*, Lateral roentgenogram (from an adult) showing great indentations on the posterior aspect of the esophagus, from tremendously enlarged right intercostal arteries which enter the aorta below its constriction.

either by the intravenous route or in a retro-arterial manner. Seventy per cent Diodrast, if injected quickly into a vein, will often remain in sufficient concentration through the circulation so that the aortic arch and its branches can be seen in serial films (Fig. 472). All too often, the dye becomes diluted and does not show the great arteries very well. Another technique is that in which visualization is obtained by introducing a polyethylene catheter into an artery of the left arm, threading it back through the left subclavian artery into the aorta, at which time the injection is made. Burford and Carson[8]

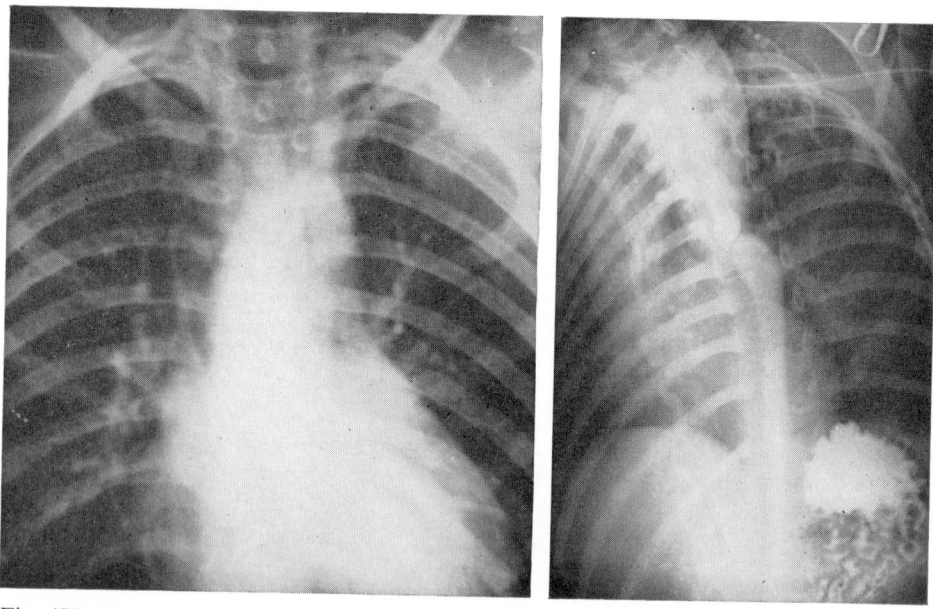

Fig. 472. Visualization of aortic obstruction by Diodrast. *Left*, From a six-year-old girl, the dye having been injected intravenously. *Right*, From a child, the opaque material having been injected in a retrograde manner on the arterial side.

and more recently Freeman et al.[11] have obtained excellent pictures of the vessels by injecting Diodrast down a neck artery, preferably the left common carotid, while temporarily obstructing the artery above the point of injection.

On many occasions I have been disappointed or have been misled by angiocardiography for study of coarctation patients. At times the dye would show the upper end of the narrowed area but did not give information regarding the length of the stricture. In other cases, when there was a complete aortic block, nothing was learned about the segment of aorta below it. Presumably, angiocardiography should be of assistance in deciding which cases are suitable for surgery and which are not, but often this is not so. This has been especially true in older patients when visualization might show an arrangement of vessels which suggested that removal of the constricted area would be feasible; when the chest is opened the vessels might be found to be rigid or fixed and surgical attack has to be abandoned.

Angiocardiography is not an essential part of a routine work-up, but it can be of value in those cases in which some special interest is aroused by unusual or inexplicable physical findings. Its greatest usefulness is probably in those patients who have an aortic block (by physical examination) but who have no "E sign" on the esophagus and no notching on the ribs; they might have either a coarctation or a hypoplasia of the entire aorta; visualization of the aorta should settle the differential point.

SELECTION OF CASES FOR SURGERY

It is our belief that almost all patients with coarctation should be operated upon at some appropriate time, provided there are no serious contraindications. Statistics now show that the mortality rates of operation can be kept reasonably low. It therefore seems best to accept these risks, which are almost certainly lower than those of letting the patient go without therapy. In an occasional case it might be wise to defer surgery if the blood pressure is at relatively safe levels. However, it is well to remember that while a child may show only slightly elevated pressures, important hypertension can appear subsequently in the teens or in adult life.

There are several *contraindications* to operation; certain coexisting conditions have been found to enormously increase operative risks. Rheumatic mitral disease of serious degree, aortic valve regurgitation of serious degree (diastolic murmur of more than grade 3 intensity, or a diastolic pressure which is appreciably lowered), serious conduction bundle defects (by EKG) and advanced myocardial damage (by clinical picture or EKG) are all contraindications to surgical attack on a coarctation.

Many persons with coarctation have congenital bicuspid aortic valves with no regurgitation or only mild leakage (grade 1 to 3 diastolic murmur, no important depression of the diastolic pressure). These persons can be operated upon with no serious increase in the risks of surgery.

The optimum ages for operation lie between ten and eighteen years. In this range the aorta is large enough to work upon with facility, has little or no degenerative change, and an anastomosis can generally be made which is sizable and satisfactory. The lumen will be large enough to carry the patient along through adult life.

Beyond eighteen to twenty years, patients begin to present conditions which greatly increase the difficulties of operation. The chest is larger, the exposure is more difficult, the aorta is more inelastic, and a higher number of aneurysms are found in the distal aortic segment or one of its connecting intercostal arteries. These and other factors make the procedures more troublesome for the surgeon and also less promising for establishing a satisfactory aortic pathway for the patient. The various difficulties are more apt to be encountered in men; in contrast, women have vessels which are softer, more elastic, and easier to work upon.

Frequently babies, in the first few months of life, have impressive symptoms and evidence of cardiovascular embarrassment from a coarctation of the aorta; in some there is a fatality. If these patients get beyond the first year, they are then apt to go through childhood without too much difficulty. This poses the question whether or not the baby who is having cardiac troubles should be operated upon. It has generally been our policy to advise against operation in this group because it appears that the vast majority of these infants can be tided over their period of embarrassment by medical means, beyond which time they do reasonably well; we believe that their best chance for a satisfactory operation will come between eight and twelve years of age. We have steered away from surgery in the infant because, while it is technically possible to work upon the tiny aorta and give it a lumen which is of normal caliber for this size of patient, there is no assurance that the growth of the anastomotic site will keep pace with that of the individual. From laboratory observations on aortic anastomoses in growing pigs, it has been found that it is possible for the lumen to enlarge reasonably well with the increase in size of the growing animal, but in some instances it lags behind somewhat. Hence, in a human baby, we generally prefer to carry along with treatment by medical means, and then perform aortic resection and anastomosis later in childhood when there is a more reasonable promise that the pathway will be large enough to be adequate during adult life. That it is possible to surgically treat coarctation in an infant has been shown by Kirklin, et al.[22] Therefore, if medical means do not seem to be sufficient to control cardiac failure in a baby, surgery can be undertaken as the indications require.

There is no definite upper age limit beyond which it is advisable to avoid surgical removal of a coarctation. However, beyond the ages of thirty or thirty-five one should be reasonably sure that the myocardium is in fairly good condition, a point which can be judged by the patient's tolerance for exercise and by the electrocardiographic tracings.

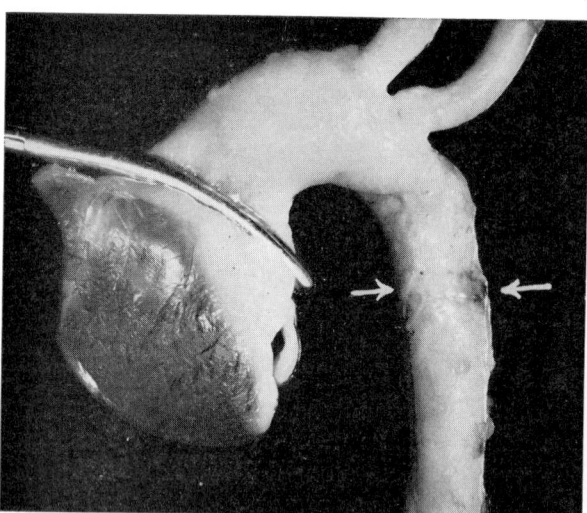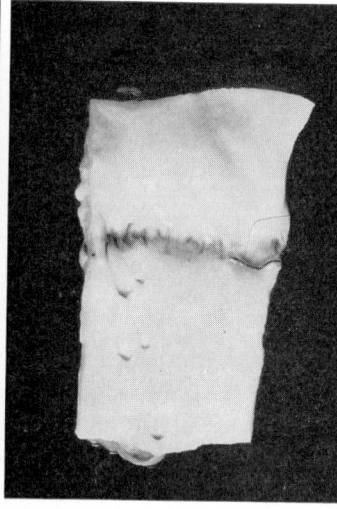

Fig. 473. Experimental division of the thoracic aorta (in a dog) followed by end-to-end anastomosis, showing the excellent healing in a vessel of this size. *Left*, Photograph of a specimen from a dog sacrificed three months after aortic suture. *Right*, The aorta opened to show the interior. The silk sutures are being covered over by endothelium which eventually gives the interior of the anastomotic line a smooth surface.

SURGICAL TREATMENT

Sympathectomy. We do not believe that sympathectomy is of any value in the treatment of hypertension which is on the basis of coarctation.

Use of the Left Subclavian Artery. Blalock and Park[4] described a form of treatment for coarctation by severing the left subclavian artery high in the chest and turning it downward for union to the segment of aorta which is distal to the obstruction. The subclavian in these patients is often of very large size, and in some instances approaches the diameter of the aortic arch, suggesting that it should provide an excellent pathway if properly joined to the distal aorta. However, there are two drawbacks to such an undertaking: (1) The severance of a subclavian artery cuts off a large number of collateral channels, the loss of which is not inconsequential. (2) The base of a subclavian artery is sometimes semi-rigid, so that attempts to turn the vessel downward result in a kinking which greatly reduces the effective size of its lumen. While the subclavian operations have given a few good results in relief of hypertension, on the whole they are very disappointing; we have abandoned them completely.

Excision of Coarctation. Primary Anastomosis

The ideal method of therapy—feasible in most instances—is excision of the coarctation and reconstruction of the pathway by bringing together the remaining ends of the aortic tube. The steps in accomplishment of these are shown in Figure 475. Technical points and general principles are well worth stressing here.

Preparation for Transfusion. Blood loss is apt to be high in these operations. The chest wall is almost always exceedingly vascular; in spite of the fact that a very large number of vessels are clamped and ligated, bleeding is considerable. It is necessary to be prepared ahead of time for constant infusion of blood during operation to com-

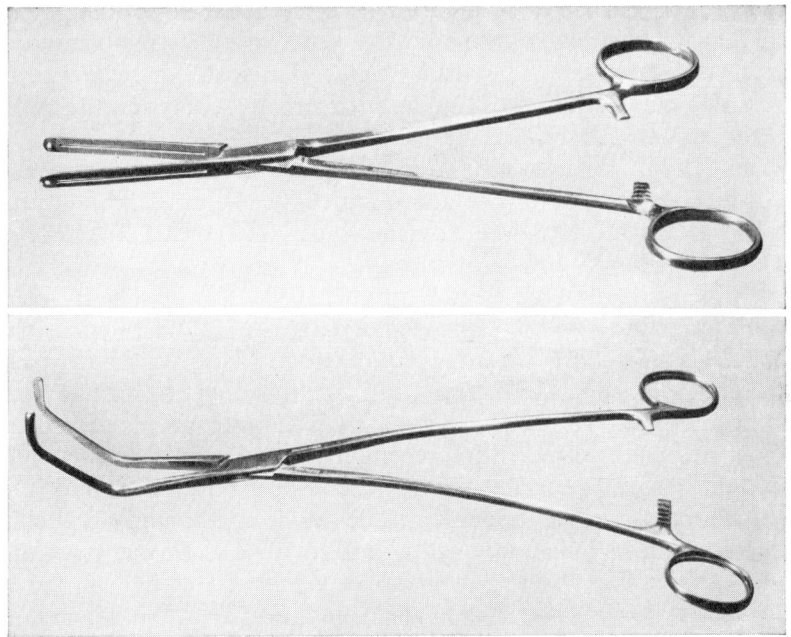

Fig. 474. Clamps used for occluding the aorta while removing coarctations from human patients. *Above,* A clamp 9 inches in length which is used on the aorta below its obstruction (a somewhat shorter clamp is used for children under six to seven years of age). The jaws and the handle have a good resiliency and therefore will not crush the aorta. The jaws have sufficient roughness of internal surface so they will not slip on the aorta. *Below,* A Satinsky (porto-caval) clamp which has been revamped (by slightly bending the tips of the jaws so that they will appropriately grasp a vessel the size and thickness of the aorta). This clamp is found to be extremely useful for applications high on the aortic arch (Fig. 478), thus allowing anastomoses to be made directly to the undersurface of the aortic arch.

pensate for this deficit. For small children, at least 1000 cc. of blood should be matched before operation. For large children or adults 2000 to 3000, or preferably 4000 cc. should be on hand.

A large cannula, or polyethylene catheter, must always be inserted in an ankle vein before beginning the thoracotomy. Through this, blood can be injected quickly and surely during any emergency.

It is always our custom to give throughout operation an infusion of 10 per cent glucose in water intravenously, which can be administered through an intravenous needle inserted into the back of the left hand. (Glucose should not be given through the ankle cannula, for fear of gumming or clogging it.)

Vascularity of Chest Wall. Transecting the subcutaneous tissues and muscles of the chest wall can be a bloody undertaking. The older and the larger the subject, the greater in size and number are the collateral channels. It can be very time-consuming to identify and doubly ligate all of these before severing them, yet a dry field must be obtained.

This stage of the operation might entail the loss of a considerable amount of blood; for compensation, appropriate amounts of blood should be given intravenously to keep the patient in a stable state.

Exposure. To give one's self the best chance to work on the aorta—which in some cases is exceedingly difficult anyway—a wide-open exposure is of considerable help. There are some surgeons who have employed only a long wound through the fourth interspace or throughout the bed of the fourth or fifth rib (after removing the same subperiosteally). We believe these to be inadequate, or certainly not optimum. A T-shaped wound in the bony cage gives an ideal view; we use it routinely in all cases. The fourth interspace is opened throughout its entire length, with posterior severance of two ribs above this and two below (in large subjects three ribs are always cut below).

Safest Progression in Liberating Aorta. In mobilizing the aorta, it is a very sound principle to avoid at first those regions which are apt to be dangerous or difficult to deal with; instead, the easiest parts of the dissection should be done initially. In this way, as one approaches the most risky areas (the upper intercostals, the coarctation, the ligamentum arteriosum) any injury or bleeding can be cared for quickly because the regional vessels have already been freed from their beds. Conversely, if one attacks the most vulnerable parts first—and sets up a hemorrhage—it is almost impossible to handle the catastrophe. Therefore, it is good procedure to start work on the various vessels by freeing up the entire left subclavian artery, carrying this down to include somewhat the anterior and posterior surfaces of the distal arch. Then attention is turned to the aorta *below* the upper two or three sets of intercostal arteries. Down at this low site, it is not difficult or too dangerous to circumvent the aorta and get a tape around it. From here the dissection can be carried up underneath the aorta, dividing any bronchial arteries. By tapes, the aorta can be pulled up slightly into the field and away from the vertebral column, which dislocation will aid in identifying and stretching out the upper thin intercostal arteries which are now freed. The coarctation area, the ligamentum arteriosum, and the under surface of the aortic arch are then cleared.

Saving Intercostal Arteries. In some cases it is necessary to doubly ligate and divide one or two sets of intercostal arteries if they come into the aorta very close below a coarctation. To get all the coarctation cut out, and in addition give enough cuff for making an anastomosis, it is occasionally essential to divide those intercostals which are close by. However, in the vast majority of cases the thin intercostal arteries can be raised from their beds and can be temporarily occluded by small serrefine clamps without hampering too much the subsequent stages of operation; in this way a maximum amount of the collateral circulation can be spared. However, it is important to emphasize that it is pointless to save intercostals if doing so compromises the establishment of a good anastomosis. The primary objective should be to make a first-rate anastomosis of full aortic size, even though some collaterals might have to be sacrificed to attain this.

Removal of Sufficient Aortic Tissue. It is important to emphasize that if these operations are going to prove successful in the relief of hypertension, it is necessary to remove *all* of the coarctation. Under the stress of operation it is quite tempting for the surgeon to cut away only the more-narrowed part of the constricted area, because he is fearful that more radical excision would lead to difficulties in approximation of the remaining aortic ends. Such a compromise is very apt to be followed by incomplete relief of hypertension. To obtain the best possible results, every effort must be made to remove *all* of the constriction and to establish a pathway which is fully the diameter of the aortic arch.

Form of Anastomosis. In bringing remaining ends of aorta together, it is wrong to attempt an anatomic repair of intima to intima, media to media, adventitia to adventitia.

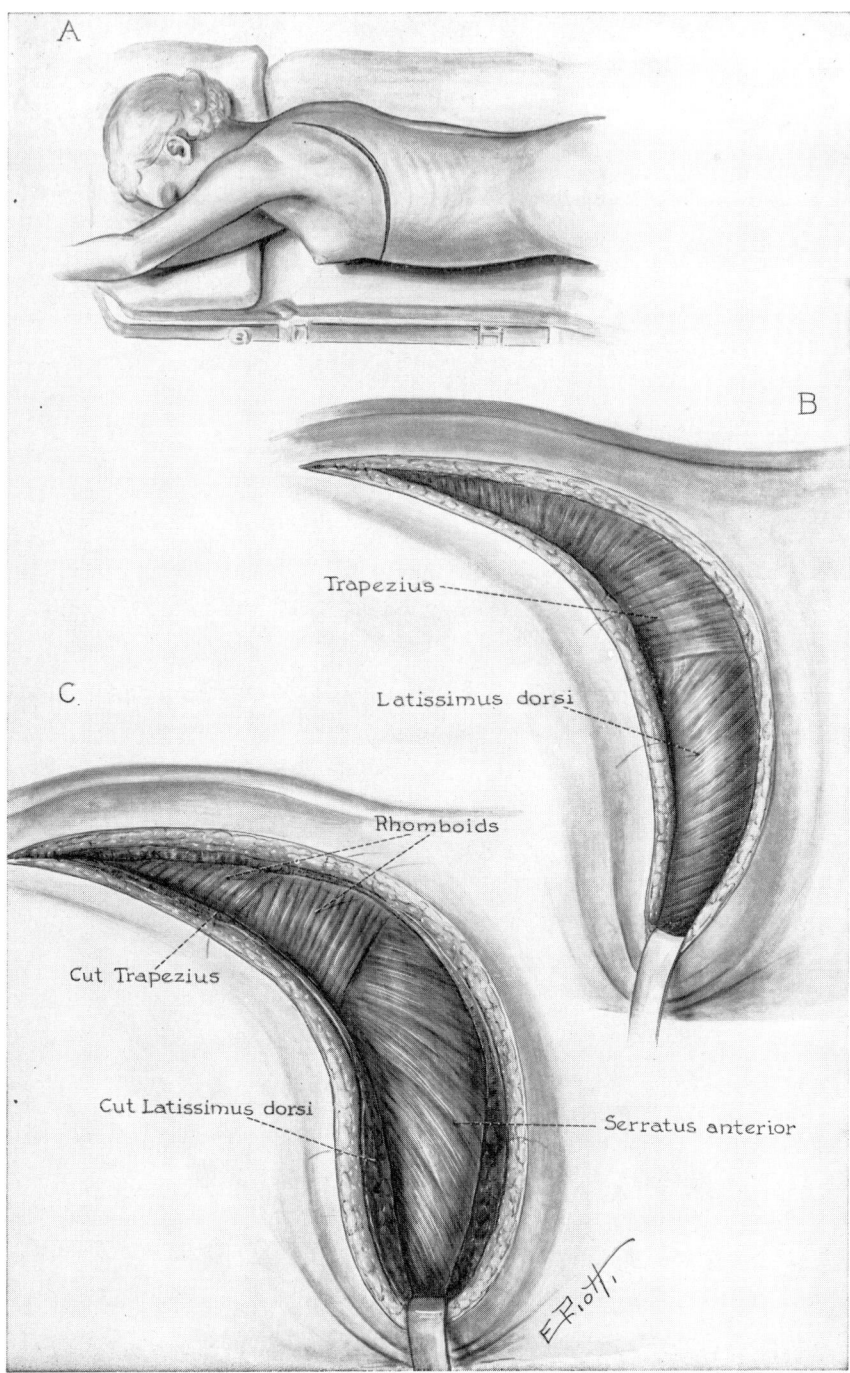

Fig. 475. Technique of mobilization of aorta and resection of a coarctation, followed by direct anastomosis. A, Position of patient on table, showing extent of the cutaneous incision medial to and below the scapula. To give adequate exposure it must run up almost to the shoulder and must extend across to the nipple line. B, The great muscles of the chest exposed. To minimize the extent of post-operative muscle atrophy, incision through the trapezius and latissimus dorsi should be made as far medial and inferior as possible. C, The next layer of muscles exposed. To minimize postoperative muscle atrophy, the rhomboids should be severed as far laterally and near the scapula as possible.

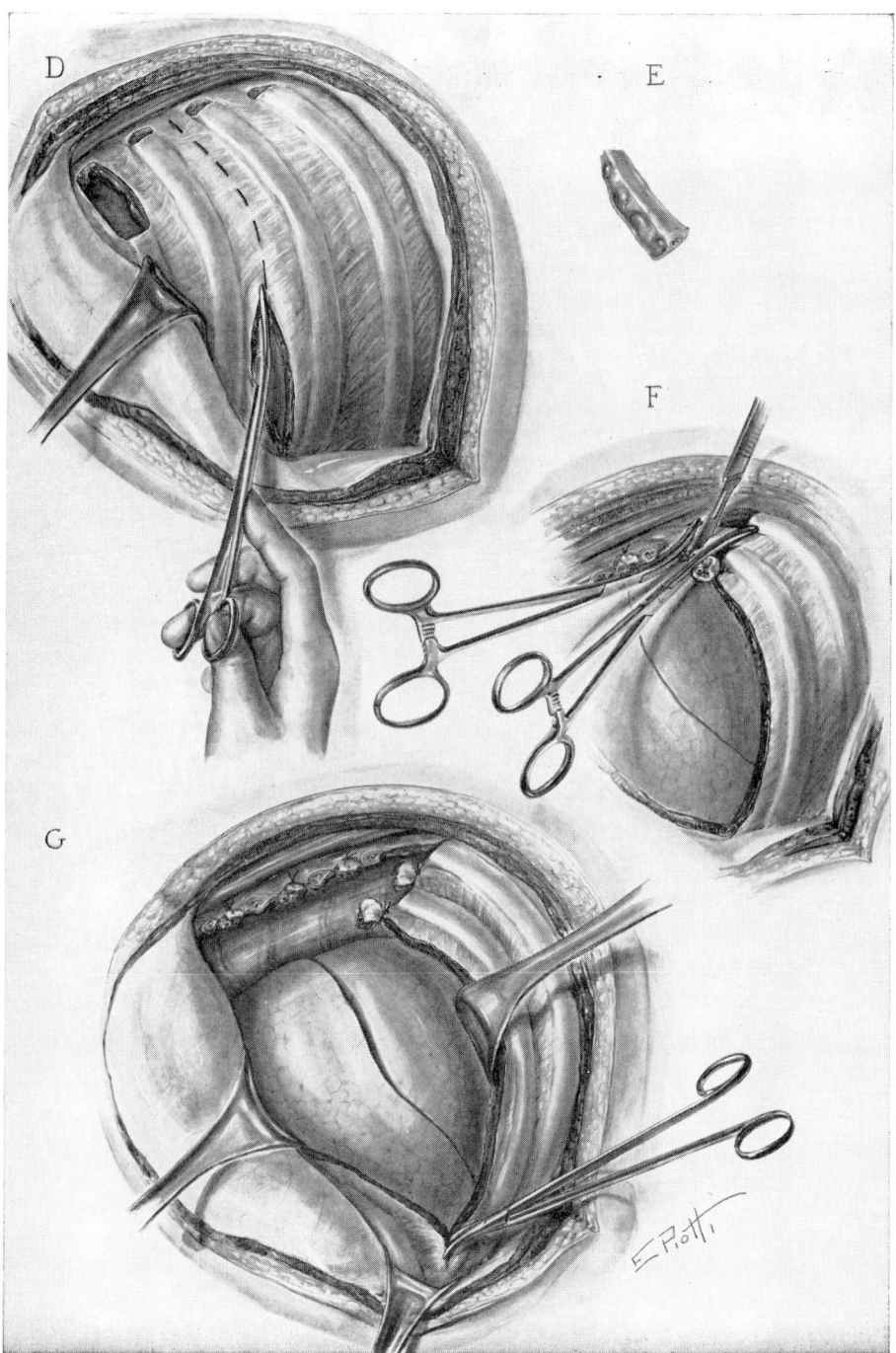

Fig. 475 (*continued*). D, External muscles of chest all divided. A short segment of the third rib, about 1 inch in length, removed. Fourth, fifth, and sixth ribs cut as far posteriorly as possible (in large subjects and in all adults the seventh rib is likewise divided). Incision being made throughout the length of the fourth interspace. E, Segment removed from the third rib. This will be saved for making four rib pegs for intramedullary struts of the lower four ribs when closing the chest. F, Division of intercostal muscle bundles. Usually one bundle above the transverse part of the wound and two bundles below it must be divided. Sometimes in very large subjects more bundles must be severed. G, Muscle bundles divided posteriorly. The incision in the fourth interspace is being continued around to (but not injuring) the internal mammary artery. This is very important in permitting the wound to open up properly.

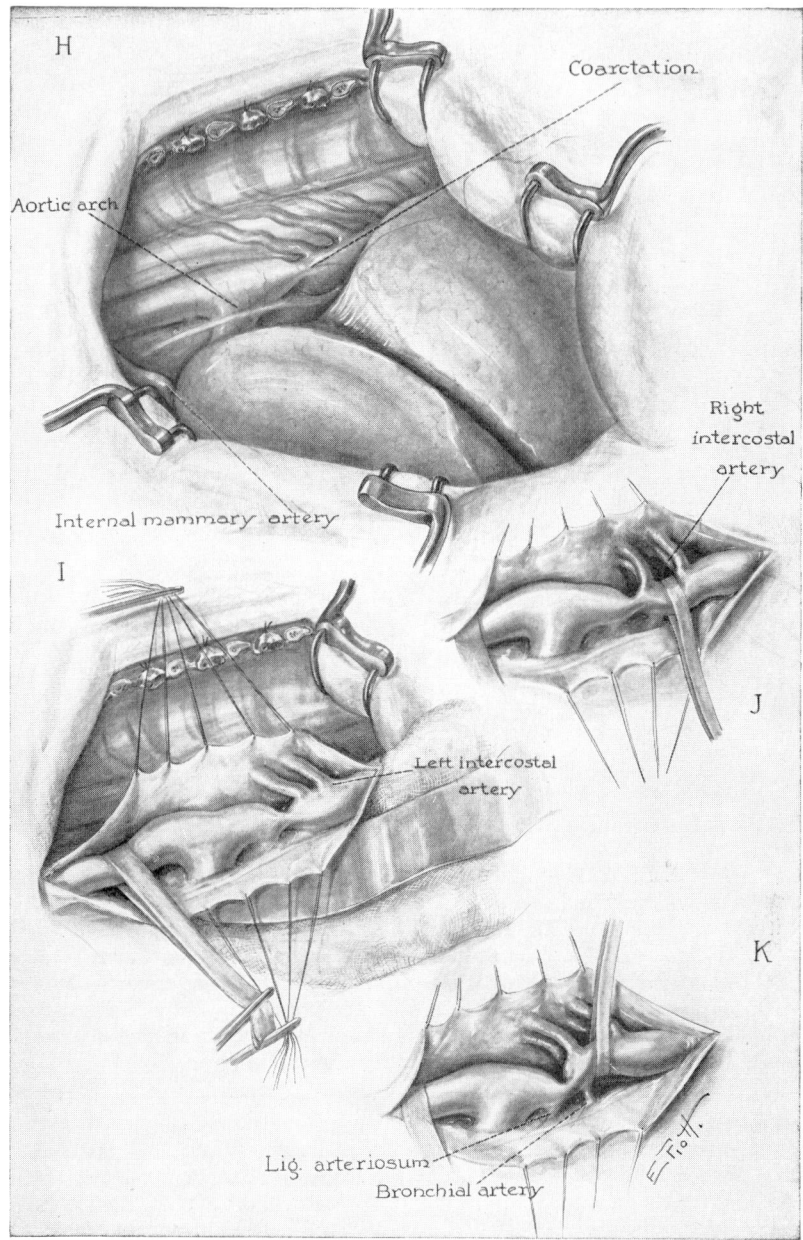

Fig. 475 (*continued*). H, Wound widely spread open and held with two self-retaining retractors, giving an excellent view of the interior of the chest. The lung collapses away. The terminal portion of the aortic arch, the descending aorta, the coarctation, and the collateral vessels can be seen. These are all overlain with the parietal pleura. I, Parietal pleura opened and dissected away from aorta and regional vessels. To save these flaps, they are held backward and forward with silk sutures. The very thin and enlarged intercostal arteries are easily damaged and must be treated very delicately. Mobilization of the great vessels begun by raising the left subclavian artery from its bed and placing a tape around it. J, Mobilization of the aorta beyond the coarctation, passing a tape around it for handling the structure. Generally, it is best to begin this mobilization at a point two or three intercostals below what is shown here; farther down, the intercostals are smaller and there is less chance of damage as the initial tape is being run around the aorta. K, Continuing mobilization of aorta by raising it from its bed and bringing into view the structures underneath it.

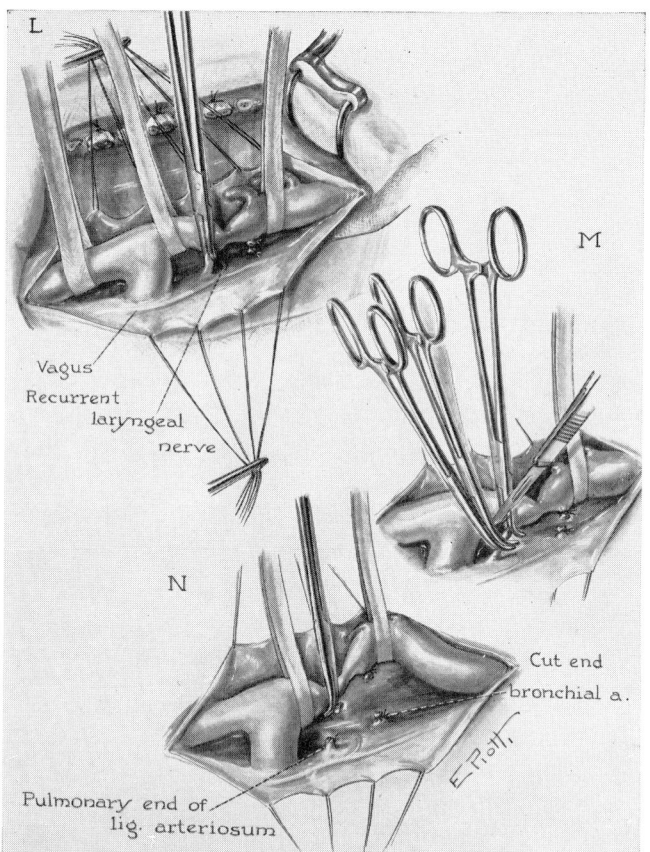

Fig. 475 (*continued*). L, Wide mobilization of the aorta has been accomplished. The bronchial artery has been doubly ligated and divided. With great care the recurrent laryngeal nerve is pushed away so that it will not be injured. The ligamentum arteriosum (or a patent ductus arteriosus) has a right-angle clamp on its aortic end. M, Ligamentum arteriosum (or patent ductus) suitably clamped at both ends, following which the structure is divided. N, Ligamentum arteriosum completely divided. Before removing the lower clamp from the ligament, the presenting end is always sewed over-and-over with a silk stitch because there is frequently a lumen in this portion of the structure. Here the pulmonary end of the ligament has been closed and the clamps removed.

(*Continued from p. 845*)

clamps are rotated toward the front of the patient and held by an assistant, who gently and constantly holds the clamps in such a manner that the ends of the aorta are brought together so that the suturing can be done without the slightest tension. The suture is begun on the deepest part of the aorta. All of the sutures are mattress stitches of 00000 Deknatel silk (on a straight needle). They include entire thickness of the wall, turning the ends of the aorta outward and bringing intima to intima. R, The function on the posterior part of the aorta has been completed. The clamps have now been rotated toward the patient's back, the assistant having gone around the table to hold these clamps. The operator continues the anastomosis as he stands to the front of the patient. The anastomosis is being continued anteriorly with the interrupted mattress stitches of silk, turning the aortic ends outwards. S, The anastomosis has been completed. The lower clamp is always removed first, so that blood can come back into the anastomotic area and test it under low pressure. If there are any serious leaks, they are quickly closed with additional sutures as necessary. T, The upper clamp has been *slowly* removed (over a period of two or three minutes). The union is water-tight. A lumen fully the size of the aortic arch has been made at the anastomosis. The flaps of pleura will now be accurately closed over the aorta, leaving a small opening 1 to 2 cm. in length at the lower end so that any fluid can escape into the pleural cavity.

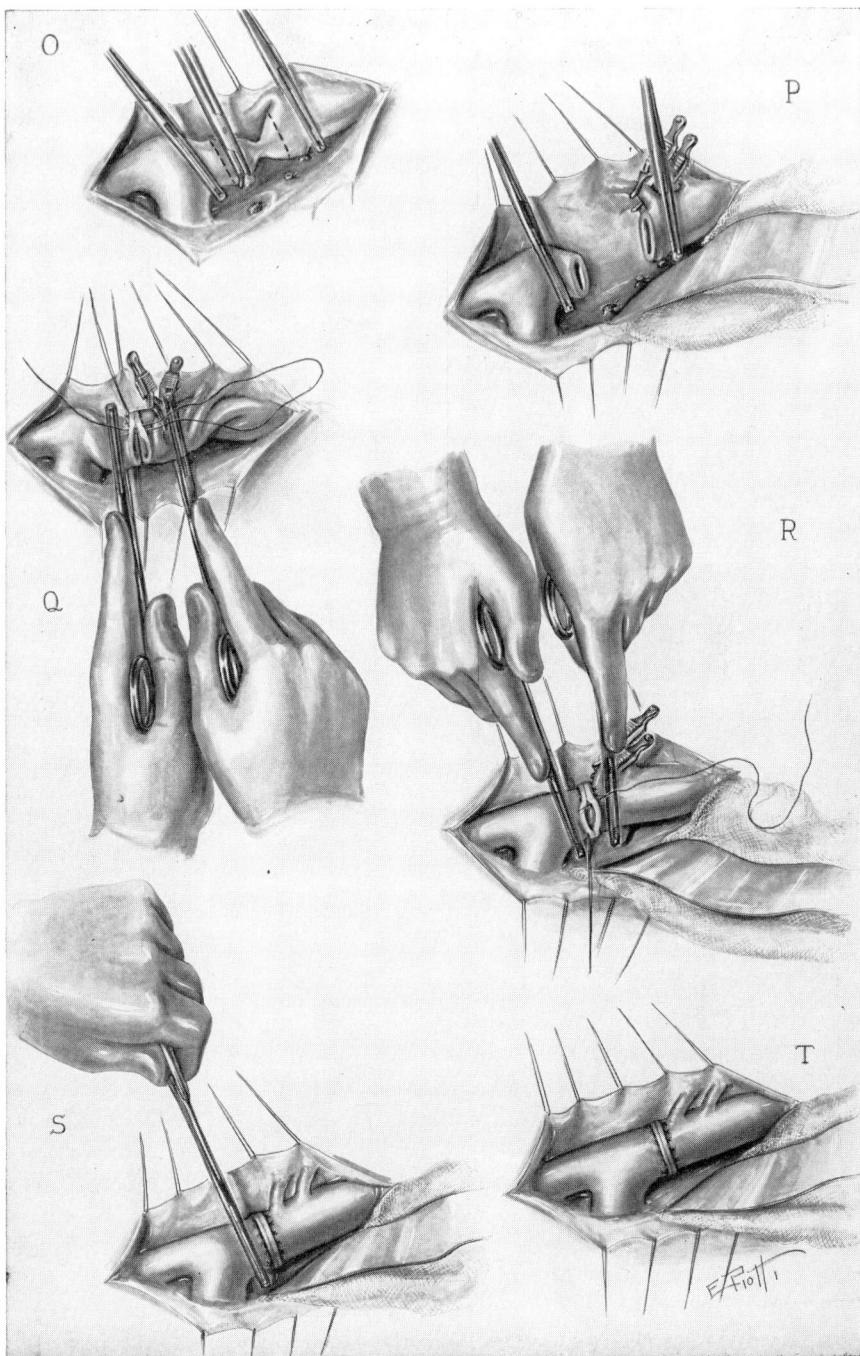

Fig. 475 (*continued*). O, Appropriate clamps applied on the aorta above and aorta below the obstruction. That segment of vessel between the dotted lines will be resected. For all coarctations which reside at a very high level it is best to use a Satinsky clamp (Fig. 478) which can be placed high on the aorta and allows operative manipulations up against the aortic arch. P, Any intercostal arteries which come into the aorta above the lower aortic clamp are temporarily occluded with serre-fine clamps. In some cases these intercostal arteries come in so close to the coarctation that it is necessary to divide them to get an adequate aortic segment to work up. Coarctation removed. Q, Aortic

(*Continued on opposite p. 844*)

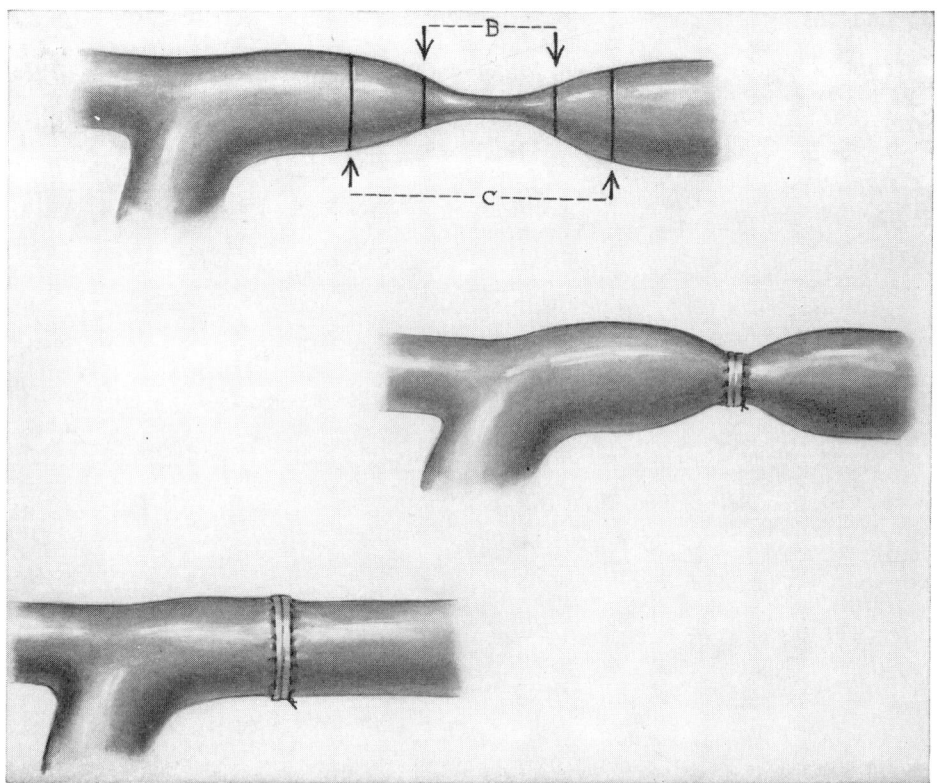

Fig. 476. Sketch to show the goal in removal of coarctations. If only the narrowest part of the constricted area, marked B, is removed, the remaining ends when brought together will give a reconstruction shown in the middle sketch. This improves the pathway, but generally is not sufficient to completely relieve hypertension. The constant aim should be to remove sufficient aorta, indicated C, so that a lumen of full size is reached above and below, giving a reconstruction shown in the lower sketch.

Though this has been advised and used by some surgeons, it is a distinctly inferior type of union and will often give way and disrupt. Overwhelming evidence indicates that the best repair is by taking mattress stitches through the entire thickness of the aortic wall, bringing intima to intima, and turning the ends of the vessel outward. We routinely make the stitches interrupted. The suture material should be 00000 Deknatel silk, carried on a straight needle, $\frac{5}{8}$ inch long.

Position of the Coarctation. The position of a coarctation has much to do with the ease or the difficulty with which it can be excised. Obviously, the surgeon's troubles are least when the block lies well beyond the arch so that a segment of the descending aorta (above the block) is available for manipulation, clamping, and sewing. Unfortunately, many obstructions are at a very high level—just beyond the origin of the left subclavian artery—and in a few cases may actually be in the distal part of the arch itself. With such high constriction, the surgeon's difficulties are tremendously increased, particularly when dealing with older subjects in whom the vessels are rigid. While high strictures should be approached with more caution and apprehension, they do not necessarily present an insuperable problem. To obtain a proximal stump it is necessary to place a clamp directly across the aortic arch and across the left subclavian artery so that the latter is partially or totally occluded temporarily (Fig. 478).

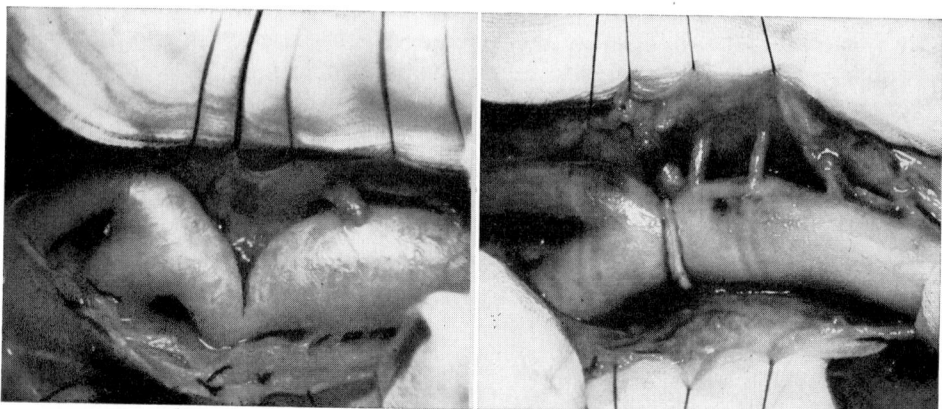

Fig. 477. *Left*, Photograph of coarctation taken at the operating table. The constricted portion of aorta can be seen, there being a medial deviation of the aorta, due to its inward retraction by the ligamentum arteriosum. *Right*, After mobilization of aorta and removal of the narrowed zone, the remaining ends have been brought together by an everting anastomosis, giving a pathway of very satisfactory size.

Anticoagulants. It is not necessary to administer Dicumarol or heparin to prevent local thrombosis. If the aorta is not damaged by instruments, and if a proper anastomosis has been performed, the danger of regional thrombosis is negligible.

Analgesia for Wound. The extensive posterior chest wound can give a great deal of pain in the postoperative period. It is of considerable help to the patient's comfort to inject, while the chest is still open, 4 to 5 cc. of Nupercaine in oil around each of the upper sixth to eighth intercostal nerves, infiltrating this material between the necks of the ribs. This provides an analgesia to the chest wall for about a week.

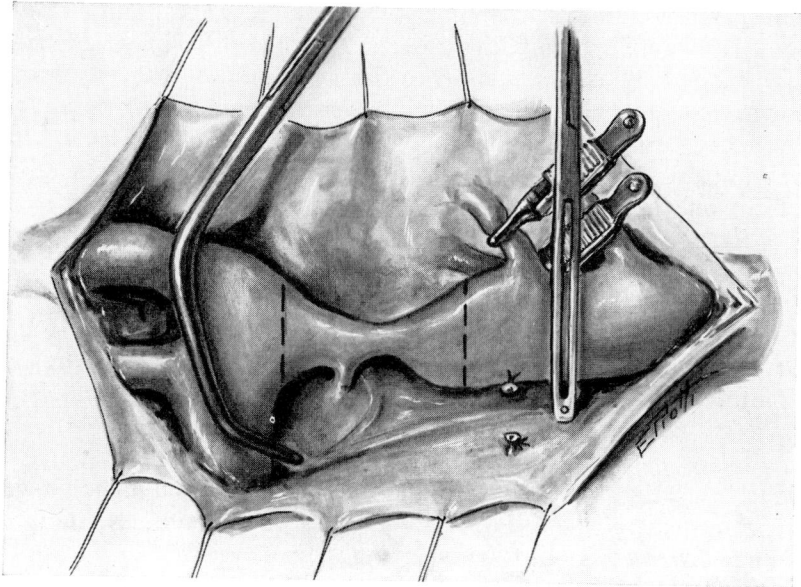

Fig. 478. Removal of coarctation which is quite close to the aortic arch. That segment of aorta which is between the dotted lines will be removed. A revised Satinsky clamp has been applied across the aortic arch and left subclavian artery so that the distal part of the arch itself is available for an anastomosis.

Chest Drainage. Because of the extensiveness of the wound, some serosanguinous fluid always accumulates in the chest after operation. It is therefore best to provide intercostal drainage by a tube for three to four days after operation.

Postoperative Activity. Generally, patients can be allowed out of bed in four or five days, and can leave the hospital in about two weeks. Their activities are graded according to their return of strength; generally they can be back to full physical activity (or work) in about five to six weeks after operation. Frequently they have some pain or discomfort in the left shoulder or side of the chest for a month or two, which from time to time might require the use of codeine. It always disappears in time. The limitation of motion in the left shoulder girdle clears up spontaneously in a few months.

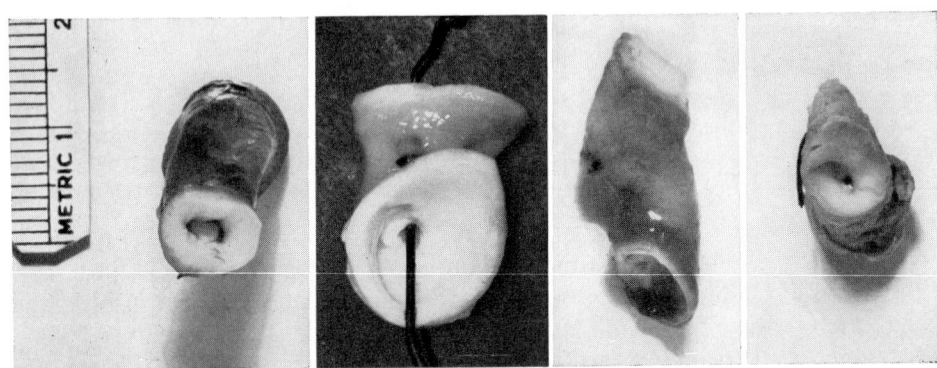

Fig. 479. Photographs of typical coarctation specimens removed at operation. Each specimen has a lumen only 2 or 3 mm. in diameter. (In some cases there is a complete block.)

Excision of Coarctation. Insertion of a Graft

Extensive laboratory work (on dogs) has shown that it is possible to transfer an aortic segment from one animal to another (of the same species) and to have it serve as an excellent pathway. Such grafts have been implanted in recipient animals and observed for periods as long as two years. The risk of dilatation or aneurysm formation appears to be almost nil. The grafts do show degenerative changes, particularly in the media, but yet they carry blood in a highly satisfactory manner. While observations from animal work do not necessarily indicate what will happen if aortic segments are transferred from one human to another, there seemed to be sufficient experimental background to justify use of grafts in human subjects to bridge large arterial gaps which cannot be treated by any other means.

Aortic segments can be collected from human beings, preferably young individuals, within four to six hours after death. If gathered aseptically they can be stored in a modified Tyrode's fluid at 3 to 4° C., and can be used any time up to five or six weeks,[17] after which they decompose and are useless. Similarly, sterile segments can be packaged in cellophane bags, frozen in carbon-dioxide ice at −50 or −55° C., and then stored at this temperature for many months. If segments happen to be contaminated during removal from a body, they can be frozen, and then sterilized by a high voltage cathode ray machine, an apparatus which is available in but few communities. Sterilized frozen segments can be kept many months before using them as grafts.

There are four general situations in which it is impossible to perform the ideal operation of excision of a coarctation and anastomosis of the remaining aortic ends. These problems (Fig. 482) are best handled by removing all of the pathologic tissue, getting back to lumina of full size above and below, and then inserting a graft.

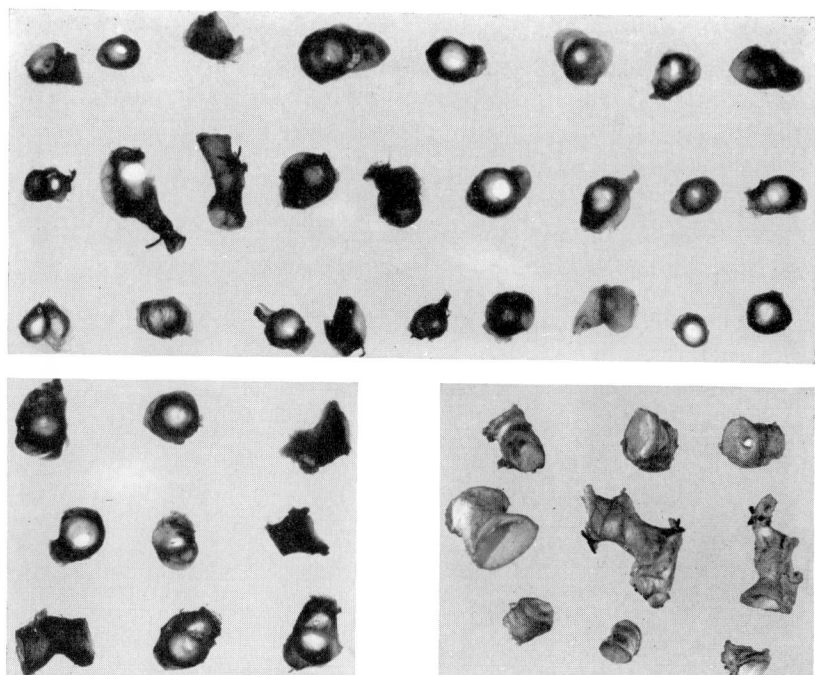

Fig. 480. Photographs of 44 specimens removed surgically from coarctation patients. These specimens are somewhat shrunken, because of their fixation in formalin.

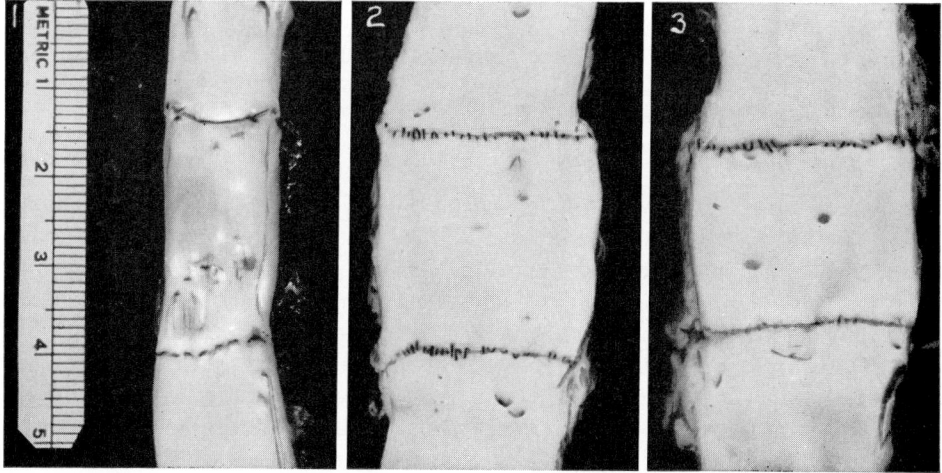

Fig. 481. Homologous aortic grafts (from dog to dog), the animals being sacrificed at varying periods of time after implantation of the grafts. 1. Graft which had been preserved one month in modified Tyrode's solution at 4° C., and then placed in the recipient animal for four months. 2. Graft which had been similarly preserved for five weeks and then implanted into a recipient animal for six months. 3. Graft which had been preserved by freezing at —55° C., kept six months, and then put into a recipient animal for twelve months.

All specimens show excellent pathways for the conduction of blood.

The need for grafting is only seldom encountered in childhood. It is frequently required for adult patients, in whom complicated pathology and technical difficulties are more frequently encountered.

While it requires fifteen to twenty minutes longer operating time, because there are two anastomotic lines to make, reconstruction by use of a graft is generally much easier than treatment by primary anastomosis because of the fact that there is no tension on the aorta or the lines of suture.

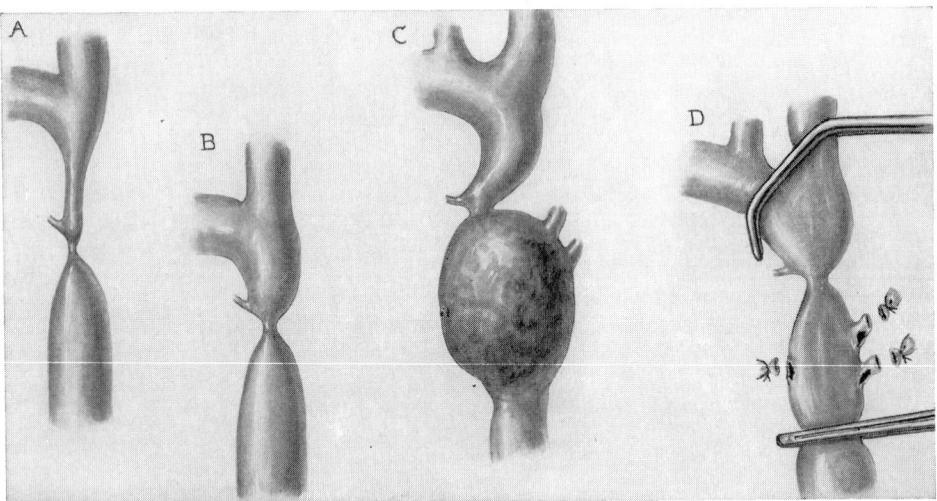

Fig. 482. Conditions for which aortic grafting might be necessary in humans. A, Situation in which there is a very long segment of constricted aorta, the removal of all of which would leave an extremely long gap. B, Fairly short segment of constriction, but aorta is rather rigid and will not allow remaining ends to be approximated. C, Situation in which there is a coarctation and also an aneurysm in the aorta (or of an intercostal artery as it joins the aorta below the block). It is generally necessary to remove the coarctation and the entire aneurysmal area. D, Condition in which there is surgical trauma to the aorta, or the branches which enter it, necessitating removal of the coarctation and a considerable portion of the aorta below this, leaving a long gap.

Record of Blood Loss

In extensive operations when there is great blood loss, it is possible to keep patients in a safe condition by viewing the amount of blood lost in the field, keeping count of the pulse and blood pressure, and replacing blood in amounts which appear to maintain the individual on a reasonably satisfactory plane. While such haphazard methods are sufficient in most instances, fatalities or serious complications can occur when replacement therapy is inadequately guided. If too much blood is infused, the cardiovascular apparatus may be embarrassed or the heart may fail; if too little blood is given, the patient may develop serious or even fatal shock. It is very desirable to keep a running account of the blood which is lost, so that appropriate amounts can be infused to keep the patient in a stable condition. Blood which is sucked out of the operative field can easily be measured in a collecting bottle, placed on the floor; that which is discarded on gauze sponges can be weighed.

In the operative field we employ only dry sponges; they are of a standard, commercial variety which uniformly weigh 8 gm. Using sponges of uniform size makes it possible to use a weighing scale[16] which is fitted with a rapidly adjustable device which can quickly compensate for the number of sponges which are being weighed. Turning

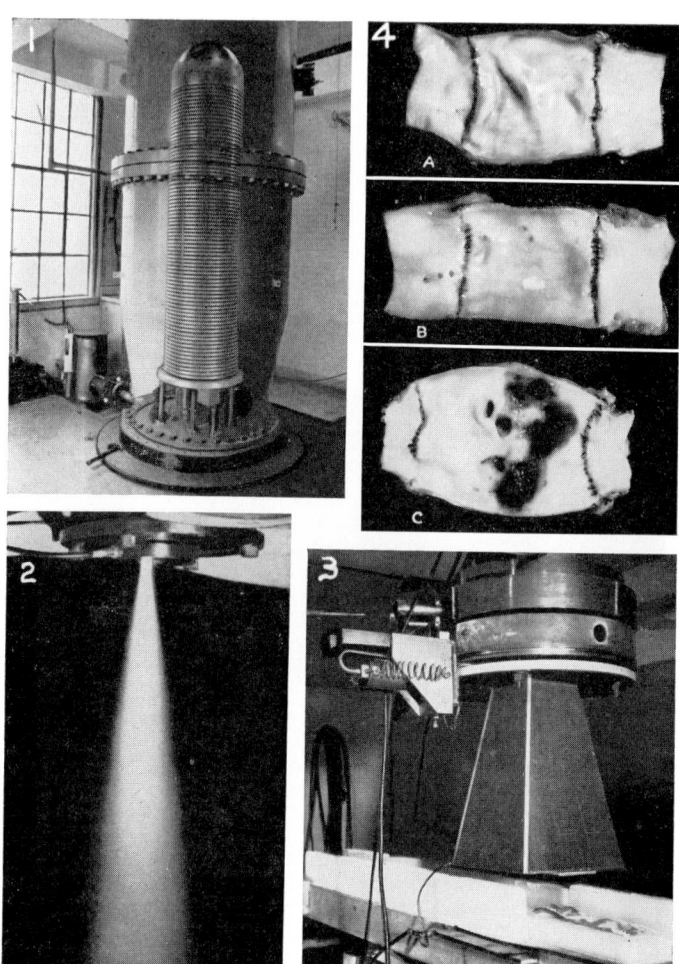

Fig. 483. Method for sterilization of infected (contaminated) aortic segments which have been removed unsterilely at autopsy. 1. Photograph of 3,000,000 volt electron-beam cathode-ray machine (at the Massachusetts Institute of Technology) used for the irradiation. 2. In the room immediately below machine shown in 1 is this electron-beam, some 50 cm. in length. 3. Electron-beam is covered by a cone-shaped shield. The frozen material to be irradiated is run along on an endless belt beneath the conical hood, thus exposing material to the irradiation for a short period of time. 4. From dogs, aortic segments which had been purposely infected, then frozen, then sterilized by electron-beam irradiation, and then stored before implanting them into recipient animals as aortic grafts. A, The graft has been irradiated with 1.5 million R.E.P. (Roentgen-Equivalent-Physical Units). Graft from dog sacrificed at one year. It is smooth and in excellent condition. B, The graft had been frozen, heavily contaminated, irradiated with 2.0 million R.E.P. Graft from dog sacrificed at five months. The graft gives an excellent aortic pathway but has several tiny calcified plaques in its wall. C, This graft had been irradiated with 3 million R.E.P. Graft from dog sacrificed at two and one-half months. There are extensive degenerative changes in the vessel wall and large thrombi on its surface. It has been found that irradiations between 1.5 and 2 million Roentgen-Equivalent-Physical Units are extremely satisfactory for sterilization of contaminated segments and that they do not produce serious damage to the arterial segment.

this adjustment will allow the scale-pointer to indicate directly the number of grams (or cubic centimeters) of blood contained in the soiled sponges.

The weighing instrument (Fig. 486) has been revamped from an ordinary dietetic model. It has a dial-face which can be turned. The outer rim (1 cm. wide) of this dial has been marked off at intervals of 8 gm. (the weight of each dry sponge); these markings are in a counterclockwise direction. The body of the instrument is fitted with a plate carrying the legend "number of sponges" and a central arrow which lies above the rim of the turnable dial-face. The platform of the scale has firmly attached to it a pan which will receive the sponges.

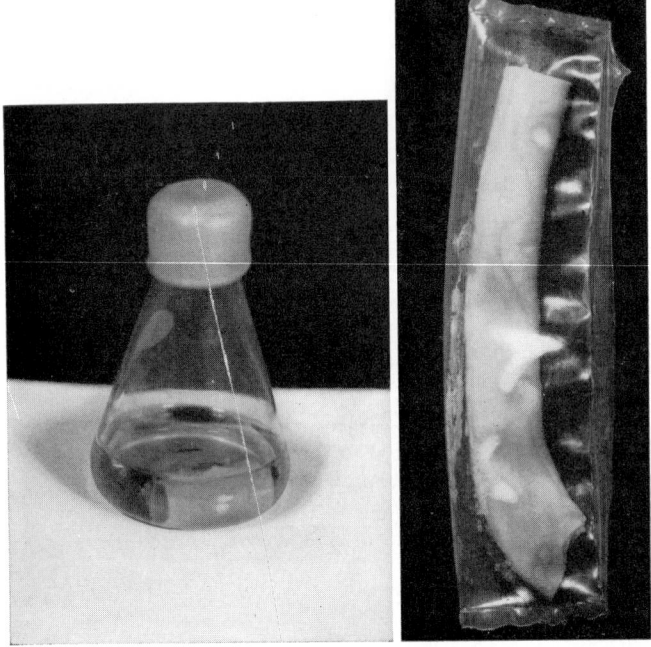

Fig. 484. *Left*, Aortic segment which has been collected aseptically from a human autopsy and stored in modified Tyrode's solution at 3 to 4° C. Vessels can be kept in this manner for five or six weeks. *Right*, Graft which had been contaminated during its removal from human autopsy, placed in a cellophane bag, frozen in carbon dioxide snow (at —55° C.) sterilized by ten seconds irradiation in an electron-beam (2,000,000 Roentgen-Equivalent-Physical Units) and kept in this frozen state until required at operation for a graft. Frozen segments can be kept for many months.

During an operation it is the duty of the circulating nurse occasionally to remove the discarded sponges from the floor bucket and weigh them on the scale which is kept on a side table. If, for instance, ten sponges have been placed in the scale pan (Fig. 486), she simply turns the face-dial so that the rim number "10" comes opposite the arrow at the top. The central pointer-hand will then directly show (on the inner row of figures) the cubic centimeters of blood in the sponges. These maneuvers take but a few minutes, they require no complicated figuring on the part of the nurse, and they can be carried out in conjunction with her manifold other duties.

It has been our practice to have the circulating nurse keep a rough balance sheet. Each time a load of sponges is weighed, the weight of the blood is listed on the record sheet. To determine the patient's total blood loss at any given moment, it is possible to glance at the bottom figure on this sheet and add to it the amount of blood which resides in the suction-apparatus bottle on the floor. Amounts of blood which have been given intravenously are also noted in an appropriate column on the record sheet. This system accomplishes two purposes: First, it allows the circulating nurse to know how much is being lost so that she can replace blood in proper amounts without having to

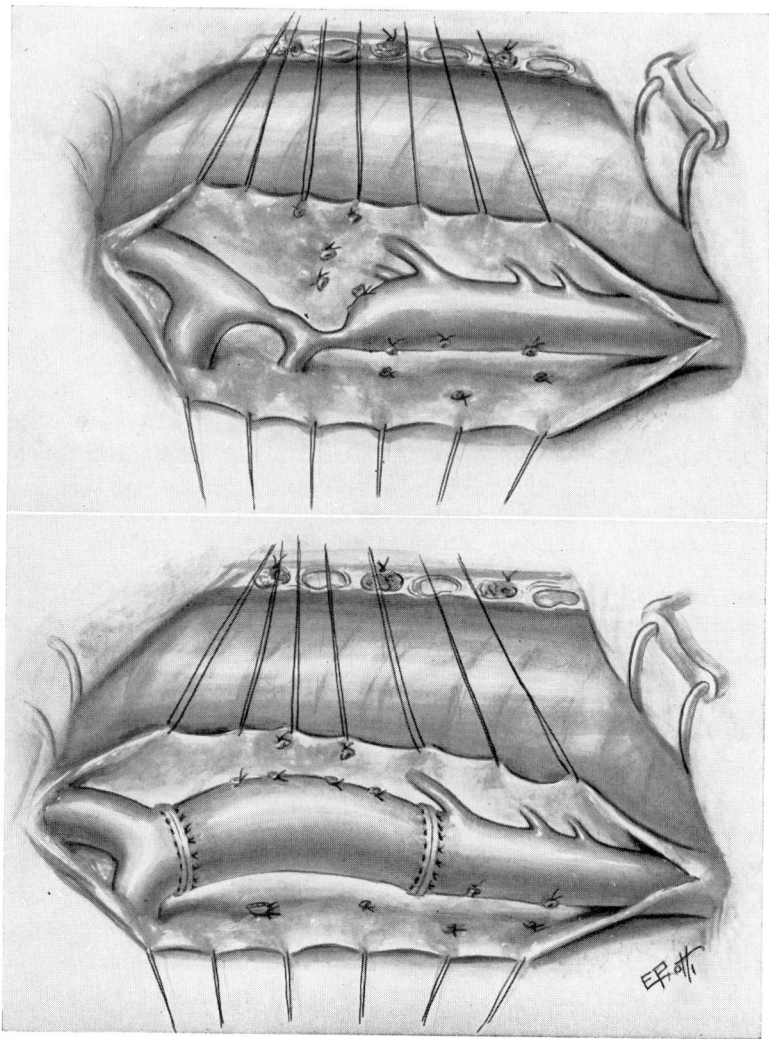

Fig. 485. *Above*, Sketch made at operation on a patient who had an elongated segment of constriction in the first portion of the descending aorta. Removal of this entire segment left a gap too long to be treated by primary anastomosis. *Below*, shows the constricted portion of aorta completely removed and replaced by a graft.

receive instructions from the surgeon or anesthetist who may be having their own troubles at some particularly critical moment. Second, it permits the surgeon to call at any time for an accounting of the blood balance; he can be told instantly how much has been lost and how much has been replaced. The general method obviously has inaccuracies and it does not account for blood which resides on the drapes, but for practical purposes it is accurate enough. The measured loss indicates the minimum amount of blood which must be replaced; as a rule somewhat larger amounts are administered, depending upon the size of the patient, the length of the operation, and other factors.

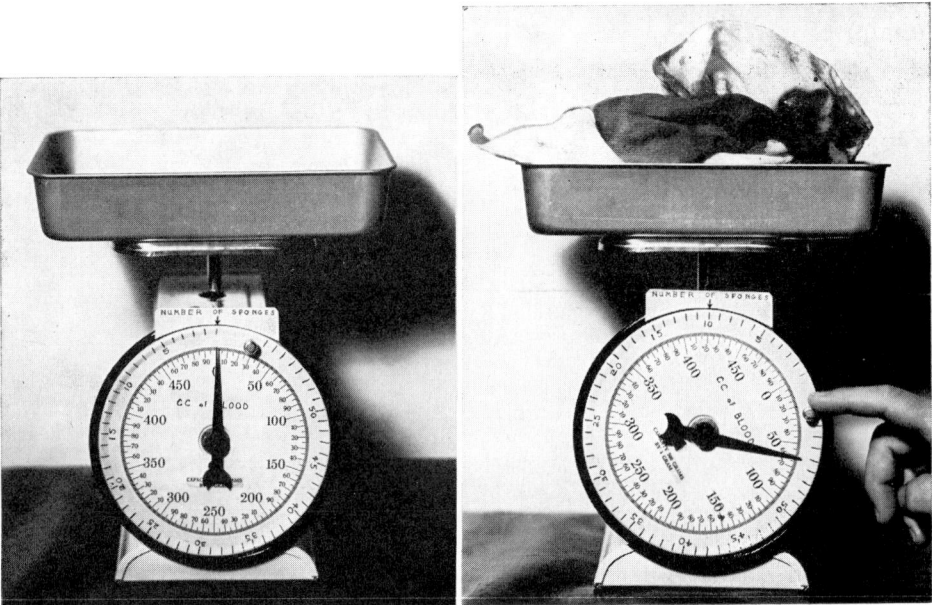

Fig. 486. *Left*, A scale (revamped from a diabetic scale) for weighing sponges which contain blood. The entire face-dial can be rotated around the shaft of the central pointer. *Right*, The weighing scale in use. Blood-soaked sponges have been put in the pan for weighing. With a finger, the face-dial is rotated so the figure indicating the number of sponges (here it is ten) comes opposite to the arrow at the top. The central pointer directly indicates that the sponges contain 62 gm. (62 cc.) of blood. (Turning the face-dial automatically discounts the weight of ten uniform-weight dry sponges.)

RESULTS OF THERAPY

Mortality Rates

The surgical treatment of coarctation has been placed on a reasonable basis, carrying low fatality rates. To date, we have operated upon 270 patients; in the first 100 of these there were 15 fatalities in the last 100 there have been but 2 deaths. This improvement is ascribed to: (1) The avoidance of operation in subjects who are known to have complicated cardiovascular conditions (noted above under Selection of Cases for Surgery; (2) the abandonment of cyclopropane anesthesia; and (3) increasing experience with the operation, giving greater facility in handling emergencies which can be encountered.

Exploratory Operation

In some patients it has been impossible to remove an aortic obstruction because: (1) The patient was tolerating anesthesia poorly. (2) The obstruction was too high in the arch. (3) The vessels were densely adherent to surrounding structures and could not be mobilized. (4) The area of constriction was a very long one, prohibiting the possibility of excision and primary aortic anastomosis. For these various reasons, the attempt at surgical removal of the aortic block had to be abandoned, only an exploratory procedure having been done. In the early part of our series, such explorations were always a disappointment to the surgical team and to the patient; much work, anxiety, and expense accomplished nothing of value except establishment of the fact that the lesion was "inoperable." Fortunately, exploratory operations have now been reduced to a much lower figure; in our last 100 operations there have been but 6 (in 2 of these it was reasonably clear before operation that the condition was not amenable to surgical therapy). This reduction is largely due to the fact that grafts are now available for the treatment of certain situations which previously we would have called inoperable.

Age of Patients Operated Upon

The series of 270 operative cases includes children and adults; the distribution according to ages has been as follows:

0–10 yrs.	46 patients
11–20 yrs.	118 patients
21–30 yrs.	74 patients
31–40 yrs.	30 patients
41–50 yrs.	1 patient
Above 50 yrs.	1 patient

For adults, technical difficulties at the operating table have generally been far greater than were those encountered in the childhood group. Fatality rates have been slightly lower in children than in adults, but the difference is not great.

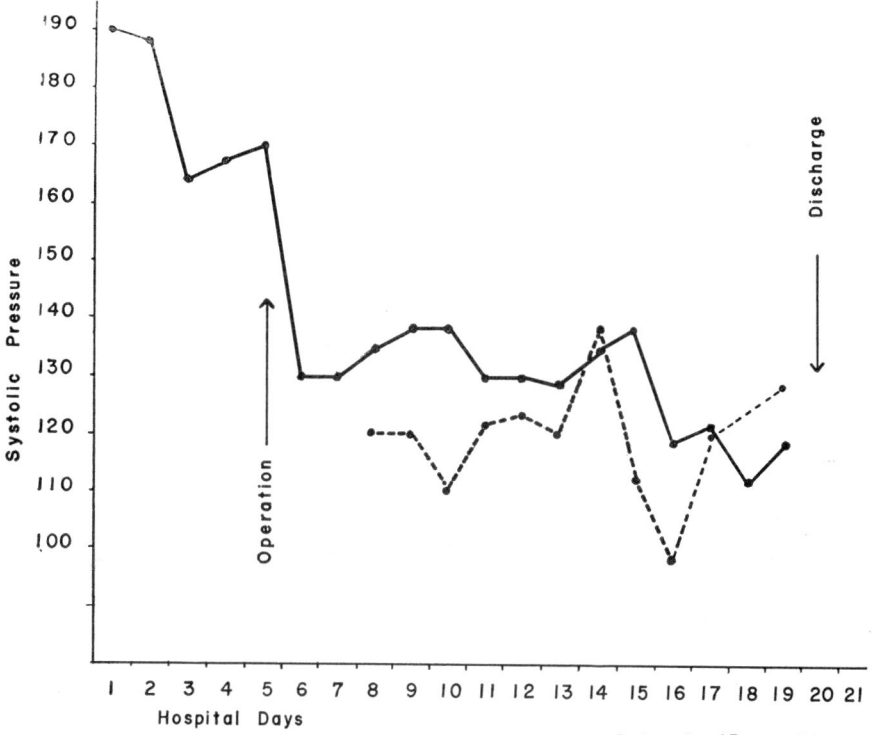

Fig. 487. Blood pressure chart from a fifteen-year-old boy with coarctation of the aorta who was treated by excision of the constricted portion and primary anastomosis of the remaining aortic ends. The solid line indicates systolic blood pressures in the arm. The dotted line indicates systolic blood pressures in the leg. Following operation there was a very satisfactory fall in the arm pressures. By the time of hospital discharge the arm pressures were normal and the leg pressures were somewhat higher than the arm values, which is a normal relationship.

Blood Pressure Changes

In evaluating postoperative states we are concerned most with objective evidence of what has been accomplished. Studies of the changes in blood pressure afford the best record of the readjustments which have been made in the circulatory system. The relief of hypertension is the main purpose of the surgical attack, and observations indicate that it is possible to reach this goal in a very high percentage of cases. Removal of an aortic block seldom gives a precipitous fall of the arm pressures. Though we have seen arm pressures return to normal within twenty-four hours in a few individuals, the more

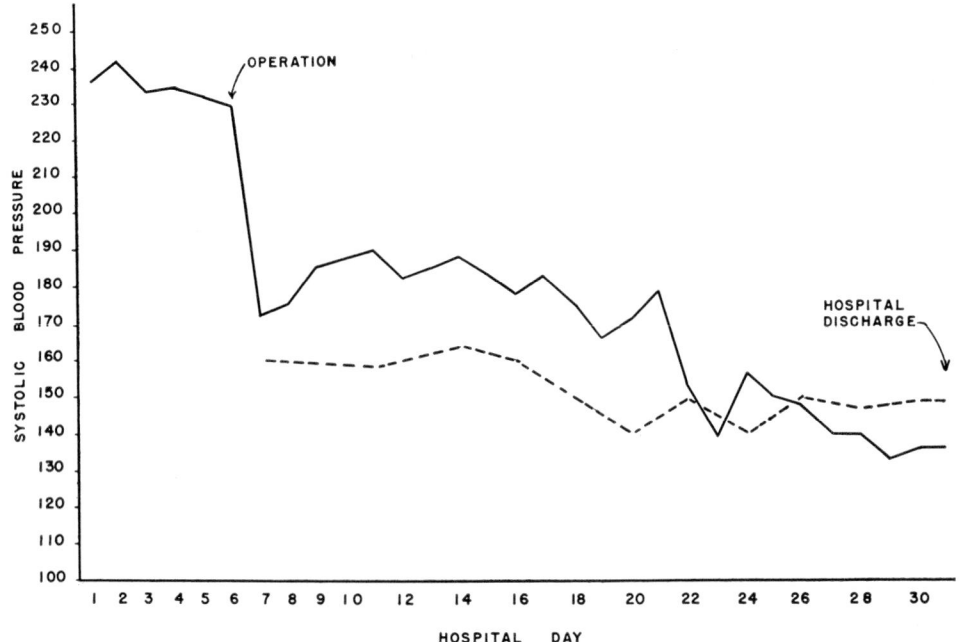

Fig. 488. Blood pressure chart from a twelve-year-old boy with marked hypertension who was treated by excision of a coarctation and primary anastomosis of the remaining ends. The solid line is the arm systolic pressure. The dotted line represents leg systolic pressures. Removal of the aortic block gives a very satisfactory relief of hypertension in the upper part of the body.

common reaction is to have a gradual distention of the vascular bed in the lower part of the body during a period of two or three weeks, and concomitant with this there is a progressive fall in the arm pressures. Generally, the maximum benefit is manifested by the end of a week or two; if relief of hypertension has not been obtained in this period it is usually wishful thinking to anticipate that it will occur in the more distant future.

Of our patients who have survived excision of a coarctation, follow-up studies have been made for periods varying from two months to as long as seven years since operation. There has been no relief of hypertension in 2 per cent of the cases, a fairly satisfactory relief of hypertension in 10 per cent, and a complete cure of hypertension in 88 per cent.

Postoperative Development of Aneurysm

Routine, long-term postoperative chest roentgenograms have not been obtained in all of our cases, but in those studies which we have made, no postoperative aneurysm has yet been found.

Postoperative Disruption

We have had only 1 death in patients following discharge from the hospital. This occurred in a twenty-two-year-old man who obtained a satisfactory relief of hypertension by removal of his coarctation. One year after operation there was sudden onset of chest pain and hemoptysis; roentgenogram showed a fist-sized mass in the chest to the left of the spine which almost certainly represented a hematoma near the operative site. With bed rest, sedation, and transfusions the bleeding subsided, but was followed a few weeks later by a fatal hemorrhage. No autopsy examination was allowed. Whether the bleeding had come from a thin intercostal artery or from the aortic suture line is unknown.

Use of Aortic Grafts

Grafting of aortic segments from one human being to another is still in the early stages of trial; hence no definite statement can be made regarding the ultimate usefulness of the technique. However considerable work has been done in this field and it is possible to sum up the observations to date.

We have employed aortic grafts in 37 patients. The age distribution of subjects and the percentage of cases in each age group requiring grafts were as follows:

1–10 yrs.	3 patients	6 per cent
11–20 yrs.	11 patients	9 per cent
21–30 yrs.	17 patients	23 per cent
31–40 yrs.	6 patients	20 per cent
Over 40 yrs.	0 patients	0 per cent

In the entire series of 270 patients treated for coarctation of the aorta, grafts were employed in 13.9 per cent of the cases. (It is quite likely that the more liberal use of grafts would have improved the results in that group of patients who, because of a poor primary anastomosis and production of a lumen of sub-optimal size at the junction, had only fair relief of hypertension.) The need for grafting in the child is uncommon; the call for it in adult patients is frequent.

Three kinds of grafts were employed: (1) Segments collected sterilely and stored in modified Tyrode's solution at 3 to 4° C., for 29 cases. (2) Segments collected sterilely, frozen in carbon-dioxide snow and stored at −50° C., for 3 cases. (3) Segments collected unsterilely (contaminated at autopsy), frozen in carbon dioxide snow, sterilized by cathode-ray irradiation, and stored at −55° C. until used, for 5 cases. There are not a sufficient number of cases or lengthy enough observations to warrant statistical analyses, but we have a distinct impression that the best results are obtained with the first method. We employ the second method *only* when there is not available material preserved by the first one. We have used the third method *only* in those instances when we have no segments which have been stored by the first two methods.

Certain statements can be made regarding aortic grafting. There has been no sepsis in any case, a fact which we believe is due to meticulous care in collecting and handling the grafts. Three patients died while still in the hospital, all from causes unrelated to the grafting. The survivors have been followed for periods of time varying from a few months to as long as five years. In no case has there been rupture of a graft. In no case has there been aneurysm formation. One subject shows roentgenographic evidence of calcification in the graft, but on clinical findings has an excellent aortic pathway. In no instance has there been any symptom or sign suggesting embolism from a graft site.

Viewed from the point of view of therapy for preexisting hypertension, the over-all picture has been very pleasing. The results can be classified as unsatisfactory in one, fair in 2, satisfactory in 2, and excellent in 29. In the "excellent" group, the arm pressures have been restored to normal.

Confirming observations previously made from aortic grafting in dogs, aortic grafts in humans tend to shrink slightly—as judged by the fact that postoperative leg pressures

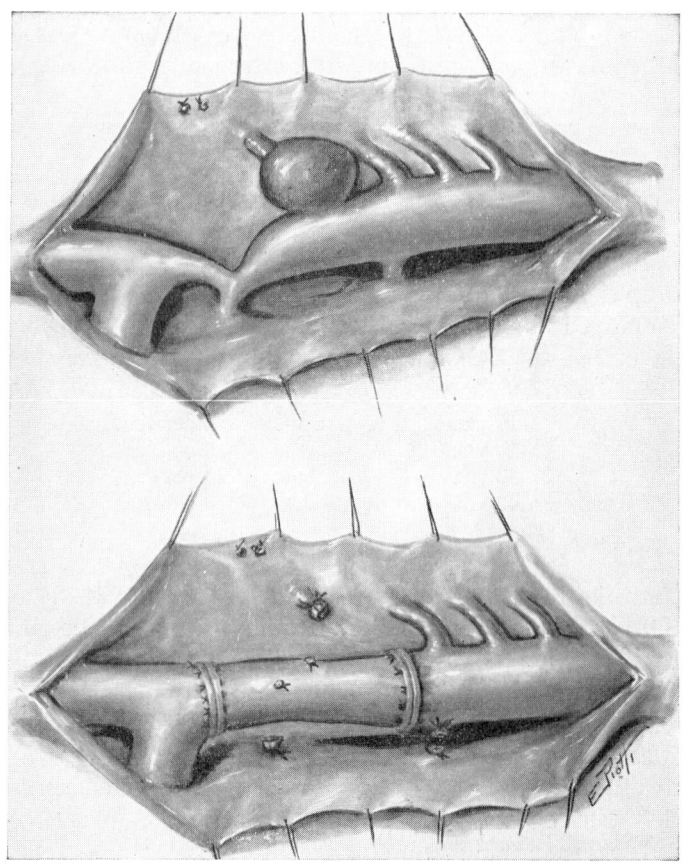

Fig. 489. Operative sketches made from a patient who had an aneurysm of an intercostal artery as it entered the aorta. The aneurysm was of tissue-paper thinness. *Above* shows the pathology encountered. *Below* shows excision of the coarctation and the portion of aorta bearing the aneurysm, filling in the gap with an aortic graft.

increase greatly over their preoperative state, but they seldom rise above the arm pressures (as is the finding when a full-sized pathway is established by excision of a coarctation and primary anastomosis of the remaining ends).

There can be no doubt that the ideal therapy for aortic coarctation is that in which the stricture is removed and a primary aortic anastomosis is made which establishes a lumen of completely normal size. However, sometimes, it is technically impossible to accomplish this; under such circumstances the use of a graft has permitted treatment of a lesion which otherwise could not have been attacked by any other surgical means. Short-term observations of these human grafts (up to five years) have been extremely gratifying; no final conclusions should be made until the patients have been followed for several decades.

Finding of Aneurysm

In 21 patients an aneurysm was found either in the aorta just beyond the constriction, or more commonly in the terminal portion of an intercostal artery just as it joined the aorta. These thin-walled lesions were considered to be a great hazard, because of the danger of rupture. It was therefore felt that they always demanded treatment.

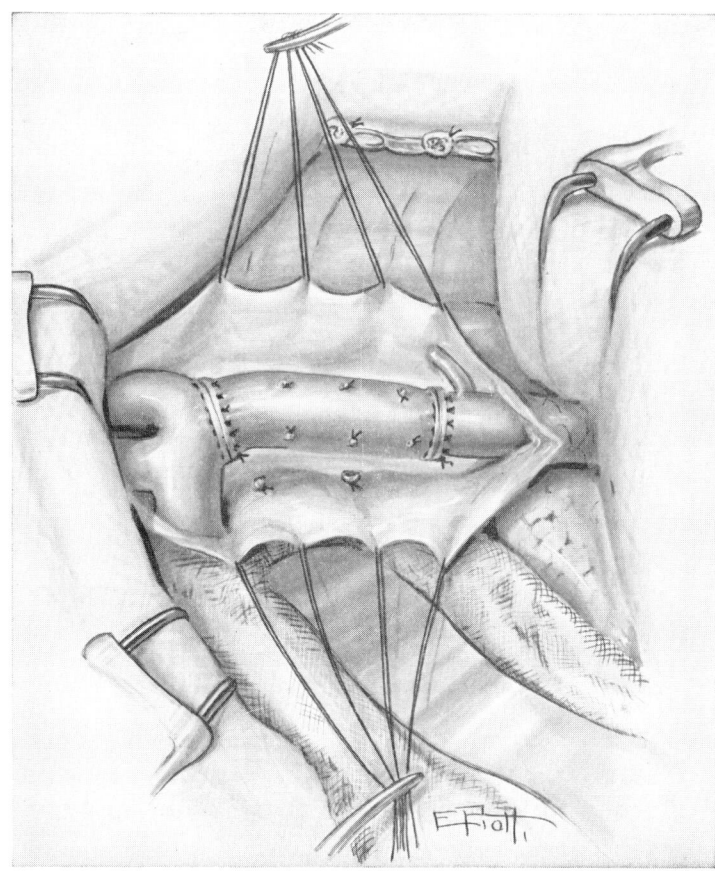

Fig. 490. Operative treatment of a child who had a fairly short aortic constriction, but during mobilization of the aorta, several intercostal vessels were damaged as these thin vessels entered the aorta. It was impossible to repair them. The coarctation and the damaged aorta were removed, the gap being filled in with a graft as shown.

Because of the thinness and friability of the adjacent aortic wall, it was never possible to treat one of the intercostal aneurysms by removal of the mass and closure of the adjacent aortic wall. The aneurysms (intercostal or aortic) were treated by: (1) Severing the intercostal artery (proximal to an aneurysm) and tucking in the aneurysmal sac with adventitial sutures, in 7 cases. (2) Excision of the aneurysmal segment of the aorta and establishment of a primary aortic anastomosis, in 3 cases. (3) Excision of the aneurysmal portion of the aorta and insertion of an aortic graft, in 11 cases.

Postoperative Paralysis

In 2 patients, aged thirty-one and fifty years respectively, there developed during operation a spinal cord damage (presumably ischemia) which left these subjects with severe nerve weakness of both legs. This distressing complication places these two adults in a far worse condition after operation (in spite of cure of hypertension) than they were in before. There was nothing at operation (in the way of shock, obliteration of intercostal arteries, et cetera) that we could blame specifically as being the cause of

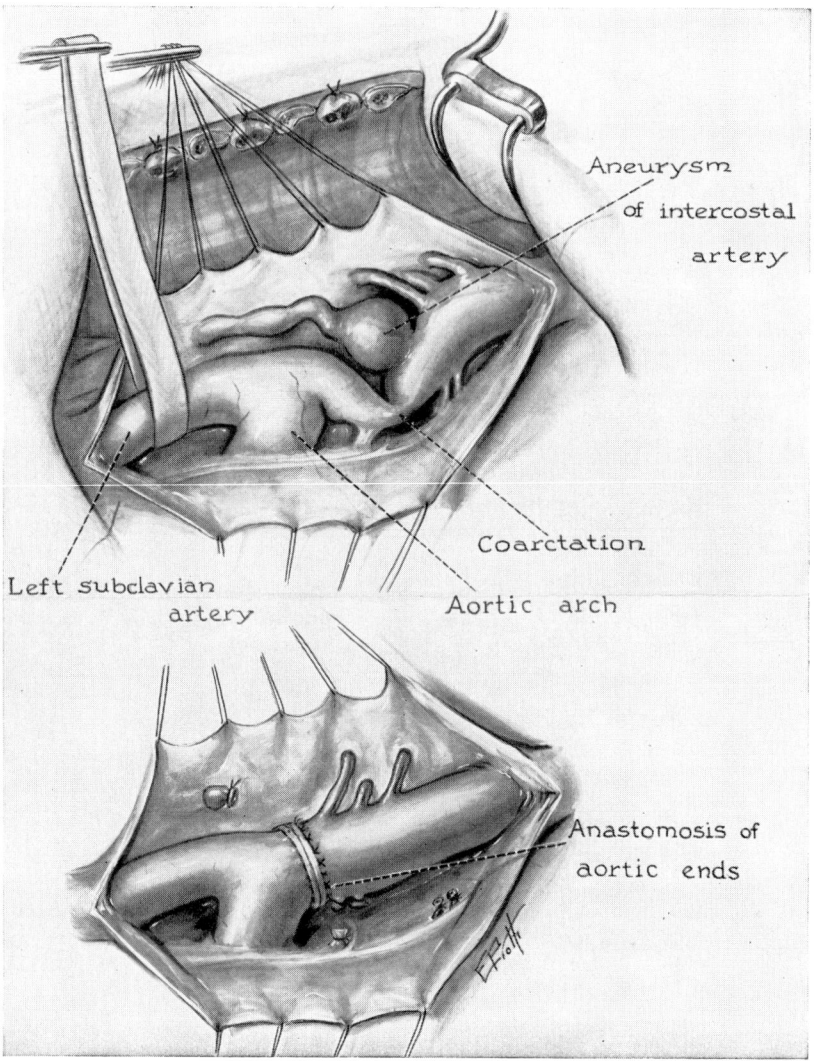

Fig. 491. Fifteen-year-old girl with coarctation of the aorta and also an aneurysm of an intercostal artery. Treatment by excision of coarctation and aneurysmal structure, there being sufficient elasticity in the remaining aorta to permit a primary anastomosis.

these disasters. There may have been some abnormality in the anterior spinal artery, sclerosis of regional vessels, or the like, which (when accompanied by the intrathoracic manipulations of the operation) accounted for a diminished flow of blood to the spinal cord. These serious complications point out again the trials and tribulations of aortic surgery in adults in comparison to the more favorable results which are obtained with procedures in childhood and in the teen-ages.

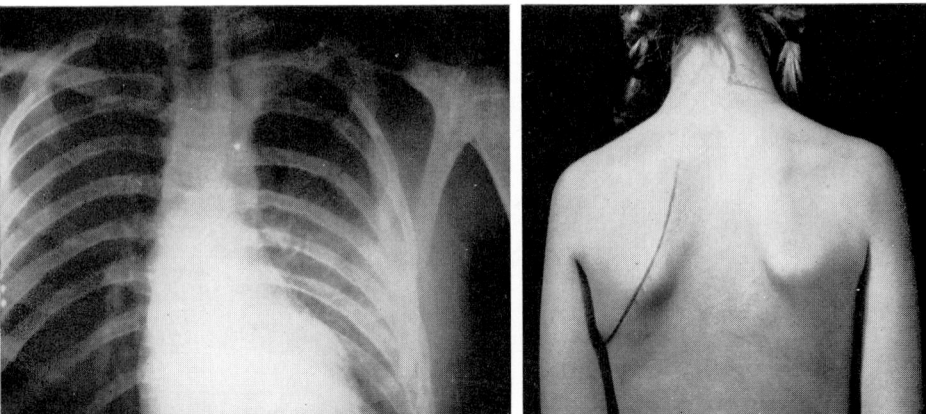

Fig. 492. *Left*, Postoperative roentgenogram of chest, showing the excellent reconstruction of the ribs which is gained by intramedullary pegging and then approximation of the rib ends with silk ties (through drill holes). *Right*, Postoperative view of wound showing position of the same and excellent healing which can be obtained.

General Observations

Following relief of an aortic obstruction there have been various findings in some—not all—patients which are worthy of note. When there have been serious headaches or epistaxes before operation, these have generally disappeared. When there have been cramps or weakness in the legs, these have vanished. Many patients have volunteered the information that their legs are warmer and now "beat" after operation, sensations

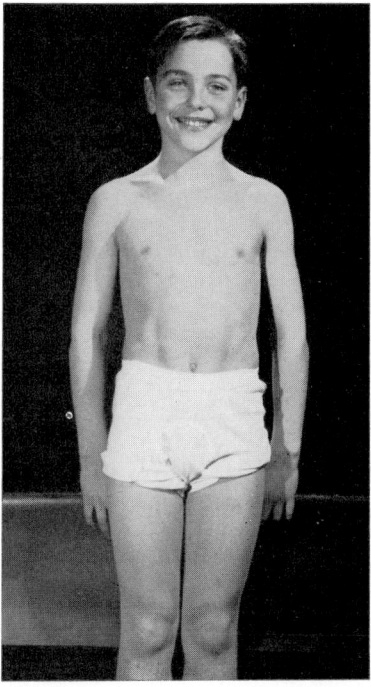

Fig. 493. Photograph of a patient three years after insertion of an aortic graft. The arm pressure at this time is 105/70. Subsequent observations show this boy to be completely well five years after insertion of the graft.

which they had not previously experienced. When there have been symptoms of cardiac embarrassment, these could be greatly improved by reducing the cardiac burden. Five of the adult females have subsequently passed through normal pregnancies and deliveries without any cardiovascular embarrassment.

While surgical therapy for coarctation of the aorta has been available only since 1944, it is now quite evident that it rests on a sound basis and has a great deal to offer most persons who are afflicted with the abnormality.

REFERENCES

1. Abbott, M. E.: Coarctation of the Aorta of the Adult Type. II. A Statistical Study and Historical Retrospect of 200 Recorded Cases with Autopsy, of Stenosis or Obliteration of the Descending Arch in Subjects Above the Age of Two Years. Am. Heart J., *3:*574, 1928.
2. Bahn, R. C., Edwards, J. E. and DuShane, J.: Coarctation of the Aorta as a Cause of Death in Early Infancy. Pediatrics, *8:*192, 1951.
3. Bing, R. J., Handelsman, J. C., Campbell, J. A., Griswold, H. E. and Blalock, A.: The Surgical Treatment and the Physiopathology of Coarctation of the Aorta. Ann. Surg., *128:*803, 1948.
4. Blalock, A. and Park, E. A.: Surgical Treatment of Experimental Coarctation (Atresia) of Aorta. Ann. Surg., *119:*445, 1944.
5. Blumgart, H. L., Lawrence, J. S. and Ernstene, A. C.: The Dynamics of the Circulation in Coarctation (Stenosis of the Isthmus) of the Aorta of the Adult Type. Relation to Essential Hypertension. Arch. Int. Med., *47:*806, 1931.
6. Bramwell, C. and Jones, A. M.: Coarctation of the Aorta: The Collateral Circulation. Brit. Heart J., *3:*205, 1941.
7. Brown, H. R., Hoffman, M. J. and DeLalla, V., Jr.: Ballistocardiograms in Coarctation of the Aorta. New England J. Med., *240:*715, 1949.
8. Burford, T. H. and Carson, M. J.: Visualization of the Aorta and its Branches by Retroarterial Diodrast Injection. J. Pediat., *33:*675, 1948.
9. Clark, R. J. and Firminger, H. I.: Coarctation of the Aorta Associated with Adams-Stokes Syndrome, Complete Heart Block and Bicuspid Calcareous Aortic Valve. New England J. Med., *240:*710, 1949.
10. Crafoord, C. and Nylin, G.: Congenital Coarctation of the Aorta and its Surgical Treatment. J. Thoracic Surg., *14:*347, 1945.
11. Freeman, N. E., Miller, E. R., Stephens, H. B. and Olney, M. B.: Retrograde Arteriography in the Diagnosis of Cardiovascular Lesions. II. Coarctation of the Aorta. Ann. Int. Med., *32:*827, 1950.
12. Friedman, M., Selzer, A. and Rosenblum, H.: The Renal Blood Flow in Coarctation of the Aorta. J. Clin. Investigation, *20:*107, 1941.
13. Furman, R. H., Kennedy, J. A. and Daniel, R. A.: Coarctation of the Aorta Complicated by Dissecting Aneurysm in Pregnancy: Report of a Case with Survival, Studied by Arteriography. Am. Heart J., *43:*765, 1952.
14. Glenn, F., Keefer, E. B. C., Speer, D. S. and Dotter, C. T.: Coarctation of the Lower Thoracic and Abdominal Aorta Immediately Proximal to Celiac Axis. Surg., Gynec. & Obst., *94:*562, 1952.
15. Gross, R. E. and Hufnagel, C. A.: Coarctation of the Aorta: Experimental Studies Regarding its Surgical Correction. New England J. Med., *233:*287, 1945.
16. Gross, R. E.: A Scale for Rapid Measurement of Blood Which Is Lost in Surgical Sponges. J. Thoracic Surg., *18:*543, 1949.
17. Gross, R. E., Bill, A. H., Jr., and Peirce, E. C., II.: Methods for Preservation and Transplantation of Arterial Grafts. Surg., Gynec. & Obst., *88:*689, 1949.
18. Gross, R. E.: Coarctation of the Aorta. Surgical Treatment in One Hundred Cases. Circulation, *1:*41, 1950.
19. Gross, R. E.: Treatment of Certain Coarctations by Homologous Grafts. A Report of Nineteen Cases. Ann. Surg., *134:*753, 1951.
20. Gross, R. E. and Stahl, N.: Treatment of Aneurysms which are Associated with Coarctation of the Aorta. In Press.
21. Keith, J. D. and Forsyth, C.: Aortography in Infants. Circulation, *2:*907, 1950.
22. Kirklin, J. W., Burchell, H. B., Pugh, D. G., Burke, E. C. and Mills, S. D.: Surgical Treatment of Coarctation of the Aorta in a Ten Week Old Infant: Report of a Case. Circulation, *6:*411, 1952.
23. Lewis, T.: Material Relating to Coarctation of the Aorta of the Adult Type. Heart, *16:*205, 1933.

24. Meeker, I. A., Jr., and Gross, R. E.: Sterilization of Frozen Arterial Grafts by High-Voltage Cathode-Ray Irradiation. Surgery, *30*:19, 1951.

25. Railsbach, O. C. and Dock, W.: Erosion of the Ribs Due to Stenosis of the Isthmus (Coarctation) of the Aorta. Radiology, *12:* 58, 1929.

26. Reifenstein, G. H., Levine, S. A. and Gross, R. E.: Coarctation of the Aorta. Am. Heart J., *33:*146, 1947.

27. Rytand, D. A.: The Renal Factor in Arterial Hypertension with Coarctation of Aorta.

J. Clin. Investigation, *17:*391, 1938.

28. Scott, H. W., Jr., and Bahnson, H. T.: Evidence for a Renal Factor in the Hypertension of Experimental Coarctation of the Aorta. Surgery, *30:*206, 1951.

29. Sealy, W. C.: Arterial Hypertension Produced by Experimental Stenosis of the Thoracic Aorta. Proc. Soc. Exper. Biol. & Med., *71:* 174, 1949.

30. Stewart, H. J. and Bailey, R. L., Jr.: The Cardiac Output and Other Measurements of the Circulation in Coarctation of the Aorta. J. Clin. Investigation, *20:*145, 1941.

CHAPTER 62

Interauricular Septal Defect

Among all the congenital abnormalities of the heart which occur as sole lesions, inter-auricular septal defects are probably the most common.

Openings in the interatrial septum allow shunting of blood from the left to the right auricle, thereby increasing the flow through the right side of the heart and through the pulmonary circulation. While there is no direct correlation between the size of a septal orifice and the duration of life, in general the smaller defects are known to be compatible with a long and active existence, while the larger ones are very apt to bring about right-sided heart failure or fatality in childhood or early adult years. There seems to be little doubt that in the average run of cases, a septal defect greatly reduces life expectancy.

It is highly desirable to close surgically the larger septal openings; cardiac invalidism and fatality should be averted if the burden on the heart can thereby be reduced. With careful clinical evaluation and with the use of modern ancillary diagnostic methods, it should be possible to select those patients who have atrial defects of great size and who might logically be expected to be in considerable danger from the abnormality. Such patients constitute a group who should be greatly benefited by adequate corrective procedures.

ANATOMIC AND PHYSIOLOGIC DATA

Anatomic Points

Interauricular defects vary in size, shape, and position; sometimes there are multiple openings in a septum. An orifice may be centrally located, but often it is situated high (near the mouth of the superior vena cava), very low (near the entrance of the inferior vena cava), or rather far forward (in juxtaposition to the ring of the tricuspid valve). One or several openings may be found; in some instances the septum has multiple fenestrations. Those defects with a total cross-sectional area less than three-quarters of a square centimeter are probably functionally insignificant. Those producing symptoms or cardiac embarrassment are usually one to several square centimeters in size; they have been found as large as 4 or 5 cm. in diameter (12 to 20 sq. cm. in area). In some cases there is an incomplete rim of septum around the opening; others have a margin around the entire circumference of the defect. Not infrequently the defect is so large that there is only a vestige of septum remaining; in effect the two auricles form a common chamber. All of these points are of tremendous interest to the surgeon because of the technical problems they pose if attempts are to be made to close the anomalous openings.

Physiologic Considerations

The basic hemodynamic abnormality in atrial septal defect is a shunting of fully oxygenated blood from the left into the right atrium. There is no cyanosis. The magnitudes of shunts, as measured by catheterization, have been found within wide limits; they have been calculated from a few liters up to 20 or more liters per minute. The pressure gradient between the two atria is never large; the huge flows therefore depend upon the tremendous size of the septal orifice.

Because of the intracardiac shunt, the flow of blood through the right side of the heart and through the pulmonary bed is much greater than that through the left ventricle. This increased flow in the pulmonary circuit can be two, three, or even four times

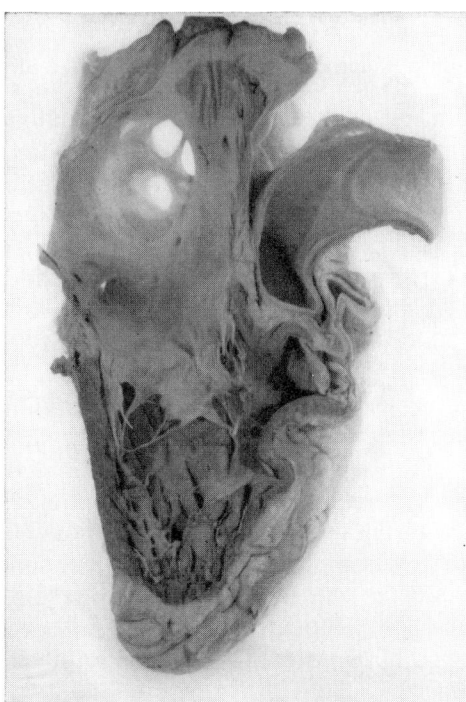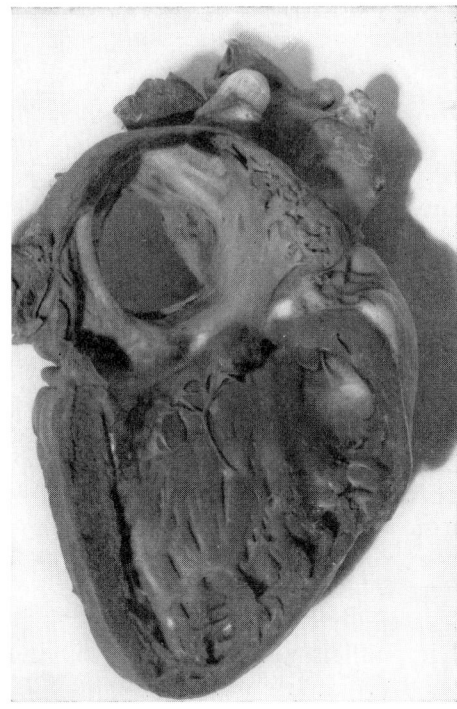

Fig. 494. Interauricular septal defects from two patients. *Left*, Small septal openings, incidentally discovered at autopsy on a sixty-year-old man; the heart was not enlarged. There had been no symptoms referable to this small lesion. There had been no cardiac physical findings or enlargement (by x-ray) during life. (Photograph by kindness of Dr. Samuel A. Levine.) *Right*, Heart of an eight-year-old girl who had had longstanding right-sided cardiac failure. Note the huge opening (4.5 × 5 cm.) in the interauricular septum. The right ventricle is greatly hypertrophied. Catheter studies had shown a left-right shunt of 16.4 liters per minute, a flow through the right ventricle of 18.5 liters per minute, and a flow through the left ventricle and periphery of 2.08 liters per minute.

that through the peripheral circulation of the body. As long as the resistance in the pulmonary vascular bed does not rise appreciably, the pressures within the right heart and the pulmonary artery are within normal limits or are elevated only slightly.

In later life an increased pulmonary vascular resistance is known to occur, thereby producing a damming up of blood in the right side of the heart, an equalization of pressures in the two auricles, and eventually a reversal of flow in the shunt so that the direction is then from right to left, a situation which produces cyanosis and almost invariably indicates a terminal course. Such a rise in the pulmonary resistance, which brings profound changes in the cardiovascular dynamics, can appear in childhood or it may be delayed until early adult life. In a few adult patients, thrombosis has appeared in various parts of the pulmonary arterial tree, which increases the backing up of blood in the right side of the heart, augments reversal of the shunt through the septal defect, and produces or increases cyanosis in the terminal stages of the patient's life. Paradoxical embolism can occur.

CLINICAL FINDINGS

Sex

It is generally agreed that there is a considerable predominance of the abnormality in females; the ratio of females to males in many series varies from two to one to as high as four to one.

Symptoms

Physical Development. While the configuration of the body may be essentially normal, those patients with the larger shunts tend to be of the asthenic type and to have some physical retardation in their physical development; in some this is a marked feature.

Complaints. Pulmonary Infections. A considerable number of children with this condition have no complaints whatsoever. A large proportion of older children and the majority of adults have dyspnea or exertion. Children are particularly prone to have frequent and severe respiratory infections superimposed upon the pulmonary congestion.

Color. Cyanosis and clubbing are absent, since the shunt is from left to right. In later stages of the picture, when there is a reversal of flow through the septum, cyanosis of some degree begins to appear and advances until exitus occurs.

Changing Picture. Some babies and small children with interauricular septal defects have serious difficulties in the first year or two, during which time life hangs in a delicate balance, but apparently some readjustments take place (which can be aided by supportive medical care) so that the critical period passes; the heart becomes somewhat smaller and the over-all picture of the child improves. Even though considerable evidence of cardiac invalidism remains, a crisis has been passed; an example of this is illustrated in Figure 496.

Cardiac Failure. Congestive heart failure, almost exclusively right-sided, is an extremely frequent finding. The onset of failure may be slow; it is very common to have the picture of right-sided embarrassment protracted over a period of many months or even several years.

Endocarditis. Superimposed, subacute bacterial endocarditis is rare, a distinct contrast to the experience with interventricular septal defects.

Rheumatic Fever. It has been said that patients with auricular septal defects are particularly prone to develop rheumatic heart disease, but no convincing statistics are available on this point; we are inclined to doubt these statements. Narrowness of the mitral orifice has been described in association with interauricular septal defect, the so-called Lutembacher syndrome. Whether the mitral valve deformity is on the basis of a congenital arrest of development or on a rheumatic scarring is usually difficult to prove. In our experience, with subjects beyond the first year of life associated mitral stenosis is quite rare.

Physical Findings

Chest Wall. Enlargement of the right ventricle from very early life, during the period of formation and active growth of the thoracic wall, not infrequently gives a permanent bony prominence and bulging of the left side of the sternum and adjacent rib cage.

Blood Pressure. The blood pressure is within a normal range, but tending to be a little lower than the average normal.

Cardiac Activity. The heart has a powerful "thrust" or activity at the apex, related to the enormous amount of blood expelled at each stroke of the right ventricle. Extrasystoles are fairly common.

Murmurs. There may be little or nothing in the way of murmur in early life, and indeed this situation can continue for many years in spite of the fact that there is a large flow of blood through an auricular septal defect. The majority of patients have a systolic murmur of moderate intensity which is heard widely over the precordium and which is most intense in the second or third interspace to the left of the sternum. This is of moderate intensity and of rather low pitch, in comparison to the high-pitched and louder murmur which is so apt to accompany an interventricular septal defect. It is believed that this seldom arises from the septal defect itself, but instead is set up by a large amount of blood rushing through a normal pulmonic valve. There may be an accompanying systolic thrill, which likewise is most intense over the pulmonic area. The second pulmonic sound is apt to be split. In some patients a mid-diastolic rumble at the apex is not an uncommon finding; such a murmur presumably comes from the septal defect alone; it does not necessarily imply the presence of another abnormality (such as a mitral stenosis).

Failure. If failure is present, the picture is almost always one of right-sided embarrassment. There is distention of the neck veins, enlargement of the liver, pallor, orthopnea, dyspnea, and possibly edema; in some cases there is late onset of cyanosis.

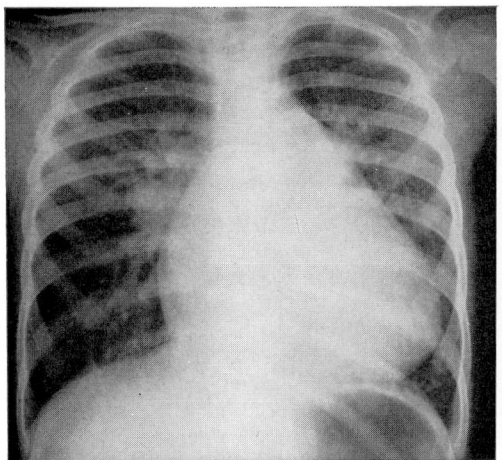 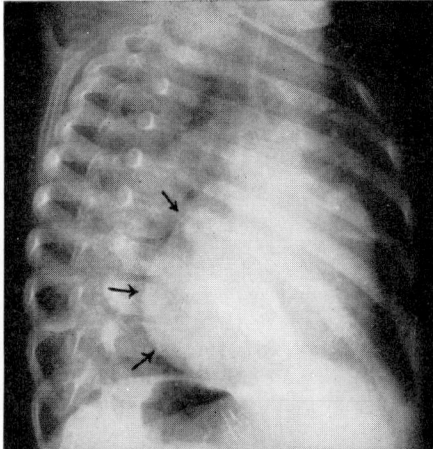

Fig. 495. Roentgenogram from a four-year-old girl with a large interauricular septal defect, subsequently proved at autopsy. *Left,* Enlargement of the heart, with particular prominence of the right auricle, the pulmonary artery, and greatly increased vascularity in the lung fields. *Right,* Oblique view to show the great enlargement of the right auricle (arrows).

Roentgenographic Findings

The main radiologic findings in advanced cases of atrial septal defect are as follows: The right auricle, the right ventricle, and the main pulmonary artery are dilated. The branches of the pulmonary artery are very large and they may pulsate markedly, while the vascular markings throughout the lungs are greatly increased, indicating a great engorgement of the lungs. The aortic arch is smaller than normal, a reflection of the reduced peripheral flow of blood.

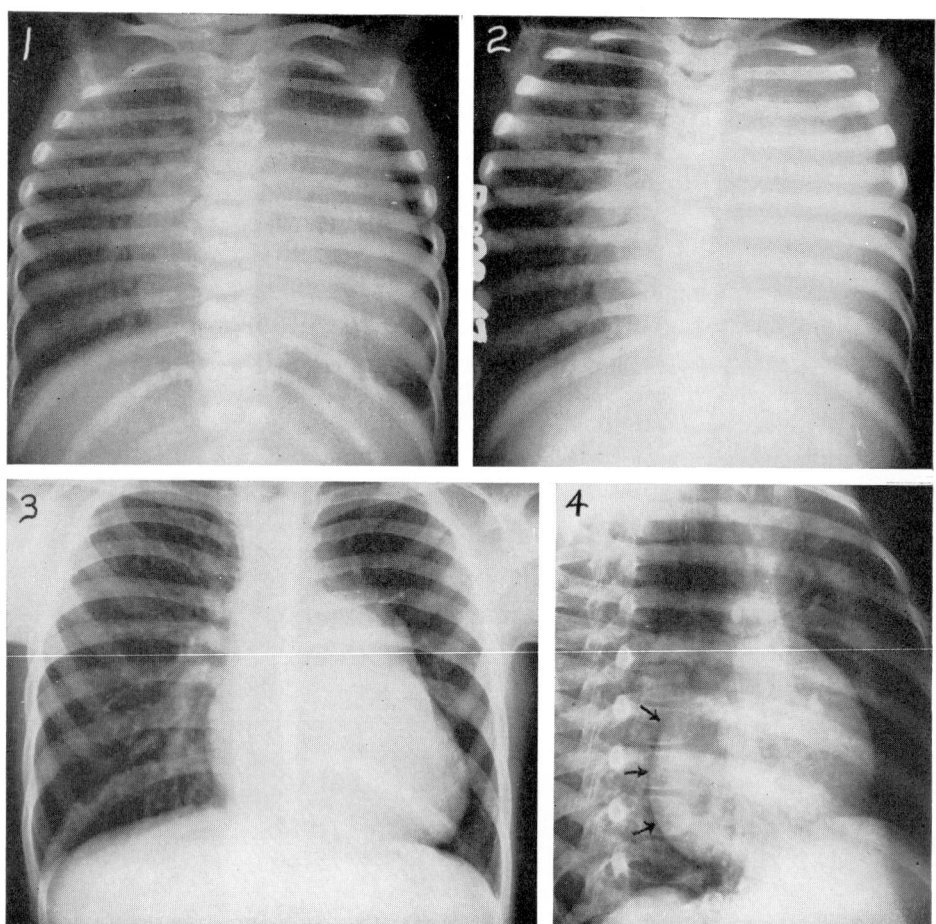

Fig. 496. Roentgenograms of a girl with interauricular septal defect; examination at several ages. 1. At four years of age, at which time the child was having marked cardiac embarrassment and obvious failure. There was tremendous enlargement of the heart and congestion in the lung fields. 2. One month later, at which time the child seemed almost *in extremis;* the cardiac enlargement had greatly advanced. Dyspnea and orthopnea were marked. The liver was greatly enlarged. Medical therapy was instituted, and following this the child gradually improved to a considerable degree. 3. Roentgenograms at eleven years of age. The heart size has become greatly reduced but it is still distinctly enlarged, has prominence of the right auricle, prominence of the pulmonary artery, enlargement of the right ventricle, and engorgement of pulmonary vessels, seen particularly well in the central part of the right lung. 4. Oblique film at same age as 3, showing great prominence of the right auricle (arrows). One year later autopsy showed a huge interauricular septal defect.

The chief findings of fluoroscopy are demonstration of pulmonary plethora and enlargement of the right ventricle. Engorgement of the lung fields can be found with patent ductus arteriosus or interventricular septal defect, but when increased pulmonary flow is combined with obvious enlargement of the right auricle, interauricular septal defect is the most tenable diagnosis.

Electrocardiographic Tracings

Right axis deviation is the rule. Incomplete, or occasionally complete, right bundle-branch block is an almost constant finding. The demonstration of this phenomenon depends on the extensive use of the unipolar electrocardiograph. Auricular enlargement is shown by very large P waves and by a widening and notching of the QRS complex. Some patients have prolongation of the A-V interval, presumably because the distortion of the bundle of His has brought about elongation of this structure.

Cardiac Catheterization

Cardiac catheterization is a most important part of the study with patients suspected of having interauricular septal defects, not only to place the diagnosis on a positive basis but also to obtain accurate measurements regarding the flow through the septal aperture. If the catheter can be passed from one auricle to the other, this is positive proof of existence of a septal defect. Sometimes it is possible by fluoroscopic observation of the tip of the catheter to gain some impression regarding the position of the septal defect, but observations of this type can be very misleading. The collection of blood from various parts of the cardiovascular system and examination of these specimens for oxygen content can give direct evidence of the direction of flow through the shunt and can indicate the extent of the flow. Samples of blood from the right auricle, right ventricle, and pulmonary artery generally show oxygen saturation of 80 to 90 per cent, which is greatly in excess of that found in the venous blood in the venae cavae.

By pressure measurements, catheter studies can give incontrovertible evidence regarding resistance in the pulmonary vascular bed, a point of considerable importance in selecting cases for surgical therapy.

SELECTION OF PATIENTS FOR OPERATION

Indications

There is as yet no clear-cut distinction between those patients who have small septal lesions which will be tolerated through a long life and those who have sizable defects which almost certainly will lead to disaster in childhood or early adult years. The smaller defects, because of the known benignity of their course, should not be subjected to the risks of operation. However, it would seem that all of the larger openings should have operative closure. Certainly, there can be no doubt that those subjects who have any important symptomatology or who have evidence of right-sided heart failure should be operated upon. Also, those subjects who have cardiac enlargement by roentgenographic study almost certainly have a sizable septal defect and probably should be operated upon, even though they have no symptoms. Finally, those subjects who, by cardiac catheterization, are shown to have left-right flows of blood of great degree are almost certainly headed for subsequent cardiac embarrassment, even though they are momentarily asymptomatic. As yet it is not known at what level the dividing line should be drawn, but probably any patient with a flow through the right ventricle which is more than 50 per cent larger than that through the left ventricle should be given the benefit of surgical correction of the septal anomaly.

Contraindications

Cardiac failure, in itself, is not a contraindication to surgery; we have operated upon children who were in severe failure at the time but who survived closure of the septal defect and were enormously benefited thereby. There are certain contraindications to operation, principal among which is a terminal picture wherein there is evidence of increased vascular resistance in the pulmonary bed which has given rise to a reversal of flow through the septal opening. It is very doubtful if closure of a septal defect at such a late hour will be tolerated or beneficial.

METHODS FOR CLOSURE OF INTERAURICULAR SEPTAL DEFECTS

Various methods have been suggested, or have been attempted, for closure of inter-auricular septal openings; they fall into five general categories: (1) Transfixion of the auricles with mattress sutures placed in the plane of the septum. (2) Invagination of atrial appendages, or the lateral wall of an auricle, to plug the defect. (3) Diversion of blood from the heart by use of a pump-oxygenator, opening the heart, and closing the defect under direct vision. (4) Temporary occlusion of the venae cavae for a few minutes, opening the auricle and repairing the defect. (5) Attachment of a rubber "well" to the right atrium, into which the auricle can be opened; working through this pool of blood the septum can be approached and its defect repaired.

1. Murray[16] has passed large mattress sutures of silk or fascia through the heart, placing these approximately in the plane of the atrial septum. Snugging-up of these sutures compresses the heart antero-posteriorly, and can partially diminish the size of the atrial opening. Although clinical improvement has been reported in several patients subjected to this procedure, no precise evidence has been presented yet to show that the shunts have actually been reduced. Certainly, the method gives no promise of closing a septal defect completely.

2. Various workers have devised methods for invaginating the atrial appendages or the lateral wall of an auricle to occlude a septal opening. Swan[21] and his co-workers have infolded both the right and left auricular appendages to the septum, occluding the defect by holding the inverted appendages in this position with mattress sutures which pass through both of the appendage tips. The use of this procedure in humans has been abandoned by Swan, because of the danger of partially obstructing orifices of the pulmonary veins. Santy et al.[20] reported the plugging of a small septal opening by in-verting the tip of an auricular appendage through it. Cohn[5] has suggested indentation of the right auricular wall towards the septum, anchoring it in this position by sewing it to the septum with sutures which have been introduced from the exterior of the heart. Bailey[1] has modified this by introducing a finger through the auricular appendage, so that the digit inside the auricular cavity could guide the placement of the sutures around the edges of the septal defect. While these various techniques of inversion of an auricular wall to the septum might be highly satisfactory for closure of centrally placed defects, it is important to remember that many septal openings in humans are located very high, very low, or very far forward, so that the inversion of an auricular wall to occlude them would almost certainly give partial obstruction of the superior vena cava, the in-ferior vena cava, the coronary sinus, or the tricuspid valve.

3. After extensive investigations on animals, considerable information has been accumulated regarding the technical designs and capabilities of various mechanical pump-oxygenators which can divert blood from the heart so that the organ can be opened temporarily. Little information is yet available concerning the use of these appliances during intracardiac operations on man. Dennis et al.[6] have reported experi-ences in the use of a mechanical heart-lung machine attached to a human, with an attempt at suture of an atrial defect under direct vision after opening the heart. To date, no successful repair has been described by this method. While enormous strides have been made in the perfection of machines for temporary diversion of blood from the heart, there is yet much to be learned concerning the various problems dependent upon the use of these during intracardiac operations in man.

4. In attempts to close septal defects in dogs under direct vision, Swan et al.[21] as well as Martin and Essex[14] have temporarily occluded the caval inflow. This drastic maneuver, while tolerated temporarily, cannot be continued for more than three or

four minutes. This length of time can be about doubled if the subject has been re-frigerated to low temperatures (below 80° F.). Using such methods of refrigeration and temporary caval compression, the human heart has been opened and atrial septal de-fects closed by Bailey[1] and by Varco and Lewis.[23] It is quite doubtful (in the presence of septal openings) whether it will be possible always to prevent embolization of air into the systemic arteries. Furthermore, this method would seem to be impractical for treat-ment of very large defects, the closure of which will almost certainly require a longer operating time.

5. A different approach to the problem has been devised by Gross et al.[10,11] using a rubber bag or "well" (Fig. 497) which can be sewed to the presenting surface of the

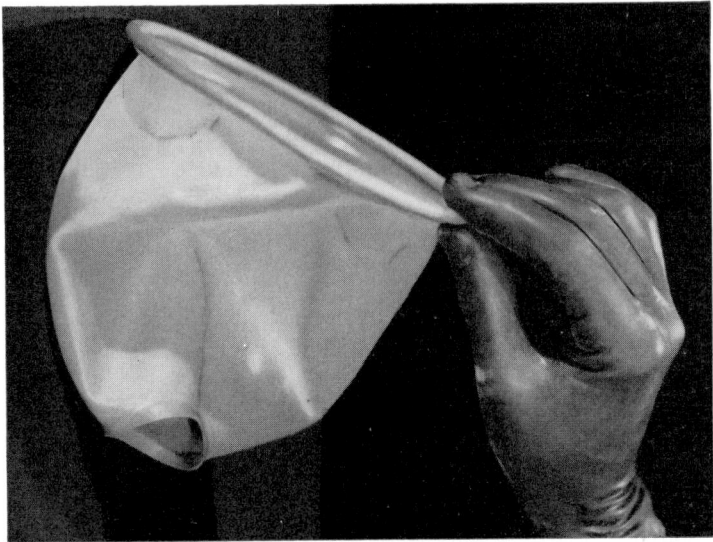

Fig. 497. Rubber "well" of size and shape for use on the human heart.

enlarged right auricle. Opening the auricle into the base of this attached appliance allows blood to rise up in the latter to a distance equal to the intra-auricular pressure, which is never very high. This rubber "well" then provides a pool of blood (kept fluid with heparin) through which fingers and instruments can be passed into the cavity of the auricle, for examination of its interior and for repair of a septal defect. The heart tolerates such an appliance with amazingly little disturbance. Attached to humans, such wells have been left open for periods longer than two hours. The operator can repair the septal defect in a deliberate, careful, and unhurried manner.

We believe that of all the methods which have thus far been proposed or used for closure of septal defects, the well technique gives the greatest promise for closure of these openings regardless of their size, shape, or position. The well method is blind, but it has learned in the laboratory that with a palpating finger the interior of an auricle can be examined thoroughly and that septal openings can be closed effectively and completely. Despite its shortcomings, the method has the enormous advantage of permitting an operation to be carried out without the least hurry. Therefore, the repair can be made accurately and with great satisfaction. It is the most versatile method yet developed for treatment of all the variations of septal anomalies which are known to occur in humans.

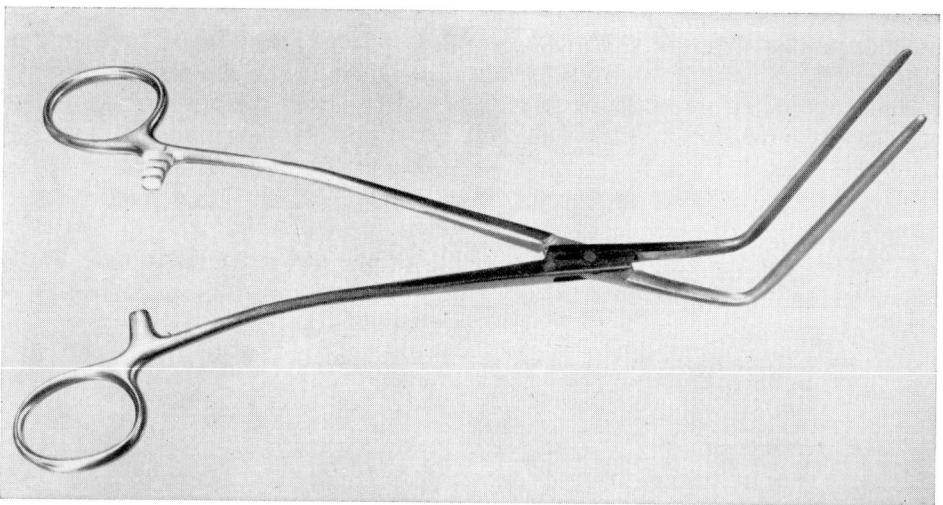

Fig. 498. Atrial clamp, to be used for isolation of a segment of the atrial wall during attachment of a rubber well to it.

RECOMMENDED SURGICAL TREATMENT

Our experience with surgical treatment of interauricular septal defects has been wholly with the well technique. We therefore wish to limit our presentation to illustration and description of this surgical procedure (Fig. 500).

Preoperative Measurements

When anticipating the use of the rubber well technique for the treatment of septal defects, the pressure in the right atrium should be determined by cardiac catheterization before operation; this pressure is an indication of the height of the column of blood which will appear in the attached well at operation. While we originally feared that a patient in cardiac failure would have such high auricular pressure that the well technique

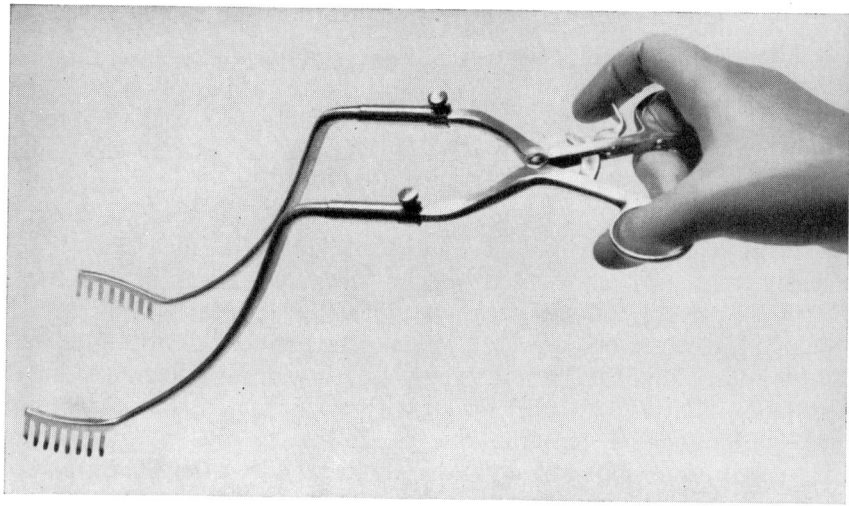

Fig. 499. Self-retaining retractor, to be inserted into an atrial well and to spread open the orifice in the lateral wall of the right auricle. When retractor is opened, the auricular wall orifice will be 5 or 6 cm. in diameter.

might not be feasible, experience in 10 human cases (4 of whom were in failure at the time of operation) has now allayed our apprehension in this regard. The preoperative range of pressures measured 4, 8, 14, 8, 14, 15, 8, 5, 6, and 4 cm. of saline respectively. Generally, the height of blood columns in the wells at operation were much lower than these figures, such reductions being dependent upon many accessory factors such as anesthesia, opening of the chest, etc.

Incision and Exposure

Exposure must be very liberal. With the patient turned so that the right side is uppermost, incision is made throughout the length of the right fifth interspace, dividing the sixth and seventh ribs posteriorly and the fifth, fourth, and third cartilages anteriorly very near their sternal junctions. Wide opening of the chest is essential. The lung is found to be heavy because of the increased amount of blood within it; the vessels supplying and draining it are greatly enlarged and engorged. Frequently, there is a marked thrill in the lung root, because of blood rushing through it. The lung is packed away posteriorly. The pericardium is split open anterior to the phrenic nerve. We are inclined to believe that the injection of procaine into the pericardium, while possibly reducing the irritability of the auricle, is too apt to give a disturbing fall in peripheral pressure; therefore we generally do not employ it as a routine measure. Bathing of the surface of an auricle with procaine can be reserved for those cases wherein the auricle seems to be particularly irritable as it is being handled. Intravenous injection of procaine amide (Pronestyl) is used only when there are frequent extrasystoles; generally it is not used.

Attachment of Rubber Well

Steps in the use and attachment of an atrial well are illustrated in Figure 500. Linen tapes should always be passed around the inferior and superior venae cavae, before attachment of the well, so that if a defect is later found very high or very low in the septum, near the orifice of either vena cava, the vessel can be raised (with the tape) and the occluding polyethylene sheet can be attached to the auricular wall just *medial* to the orifice of the cava. This makes sure that all caval blood is thereby diverted into the right auricle.

It is rather important to place the well as far inferiorly and posteriorly as possible because this will give the best positioning for the transauricular approach to the defect in the septum in most cases. It is possible to make a water-tight junction between the lower rim of the rubber well and the isolated segment of auricular wall. To sew this rubber appliance into place requires about fifteen minutes. We have had no difficulty with the attachment of a well to the auricle of a human; the union can always be made leak-proof. When the atrial clamp is removed and blood is allowed to flow up into the well, an intravenous infusion of a similar amount of blood should be given rather rapidly to compensate for that which is "lost" into the appliance (100 to 300 cc., depending upon the size of the subject). Beyond this point, transfusion is necessary only in small amounts; the indications for its use are judged by the level of the peripheral arterial pressure.

The hole in the lateral auricular wall (where it is attached to the base of the rubber well) is now spread by placing within it an expanding, self-retaining retractor (Fig. 499). This gives an entryway of 5 or 6 cm. in diameter, which is adequate for working in the auricular cavity.

There must be constantly at hand on the operating table a solution of anticoagulant

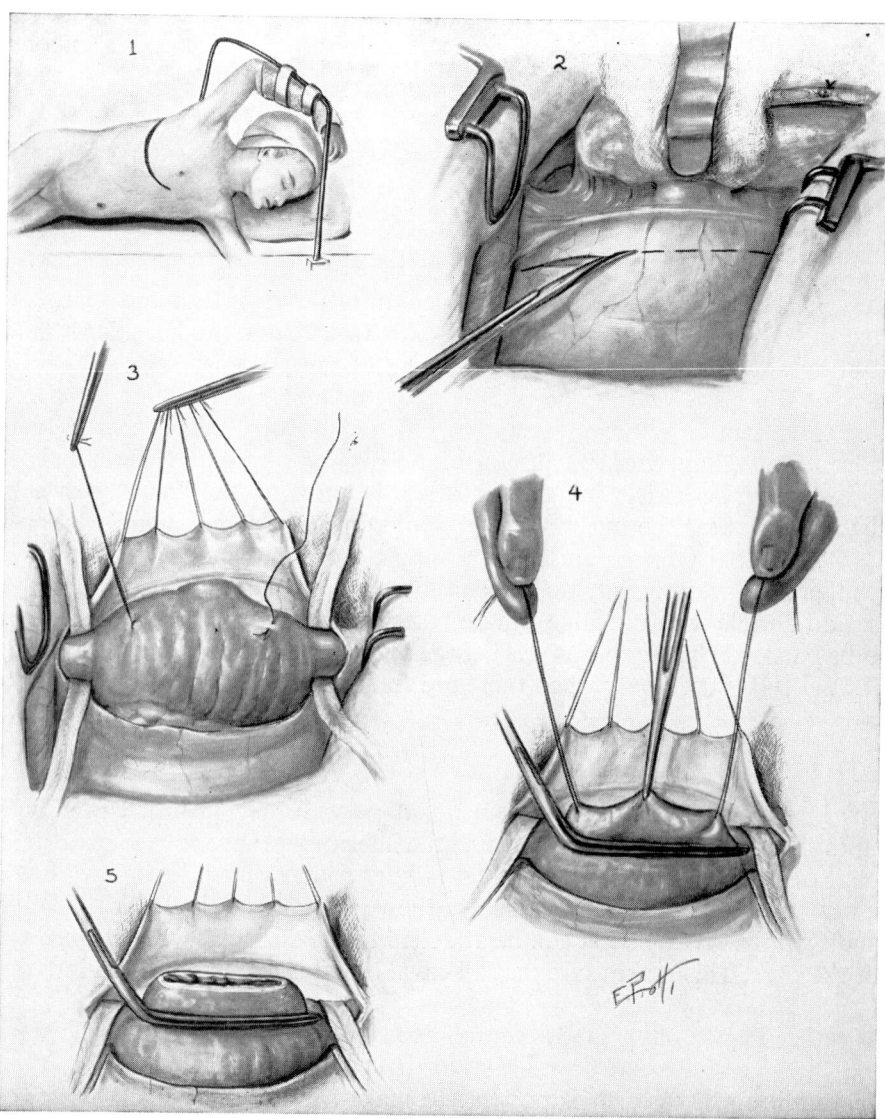

Fig. 500. Use of an atrial well to explore the interior of the right auricle and to repair an inter-auricular septal defect. 1. Position of patient on table, lying on left side, with the right arm suspended upward. Position of incision is shown. 2. The chest has been entered throughout the entire length of the fifth interspace. Fifth and sixth ribs have been divided posteriorly. Fifth, fourth, and third cartilages have been severed anteriorly very near to the sternum. Self-retaining retractor in place. The lung is retracted posteriorly. Great engorgement of pulmonary veins is usually evident (just below the tip of the malleable retractor). Pericardium being opened along the dotted line, in front of the phrenic nerve. 3. Pericardium opened, the posterior flap is held upward with traction sutures. Inside the pericardial sac, linen tapes have been passed around the inferior and the superior vena cava. (This step is made in the event of finding a septal defect which is very close to the orifice of either cava. It will be necessary to raise the vena cava by traction so that sutures bringing into place a plastic sheet can be run *medial* to the cava, thereby directing all caval blood into the right auricle, Fig. 502.) Two traction sutures being placed in the wall of the auricle. 4. Pulling upward on traction suture so that the atrial clamp can be suitably placed on the auricular wall. The heel of this instrument should extend as far posteriorly and inferiorly as possible (over the orifice of the inferior cava) for best positioning of the rubber well. 5. Auricular wall opened.

(40 mg. of heparin in 100 cc. of 0.85 per cent sodium chloride). We have used weaker heparin solutions, but believe that this concentration is probably better. One to two hundred cubic centimeters of the mixture will be required, depending upon the length of time the well is kept open. The second assistant is instructed, and has as his main duty, to squirt a few cubic centimeters of this material into the blood within the well

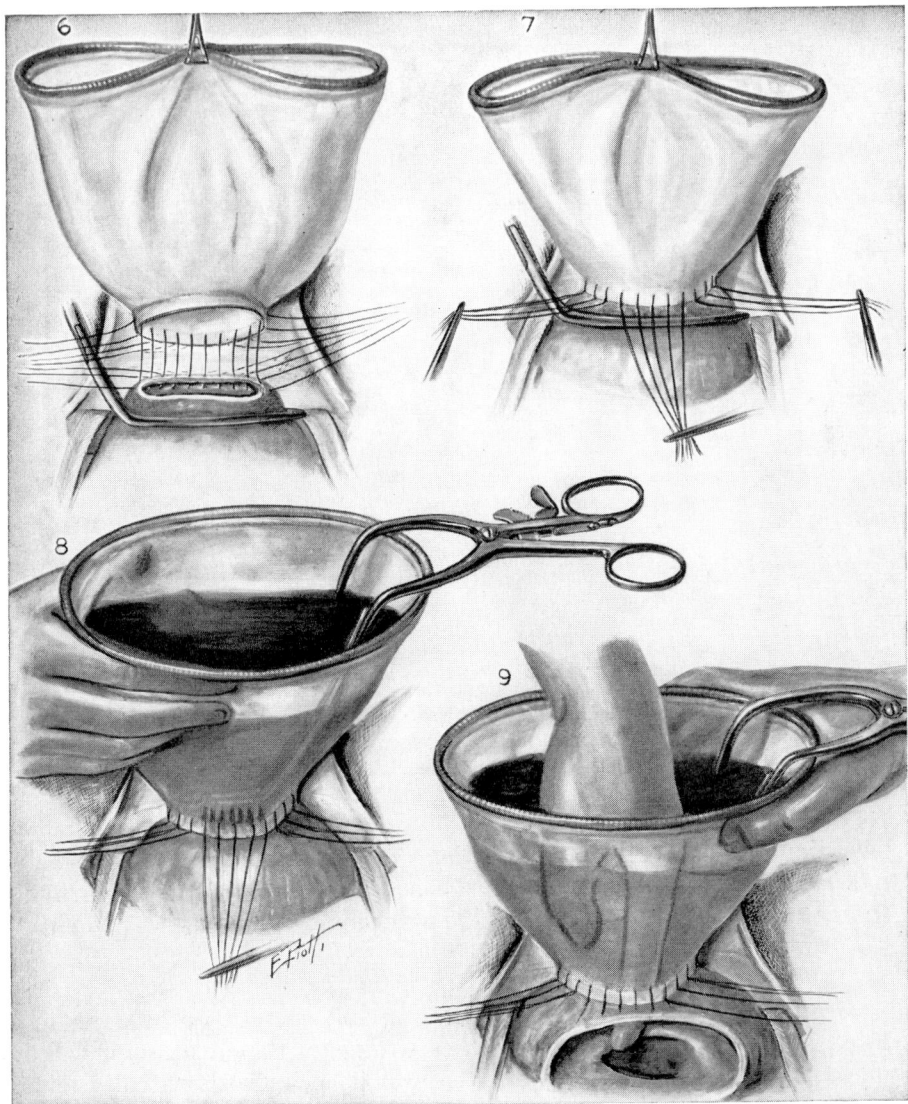

Fig. 500 (*continued*). 6. Rubber well being brought into place, silk sutures being taken through the auricular wall and grasping the lower rim of the rubber well. Sutures of 0000 Deknatel silk. 7. All stitches in place and tied. These silks are divided into four quadrants and the ends caught in hemostats as shown. 8. Atrial clamp removed, allowing blood to rush up into the well, to a distance equal to the intra-auricular pressure. Pulling on the anterior and posterior hemostats (which hold the silk sutures) will pull open the orifice of the auricular wall and facilitate introduction of the self-retaining retractor which is shown here in place. Spreading of the retractor gives an opening in the auricular wall 5 to 6 cm. in diameter (depending upon the size of the subject and the auricle). 9. Hand introduced through the pool of blood in the well, running a finger inside of the auricle, palpating the edge of the septal defect.

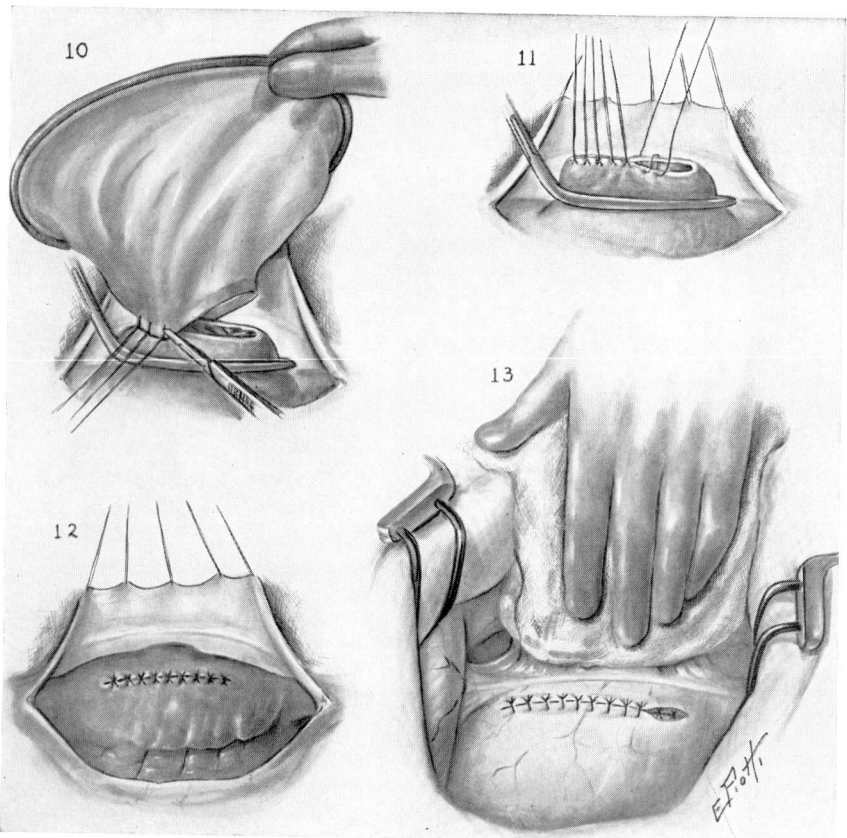

Fig. 500 (*continued*). Method of removal of the auricular well after completion of the intra-cardiac procedures. 10. Atrial clamp reapplied, taking care that this does not impinge on the coronary vessels. Rubber well being removed by cutting the silk sutures away from its base. 11. Closure of the auricular wall with interrupted figure-of-eight silk stitches. 12. Auricle closed. 13. Repair of pericardium, leaving a small slit above for the escape of any excess pericardial fluid.

every few minutes; this will prevent clotting of blood at all times. Occasionally the operator's gloves should be rinsed with the heparin solution. Any fibrin film which might form around the upper margins of the well should be wiped away with a piece of gauze.

It is possible to keep a well open for an indefinite period of time, certainly long enough to carry out the intracardiac exploration and operative procedures in an unhurried and in a deliberate manner. The heart tolerates these exposures without embarrassment; it just keeps beating on while the well is open. Cardiovascular adjustments can apparently be made without much difficulty, even if patients had previously been in heart failure. The size of the defect, the position of the same, and the availability of marginal shelf around the opening will determine the length of time during which the heart must be kept open for the repair; this will vary from case to case. Generally we have been able to accomplish all that is desired in thirty to forty-five minutes. The longest we have kept a well open in humans was two hours and five minutes! *There need be no haste during the intracardiac manipulations.* The examination of the interior of the auricle and the performance of the various steps in closure of the septal defect can be made carefully and in an effective manner.

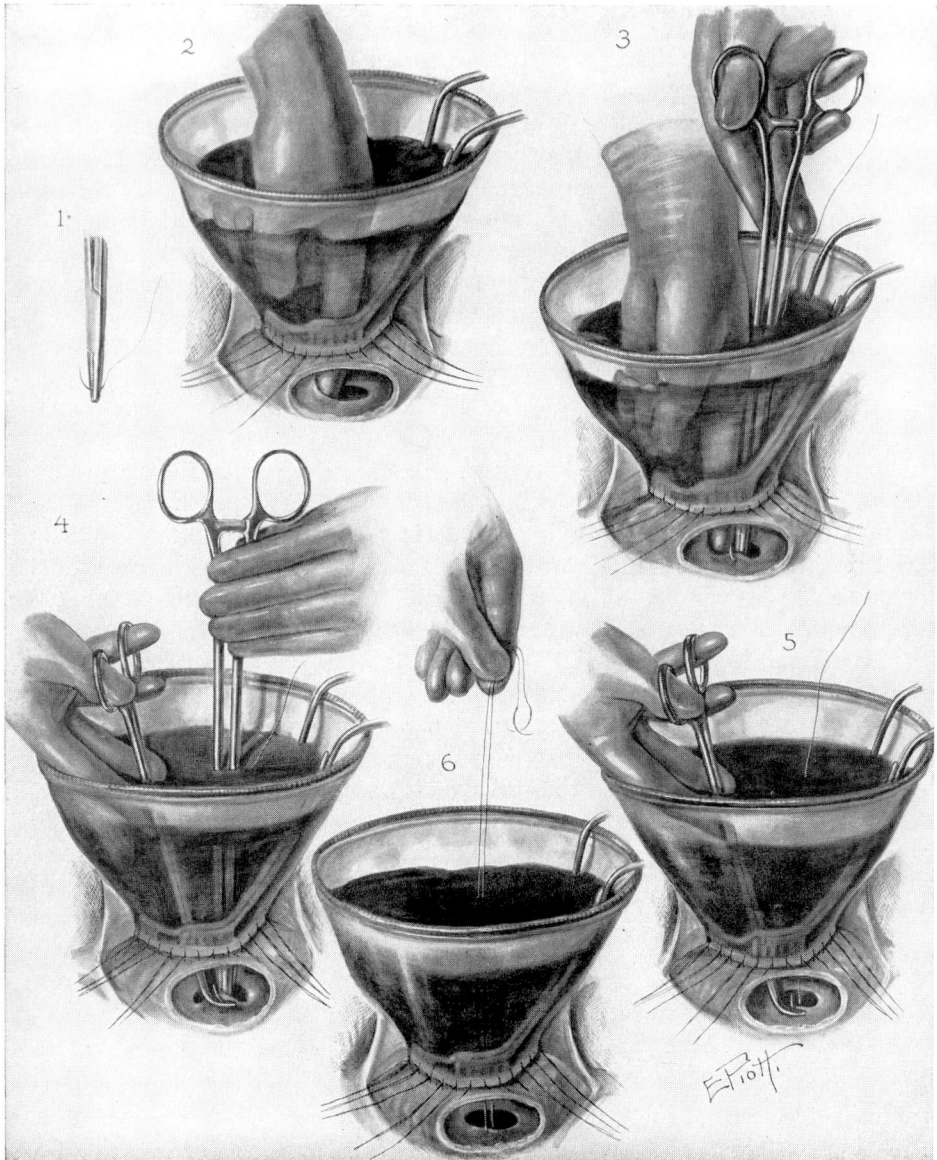

Fig. 501. Method of placing sutures in the edge of a septal defect, working through an atrial well. 1. Atraumatic needle carrying No. 000 Deknatel silk. Position of needle in needle-holder. 2. Left index finger exploring the septal defect and identifying its margin. 3. With the right hand, a 10-inch long, diamond-jawed needle-holder carries the needle into place, grasping 3 or 4 mm. of the septal edge. 4. The needle-holder is given to an assistant who keeps upward traction on it. The presenting point of the needle is palpated with left index finger and grasped with a right angle clamp. 5. Original needle-holder removed; right angle clamp still grasping the needle. 6. Needle recovered. When a septal closure is to be made by direct suture, the 30-inch threads should carry an atraumatic needle at either end to facilitate placement of suture through both sides of the septal margins.

Examining Interior of Auricle

By introducing the lower part of the hand into the well and passing the fingers into the interior of the auricular chamber, it is possible to identify very accurately the orifice of each vena cava, the tricuspid valve, the coronary sinus, and the auricular septum. The defect can be palpated; observations can be made regarding its position, size, shape, and surrounding marginal tissues. If there was any previous question about the presence of a mitral valve stenosis, a finger can be passed directly through into the left auricle and the orifice of the mitral valve examined. It is very important to palpate the posterior wall of the auricle, a point of particular importance when there is a "common chamber." If no ridge of septal tissue exists posteriorly, the entrances of the right pulmonary veins must be accurately recognized so that any reconstruction of the septum can be made in a way which assures that all the pulmonary veins will be directed thereby into the left auricular cavity.

Closure of Septal Defects

In employing an auricular well several methods are available for closure of septal defects; we have come to believe that only the last two will find wide use and effectiveness in treatment of humans. (1) It is possible to sew onto the septum organic tissues such as a resected tip of an auricular appendage or a piece of pericardium, anchoring the material with interrupted silk stitches to the septum around the periphery of the defect. (In animals, these gave extremely good closures but the softness of the materials made them difficult to handle.)

(2) It is possible to bring into place two rigid plastic discs, of the Hufnagel[12] type, so constructed that the discs can be screwed together by virtue of a central core and thread which they possess; after one is placed on the left of the septum and the other on the right of the same, the two are screwed together so that they completely occlude the septal opening. Such discs can be made in a variety of sizes, from one to many centimeters in diameter; they are machined from Lucite or Kel-F. They are accepted in an extraordinarily satisfactory manner by the heart and they are subsequently incorporated into the substance of the septum. While they have worked extremely well in dogs where there is a good rim of septum around the entire periphery of an artificially made septal defect, we have had fatalities when they were employed in humans. In humans there is apt to be an incomplete rim of marginal tissue, with insufficient substance to hold on to. The buttons are apt to work loose and drop into either of the auricular cavities. While such discs have the great advantage that they can be positioned within a few minutes, we are inclined to think they will seldom be useful in man except for closure of smaller defects when one is assured that there is a good rim around the entire opening for the button to grasp.

(3) From animal experiments[10,11] it has been shown that sheets of plastic material such as Nylon* or polyethylene can be cut to appropriate size and then sewed directly to the septum with interrupted stitches around its entire periphery; thus firmly anchored, the plastic material completely covers the septal opening. Nylon sheets* are available in thicknesses of 0.81 mm. and 0.13 mm. Polyethylene sheet† is available in thicknesses of 1.52 mm. and 0.51 mm., the latter being most suitable. Nylon and polyethylene sheets are sufficiently soft and pliable so that they can be cut readily by scissors to desired size

---

* Sold as Fe 1044 by the Polymer Corporation of Pennsylvania, Reading, Pennsylvania.
† Sold as "Type M" polyethylene sheeting by the Plax Corporation, Hartford, Connecticut.

and shape at the operating table, yet they are stiff enough to manage easily. The materials can easily be pierced by needles. They cannot be autoclaved; they must be sterilized by immersion in antiseptics (we prefer aqueous Zephiran, 1:1000, for twenty-four hours). The rapidity with which these foreign materials are covered is striking. Within a few hours after operation they are overlain by a fine layer of thrombus a millimeter or two in thickness. In a few weeks there is conversion of this thrombus to a fibrous covering, this

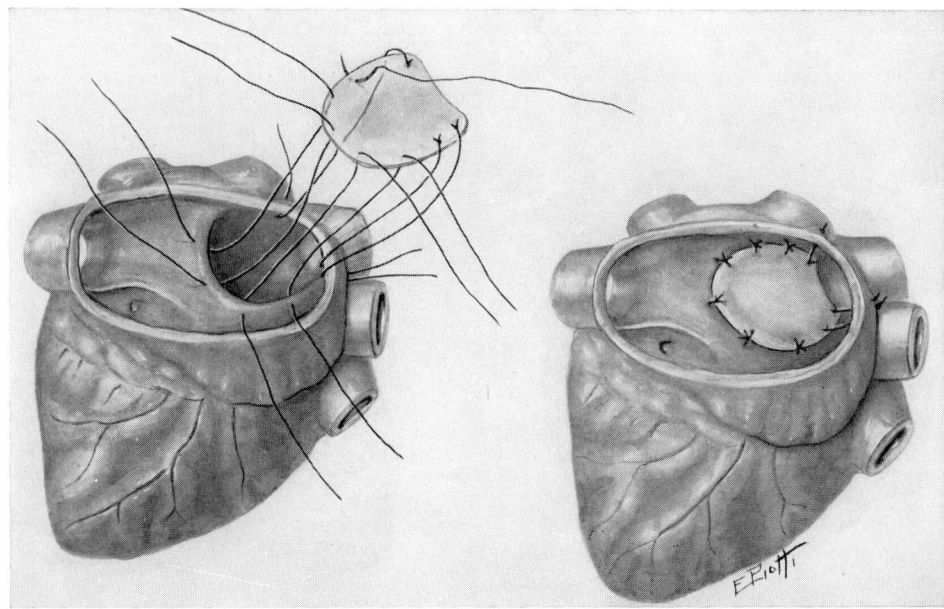

Fig. 502. Method of closure of interauricular septal defect by the onlay of a piece of polyethylene sheet. *Left*, A high septal defect with a good margin of septal tissue anterior and inferior to it, but no edge of septal tissue above and posteriorly near the orifice of the superior vena cava. Working through a rubber well (omitted here for purposes of clarity) the polyethylene sheet has been cut to appropriate size and shape, silk sutures have been taken through the periphery of the plastic material, and each has grasped tissue of the septum at an appropriate spot. Above and posteriorly, where there is no septal edge, silk threads have been run out through the auricular wall in a way which will subsequently draw the plastic sheet *medial* to the orifice of the superior vena cava, thereby directing all caval blood into the right auricle. *Right*, Plastic sheet drawn into place. The silks have been tied down and the excess cut off. Those silks which pierce the auricular wall have been tied externally. A complete closure of the septal opening.

change starting at the periphery and progressing toward the center. Endothelium grows in and completes the encasement in four to six weeks. Beyond six to eight weeks the plastic sheets are buried in a tough fibrous layer which blends imperceptibly with the surrounding septum. The plastic material always becomes sequestrated within the septum; in no instance in the laboratory have we seen formation of a cyst around it. From experimentation we have come to prefer polyethylene over Nylon; it gives less reaction in surrounding tissue.

(4) It is possible to close some septal openings by direct suture. Just how large an opening can be obliterated in this manner is open to debate. When there is very thick substance in the marginal tissues, stitches will hold sufficiently to permit pulling together of edges which are widely apart. Conversely, when septal edges are thin (as is so often the finding in humans), they will not accept much pull from stitches without

tearing. Therefore, we feel that it is seldom wise to attempt direct suture of a defect which is larger than 1 or possibly 1.5 cm. in width.

Suture Material. For all intracardiac suturing, 000 Deknatel silk 30 inches in length is used; at either end is an atraumatic curved needle 1.5 cm. long. It is essential that the silk be swedged to the needle; if at any time a needle is lost in an auricle, it can be retrieved instantly by pulling on the free end of the silk which runs up outside the well. It is also important to have available 30-inch sutures which are swedged onto two straight needles, about 4 cm. in length, these to be used in any part of the operation at

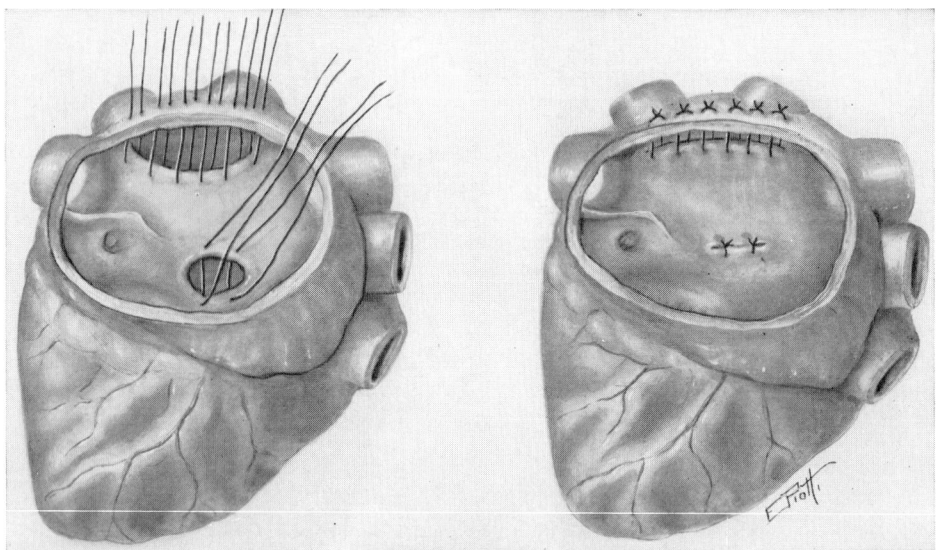

Fig. 503. Closure of septal defect in one patient by direct closure, the orifices being rather narrow and the marginal septal tissue being thick enough to permit direct approximation. *Left,* The two septal openings. The smaller one measured 1.5 × 1 cm. The larger, posterior one measured 3.5 cm. long and 1 cm. wide; there was no edge of septal tissue on the posterior auricular wall. The silk sutures were placed as shown for closure of the smaller anterior defect. For closure of the larger, posterior opening, mattress stitches were taken in a way which grasped the available septal edge and the silks were directed out through the posterior auricular wall to the right of the right pulmonary veins. *Right,* Silk stitches snugged up. The anterior opening is closed. The posterior opening is closed in a way which brings the septum to the posterior wall of the auricle in a position so that all of the pulmonary vein blood has been directed into the left auricle.

which one finds an incomplete septal edge and it is desired to place sutures in such a way that they are run out through the auricular wall. Straight needles can be passed out through the cardiac wall, and subsequently tied externally.

Placement of Sutures, Working Through a Well. To take stitches in a septum (to close an opening by direct suture or to anchor in place a piece of plastic sheet) might seem to present formidable problems of technique. However, with practice in the animal laboratory one can learn to carry out the manipulations of placement and tying of stitches in the depth of a pool of blood. Even though the operator cannot see what is being done, the stitches can be placed and tied accurately by "feel" (Fig. 501). With the left index finger, the margin of the septal defect is palpated; the right hand manipulates the 10-inch long holder carrying the needle. The tip of the needle-holder is passed through the septal opening and the needle is made to pierce the septal tissue, 3 or 4 mm. back from its edge, guiding this maneuver with the left index finger tip. The needle-holder is then given to the assistant, who carefully maintains the upward traction and impalement of the needle. With his right hand, the operator passes down into the auricle a right-angle clamp; under guidance by the left index finger, the right-angle clamp grasps the tip of the needle. The assistant releases the original needle-holder; the operator pulls up the needle (with his right-angle clamp). Working in this way, any desired number of stitches can be placed.

Closure of Large Defects by Polyethylene Sheet. For the larger defects, when one elects to sew a sheet of plastic material into place (Fig. 502), the sheet is cut to appropriate size and shape, making it slightly larger than the septal opening, but avoiding making it too large (a common tendency). This is then grasped with a hemostat at one edge and is held in a horizontal plane just above and to one side of the upper rim of the well; it is held constantly in this position by the second assistant while all of the sutures are being put in place. A stitch is taken by piercing the edge of the plastic material; then this needle grasps a margin of septal tissue in that area where the corresponding portion of plastic will later come to lie. Progressing in an orderly fashion, either in a clockwise or a counter-clockwise direction, separate silk sutures are taken and are individually allowed to drape over the side of the well in a radial fashion, clamping with a hemostat the two ends of each silk. These steps must be carefully done and no one on the team should be allowed to interfere with or to move the silks; with this precaution they will not become intermixed or tangled. After all of the stitches have been taken, the plastic sheet can be run down slowly through the pool of blood into the auricle and brought up against the septum, tightening up the various silks around the periphery as the plastic sheet is lowered into place. When the plastic is against the septum, the silks are picked up one by one, and are tried. It is best to tie the silks in a progressive manner, continuing around in a clockwise or counter-clockwise direction. This will minimize the possibility of mixing up the threads. After all of the stitches have been tied, the excess silk is now cut off; each silk is raised and kept taut by the assistant, thus allowing the operator by palpation with his left index finger to identify the strand at the bottom of the auricular cavity and thereby permitting guidance of scissors into place so that the silks can be cut close to their knots.

In those cases in which there is an incomplete margin of septal tissue around the septal opening, the plastic sheet can be brought directly against the external auricular wall by silk stitches which grasp the edge of the polyethylene and then pass out through the auricular wall; these silks can be tied subsequently outside of the auricle. If there is no edge of septal tissue antero-superiorly, such sutures must be run out through the auricular wall immediately to the left of the base of the auricular appendage, on the antero-superior surface of the heart. If there is no marginal tissue near the opening of the superior (Fig. 502) or the inferior vena cava, these transfixing stitches must be run out through the auricular wall *medial* to the base of the vena cava, so that all cava blood is directed into the right auricle when the prosthesis is brought into place. Finally, if there is no edge of septal tissue posteriorly, the plastic sheet must be brought against the posterior wall of the auricle and the stitches carefully placed so that they come out of the auricular wall to the right of the right pulmonary vein, thereby insuring that the plastic will be brought into place so that all blood from the lung is directed into the left auricle.

Closure of Small or Narrow Defects by Suture. In instances in which direct suture is to be employed (which will probably be in a minority of cases), an appropriate number of stitches can be placed, grasping the edges of the septum (Fig. 503). These strings emerge from the well and are left draped over the sides thereof; the free ends of each silk are held together by a hemostat. These silks must not be disturbed in any way which will permit them to be intertangled or mixed. After all of the sutures are placed, they can then be snugged up and the extra silk cut off.

Removal of the Well. After the intracardiac explorations and manipulations have been completed, the well is removed by withdrawing the self-retaining retractor, by replacement of an atrial clamp across the auricle (making sure that this clamp does not come too close to the coronary vessels) to shut off the base of the well from the general auricular cavity, and then cutting the various silk sutures that have anchored the rubber appliance to the heart. The lateral auricular wall is closed with interrupted figure-of-eight stitches of 0000 Deknatel silk. The pericardial sac is now closed loosely; an opening 8 to 10 mm. in length should be left in the pericardium, preferably at its upper end, so that any excess accumulation of fluid in the pericardial sac can escape into the pleural cavity.

The pleural space should always be drained by a large intercostal catheter, fitted with several holes, so that any fluid or blood in the pleural sac can be evacuated either by intermittent aspiration or by dependent drainage (using a water seal). The tube can generally be removed in three or four days.

Postoperative Measures

Renal Function. In some of these patients there has been a distinct oliguria (without evidence of renal damage) for the first few days after operation. The retention of fluids probably gives a hypervolemia; this might embarrass the circulation and put the heart on the verge of failure in the first few days after operation. It appears highly important to make sure that the kidneys are eliminating properly and that excessive intake of fluids (by parenteral routes) is avoided. To accomplish the former, we believe it to be helpful to give 50 per cent glucose intravenously immediately at the end of operation and possibly to repeat this three or four times during the first twenty-four hours, giving 25 to 100 cc. each time, depending on the size of the patient and the urgency which seems to be required in getting the kidneys excreting properly. In the administration of any parenteral fluids for the first few days, it is safer to keep the patient distinctly on the "dry" side; this will be quickly and safely corrected by the patient when fluids and nourishment can be taken by mouth.

Hemolysis. With an open well, the exposure of circulating blood to the dry air of the room, to the lower temperature of the room air, to the manipulations of fingers and instruments, etc., apparently damages red blood cells so that they will disintegrate prematurely. In some subjects there have been marked declines in the red-cell counts and hemoglobin values several days after operation (which cannot be accounted for on the basis of any blood loss into the pericardium or pleural cavity). The counts can fall to 2 or 3 million. Such excessive destruction of erythrocytes is ended by seven to ten days after operation. During the first postoperative week, a red blood count or hemoglobin determination should be made daily so that any significant anemia can be detected quickly and can be treated appropriately by transfusion of blood or packed red cells.

RESULTS OF OPERATION

Experience with the closure of septal defects in man is limited, but there is excellent promise that these congenital abnormalities can be treated with a reasonable degree of success. Ten children have been operated upon in our clinic. They ranged in age from five to sixteen years. Four of them were in right-sided failure prior to operation. There have been 6 fatalities. Three of these deaths were directly related to the use of plastic (screw-on) discs of the Hufnagel type; each of these worked loose and led to fatality in

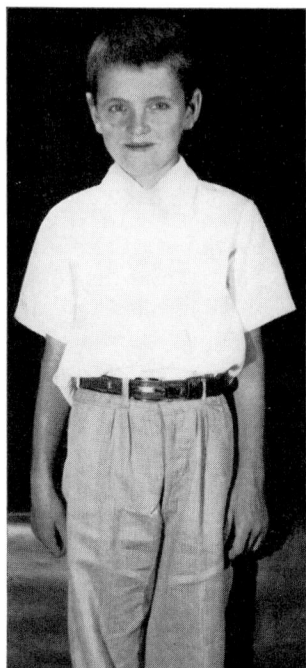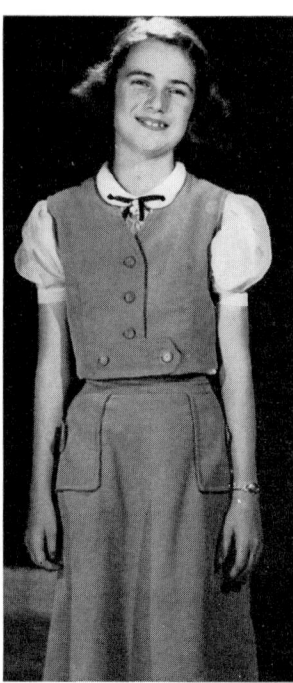

Fig. 504. Two children, six months after closure of septal defects. The boy on the left had a closure by an onlay of polyethylene sheet (Fig. 502). Postoperative catheterization shows that the septal defect is completely closed. The girl on the right had a closure of two septal openings as shown in Figure 503. Before operation her liver had been enlarged and her physical activities had been limited. Her liver is now normal in size and she enjoys completely normal physical exercise and sports.

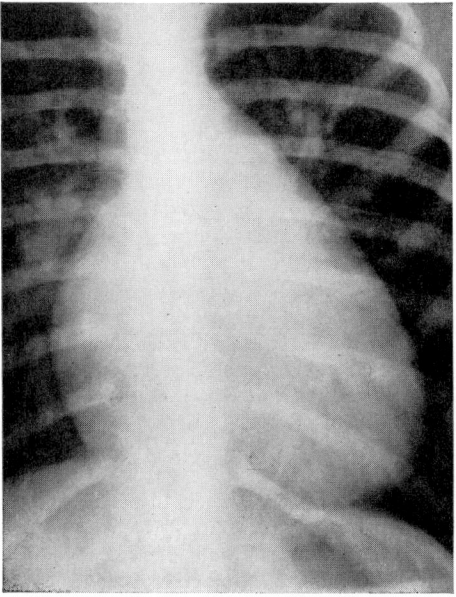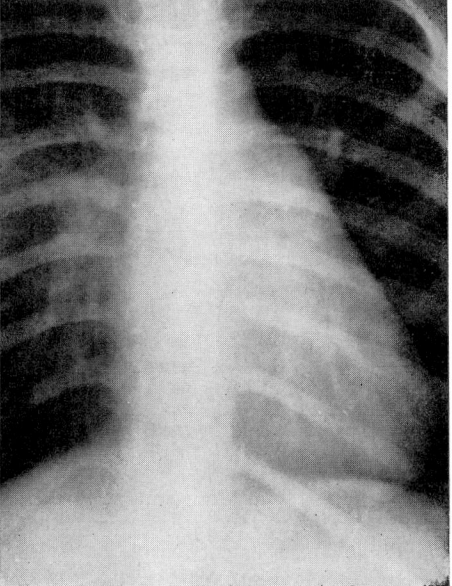

Fig. 505. Heart film from a five-year-old girl who had surgical closure of an interauricular septal defect. *Left*, Film before operation. *Right*, Film three weeks after operation showing diminution, in size, particularly of the right side of the heart and the pulmonary artery.

a few days or few weeks. The fourth death occurred following the use of a plastic sheet which had been sewn into place; inadvertently the sheet was cut too large and it therefore extended down over the annulus of the tricuspid valve, underneath which a thrombus formed which partially blocked the tricuspid orifice. Of the four patients who survived, three have had defects closed by the onlay of a plastic sheet (Fig. 502) anchored into place with silk sutures, while one child had the defects (two openings) closed by silk-suture approximation of the edges (Fig. 503).

It has been amazing to see the rehabilitation in the surviving children. Where there had previously been evidence of right-sided failure (with greatly enlarged liver and marked limitation of activities) the liver has receded to normal and the children have been able to carry on any form of exercise in a completely uninhibited way.

There seems to be little doubt that the method of approaching the interior of an auricle by the use of a rubber well has great usefulness. The technique is certainly a very practical one. The appliance apparently can be left in place for a rather indefinite period of time, permitting intracardiac manipulations to be carried out with great precision and accuracy. Large interauricular septal defects of any shape or position can be closed by the use of a plastic sheet, accurately sewn into place and anchored with silk stitches around its periphery. Small defects can be closed by direct suture.

REFERENCES

1. Bailey, C. P.: Personal Communication.
2. Barber, J. M., Magidson, O. and Wood, P.: Atrial Septal Defect with Special Reference to the Electrocardiogram, the Pulmonary Artery Pressure, and the Second Heart Sound. Brit. Heart J., 12:277, 1950.
3. Bedford, D. E., Papp, C., and Parkinson, J.: Atrial Septal Defect. Brit. Heart J., 3:37, 1941.
4. Brannon, E. S., Weens, H. S. and Warren, J. V.: Atrial Septal Defect. Study of Hemo-dynamics by the Technique of Right Heart Catheterization. Am. J. M. Sc., 200:480, 1945.
5. Cohn, R.: An Experimental Method for the Closure of Interauricular Septal Defects in Dogs. Am. Heart J., 33:453, 1947.
6. Dennis, C., Spreng, D. S., Jr., Nelson, G. E., Karlson, K. E., Nelson, R. M., Thomas, J. V., Eder, W. P. and Varco, R. L.: Development of a Pump-Oxygenator to Replace the Heart and Lungs; An Apparatus Applicable to Human Patients, and Application to One Case. Ann. Surg., 134:709, 1951.
7. Dexter, L., Haynes, F. W., Burwell, C. S., Eppinger, E. C., Sosman, M. C. and Evans, J. M.: Studies of Congenital Heart Disease. III. Venous Catheterization as a Diagnostic Aid in Patent Ductus Arteriosus, Tetralogy of Fallot, Ventricular Septal Defect, and Auricular Septal Defect. J. Clin. Investigation, 26:561, 1947.
8. Dodrill, F. D.: A Method for Exposure of the Cardiac Septa. J. Thoracic Surg., 18:652, 1949.
9. Dow, J. W. and Dexter, L.: Circulatory Dynamics in Atrial Septal Defect. J. Clin. Investigation, 29:809, 1950.
10. Gross, R. E., Pomeranz, A. A., Watkins, E., Jr. and Goldsmith, E. I.: Surgical Closure of Defects of the Interauricular Septum by Use of an Atrial Well. New England J. Med., 247:455, 1952.
11. Gross, R. E., Watkins, E., Jr., Pomeranz, A A. and Goldsmith, E. I.: A Method for Closure of Interauricular Septal Defects. Surg., Gynec. & Obst. 96:1, 1953.
12. Hufnagel, C. A. and Gillespie, J. F.: Closure of Interauricular Septal Defects. Bull. Georgetown Univ. M. Center, 4:137, 1951.
13. Ingraham, F. D., Alexander, E., Jr. and Matson, D. D.: Synthetic Plastic Materials in Surgery. New England J. Med., 236:362, 1947.
14. Martin, W. B. and Essex, H. E.: Experimental Production and Closure of Atrial Septal Defects, with Observations of Physiologic Effects. Surgery, 30:283, 1951.
15. Miller, B. J., Gibbon, J. H., Jr. and Gibbon, M. H.: Recent Advances in the Development of a Mechanical Heart and Lung Apparatus. Ann. Surg., 134:694, 1951.
16. Murray, G.: Closure of Defects in Cardiac Septa. Ann. Surg., 128:843, 1948.
17. Nadas, A. S. and Alimurung, M. M.: Apical Diastolic Murmurs in Congenital Heart Disease. The Rarity of Lutembacher's Syn-

drome. Am. Heart J., *43*:691, 1952.
18. Patten, B. M.: Developmental Defects at the Foramen Ovale. Am. J. Path., *14*:135, 1938.
19. Roesler, H.: Interatrial Septal Defect. Arch. Int. Med., *54*:339, 1934.
20. Santy, P., Bret, J., and Marion, P.: Communication inter-auriculaire traitée par invagination transeptale de l'auricule gauche dans l'auricule droite. Lyon chir., *45*:359, 1950.

21. Swan, H., Maresh, G., Johnson, M. E. and Warner, G.: The Experimental Creation and Closure of Auricular Septal Defects. J. Thoracic Surg., *20*:542, 1950.
22. Uhley, M. H.: Lutembacher's Syndrome and a New Concept of the Dynamics of Interatrial Septal Defect. Am. Heart J., *24*:315, 1942.
23. Varco, R. and Lewis, J.: Personal Communication.

CHAPTER 63

Tetralogy of Fallot

Among the various congenital abnormalities of the heart and great vessels which give rise to cyanotic states, the tetralogy of Fallot assumes greatest importance because it is the most common and also because it can be alleviated by surgical measures. Such malformations of the heart and great vessels have been recognized and extensively described by many writers, even before the time of Fallot who made his classic description of the pathologic anatomy in 1888. From this focus on the postmortem findings, attention gradually turned to more accurate recognition of these states during life so they could be separated from other forms of cyanotic congenital heart disease. The various pathologic and clinical observations were of value in clearly delineating the picture and the life history of the condition, but they added nothing for the treatment of humans affected with the malady. It remained for the brilliant interpretations of Taussig to emphasize the abnormal physiology, showing that the cyanotic state was due partially to intermixture of venous and oxygenated blood (by over-riding of the aorta) and to the insufficient flow of blood through the lungs (because of the pulmonic obstruction). This shift of attention from the anatomic deformities to the physiologic aberrations, permitted Taussig to see that it might be possible by some surgical maneuver to increase the flow of blood into the lungs and thereby improve the patient's condition. With this suggestion, Blalock was able to devise ingenious shunts which could divert incompletely oxygenated blood from the arterial system into the pulmonary circuit, so that more oxygen could be picked up. Subsequently, Potts and his co-workers introduced technical variations of this principle for producing a shunt from the aortic system into the pulmonary bed. More recently, Brock and others have made a direct attack on one portion of the tetralogy, by relieving the block which exists at the pulmonary valve or in the infundibulum below it.

PATHOLOGIC ANATOMY

The main features of these cardiovascular abnormalities include the following defects or secondary changes: There is obstruction in the right ventricular outflow tract. This may be in the valve itself, the cusps of which are fused, there being a central tiny orifice. The dome-shaped valve may be somewhat thicker than normal, but this is apt to be a minor change. The pulmonary artery and its branches are smaller than normal, are thin-walled, and of course carry a much reduced flow of blood. In an occasional case there is complete obstruction (atresia) at the pulmonic valve; in such an instance the pulmonary artery is exceedingly tiny (and may be so small that it is difficult or impossible to make any surgical shunt to it).

Not infrequently, the obstruction lies in the infundibular area, at a variable distance below the valve. This may have a funnel-shaped configuration or, less commonly, appear as a thick shelf or partial diaphragm; in either form the obstructing tissue is an intermixture of muscle and fibrous substance. Rather frequently the entire outflow tract, including the surrounding musculature of the conus, is small and underdeveloped (a situation making any surgical enlargement of this area impractical).

The incidence of the two varieties of obstruction (valvular versus infundibular) is open to debate; the matter is of considerable interest to those surgeons who desire to treat directly this portion of the malformation. Statistics on the point vary greatly with the age-groups of patients studied and whether the data has been gathered from autopsy or surgical observations. It is rather widely agreed that in the great majority of cases of tetralogy, the obstruction is infundibular in position; this is in distinct contrast to the findings in cases of "pure" pulmonic stenosis (in absence of tetralogy) in which the valvular form is much more common.

A defect occurs in the upper portion of the interventricular septum, immediately beneath the pulmonic and aortic valves; indeed the aorta is generally positioned in such a way that it straddles the upper part of this septal opening. There is always some degree of dextro-position or over-riding of the aorta so that it receives blood directly from both the left and the right ventricles.

From case to case, there are marked variations in the combinations which occur in relation to pulmonary obstruction and aortic over-riding. One subject might have little pulmonic obstruction and much over-riding; another may have the reverse; all degrees of intermixture of the two lesions can be seen. These are points of practical interest which have much to do with the success or the disappointment which follows surgical attempts to relieve the cardiovascular symptoms.

Because of its overwork, brought about by obstruction in the ventricular outflow tract, and also because of the fact that blood must be pumped at a pressure higher than normal to help to support the pressure in the aorta, the right ventricle becomes hypertrophied and often approaches, or can even exceed, the thickness of the left one.

There are several minor abnormalities which can be found in combination with the major defects, among which are interauricular septal openings, patency of the ductus arteriosus, or a right-sided aortic arch (which occurs in approximately 20 per cent of patients).

With the passage of years, nature attempts to build up collateral channels to get an increased amount of blood into the lungs. The bronchial arteries can become enlarged and form an important part of such accessory pathways. Myriads of small subpleural vessels around the hili of the lungs dilate and proliferate; these can be exceedingly numerous and appear as medusa-like fans or networks at the lung roots and in adjacent portions of the mediastinum and chest wall. The lung may become adherent to the parietal pleura (in adolescent or early adult life); collateral channels become established across this preexisting barrier. The development of all such accessory pathways allows more blood to enter the lungs and can bring amelioration of symptoms in late childhood or early adult life. The presence of these vessels can make surgical dissection of the lung root a complicated and troublesome affair.

CLINICAL PICTURE

History

Generally, these children are cyanotic from birth, but in some the color can be fairly good in early life during such time as the ductus remains open and provides a fairly good pulmonary flow. Cyanosis varies from mild to severe, depending upon the combination and degree of the defects which contribute to the total cardiovascular derangement; in some it is quite mild and in others it is very deep, there being all grades in between. Cyanosis is a constant finding; it is increased during crying, straining, or exercise.

Tolerance for physical exercise varies from mild disability to great limitation of activity. Beyond the first few years of life, squatting is commonly seen, the cause for assumption of this position being poorly understood. Dyspnea is common and is greatly exaggerated during exercise. Attacks of fainting or more prolonged periods of loss of consciousness are frequently seen in the more severe cases, particularly in the first few years of life.

The sluggishness of the circulation, the reduced pressure in the peripheral bed, and the increased viscosity of the blood, all contribute to the formation of spontaneous intravascular thromboses, which castastrophe is particularly apt to be brought on during times of dehydration (bouts of diarrhea, respiratory infection, and the like). Such clotting is especially prone to appear in the central nervous system; there can be extensive neurologic damage or even fatality.

Parents frequently complain that the child eats poorly; the youngster has learned that ingestion of large meals causes cardio-respiratory distress.

Superimposed *Streptococcus viridans* infection is very rare.

Physical Findings

On examination there is a variable degree of cyanosis which can be anything from mild to marked, and which is increased during physical activity. There is suffusion of the scleral vessels. The patient generally has rather slow and laggard movements. There is clubbing of the nails of the toes and fingers. The heart is not enlarged, or is only slightly so. There is generally a systolic murmur of mild or moderate intensity over the central portion of the precordium, and a diminution or absence of the second pulmonic sound. The systolic pressure is generally low. While the general physical development may be fairly good, the vast majority of subjects are thin, frail, and physically retarded.

Laboratory Data

There is an increase in the red blood count; it is commonly 6 or 7 million, and may rise to 8 or even 9 million. The hemoglobin values are elevated, ranging up to figures nearly twice normal. The hematocrit is high, is commonly between 60 and 70 per cent, and in very severe cases may be as high as 80 or 85 per cent. The oxygen saturation of the arterial blood is reduced at rest, and falls still further during exercise.

Electrocardiographic Tracings

There is always a marked right axis deviation. This is a point of considerable importance in differentiation from a tricuspid stenosis (or atresia), which can give quite a similar clinical picture, but which always has a left axis deviation in the electrocardiogram.

Prognosis

As one views a large series of patients with tetralogy, it appears that the most severely deformed die off in the first year, that there can be critical periods during which life hangs in the balance between six and twenty-four months of age, that there are a scattering of fatalities through the childhood years, with a large peak of deaths around the age of puberty, and with a minority of subjects living into early or even to mid-adult life. The average duration of life in Abbott's series was twelve years. While life expectancy is obviously cut short in all subjects, it is unwise to make specific statements

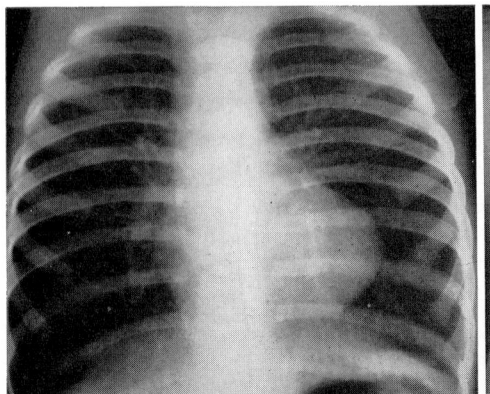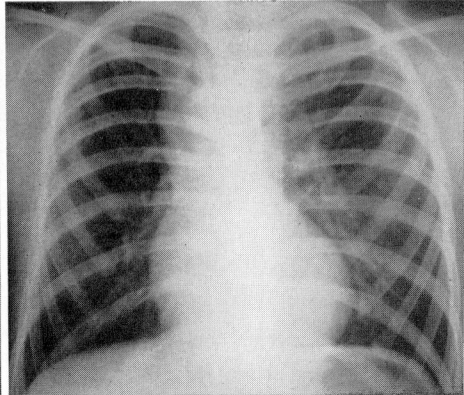

Fig. 506. Roentgenograms from typical cases of tetralogy of Fallot. *Left*, nine-year-old boy. Enlargement of the right ventricle, which raises the apex of the heart up above the diaphragm. Narrowness of the waist of the heart, from a small pulmonary artery. Increased radio-lucency of the lung fields, indicating diminished pulmonary blood flow. Aortic arch on patient's left. *Right*, seven-year-old girl. Enlargement of right ventricle, a very small pulmonary artery, only questionable evidence of diminution in pulmonary vascular markings. The aortic arch is on patient's right.

to a family regarding the prognosis for any particular child. The less severely deformed generally go through childhood without any great threat to life. The badly deformed patients can die at any time from cardiac failure, from overwhelming pulmonary infection, or from cerebral accident, but it is common to see youngsters desperately ill and blue and yet they hang on and survive in an amazing manner.

ROENTGENOGRAPHIC AND CATHETERIZATION DATA

There are certain features of fluoroscopic and film studies by which the tetralogy can generally be recognized, though from the outset it must be admitted that the ramifications of congenital cardiovascular cyanotic anomalies are so great that errors in roentgenographic diagnosis are not uncommon.

The heart is seldom enlarged, certainly the over-all size is never increased greatly; it may be subnormal in transverse dimension. It is generally possible to identify selective enlargement of the right ventricle, which raises the apex of the heart from the diaphragm, giving the so-called boot-shaped or sheep-nose configuration. The waist of the heart is narrowed. The pulmonary artery is small and has a markedly reduced pulsation. In the left anterior oblique view, there is an increased clarity in the aortic window, brought about by the smallness of the pulmonary artery and its branches. In about one-fifth of cases, the aortic arch is on the right side. The pulmonary fields have an increased radio-lucency, indicative of a diminished flow in the pulmonary bed; the lung hili have reduced pulsations.

Visualization of the heart and great vessels by radiopaque materials injected into the venous circulation show enlargement of the right ventricle, a right-left shunt within the heart through the septal defect, the early appearance of dye in the ascending aorta because of the over-riding of this vessel, and a diminished flow of blood through the lung fields.

Cardiac catheterization studies can give considerable evidence regarding the anomalies at hand. A catheter might be run through the septal defect and into the left side of the heart. Generally, it can be passed from the right ventricle directly into the ascending aorta, giving evidence of the over-riding. It may or may not be possible to introduce the catheter into the pulmonary artery. Pressure measurements from various positions in the pulmonary artery and right ventricular outflow tract can at times give information regarding the exact position of the pulmonic obstruction (valvular or infundibular) and also give some impression regarding the position and degree of the obstruction. By complicated formulas, the extent of the cross shunts, the peripheral flow, and the pulmonary flow can be determined; in some instances there are so many variables that such physiologic calculations are unreliable.

SELECTION OF CASES FOR OPERATION
Most Patients Should Be Operated Upon

Not all patients with tetralogy of Fallot should be operated upon. Those who have only faint cyanosis and only mild limitation of activity can be treated expectantly and operation deferred. In some of these, the symptoms improve with the passage of time, presumably due to the spontaneous development of collateral flow into the lungs. Conversely, some develop more severe symptoms in subsequent years and operation becomes desirable.

The vast majority of tetralogy patients have important symptomatology for which surgical alleviation should be offered. Unfortunately, many lay people have the impression, or the hope, that the cardiovascular abnormality can be miraculously and completely cured by surgical means. They must be informed that, while the situation cannot be made perfect, there is good likelihood of improving it. Before operation it is best to explain to the parents and relatives that the defect is a combination of abnormalities, some of which cannot be attacked but a portion of which can be helped or compensated for by surgical maneuvers In those cases in which symptoms have been very mild, the family sometimes prefers to avoid the risks and tribulations of surgery, which cannot completely correct the condition, whereas for those patients who have had marked symptoms there is almost always an acceptance of any gain which the surgeon can provide.

Surgical Results Unpredictable

Prior to operation, it is almost impossible to predict exactly what sort of a result will be forthcoming from surgery; the family should be informed of this. Some patients will have a result which is brilliant and is very pleasing to the surgeon, patient, and family. In others, the gains are not so marked but are still quite worth while. In a small minority, nothing is accomplished by operation; indeed the situation might actually be made worse because the heart is thrown into failure. Such great variations in surgical results are due to the tremendous range of combinations and extents of defects which can be found in the hearts. When pulmonary obstruction is high and over-riding of the aorta is minimal, the outcome of surgery will be striking. When there is a minimal degree of pulmonary obstruction and extensive aortic over-riding, the results of surgery are apt to be disappointing. It is generally impossible by clinical findings, by catheterization studies, or by angiocardiography, to identify with any degree of accuracy what proportion of the total clinical picture is caused by each of the anatomic deformities. Furthermore, none of these three studies gives reliable information regarding the result which can be anticipated by surgery. In spite of all these uncertainties, there are some factors which indicate types which are favorable for surgery, and there are some which suggest that technical difficulties of surgery will be high, that operative risks will be great, or that postoperative results might be poor. Favorable factors are: an age above four or five years of age, a pulmonic systolic murmur which is prominent, and a markedly diminished pulmonary flow as noted by roentgenographic, angiographic, or catheter study. Factors which make one apprehensive about accepting a case for surgery are: absence or faintness of a systolic murmur, smallness of a child (under two or three years), and peculiarities in the various findings of roentgenographic, catheterization, or angio-cardiographic study which might indicate important deviations from the common tetralogy picture.

Avoidance of Early Surgery

There is frequent and constant pressure from distraught parents for surgical allevi-ation of cyanotic states in babies. It has now become well recognized that these opera-tions in the first few years of life give much higher fatality rates, bring greatly increased technical difficulties at operation because of the smallness of the vessels which have to be dealt with, and are followed by more frequent postoperative disappointments. Therefore, as a general policy, it is best, whenever possible, to defer operation until the child is beyond three or more years of age. In spite of the precarious state of a baby or small child, it is generally possible to tide the youngster along until an age which is more favorable for operation. If it is found subsequently that the child is doing very poorly, the decision may have to be reversed and earlier operation resorted to, in spite of its high risks, greater technical difficulties, and lower promise of relief.

Optimum Ages for Operation

The optimum ages for surgical alleviation of the tetralogy of Fallot lie somewhere between four and fourteen years, but these are by no means sharply set limits. Excellent results have at times been obtained in younger and in older subjects.

SURGICAL TREATMENT

Prevention of Dehydration Essential

Dehydration must be avoided during the night before operation; the practice of limiting intake of food or fluid prior to surgery may be disastrous for these patients. When the hematocrit is very high, withholding fluids can produce intravascular throm-bosis. Adults or older children should be allowed water in unrestricted amounts up to one hour before surgery. For smaller children who appear to be cantankerous or nega-tivistic, it is generally best to give a slow-drip intravenous infusion during the early morning hours before operation is undertaken.

Methods for Surgical Correction

Two general methods are available for alleviation or correction of portions of the tetralogy picture. *First*, an opening can be made from a branch of the aorta to the pulmonary artery by the Blalock technique or the same result can be accomplished by direct anastomosis between the aorta and a pulmonary artery by the Potts modification. Creation of a shunt does not alter the underlying anatomic abnormalities; indeed it adds one more. In spite of such theoretical objections, these procedures have become well standardized, have been widely used, and have been recognized universally as bringing beneficial results. Second, it is possible to correct partially one of the anomalies by opening up the stenotic area in the pulmonic valve (or in the infundibulum below it); theoretically this is more desirable than a shunting operation because instead of adding another load, it cuts down on the number of abnormalities. Enlarging the pulmonary outflow tract is a rational procedure because, not only is more blood permitted to enter the lungs, but by reducing the pressure in the right ventricle there is less tendency to

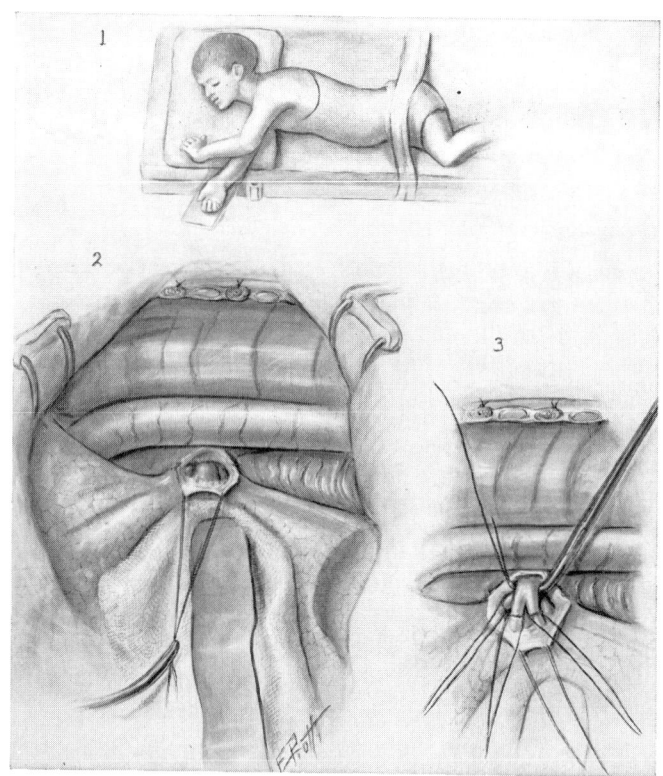

Fig. 507. Steps in establishment of a modified Potts aorta-pulmonary anastomosis. 1. Position of child on the table. 2. Incision throughout entire length of the fourth interspace; fourth and fifth ribs divided posteriorly. Lung held forward. After opening the pleura over the lung root, traction sutures as shown help to hold the lung out of the way and also attenuate the lung root and thereby aid in the subsequent dissection. 3. Pulmonary artery and its branches freed from their bed. Encircling threads of heavy braided silk around peripheral branches of the vessel. Similar thread being drawn around proximal portion of the left pulmonary artery.

force poorly oxygenated blood out into the over-riding aorta. Both factors contribute to a reduction of cyanosis. Unfortunately, attempts at removal of an obstruction in the outflow tract of the right ventricle (in cases of tetralogy) have always carried higher mortality rates than shunting operations; this is particularly true when blocks are in the infundibular region. If the surgeon attempts to perform pulmonary valvulotomy (or infundibulectomy) and has a fatality on the table, it invariably leaves the feeling that the patient might have survived if the heart itself had been left untouched and a shunt had been established.

We prefer to leave the decision regarding which method will be used until the chest is opened and the local findings can be evaluated. If by inspection and palpation the pulmonic obstruction is in the valve, a valvulotomy is done since this can be accomplished without too much difficulty, and with a rather high promise of survival. If, however, the block is found to be infundibular in position, the high risks of attack on this are avoided, and a shunt is made.

Operative Approach

For establishment of shunts, surgeons have varied in their selection of which side of the chest to enter, basing their choice upon the size of the patient, upon the side which carries certain of the great arteries in the superior mediastinum, or upon the side upon which the descending aorta resides. We have abandoned all such considerations and now open the left side of the chest in all subjects. This allows us to perform either a valvulotomy or to make a shunt, whichever seems most desirable. If a shunt is to be made, we have a marked preference for the Potts type of aorto-pulmonary unions. If the descending aorta is on the left, a Potts anastomosis is made, but if the aorta happens to be on the opposite side, the left subclavian artery is turned down for union to the left pulmonary artery by the Blalock method.

With the patient on the table and the left side uppermost, the left arm is extended forward and upward alongside of the head, the chest skin is prepared and draped well beyond the midline posteriorly and anteriorly, and a long incision is made over the fourth interspace from the nipple line well around to the medial border of the scapula, curving the posterior end up somewhat toward the shoulder. The chest is entered throughout the entire length of the fourth interspace. It is now possible to inspect and palpate the presenting portions of the heart and the first part of the pulmonary artery,

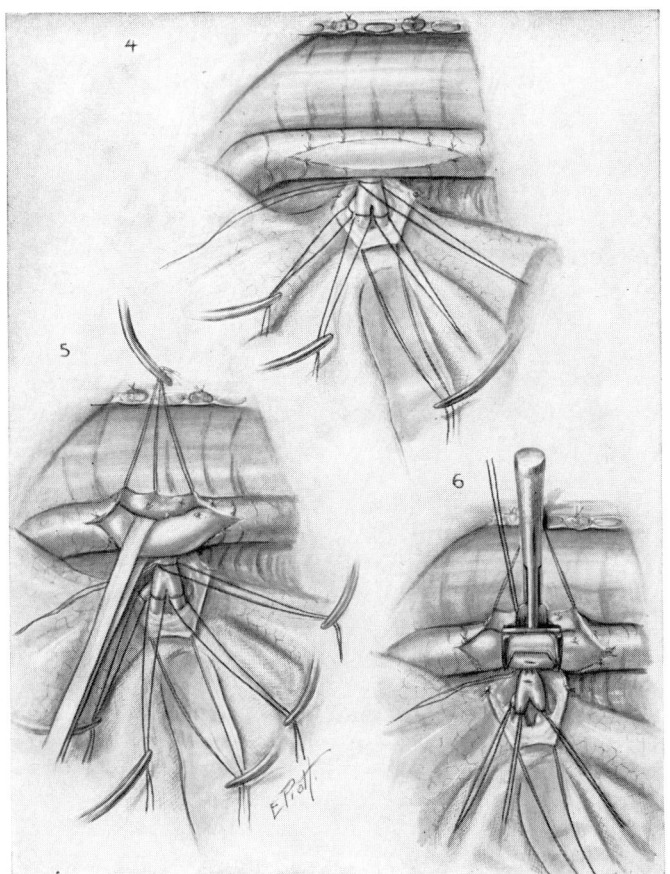

Fig. 507 (*continued*). 4. Encircling ligatures all in place. A fine "pull-out" string passes around the thread on the main pulmonary artery. Pleura over aorta opened. 5. Flap of pleura held back with sutures. The aorta is handled with a linen tape, which facilitates holding it up and freeing it from its bed. Intercostal arteries (two or three sets) divided. 6. Potts aorta clamp in place, allowing some flow of blood down the vessel, but isolating a segment for the anastomosis. Encircling ligatures snugged up on the pulmonary artery and its branches; the threads from the main artery are passed up behind the Potts clamp. The vessels lie in right-angle juxtaposition to each other. Opening made in each vessel.

894   THE SURGERY OF INFANCY AND CHILDHOOD

opening the pericardium, if necessary, to gain additional information. If the obstruction in the right ventricular outflow tract appears to be in the valve (as determined by feeling a jet through the center of the valve and by the ability to stop this thrill by local inward pressure of the pulmonary artery wall against the valve), direct valvulotomy should be decided upon. To facilitate this, the patient can be turned backward somewhat (the drapes having been arranged beforehand to permit this) and the fourth and third costal cartilages are divided very near the sternum. For pulmonary valvulotomy by the Brock technique, details are listed in Chapter 64. If the obstruction appears to be in the infundibular region, we much prefer to proceed with establishment of a shunt. To get adequate exposure for this, the patient is not turned, nor are the cartilages cut; instead, the fourth and fifth ribs are divided posteriorly, thus allowing them to be spread widely.

Potts Type Anastomosis

For establishment of a Potts form of union, steps are shown in Figure 507; these include certain slight modifications which seem to be of some advantage. We have found

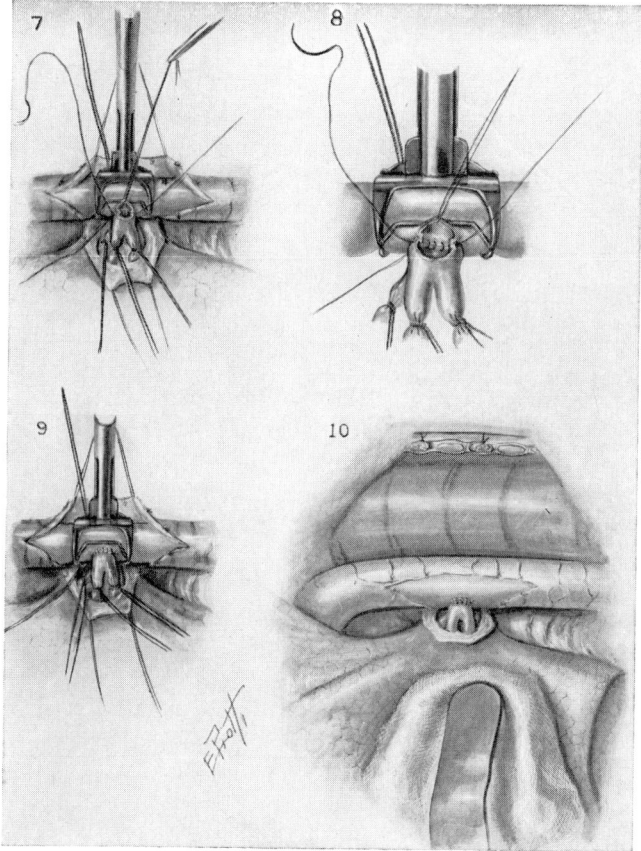

Fig. 507 (*continued*). 7. To give better exposure, the anterior flap of the aorta wall is held up with a fine suture. Anastomosis being made along medial wall by an over-and-over continuous suture of 00000 Deknatel silk. 8. Anastomosis completed along the back wall. 9. Anastomosis carried along lateral wall, turning edges of the vessels outward. In removing the encircling ligatures from the pulmonary artery, the fine pull-out thread will be helpful in retrieving the deep one. 10. Anastomosis completed. The advantage of performing the anastomosis in this way is that there will be no angulation of the pulmonary artery as the lung is expanded.

that attempts to anastomose the aorta and left pulmonary artery (as originally described by Potts) while having the vessels lie parallel to each other were often followed by kinking and partial blockage of the pulmonary artery when the lung was expanded at the end of operation. Because of such disappointments, we feel it is better to keep the pulmonary artery *at right-angles to the aorta*, a relation which it retains when the lung is expanded. When the aorta and pulmonary artery are opened, it is best to cut out from them a small elliptical or circular disc, rather than merely make a slit in each vessel; it is believed that this gives a stoma which is much more apt to remain open. Constant precaution must be taken to avoid making an anastomosis of too large size, an error which will overtax the heart and lead to its failure. The orifice should be made no more than 4 or 5 mm. in diameter. When the obstructing clamp and temporary ligatures are removed from the aorta and the pulmonary artery, a continuous thrill is set up in the pulmonary artery, indicating that blood is flowing into this vessel. From this point onward the patient's status generally improves and apprehension regarding his condition subsides.

Blalock Anastomosis

When the descending aorta is found to be on the opposite (right) side, a Blalock type of shunt must be made, for which freeing of the innominate artery and extensive mobilization of its subclavian branch will provide a vessel of adequate length to reach down to the pulmonary artery (Fig. 508). The subclavian artery is ligated as high as possible at the thoracic outlet and a serrefine clamp is placed on its origin, after which the artery is divided just proximal to the ligature. The pulmonary artery having been mobilized from its bed can now be tented upward somewhat. As a routine measure, the inferior pulmonary ligament should always be divided, to allow the lung to rise in the thorax and thereby move the pulmonary root toward the subclavian artery. It is generally possible to perform an end-to-side anastomosis between the subclavian and pulmonary arteries, but in an occasional case there is a considerable gap between these two structures; it becomes necessary to divide the pulmonary artery and perform an end-to-end union between the subclavian and the distal part of the left pulmonary artery. While this procedure has been found to be reasonably satisfactory, it is not as desirable as an end-to-side type of shunt which directs blood into both lungs. Rather than have an assistant hold clamps which stabilize the pulmonary artery and the severed end of the subclavian in relation to each other, we have found that it gives a much clearer field and is more satisfactory if the vessels are held together with two or three fine interrupted silk stitches taken in the adventitia of the vessels; these constantly hold the two vessels in proper alignment so the anastomosis can then be performed without the slightest tension on the stitches. An everting type of union is desirable if it can be made; generally a continuous everting mattress stitch of 00000 Deknatel silk is employed. In some cases we have placed a continuous everting mattress stitch medially but have used interrupted mattress stitches laterally.

Use of Plasma

During operations for establishment of shunts, it is our policy to avoid transfusion of blood if possible since the patient has red cells which soon will be superfluous if a good shunt is obtained. We therefore prefer to infuse only plasma, giving such amounts as are necessary to keep the peripheral pressure at an adequate level. In some patients, injection of ephedrine helps to support the blood pressure. Transfusion of blood is given only if the loss of blood has been great, which is seldom the case.

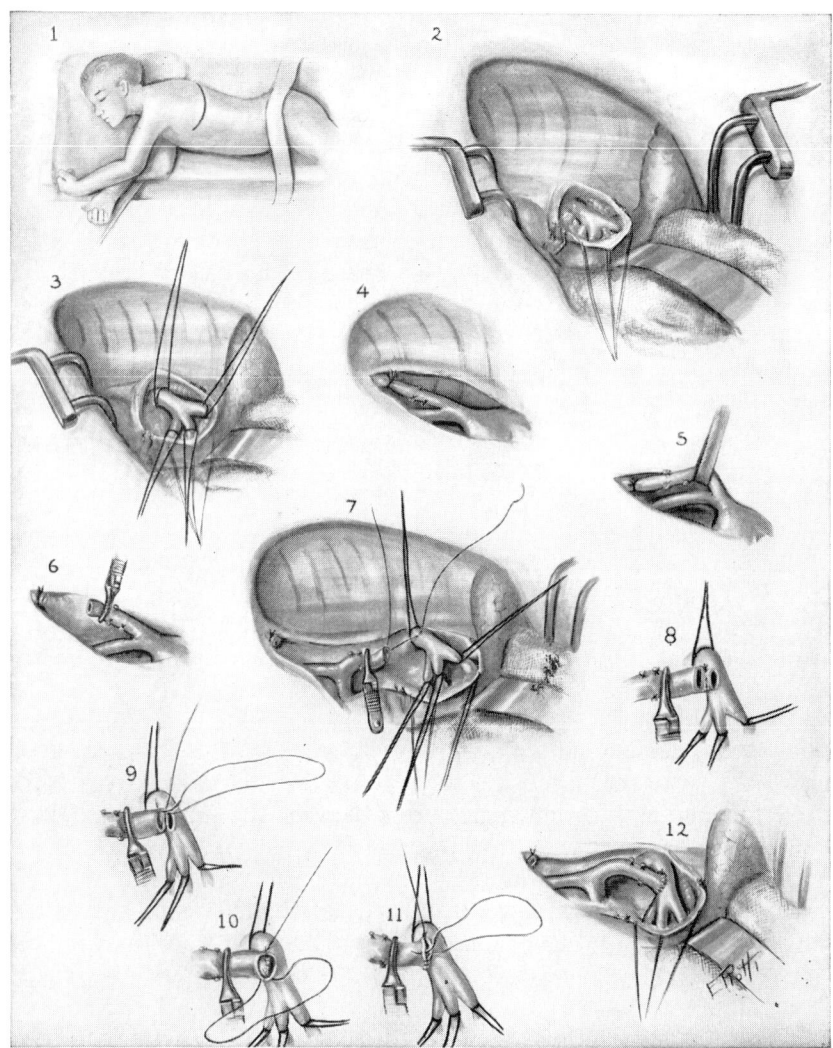

Fig. 508. Method employed for construction of subclavian-pulmonary artery anastomosis by the Blalock principles. 1. Position of child on the table. 2. Incision throughout the length of the fourth interspace, dividing the fourth and fifth ribs posteriorly. Lung root opened; the traction sutures on its pleural edge help to hold the lung down and also to attenuate the root vessels. 3. Left pulmonary artery and its branches isolated and encircled with temporary ligatures of large braided silk. 4. Dissection in apex of the thorax, exposing the innominate artery and the left subclavian artery which arises from it. Small branches of the subclavian have been divided. The subclavian has been ligated as far distally as possible. 5. Tape around the subclavian (sometimes around the innominate) an aid in freeing these vessels. 6. Serrefine clamp on the subclavian, after which the artery is divided. 7. Subclavian artery turned downward. Several sutures will be taken through the adventitia of the subclavian and pulmonary arteries. Snugging up and tying these will bring and hold the vessels together, so there will be no tension during performance of the anastomosis. 8. Vessels held together by the adventitial stitches. A disc has been cut out of the pulmonary artery wall. 9. Beginning of the anastomosis, employing 00000 Deknatel silk. 10. Back row completed, as an over-and-over stitch. 11. Continuing the anterior portion of the union, turning the edges of the vessel outward. Interrupted mattress stitches may be used here if preferred. 12. Anastomosis completed.

Pleural Drainage

To give maximum expansion of the lung, it is best to keep the pleural cavity as dry as possible after operation by use of an intercostal catheter, which is kept in place and on constant suction (or on dependent drainage) for two or three days.

Postoperative Handling

Hematocrit Level. During thoracotomy for establishment of an anastomosis, enough blood has usually been lost to reduce appreciably the red blood count by the end of operation. However, in some subjects in whom the hematocrit has been very high, it is necessary to withdraw additional amounts of blood to combat the polycythemia. At the termination of operation, a hematocrit determination is made; if it is higher than 55 per cent, phlebotomy is done to reduce the figure to somewhere between 50 and 55 per cent; this minimizes the chance of developing an intracranial thrombosis or a clot at the pulmonary anastomosis.

Maintenance of Arterial Pressure. Immediately after, and during the first 12 to eighteen hours following establishment of a shunt, efforts should be made to keep the arterial pressure at a level high enough to insure a good flow of blood through the shunt and into the lungs. If the arterial pressure falls, it can be supported by a slow infusion of fluids containing nor-epinephrine or Neo-synephrine.

Oxygen Tent. Following operation an oxygen tent should be employed, generally for several days, until such time as the patient's color is reasonably good, his condition is stable, and the cardiovascular apparatus is adjusted in a satisfactory manner.

Fluid Balance. During the first day or two after operation, overhydration must be guarded against assiduously because the unstable cardiovascular system, attempting to compensate for its many abnormalities, can be thrown into irretrievable failure if the blood volume is pushed beyond safe limits. As a general rule, it is much safer to keep patients slightly dehydrated for the first twenty-four or forty-eight hours. The use of intravenous fluids should be abandoned as soon as possible, because it is much safer to have the patient take fluids by mouth and in this way avoid embarrassment of the cardiovascular apparatus.

RESULTS OF THERAPY

It is rather difficult to compare mortality rates from various clinics because there are marked differences in selections of patients for operation. Surgical procedures in the milder or moderate forms of tetralogy are followed by rather low mortality rates, whereas operation on seriously maimed individuals can greatly increase mortality figures.

Results of Shunt Operations

In most large series of cases, the mortality rates have been from 4 to 8 per cent for patients over three years of age and from 20 to 30 per cent for children younger than this. In the Children's Hospital series, 181 patients have been operated upon by a shunting procedure either by a Blalock or Potts type up to December 31, 1952. In the last three years of this work, there were 135 cases and 15 surgical deaths (fatalities from all causes while in the hospital) giving a total mortality rate of 11 per cent; for patients under three years of age the figure was 30 per cent and for those over three years of age it was 7.1 per cent.

The postoperative results in patients who survived shunting operations are not uniformly bright but on the whole have been exceedingly satisfactory. A few individuals have not been able to stand the additional burden placed on the heart, even though the shunt was not of excessive size; the heart has bordered on failure or lapsed into complete incompetency in spite of all efforts to avoid this. Failure may appear within a few days after operation, but in some instances is delayed in onset for many months. Generally, if there has been no evidence of failure within five or six months, the patient will probably not have much risk of this sort thereafter.

In some patients the over-all picture is one of fair improvement, possibly not as much as the surgeon and patient would like to see, but yet the gains have been sufficiently great to make the operation worthwhile. In the vast majority of cases the improvement is dramatic and sustained. The cyanosis largely disappears, the clubbing becomes minimal, and the activity of the individual is greatly increased; physical effort can be carried on in an unhampered way. Of great importance is the reduction in red blood count and hemoglobin to safe levels, thereby removing the threat of vascular thomboses and brain damage. It is very pleasing to see a child who was previously blue, sluggish, dyspneic, and extremely limited, now take a new lease on life; the color is vastly better and the youngster is able to enjoy activities which rehabilitate him in an astounding way. Unfortunately, relief of the cyanotic state throws these patients over into a group where *Streptococcus viridans* infection becomes a real threat. Many such complications have already been reported.

If an anastomosis has been successfully established between the aortic and pulmonary systems and this stoma remains open for a few weeks after operation, there is relatively little chance of having it close off thereafter. In an occasional patient subsequent thrombosis or contracture does occur so that the shunt largely or completely disappears, and there is a return of cyanosis and limitation of activity which existed prior to operation. In such instances a further shunting operation can be done either by reexploration of the operative site or preferably by entering the opposite side of the chest and making an anastomosis of an appropriate sort in a new and undisturbed field.

Results with Valvulotomy or Infundibulectomy

In direct attack on an obstruction in the pulmonary valve (or infundibulum) for patients with tetralogy, Brock has reported 7 deaths in 39 cases, though the latter part of the series would tend to indicate much more favorable results than the total figures show. In a similar handling of the problem, Glover and Bailey reported fatality in 7 out of 30 patients. Of those patients who survived operation, the over-all picture seems possibly to be a little bit better than in others who had had shunting operations, this being particularly true when the obstruction had been of a valvular type.

Tricuspid Atresia

Tricuspid stenosis or atresia can occur in combination with a variety of malformations, foremost among which are interauricular septal defect, pulmonary stenosis, and hypoplasia of the right ventricle. There is cyanosis, but a left-axis deviation in the electrocardiogram. If the interauricular septal defect is small, there may be a damming up of blood behind the heart, the liver becoming greatly enlarged. Operative treatment of the condition by establishment of an aorto-pulmonary shunt has given beneficial results, but carries a much higher fatality rate than for the tetralogy; furthermore, cardiac failure subsequently supervenes in a considerable proportion of cases. In 2 cases we have combined a shunt with operative enlargement of the auricular defect, hoping by the latter step to increase the size of the avenue allowing blood to escape from the right side of the heart; after this, clinical improvement has been dramatic.

REFERENCES

1. Bahnson, H. T. and Ziegler, R. F.: A Consideration of the Causes of Death Following Operation for Congenital Heart Disease of the Cyanotic Type. Surg., Gynec. & Obst., 90:60, 1950.
2. Bing, R. J., Vandam, R. D., Handelsman, J. C., Campbell, J. A., Spencer, R. and Griswold, H. E.: Physiological Studies in Congenital Heart Disease. VI. Adaptations to Anoxia in Congenital Heart Disease with Cyanosis. Bull. Johns Hopkins Hosp., 83: 439, 1948.
3. Blalock, A.: Surgical Procedures Employed and Anatomical Variations Encountered in the Treatment of Congenital Pulmonic Stenosis. Surg., Gynec. & Obst., 87:385, 1948.
4. Brock, R. C.: Direct Cardiac Surgery in the Treatment of Congenital Pulmonary Stenosis. Ann. Surg., 136:63, 1952.
5. Campbell, M. and Reynolds, G.: Physical and Mental Development of Children with Congenital Heart Disease. Arch. Dis. Childhood. 24:294, 1949.
6. Fatti, L. and Gilroy, J. C.: Thoracoscopy as Aid to Diagnosis in Congenital Heart Disease. Brit. Heart J., 11:398, 1949.
7. Glover, R. P., Bailey, C. P. and O'Neill, T. J. E.: Surgery of Stenotic Valvular Disease of the Heart. J.A.M.A., 144:1049, 1950.
8. Humphreys, G. H., II.: Diagnosis and Treatment of Congenital Cyanotic Heart Disease. Bull. N. Y. Acad. Med., 23:283, 1947.
9. Josephs, H. W.: Mechanism of Reduction of Red Cells and Hemoglobin Following Operation for Tetralogy of Fallot. Bull. Johns Hopkins Hosp., 86:1, 1950.
10. Perkins, G. B., Hammond, M. M., Dwan, P. F. and Shapiro, M. J.: Tetralogy of Fallot; Analysis of 41 Cases of Patients Treated Surgically at the University of Minnesota Hospitals. J. Pediat., 35:401, 1949.
11. Potts, W. J., Smith, S. and Gibson, S.: Anastomosis of the Aorta to a Pulmonary Artery. J.A.M.A., 132:627, 1946.
12. Potts, W. J.: Aortic-Pulmonary Anastomosis for Pulmonary Stenosis. J. Thoracic Surg., 17:223, 1948.
13. Potts, W. J. and Gibson, S.: Aortic-Pulmonary Anastomosis in Congenital Pulmonary Stenosis. J.A.M.A., 137:343, 1948.
14. Potts, W. J. and Smith, S.: New Surgical Procedures in Certain Cases of Congenital Pulmonary Stenosis. Arch. Surg., 59:491, 1949.
15. Potts, W. J.: Surgical Treatment of Congenital Pulmonary Stenosis. Ann. Surg., 130: 342, 1949.
16. Rich, A. R.: A Hitherto Unrecognized Tendency to Development of Wide-Spread Pulmonary Vascular Obstruction in Patients with Congenital Pulmonary Stenosis (Tetralogy of Fallot). Bull. Johns Hopkins Hosp., 82:389, 1948.
17. Taussig, H. B.: Diagnosis of Tetralogy of Fallot and Indications for Operation. J. Thoracic Surg., 16:241, 1947.
18. Taussig, H. B.: Tetralogy of Fallot; Especially the Care of the Cyanotic Infant and Child. Pediatrics, 1:307, 1948.
19. Taussig, H. B.: Analysis of Malformations of the Heart Amenable to a Blalock-Taussig Operation (George Brown Memorial Lecture). Am. Heart J., 36:321, 1948.
20. Taussig, H. B., King, J. T., Bauersfeld, S. R. and Padbamati-Iyer, S.: Results of Operation for Pulmonary Stenosis and Atresia (Report of 1000 Cases). Tr. A. Am. Physicians, 64:67, 1951.
21. Ziegler, R. F.: The Cardiac Mechanism during Anaesthesia and Operation in Patients with Congenital Heart Disease and Cyanosis. Bull. Johns Hopkins Hosp., 83:237, 1948.

CHAPTER 64

Congenital Pulmonary Stenosis

Some of the congenital obstructions in the pulmonary outflow tract are now amenable to surgical therapy, owing to the brilliant work of Brock of London. These abnormalities can appear in several forms in or near the pulmonic valve, producing a bottleneck, and greatly impeding the flow of blood into the pulmonary circuit. The malformations are not difficult to recognize. Some of them are minimal and do not require surgical therapy, whereas the majority give a high degree of obstruction which makes operative intervention quite desirable.

The term "pure" or "isolated" is often applied to this form of pulmonic stenosis to differentiate it sharply from that combination of defects known as the tetralogy of Fallot (in which there is pulmonary stenosis, overriding of the aorta, an interventricular septal defect, and right ventricular hypertrophy).

PATHOLOGIC CONSIDERATIONS

Obstructions can be found in various parts of the outflow tract of the right ventricle. They can be in the pulmonary artery itself, in the pulmonary valve, in the valve ring, or in the infundibulum; these are all indicated in Figure 509. While infundibular types of stenosis occur rather frequently with tetralogy of Fallot, they are seen in only a minority of patients who have "pure" pulmonic lesions.

Fortunately, from the surgeon's standpoint, the most common obstruction is in the valve itself, there being no individual leaflets; instead the cusps are fused and form a conical or dome-shaped membrane with a small central orifice which may be no more than a few millimeters in diameter (Fig. 509, 1). This curved diaphragm is not particularly rigid or tough, though it may be slightly thickened toward its central edge. In older patients, the small orifice may carry warty vegetations; exceptionally the valve may be calcified. The structure is always thin enough so that it can be pierced readily and can be cut with the blade of a knife. With this form of block, the pulmonary artery is almost invariably dilated greatly.

Constrictions are occasionally seen in the pulmonic valve annulus or in the tissues immediately proximal to it (Fig. 509, 2). The valve leaflets are normal, but these and the first part of the pulmonary artery are very apt to be smaller than normal; the entire outflow channel is somewhat narrowed, giving a situation which is exceedingly difficult to remedy by operative means.

In a distinct minority of cases, stenosis occurs in the infundibulum. It might be of a *diaphragmatic* character, and consist of fibrous and muscular tissue, located at a variable distance below the valve; the shelf-like structure of the deformity makes it possible to cut away some of it surgically. Between this shelf and the pulmonary valve is an "infundibular chamber" of variable size. This chamber has an external cardiac wall of variable thickness; it may be quite thin, or it can be thick and muscular. It assumes surgical importance because, if large enough, it provides an avenue of approach (the pressure within it being low) through which the operator can work downward and come upon the constricted area from its distal aspect. Infundibular stenoses can also be long and *funnel-like*, making a situation which is quite difficult for the surgeon to treat by incision, excision, or dilatation. While pulmonic obstruction might be valvular or intundibular, in rare instances these two forms can coexist.

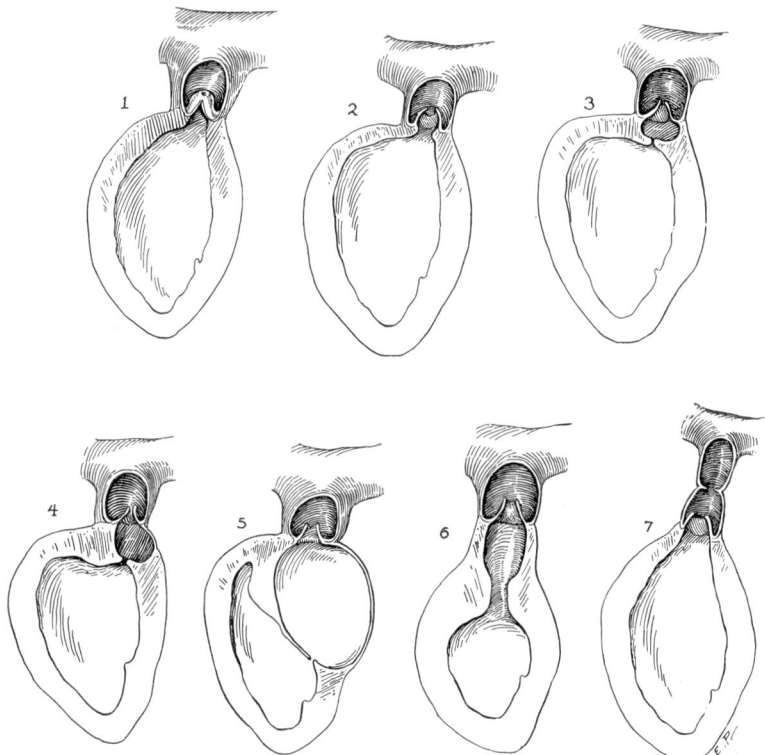

Fig. 509. Types of congenital obstruction in the pulmonary outflow tract. 1. Obstruction of a valvular type in which the leaflets are fused, presenting a small central orifice. The pulmonary artery is generally quite dilated. This valvular form of block is most amenable to surgical therapy. 2. A constriction in the annulus, at the base of the valve, exceedingly difficult to treat. 3. An infundibular type of block which is immediately below the valve. There is not enough of a chamber above this to enter the heart above the obstruction. The valve ring, valve, and pulmonary artery are apt to be smaller than normal, making this situation somewhat difficult to treat. 4. Infundibular block a little farther separated from the valve, but still with a chamber above it insufficient to work through. The pulmonary valve ring, valve, and pulmonary artery are essentially normal in size. 5. Infundibular diaphragm with a chamber above it which is large enough to enter and to work downward to excise a piece of the diaphragm. 6. Infundibular fusiform type of obstruction which is exceedingly difficult to cut, dilate, or enlarge in a satisfactory manner by operative means. 7. Obstruction in the main pulmonary artery.

With any of the anomalies which have been described, that portion of the right ventricle which is proximal to the obstruction becomes hypertrophied and dilated, because of the overwork of this part of the heart.

With any of the obstructions, pressure in the pulmonary artery is always much lower than normal; the pulmonary artery is seldom normal in size. When accompanying a valvular block, the vessel almost always, for some poorly understood reason, is dilated strikingly, whereas with the blocks below the valve the artery tends to be diminished in size.

In slightly less than half of the cases, obstruction of the pulmonary outflow tract is the only anomaly within the heart; in the remainder there is an associated defect, either in the interauricular or interventricular septum. Interventricular openings are probably somewhat more common than are interauricular ones, but these associated malformations seem to vary greatly in incidence in different series of cases. While valvular stenosis commonly exists without a septal defect, infundibular stenosis rarely is found as an isolated lesion without patency of the septa.

CLINICAL FINDINGS

Constrictions in the pulmonary outflow tract can vary so widely in their degree of obstruction that one finds symptomatologies which range from mild to severe. With high grades of block, difficulties can appear early in infancy or childhood, whereas with lesser obstructions there may be little or no trouble until the teen-ages or even adult life. Indeed, a few of the malformations are so mild that they can be tolerated through a rather long life.

Complaints

In the presence of a pure pulmonic obstruction (with no associated septal defect), the patient shows relatively little or no distress when at rest or at mild activity. With increasing exercise, the flow of blood through the circulation becomes held up at the bottleneck, and symptoms appear. These are largely in the form of dyspnea, palpitation, and weakness. There is no true cyanosis, since the arterial blood is completely saturated with oxygen. The flow through the entire peripheral system is so slowed that blood lingers in the capillary bed; oxygen in amounts greater than normal is removed from the red cells, thus giving rise to a faint dusky appearance of the lips and nailbeds, the so-called "peripheral" cyanosis. Clubbing is absent or minimal; polycythemia is unusual. Squatting is quite rare, a notable contrast to the finding in cases of tetralogy. Dyspnea can occur in paroxysms, and is a warning of approaching dissolution. A history of fainting attacks is especially an ill omen. In the presence of failure, the liver is greatly enlarged, and possibly pulsating. When failure begins to appear, complete collapse and death are very apt to supervene shortly thereafter, unless averted by timely surgical valvulotomy.

In those cases in which there is a pulmonic obstruction plus a septal defect, the clinical picture is much the same, except for the addition of generalized cyanosis, which is apt to diminish (or disappear) during rest, and become intensified during exercise. Clubbing can be found. The high pressure in the right side of the heart produces a right-to-left shunt; the intermixture gives a reduction in oxygen saturation of the arterial blood. Although cyanosis of this origin can be present from birth, it is more apt to develop insidiously and come on during the early years of childhood. The cyanosis is seldom as great as that seen in the more striking cases of tetralogy of Fallot. Squatting is sometimes seen.

Physical Examination

The outstanding finding is a very loud blowing or harsh murmur, generally accompanied by a thrill, systolic in time, which is most intense in the second or third interspace to the left of the sternum. The second pulmonic sound is absent or is greatly diminished. This prominent murmur in the pulmonary region generally covers or masks any murmur which might be originating from a septal defect. Squatting is sometimes seen in those cases where there is cyanosis. The heart may show a variable degree of enlargement;

if this is marked, it suggests that the heart is in failure or verges on it. Enlargement of the liver is found when the right ventricle has been embarrassed.

Electrocardiographic Tracings

There is marked evidence of a right axis deviation and either right ventricular hypertrophy or right bundle branch block.

ROENTGENOGRAPHIC DATA

By film and fluoroscopic studies the right ventricle is always enlarged, at times greatly so. There is a diminished pulsation in the pulmonary artery and its branches, as well as in the hili of the lungs. The main pulmonary artery might be normal or smaller than normal, but frequently it is tremendously dilated. The latter finding is a particularly

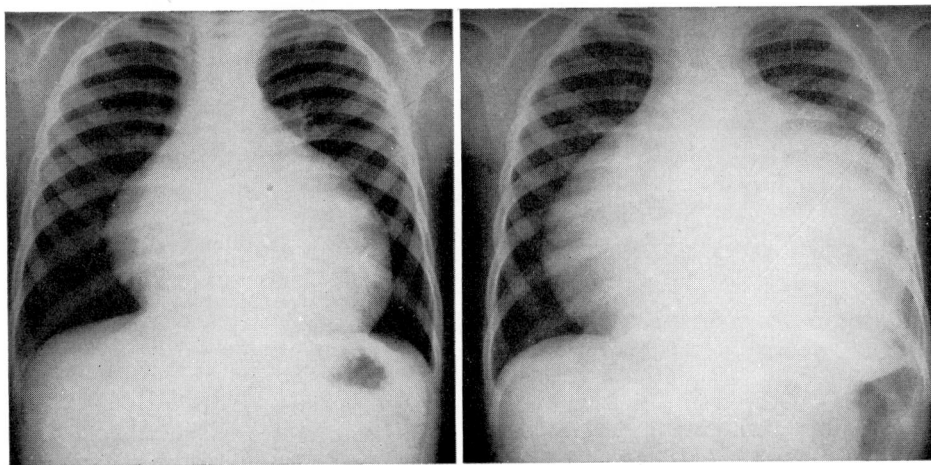

Fig. 510. *Left*, Film from child six years of age, with marked cardiac enlargement. Pulmonary stenosis proved by catheterization, the right ventricle pressure being 200 mm. Hg. Only minimal symptoms at this time. *Right*, Two months later, the child in failure. Massive cardiac enlargement and pericardial effusion.

happy one, since it usually implies that the obstruction is valvular and hence very favorable for surgical relief. The auricles are not enlarged, unless there is an associated interauricular septal defect, or unless impending failure of the right ventricle allows blood to dam up in the right auricle and distend this chamber.

Visualization of the right side of the heart and the pulmonary artery by angio-cardiography is not always necessary, but is sometimes helpful. Because of retardation in flow, the dye remains longer than normal in the right side of the heart, the pulmonary artery, and in the lung fields. The right ventricle is more capacious than normal. A small or normal artery generally suggests an obstruction in the infundibular region, whereas a greatly dilated artery is more commonly indicative of a valvular type. Sometimes the point of obstruction can be visualized if an exposure happens to be taken at precisely the right moment, and the patient turned at an appropriate angle. Early appearance of dye in the left auricle or left ventricle (prior to the time that it has been able to reach these by way of the pulmonary circuit) is good evidence of a septal defect. Absence of dye in the ascending aorta, prior to the time that the material comes through the left side of the heart, rules out any overriding of the vessel.

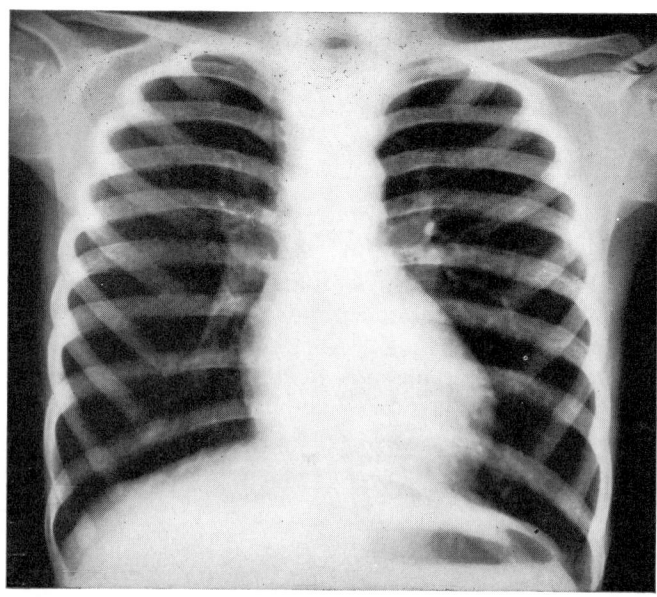

Fig. 511. Film from six-year-old girl with limitation of activities and right ventricular preponderance by electrocardiogram. The pulmonary artery is smaller than normal. At exploratory operation the main pulmonary artery was hypoplastic (Fig. 509, 7), the pulmonary infundibulum and pulmonary valve being normal.

CATHETERIZATION STUDIES

Cardiac catheterization studies are highly desirable in all patients with obstruction of the pulmonary outflow tract. While this is not necessary in all patients to establish a diagnosis, in some it is an important feature in differentiating this pathology from other types of congenital heart disease. Pressure measurements provide a preoperative basal figure with which postoperative values can be compared later to see how much has been gained by surgical therapy.

There is generally little or no difficulty in passing a catheter into the right ventricle and through its outflow tract, since the catheter tends to be carried in the blood stream and its tip can be directed through the smallest of orifices which are generally conical in shape when approached from the proximal side. With the catheter placed well up into the pulmonary artery, a great deal can be learned as it is withdrawn. Pressure in the pulmonary artery is markedly reduced; as the catheter is withdrawn proximal to the obstruction, the recorded pressure rises sharply; the difference between these two values indicates the degree of obstruction. The systolic pressure in the right ventricle (normally 25 to 30 mm. of mercury) is always elevated, and may even exceed 200 mm. of mercury. Under fluoroscopic visualization, the tip of the catheter can be observed as it is pulled back; at that point where a marked rise in pressure occurs, fluoroscopic identification of the catheter tip can usually indicate the position of the obstruction. If there is any coexisting septal defect, it might be possible to pass the catheter through it; physiologic measurements almost invariably show a shunt from right to left.

Findings from a typical case of pulmonic stenosis and patent foramen ovale in a nine-year-old boy gave the following:

SITE	O₂ CONTENT Vol. %	% O₂ Sat.	PRESSURE mm. Hg
Superior vena cava	9.9	65	8–5
Inferior vena cava	9.4	61	9–6
Right auricle—low	10.0	66	8–4
Right auricle—high	9.5	62	10–7
Right ventricle	10.3	67	90–10
Right ventricle—outflow	9.7	63	86–16
Main pulmonary artery	9.8	64	25–17
Left pulmonary artery	10.3	67	22–10
Left auricle	13.6	88	9–2
Left pulmonary vein	14.0	91	15–10

From a representative group of children, all subsequently proved at operation to have pulmonary stenosis, the following figures were obtained at catheterization:

PATIENT	AGE	RIGHT VENTRICULAR PRESSURE (mm. Hg)
J. W.	9 yrs.	70–0
J. M.	8 yrs.	92–10
A. S.	10 yrs.	140–8
D. C.	4 yrs.	220–5
W. U.	8 yrs.	190–10
K. B.	9 yrs.	200–8

INDICATIONS FOR OPERATION

Not all patients with obstruction of the pulmonary outflow tract require operation. There are some with minimal degrees of block who tolerate the anomaly in a reasonably satisfactory way and hence should not be subjected to the risks of operation. These patients should be reexamined from time to time, for a few of them might subsequently develop findings which make operation desirable. There can be no question about the advisability of surgery for those with important symptoms. Dyspnea, cardiac enlargement, or evidence of increasing cardiac fatigue are all positive indications for surgical therapy.

There remains a considerable group of patients, particularly in childhood, who have very little in the way of symptomatology and concerning whom there can be debate regarding the pros and cons of surgery. In such a dilemma, cardiac catheterization and determination of the right ventricular pressure is of great help in appraising the cardiac status. If right ventricular pressure is increased to only a mild or moderate degree, it is best to defer operation, but if it is above 75 or 80 mm. of mercury, there is such a high chance of subsequent embarrassment or failure of the right side of the heart that we prefer to advise operation, even though there be no symptoms at the moment. When marked elevations of pressures are found (150 to 200 or more), operation is imperative, because right ventricular collapse can take place at any time, and can do so precipitously. It is much better to operate while a myocardium is still in good state of compensation, rather than wait until it is damaged irretrievably. Some cardiologists have preferred not to use the right ventricular pressure as the guide in the decision for or against therapy, but instead have depended more upon the electrocardiogram, feeling that any change from right-sided hypertrophy to right-sided strain is a clear indication for operation.

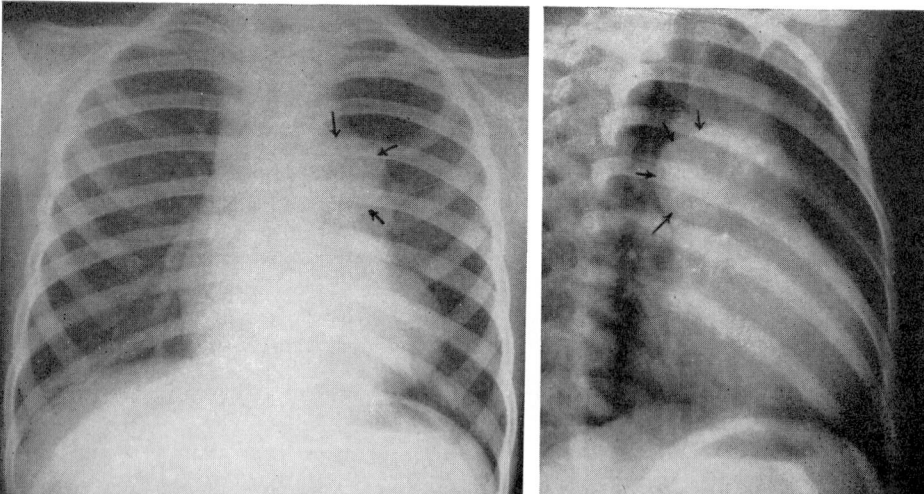

Fig. 512. *Left,* Eleven-year-old boy with congenital stenosis of pulmonary valve, enlargement of the right ventricle, and great dilatation of the pulmonary artery (arrows) beyond the valvular obstruction. *Right,* Lateral view shows the markedly dilated pulmonary artery (arrows). In the presence of obstruction in the pulmonary outflow tract, prominent dilatation of the pulmonary artery usually implies that the obstruction is in the valve itself—a situation very favorable for operative relief.

SURGICAL TREATMENT
Choice of Procedure

Any form of shunting operation such as a Blalock-Taussig or a Potts procedure should be avoided in the treatment of these cases; this is in contrast to the beneficial effects of a shunt on the tetralogy of Fallot. For pure pulmonic stenosis, an artificial shunt gives absolutely no relief; the right ventricle is still pumping against an obstruction and

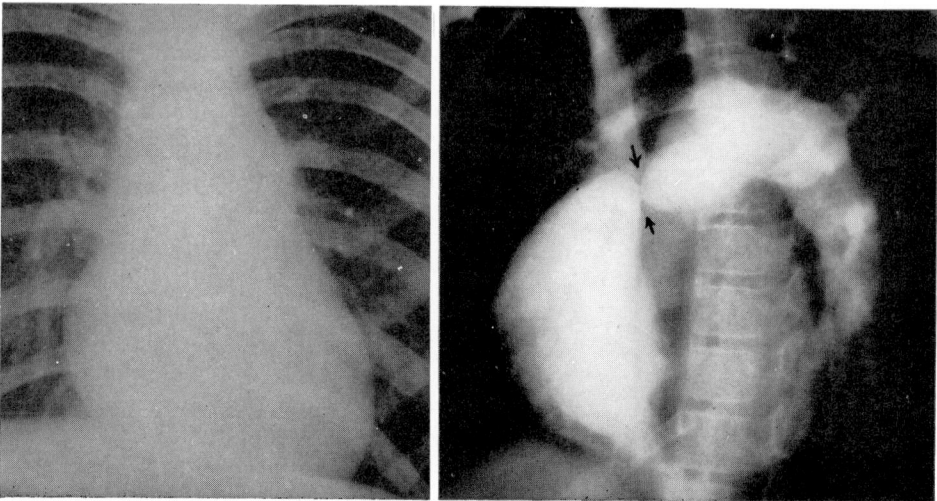

Fig. 513. Roentgenographic findings from a six-year-old girl with congenital obstruction at the pulmonic valve. *Left,* Roentgenogram showing some enlargement of the right side of the heart and a prominent dilatation of the pulmonary artery beyond the valvular obstruction. By fluoroscopy this dilated vessel had a reduced pulsation. *Right,* Visualization of the right ventricle and the pulmonic outflow tract, showing well marked constriction at the valve (arrows) and a great dilatation of the pulmonary artery beyond this.

will fail. While the combination of pulmonic obstruction and septal defect (either between the auricles, or especially between the ventricles) can be helped somewhat by providing a shunt and recirculating incompletely oxygenated blood back through the lungs, such handling is still rather poor because the right ventricle continues to be overworked. The best therapy for a pulmonic obstruction (whether or not there is an associated septal defect) is by direct attack on the obstruction and enlargement of the ventricular outflow tract.

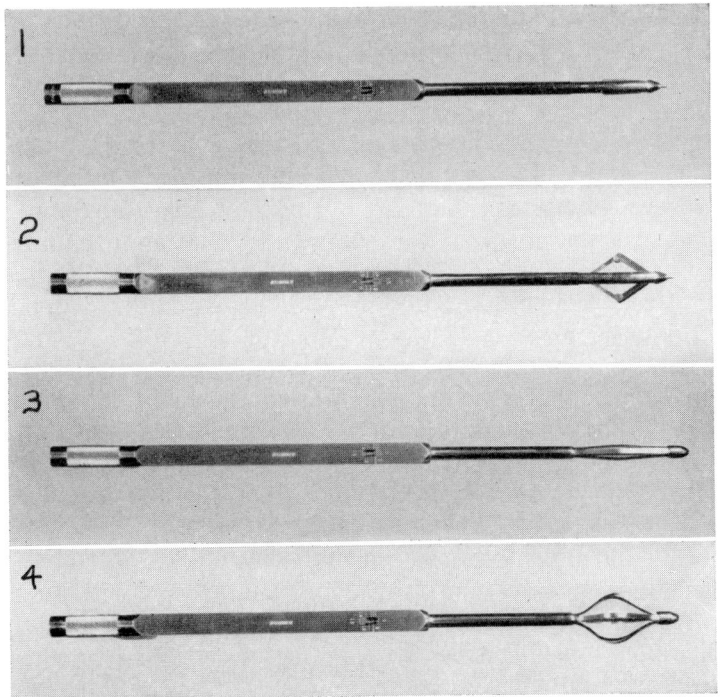

Fig. 514. Potts pulmonary valvulotome and dilator. These instruments have great advantage in that (in a closed position) each can be introduced through a small orifice in the ventricular wall and then be opened after it is in the chamber of the heart, thereby reducing the amount of blood lost through the ventricular incision. 1 and 2. The valvulotome in closed and open positions. 3 and 4. The dilator in closed and open positions.

Anesthesia. Drugs

For pulmonary valvulotomy, or infundibulectomy, we have found it most suitable to operate under ether anesthesia, with an intratracheal tube, and a closed system.

The question is constantly raised concerning the advisability of using a drug to reduce irritability of the heart during manipulations of it. We employed Pronestyl (procaine amide) in about half of our cases but have often felt that it was a factor in producing serious fall of peripheral arterial pressure. We now use it but rarely; it is given only if there have been frequent extrasystoles before operation or ventricular tachycardia during the procedure. While some have advocated the injection of procaine into the pericardium before opening it, we have abandoned this.

Exposure

The operative exposure is a left, antero-lateral one, through the fourth interspace, carrying the incision from the posterior axillary line to the very edge of the sternum.

The fourth and third costal cartilages are divided so the ribs can be spread apart widely. In some patients a better angle of approach to the pulmonary conus and pulmonary artery is provided by also dividing the fifth cartilage.

Procedure

Everything for the intracardiac procedure should be in complete readiness before the pericardium is opened; there should be no delay after this sheath is slit. In some individuals the opening of a pericardium does not particularly affect the cardiac action, whereas in others who are on the verge of failure, release of this envelope allows the heart to dilate; its beat becomes feeble and failure is imminent. Therefore, it is best to be well prepared to go directly ahead with the intracardiac manipulations as soon as the pericardium is entered

The pericardium is opened extensively in front of the phrenic nerve. Its anterior flap is grasped with several half-length clamps, which the assistant holds upward tautly, a movement which tends to roll the heart out of the mediastinum and into a position which is optimum for the operator to work upon it. A rapid inspection and palpation should now be done to gain accurate information regarding the position of the block. If the obstruction is a valvular one, a finger pressed lightly on the main pulmonary artery can feel a central jet of blood as it emerges from the tiny orifice of the valve. Pushing with the finger and momentarily inverting the pulmonary artery wall toward the apex of the valve, the jet and thrill can be made to disappear. With an infundibular stenosis one is not so apt to find the central jet or rush of blood in the pulmonary artery; the thrill cannot be shut off by inverting the pulmonary artery wall against the valve; the most intense thrill will be felt somewhere down over the conus or on the presenting surface of the right ventricle. If an infundibular obstruction is an appreciable distance below the valve annulus, one finds the bulging of a thin-walled so-called infundibular chamber above this. A probe can be inserted through this chamber, directed downward, and the infundibular area examined blindly but reasonably satisfactorily.

Before entering the right ventricle, two stay sutures of heavy braided silk are passed through the wall of the conus, taking these through the entire thickness of the musculature, and placing them in such a way that they avoid coronary vessels. Between the stay sutures, a short nick is made into the musculature, carrying this through only about three-quarters of the thickness of the ventricular wall. The cutting instrument to be used can now be pushed bluntly through the thin remaining portion of muscle and directed into the ventricle. For a valvular stenosis, the instrument is maneuvered upward to engage and slit open the valve. It is possible to push upward for a short distance a diaphragmatic valve without actually cutting it; to insure an adequate incision, the valvulotome must be advanced well into the pulmonary artery. Usually, one is aware of a sudden release in resistance as the valve edges are severed, but it is important to check the position of the instrument by digital palpation of it in the artery beyond the valve.

It is now advisable to introduce some sort of a dilating instrument to make sure that the valve flaps are spread apart adequately and an orifice of suitable size has been established. We have generally been most satisfied with introduction of a half-length clamp into the ventricle, directing this up through the valve; rapidly opening the instrument will spread the valve cusps. With this crude spreader, one can get a reasonably good "feel" of how much the valve has given and how large an orifice has been made.

With knives or dilators (of the Potts type) carrying retractable blades, the hole in the ventricular wall can be kept very small, and loss of blood can be minimized.

The intracardiac manipulations are almost always accompanied temporarily by extrasystoles, dropping beats, or faltering rhythm. After a valve has been cut and dilated, and the instruments have been withdrawn, the stay sutures are quickly crossed for hemostasis; the heart regains its forcefulness and regularity of beat. If there is any

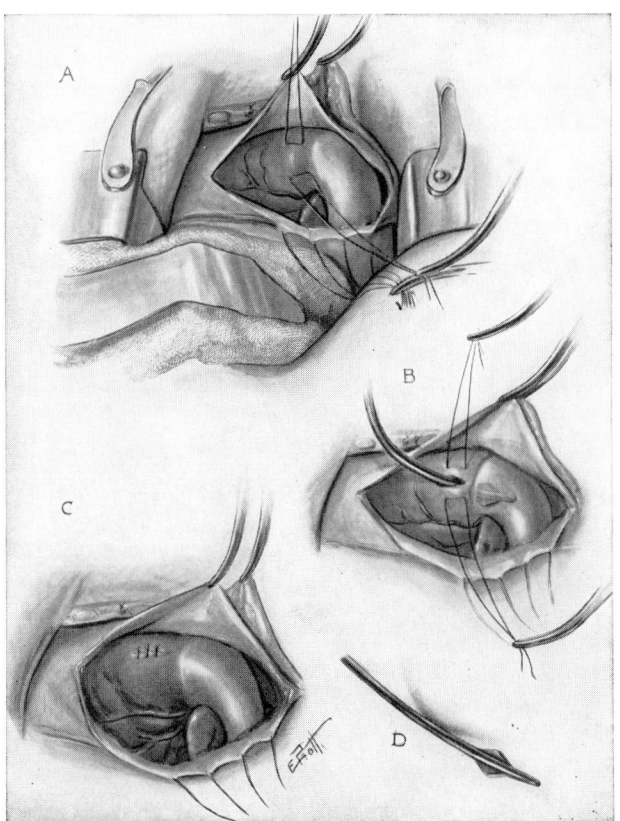

Fig. 515. Operative treatment of a valvular pulmonic stenosis by the Brock technique. A, Exposure through the left side of the thorax, with an incision in the fourth intercostal space, dividing the fourth and third costal cartilages. The pericardium has been opened and its flap retracted. Stay sutures of heavy silk placed in the pulmonary conus, keeping these away from coronary vessels. B, Incision of the myocardium in the right pulmonary conus. A Brock knife is being passed upward and directed through the valve to slit and enlarge its orifice. C, Closure of the cardiac musculature with interrupted silk sutures. D, The working end of a Brock knife. The shaft is malleable and can be bent to that conformity which is most suited for the size of a heart and the presenting angle of the pulmonary artery. The leading tip passes through the valve orifice and acts as a guide when the cutting blades come up to and pierce the narrowed valve. If preferred, Potts instruments with retractable blades can be used.

weakening which seems to be of importance, the direct injection of epinephrine will usually restore the cardiac vigor. Of greater usefulness is the injection of 3 to 5 cc. of 10 per cent calcium chloride into the pulmonary artery; this generally has a very beneficial effect in strengthening the cardiac contraction, or even in helping to reestablish a beat if there has been a cardiac standstill. The incision of the ventricle is now closed with interrupted silk stitches; the wound can be made completely dry. The stay sutures are withdrawn.

For infundibular obstructions the methods of treatment are not nearly as satisfactory as are those for dealing with a valvular form of block. If the infundibular constriction is long and narrow, the insertion of a blade and cutting of the sides of the canal may allow the pathway to open up somewhat, but this is often unsatisfactory and leaves much to be desired; furthermore, one never knows how much regional scarring and contracture will appear here later. When an infundibular block has a diaphragmatic form, much can be accomplished by entering the infundibular chamber, and directing a valvulotome proximally to cut the obstructing shelf; this can then be stretched as desired. In some instances it is possible to cut out and remove a portion of a shelf, using a small double-acting bone rongeur or a specially devised instrument as the Brock resector.

Prompt Action Often Essential

It is highly important to emphasize that if a heart is acting badly and seems to be on the verge of failure or cardiac standstill before obstruction is relieved, it is completely wrong to delay the attack in the hope that the cardiac status can be improved by supportive measures. There is nothing so effective in restoring satisfactory cardiac action as proceeding immediately and removing the obstruction; these are maneuvers which can be done in a minute or two. It is amazing to see a heart which appears to be just about giving its last stroke, when a bold insertion and rapid use of a valvulotome bring back a vigorous beat very promptly.

Changes Observed

After release of an obstruction, one can usually sense by digital palpation of the pulmonary artery that the pressure within it has increased, the turbulence has changed, and that the flow in the vessel has been greatly augmented. In many cases, direct manometric readings from the pulmonary artery, before and after removal of a block, will show an appreciable rise in pressure. However, not too much reliance can be put upon such tracings from the pulmonary artery, because so many factors have come into play (such as shock, change in size of the pathway, variation in blood volume either by blood loss or by transfusion) that there is great instability for a few minutes. The pressures are a poor index of what has been accomplished (or not accomplished) in treating the pulmonary lesion. In a few patients we have inserted a small polyethylene catheter into the right ventricle and have made continuous readings before, during, and after the intracardiac manipulations, hoping we could get an indication of what was being accomplished. Here again, so many momentary factors come into play that very little was gained by these observations. Certainly, if the right ventricular pressure remains elevated, it could be assumed that the obstruction was incompletely relieved. Conversely (as was so often the case) pressure in the ventricle fell, and we could not be sure whether this was due to relief of obstruction or to temporary shock.

Pericardial Closure

The pericardium should never be closed completely, for fear that accumulation of fluid within it might give cardiac tamponade in the postoperative period. An opening 8 to 10 mm. in length should be left at one end, preferably at the upper angle, so that any excess fluid can escape into the pleural cavity.

RESULTS OF OPERATION

In many clinics mortality rates have been amazingly low with these operations. This is particularly true when dealing with the valvular type of stenosis; fatalities generally run higher when dealing with the more complicated infundibular obstructions. In 25 cases operated upon by Humphreys,[11] there were 9 with the valvular type of obstruction and 16 with an infundibular form; 5 of the patients had interauricular septal defects and 11 had interventricular openings; in his entire series there was one fatality. Dammann[8] stated that 33 patients had been operated upon by the Brock technique at the Johns Hopkins Hospital; there were 5 deaths. Potts and Riker[15] reported 13 pulmonary valvulotomies, with one death; included in the group were 5 patients under a year of age, two being 23 and 39 days old respectively. Brock[5,6] operated upon 43 patients with pure pulmonary valvular stenosis, with 9 deaths. In our own series of 20 cases, including both valvular and infundibular types, there have been 2 fatalities.

Postoperative observations on patients clearly indicate, as one would expect, that the abnormality cannot be completely corrected; it can only be alleviated. However, great gains can be demonstrated both by subjective and objective means. The murmur changes but little; it usually becomes somewhat more coarse and lower pitched in character; actually it may be more intense than it was prior to operation. Subjective symptoms ar e diminished greatly. The individual is able to undertake physical activities which before were impossible, or at least can undertake them with much less in the way of cardiac palpitation, fatigue, and dyspnea. When there has been cyanosis because of a right-left shunt through a septal defect, this either disappears or is greatly improved. Objectively, the best measurements come from cardiac catheterization which can show an immediate and striking reduction of right ventricular pressure which, while not approaching normal, is far below the preoperative level.

In the hands of many surgeons these operations have been found to be extremely worthwhile and beneficial. Even though the patient cannot be returned to normal, so much can be accomplished that the operation has been found to be of importance and satisfaction. The over-all results following operations for valvular types of obstruction are distinctly better than those for infundibular blocks.

REFERENCES

1. Allanby, K. D. and Campbell, M.: Congenital Pulmonary Stenosis with Closed Ventricular Septum. Guy's Hosp. Rep., 98:18, 1949.
2. Blalock, A. and Kieffer, R. F., Jr.: Valvulotomy for the Relief of Congenital Valvular Pulmonic Stenosis with Intact Ventricular Septum. Ann. Surg., 132:496, 1950.
3. Brecher, G. A. and Opdyke, D. F.: The Relief of Acute Right Ventricular Strain by the Production of an Interatrial Septal Defect. Circulation, 4:496, 1951.
4. Brock, R. C.: The Surgery of Pulmonary Stenosis. Brit. Med. J., 2:399, 1949.
5. Brock, R. C.: Congenital Pulmonary Stenosis. Am. J. Med., 12:706, 1952.
6. Brock, R. C.: Direct Cardiac Surgery in the Treatment of Congenital Pulmonary Stenosis. Ann. Surg., 136:63, 1952.
7. Campbell, M. and Hills, T. H.: Angiocardiography in Cyanotic Congenital Heart Disease. Brit. Heart J., 12:65, 1950.
8. Dammann, J. F., Jr.: Congenital Malformations of the Heart Amenable to Surgery South. M. J., 44:915, 1951.
9. Dow, J. W., Levine, H. D., Elkin, M., Haynes, F. W., Hellems, H. K., Whittenberger, J. W., Ferris, B. G., Goodale, W. T., Harvey, W. P., Eppinger, E. C., and Dexter, L.: Studies of Congenital Heart Disease. IV. Uncomplicated Pulmonary Stenosis. Circulation, 1:267, 1950.
10. Engle, M. A. and Taussig, H. B.: Valvular Pulmonic Stenosis with Intact Ventricular Septum and Patent Foramen Ovale. Circulation, 2:481, 1950.
11. Humphreys, G. H., II.: Personal Communication.
12. Johnson, R. P. and Johnson, E. E.: Congenital Pulmonic Stenosis with Open Foramen Ovale in Infancy. Am. Heart J., 44:344, 1952.
13. Muller, W. H. and Longmire, W. P., Jr.: The Surgical Treatment of Pure Pulmonic Stenosis. Surgery, 30:275, 1951.
14. Potts, W. J., Gibson, S., Riker, W. L. and

Leininger, C. R.: Congenital Pulmonary Stenosis with Intact Ventricular Septum. J.A.M.A., *144*:8, 1950.

15. Potts, W. J. and Riker, W. L.: Surgical Treatment of Pulmonary Stenosis with Intact Interventricular Septum. Arch. Surg.,

62:776, 1951.

16. Sellors, T. H. and Belcher, J. R.: Surgical Relief of Congenital Cyanotic Heart Disease, Late Results in 72 Cases. Lancet, *2*:887, 1950.

CHAPTER 65

Vascular Anomalies in the Thorax Producing Compression of the Trachea or Esophagus

Many vascular malformations in the superior mediastinum have little or no clinical significance, but others assume importance because an abnormal or displaced vessel can compress the trachea or esophagus (or both) and give partial obstruction of these vital pathways. Since methods are now available for thoracic exploration of even the smallest subjects, a new field of surgical endeavor is opened whereby it is possible to correct or readjust such malformations and bring relief of the esophageal or tracheal disturbance. While these abnormalities were once of interest only to anatomists and pathologists, it is now desirable to recognize them during life so that corrective measures can be instituted whenever necessary.

Arterial derangements within the thorax are common, are complex, and can assume many diverse forms; these facts are at once apparent if one reviews the extensive literature which has accumulated. It would require a presentation of monographic size to list and describe all the anomalies which have been encountered. It is intended to present herewith only those which have been found at the operating table when attempting to relieve an existing tracheal or esophageal compression.

While additional types of anomalies may be found to be amenable to therapy in the future, at the present time at least five different malformations should be described, for in each category surgery has much to offer in the treatment of the patient. These include *double aortic arch, right aortic arch with a left ligamentum arteriosum, anomalous innominate artery, anomalous left common carotid artery,* and *aberrant subclavian artery.* Endoscopic visualization of the interior of the esophagus or trachea gives valuable information in some cases. The investigation of these subjects should include fluoroscopic and film studies of the esophagus and trachea by contrast media. Data gathered from roentgenologic examinations usually give a fairly clear idea of the type of vascular anomaly which is present. The following sections are based on the study and surgical care of 57 babies and children with such vascular deformities.

DOUBLE AORTIC ARCH

Pathologic Anatomy

While the normal human being has an aortic arch which passes anterior and to the left of the trachea and then proceeds as the descending aorta, occasional subjects are born with a double aortic arch. The ascending aorta bifurcates into two branches, one of which passes in front of and to the left of the trachea, while the other progresses to the right and to the posterior aspect of the esophagus, both limbs then joining to form a descending aorta. In the great majority of cases, the left (anterior) arch is the smaller of the two, and obviously is the one which must be divided at any surgical undertaking. In a minority of cases, the right (posterior) arch is the smaller of the two and hence is the one which should be severed. In occasional instances a double aortic arch may appear in combination with a descending aorta which lies to the right of the vertebral column (Fig. 521).

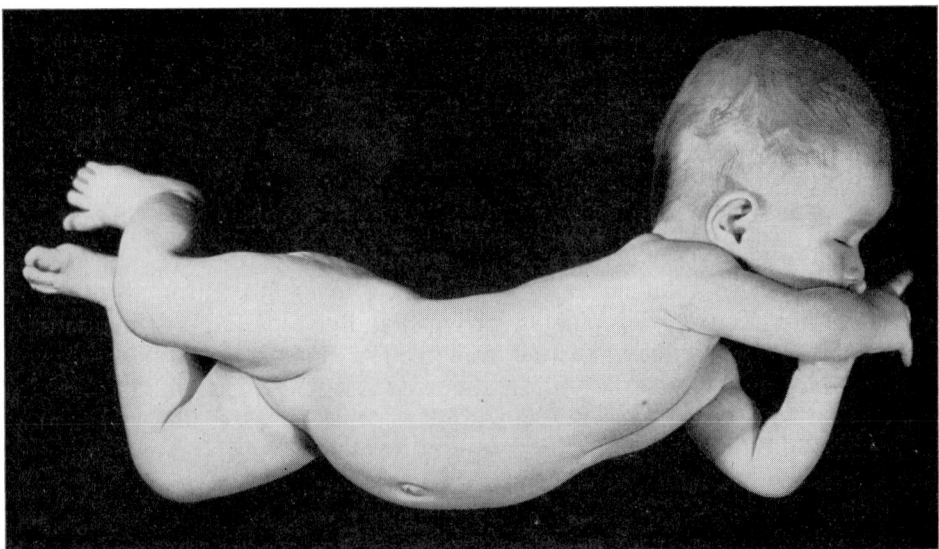

Fig. 516. Baby with anterior compression of the trachea, showing the marked tendency to hold the head in hyperextension (which improves the airway).

Clinical Picture

It is possible to have a double aortic arch with little or no attendant difficulty, provided the space between the two limbs is relatively large and the encircled trachea and esophagus are thereby given sufficient room. However, most subjects with this anomaly have very little space between the two arches; the esophagus and particularly the trachea are greatly compressed. While a bifid arch is compatible with a long life and relatively minor symptoms, the anomaly is usually a serious one, often leading to fatality within the first year or two of life, because of extreme tracheal obstruction and because of superimposed pulmonary infection which these youngsters are so prone to develop.

Most humans with a double aortic arch have enough difficulties to come to the attention of a physician during infancy. There may be mild to moderate hesitation in swallowing. Of greater importance are the alarming symptoms which come from tracheal narrowing. The respiratory rate may be increased. The baby or child obviously works hard to obtain an adequate exchange of air, an effort which requires use of the accessory muscles of respiration. During inspiration there may be intercostal and suprasternal retraction. A loud wheeze can be heard by stethoscopic auscultation, but usually the noise is great enough to be heard with the unaided ear many feet or yards away. There is apt to be a "crowing" type of respiration, with a marked inspiratory and expiratory stridor. At times there is a rattling or gurgling noise from the lower airway, but even when all fluid can be cleared from the passages, there is a residual noise which is highly suggestive of an obstruction somewhere below the epiglottis. Respiratory distress is often made worse during or immediately after the swallowing of milk or food. These babies have a strong tendency to lie with the head in hyperextension (Fig. 516), because this position attenuates the trachea and pushes away from its anterior surface any structure which is impinging upon it. If the examiner forcibly flexes the head, the exchange of air is reduced or may even be completely cut off, though the movements of the thorax continue. Superimposed upon the tracheal obstruction may be infection or pneumonia which complicates the picture and makes the condition of the child more grave. Respiratory symptoms may be serious enough to demand oxygen therapy.

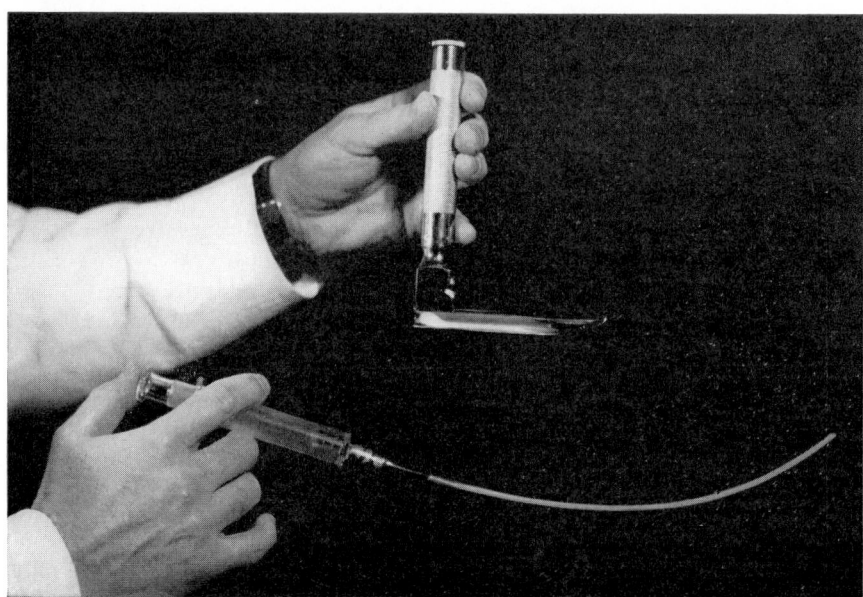

Fig. 517. Simple instruments for making tracheograms. *Above*, Laryngoscope. *Below*, Syringe (filled with Lipiodol) fitted with a plastic tube for injecting the material into the larynx. This can be done without anesthesia in babies under a year of age.

Roentgenologic Findings

By roentgenologic examination, important data can be gathered in several ways (Fig. 518). Simple films of the chest might show pneumonitis, but they can also give additional evidence suggesting tracheal blockage. During inspiration there may be poor or irregular aeration of the lungs, whereas during exhalation the lungs may be hyper-aerated. Lateral films, if made at precisely the correct exposure, can outline the trachea because of the air which it contains. The upper trachea is of normal caliber, but the lower portion has a marked reduction of its lumen and is displaced forward. A swallow of barium shows indentation of the posterior wall of the esophagus at the level of the third or fourth thoracic vertebra, this defect being horizontal or nearly so. Injection of Lipiodol into the trachea gives clear delineation of this structure. Antero-posterior films show a definite compression of both sides of the trachea in its lower third, but lateral views show the constriction more strikingly. This narrowing is at a level close to that where the defect was previously found on the posterior wall of the esophagus. This combination of a posterior esophageal compression and an anterior tracheal defect (in the absence of a demonstrable mediastinal mass) is almost certain proof of some sort of an encircling "vascular ring." By various roentgenographic changes, particularly from the size of the posterior esophageal indentation, it is usually possible to predict

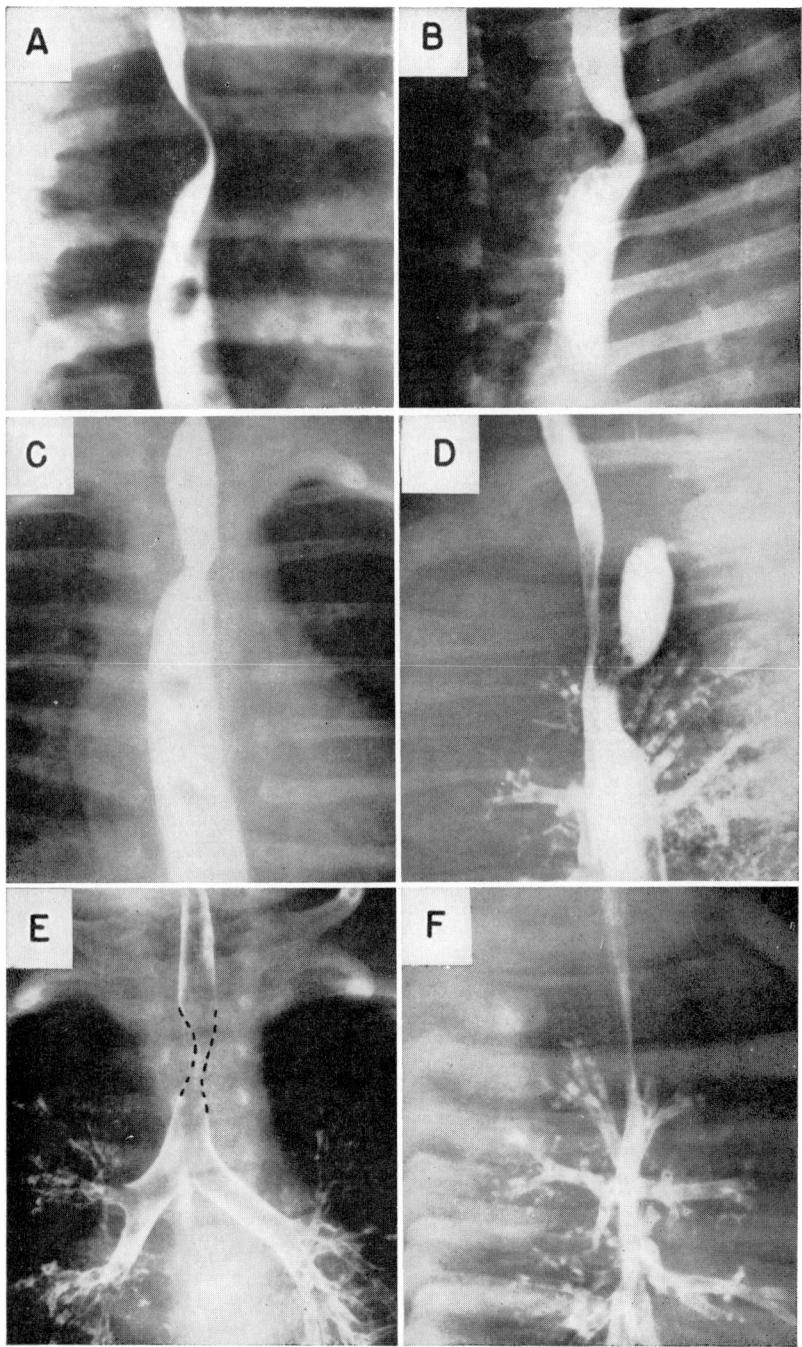

Fig. 518. Typical roentgenographic findings from several cases of double aortic arch. A, Lateral view, with large posterior compression of esophagus. B, Lateral view from baby with smaller posterior indentation of esophagus. C, A-P view with moderate indentation of both sides of esophagus. D, Combined tracheogram and esophagogram. Trachea is quite narrowed while posterior wall of esophagus is compressed at slightly lower level. E, Visualization of trachea by Lipiodol. There is compression of both sides of trachea. F, Lateral view of trachea, showing marked narrowing.

the relative size of the two arches. Intravenous injection, or retro-arterial injection, of Diodrast will outline the arch system, but this is seldom necessary; it gives excellent visualization of the arches, but it would not change the therapeutic attack in any given case.

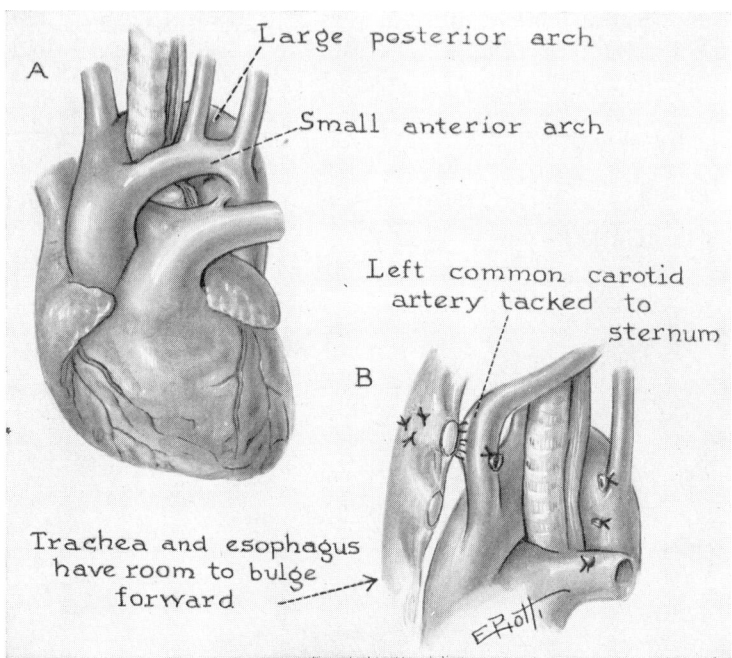

Fig. 519. Double aortic arch with large posterior limb and smaller anterior limb. Of 21 cases with double aortic arch, 9 had this configuration. A, Anatomic arrangements producing constriction of esophagus and trachea. B, Surgical alleviation of condition. Ligamentum arteriosum has been divided to allow pulmonary artery to fall forward. Small anterior aortic arch has been divided to break constricting ring. Left common carotid artery has been tacked forward to back of sternum, so that it will not press upon anterior surface of trachea.

Surgical Therapy

Surgery has much to offer these patients, because division of one arch provides more room for the esophagus and particularly for the trachea. When the chest is opened, it is vitally important to expose adequately (by removing the thymus), and to trace out in detail, all the major vessels so that one can be quite sure of the anatomic arrangements which are present. It is especially important to determine which of the two arches is the smaller, so that this one can be selected for division, thereby leaving the larger one as an adequate pathway for the distribution of blood. If the posterior arch is the smaller of the two, it can be exposed in the posterior mediastinum, and can be doubly ligated and cut (Fig. 522). This completely relieves all esophageal and tracheal constriction and it also gives the vascular system a normal configuration. More commonly, it is the anterior arch which is smaller and thus is the one which must be severed (Fig. 519). When this is done the remaining vascular system, while not anatomically normal, is physiologically sufficient. The procedure will give sufficient room for the esophagus and trachea, which can now bulge forward and to the left.

Presumably a left (anterior) arch could be cut proximal to the origin of the left common carotid artery. However, it is probably wise to avoid this segment which is apt to be large and also rather short, both of which are factors which make it difficult to divide it with safety. Attempting a division in this area for one of these patients led to uncontrollable hemorrhage and fatality; we are reluctant to ever try it again. Furthermore, if this arch is divided to the right of (proximal to) the origin of the left common carotid artery, any subsequent flow of blood into the carotid must depend entirely upon the intercommunication of the two limbs as they join to form the descending aorta. In some cases this orifice is quite small and might lead to an insufficient distribution into

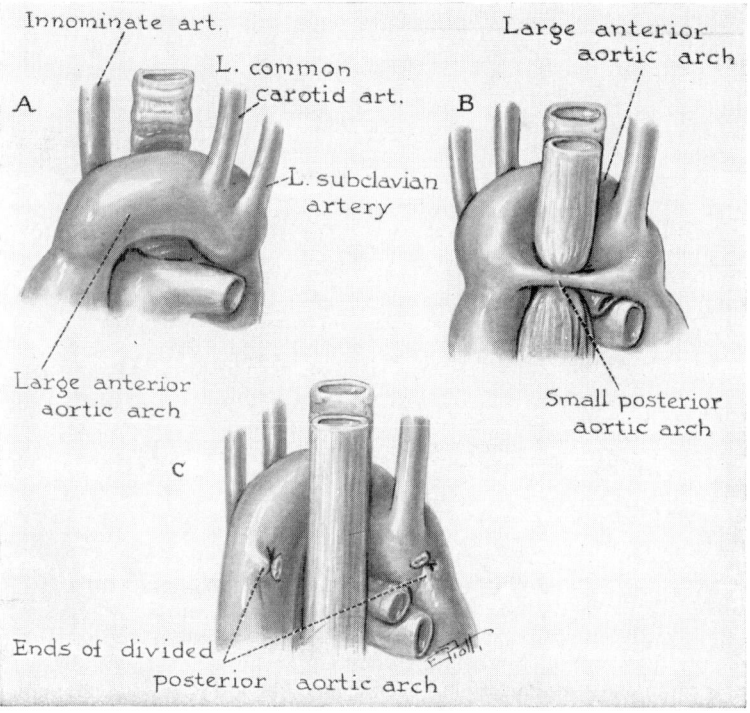

Fig. 520. Double aortic arch with large anterior limb and smaller posterior limb. Of 21 cases with double aortic arch, 4 had this configuration. A and B, Anterior and posterior views of anatomic arrangements, showing encirclement and constriction of trachea and esophagus. C, Surgical cure of condition by complete division of smaller posterior arch.

the left common carotid artery. Hence, a proper supply to the left common carotid artery is best provided by dividing the left (anterior) arch between the origins of the left common carotid and the left subclavian artery as shown in Figure 519. This has become our standard procedure. After the arch has been cut in this way, one finds that the remnant of the left arch will course upward and will continue into the left common carotid artery and that these will press against the anterior surface of the trachea like a taut elastic band. It is important to recognize this and to provide forward displacement of this vascular channel by taking several mattress stitches of silk (00 or 000 Deknatel), grasping only the adventitia or surrounding tissues, and carrying them forward as stitches which pierce the substance of the sternum. When these sutures are tied up with sufficient tension, the vessel is drawn forward so that it no longer touches the trachea at any point.

In some cases the pulmonary artery has been held in a retrodisplaced position by virtue of its attachment, through the ligamentum arteriosum, to the aorta. This ligament should be divided, to allow the pulmonary artery to fall forward. While this additional step seemed to have little value for some patients, it has certainly been worth while for others.

In those rare cases with a double aortic arc and a right descending aorta, the smaller arch has coursed to the left and posterior aspects of the trachea and esophagus (Fig. 521). Under these conditions, we have severed this left arch in its retro-esophageal portion, but also divided the first part of the subclavian artery and furthermore cut the ligamentum arteriosum which was a taut element in the constricting ring.

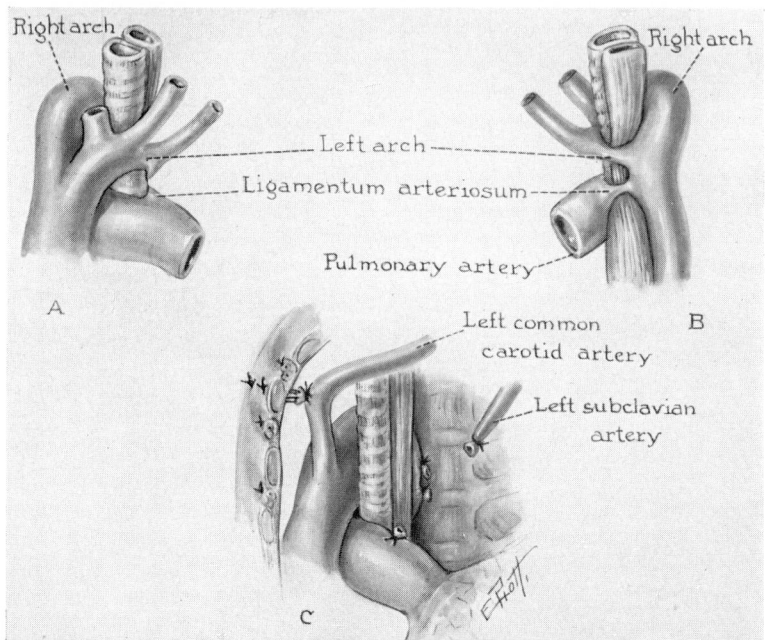

Fig. 521. Double aortic arch, combined with right descending aorta. Of 21 cases with double aortic arch, 8 had this combination. In 2 cases there was no lumen in that portion of left arch which lay behind the esophagus; in the other 6 instances, this segment was patent. A and B, Anterior and posterior views showing anatomic arrangements which give constriction of trachea and esophagus. C, Surgical relief of condition by division of ligamentum arteriosum, division of left arch (posteriorly), division of left subclavian artery, and tacking left common carotid forward so that it is pulled away from trachea. All these steps give more room for the esophagus and trachea.

Results of Therapy

Of the 21 patients with double aortic arches who have come to operation, 13 had the aorta descending on the left and 8 on the right. Of the 13 with a left descending aorta, there were 9 in whom the left (anterior) arch was the smaller of the two and was accordingly divided, and there were 4 in whom the smaller right (posterior) limb was sectioned. In the 8 patients who had double arches and a right descending aorta, it was always the left (posterior) one which was divided. These 21 patients ranged in age from one month to two years. There have been 5 deaths; 2 from hemorrhage at the operating table, 1 from cerebral edema the day following surgery (the child had been dangerously ill and was in an oxygen tent for four months before coming to this hospital), and 2 from pneumonia three and ten days after operation. The 16 surviving patients have been followed for varying lengths of time (up to seven years) since operation; they have had extraordinary relief of symptoms. Usually, a marked improvement in the airway has

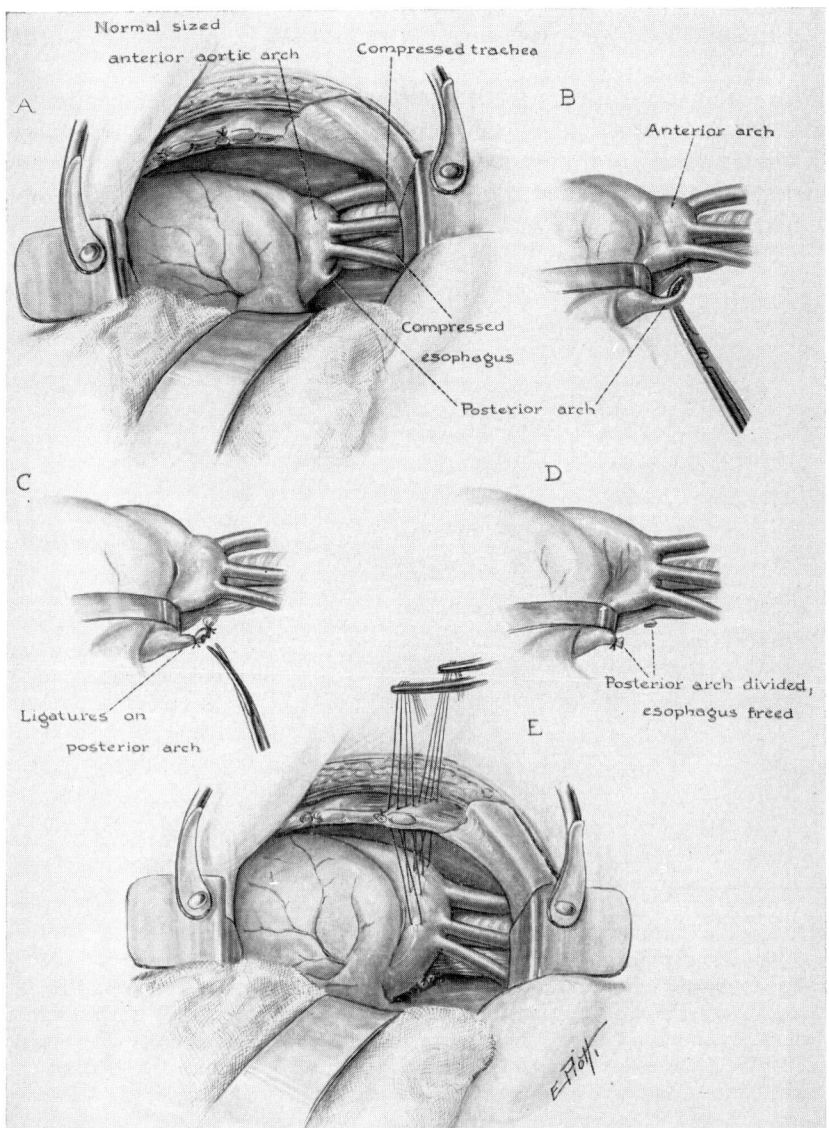

Fig. 522. Steps in division of a double aortic arch, when the posterior limb is the smaller of the two (as in Fig. 520). Exploration through left antero-lateral, transpleural approach. A, View in the chest, after removal of the thymus. B, Identification and liberation of small posterior arch. C, Double ligation and division of posterior limb. D, Back arch severed. E, Anterior arch grasped with silk sutures through its adventitia (and pericardial reflections). These sutures are then passed through the sternum. When they are drawn up and tied, the arch and its branches will be pulled forward away from the trachea, relieving all pressure therefrom.

been noted immediately after operation. In all cases, the exchange has obviously been more free and the subject has not had to use the accessory muscles of respiration for ordinary activity. Intercostal and suprasternal retractions have disappeared and the stridor has usually vanished. In a few subjects the respiratory sounds are quiet during resting periods, but are a little more prominent than normal during times of severe straining, crying, or other marked exercise. While complete follow-up tracheogram studies over long periods of time have not been made, the impression is that the tracheal airway is markedly improved soon after operation, but that some deformity persists in the cartilages. However, it is reasonable to assume that the removal of all external pressure will now allow the trachea to grow in a more normal way during future years. Long-term studies over a decade or more will probably be required to give conclusive data regarding the ability of the trachea to reform in a satisfactory manner.

To date, the over-all results in surviving patients have been exceedingly dramatic and have proved beyond doubt that the operative attack on this vascular abnormality has great merit. This does not imply that all humans with a double aortic arch require operation, because there are doubtless a few subjects who tolerate the condition in a reasonably satisfactory way through a long life. However, it appears that most infants and young children with this abnormality are very apt to develop serious or fatal complications. Hence it becomes highly desirable to undertake surgical correction if adequate surgical facilities are available.

RIGHT AORTIC ARCH WITH LEFT LIGAMENTUM ARTERIOSUM
Pathologic Anatomy

In the development of the human embryo it is the left fourth branchial arch which persists and gives rise to the definitive aortic arch in postfetal life. If, however, the left fourth arch disappears and the right one assumes the role of the main arterial channel leading from the heart, the subject is born with an arch which ascends, passes to the right of the trachea and esophagus, and then continues as a descending aorta which may lie either to the left or the right of the vertebral column. A right arch in itself causes relatively minor disturbances, though it has been known to press on the right main bronchus or one of its branches and has led to pathologic changes in the lung. Of greater importance than the position of the arch itself is the location of the ligamentum arteriosum (or patent ductus), which must connect the pulmonary artery with the first portion of the descending aorta. In some instances the ligamentum may be a harmless structure because it lies anterior to, and to the right of, the trachea. More commonly, the ligamentum arteriosum passes to the left of the trachea and then around behind the esophagus to reach the aorta, thus completing a "ring" which constricts the esophagus and especially the trachea (Fig. 524). If this ring is sufficiently large, the functions of the esophagus and trachea are not altered to any important degree, but if the ligament is taut, the space within the encircling structures is so small that the incarcerated esophagus and especially the trachea are greatly disturbed.

Clinical Picture

With this anomaly, symptoms can develop which are quite similar to those which are produced by a double aortic arch, but generally they are not quite so severe. As a rule, the onset of complaints is more apt to be delayed until a little later in life; (the average age of our double-arch patients was under six months, whereas most of those with a right arch and left ligamentum arteriosum were several years older). There may be a crowing type of respiration, some intercostal and suprasternal retraction, possibly recurrent pulmonary infection, and occasionally some hesitation in swallowing. Respiratory symptoms tend to be aggravated during deglutition.

Roentgenologic Findings

Films of the chest may show pulmonary infection if the patient is seen during the time of such a complication. There is a prominent shadow (the right arch) projecting

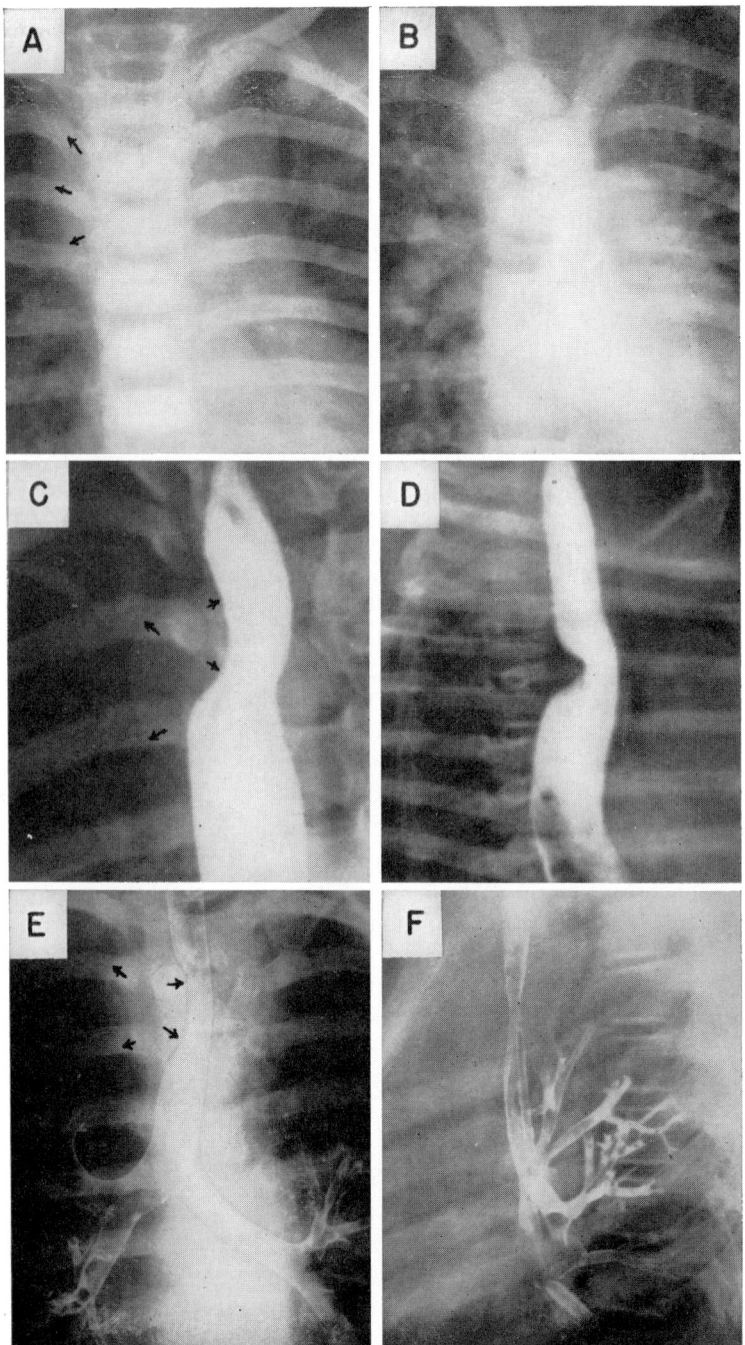

Fig. 523. Typical roentgenograms from cases of right aortic arch with left (posterior) ligamentum arteriosum (compare Fig. 524). A, Plain film showing arch to patient's right (arrows). B, Angiogram visualizing arch passing to patient's right instead of to left. C, A-P view of esophagus with slight indentation on patient's left and larger compression on right, latter being caused by aortic arch (arrows). D, Lateral view of esophagus with deep and narrow posterior indentation which is made by ligamentum arteriosum. E, A-P film of trachea, with compression of its right side by aortic arch (arrows). F, Lateral view of trachea, showing marked narrowing.

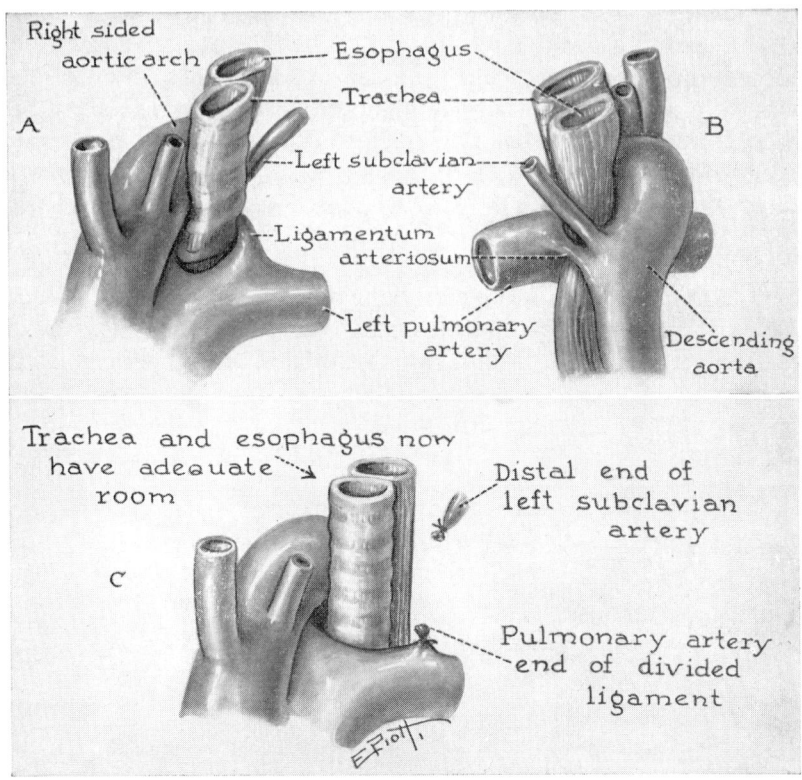

Fig. 524. Right aortic arch with left-posterior ligamentum arteriosum. Fifteen cases of this sort have been treated. A and B, Anatomic arrangements with constriction of esophagus and trachea. Left subclavian artery and ligamentum arteriosum sometimes arise close to one another from the aortic wall and these two taut structures have a tendency to pull out the aortic wall into sort of diverticulum. C, Surgical alleviation of anomaly. Ligamentum arteriosum and first part of left subclavian artery have been divided, thus allowing esophagus and trachea to displace posteriorly and to patient's left.

from the right of the superior mediastinum (Fig. 523). During inspiration there may be incomplete aeration of the lungs, and during expiration there may be hyperaeration, indicative of an obstruction somewhere above the carina. Lateral films of the thorax, if correctly exposed, can outline the air-filled trachea; the upper portion of this is normal, whereas the lower segment is distinctly narrowed. Instillation of Lipiodol into the trachea gives better visualization; there is a slight and rather elongated indentation of the right wall of the trachea (imposed by the adjacent aortic arch), indentation of the anterior surface of the trachea (where the pulmonary artery is pulled against it), and a depression on the left side of the trachea (from the ligamentum arteriosum). With a swallow of barium one finds (at the same level as the tracheal defects) that the esophagus has a narrow but deep constriction on its left-lateral and posterior surfaces. Above this posterior notching of the esophagus, it is sometimes possible to identify a separate defect, passing obliquely upward and to the left, caused by the left subclavian artery which arises from the aorta and passes behind the esophagus to reach the left apex of the chest. By fluoroscopic and simple film studies, it is usually possible to recognize accurately this combination of anomalies, but in some instances it has been almost impossible to differentiate this from a double aortic arch with a right descending aorta.

If conclusive evidence is desired prior to operation, angiography will visualize the aortic pathway and can lead to a positive recognition cf the type of pathology which actually exists. Such study in several cases has provided excellent delineation of the vascular structures, but from a practical standpoint angiography is seldom required because it is possible to recognize the esophageal and tracheal compression by more simple means and to proceed forthwith to surgical alleviation (the surgical approach being the same, regardless of the type of pathology).

Surgical Therapy

Treatment of this condition is obviously one of alleviation and not of cure, because it is impossible to shift the aortic arch from its right-sided bed (Fig. 525). Operation includes the identification, the liberation, and the division of the ligamentum arteriosum, so that the constricting "ring" is broken. When this is properly performed, the pul-

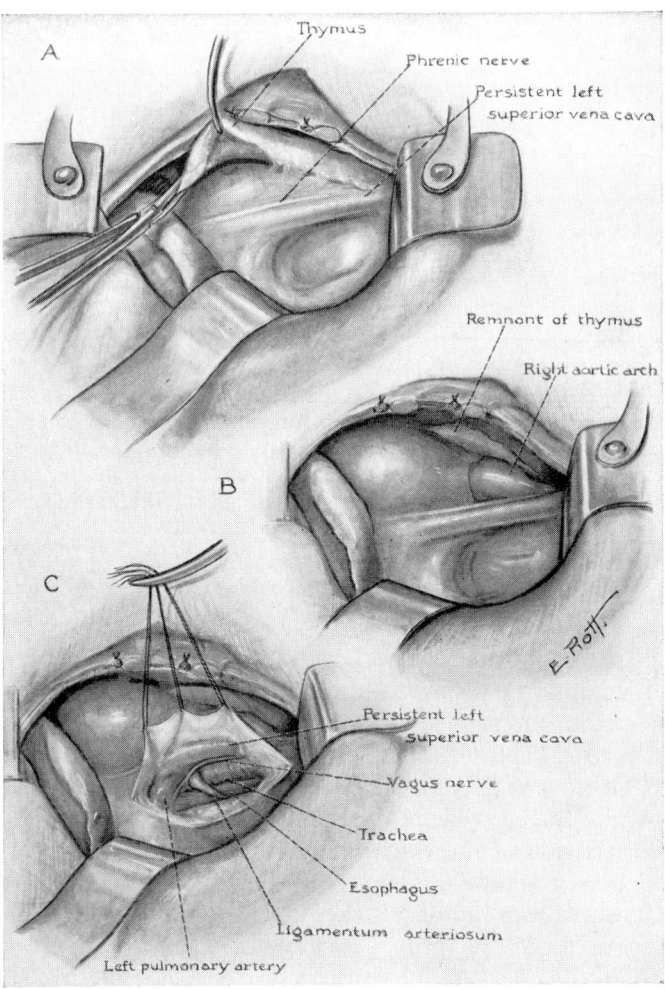

Fig. 525. Details of treatment in a child who had a right aortic arch and a left ligamentum arteriosum (see Fig. 524). Left antero-lateral transpleural approach. A, Thymus gland being dissected away. (This patient had double superior venae cavae, the left one of which shows here.) B, Most of thymus excised, allowing view of the aortic arch on right. C, Pleura opened posteriorly, to allow entrance to posterior mediastinum.

monary artery falls forward into a more normal position and sufficient room is given for the esophagus and the trachea to drop backward and to the left. Whenever the left subclavian artery is found behind the esophagus, it should also be cut. This step (while not so important as the severance of the ligament) helps somewhat to release the constricting mechanism.

In undertakings of this sort, great care must be exercised in the recognition of all of the regional vessels so that the exact components of the anomalous situation are known before any structure is divided. It is possible to accomplish this by opening into the anterior mediastinum (after removal of the thymus) and also by entering the posterior mediastinum (behind the vagus nerve). It is difficult but important to identify the left recurrent laryngeal nerve, which takes off from the vagus, courses closely around beneath the ligamentum arteriosum and then proceeds upward, quite adherent to the esophagus. In all subjects it has been possible to find this nerve and leave it uninjured.

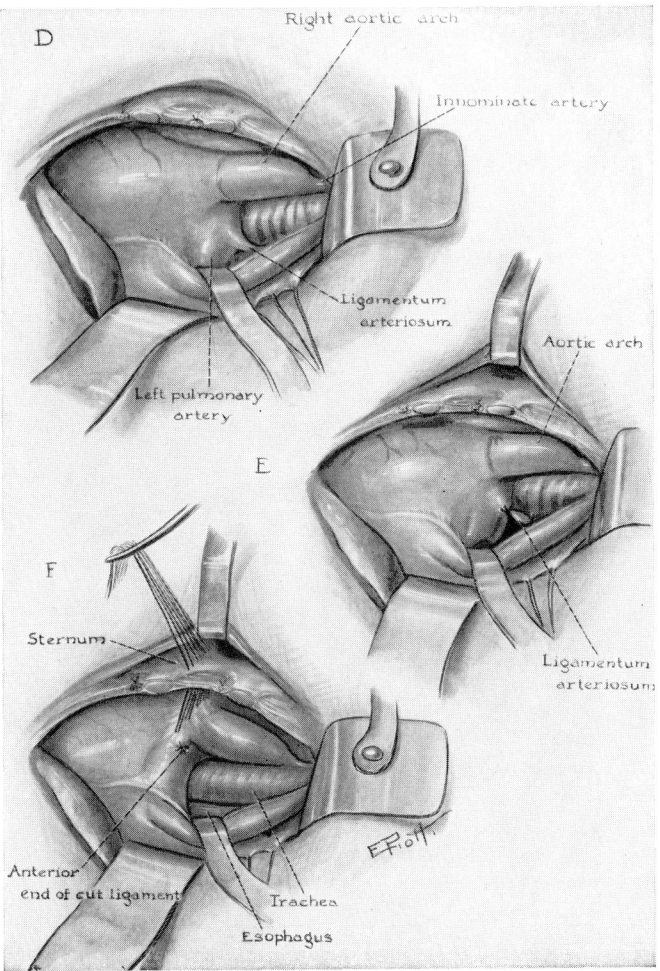

Fig. 525 (*continued*). D, Ligamentum arteriosum identified. E, Ligament doubly ligated. F, Ligament has been severed. Stitches taken through pericardial attachments at base of aorta and pulmonary artery; these sutures are then passed through the sternum. When they are tightened, they will pull vascular structures away from front surface of trachea.

Results of Treatment

Fifteen patients with this anomaly have been operated upon, the youngset two months and the oldest twelve years of age; there have been no deaths. The results in all subjects have been those of striking improvement. The children have shown complete disappearance of any preexisting dysphagia and there has been marked alleviation of the respiratory distress which all had prior to operation. In one twelve-year-old child, repeat tracheograms at the end of a year showed rather disappointing growth of the tracheal rings in the involved area. While it is possible that this portion of the trachea can still grow until the time that the patient reaches maturity, this case emphasizes the desirability of carrying out operations much earlier in life, so that prompt removal of the external pressure will give the trachea the best possible chance to enlarge during the remaining childhood years.

Roentgenologists and cardiologists have long known that a rather large number of patients possess a right aortic arch and have few symptoms therefrom. Presumably, these have had either a ligamentum arteriosum in front of the trachea or else the ligament has passed to the left of the trachea and has been very long and lax. There are many humans with a right aortic arch who do not require any operative intervention, but it is important to recognize those occasional individuals who have a high degree of tracheal narrowing, because it is in this group that surgical attack is a procedure of great value. If such surgery is undertaken, the best long-term results will probably follow those operations which are performed early in life, before the tracheal wall has been permanently deformed.

ANOMALOUS INNOMINATE ARTERY

Pathologic Anatomy

The innominate artery can originate at a point farther along on the arch than normal; when it does so, it must wind around the anterior surface of the trachea as it courses upward and to the right to reach the right apex of the thorax (Fig. 527). If the vessel is long and lax, it will probably not give rise to important symptoms; conversely,

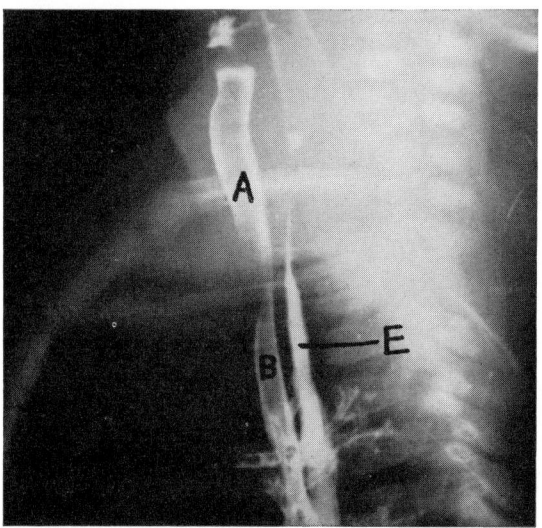

Fig. 526. Roentgenographic visualization of a trachea, compressed on its anterior surface by an anomalous innominate artery. Between A and B can be seen the tracheal compression. The esophagus (E) when filled with barium was found to be normal.

a large and tight vessel can compress the trachea to a serious degree. While the pathology is seemingly only a minor variation from normal and would appear to be of little consequence, the severity of symptoms which can accompany it was emphasized by the first baby who came to the author's attention.

Clinical Picture

This four-month-old girl had been hospitalized elsewhere since birth because of dyspnea, inspiratory and expiratory crow of considerable degree, intercostal and suprasternal retraction, pallor, and on at least two occasions there had been frank pneumonia. At times the respiratory distress was marked enough to require the use of an oxygen tent, which on one occasion was employed for as long as two weeks. The baby had a marked tendency to hold the head in hyperextension—a position which apparently improved the exchange of air. When the head was forcibly pushed forward in direct alignment with the body, the exchange of air obviously diminished. When the head was further pushed forward by the examiner to a position of flexion, the exchange of air was completely shut off, though the respiratory motions continued and the struggling baby became fussy and apprehensive. In contrast, when the head was placed again in marked extension, the airway was improved. The child had no hesitancy in swallowing. The respiratory symptoms were not made worse by feeding.

Roentgenologic Findings

By roentgenographic study, the esophagus is entirely normal. The aortic arch is normal in size and position. Films of the trachea (without contrast medium) may show little in the antero-posterior projection, but lateral views suggest a narrowing in its lower third. Visualization with Lipiodol clearly indicates that the posterior surface of the trachea is normal, whereas the anterior one has a long and pronounced indentation, with rather ill defined upper and lower limits. It may be exceedingly difficult or indeed impossible to determine whether the innominate artery or the left common carotid artery (described in the next section) is at fault, but in some instances the obliquity of the tracheal defect suggests one or the other. In the absence of any anterior, mediastinal

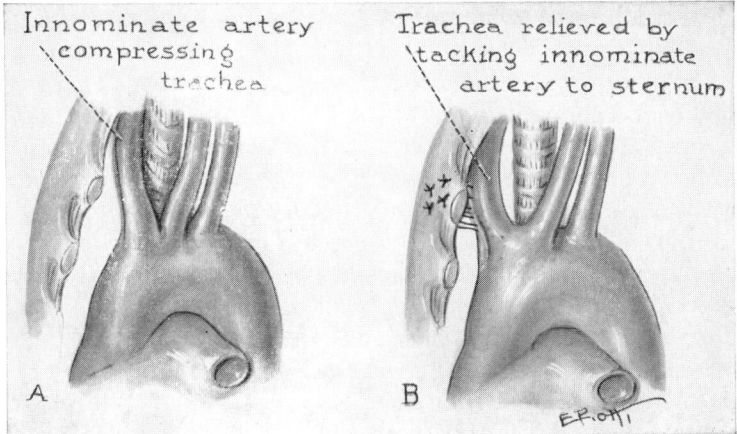

Fig. 527. Anomalous innominate artery which compresses front of trachea. Seven patients with this condition have been treated. A, Anatomic peculiarity of innominate artery, in which the vessel has origin from aortic arch farther to patient's left than normal. As it courses upward toward right apex of chest, vessel winds around and indents front of trachea. B, Surgical correction of condition by pulling vessel forward so that it no longer touches trachea.

shadow (such as cyst or neoplasm), a filling defect certainly suggests some abnormal blood vessel in the region. Any narrowing of a trachea which hints the presence of an abnormal blood vessel can also raise the question whether the diminished lumen is dependent upon incomplete development of the tracheal cartilages. Data on this point can be gathered by serial observations throughout the respiratory cycle. If the trachea defect is due to some external pressure, it will remain fixed during the respiratory cycle, but if a defect is due to deficient cartilaginous rings, the caliber of the trachea will diminish during expiration.

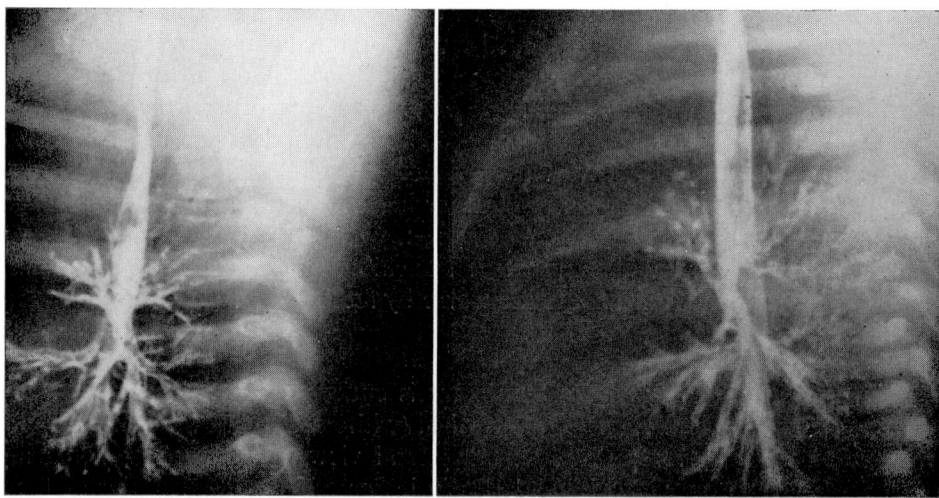

Fig. 528. Lateral tracheograms from a patient to show the beneficial effects of surgically displacing an innominate artery away from the trachea. *Left*, Before operation, showing the marked narrowing of the trachea. *Right*, After operation, there is a normal-sized airway.

Surgical Therapy

Upon exploration of the thorax it is possible to view this region clearly after dissecting off and discarding the thymus. The aortic arch is normal in size, position, and direction. The vessels arising from it are not unusual, except for the fact that the innominate artery takes off from the arch a bit farther to the patient's left than is normal; indeed it is apt to have a common origin with the left carotid artery (Fig. 527). The vessel can be seen wrapped around the anterior surface of the trachea, giving a decided indentation of the same. While it might be possible to relieve quickly the respiratory distress by cutting the artery, such a step is so fraught with the danger of brain damage that it should never be done. The trachea can be freed of the oppressing vessel by dislocating the latter into a more anterior position. This can be accomplished with four or five silk sutures (00 or 000 Deknatel), grasping merely the adventitia, placing some of them well up toward the superior aspect of the vessel and others well down toward its base. These silks are then threaded onto large cutting needles which are thrust through the sternum at suitable points. Tightening and tying the mattress stitches at appropriate tension will draw the innominate artery forward so that it is completely lifted off the trachea. These maneuvers are relatively easy to perform. The stitches must not enter the lumen of the vessel, nor indeed must they go far enough into the vessel wall to cause any damage thereto. Sufficient pull can be obtained by grasping only the adventitial structures and by distributing the pull through a number of stitches.

Results of Treatment

The results of this simple undertaking have been extremely gratifying. Seven patients, all under one year of age, have been operated upon. The first patient had previously been hospitalized for four months; she was discharged eight days after operation, completely relieved of symptoms. She has been well in every respect during the five years since operation. The other patients have been likewise fully cured of their respiratory complaints.

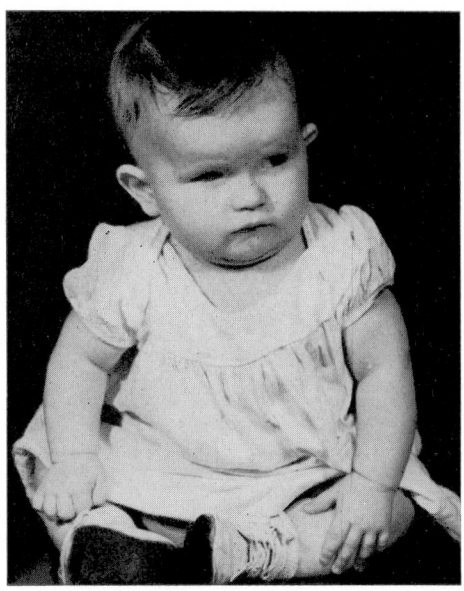

Fig. 529. Child who had marked tracheal obstruction from an anomalous innominate artery. There had been crowing and marked hyperextension of the head. This photograph was taken ten days after operation, the child being completely relieved of symptoms.

ANOMALOUS LEFT COMMON CAROTID ARTERY

Pathologic Anatomy

This malformation is probably of considerable rarity. It is somewhat akin to the anomalous innominate artery which was described in the last section, in that the vessel is normal in size and distribution but has an origin which is slightly unusual (Fig. 530). It branches off the aortic arch more to the patient's right than is customary; it must therefore wind around the anterior surface of the trachea as it courses upward and to the left, to reach the left apex of the chest.

Clinical Picture

The symptoms produced will obviously depend upon the degree of pressure which is exerted against the front of the trachea.

We have encountered two cases of this sort, in neither of which was there any disturbance in swallowing, but in both of which there was moderate respiratory distress, some crowing during respiratory movements, dyspnea of mild to moderate degree, and several bouts of pulmonary infection. These subjects were both under one year of age.

Roentgenologic Findings

By roentgenographic examination, the findings are quite similar to those which have been described for an anomalous innominate artery. The esophagus is normal by barium study. The aortic arch is normal in size and position. The trachea has a posterior wall which is sharp, distinct, and of normal contour, whereas the anterior surface shows a rather long indentation or filling defect. (There is no anterior mediastinal cyst or tumor to account for these changes.) Appropriate fluoroscopic or film studies taken at various angles might show that the defect is a grooved one, running upward and obliquely to the left, which finding strongly suggests that the indentation is due to an anomalous left common carotid artery. However, it may be difficult to see that such obliquity exists and hence the exact identification of the offending vessel may be impossible.

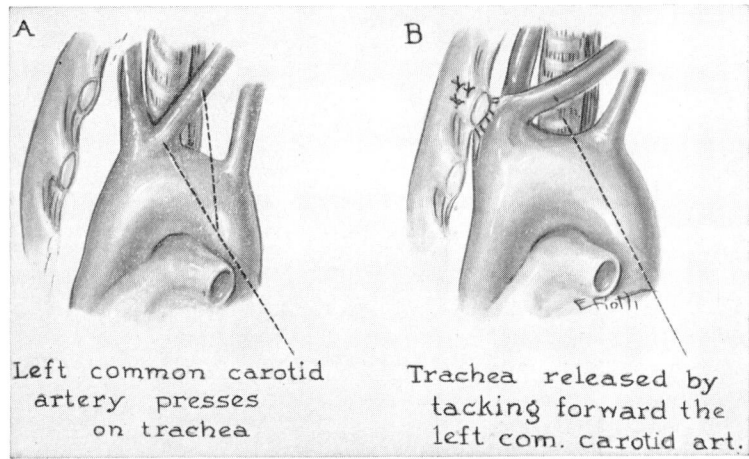

Fig. 530. Anomalous left carotid artery, compressing trachea. Two patients with this condition have been treated. A, Anatomic arrangements showing left common carotid artery with origin farther to patient's right than normal. To reach left apex of thorax, vessel winds around front of trachea and indents it. B, Surgical correction by dislocating left common carotid artery forward and thereby taking all pressure off trachea.

Surgical Treatment

The surgical treatment of this condition (Fig. 530) is similar to that described for an anomalous innominate artery. The carotid impinges against the trachea and doubtless this pressure could be removed by severance of the vessel, but the high chance of cerebral ischemia militates against such a step. A preferable therapy consists of pulling the carotid artery forward with mattress stitches which are anchored through the substance of the sternum; appropriate tension applied through such sutures can draw the vessel anteriorly so that it no longer has any contact with the trachea.

Results of Therapy

Two patients have been subjected to this procedure. Both youngsters have had complete relief of respiratory distress.

ABERRANT SUBCLAVIAN ARTERY
Pathologic Anatomy

"Dysphagia lusoria" has long been known to come from an aberrant subclavian artery (Fig. 532) which presses upon the esophagus, fascinating descriptions of the clinical picture and the related pathology having been given clearly by Bayford in 1794.[1] Normally, the right subclavian branches from the innominate, but it is not uncommon for it to take off independently from the distal part of the aortic arch. It ascends and must deviate to the right to reach the right apex of the chest. In rare instances the artery has been described as passing in front of the trachea, in a higher percentage of cases it runs between the trachea and esophagus, but in the vast majority of subjects it courses behind the esophagus. (In the series summarized here, there was one patient who had a right aortic arch but with no constriction fron a ligamentum arteriosum, the ligament being in front of and to the right of the trachea, but there was hesitancy in swallowing because a left subclavian artery ran upward and to the left, behind the esophagus.)

Clinical Picture

Aberrant right subclavian arteries have been recognized frequently by radiologists who have seen them during the esophageal portion of gastrointestinal examinations; in a very high percentage of these subjects there has been no important disturbance in the swallowing mechanism. However, in a few humans the subclavian artery can stretch sufficiently taut around the esophagus so that the peristaltic wave in the latter is altered and the patient experiences a hesitation in swallowing which may be bothersome and annoying. In babies, delay in swallowing can be found even in the early months of life. The child is hungry and eager for food, will suckle, and start to swallow in an apparently normal way but will then have difficulty in getting the bolus started along the esophageal pathway. Some of the food or milk might pass downward, while the remainder stays in the pharynx for a considerable length of time, or is expectorated. Some of these patients have no delay in swallowing milk or other fluids, but they encounter difficulties when solid or semi-solid food is added to the diet. Conversely, there have been several instances in which solid food was taken with alacrity but fluids were taken only with hesitation. This disturbed swallowing is not accompanied by manifestations of pain, but a young child or baby obviously has some sort of distress; after several attempts of swallowing there may be temporary refusal to try it again. The amount of food or milk taken at any one sitting might be relatively small, but as a rule the general nourishment of the individual does not suffer, because the mother usually learns that a sufficient intake over a twenty-four-hour period can be attained by giving the feedings in small amounts and offering them frequently. These children have no respiratory distress between feedings, but there may be some aspiration of material while attempting to swallow, so that gurgling or noisy respirations appear at such times.

Roentgenologic Findings

By roentgenologic examination the abnormality can be identified quickly and with a high degree of accuracy (Fig. 531). The aortic arch is normal in size, position, and direction. The trachea shows no abnormality, and indeed in most cases the absence of respiratory symptoms does not lead to a detailed examination of the airway. With a swallow of barium, the lateral projection reveals a defect of rather small caliber on the posterior wall of the esophagus at the level of the third or fourth thoracic vertebra. On antero-posterior view, this indentation runs obliquely upward and toward the patient's right, the direction and position of the defect being in a line from the distal part of the aortic arch to the right apex of the chest. There is usually little or no ballooning of the esophagus above this area, but a delay in the passage of the barium is commonly observed.

Surgical Treatment

The surgical undertaking for the alleviation of dysphagia lusoria is a rather simple one (Fig. 532); it consists merely of exploration of the posterior mediastinum, freeing

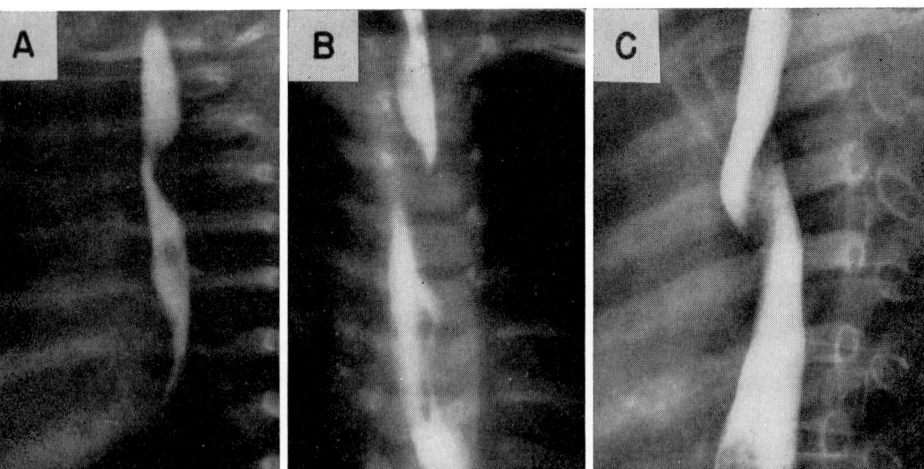

Fig. 531. Roentgenograms from patient with aberrant right subclavian artery (compare Fig. 532). A, Lateral view with barium swallow showing filling defect on posterior surface of esophagus, high in thorax. B, A-P view of oblique posterior esophageal defect. C, Oblique view of esophagus, showing winding defect caused by aberrant right subclavian artery. (There was no concomitant deformity of trachea.)

the anomalous subclavian artery from its bed, doubly ligating and dividing it. There need be no hesitancy about severing the first part of a subclavian artery because there is sufficient supply through collateral blood-flow to the second and third portions of the vessel to give an adequate supply to the corresponding arm.

Results of Therapy

In our series of 12 surgically treated cases, there were 11 with an aberrant right subclavian and one with the offending vessel on the left. These patients varied in age from three weeks to six years. All subjects survived this surgery, and in each instance

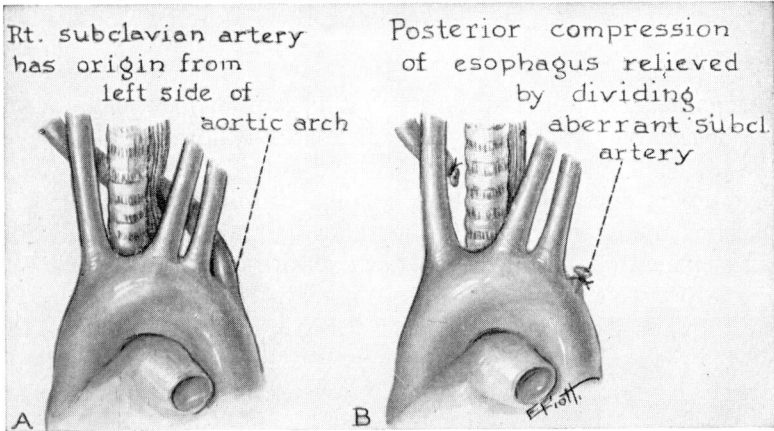

Fig. 532. Aberrant right subclavian artery. Twelve patients with such an anomaly have been treated. A, Anatomic arrangement. Instead of arising from the innominate artery, the right subclavian branches from the distal part of the aortic arch and runs behind the esophagus, upward and toward the patient's right. B, Surgical correction of the condition, by double ligation and division of the subclavian.

there was complete disappearance of the symptoms which had existed prior to the undertaking. (One child, who was known to be mentally deficient before operation, died after hospital discharge.)

TECHNICAL CONSIDERATIONS OF OPERATION

Some general statements might be of value for those who are interested in the technical aspects of these surgical endeavors.

Preparation for Surgery

If pulmonary infection is present, as is so frequently the case in the first four types of anomalies above described, adequate preoperative management should include control of this before undertaking surgery. Appropriate chemotherapy, administration of oxygen as required, and the use of a steam room in some cases, are important elements in preoperative care.

For the administration of fluids or blood which might be required from time to time, it is wise to insert a cannula or a plastic catheter into an ankle vein. Such a precaution becomes a great asset during operation because it facilitates the intravenous injection of fluids, which under some circumstances might have to be given quickly. Furthermore, the inlying vein catheter provides an extremely useful avenue for supplying nourishing fluids during the early postoperative period.

Anesthesia

Anesthesia in all these subjects must be with a closed system, using ether or cyclopropane. In all cases, an intratracheal tube, preferably of soft polyethylene, should be employed. Such a tube is essential for the maintenance of an adequate airway, particularly in the first four types of anomalies described, in each of which the trachea is markedly narrowed and an adequate exchange might not be obtained until a tube is passed down beyond the obstructed point.

Surgical Approach

In all these cases, regardless of the type of vascular anomaly which is being treated, the operative attack has been through a left antero-lateral incision with a transpleural approach. The incision is made below the breast, the chest is entered throughout the length of the third interspace, and the third and second costal cartilages are severed. The left lung is temporarily collapsed during operation, and is expanded immediately thereafter. This approach gives an admirable view of the superior mediastinum from its left, lateral aspect. While it is possible that a right-sided opening might be satisfactory for some of the anomalies, a thorough consideration of the various problems leads to the firm conviction that it is better to expose all these malformations from the left side. In the first four types of anomalies described (double aortic arch, right arch with left ligament, anomalous innominate artery, anomalous left common carotid artery), the anterior mediastinum must be opened and structures liberated in an adequate fashion so that all the important vessels can be viewed, palpated, and accurately identified. To accomplish this, the thymus gland can be readily dissected from its bed (after opening the parietal pleura), carrying the dissection upward and avoiding the innominate veins; about three-quarters to seven-eighths of the thymus can be cut off and discarded. This removal can be completed without perforating the right pleural sac. With some types of anomaly, such as a double arch or a right arch with a left ligament, it is necessary to make a separate opening into the posterior mediastinum to identify structures in that region. This is done by incising the parietal pleura parallel to and behind the vagus nerve, dislocating this nerve forward so that it is left uninjured. The posterior mediastinal exploration can be carried to the midline and even to the right of the vertebral column. This dissection must be made slowly, carefully, and with due concern for the tragedy that would result from damage to any of the large vessels which could give uncontrollable hemorrhage. In all cases (when posterior mediastinum dissection has been necessary) we have been able to indentify the thoracic duct and leave it undisturbed.

In those cases in which operation is performed for division of an aberrant subclavian artery, no entry is required into the anterior mediastinum, but the posterior mediastinum is entered through a longitudinal incision behind the vagus nerve. With this opening, it is possible to dissect down behind the aortic arch, to identify the subclavian, and to divide it.

All Constricting Elements Must Be Divided

Great emphasis must be laid upon the fact that constrictions of the esophagus and trachea are not caused solely by the vessels or ligaments which compress them, but that *the constriction is likewise produced by fibrous bands or sheaths which accompany these vessels and ligaments.* Hence it is not only important to divide the appropriate vessel or ligament, but *it is likewise essential to cut any strands or bands of tissue which accompany them*; failure to do so will give only partial release of an incarcerated esophagus or trachea.

Chest Closure

Following completion of the mediastinal portion of one of these procedures, the chest wall is closed tightly, and all air is aspirated from the pleural cavity with a catheter which is then withdrawn just before the skin is sutured. It has never been found necessary to tap the chest following operation; in some instances small amounts of pleural fluid have accumulated which subsequently disappeared spontaneously.

Postoperative Measures

For those children who have had division of a subclavian artery, no special treatment is necessary following operation; fluids can be swallowed as soon as there is recovery from anesthesia. In all the other malformations, there has been a preexisting tracheal obstruction, there has been manipulation of the trachea during mediastinal exploration, and there has been some trauma to the interior of the trachea from the intratracheal tube. In all these cases, very close postoperative supervision for forty-eight to seventy-two hours is essential. Appropriate chemotherapy is given to control any infection which might be lurking in the respiratory tract. Oxygen is administered to most patients for several days. It has been customary to place the subjects in an oxygen tent with a very moist atmosphere (produced by constant nebulization of water into the enclosure) because of its beneficial effects in reducing any irritation which is present in the glottis, larynx, or trachea. Beyond the first few days, fluids and milk can be offered as tolerated and can be rapidly increased in amount to supply adequate caloric and fluid intake. Hospitalization has seldom run beyond eight or ten days following operation.

REFERENCES

1. Bayford, D.: An Account of a Singular Case of Deglutition. Mem. M. Soc. London, *2:* 275, 1794.
2. Congdon, E. D.: Transformation of the Aortic Arch System During the Development of the Human Embryo. Contributions to Embryology, No. 14. Carnegie Institution of Washington, 1922.

3. Copleman, B.: Anomalous Right Subclavian Artery. Am. J. Roentgenol., *54*:270, 1945.

4. Faber, R. K., Hope, J. W. and Robinson, F. L.: Chronic Stridor in Early Life. J. Pediat., *26*:128, 1945.

5. Gross, R. E.: Surgical Relief for Tracheal Obstruction from a Vascular Ring. New England J. Med., *233*:586, 1945.

6. Gross, R. E.: Surgical Treatment for Dysphagia Lusoria. Ann. Surg., *124*:532, 1946.

7. Gross, R. E. and Neuhauser, E. B. D.: Compression of the Trachea by an Anomalous Innominate Artery. An Operation for its Relief. Am. J. Dis. Child., *75*:570, 1948.

8. Gross, R. E. and Neuhauser, E. B. D.: Compression of the Trachea or Esophagus by Vascular Anomalies. Surgical Therapy in 40 Cases. Pediatrics, *7*:69, 1951.

9. Holzapfel, G.: Ungewöhnlicher Ursprung und Verlauf der Arteria subclavia dextra. Anat. Hefte, *12*:369, 1899.

10. Neuhauser, E. B. D.: The Roentgen Diagnosis of Double Aortic Arch and Other Anomalies of the Great Vessels. Am. J. Roentgenol., *51*:1, 1946.

11. Potts, W. J., Gibson, S. and Rothwell, R.: Double Aortic Arch; Report of Two Cases. Arch. Surg., *57*:227, 1948.

12. Sprague, H. B., Ernlund, C. H. and Albright, F.: Clinical Aspects of Persistent Right Aortic Root. New England J. Med., *209*: 679, 1933.

13. Wolman, I. J.: Syndrome of Constricting Double Aortic Arch in Infancy. Report of Case. J. Pediat., *14*:527, 1939.

CHAPTER 66

Thyroglossal Cysts and Sinuses

Midline cervical cysts and sinuses arising from the thyroglossal duct are often encountered in childhood. These lesions are of importance because of disfigurements which they produce and because they may be the seat of recurrent inflammatory disease. During the thirty-five-year period from 1916 through 1950, 309 patients with these malformations have been observed at the Children's Hospital; 215 of these were operated upon.

EMBRYOLOGY

In embryos between 1.5 and 2.5 mm., the thyroid anlage appears as a midline structure projecting downward between the first and second branchial arches. The stalk of this has an attachment at the *tuberculum impar*, which later becomes the *foramen cecum*. The thyroid anlage descends in the neck but maintains its superior connection by the attenuated thyroglossal duct. Toward the latter half of the second month, the developing hyoid bone divides the thryoglossal duct into upper and lower portions which subsequently atrophy and disappear by the end of the eighth week. Rests of cells may remain anywhere along this tract and give rise to postnatal development of cysts. By pressure necrosis of the overlying skin or by suppuration during a superimposed inflammation, such a cyst may attain an external cutaneous opening and thereby be transformed into a fistula.

PATHOLOGY

Thyroglossal cysts are lined by an epithelium which is usually columnar or ciliated, but which may be squamous in type. Like the cysts, sinuses may have rather flattened epithelial lining, but not uncommonly there are small slit-like or irregularly branching side pockets extending out for several millimeters into surrounding tissues. A cyst or sinus usually contains some mucoid material which has been secreted by its membrane; but if squamous cells form a part of the epithelial lining, yellow grumous or pasty material may be found in the lumen. Varying degrees of acute and chronic inflammation are found in the walls, particularly in the sinuses.

Microscopic sections of the central part of the hyoid bone from these cases often show an irregular or branching epithelium-lined tract within the substance of the bone or its periosteum. It may be utterly impossible to detect this abnormality by gross inspection, palpation, or probing. Likewise, study of soft tissues removed *en bloc* above or below the hyoid bone, and yet above the gross cyst or sinus, often shows tracts of microscopic size which were unsuspected by the surgeon. Therefore, the thorough operator must always remove a block of tissue upward as far as the foramen cecum and must remove the central part of the hyoid bone, even though he cannot see or feel any tract in these structures.

CLINICAL FINDINGS

In approximately 65 per cent of our patients the lesions were cysts; in about 15 per cent they were cysts and an associated sinus; in about 20 per cent they were sinuses alone. When a sinus and a cyst coexist, they do not necessarily connect with one another. In some cases a midline cyst has been present for a considerable period of time before it subsequently attains a cutaneous opening.

A Thyroglossal Cyst may be found anywhere in the midline of the neck from the submental area downward to the suprasternal notch. They are most common halfway between these extremes, in juxtaposition to the hyoid bone. The cyst may be as small as a pea, or as large as a flattened golf ball. An average one is 1 to 2 cm. in diameter. In general, the cysts are smoothly rounded and have a well defined border, but the larger ones are apt to be compressed by overlying skin or fascia. The larger cysts can

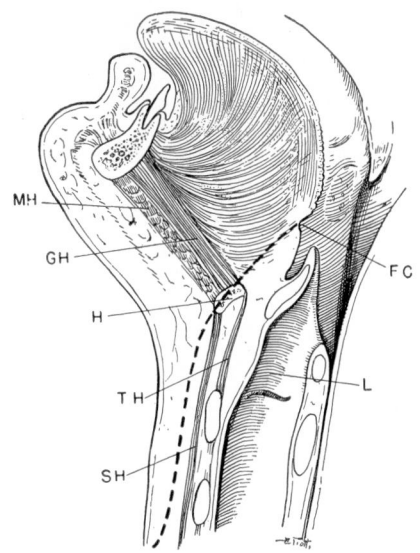

Fig. 533. Sagittal section through the tongue, larynx, and neck, showing the position of structures related to thyroglossal cysts and sinuses, which may occur anywhere along the dotted line. FC, foramen cecum; GH, geniohyoid muscle; H, hyoid bone; L, larynx; MH, mylohyoid muscle; SH, sternohyoid muscle; TH, thyrohyoid membrane.

be moved but little; the smaller ones can be displaced slightly upward and downward and also from side to side. They are anchored to the hyoid bone and deep tissues. They are seldom attached to the skin unless there has been superimposed infection. As a rule they are non-tender, unless there is concurrent inflammation. If a cyst is freely movable it may not ride directly in the midline, but can slide off slightly to one side of the trachea or larynx. Because of the overlying cervical fascia, the cysts usually do not transilluminate well, in spite of the fact that they generally contain clear fluid. In rare cases, pressure on a cyst will express a small amount of fluid into the throat by way of a channel leading to the base of the tongue.

Intra-Oral Swellings. The vast majority of thyroglossal cysts appear on the exterior of the neck. We have seen 3, 1 cm. or more in diameter, which presented as swellings in the mouth, near the foramen cecum; the excision was performed through the mouth.

Thyroglossal-Duct Sinuses open in the midline anywhere from the suprasternal notch upward to a position just in front of the hyoid bone. In most cases careful palpation of the neck will reveal a cord of tissue running upward in the deep structures of the neck; an attachment to the hyoid bone can often be made out. The cutaneous openings are from 1 to 3 mm. in diameter. The skin around the opening usually shows some de-

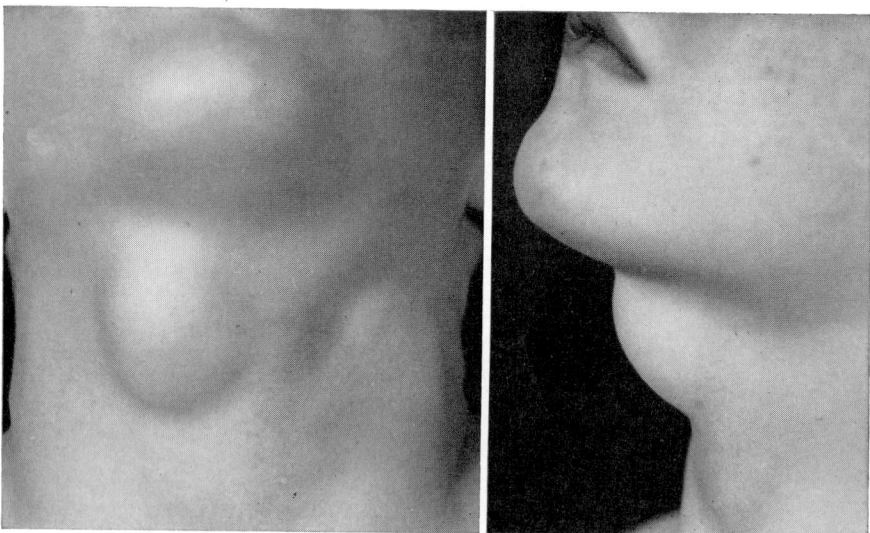

Fig. 534. Five-year-old girl with a thyroglossal cyst which had been present for three years. In the anterior view the cyst is seen to be displaced slightly from the midline.

gree of low-grade inflammation. From time to time, droplets of fluid, which are either thin or mucoid, clear or cloudy, colorless or yellowish, may exude from the sinus. Yellowish fluid may represent purulent exudate or else a discharge of cells which have been desquamated from the lining of the tract.

Superimposed Infection. Of our series of 309 patients, 35 per cent had a history or current physical findings of superimposed infection, with spontaneous or operative drainage of the same.

Age of Patients. All of our patients were under 13 years of age, but it would be misleading to suggest that thyroglossal duct anomalies are entirely pediatric problems.

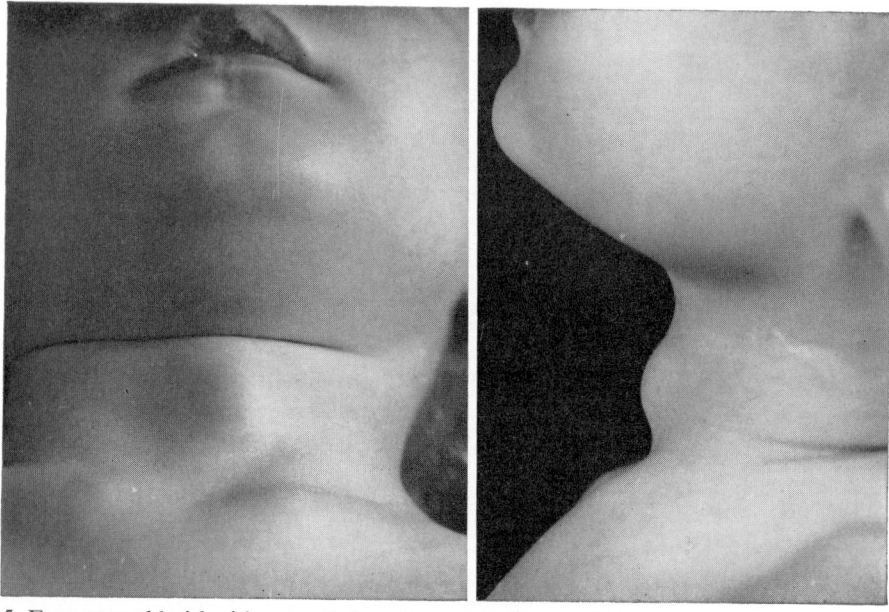

Fig. 535. Four-year-old girl with a small, low, thyroglossal cyst which had been present for one year.

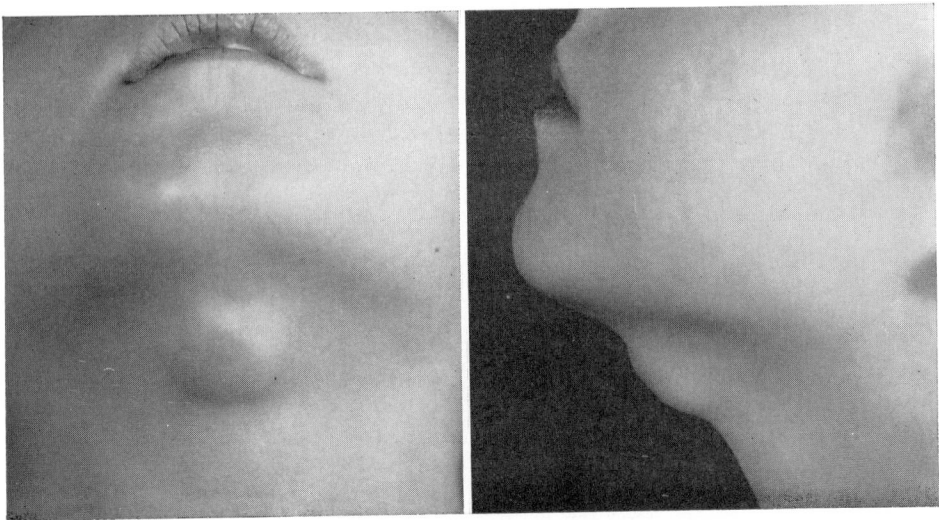

Fig. 536. Rather high thyroglossal cyst.

Indeed, the majority of papers on the subject have been based on series of adult cases. Reviewing 110 of our records to analyze the age distribution of subjects, the chart (Fig. 540) has been constructed. The lesions were first noticed by the parents in 30 per cent of cases during the first year, in 45 per cent from the first to the fifth year, and in the remainder of the cases after this age. In most instances there was a lapse of many months or years before treatment was sought.

Sex Distribution. Thyroglossal duct sinuses and cysts appear with about the same frequency in girls and boys.

DIFFERENTIAL DIAGNOSIS

Submental Adenitis usually gives no difficulty in the differential diagnosis, because the origin of infection from the teeth, the lower lip, or the chin is obvious. Furthermore,

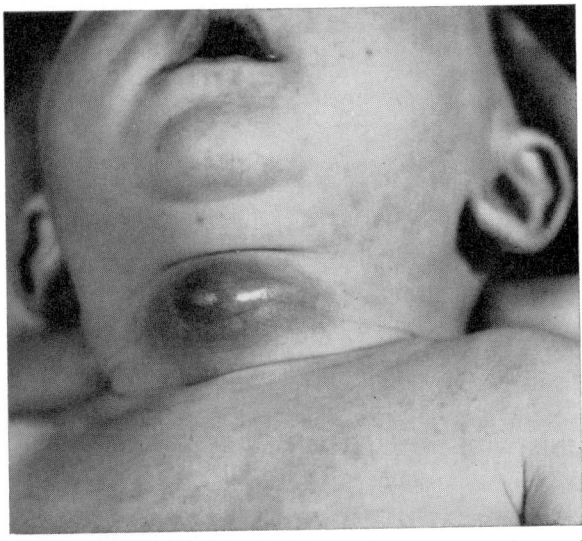

Fig. 537. Baby with a thyroglossal cyst and superimposed abscess formation.

these inflammatory lesions in the submental area are more anterior in location than is usually the finding with remnants of the thyroglossal system.

Branchiogenic Cysts should rarely give difficulty in differentiation; they have a more lateral position, tending to occur along the anterior border of either sternomastoid muscle. While a thyroglossal cyst may slide off slightly to one side of the neck, it is seldom displaced far enough to be confused with a branchiogenic cyst. *Branchiogenic sinuses* always have a lateral cutaneous opening, while thyroglossal sinuses invariably open in the midline.

Suppurative Lesions, usually tuberculous, arising in the mediastinum which have dissected upward and discharged through the skin can be confused with a thyroglossal

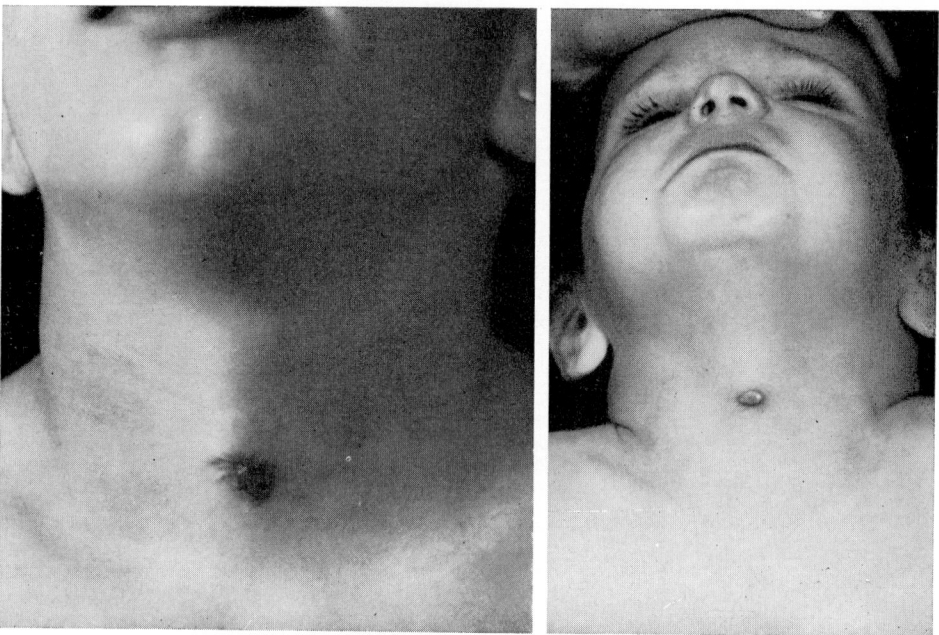

Fig. 538. Two children with persistently draining thyroglossal sinuses.

sinus which has a cutaneous opening below the level of the thyroid isthmus. It is therefore obvious that every patient with a sinus which opens very low should be examined roentgenologically to exclude the possibility of tuberculosis of the lungs or of the mediastinal lymph nodes.

Lipomas of the neck are very rare. They tend to be slightly lobulated and less spherical than the thyroglossal cysts and on the basis of this finding can usually be differentiated therefrom.

Dermoid or *Sebaceous Cysts* in the midline of the neck are attached to the overlying skin, in contrast to a thyroglossal cyst, which has a deep anchorage.

Ectopic Thyroid Gland is a rare but important anomaly to bear in mind. All of the thyroid substance resides in a high, midline position, in front of the hyoid bone; no thyroid exists in the usual location of the organ. By physical examination it is impossible to distinguish this from a thyroglossal cyst; at the operating table, the differentiation can be made very quickly by inspection or by incision of the presenting mass.

Midline Cervical Clefts, examples of which are shown in Figure 542, have sometimes been confused with thyroglossal sinuses. We have seen 6 of these anomalies which arise from improper midline fusion of the lateral branchial masses. They are characterized by a vertical, raw and reddened, slightly depressed zone, one to several centimeters long and 4 to 6 mm. in width. At the upper or lower poles of such a vertical, weeping area, there may be a slightly rounded protuberant nubbin of tissue or else a sinus which plunges upward or downward in the midline of the neck. It is exceedingly difficult to treat these lesions with satisfaction. Excision of them demands a vertical elliptical incision. If this is repaired by a vertical suture of subcutaneous tissues and skin, a midline

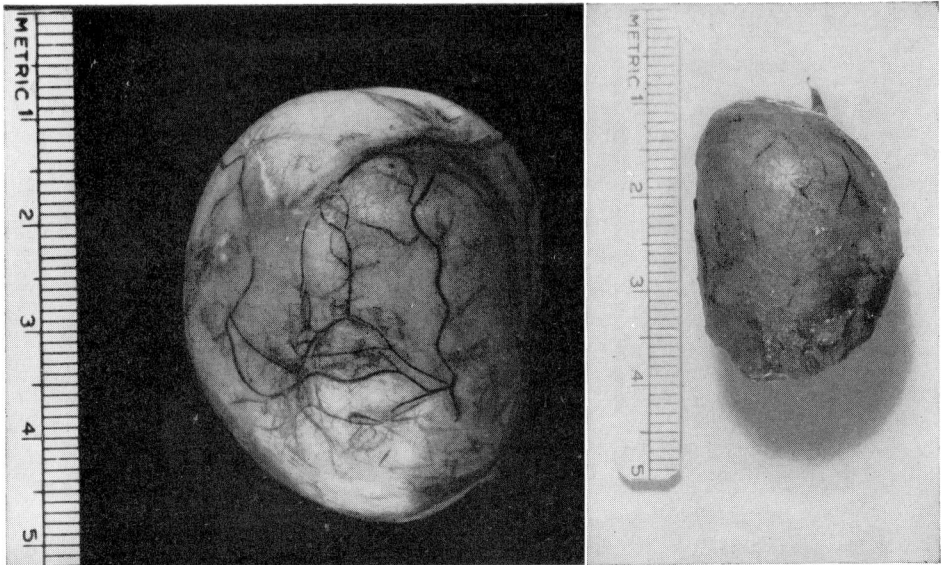

Fig. 539. Photographs of surgically excised thyroglossal cysts.

unsightly and contracting *web* almost always appears some months later which is exceedingly unsatisfactory from the cosmetic point of view and which is extremely difficult to repair by secondary operation. Our most promising results in the treatment of these midline clefts has been the vertical, elliptical excision of the lesion, followed by a lateral cut on one side at the upper pole and a lateral cut on the other side of the neck at the lower pole of the wound. Diamond-shaped flaps of skin can then be rotated and sutured in a Z fashion. The cosmetic results are reasonably good.

TREATMENT

Indications for Operation

It is probably unnecessary to remove all thyroglossal cysts. Tiny lesions, less than 5 to 6 mm., have been known to lie dormant for many years and give no trouble; it hardly seems worth while removing them. Larger ones are disfiguring and are very apt to become infected; it is best to remove all of these. Of our 309 patients, only 215 have been subjected to surgery. During the last ten years we have found ourselves tending toward surgical removal in the vast majority of cases, 95 per cent of all patients having been operated upon. We have always advised excision of thyroglossal sinuses because they are so apt to be the seat of recurring infection.

In occasional patients an infected and suppurating cyst must be incised and drained, as an initial procedure. Under such circumstances, it is generally best to let the regional induration subside for at least several weeks before undertaking removal of the lesion.

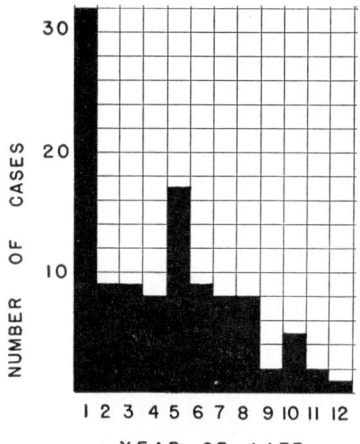

Fig. 540. Chart showing ages at which symptoms were first noticed (in a group of 110 patients) with thyroglossal cyst or sinus. Seventy-six per cent of the patients had symptoms before they were six years of age.

We do not believe in the treatment of thyroglossal sinuses or cysts by the use of sclerosing or cauterizing agents, because it is unreasonable to expect that injected fluids will reach all the epithelial-lined side pockets that can be found on histologic examination of many specimens.

Techniques of Operation

In children, operative removal of a thyroglossal cyst or sinus must always be done under general anesthesia. With the patient on the table in a semi-sitting position, the head is extended to the maximum. Midline vertical incision must never be used because

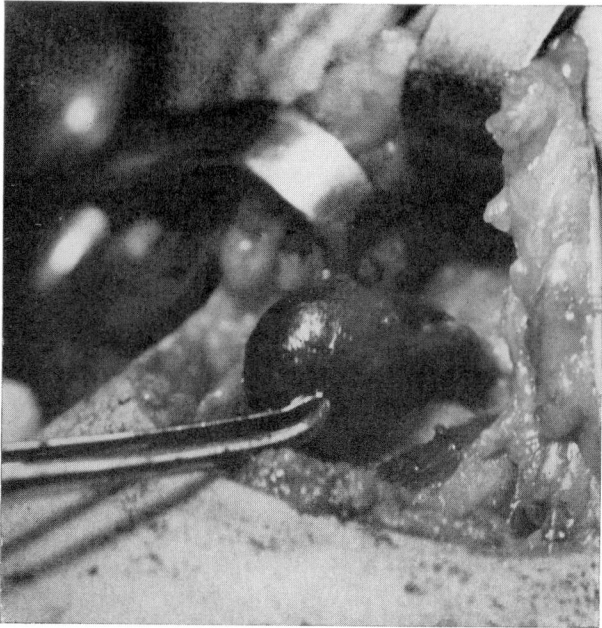

Fig. 541. Operating-table photograph of a dissected mass which was thought to be a thyroglossal cyst, but which proved to be an ectopic thyroid gland. It is attached at the hyoid bone.

the subsequent scar is unsightly and a midline contracture may appear which is extremely difficult or impossible to eradicate. A transverse incision should always be made and great care employed in the selection of the site of the incision, to make sure that it exactly falls in a fold of the neck and extends with equal distance to each side of the midline. The incision can rarely be shorter than 2 cm. if good exposure is to be obtained in the deeper portions of the neck, and it may have to be twice this length if the child is large or the cyst is big. If a cutaneous sinus is present, a transverse elliptical incision is made so as to include the cutaneous orifice. Freeing the cyst or sinus usually offers no difficulty unless there has been severe inflammation in the regional tissues.

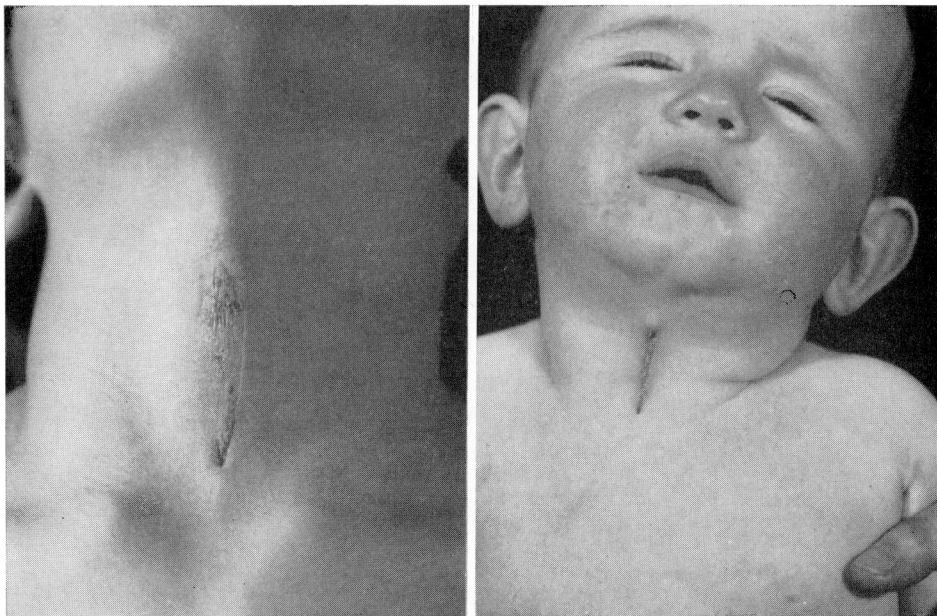

Fig. 542. Two children with midline cervical clefts. These are believed to be unrelated to thyroglossal anomalies, but arise from improper fusion of the branchial arches as they meet in the midline.

For the inexperienced operator there is often a temptation to remove the presenting cyst or sinus only as far as the hyoid bone. There are doubtless some cases in which this incomplete procedure will result in permanent cure. However, we and others have learned that to do this leads frequently to recurrence. Therefore, it cannot be emphasized too strongly that proper treatment always includes removal of about 1 cm. of the hyoid bone and in addition a block of tissue up to the base of the tongue, a procedure so clearly described and advocated by Sistrunk.[8] This more extensive operation increases the operative time but little; if it is routinely used, recurrences are very rare.

The hyoid bone can be cut with a scalpel in patients less than two or three years of age, but it must be severed with bone cutters in older subjects. In Figure 543, 7, the hyoid bone has been severed on both sides and traction on the cyst will pull forward the centrally freed portion of hyoid bone. One blade of the scissors can then be pushed inward as far as the thyrohyoid membrane and a circular cut of all the muscles can be rapidly made, so that a fringe of musculature is left on the centrally placed block of tissue. If one does not know the regional anatomy well, there may be some hesitation in the depths of the wound, for fear of entering the mouth. However, the thyrohyoid membrane is a distinct grayish yellow structure, in contrast to the red muscles superficial to it; it can

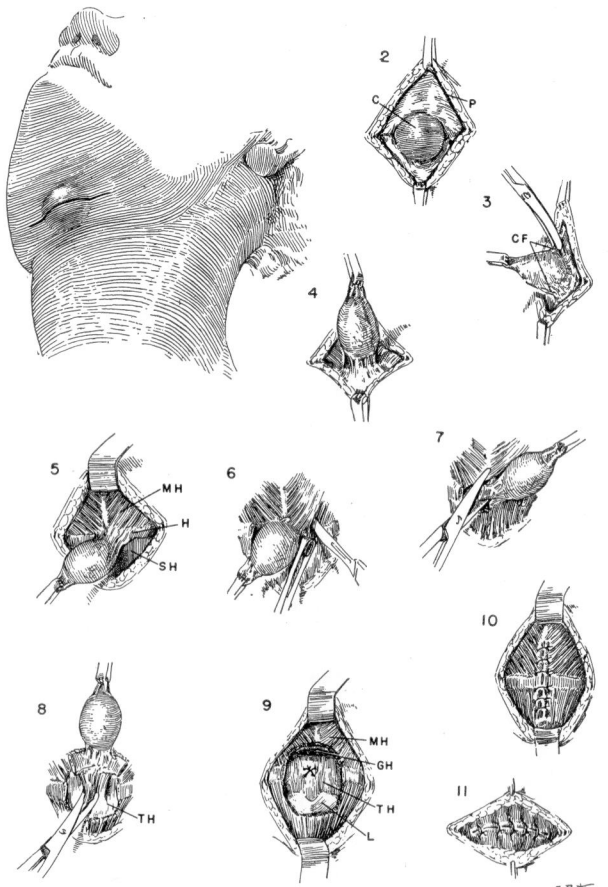

Fig. 543. Technique for removal of a thyroglossal cyst. 1. Head well extended. Transverse incision. 2. Skin and platysma incised. 3. Cyst raised, overlying cervical fascia being cut. 4. Cyst raised from its bed. 5. Hyoid bone identified. 6. Hyoid bone being cut. 7. Circular cut being made in muscles above and below hyoid bone. 8. Block of tissue raised in wound, attached only by a stalk which is now being severed. 9. Excision completed. 10. Muscles approximated in midline. (The muscles are left open if such a closure gives too much tension.) The ends of the hyoid bone are never joined. 11. Closure of platysma muscle.

be identified readily and it is easily dissected from the overlying musculature. Rather than make many cuts through the muscles to get down to this membrane, it is best to puncture entirely through the muscles at one point, and then to sweep the scissors around, severing a full thickness of musculature in each cut. When the block-excision of tissue has been adequate in extent, substance only a few millimeters thick separates the operative field from the mouth.

In closure of the wound, no attempt need be made to approximate the ends of the hyoid, and even if they do not abut against one another no subsequent derangement in the action of the local muscles will be noticed. If hemostasis has been adequate, it is not necessary to drain the wound.

This general technique is also used in the excision of a thyroglossal sinus. The tract must be followed upward, and even though a cord cannot be palpated, a complete block of tissue 8 to 10 mm. in diameter must be removed all the way to the base of the tongue, invariably excising the central portion of the hyoid bone.

Precautions Concerning Ectopic Thyroid

A word of caution must be given concerning the removal of an ectopic thyroid gland which can be mistaken for a thyroglossal cyst. There may be no thyroid in the usual location of the gland, the only thyroid tissue the patient possesses being situated as a small, midline, spherical mass, a centimeter or two in diameter, just in front of the hyoid bone. If this is removed (believing it to be a thyroglossal cyst), the patient will be thrown into myxedema. To avoid such an unfortunate experience, two rules should be adopted. First, if there is any question about the nature of a "cyst," *it should be opened before completely detaching it from its bed and its blood supply*. Second, if high, midline thyroid tissue is found, *it should not be removed without ascertaining that a normally placed thyroid gland is also present*. It will usually be found impossible to dissect downward from the high neck wound to obtain this information; hence it is justifiable to make a small transverse midline incision 1.0 to 1.5 cm. long over the thyroid isthmus to expose and positively identify the thyroid gland. Making this second exploratory incision is far preferable to producing myxedema by blindly and unhesitatingly removing a high ectopic thyroid gland.

We have encountered three of the above mentioned abnormalities in which all of the thyroid lay as a small rounded mass just anterior to the hyoid bone. The first of these was inadvertently removed, believing it to be a tense cyst. On opening the specimen, it was found to be entirely normal, solid thyroid substance; the patient has required thyroid feedings for the eighteen years she has been followed since that time. In the other two, the nature of the mass was recognized at the operating table. Inspection showed that blood vessels entered both sides of the structure. Therefore, the mass was cut in the mid-sagittal plane, and either half was turned outward and tucked beneath the ribbon muscles of the neck. In this way the blood supply was preserved and cosmetic results were excellent because the mass of tissue had been pushed back to both sides where it was not noticeable.

RESULTS OF TREATMENT

Three of our patients were successfully treated by intra-oral procedures, since the cysts presented in the mouth at the base of the tongue. In 27 cases, early in the series, incomplete operative procedures were done, in which a portion of the hyoid bone was not resected or insufficient tissue was removed above the hyoid bone. Eighteen of these have shown no evidence of recurrence, but the other 9 have had subsequent formation of a cyst. Seven of the recurrences were subjected to secondary or tertiary procedures before a final cure was obtained, and 2 patients refused to have additional treatment.

For 188 patients an operation was performed which was thought to be thorough and complete. Of these, 181 were cured and 7 had a recurrence of a cyst or sinus for which secondary operation was performed. In most of these, presumably some side tract of a sinus had been missed at the first operation. In at least 2 of them, fluid discharged postoperatively from the wound and was proved subsequently to be submaxillary in origin; apparently the border of the submaxillary gland had been injured by too-extensive dissection.

The over-all results show clearly that it is possible to cure nearly all patients with a thyroglossal cyst or sinus, provided the lesion is removed by block dissection, always including the central part of the hyoid bone in the tissue which is excised.

REFERENCES

1. Gross, R. E. and Connerley, M. L.: Thyroglossal Cysts and Sinuses. A Study and Report of 198 Cases. New England J. Med., *223:*616, 1940.

2. Hendrick, J. W.: The Management of Thyroglossal Tract Cysts and Fistulas. Texas State J. Med., *32:*34, 1936.

3. Hoover, W. B.: Clinical Conditions Arising from Anomalies or Maldevelopments of the Branchial Arches and Clefts. Ann. Otol., Rhin. & Laryng., *50:*834, 1941.

4. Hubert, L.: Thyroglossal Cysts and Sinuses. Analysis of Forty Three Cases. Arch. Otolaryng., *45:*105, 1947.

5. Jenkins, H. B.: Fistula of Submaxillary Gland Following Excision of Thyroglossal Cyst. Am. J. Surg., *70:*118, 1945.

6. Marshal, S. F. and Becker, W. F.: Thyroglossal Cysts and Sinuses. Ann. Surg., *129:*642, 1949.

7. Nachlas, N. E.: Thyroglossal Duct Cysts. Ann. Otol., Rhin. & Laryng., *59:*381, 1950.

8. Sistrunk, W. E.: The Surgical Treatment of Cysts of the Thyroglossal Tract. Ann. Surg., *71:*121, 1920.

9. Ward, G. E., Hendrick, J. W. and Chambers, R. G.: Thyroglossal Tract Abnormalities— Cysts and Fistulas; Report of 105 Cases from Johns Hopkins Hospital Observed During Years 1926 to 1946. Surg., Gynec. & Obst., *89:*727, 1949.

CHAPTER 67

Cysts, Sinuses, and Other Anomalies of the Branchial Apparatus

One of the many interesting chapters in the study of surgical problems in childhood is concerned with congenital abnormalities of the face and neck arising from the branchial apparatus. The various aspects in development, diagnosis, and treatment of cervical cysts and fistulas have been stressed from time to time by many different authors. Our material includes 308 cases observed in infants and children during the twenty-five-year period ending December 1950.

EMBRYOLOGY

In the first two or three weeks of embryonic life there develop on either side of the neck four, and possibly five, *branchial clefts* which run almost parallel to one another, coursing obliquely downward, forward, and somewhat medially. These external depressions or grooves separate the adjacent structures into six rounded *branchial arches* which ultimately form the neck and lower part of the face. Each external groove is matched internally by a corresponding outpocketing of the foregut, the two portions of this compound structure being separated by a membrane which is lined externally by ectodermal tissues and internally by an entodermal layer. In fish, the internal pouch and external cleft normally communicate with each other to form the gill apparatus. In the human, the dividing membrane does not normally rupture at any time, though a few observers believe that the membrane of the second cleft does occasionally perforate. While most of these embryonic structures disappear, the first pouch persists in the form of the eustachian tube, middle ear, and mastoid cells and the first cleft forms the external auditory canal, while its membrane becomes the tympanic membrane.

As an integral part of each branchial arch, the vascular system acquires an aortic branch, the artery in each instance coursing along in an antero-posterior direction. With degeneration of the branchial arches, many of these blood vessels undergo regressive changes; the first and second aortic arches disappear. However, certain portions of these primitive arterial channels persist and are represented in the fully formed vascular system. The third aortic arch forms the base of the internal carotid, and the fourth aortic arch on the right forms the base of the subclavian, while on the left it is transformed into the arch of the aorta.

The first branchial arch gives rise to that part of the face which includes the lateral portion of the upper lip, the cheek, the maxilla, and the mandible, as well as the tragus and helix of the ear. *Meckel's cartilage*, within the first arch, is the precursor of the mandibular bone. From the second arch arises the antitragus and antihelix of the ear and in addition the lesser wing of the hyoid bone. From the third arch arises the greater wing of the hyoid bone which later fuses anteriorly with the same structure of the opposite side to form the body of the hyoid bone.

The above brief resume is of importance in attempting to discover the relationship of cervical fistulas and cysts to the embryonic structures of the neck. Wenglowski[20] made a very intensive study of the subject and proposed the idea that cervical fistulas are not derived from the branchial clefts, but rather that they originate from the thymic "duct"; this anlage of the thymus gland is an elongated structure which extends downward and forward from the third pouch. We are inclined to agree with Shedden[17] and others, however, that there is really little to support Wenglowski's theory. Since certain structures of the neck are definitely identified with, or are derived from, parts of the primitive branchial arches, we are now able to use these landmarks and can plot on the human child what would be the relative course of the primitive branchial apparatus. The constancy of the location of the cervical fistulas in relation to what would be the course of the upper branchial clefts forces us to believe that these congenital defects actually represent a persistence of one of these branchial structures.

Assuming that a cervical fistula arises from a branchial cleft, which one of these grooves is the precursor of the congenital anomaly? Some authors have stated that any of the clefts may give rise to one of these fistulas, but obviously this is not true. At once we can rule out the fourth and fifth clefts as precursors of these fistulas because it would be necessary for such a tract to course below the corresponding fourth branchial artery, or its derivative, namely, the aortic arch on the left or the subclavian artery on the right. Inasmuch as no fistula has ever been reported in these positions, the fourth and the fifth clefts can be ruled out as the responsible embryologic structures.

If the tract were derived from the third cleft, it would have to course postero-inferiorly to the glossopharyngeal nerve which runs in the third arch. There are insufficient data, from published cases and from our own material, to state definitely whether or not a branchial fistula courses behind this nerve in any appreciable number of cases, but it is our impression that such a position is not commonly encountered. Another relationship, which should exist if the fistula were developed from the third pouch and arch, would bring the tract lateral to the internal and external carotid arteries. Again, it is our belief that such a course for the fistula is not a common one.

If a cervical fistula should develop from the second branchial cleft, it would have to assume a position so as to lie *between* the internal carotid and external carotid arteries. Such a position is one which is often encountered. Furthermore, the internal end of what was the primitive second pouch lies somewhere within the tonsillar fossa. This coincides closely with what we have been able to determine at operation, for in those patients who have a complete tract, the inner orifice is usually found near the base of the tonsil or along the posterior tonsillar pillar. We are led to conclude, therefore, that the great majority of congenital fistulas of the neck are actually derived from the second branchial cleft and pouch.

Regarding the congenital anomalies possibly derived by persistence of the first cleft, we have less accurate knowledge. Since it is known that the first pouch and cleft lead to the formation of the eustachian tube and external auditory canal, it is logical to believe that any persisting sinus which might communicate with either of these structures must arise from the first cleft. In one child we have seen a small cutaneous orifice just beneath the mandible and an inch anterior to the angle of the jaw. On dissection a sinus was found which ran upward and backward to enter the external auditory canal. This is the only instance of its kind which has come to our attention, but it probably represents an irregularity of first cleft development.

The different portions of the ear arise from six small nodules which originate from the first and second branchial arches (Fig. 544). The three nubbins which are derived from the first arch subsequently form the helix and tragus of the ear, while the three rounded nodules from the second arch give rise to the antihelix and antitragus. While we can offer no proof to support the contention, it appears likely that the sinuses opening on the ear or just in front of the ear arise because of incomplete fusion of these adjacent lobules.

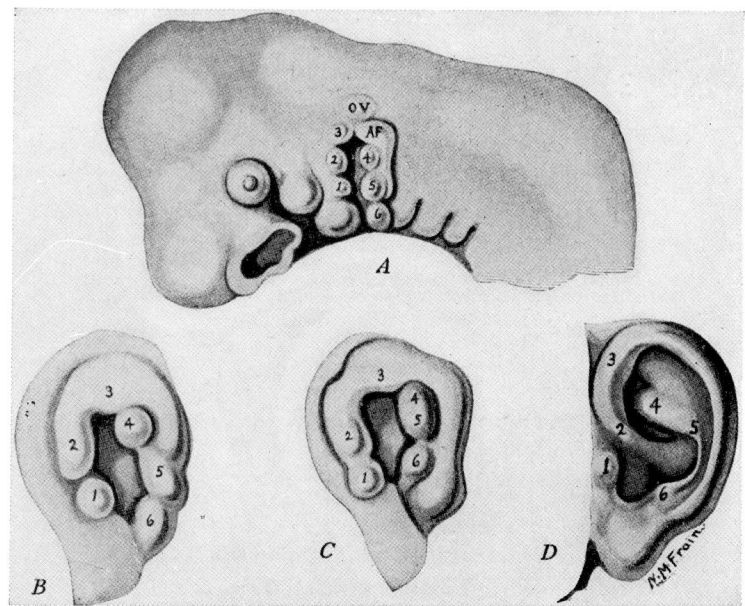

Fig. 544. Stages in development of the external ear, adapted from His and from Arey's Developmental Anatomy. A, 11 mm. B, 13.6 mm. C, 15 mm. D, Adult. 1, 2, 3. Elevations on the first branchial arch. 4, 5, 6. Elevations on the second arch. AF. Auricular fold. OV. Otic vesicle. 1. Tragus. 2, 3. Helix. 4, 5. Antihelix. 6. Antitragus. Small congenital fistulas opening on the ear or just in front of the tragus probably represent a failure of fusion of two adjoining elevations.

Regarding those rare cases in which there is a small cutaneous lobule and cartilage in the anterior triangle of the neck, there appears to be a definite relationship to the branchial arch system. This malformation must represent the anomalous formation of cartilage which in fish is a normal structure in the gill arches.

In rare instances, the lateral branchial arches from the two sides might not fuse properly in the midline, giving rise to a midline cyst or particularly a cleft (Fig. 551).

CLINICAL DATA

In reviewing the records of the Boston Children's Hospital, we find a total of 308 cases in which there was a cyst, fistula, or cartilaginous cutaneous tab of the neck, or a fistula or tab of the face or ear, all of which were believed to have been derived from the branchial apparatus. These cases may be grouped as follows:

Lateral cervical fistulas

Right	65
Left	58
Bilateral	25
Total	148

Lateral cervical cysts

Right	12
Left	11
Bilateral	3
Total	26

Cervical cutaneous tabs containing cartilage

Right	4
Left	9
Bilateral	4
Total	17

Midline cervical anomalies

Cysts	3
Clefts	6
Sinuses	2
Total	11

Auricular or preauricular cysts or sinuses

Right	15
Left	17
Bilateral	12
Total	44

Preauricular tabs containing cartilage

Right	21
Left	20
Bilateral	21
Total	62
Grand Total	308

Of these 308 patients, 261 had some operative treatment. In each of the remaining patients there has been no operation because the fistula or cyst was so small that the insignificant symptoms did not warrant a surgical procedure, or else some other illness was present which made it advisable to defer operation. In the group of cases operated upon, the following numbers are found in each class:

PATIENTS TREATED BY OPERATION

Lateral cervical fistulas	117
Lateral cervical cysts	22
Cervical tabs containing cartilage	15
Midline branchiogenic anomalies	11
Auricular or preauricular sinus or cyst	39
Preauricular tab	57
Total	261

Branchial Fistulas

Branchial fistulas, sometimes called lateral cervical fistulas, or persistent branchial clefts, present a considerable variety of clinical findings. The tract in a given case may be *complete*, that is, it courses through the tissues of the neck and possesses an internal, as well as an external opening. In those cases in which the tract is *incomplete*, only a portion of such sinus is present, usually, the orifice on the skin and a sinus extending a short distance into the deep structures of the neck.

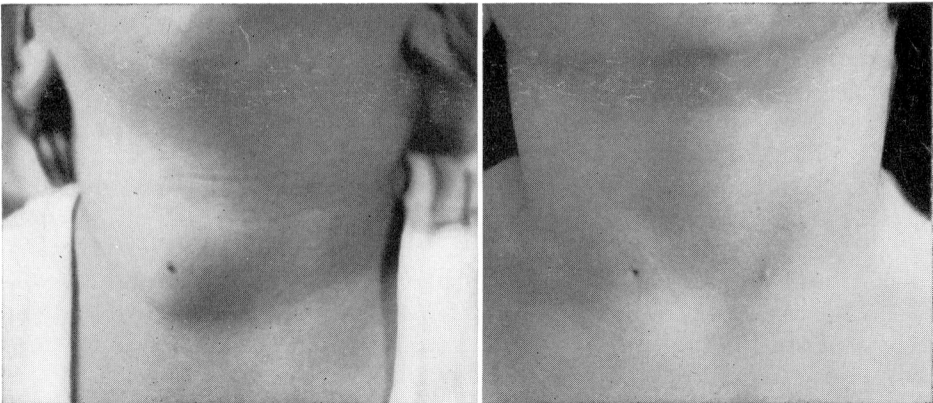

Fig. 545. Two children with branchiogenic sinuses. *Left,* Just beneath the cutaneous orifice is also a small branchiogenic cyst. *Right,* Two small cervical fistulas from which clear mucoid material occasionally oozed.

When a sinus opens externally, as it does in the majority of cases, this orifice may be anywhere along the anterior border of the sternocleidomastoid muscle, but most commonly it is seen along the lower third of this structure. The opening has a variable size, usually not greater than a millimeter or two in diameter, and often will admit only the smallest probe. A discharge of mucoid material is commonly the presenting symptom and in more than half of the cases is noticed since birth, though its appearance may be delayed until the child is several years of age.

The sinuses are lined by stratified squamous epithelium, by ciliated or non-ciliated columnar epithelium, possibly showing secretory activity, and similar to that of the respiratory tract. The lining membrane may have deep crypts or infoldings of great irregularity. Lymphoid tissue is commonly found in the walls.

Secondary infection is a frequent complication of a branchial fistula; when this occurs the character of the discharge changes to a purulent one and there are signs of inflammatory reaction around the cutaneous orifice and even in the deeper structures

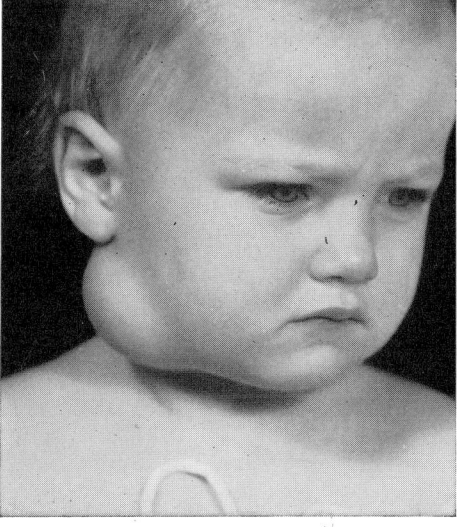

Fig. 546. A typical branchiogenic cyst. These always lie in front of the sternocleidomastoid muscle.

of the neck. When infection has once entered a sinus of this sort, recurring attacks of inflammation are common until the entire tract has been excised.

Merely because a discharge from a branchial fistula is yellow does not mean that there is infection. Frequently these lesions are described as having a purulent exudate, whereas a microscopic examination of the material shows it to be only squamous epithelial cells which have been desquamated from the lining of the sinus.

A draining sinus from a tuberculous lymphadenitis which has undergone necrosis might be confused with a branchial fistula. The character of the discharge, the presence of multiple cutaneous openings, and the presence of enlarged, matted lymph glands in the tuberculous lesion are sufficient to differentiate it from a branchial fistula.

X-ray examination of a cervical sinus is of some interest, but is unreliable as an aid to diagnosis or in determining the extent of the tract. It has been our experience that injection of a sinus with Lipiodol or other opaque substance may not be easy, for the caliber of the tract varies greatly and in many places may be so small as to militate against complete filling. Thus the x-ray picture does not always give a true idea of the entire extent of the tract.

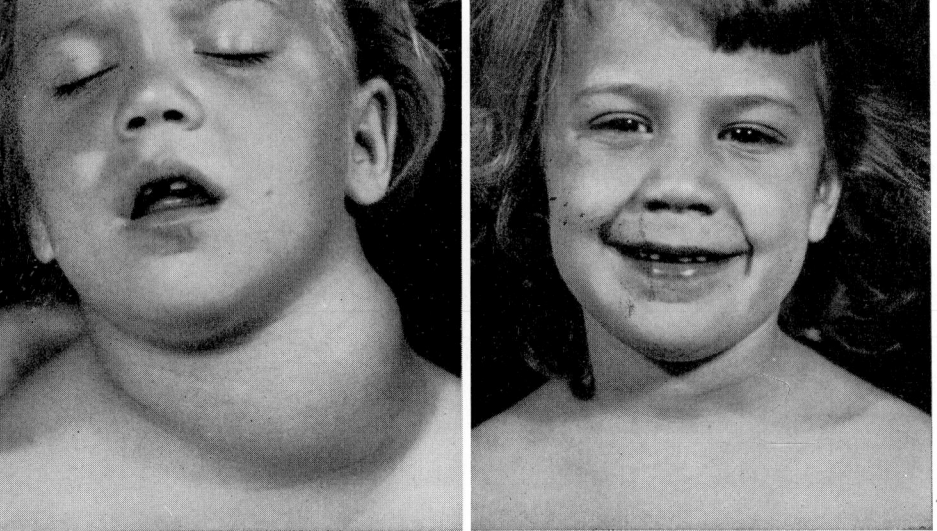

Fig. 547. *Left*, A branchiogenic cyst which was larger than average. *Right*, Photograph six months after operative removal, showing satisfactory cosmetic result.

Lateral Cervical Cysts

These are variously called lateral cysts of the neck, branchial cysts, or congenital cysts of the neck. They appear in the anterior triangle and are never seen behind the sternocleidomastoid muscle. They are prone to lie higher in the neck than is the cutaneous opening of a branchial fistula. While a cyst may be found anywhere along the anterior border of the sternocleidomastoid muscle from the manubrial notch to the angle of the jaw, it is more apt to be located opposite the middle third of this muscle. This is particularly true of a large cyst which is probably displaced by its mere size to this less constricted region.

Branchial cysts vary considerably in size. The smaller ones are little more than 1 cm. in diameter, the average is twice or three times this size, while the largest may be 4 or 5 cm. in diameter. Since our series is composed only of children under twelve years of age, we have not encountered the larger cysts of adolescent or adult life which have been described in the literature.

Cysts may be lined by squamous or columnar epithelium. Acute and chronic inflammatory changes are often seen in the walls. Lymphoid accumulations are commonly encountered in the adjacent tissues.

The cysts vary in elasticity, according to the amount of fluid they contain and the degree of pressure under which this is held. Such a mass usually has only very slight mobility because of its attachments to surrounding structures; particularly is it anchored if previously it has been the focus of infection. As a rule, a cyst transmits light poorly because of the thickness of its wall and the overlying platysma and skin. Such a cyst does not usually have progressive enlargement. It may vary in size from time to time

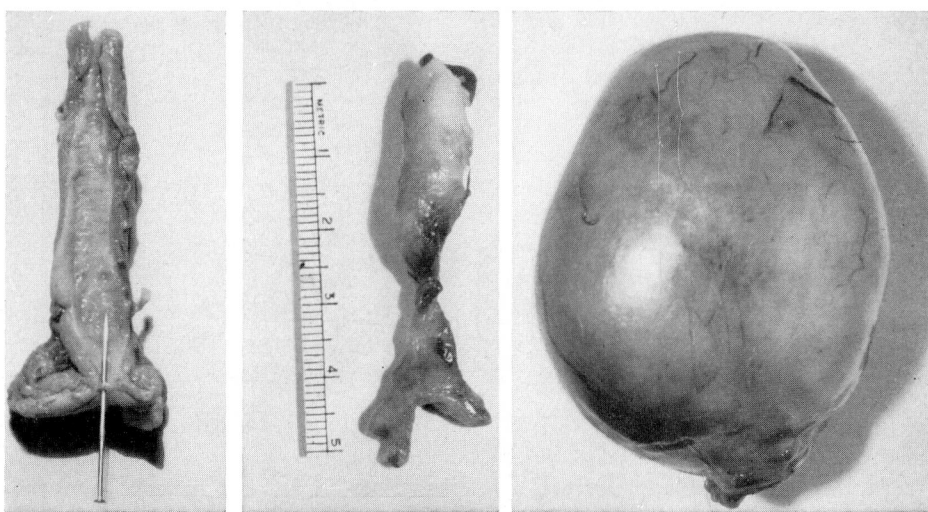

Fig. 548. *Left* and *middle*, Excised branchiogenic sinuses. *Right*, Branchiogenic cyst from a twelve-year-old girl.

in a given patient, this phenomenon being due either to a spontaneous external discharge of its contents through an associated cutaneous fistula or else to an internal drainage of the cyst fluid to the throat by way of a small pharyngeal communication.

Because of an opening into the pharynx or onto the skin of the neck, bacteria often enter a branchial cyst and cause suppuration. If a patient is seen for the first time during an acute inflammatory period, it may be difficult to differentiate the condition from suppurative cervical lymphadenitis unless attention is paid to the history of a swelling which long preceded the inflammatory symptoms.

While the diagnosis of a branchial cyst is usually made with little difficulty, there are occasional cases in which the true nature of the lesion might be overlooked for many months, particularly if there have been recurring inflammatory changes to suggest a diagnosis of tuberculosis. To aid in this differentiation, Wangensteen[18] has suggested making a roentgenogram of the neck after the injection of an iodized solution into the cyst. The finding of a smooth-walled cavity is practically diagnostic of a branchial cyst, whereas an irregular wall is more indicative of tuberculous or other suppurative lesion.

Aside from its local manifestations, a branchial cyst may give rise to symptoms by a reflex mechanism when there is pressure on the vagus nerve. Isolated cases have been reported in which manipulations of a branchial cyst, or probing of a fistula, would produce vagal irritation such as coughing, nausea, or variation in the heart rate.

Cartilaginous Rests of the Neck

These peculiar pedunculated or sessile tabs (Fig. 550) on the neck have been occasionally reported in the literature and have been particularly commented upon by Nieden and Asbeck.[13] They may appear as an irregular mass of cartilage, several millimeters in greatest diameter, lying in the subcutaneous tissues of the neck, usually just in front of the lower third of the sternocleidomastoid muscle. In other cases they assume

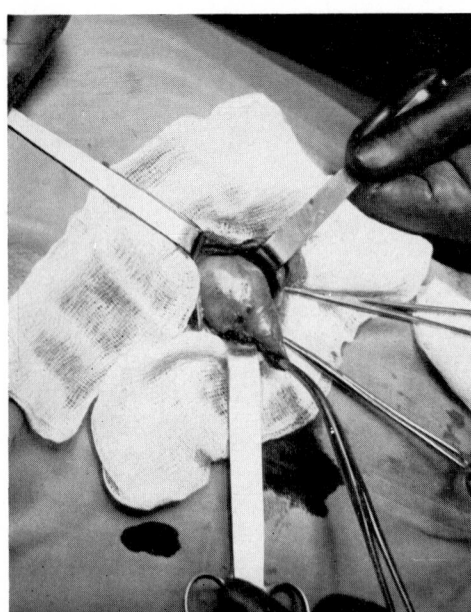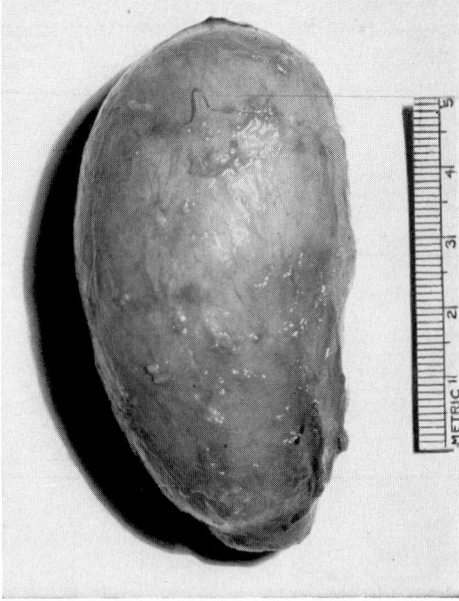

Fig. 549. *Left,* Operating-table photograph of a branchiogenic cyst being removed from the neck *Right,* The specimen.

the form of an external pedunculated mass from 4 to 6 mm. in diameter and 0.5 to 2 cm. in length; when such tabs are bilateral they are rather reminiscent of the bells of a goat's neck.

These tabs, as well as the subcutaneous cartilaginous rests, contain a small bit of cartilage which extends beyond the base of the lesion and reaches several millimeters into the superficial tissues of the neck. In none of these cases has there been any associated external fistulous opening, and indeed we have been unable to discover any tract with a lumen either in the tab itself or leading upward in the neck. In some of the cases there is a cord of fibrous tissue passing upward a few centimeters along the medial border of the sternocleidomastoid muscle, but we have not found one leading up to the pharynx.

Midline Cervical Clefts or Cysts of Branchiogenic Origin

While most midline anomalies arise from thyroglossal duct abnormalities, there are a few rare ones that do not; they arise from improper midline fusion of the two sides of branchial arches. If this mal-union occurs in the lower arches, a small midline cyst can occur below the suprasternal notch, in front of the menubrium or upper part of the sternum (Fig. 552). If the improper fusion occurs at a higher level, there is a long, midline, vertical cleft, lined by a weeping reddened membrane, from the lower or upper end of which a tiny sinus may plunge for a short distance into the deeper structures of the neck (Fig. 551).

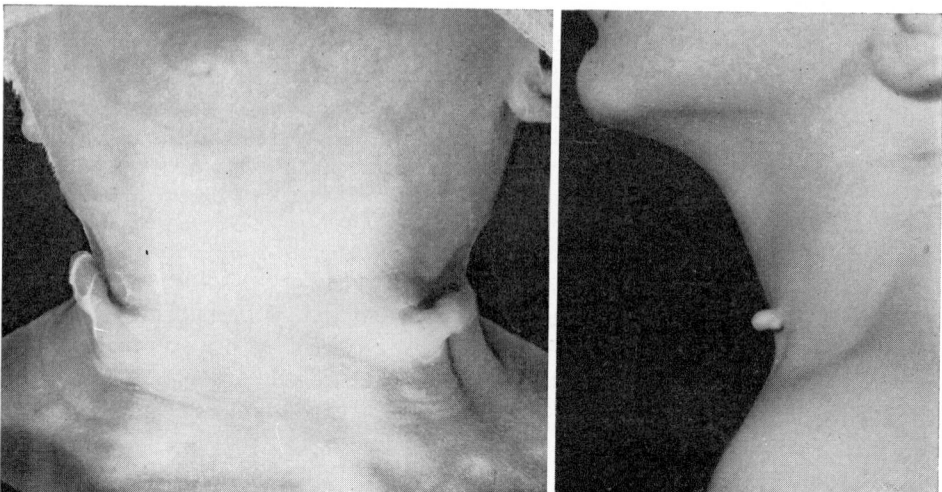

Fig. 550. Two children with cutaneous cervical tabs. *Left,* Bilateral anomalies in a baby. *Right,* Unilateral lesion in a boy.

Preauricular and Auricular Fistulas

Little attention has been given to this subject in the literature. These small fistulas may open on the helix, on the tragus, and occasionally on the lobule; most commonly they open immediately in front of the ear. The external orifice of such a sinus is little more than a millimeter in diameter and the tract, which leads forward for no more than 1 or 1.5 cm., never has an internal opening in the mouth. The amount of mucoid discharge is never very great, for in so short a tract there can be only little secretory epithelium. While these small sinuses often pass without notice, it has been our experience that they may be very troublesome, and indeed may be quite disfiguring, because they are quite apt to become infected and serve as a focus for recurring inflammation. The few sinuses which we have seen on the ear proper have never shown any evidence of infection, but the ones anterior to the ear are quite prone to become infected.

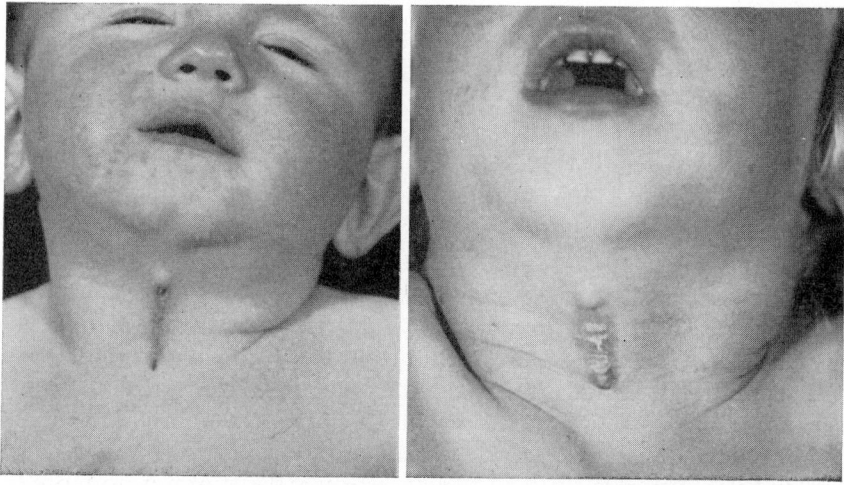

Fig. 551. Midline cervical clefts in two children. Presumably, the defect is caused by improper fusion of branchial arches as they meet in the midline.

Preauricular Tabs

These small anomalous tabs, quite similar to those described above which occur in the neck, are tiny structures but a few millimeters in length, often containing cartilage, lying just in front of the ear (Fig. 554).

TREATMENT

Branchial Fistula

Because of the very high incidence of secondary infection in such tracts it has been our practice to advise excision for all branchial fistulas.

There have been several proposals for the treatment of branchial cysts of fistulas by the injection of various sclerosing agents. We have had no experience with this method of therapy and have not used it because of strong theoretical objections. From experience we find it is very difficult to inject Lipiodol so as to fill an entire tract; it seems equally improbable that a sclerosing agent can be injected so that it will reach all of the crypts and folds which generally are present in the wall of such a sinus. Furthermore, a sclerosing agent strong enough to destroy a thick portion of the membrane might easily perforate the wall where the lining is thin.

The surgical removal of a branchial fistula may be quite a simple procedure if the tract is short and does not extend deeply into the neck, but if the sinus reaches up to the pharynx, the neck dissection becomes a major operation. The type of incision is of considerable importance from the standpoint of cosmetic result. Some authors have advocated an incision running parallel to the anterior border of the sternocleidomastoid muscle. This gives an excellent exposure for the surgeon, but it is very apt to give a web-like, unsightly scar; therefore it should always be avoided. From the cosmetic angle, it is far better to make a transverse incision, made elliptical around the cutaneous orifice; the closure of such a wound (in the direction of the neck folds) gives a scar with extremely little disfigurement. If the tract is a short one, such an incision gives an adequate exposure, but if the dissection must be carried up to the tonsillar fossa, a second incision, parallel to the first one, can be made higher up and more posteriorly, just beneath the angle of the jaw. This combination has well been called a "stair-steps incision." When each of these wounds is carefully sutured, by accurately bringing together the platysma muscle and then suturing the skin with fine material, the resulting scars are almost invisible. In the vast majority of cases, we have been able to complete the entire dissection through one wound; only rarely has it been necessary to employ the double openings.

A branchial sinus courses lateral to the internal jugular vein and also lateral to both the internal and external carotid arteries until it turns into the pharyngeal wall when it passes between the internal and external carotid arteries. The tract lies beneath the posterior belly of the digastric muscle. As the pharyngeal wall is approached, it is sometimes desirable to have an assistant place a finger in the mouth and push against the pharyngeal wall on the same side as that on which the operation is being done. Now palpating in the depths of the wound, the operator can feel the assistant's finger in the pharynx and can thereby judge how much further the dissection can be carried without perforating the pharyngeal wall. When the tract has been freed to within 2 or 3 mm. of the pharynx, it is tied off and cut across with a carbolized knife. Various procedures have been devised to turn the remaining small stump inward so that it will empty into the throat, but this does not appear to be necessary if the stump is no more than a few millimeters long. During the course of these dissections, it is well to make a practice of always identifying the spinal accessory nerve. We have routinely taken this precaution and in no case has it been severed.

After all bleeding points have been ligated, the wound is closed by accurately approximating the platysma and subcutaneous fat with interrupted sutures of fine silk or catgut. The skin is closed in an appropriate fashion; we prefer interrupted silk of 00000 Deknatel, taking great care to establish nice approximation of the skin edges.

Branchial Cyst

The removal of a branchial cyst involves essentially the same operative problems as does a fistula, for in most cases there is a tract from the skin to the cyst, or from the cyst upward to the pharynx. Too much attention must not be focused on the cyst, to the neglect of an associated fistula, because an incomplete operation is apt to be followed by recurrence of the anomaly.

The above considerations are, of course, only applicable in those cases in which there is little or no infection at the time operation is undertaken. In an appreciable number of patients, suppuration is present and there is incomplete drainage by a small cutaneous orifice, or indeed there may be no external discharge at all. In such cases adequate incision and drainage must be performed, deferring removal of the underlying lesion until a second operation, when infection is minimal or has entirely disappeared.

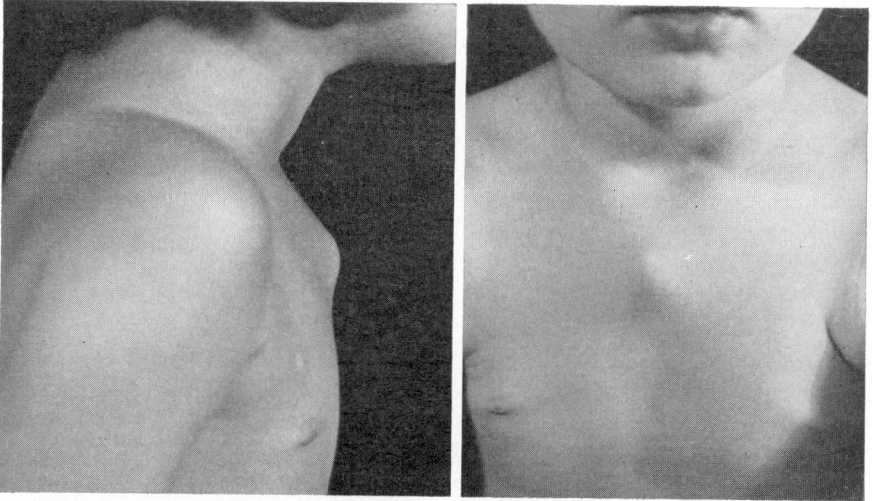

Fig. 552. Rare, midline presternal cyst, believed to be caused by improper midline fusion of the lowest pair of branchial arches.

Tabs or Cartilaginous Rests of the Neck

Treatment of the external tabs or the subcutaneous cartilaginous rests of the neck is a simple undertaking, for the mass can be excised easily with an elliptical piece of skin, including with it that tissue which extends for a little distance into the neck. Generally these malformations do not have associated sinuses which run upward to the pharyngeal wall; hence the dissection involved only the superficial planes of the neck.

Midline, Vertical, Cervical Clefts

These anomalies (Fig. 551) are easy to excise but are extremely difficult to treat in any way which gives a pleasing cosmetic result. To sew up the wound vertically, even

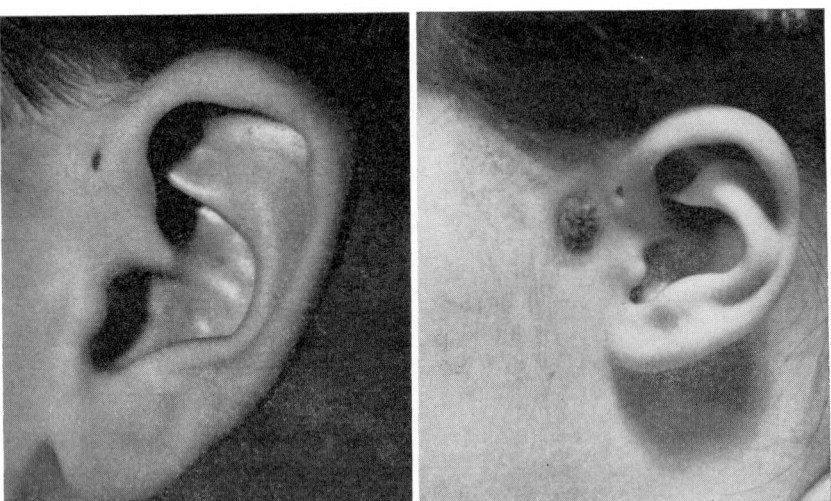

Fig. 553. Preauricular sinuses. *Left,* Uninfected sinus just in front of helix *Right,* Preauricular sinus which has been the seat of recurring infection and abscess formation.

if this is combined with postoperative irradiation of the wound, is followed by keloid and a contracting web-like scar which is usually more disfiguring than the original lesion. To sew up the vertical wound in a transverse manner has not been satisfactory. The best results, and these are not too desirable, have been obtained by using the vertical wound as the central part of a Z by making appropriate cuts from either end out to the sides; the flaps are then rotated and interlocked so that the closure gives a horizontal line, from either end of which an oblique line runs upward (and downward) to the mid-line of the neck.

Preauricular Tabs cause no concern in therapy. They can be excised easily with an elliptical incision around their base.

Preauricular or Auricular Sinuses

The small sinuses of the helix, tragus, and lobule of the ear have rarely given enough symptoms to warrant surgical intervention, but in those cases in which it has been

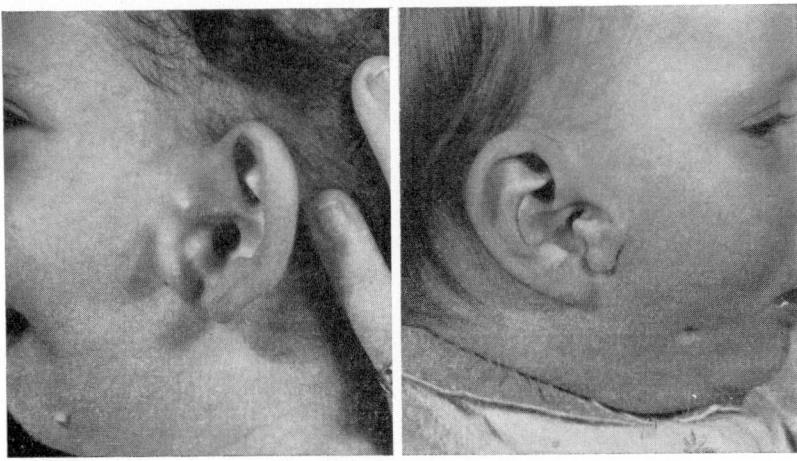

Fig. 554. Preauricular tabs in two children. *Left,* Single tab (they appeared bilaterally). *Right,* Irregular preauricular tab, deformity of external auditory canal, and a facial sinus, all of which are malformations related to the first branchial arch and cleft.

desirable to improve the cosmetic appearance, the shortness of the tract has made excision a simple matter.

A sinus in front of the ear is very apt to be troublesome, for they seem to be particularly prone to infection. This recurring abscess formation often leads to a very disfiguring scar which is difficult to excise because of the subjacent facial nerve. We have attempted destruction of some of these short tracts by insertion of a needle or wire and passing a coagulating current through it; the results have been very poor. An uninfected preauricular sinus can usually be excised with an elliptical incision which slopes downward and forward, closing the wound by appropriate sutures. An infected preauricular sinus (abscess) which does not respond to incision and drainage plus chemotherapy, is best treated by opening it up widely, curretting away all lining, and packing open the wound with gauze for five or six days. After the gauze is removed, there remains a disagreeable looking crater but this has an amazing way of filling in spontaneously and flattening out to give in the end a fair cosmetic result.

REFERENCES

1. Adams, W. S.: A Branchial Cleft Appearing as a Post-tonsillar Abscess. J. Laryng. & Otol., *61*:552, 1946.
2. Bailey, H.: Clinical Aspects of Branchial Fistulae. Brit. J. Surg., *21*:173, 1933.
3. Baumgartner, C. J.: Branchial and Thyroglossal Duct Cysts and Fistulas in Children. Surg., Gynec. & Obst., *56*:948, 1933.
4. Blassingame, C. D.: Congenital Cysts and Fistulae about the Head and Neck. Ann. Otol., Rhin. & Laryng., *56*:395, 1947.
5. Carp, L.: Branchial Fistula—Its Clinical Relation to Irritation of the Vagus. Surg., Gynec. & Obst., *42*:772, 1926.
6. Christopher, F.: The Surgical Treatment of Lateral Cervical Fistulae. Surg., Gynec. & Obst., *38*:329, 1924.
7. Ewing, M. R.: Congenital Sinuses of the External Ear. J. Laryng. & Orol., *61*:18, 1946.
8. Hoover, W. B.: Clinical Conditions Arising from Anomalies or Maldevelopments of the Branchial Arches and Clefts. Ann. Otol., Rhin. & Laryng., *50*:834, 1941.
9. Hyndman, O. R. and Light, G.: The Branchial Apparatus: Its Embryologic Origin and the Pathologic Changes to Which it Gives Rise, with Presentation of a Familial Group of Fistulas. Arch. Surg., *19*:410, 1929.
10. Josa, L.: Ueber Fisteln des ersten Kiemenbogens. Zentralbl. f. Chir., *63*:1760, 1936.
11. Meyer, H. W.: Congenital Cysts and Fistulae of the Neck. Ann. Surg., *95*:1, 1932.
12. Neel, H. B. and Pemberton, J. deJ.: Lateral Cervical (Branchial) Cysts and Fistulas. A Clinical and Pathologic Study. Surgery, *18*: 267, 1945.
13. Nieden, H. and Asbeck, C.: Kongenitale Knorpelreste am Halse und ihre Beziehung zu den seitlichen Halsfisteln. Beitr. z. klin. Chir., *153*:47, 1931.
14. Nylander, P. E. A.: Beiträge zur Kenntnis der kongenitalen Halsfisteln und Zysten. Arb. a. d. path. Inst. der Universtät Helsingfors, *5*:114, 1927.
15. Parkinson, S. N.: Branchiogenous Carcinoma in a Child. Am. J. Dis. Child., *61*:1272, 1941.
16. Peterson, E. W.: Tumors of the Neck. Special Reference to Congenital Cysts and Fistulas. Am. J. Surg., *61*:350, 1943.
17. Shedden, W. M.: Branchial Cysts and Fistulae. New England J. Med., *205*:800, 1931.
18. Wangensteen, O. H.: Differentiation of Branchial from Other Cervical Cysts by X-ray Examination. Ann. Surg., *93*:790, 1931.
19. Ward, G. E., Hendrick, J. W. and Chambers, R. G.: Branchiogenic Anomalies. Results of Seventy Cases Observed at the Johns Hopkins Hospital between 1926 and 1946. West. J. Surg., *57*:536, 1949.
20. Wenglowski, R.: Ueber die Halsfisteln und Cysten. Arch. f. klin. Chir., *98*:151, 1912.

CHAPTER 68

Cystic Hygroma

Cystic hygroma is an endothelium-lined, fluid-containing lesion of lymphatic origin which is encountered most often in infancy and childhood. Dowd[3] collected 91 cases which had been published prior to 1913. Vaughn[19] added to this review, collecting all cases up to 1934, bringing the total to 155. Goetsch,[6] in 1938, made an excellent pathologic study of 12 personally observed cases. Our own material includes 112 examples of the lesion in infants and children, seen up through December 1950.

Cystic hygromas have been described in various regions of the body, particularly in the axilla and chest wall and less frequently in the groin. The cervical lesions are by far the most common and constitute probably four-fifths of all hygromas which have been studied.

PATHOLOGY

Macroscopic Picture

The hygromatous cyst is a rounded, ovoid, or smoothly lobulated sac which is thin-walled and translucent. The paper thinness of the walls and the fluid content of the sac impart to the specimen a soft consistency. The structure is occasionally monolocular, but there may be side pockets separated by fibrous septa which freely communicate with the main cavity. Thus, a puncture of any one of the accessory chambers results in a collapse of the entire structure. In some specimens, there are closely adherent, thin-walled cysts which do not possess openings between their lumina; there is a multilocular configuration. The walls of the cysts have a very low vascularity, and the blood vessels which are present are always quite small. The cyst fluid is characteristically thin, clear, and usually colorless though it may possess a very slight yellowish tinge. Occasionally there may be old or recent hemorrhage into cyst cavities.

Microscopic Findings

The fibrous wall is composed of connective tissue of variable cellularity. Collagen may be abundant and compact, or may be scanty and have a myxomatous appearance. Even in the absence of infection, there are isolated lymphocytic cell infiltrations, and it is not uncommon to encounter lymphoid follicles with germinal centers. Blood vessels are mostly of capillary or arteriolar size; larger channels are seldom seen. A thin layer of flattened endothelial cells lines the cystic spaces. Occasionally a blood vessel, nerve, or small muscle-bundle traverses a crypt or outpocketing of the main cyst cavity, and in each instance this structure is covered by a layer of endothelial cells.

Goetsch[6] has added greatly to our understanding of the pathology of these lesions, particularly in reference to the manner of growth and propagation of hygromas. According to his concept, there are narrow outgrowths or cords of endothelial cells which insinuate themselves between muscle bundles, nerve fibers, and other anatomic structures of the region. While these cords are at first solid, they later acquire a lumen by the accumulation of a lymph-like fluid which forces apart the walls to form an endothelial lined sac, which either abuts against the main cyst cavity or else attains a communication with it. The continued collection of fluid in one of these side pockets or daughter cysts enlarges the wedge between anatomic structures of the region. These structures become surrounded and enveloped, so that eventually a muscle bundle, a blood vessel, or nerve becomes separated from its supporting tissues and is covered by a layer of endothelial cells. In this way a small strand of muscle or an artery is made to *traverse* the cavity of a hygroma and it may be atrophied by pressure from the surrounding fluid.

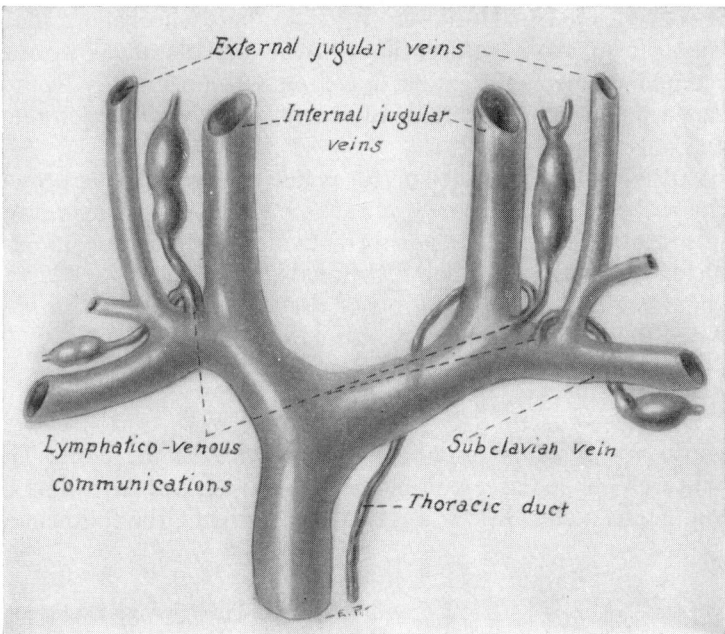

Fig. 555. Sketch showing position of the lymphatic buds of the neck and their communications with the venous system as found in the embryo of a monkey (*Macacus nomestrinus* Linn) (after McClure and Silvester).

ETIOLOGY

In studying the etiology of cystic hygromas it is tempting to group them with the lymphangiomas found in the neck and in other regions of the body. Lymphangiomas are often encountered in skin and subcutaneous fat or superficial tissues, particularly in the lip, axilla, anterior chest wall, arms, or legs. There is little objection to the classification of hygromas with such lesions, regarding them as cystic or cavernous lymphangiomas. Indeed, some pathologists have freely used the terms "hygroma" and "cavernous lymphangioma" as being synonymous and can offer histologic material to support this view. However, there are two principal reasons for objecting to this grouping together of the two conditions. First, lymphangiomas of the lip, hands, feet, etc., rarely develop cystic cavities more than a few millimeters in diameter. While these lesions may be massive and very extensive, they never develop cystic spaces several centimeters in diameter as are seen in the hygromas. Second, the rather sharply defined areas in which hygromas are found in the neck and, less commonly, in the groin or retroperitoneal spaces, lead one to connect their origin with two known embryologic structures which are present in these two regions, namely, the *lymphatic sacs* of the *neck* and the *iliac areas*.

According to Sabin[17] there arises from the jugular vein a small, endothelium-lined outpocketing which subsequently becomes detached from the vein and develops as the primitive *lymphatic sac* or *bud*. This structure is paired and is found on either side of the neck. At about the same stage of fetal life there are other similar buds which arise in relation to the large pelvic veins. Less important centers for the development of these lymphatic anlagen are found along the dorsal aspects of the abdomen and thorax. Arising from these buds, particularly from the large cervical ones, the growing lymphatic vessels coalesce and become a unified, anastomosing system which later acquires permanent communication with various veins.

This view is challenged by Huntington[10] and others who believe that the endothelium-lined lymph sacs of the neck and other portions of the trunk do not arise as offshoots of the venous system, but rather that they develop directly from mesenchymal tissues and then, after a period of ramification and coalescence, acquire unions with the venous channels.

Whichever of these two views is correct is not pertinent to the present discussion. Suffice it to say that there is agreement among embryologists concerning the presence of the jugular and other lymphatic sacs in human fetuses. The positions of these embryologic structures—and the similar locations of hygromas—appear to leave little doubt that a pinching off or sequestration of tissue from one of them gives rise to an endothelium-lined lesion which we know as a "hygroma."

CLINICAL DATA

Hygromas do not occur at random in any portion of the body. They are found mostly in certain well defined areas, principally in the neck or extending from the neck into closely contiguous zones. In our series of 112 patients, the following locations are noted:

Left side of neck	52 (In 2 the hygroma extended into the mediastinum)
Right side of neck	39 (In 1 the hygroma extended into the cheek and tongue. In 1 it extended into the mediastinum. In 1 it extended into the right axilla.)
Both sides of neck, extension into tongue	7
Posterior neck	2
Right parotid area	1
Left shoulder	1
Mediastinum	3
Right axilla	1
Left axilla	1
Right thigh	2
Left pectoral area	2
Right pectoral area	1
Total	112

Most hygromas appear in the neck, especially in the posterior triangle, behind the sternocleidomastoid muscle, occupying the supraclavicular fossa or extending over toward the crest of the shoulder. In a much smaller proportion of cases, the cyst may occupy the anterior cervical triangle; but when it does so, there is a tendency for it to lie in a high position just beneath the angle of the jaw or to overlie the ramus of the mandible. In those which have a high position, there is a strong tendency for the lesion

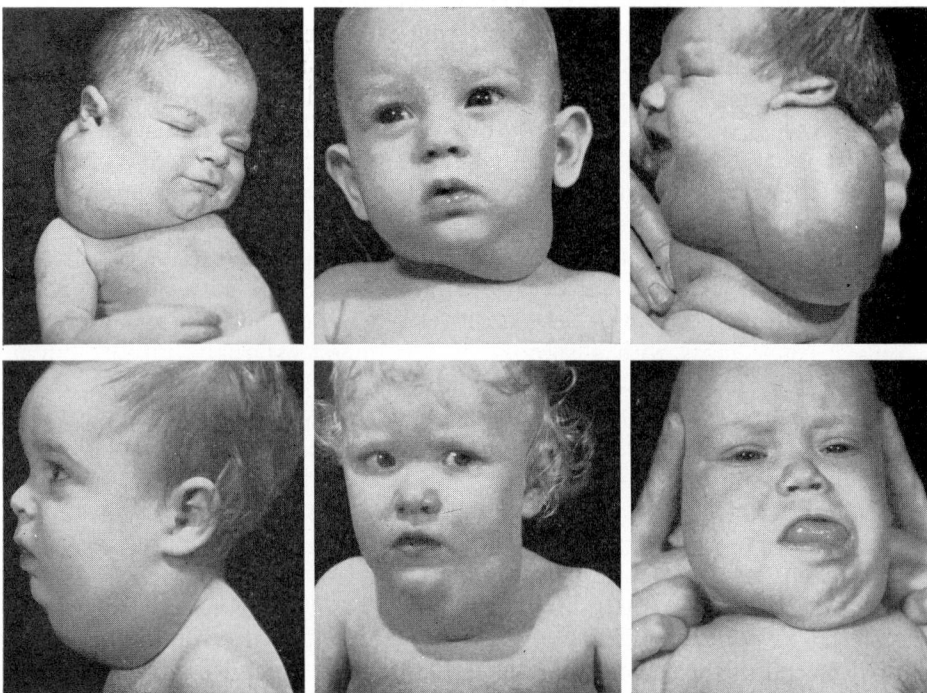

Fig. 556. Photographs of six patients with cystic hygroma of the neck, showing some characteristic lesions.

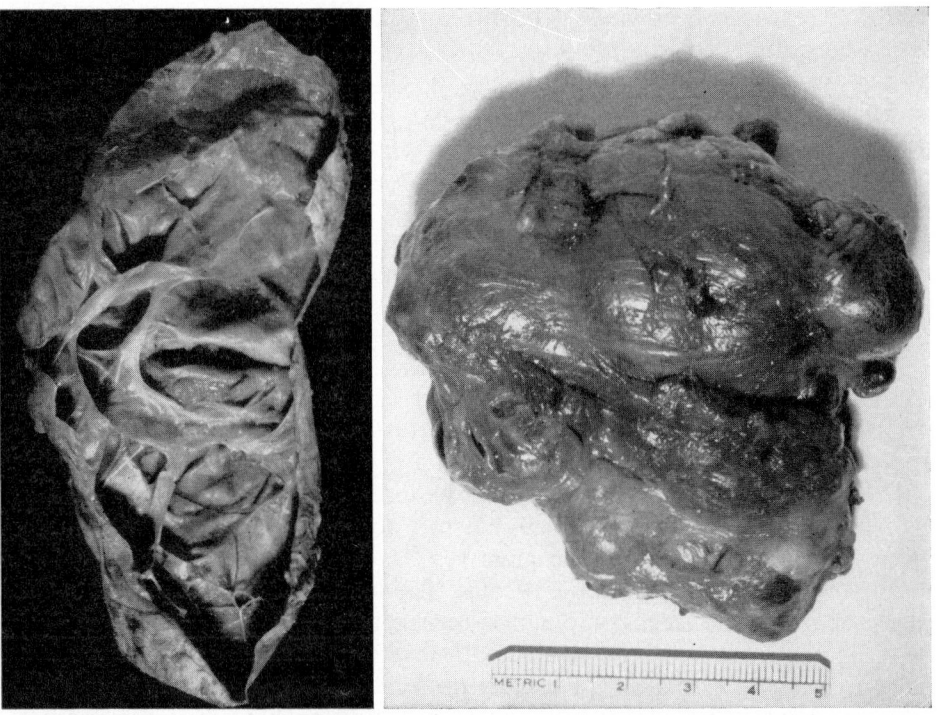

Fig. 557. *Left*, Multilocular cystic hygroma from the neck. *Right*, 88 gram, cervical hygroma from a year-old child.

to project upward in such a way that the musculature of the floor of the mouth is in-filtrated and greatly distorted. In a few striking examples of the condition, a massive cystic structure may completely fill the lateral hollow of the neck and extend from the side of the head well down to the tip of the shoulder, and it may even bulge to the sub-clavicular fossa and the axilla anteriorly or to the spine of the scapula posteriorly.

The size of a mass does not bear any definite relationship to the age of the patient or to the duration of the lesion. Indeed, we have encountered some of our largest speci-mens in infants only a few weeks of age. The smallest cyst in our series was about 5 cm. in length and 4 cm. in diameter. Commonly they are described as "lemon" size, less often they are "orange" size, and occasionally the mass is large enough to efface the normal contour of the neck on the affected side. When the lesion is small, there appears to be only a single mass with a smooth, well rounded external contour; but in the larger growths a faintly lobulated surface indicates multilocular development. The cyst is usually not tense, and it commonly has a limpid consistency and poorly defined borders. While the overlying skin is essentially normal in texture, it may vary somewhat from its usual pinkish color and have a slightly bluish cast imparted to it by the underlying fluid. The thinness of the cyst wall and the clear colorless nature of the entrapped fluid permit the mass to be easily transilluminated. This latter finding occasionally is altered if there has been hemorrhage into a cyst cavity.

The local swelling is usually noted early in life. In our series, 65 per cent were noted at birth, 80 per cent were discovered within the first year, and 90 per cent were present by the end of the second year. The oldest age in which we have seen initial de-velopment of hygroma swelling was fourteen years. It is very rare to have initial appear-ance in adult life.

Males and females are affected in about the same frequency, our proportions being 60 to 52. Reference has been made in the literature to the tendency of the lesion to occur in the first-born child of a family, but our material shows no evidence to support this view.

X-ray examination of a cervical hygroma seldom gives additional information of value. The soft tissue swelling gives a shadow of rather uniform density with poorly defined borders. The exact extent of the cavities can be demonstrated better by the injection of iodized oil, or better still an aqueous iodide solution, into the cyst as sug-gested by MacGuire[12] and by Vaughn.[19] Roentgenologic examination may aid in show-ing lateral displacement of the trachea, forward displacement of the upper esophagus or pharynx, or an extension of a hygroma into the mediastinum.

SYMPTOMS AND SIGNS

As might be expected, most cystic hygromas of the neck give little in the way of troublesome symptoms. Pain or local discomfort is rarely encountered unless secondary infection has occurred. The tendency for such a cyst to lie in a superficial plane of the neck permits it to bulge outward and thus be directed away from the important and deeply-lying cervical structures. Hence it is rare to have interference with the normal functions of the brachial plexus, the great vessels, the esophagus, or the trachea. The larger hygromas may be bothersome because they limit the free movements of the head and neck. In short, the chief complaint is related primarily to the presence of a lump or the disfigurement which is associated with it. While the softness of the mass and its tendency to outward displacement usually protect the deep structures from damage, a few patients have had definite tracheal compression or have had interference with mastication by protrusion of the cysts into the floor of the mouth. Such babies can present most distressing pictures; they are unable to swallow properly, they have great difficulty in breathing, and they are constantly in danger of aspiration pneumonia.

The local mass can be present for variable lengths of time before medical attention is sought. Some patients are directly referred by the obstetrician who has noticed the lesion at birth. It is not uncommon, however, to learn that a mass has been present for many months or even several years, because the rather innocuous appearance of the smaller lesions may excite little curiosity or anxiety. It is characteristic of some hygromas to lie dormant or to increase in size only slowly over a long period of time and then to have a sudden augmentation in size which brings the patient to a physician.

In a few patients we have noted a relationship between the presence of an upper respiratory infection and the concurrent, sudden enlargement of a previously existing cystic hygroma. Apparently the infection has led to plugging or partial obstruction of the

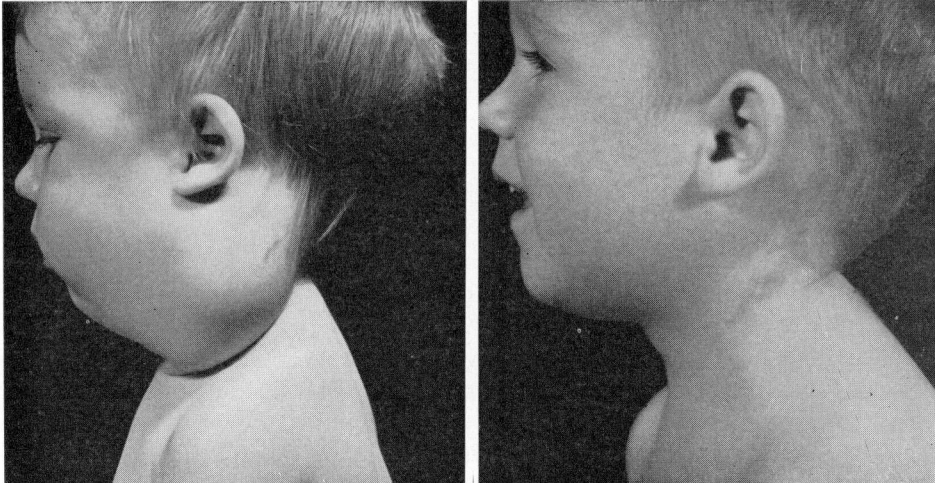

Fig. 558. *Left*, Hygroma of neck in a two-year-old boy. *Right*, Photograph two years after removal.

normal lymphatic channels so that there is a backing up of lymph in the hygroma which causes it to enlarge. While we have no microscopic proof that there are communications between a hygroma and the normal lymphatic channels of the neck, these isolated observations make us feel that such anastomoses do actually exist in some subjects.

If suppuration occurs within the cyst cavities, the outlook is extremely poor because a spreading, suppurative lesion of the neck may be exceedingly difficult to treat.

TREATMENT

In the treatment of cystic hygromas, several forms of therapy are available. To present the factors in favor of or against a given method, it is advisable to consider the various therapeutic procedures individually.

Expectant Treatment

Some authors, notably Fraser,[5] have advised that surgical attempts aimed at removal should be withheld for an indefinite period because of the tendency of a hygroma to undergo spontaneous regression. This proposal cannot be supported by our observations, for in children who have been followed for several years we have yet to see a patient in whom there has been a spontaneous disappearance of the mass. It is true that the cyst, or cysts, can decrease in size from time to time, but they will again refill, and, in general, we have found that there is always a progression in size if the patient is followed over a long period of time. Our experience does not permit us to endorse the idea of "expectant treatment," and indeed there is much to be said against it because the tendency of a hygroma to undergo suppuration during respiratory infections makes it desirable that this serious complication be avoided by early excision of the cystic mass.

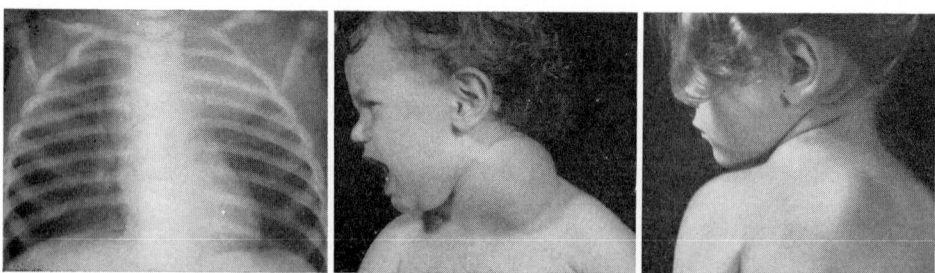

Fig. 559. Fourteen-month-old girl with hygroma of thorax, neck, and back. *Left*, Roentgenogram showing the intrathoracic portion. *Middle*, The cervical part. *Right*, Photograph two years after removal of thoracic and cervical lesions, showing development of cyst over scapula.

Spontaneous Regression Following Infection

If suppuration occurs in a hygroma, and the patient does not die of generalized sepsis, there is a strong likelihood that the hygroma will be partially or largely destroyed by the inflammatory process. We have seen two examples of this in which, following tonsillitis and an upper respiratory infection, the purulent exudate which collected in hygromas required incision and drainage. Subsequent to the disappearance of the sepsis and the healing of the wound there has been no recurrence of these two cystic lesions in a period of five years during which they have been followed.

Aspiration

As early as 1839, Arnott advocated the use of aspiration of large cysts in small infants who might not be able to stand the insults of a surgical procedure. In only one instance have we attempted this and, after multiple needlings, the stagnant fluid within the cyst became infected. We have, therefore, discouraged the use of the procedure and would advise it only as an emergency measure for relief of pressure symptoms such as might occur because of displacement of the larynx or compression of the great neck vessels.

Injection of Sclerosing Agents

This has been suggested by MacGuire[12] and others. Harrower[9] has advocated the use of sodium morrhuate because he felt that open operation carried too high a mortality rate. In his patient, 2 cc. of 5 per cent soldium morrhuate was injected into the swelling. On the following day the mass had increased to one and a half times its previous size, but on the third day it began to shrink. Six days later a second such treatment was given and, though there was some local reaction, the mass had entirely disappeared in a month.

After a study of pathologic material, it would seem that the thinness of the lining of a hygroma would make the lesion almost ideal for injection therapy, because the sclerosing agent could be easily diffused through the fluid medium and would not have

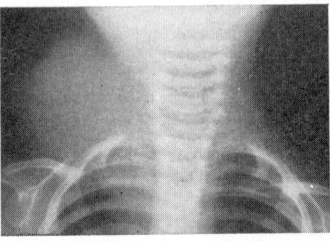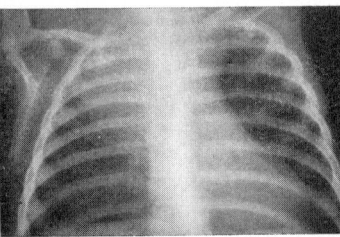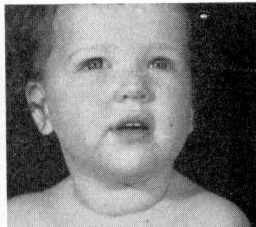

Fig. 560. Case with cervical hygroma having an intrathoracic extension. *Left*, Film showing the mass in neck. *Middle*, Film showing the portion within the thorax. *Right*, Photograph following removal of multilocular hygromas.

to penetrate deeply to destroy the cyst lining. However, a word of caution must be inserted regarding this method of therapy. A hygroma is apt to dissect downward to the large vessels of the neck and to partially or completely surround them. If, under such conditions, a necrotizing agent is introduced into the sac, it is possible to damage or thrombose the internal jugular vein or carotid artery. Furthermore, the introduction of a sclerosing fluid into the sac may be disastrous in certain cases in which there happens to be a communication between the hygroma and the venous system. What appeared to be such a connection was well demonstrated in Vaughn's patient who was studied roentgenographically after the injection of iodized oil into the hygroma.[19] X-ray plates taken immediately showed clearly the outlines and extent of the cystic swelling, but a plate one-half hour later showed complete disappearance of the opaque medium which presumably had run off into some neighboring vein. It is not difficult to contemplate the possible complications if a sclerosing solution had been introduced into this lesion. The likelihood of having small lymphatico-venous anastomoses makes us fearful of using injection treatment in any case.

Radium or Roentgen Ray Irradiation

New,[16] in 1924, was the first to treat a hygroma successfully with radium. Figi[4] has been the principal proponent of radium therapy. He treated 12 patients, employing from 3000 to 7000 milligram hours of radium (applications made at a distance of

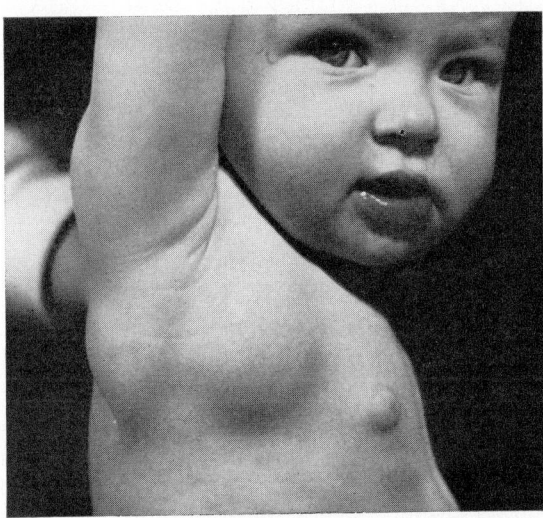

Fig. 561. Child with hygroma of axilla.

2.5 cm., using 2 mm. lead screening). These were repeated at intervals of two or three months, giving the patients an average of four treatments. Seven of these patients died of sepsis which had sprung up in the lesion; 4 of the patients had been infected prior to the first application of radium. Of the 5 patients who survived, 3 were entirely cured and 2 were much improved.

Our own experiences with x-ray irradiation in a few cases—either with or without surgery—has been most discouraging. We believe that irradiation has very little to offer except possibly to help kill off any small bits which have been left in an operative field, or to treat those portions of hygroma which widely infiltrate the musculature of the tongue.

Surgical Excision

The removal of a hygroma by surgical dissection has proved to be the most satisfactory method of treatment. Many surgeons have evaded this undertaking believing that a young subject does not take an anesthetic well, that the dissection is tedious and difficult, and that the attendant mortality is high. Contrary to these statements, it has been our experience that a child, even a newly born infant, will tolerate ether anesthesia nicely if it is administered by a capable anesthetist, that the excision of a hygroma can be performed with thoroughness if care is exercised, that the resulting mortality is low, and that permanent cure can be expected in the vast majority of cases.

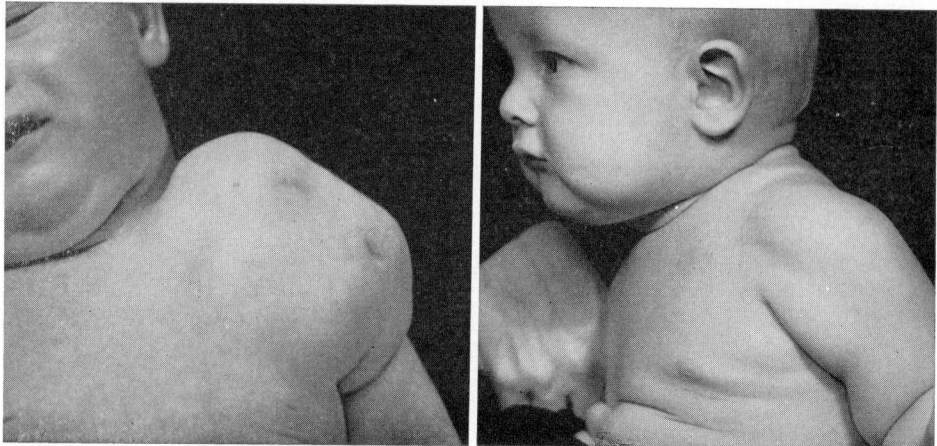

Fig. 562. *Left*, Cystic hygroma of shoulder. *Right*, Photograph following excision of the hygroma.

In general, the skin incision should be made in a direction which will later correspond to the normal folds of the neck. If the mass is relatively small, none of the over-lying skin need be cut away; if a hygroma is large, it may be desirable to remove an elliptical portion of skin so that there will not be too much excess tissue when the cutaneous flaps are later brought together. It is not necessary, however, to plan on an accurate adjustment of the skin flaps to remove all wrinkles at the time of the wound closure; it has been amply demonstrated that large and unsightly cutaneous folds will disappear rapidly and a pleasing contour of the neck will be reestablished in a few months. The dissection and removal of a hygroma is not difficult if patience is exercised and haste is avoided. The overlying skin, though tense and thin, will readily separate from the underlying cyst. If the wall of the cyst is closely followed, blunt dissection will disclose a plane of cleavage leading around the greater portion of the mass. When proper planes of cleavage are found and followed, little bleeding is encountered, for vessels running to the hygroma are quite small in size and few in number. In general, a large unilocular cyst is easier to dissect than is a small, multilocular lesion which is apt to be very adherent to surrounding structures.

A cyst wall is little more than tissue paper in thickness and tends to tear easily, hence it is important not to grasp it with instruments but rather to hold it with the gloved hand or with a piece of moist gauze. Every effort should be made to keep the cyst intact, for as long as this is done the borders of the structure are readily definable; once the mass has collapsed, there may be prolongations outward between the muscles or vessels of the neck which are then difficult to remove. Such islands of tissue which are left behind are apt to act as foci for recurrence, hence, meticulous technique should be employed to avoid leaving bits of the endothelial lining in the field.

The removal of a hygroma generally leads the operator extensively into the deeper planes of the neck for it is the nature of the lesion to possess projections along the great vessels, between muscle bellies, along the brachial plexus, into the axilla, or downward over the surface of the apical pleura. Such behavior at once implies that care must be employed to insure that all of the contiguous and important structures of the neck are left uninjured. The internal jugular vein, carotid arteries, and branches of the brachial plexus are all large enough so that they can be easily identified and avoided, but the hypoglossal nerve and the lower filaments of the facial nerve are apt to be overlooked and severed, thus giving distressing deformity. Mason and Baker[14] have recommended that for tumors high in the parotid region it is safer to incise the skin well up behind the ear and first expose the facial nerve, so that it can be identified along its entire course as the subsequent dissection proceeds anteriorly. In affirming this teaching, we would also add that whenever the dissection carries one in front of the sternomastoid muscle it is best to identify the spinal accessory nerve immediately so that it can be isolated and retracted to the upper border of the operative field and left uninjured.

The wound should be closed so that the edges of the platysma muscle are approximated. If this is done, there will be little tendency for separation of the skin margins; the resulting cutaneous scar will be minimal and almost invisible. *These wounds should always be drained.* There is a strong tendency for fluid or serum to accumulate under the skin flaps, and if this is not allowed to escape quickly, new smooth-walled cysts will be formed.

In most cases the hygroma can be removed completely at a single operation. However, in an infant a few weeks of age with a very extensive growth, in whom operation is imperative because of respiratory distress, it is sometimes best to plan a multiple-stage procedure, removing only a portion of the growth at each sitting.

RESULTS OF THERAPY

The operative mortality should be low. In our 112 patients, surgical removal of hygroma was performed in one or more stages with 6 deaths. The causes of death were: shock in 1, postoperative hemorrhage in 2, spreading sepsis in 2, pneumonia in 1.

In 6 patients there has been partial or complete facial paralysis when attempts were made to remove completely a hygroma which extended up into the parotid area. We are now convinced that it is preferable to leave some tissue in this area, rather than to accept the risks of facial nerve damage by too extensive a dissection.

For about two-thirds of our patients it has been possible to remove hygromas completely at one operation. In the remaining cases, the extent of the lesion or the weakened condition of the patient made it necessary to employ multiple-stage excision. In the vast majority of these it has been possible to remove eventually all of the hygromatous tissue, but in several instances some substance still remains and will require further therapy.

REFERENCES

1. Arnold, J.: Zwei Faelle von Hygroma colli cysticum congenitum und deren fragliche Beziehung zu dem Ganglion Intercaroticum. Arch. f. path. Anat., *33*:209, 1865.
2. Bailey, H.: The Clinical Aspects of Branchial Cysts. Brit. J. Surg., *10*:565, 1923.
3. Dowd, Charles N.: Hygroma Cysticum Colli, Its Structure and Etiology. Ann. Surg., *58:* 112, 1913.
4. Figi, F. A.: Radium in the Treatment of Multilocular Lymph Cysts of Neck in Children. Am. J. Roentgenol., *21:*473, 1929.
5. Fraser, John: Surgery of Childhood. Vol. 2, p. 616. William Wood and Company, New York, 1926.
6. Goetsch, E.: Hygroma Colli Cysticum and Hygroma Axillare; Pathologic and Clinical Study and Report of Twelve Cases. Arch. Surg., *36:*394, 1938.
7. Gross, R. E. and Goeringer, C. F.: Cystic Hygroma of the Neck. Report of 27 Cases. Surg., Gynec. & Obst., *69:*48, 1939.
8. Gross, R. E. and Hurwitt, E. S.: Cervicomediastinal and Mediastinal Cystic Hygromas. Surg., Gynec. & Obst., *87:*599, 1948.
9. Harrower, J. G.: Treatment of Cystic Hygroma of the Neck by Sodium Morrhuate. Brit. M. J., *2:*148, 1933.
10. Huntington, G.: Lymphatic Vessels of the Cat. Mem. Wister Inst., Philadelphia, 1911.
11. Luschka, H.: Ueber die Drusenartige Natur des sogenannten Ganglion Intercaroticum. Arch. f. Anat. u. Physiol., *4:*405, 1862.
12. MacGuire, D. P.: Cystic Hygroma of the Neck. Arch. Surg., *31:*301, 1935.

13. Martin-Lelong: Cystic Lymphangioma at the Base of the Neck with Intrathoracic Prolongation Revealed by Roentgenogram. Bull. Soc. pédiat. de Paris, *31:*310, 1933.
14. Mason, S. T. and Baker, L. W.: Cystic Hygroma. S. Clin. North America, *11:*1090, 1931.
15. McClure, C. F. W. and Silvester, C. F.: A Comparative Study of the Lymphaticovenous Communications in Adult Mammals. Anat. Rec., *3:*534, 1909.
16. New, G. B.: Hygroma Cysticum Treated with Radium. S. Clin. N. America, *4:*527, 1924.
17. Sabin, F. R.: In Keibel, F. and Mall, F. P.: Manual of Human Embryology, Vol. 2, p. 709. J. B. Lippincott Co., Philadelphia, 1912.
18. Thompson, J. E. and Keiller, V. H.: Lymphangioma of the Neck. Ann. Surg., *77:*385, 1923.
19. Vaughn, A. M.: Cystic Hygroma of the Neck. Am. J. Dis. Child., *48:*149, 1934.
20. Von Herepy-Casabanyi, G.: Bilateral Lymphangioma Cavernosum in the Neck. Zentralbl. f. Chir., *54:*1672, 1927.
21. Wernher, A.: Die angeborenen Kysten-Hygrome und die ihnen verwandten Geschwuelste in anatomischer, diagnostischer, und therapeutischer Beziehung. G. F. Heyer, Giessen, 1843, p. 76.
22. Wenglowski, R.: Ueber die Halsfisteln und Cysten. Arch. f. klin. Chir., *98:*151, 1912.
23. Winslow, R.: Cystic Hygroma and Other Tumors of Infancy. Surg., Gynec. & Obst., *25:*428, 1917.

CHAPTER 69

Wringer Injuries of the Arm

With the modern age of electrification of home equipment and with the American fondness for mechanical gadgets, literally millions of housewives have provided themselves with electric washing machines, most of which carry some sort of an apparatus for partially drying the clothes. Machines of more recent manufacture accomplish the drying by spinning clothes centrifugally in a whirling drum. Most of the older machines were equipped with a power-driven open wringer, through which individual pieces of clothing could be passed and squeezed. An open wringer of this sort is a potential source of injury to the curious child who fingers the turning rollers, gets his hand caught, and then has his arm dragged relentlessly into the appliance, thereby sustaining a crushing injury of the forearm or upper arm and possibly the axilla. Through 1951, 142 patients with injuries of this type were treated at the Boston Children's Hospital. The following remarks are based on a summary of this material.

THE INJURY

This accident not infrequently occurs during the first weeks of possession of the power-driven washing machine, for it is at this time that the child is most fascinated by the turning rollers, and the mother is least aware of their potential danger. As the hand and arm are drawn unmercifully into the power-driven squeezers, the soft tissues almost invariably sustain considerable damage. Less trauma will occur if the mother remains calm and simply strikes the safety-release bar. All too often, she forgets to do this and instead applies counter-traction to the child, or else reverses the direction of the rollers; the arm is subjected to a more extensive injury or to a second crushing. If the arm is flexed strongly at the elbow when the forearm is drawn into the roller, the latter will churn in the antecubital fossa, giving a maximum injury to the skin and subcutaneous tissues in this area. If an arm is relatively straight when it is drawn into the rollers, the entire limb will enter the appliance and the turning rollers will give maximum damage as they churn in the axilla.

There are certain factors which tend to make wringer injuries more extensive, and others which tend to give lesser degrees of damage. More severe traumas are caused when the rollers are set to give maximum compression, when the arm is of a large subject, when there has been a forcible attempt to pull the arm out of the rollers in a direction opposite to their rotation, and when the churning in the antecubital fossa or axilla has been particularly long. Less extensive injuries tend to be caused when the rollers have been under lesser spring-tension, when the arm is of a small individual, when there has been no forcible attempt to pull the arm out of the roller mechanism, and when the safety-release bar has been quickly pressed to reduce the amount of churning on the arm.

To the injured child and its mother, the experience of a wringer arm injury is terrifying, and the vast majority of these patients are taken immediately to a physician for treatment. On examination the arm may be found to be diffusely swollen, or to be

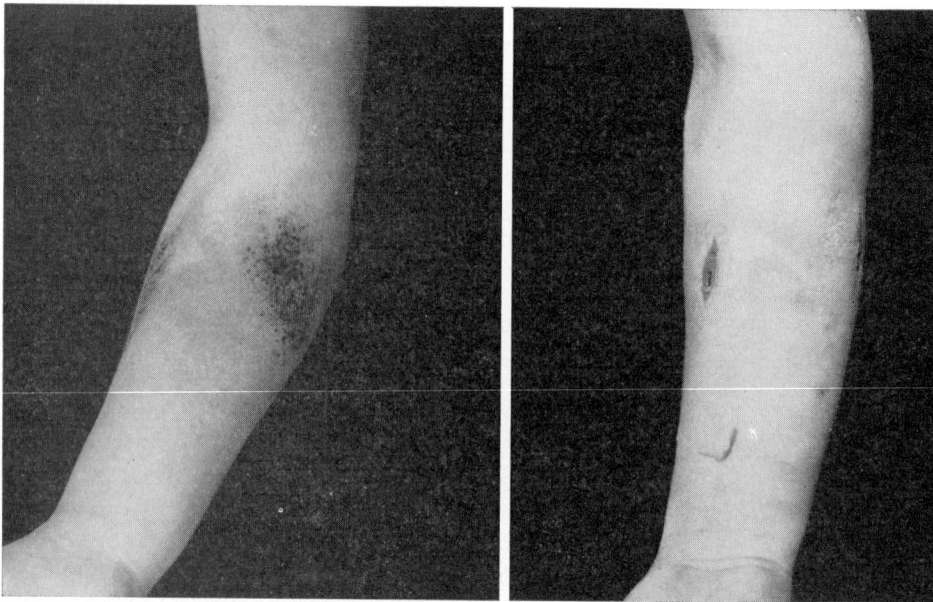

Fig. 563. *Left*, Appearance of injury to a forearm from a power-driven wringer accident. Photograph two days after accident, showing the swelling, principally composed of subcutaneous collection of fluid or blood. Impending necrosis of overlying skin. *Right*, Following incision and drainage, with evacuation of subcutaneous clot. The skin has been allowed to drop back onto its bed and has thereby retained its viability.

ecchymotic in some areas, particularly in the antecubital fossa or the axilla. There may be some minor abrasions. Seldom is there laceration or avulsion of skin. The initial examination by the physician may give the impression that the injury is a minor one, but it is well to bear in mind that this is often extremely misleading. During the subsequent twenty-four to thirty-six hours, skin which previously looked viable can begin to change color and show signs of dying. There can be subcutaneous accumulations of transudate or blood which raise the skin from its bed and rupture the nutrient blood vessels; if allowed to progress these can give subsequent sloughing of the regional

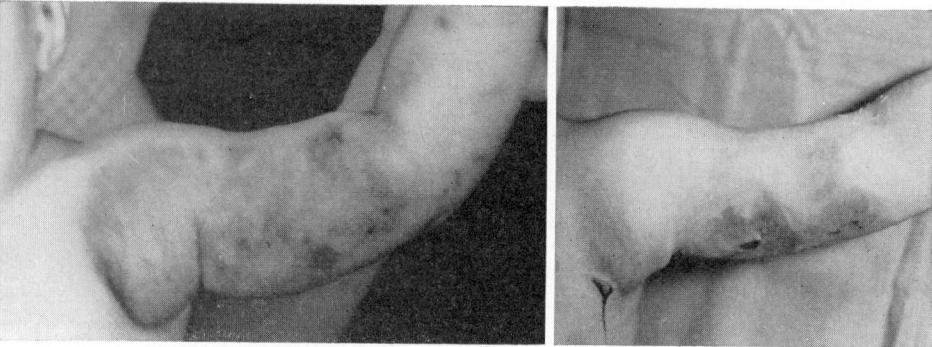

Fig. 564. *Left*, Appearance of arm forty-eight hours after injury by a power-driven clothes wringer There is diffuse ecchymosis of the upper arm and axilla. Subcutaneous collection of fluid and blood beneath these regions, and impending necrosis of wide areas of skin. *Right*, Appearance of arm following incision and drainage of upper arm and of the axilla, allowing the skin to drop back onto its nutritive bed. All of the skin survived.

skin. What at first appeared to be a minor injury can within a few days advance to an alarming situation. Therefore, it is never wise to give a prognosis before the end of twenty-four or forty-eight hours, when the full extent of the injury can be determined. The hand, being somewhat thin, seldom receives serious crushing. The skin on the volar aspect of the forearm, in and below the antecubital fossa, and in the axilla, is the area which most frequently receives extensive damage. Destruction of muscles in the forearm or upper arm is rarely marked, but we have seen serious ischemic scarring and contraction of forearm muscles in two cases and severe damage to upper arm muscles in another child (Fig. 566). In two of our patients there was crushing or disruption of nerves. The bones usually escape injury, but it is probably wise to make a roentgenographic examination in every case. In our 142 patients, fractures of minor importance were found in 4. There was one greenstick fracture of the humerus and one of the clavicle; there were 2 linear cracks through the base of the first or fifth metacarpal bones.

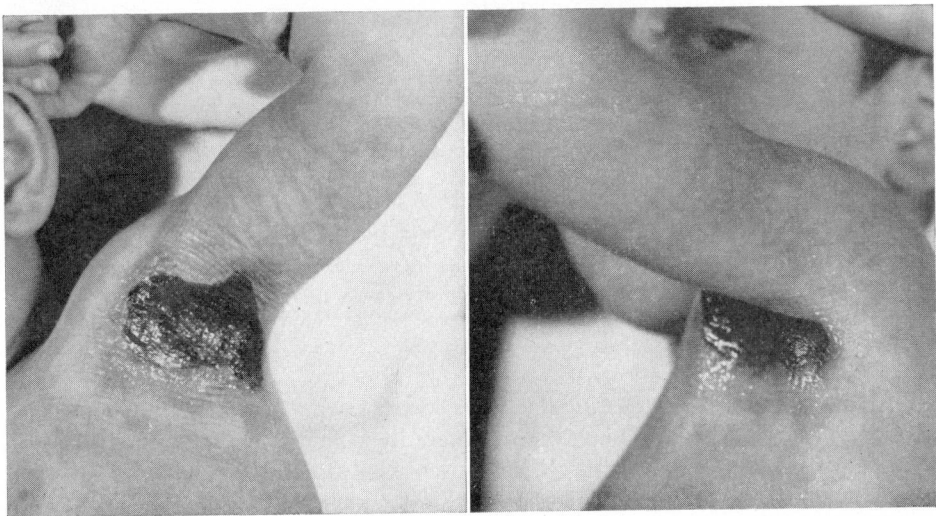

Fig. 565. Wringer injury of the axilla. The churning rollers caused extensive necrosis in the armpit. The granulating area shown here was subsequently covered by a Thiersch graft.

TREATMENT

It is our policy to hospitalize all children with wringer arm injuries for a day or two. Obviously, this might not be necessary in some of the less extensive cases, but if close observation cannot be made at home or in the physician's office, too frequently does one find progressing damage which could have been avoided or minimized with proper therapy from the start. Adequate sedation is essential. The injured part should be thoroughly cleansed with some mild antiseptic such as an aqueous Zephiran or Phisoderm, and the injured part thoroughly encased in a sterile and compression bandage. Wherever the skin seems to have been mashed or churned, it should be covered with a greasy dressing, such as a petrolatum strip or tulle gras which has been impregnated with petrolatum, this being covered with sterile gauze. The entire arm is then wrapped in a roller bandage and over this an elastic Ace bandage is applied from the hand to the axilla. The compression over the injured areas will tend to minimize and localize the collection of fluid and oozing of blood into the tissues. It will tend to keep the skin compressed against the underlying structures which supply nourishment, thereby minimizing subsequent sloughing of skin. Even though the injury is located in the upper arm, the hand and forearm are included in the compression bandage to prevent these from swelling. With the child in bed, and kept quiet by appropriate drugs, the arm should be elevated so that it is raised above the level of the shoulder to promote drainage and to minimize accumulation of fluid in the damaged parts.

Once or twice a day the dressing should be taken down to determine the extent of the injury and any progression of the same. This should be done under sterile precautions and a sterile compression bandage reapplied. If, at the end of thirty-six or forty-eight hours, it is evident that there is no important subcutaneous collection of fluid or blood, and that there is no impending necrosis of skin, the child can be discharged and cared for at home.

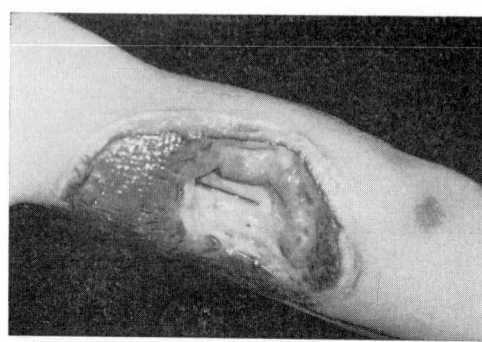 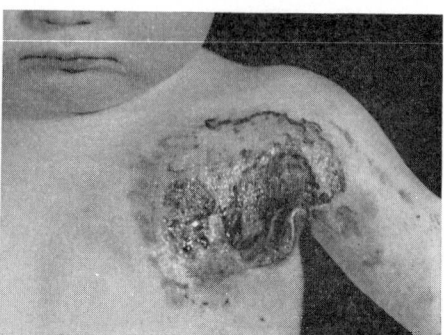

Fig. 566. *Left*, Extensive injury to upper arm from an electric clothes wringer. There has been loss of skin, muscle, and radial nerve. The humerus is exposed. *Right*, Severe injury of the upper arm and axilla from a power-driven clothes wringer. The sloughing of the axillary skin subsequently required application of a skin graft.

One of the greatest dangers in a wringer injury is the gradual pocketing of transudate or blood in the subcutaneous tissues which, by raising the skin and thus separating it from its blood supply, can lead to necrosis of the integument. Therefore, in the examinations which are made from time to time within the first few days, one should particularly have in mind the detection of any such accumulation. If they appear, it is highly important to incise and drain them so that all fluid or clot can be evacuated, thereby allowing the skin to fall back onto a nutritive bed and thus retain its viability. If at the time of such surgical drainage the interior of the cavity can be made quite dry, it is permissible to close the skin wound; if there appears to be a continuing ooze of fluid or blood, it is best to leave a small drain in the wound, so that any material can come out into the sterile dressing, thereby permitting the skin to rest continually against the underlying tissues and to have the best chance of survival.

In some instances, there is sloughing of skin in the antecubital fossa or the axilla which has been brought about by excessive churning or crushing from the rollers, or else there has been ischemia because underlying collections of fluid have not been drained properly. Whenever there is loss of skin from either of these causes, the area should be allowed to granulate for a week or two and then covered with a Thiersch graft.

Results of Therapy

In our group of 142 patients who were treated for wringer injuries of the arm the following results were obtained:

About 60 per cent of the patients had simple abrasions and contusions. They were all seen within twelve hours after the accident and were admitted to the hospital for a day or two of observation. Each recovered completely without a demonstrable scar or impairment of function.

About 20 per cent of the patients were also seen within twelve hours after the accident and were admitted to the hospital, but in this group the compression injury had been more extensive. There were subcutaneous effusions or hemorrhages which required incision and drainage for release of entrapped fluid. One of these patients subsequently required skin grafting for covering a devitalized area of the upper arm; all of the others recovered completely, the only residuum being the small scars from the drainage incisions.

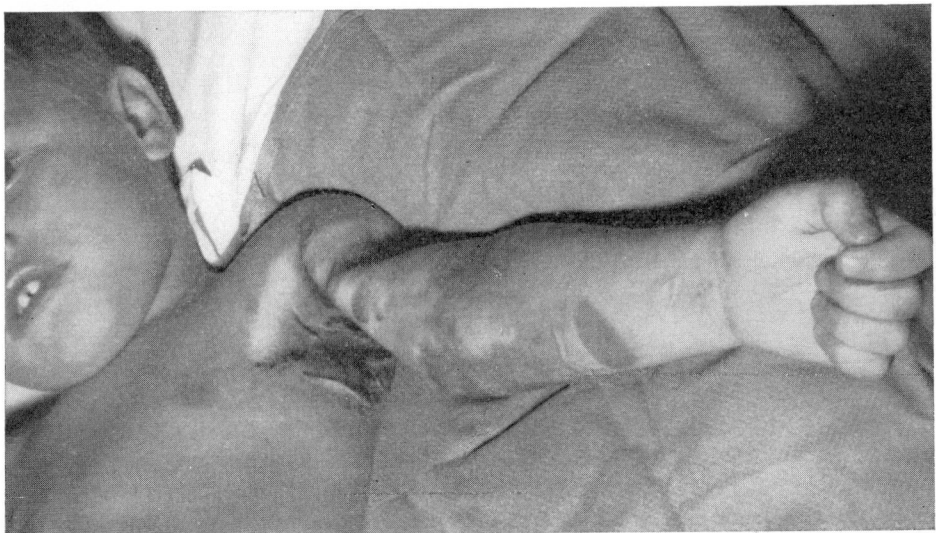

Fig. 567. The most severe wringer injury we have seen. (Child treated after period covered in statistics of this chapter.) Photograph taken immediately after admission to the hospital, within an hour after the accident; the hand is already pale. There was extensive vascular injury, requiring amputation of the arm.

About 20 per cent of the patients could be classified in a neglected group; either they had not been seen by a physician previously, or else the therapy which had been given seemed to be distinctly inadequate. The patients initially came to the hospital from two days to six months following their injury. All children in this group had necrosis and sloughing of skin and all required grafting of skin to cover denuded areas.

From our observations we are convinced that the vast majority of children with wringer injuries of the arm should be hospitalized for a day or two, because so frequently the injury appears to be more extensive at the end of twenty-four or forty-eight hours than it did at the time of the initial examination. When subcutaneous collection of fluid or blood is not released by operative means, there is apt to be a necrosis of overlying skin which requires subsequent grafting to replace the integument and there is apt to be contracture which requires physiotherapy for long periods of time. Conversely, when careful observation shows that transudate or blood is accumulating in the subcutaneous spaces, surgical release of such fluid will avoid or will minimize the loss of skin and will also shorten the convalescence.

Index

Numbers in *italics* refer to pages with illustrations.